THERAPEUTICS of PARKINSON'S DISEASE and OTHER MOVEMENT DISORDERS

THERAPEUTICS of PARKINSON'S DISEASE and OTHER MOVEMENT DISORDERS

Edited by

MARK HALLETT

National Institute of Neurological Disorders and Stroke, Bethesda, MD, USA

and

WERNER POEWE

Department of Neurology, Medical University of Innsbruck, Austria

2008

WILEY-BLACKWELL

A John Wiley & Sons, Ltd., Publication

Library of Congress Cataloguing-in-Publication Data

Therapeutics of Parkinson's disease and other movement disorders/edited by Mark Hallett and Werner Poewe.
  p. ; cm.
  Includes bibliographical references and index.
  ISBN 978-0-470-06648-5
1. Parkinson's disease–Treatment. 2. Movement disorders–Treatment. I. Hallett, Mark, 1943- II. Poewe, W.
  [DNLM: 1. Parkinson Disease–therapy. 2. Movement Disorders–therapy.
WL 359 T3974 2008]
  RC382.T43 2008
  616.8′33–dc22   2008022144

ISBN: 9780470066485

A catalogue record for this book is available from the British Library.

Typeset in 9/11 pt. Times by Thomson Digital, India

Printed and bound in Great Britain by CPI Antony Rowe, Chippenham, Wiltshire.

Contents

PART I   PARKINSON'S DISEASE AND PARKINSONISM

PART V DRUG-INDUCED MOVEMENT DISORDERS

PART VI ATAXIA AND DISORDERS OF GAIT AND BALANCE

PART VII RESTLESS LEGS SYNDROME

PART VIII PEDIATRIC MOVEMENT DISORDERS

PART IX PSYCHOGENIC MOVEMENT DISORDERS

Preface

Over the past few decades the field of neurology has seen spectacular developments in diagnostic techniques, most vividly exemplified by modern neuroimaging and molecular genetics. Although not always at the same speed this evolution has gone hand in hand with an enlarging armentarium of effective therapies to treat neurological disease. This is particularly true for the field of movement disorders, where one of the most exciting success stories of modern translational research in neuroscience unfolded more than 40 years ago: the discovery of dopamine deficiency in the striatum of patients with Parkinson's disease and the subsequent introduction of levodopa as a dramatically effective therapy of this hitherto devastating illness. Since then the therapeutic options for Parkinson's disease have grown exponentially, often making treatment decisions difficult. Moreover, there are now numerous therapies for other movement disorders with substantial impact on patients. While many therapies remain symptomatic, a number normalize the condition such as de-coppering in Wilson's disease and levodopa in dopa-responsive dystonia.

While there are a number of textbooks on movement disorders, none so far has emphasized treatment, and this current work attempts to fill this gap. Practitioners want and need practical detailed advice on how to treat patients. We have recruited a team of experts who have attempted to deal with most situations. Wherever available, chapter authors have used evidence from randomized controlled clinical trials to develop practical recommendations for every day clinical practice. As is the case for all of medicine there are many situations in the treatment of movement disorders where evidence from controlled trials is either insufficient or open to interpretation. We have therefore deliberately encouraged the expert authors to share with the reader their personal clinical acumen and therapeutic wisdom. Summary tables and algorithms are part of many chapters and will hopefully serve as a quick reference guide for practical treatment decisions in many different circumstances. Of course, each patient presents unique circumstances, so physicians will need to use their judgement every step of the way, but having expert guidance should at least set the general direction.

We are grateful to the movement disorder experts whom we have recruited from all over the world to bring their knowledge to this textbook. We appreciate their expertise and patience with our compulsive editing, as we have tried to give a uniform style to the recommendations, and occasionally added our own opinions.

We have tried to be up to date, but medications and other treatment options may change. New agents appear and some may even be withdrawn because new adverse effects surface. So, we hope that this book and its advice will be a helpful guide, but physicians must continue to be alert to any changes in practice that might arise.

MARK HALLETT
WERNER POEWE

Contributors

PRATIBHA G. AIA

Department of Neurology, Emory University School of Medicine, Atlanta, GA, USA

RICHARD P. ALLEN

Neurology and Sleep Medicine, Johns Hopkins University, Baltimore, MD, USA

HAGAI BERGMAN

The Interdisciplinary Center for Neural Computation, and the Eric Roland Center for Neurodegenerative Diseases, Department of Physiology, The Hebrew University, Hadassah Medical School, Jerusalem, Israel

KEVIN M. BIGLAN

University of Rochester Medical Center, Movement and Inherited Neurological Disorders (MIND) Unit, Rochester, NY, USA

TOMAS BJÖRKLUND

CNS Disease Modelling Unit, Department of Experimental Medical Science, Wallenberg Neuroscience Center, Lund University, Lund, Sweden

BASTIAAN R. BLOEM

Parkinson Center Nijmegen (ParC), Radboud University Nijmegen Medical Center, Department of Neurology (HP 935), Nijmegen, The Netherlands

GEORGE J. BREWER

Departments of Human Genetics and Internal Medicine, University of Michigan Medical School, Ann Arbor, MI, USA

JONATHAN M. BROTCHIE

Toronto Western Research Institute, Toronto Western Hospital, 399 Bathurst Street, Toronto, ON, Canada

PATRIK BRUNDIN

Neuronal Survival Unit, Department of Experimental Medical Science, Wallenberg Neuroscience Center, Lund University, Lund, Sweden

FRANCISCO CARDOSO

Neurology Service, Internal Medicine Department, Federal University of Minas Gerais, Belo Horizonte, MG, Brazil

LESLIE J. CLOUD

Department of Neurology, Emory University School of Medicine, Atlanta, GA, USA

CYNTHIA L. COMELLA

Department of Neurological Sciences, Rush University Medical Center, Chicago, IL, USA

GÜNTHER DEUSCHL

Department of Neurology, Christian-Albrechts-University Kiel, Universitätsklinikum Schleswig-Holstein, Kiel, Germany

DIRK DRESSLER

Department of Neurology, Hannover Medical School, Hannover, Germany

RODGER J. ELBLE

Department of Neurology, Southern Illinois University School of Medicine, Springfield, IL, USA

SHLOMO ELIAS

Department of Physiology, The Hebrew University, Hadassah Medical School, Jerusalem, Israel

CHRISTINE D. ESPER

Department of Neurology, Emory University School of Medicine, Atlanta, GA, USA

STEWART A. FACTOR

Department of Neurology, Emory University School of Medicine, Atlanta, GA, USA

SUSAN H. FOX

Movement Disorders Clinic MCL7 421, Toronto Western Hospital, Toronto, ON, Canada

STEVEN J. FRUCHT

Department of Neurology, Columbia University Presbyterian Hospital, New York, NY, USA

OSCAR S. GERSHANIK

Department of Neurology, Centro Neurologico-Hospital Frances, & Laboratory of Experimental Parkinsonism, ININFA-CONICET, Buenos Aires, Argentina

ALEXANDER C. GEURTS

Department of Rehabilitation Medicine, Radboud University Nijmegen Medical Center, Nijmegen, The Netherlands

NIR GILADI

Movement Disorders Unit, Parkinson Center, Department of Neurology, Tel-Aviv Sourasky Medical Centre, Sackler School of Medicine, Tel-Aviv University, Tel-Aviv, Israel

CHRISTOPHER G. GOETZ

Department of Neurological Sciences, Rush University Medical Center, Chicago, IL, USA

DAVID GRABLI

Fédération du Système Nerveux, Salpêtrière Hospital, Assistance Publique Hôpitaux de Paris, Université Paris 6 – Pierre et Marie Curie and INSERM U679, Paris, France

MARK HALLETT

Human Motor Control Section, National Institute of Neurological Disorders and Stroke, National Institutes of Health, Bethesda, MD, USA

SHARON HASSIN-BAER

Movement Disorders Clinic, Department of Neurology, Sheba Medical Center, Sackler School of Medicine, Tel-Aviv, Israel

ERIKA L.F. HEDDERICK

Pediatric Neurology, Harriet Lane Children's Health Building, Baltimore, MD, USA

BIRGIT HÖGL

Department of Neurology, Innsbruck Medical University, Innsbruck, Austria

SHU-CHING HU

Department of Neurology, University of Washington, Seattle, WA, USA

ZVI ISRAEL

Department of Neurosurgery, The Hebrew University, Hadassah Medical School, Jerusalem, Israel

JOSEPH JANKOVIC

Parkinson's Disease Center and Movement Disorders Clinic, Baylor College of Medicine, Department of Neurology, Houston, TX, USA

REGINA KATZENSCHLAGER

Department of Neurology, Danube Hospital / SMZ-Ost, Vienna, Austria

CHRISTOPHER KENNEY

Parkinson's Disease Center and Movement Disorders Clinic, Baylor College of Medicine, Department of Neurology, Houston, TX, USA

DENIZ KIRIK

CNS Disease Modelling Unit, Department of Experimental Medical Science, Wallenberg Neuroscience Center, Lund University, BMC A11, Lund, Sweden

THOMAS KLOCKGETHER

Department of Neurology, University Hospital Bonn, Bonn, Germany

MARTIN KÖLLENSPERGER

Research Laboratory, Clinical Department of Neurology, Innsbruck Medical University, Innsbruck, Austria

ANTHONY E. LANG

Movement Disorders Clinic, Toronto Western Hospital, Toronto, ON, Canada

KEVIN MCNAUGHT

Department of Neurology, Mount Sinai School of Medicine, New York, NY, USA

SHYAMAL H. MEHTA

Movement Disorders Program, Department of Neurology, Medical College of Georgia, Augusta, GA, USA

HANS-MICHAEL MEINCK

Department of Neurology, University of Heidelberg, Heidelberg, Germany

JONATHAN W. MINK

Child Neurology, University of Rochester Medical Center, Rochester, NY, USA

ASUKA MORIZANE

Neuronal Survival Unit, Department of Experimental Medical Science, Wallenberg Neuroscience Center, Lund University, Lund, Sweden

C. WARREN OLANOW

Department of Neurology, Mount Sinai School of Medicine, New York, NY, USA

ELIZABETH PECKHAM

National Institute of Neurological Disorders and Stroke, National Institutes of Health, Bethesda, MD, USA

WERNER POEWE

Department of Neurology, Medical University of Innsbruck, Innsbruck, Austria

OLIVIER RASCOL

Laboratoire de Pharmacologie Médicale et Clinique, Faculté de Médecine, Toulouse, France

EMMANUEL ROZE

Fédération du Système Nerveux, Salpêtrière Hospital, Assistance Publique Hôpitaux de Paris, Université Paris 6 – Pierre et Marie Curie and INSERM U679, Paris, France

KLAUS SEPPI

Department of Neurology, Medical University of Innsbruck, Innsbruck, Austria

KAPIL D. SETHI

Movement Disorders Program, Department of Neurology, Medical College of Georgia, Augusta, GA, USA

HIROSHI SHIBASAKI

Takeda General Hospital, Ishida, Fushimi-ku, Kyoto, Japan

IRA SHOULSON

University of Rochester Medical Center, Clinical Trials Coordination Center, Rochester, NY, USA

HARVEY S. SINGER

Pediatric Neurology, Harriet Lane Children's Health Building, Baltimore, MD, USA

PHILIP D. THOMPSON

University Department of Medicine, University of Adelaide; Department of Neurology, Royal Adelaide Hospital, Adelaide, Australia

MARIE VIDAILHET

Fédération du Système Nerveux, Salpêtrière Hospital, Assistance Publique Hôpitaux de Paris, Université Paris 6 – Pierre et Marie Curie and INSERM U679, Paris, France

JENS VOLKMANN

Ltd. Oberarzt der Neurologischen Klinik, Christian-Albrechts-Universität zu Kiel, Kiel, Germany

GREGOR K. WENNING

Department of Neurology, University Hospital of Innsbruck, Innsbruck, Austria

S. ELIZABETH ZAUBER

Department of Neurological Sciences, Rush University Medical Center, Chicago, IL, USA

Part I

PARKINSON'S DISEASE AND PARKINSONISM

1

The Etiopathogenesis of Parkinson's Disease: Basic Mechanisms of Neurodegeneration

C. Warren Olanow and Kevin McNaught

Department of Neurology, Mount Sinai School of Medicine, New York, USA

INTRODUCTION

Parkinson's disease (PD) is a slowly progressive, neurodegenerative movement disorder characterized clinically by bradykinesia, rigidity, tremor and postural instability (Lang and Lozano, 1998; Lang and Lozano, 1998). PD is the second most common neurodegenerative illness (after Alzheimer's disease), and both incidence and prevalence rates increase with aging. As life expectancy of the general population rises, both the occurrence and prevalence of PD are likely to increase dramatically (Dorsey et al., 2007). Levodopa is the mainstay of current treatment, but long-term therapy is associated with motor complications and advanced disease is associated with non-dopaminergic features such as falling and dementia, which are not controlled with current therapies and are the major source of disability. These trends underscore the urgent need to move beyond the present time of symptomatic treatment to an era where neuroprotective therapies are available that prevent or impede the natural course of the disorder (Schapira and Olanow, 2004). The achievement of this goal would be facilitated by deciphering the factors that underlie the initiation, development and progression of the neurodegenerative process.

The primary pathology of PD is degeneration of dopaminergic neurons with protein accumulation and the formation of inclusions (Lewy bodies) in the substantia nigra pars compacta (SNc) (Forno, 1996). However, it is now appreciated that neurodegeneration with Lewy bodies or Lewy neurites is widespread and can be seen in noradrenergic neurons in the locus coeruleus, cholinergic neurons in the nucleus basalis of Meynert, and serotonin neurons in the median raphe, as well as in nerve cells in the dorsal motor nucleus of the vagus, olfactory regions, pedunculopontine nucleus, cerebral hemisphere, brain stem, and peripheral autonomic nervous system (Forno, 1996; Braak et al., 2003; Zarow et al., 2003). Indeed, non-dopaminergic pathology may even predate the classic dopaminergic pathology (Braak et al., 2003). Pathology in PD is thus widespread and progressive, but still specific in that some areas, such as the cerebellum and specific brain stem nuclei are unaffected by the disease process.

It now appears that there are many different causes of PD (Table 1.1). Approximately 5–10% of all cases of the illness are familial and likely genetic in origin, but most cases occur sporadically and are of unknown cause. Most recent attention has focused on genetic causes of PD based on linkage of familial patients to a variety of different chromosomal loci (PARK 1-11). Mutations in six specific proteins (α-synuclein, parkin, UCH-L1, DJ-1, PINK1 and LRRK2) have now been identified (Hardy et al., 2006). Further, mutations in LRRK2 have now been identified to be present in some late-onset PD patients with typical clinical and pathological features of PD and no family history (Gilks et al., 2005). Indeed, as many as 40% of North African and Ashkenazy Jewish PD patients carry this mutation (Ozelius et al., 2006; Lesage et al., 2006). However, a genetic basis for the vast majority of sporadic cases is far from established. In sporadic PD, epidemiologic studies suggest that environmental factors play an important role in development of the illness (Tanner, 2003). Further, two large genome-wide screens have failed to identify any specific genetic abnormality (Elbaz et al., 2006; Fung et al., 2006). The cause of PD thus remains a mystery. A widely held view is that environmental toxins might cause PD in patients who are susceptible because of

Therapeutics of Parkinson's Disease and Other Movement Disorders   Edited by Mark Hallett and Werner Poewe
© 2008 John Wiley & Sons, Ltd.

Table 1.1 Genetic and sporadic forms of Parkinson's disease.

Locus	Chromosome location	Gene product and properties	Mutations	Age of Onset (yr)	Clinical spectrum	Pathological features
Autosomal Dominant PD						
PARK 1&4	4q21–q23	α-Synuclein	Point mutations (A53T, A30P and E46K)	Range: 30–60	Levodopa-responsive; rapid progression; prominent dementia	Neuronal loss in the SNc, LC and DMN
		140 amino acids/ 14 kDa protein	Duplication	Mean: 45	E46K and multiplication cases demonstrate overlap with dementia with Lewy bodies	Lewy bodies are rare and tau accumulation occur in some A53T cases. Extensive Lewy bodies in E46K and multiplication cases
		Localized to synaptic terminals	Triplication			Triplication cases demonstrate degeneration in the hippocampus, vacuolation in the cortex and glial cytoplasmic inclusions
		Function: Unknown. Possibly play a role in synaptic activity				
PARK 8	12p11.2–12q31.1	Dardarin/LRRK2	Missense	Range: 35–79	Typical PD features; slow progression; dementia present; features of motor neuron disease reported	SNc degeneration
		2482/2527 amino acids		Mean: 57.4		Some cases show extensive Lewy bodies; some do not have Lewy bodies
		Function: Unknown. May be a protein kinase				Also, intranuclear inclusions, tau-immunoreactive inclusions and neurofibriallry tangles are present

					Typical PD	
PARK 5	4p14	Ubiquitin C-terminal hydrolase L1 230 amino acids/ 26 kDa protein Neuron specific protein Function: De-ubiquitinating enzyme (possible E3 activity also)	Missense mutation (193M)	49 and 50	Typical PD	Lewy bodies reported in a single case
Autosomal Recesive PD						
PARK 2	6q25.2-q27	Parkin 465 amino acids/ 52 kDa protein Expressed in cytoplasm, golgi complex, nuclei and processes Function: E3 ubiquitin ligase	Deletions Point mutations Multiplications	Range: 7-58 Mean: 26.1	Levodopa-responsive and severe dyskinesias; foot dystonia; diurnal fluctuations; hyperreflexia; slow progression	Selective and severe destruction of the SNc and LC Generally Lewy body-negative
PARK 6	1p35-1p36	PINK 1 581 amino acids/ 62.8 kDa protein Localized to mitochondria Function: Unknown. May be a protein kinase	Missense Truncating	Range: 32-48	Levodopa-responsive; slow progression	Neuropathology not yet determined

(*Continued*)

Table 1.1 (*Continued*).

Locus	Chromosome location	Gene product and properties	Mutations	Age of Onset (yr)	Clinical spectrum	Pathological features
PARK 7	1p36	DJ-1	Deletion	Range: 20–40s	Levodopa responsive; dystonia; psychiatric disturbance; slow progression	Neuropathology not yet determined
		189 amino acids/ 20 kDa protein More prominent in the cytoplasm and nucleus of astrocytes compared to neurons Function: Unknown. Possible antioxidant, molecular chaperone and protease	Truncating Missense	Mean: mid 30s		
Sporadic PD	—	—	—	Mean: 59.5 yr	Insidious onset and slow progression. L-DOPA-responsive.	Neurodegeneration with Lewy bodies in the SNc, LC, DMN, NBM, etc

their genetic profile, poor ability to metabolize toxins, and/ or advancing age (Hawkes, Del Tredici and Braak, 2007).

Several factors have been implicated in the pathogenesis of cell death in PD, including oxidative stress, mitochondrial dysfunction, excitotoxicity, and inflammation (Wood-Kaczmar, Gandhi and Wood, 2006; Olanow, 2007). Interest has also focused on the possibility that proteolytic stress due to excess levels of misfolded proteins might be central to each of the different etiologic and pathogenic mechanisms that could lead to cell death in PD (Olanow, 2007). Finally, there is evidence that cell death occurs by way of a signal-mediated apoptotic process. Each of these mechanisms provides candidate targets for developing putative neuroprotective therapies. However, the precise pathogenic mechanism responsible for cell death remains unknown, and to date no therapy has been established to be neuroprotective (Schapira and Olanow, 2004). Indeed, it remains uncertain if any one or more of these factors is primary and initiates cell death, or if they develop only secondary to an alternative process.

In this chapter, we consider those etiologic and pathogenic factors that have been implicated in PD, based on genetic and pathological findings, and consider how they might contribute to the various familial and sporadic forms of PD (Figure 1.1).

AUTOSOMAL DOMINANT PD

α-Synuclein

The first linkage discovered to be associated with PD was located at chromosome 4q21–q23 (PARK 1&4). Genetic analyses showed A53T and A30P point mutations in the gene that encodes for a 140 amino acid/14 kDa protein known as α-synuclein (Polymeropoulos et al., 1996; Polymeropoulos et al., 1997). Subsequently, an E46K mutation in α-synuclein was reported in another family with autosomal dominant PD (plus features of dementia with Lewy bodies) (Zarranz et al., 2004), but no other point mutation has subsequently been found. In recent years, duplication (three copies) and triplication (four copies) of the normal α-synuclein gene have also been found to cause autosomal dominant PD (Chartier-Harlin et al., 2004; Farrer et al., 2004; Ibanez et al., 2004; Miller et al., 2004; Singleton et al., 2003).

Familial PD caused by α-synuclein shares many features with common sporadic PD, but patients tend to have a relatively early age of onset (mean in the 40s) and high occurrence of dementia. Also, patients with duplication/ triplication of the α-synuclein gene tend to present with a dementia with Lewy bodies (DLB) pattern rather than more conventional PD. Pathological studies show a marked increase in α-synuclein levels with protein aggregation in various brain regions (Singleton et al., 2003; Duda et al.,

2002; Kotzbauer et al., 2004). However, this is often in the form of Lewy neurites rather than Lewy bodies. In patients with the A53T mutation, Lewy bodies are rarely present and there is a marked accumulation of α-synuclein and tau in the cerebral cortex and striatum (Duda et al., 2002; Kotzbauer et al., 2004). Also, patients with triplication of the normal α-synuclein gene have vacuoles in the cortex, neuronal death in the hippocampus and inclusion bodies in glial cells (Singleton et al., 2003). These findings show that there are significant differences between the pathology that occurs in the α-synuclein-linked familial PD and common sporadic PD.

α-Synuclein, so called because of its preferential localization in synapses and the region of the nuclear envelope (Jakes, Spillantini and Goedert, 1994; Maroteaux, Campanelli and Scheller, 1988), is diffusely expressed throughout the CNS (Solano et al., 2000). It is a member of a family of related proteins that also include β- and γ-synucleins (Goedert, 2001). α-Synuclein is enriched in presynaptic nerve terminals and associates with lipid membranes and vesicles. The normal function of α-synuclein is unknown, but there is some evidence that it plays a role in synaptic neurotransmission, neuronal plasticity and lipid metabolism. Since the discovery of α-synuclein-linked familial PD, there has been a great deal of effort aimed at deciphering how mutations in this protein induce neurodegeneration. The dominant mode of inheritance suggests a gain of function. Wild-type α-synuclein is monomeric and intrinsically unstructured/natively unfolded at low concentrations, but in high concentrations it has a propensity to oligomerize and aggregate into β-pleated sheets (Conway, et al., 1998; Weinreb et al., 1996). Mutations in the protein increase this potential for misfolding, oligomerization and aggregation (Conway, Harper and Lansbury, 1998; Weinreb et al., 1996; Caughey and Lansbury, 2003; Conway et al., 2000; Lashuel et al., 2002;Li, Uversky and Fink, 2001; Pandey, Schmidt and Galvin, 2006). Oligomerization of α-synuclein produces intermediary species (protofibrils) that form annular structures with pore-like properties that permeabilize synthetic vesicular membranes in vitro. It has been suggested that protofibrils are the toxic α-synuclein species that are responsible for cell death. It is also possible that protein aggregation itself can interfere with critical cell functions and promote apoptosis.

It is possible that the cytotoxicity associated with mutant/ excess α-synuclein involves interference with proteolysis and autophagy. Wild-type α-synuclein is a substrate for both the 26S and 20S proteasome and is preferentially degraded in a ubiquitin-independent manner (Bennett et al., 1999; Liu et al., 2003;Tofaris, Layfield and Spillantini, 2001). In vitro and in vivo studies have demonstrated that mutant α-synuclein, which misfolds, oligomerizes and aggregates, is resistant to UPS-mediated degradation and

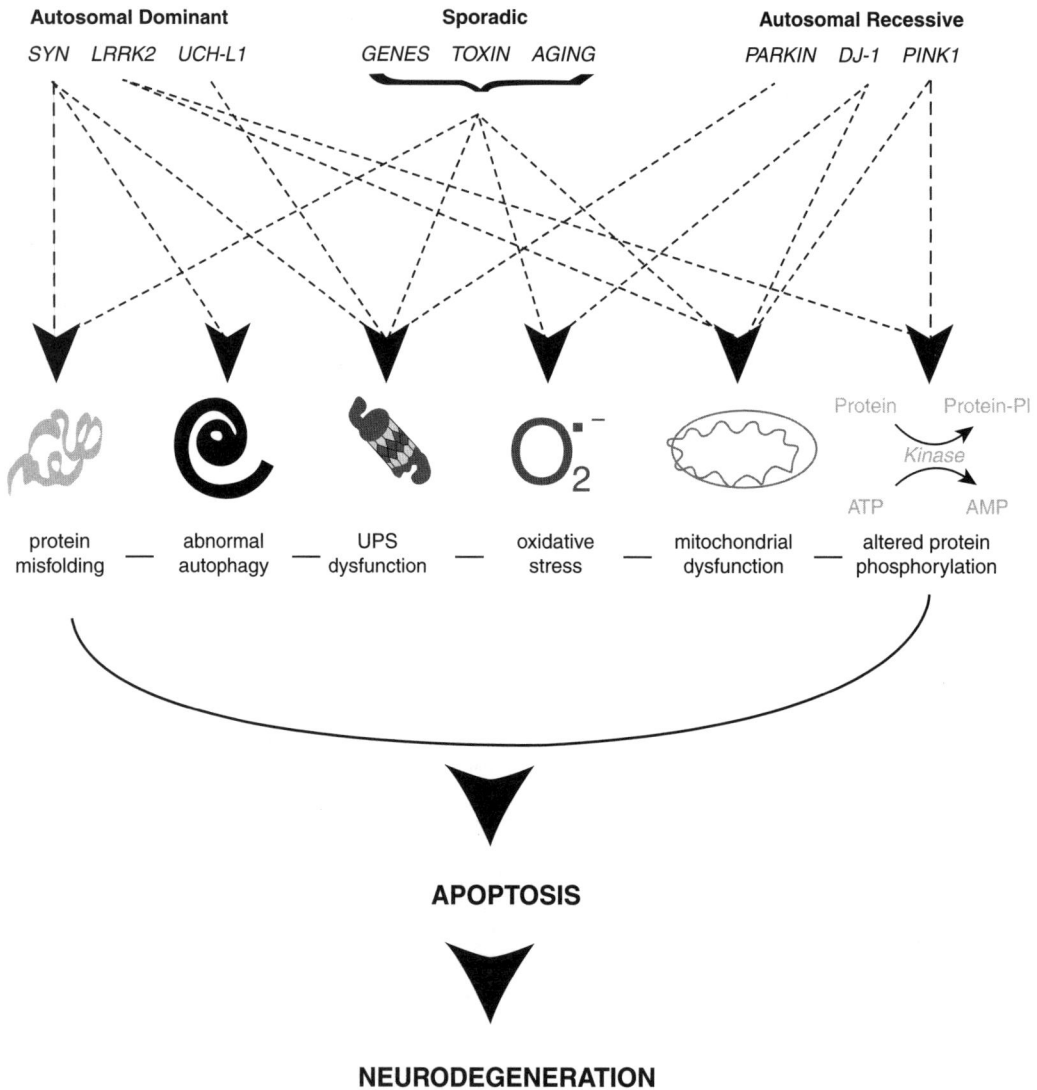

Figure 1.1 Schematic illustration of different forms of PD and factors that are thought to be associated with the development of cell death and that might be candidates for putative neuroprotective therapies.

also inhibits this pathway and its ability to clear other proteins (Snyder *et al.*, 2003; Stefanis *et al.*, 2001; Tanaka *et al.*, 2001). As a result, there is accumulation of a wide range of proteins, in addition to α-synuclein, in cells expressing mutant α-synuclein. High levels of undegraded or poorly degraded proteins have a tendency to aggregate with each other and other proteins, form inclusion bodies, disrupt intracellular processes, and cause cell death (Bence

Sampat and Kopito, 2001). Recent studies indicate that α-synuclein can also be broken down by the 20S proteasome through endoproteolytic degradation that does not involve the –N or –C terminus (Liu *et al.*, 2003). This type of degradation yields truncated α-synuclein fragments, which are particularly prone to aggregate, promote aggregation of the full-length protein, as well as other proteins, and cause cytotoxicity (Liu *et al.*, 2005). Thus, it is reasonable to consider that alterations in the α-synuclein gene can interfere with the clearance of unwanted proteins, and that this defect may underlie protein aggregation, Lewy body formation and neurodegeneration in hereditary PD (Olanow and McNaught, 2006). α-Synuclein can also be degraded by the lysosomal system, and mutations in the protein are associated with impaired chaperone-mediated clearance by autophagy which also promotes accumulation and aggregation of the protein (Cuervo et al., 2004; Lee et al., 2004).

Numerous studies, employing a variety of approaches, have examined the effects of expressing PD-related mutant (and wild-type) α-synuclein in transgenic animals (Fernagut and Chesselet, 2004). Expression of mutant (A53T, A30P) or wild-type α-synuclein in transgenic Drosophila (Feany and Bender, 2000), or the adenoviral-mediated expression of A53T mutant or wild-type α-synuclein in the SNc of adult non-human primates (common marmosets) (Kirik et al., 2003), causes selective dopamine cell degeneration. Interestingly, overexpression of A53T, A30P or wild-type α-synuclein causes inclusion body formation, but does not cause neurodegeneration in transgenic mice (Fernagut and Chesselet, 2004). In addition, some species normally express the mutant form of α-synuclein with a threonine in the alanine position, yet do not show aggregation as is found in PD patients (Polymeropoulos et al., 1997), possibly because α-synuclein is degraded differently in these species.

The relative roles of the UPS and lysosomal systems in the degradation of wild-type and mutant α-synuclein has not been clearly defined, and it is possible that defects in either the proteasomal or lysosomal systems could contribute to the accumulation of α-synuclein and other proteins. It is also noteworthy that not all carriers of point mutations in α-synuclein develop PD, suggesting that additional factors, such as environmental toxins, might be required to trigger the development of PD in individuals carrying mutations in α-synuclein.

It is noteworthy that α-synuclein accumulates in patients with sporadic PD (see below), suggesting that this protein might also have relevance to the cause of cell death in these cases. In support of this concept, it is noteworthy that knockdown of α-synuclein prevents dopaminergic toxicity associated with MPTP (Dauer et al., 2002). Heat shock proteins act to promote protein refolding and also as chaperones to facilitate protein clearance through the proteasome or autophagal systems. Indeed, it has been found that overexpression of heat shock protein prevents dopamine neuronal degeneration in Drosophila that overexpress wild-type or mutant α-synuclein (Auluck et al., 2002). Similarly the naturally occurring benzoquinone ansamycin, geldanamycin, prevents aggregation and protects dopamine neurons in this model (Auluck and Bonini, 2002). Geldanamycin binds to an ATP site on HSP90, blocking its normally negative regulation of heat shock transcription

factor 1 (HSF1), thus promoting the synthesis of heat shock protein (Whitesell et al., 1994). These studies offer promising targets for candidate neuroprotective drugs for PD. It also possible that agents that can prevent or dissolve α-synuclein aggregates such as β-synuclein or immunization with α-synuclein might be protective in PD (Hashimoto et al., 2004; Masliah et al., 2005), although it has not yet been shown that these strategies can provide protective effects in model systems.

UCH-L1

An I93M missense mutation in the gene (4p14; PARK 5) encoding ubiquitin C-terminal L1 (UCH-L1), a 230 amino acid/26 kDa de-ubiquitinating enzyme, was associated with the development of autosomal dominant PD in two siblings of a European family (Leroy et al., 1998). The parents were asymptomatic, suggesting that the gene defect causes disease with incomplete penetrance. The affected individuals had clinical features that resemble sporadic PD, including a good response to levodopa, but the age (49 and 51) of onset was relatively early. Postmortem analyses on one of the siblings revealed Lewy bodies in the brain (Auberger et al., 2005). Genetic screening studies have failed to detect UCH-L1 mutations in other families with PD, suggesting that this mutation is either very rare, or not a true cause of PD (Wintermeyer et al., 2000). Interestingly, several studies have found that the UCH-L1 gene is a susceptibility locus in sporadic PD and that polymorphisms, such as the S18Y substitution, confers some degree of protection against developing the illness (Maraganore et al., 2004). However, another study failed to find any association between UCH-L1 polymorphisms and PD (Healy et al., 2006).

UCH-L1 is expressed exclusively in neurons in many areas of the CNS (Solano et al., 2000), and constitutes 1–2% of the soluble proteins in the brain (Solano et al., 2000; Wilkinson, Deshpande and Larsen, 1992; Wilkinson et al., 1989). UCH-L1 is responsible for cleaving ubiquitin from protein adducts to enable the protein to enter the proteasome. Mutations in UCH-L1 cause a reduction in de-ubiquitinating activity in vitro and result in gracile axonal dystrophy (GAD) in transgenic mice (Leroy et al., 1998; Nishikawa et al., 2003; Osaka et al., 2003). Further, toxin- or mutation-induced inhibition of UCH-L1's activity leads to a marked decrease in levels of ubiquitin in cultured cells and in the brain of GAD mice (Osaka et al., 2003; McNaught et al., 2002), and degeneration of dopaminergic neurons with protein accumulation and the formation of Lewy body-like inclusions in rat ventral midbrain cell cultures (McNaught et al., 2002). Therefore, it is possible that a mutation in UCH-L1 alters UPS function leading to altered proteolysis and ultimately cell death. It also appears that UCH-L1 has E3 ubiquitin ligase activity, but it remains unclear if the PD-related mutation alters this function of the protein (Liu *et al.*, 2002).

LRRK2

LRRK2 mutations are now thought to be the commonest cause of familial PD. Several missense mutations in the gene (12p11.2–q13.1, PARK 8) encoding a 2527 amino acid/ ≈250 kDa protein called dardarin or LRRK2 (leucine-rich repeat kinase 2) can cause an autosomal dominant form of PD with incomplete penetrance (Funayama *et al.*, 2002; Paisan-Ruiz *et al.*, 2004; Zimprich *et al.*, 2004). This gene defect has been found in several families from different countries, and it is estimated that the mutation could account for 5% or more of familial PD cases (Farrer, 2006), although this percentage is significantly higher in north African arabs and Ashkenazi Jews perhaps reflecting a founder effect (Ozelius *et al.*, 2006; Lesage *et al.*, 2006). Not all individuals who carry these mutations develop parkinsonism, suggesting the possible requirement of other etiological factors to act as a trigger for the illness (Di Fonzo *et al.*, 2005).

The clinical spectrum of LRRK2-linked PD can be similar to sporadic PD, with an age of onset ranging from 32 to 79 years. Pathologically, most have a PD-like picture, but there can be considerable variability even within family members who carry the same mutation (Zimprich *et al.*, 2004; Wszolek *et al.*, 2004). While all subjects with LRRK2-linked familial PD have nigrostriatal degeneration, some have nigral Lewy bodies and some do not, some have a DLB picture with extensive cortical Lewy bodies, and some have tau-immunoreactive glial and neuronal inclusions resembling tauopathies such as progressive supranuclear palsy. Interestingly, some patients with this mutation have a late-onset form of PD with no family history and clinical and pathologic features typical of sporadic PD. It has been estimated that the LRRK2 mutation might account for as many as 7% of familial cases and 1.5–3% of cases of sporadic PD (Di Fonzo *et al.*, 2005; Gilks *et al.*, 2005; Nichols *et al.*, 2005).

LRRK2 protein is expressed throughout the brain (Paisan-Ruiz *et al.*, 2004; Simon-Sanchez *et al.*, 2006), but its normal function is unknown. It is a large protein that is bound to the outer mitochondrial membrane. Based on its molecular structure, it has been suggested that LRRK2 might be a cytoplasmic kinase in the MAP kinase family (Paisan-Ruiz *et al.*, 2004; Zimprich *et al.*, 2004). It is also not known how mutations in LRRK2 alter the structure and function of the protein or how these might lead to cell death. It is now appreciated that LRRK2 has kinase (West, Moore and Biskup, 2005) and GTPase (Li *et al.*, 2007) activities, and that mutations are associated with enhanced GTP binding and kinase activities that are linked to toxicity (West *et al.*, 2007). Indeed, knockdown of kinase activity leads to reduced toxicity in model systems (Greggio *et al.*,

2006; Smith *et al.*, 2006). It is therefore possible that PD-related LRRK2 mutations might be due to an increase in kinase activity leading to altered phosphorylation of substrate proteins (West, Moore and Biskup, 2005).

AUTOSOMAL RECESSIVE PD

Parkin

A hereditary form of PD, autosomal recessive juvenile parkinsonism (AR-JP) was first described in Japanese families, and is linked to chromosome 6q25.2–q27 (PARK 2) (Matsumine *et al.*, 1997). This locus was found to host the gene that encodes for a 465 amino acid/52 kDa protein called parkin (Kitada *et al.*, 1998). It is now appreciated that many deletions, point mutations, and mutations that span the entire parkin gene can cause familial PD (Hattori and Mizuno, 2004). Some estimates suggest that parkin mutations might account for as many as 50% of early-onset (<45 years) familial cases of PD (Lucking *et al.*, 2000). It is noteworthy, though, that parkin mutations can also be associated with late-onset (≥60 years old) hereditary PD (Foroud *et al.*, 2003).

Clinically, AR-JP is similar to common sporadic PD, but there are notable differences. Patients with parkin mutations tend have a very early age of onset, ranging from 7 to 72 years (average, 30 years), and demonstrate a rather slow rate of progression. The neuropathology of patients with parkin mutations differs from sporadic PD in that neurodegeneration is restricted to the SNc and LC, and Lewy bodies are largely absent (Mori *et al.*, 1998), although a few have been noted in a few older patients with parkin-linked autosomal PD (Farrer *et al.*, 2001; Pramstaller *et al.*, 2005).

Parkin is expressed in the cytoplasm, nucleus, golgi apparatus and processes of neurons throughout the CNS (Horowitz *et al.*, 2001). Several studies have shown that parkin is an E3 ubiquitin ligase (Imai *et al.*, 2001; Imai *et al.*, 2000; Shimura *et al.*, 2000; Shimura *et al.*, 2001; Zhang *et al.*, 2000) which contains a RING finger domain (comprising two RING finger motifs separated by an in-between-RING domain) at the C-terminus. The protein also contains a central linker region and a ubiquitin-like domain (UBL) at the N-terminus. Parkin acts in conjunction with several E2 enzymes, Ubc6, UbcH7 and UbcH8, to ubiquitinate a variety of substrates. These include synphilin-1, CDCrel-1, parkin-associated endothelin receptor-like receptor (Pael-R), an O-glycosylated isoform of α-synuclein (αSp22), cyclin E α/β-tubulin, p38 subunit of the aminoacyl-tRNA synthetase complex, and synaptotagmin X1. Interestingly, parkin may polyubiquitinate proteins with linkages at lysine 48 (K48) or lysine 63 (K63) (Lim *et al.*, 2005). Parkin has been shown to interact through its UBL domain with the 26S proteasome Rpn10/S5a subunit, and along with Rpt5/S6′, plays a role in the recognition of ubiquitinated substrates by the PA700 proteasome activator

(Pickart and Cohen, 2004; Sakata *et al.*, 2003). Parkin also interacts with a protein complex containing CHIP/HSP70 which promotes parkin's activity (Cyr, Hohfeld and Patterson, 2002) and with proteasomal subunits (Dachsel *et al.*, 2005).

Precisely how parkin induces pathology in familial PD is not known, but could relate to a loss of E3 ubiquitin ligase activity with consequent impairment in the ubiquitination of its protein substrates. Levels of parkin, and its enzymatic activity, are decreased in the SNc and LC in AR-JP (Shimura *et al.*, 2000; Shimura *et al.*, 2001;Cyr, Hohfeld and Patterson, 2002; Shimura *et al.*, 1999). This defect may thus underlie the accumulation of undegraded parkin substrates, including Pael-R and αSp22, found in these brain areas in PD (Imai *et al.*, 2001; Shimura *et al.*, 2001). It has been shown that normal parkin prevents endoplasmic reticulum dysfunction and unfolded protein-induced cell death following overexpression of Pael-R in cultured cells and *Drosophila* (Imai *et al.*, 2001; Imai, Soda and Takahashi, 2000; Yang *et al.*, 2003). So, it is reasonable to consider that accumulation of undegraded substrate proteins disrupts intracellular processes leading to neurodegeneration in familial PD.

Interestingly, parkin mutations in transgenic mice do not cause nigrostriatal degeneration (Goldberg *et al.*, 2003; Itier *et al.*, 2003; Perez and Palmiter, 2005; Von Coelln *et al.*, 2004). Further, the frequency of point mutations, deletions and duplications of parkin is similar in AR-JP (3.8%) and normal controls (3.1%) (Lincoln *et al.*, 2003). Taken together, these observations raise the possibility that additional factors, for example exposure to environmental substances or other gene alterations, might be necessary to trigger the development of parkinsonism in individuals carrying parkin mutations.

DJ-1

Missense and deletion mutations in the gene (chromosome 1p36, PARK 7) that encodes for a 189 amino acid/20 kDa protein called DJ-1 is responsible for an autosomal recessive early-onset form of parkinsonism (Bonifati, Oostra and Heutink, 2004; Bonifati *et al.*, 2003; Nagakubo *et al.*, 1997; van Duijn *et al.*, 2001). Since no additional mutations in DJ-1 have been reported, it is likely that this defect accounts for only a very small percentage of early-onset cases (Lockhart *et al.*, 2004). Clinically, DJ-1-linked PD is similar to parkin-related PD, namely early onset of symptoms (age 20–40 years), slow progression, presence of dystonia, levodopa-responsiveness, and the common occurrence of psychiatric disturbance. The neuropathological features of DJ-1 are not yet known.

In the CNS, DJ-1 is more prominent in astrocytes than neurons, and is present in the cytosol, nucleus and mitochondria of cells (Bandopadhyay *et al.*, 2004; Shang *et al.*, 2004).

The normal function of DJ-1 is not known, but there is evidence to suggest that it acts as a sensor of oxidative stress and proteasomal damage (Taira *et al.*, 2004; Yokota *et al.*, 2003). Additionally, the molecular structure and *in vitro* properties of DJ-1 indicate that it might act as a molecular chaperone and a protease (Lee *et al.*, 2003; Olzmann *et al.*, 2004; Wilson *et al.*, 2004). Interestingly, DJ-1 interacts with parkin, CHIP and HSP70, suggesting a link to these proteolytic systems (Moore *et al.*, 2005).

The mechanism by which mutations in DJ-1 induces pathogenesis is unknown. The recessive pattern of inheritance raises the possibility that the mutations induce a loss of function of the protein. The PD-related mutations (e.g., L166P) destabilize and inactivate the protein, impair its proteolytic activity, and promote its rapid degradation by the proteasome (Olzmann *et al.*, 2004; Moore *et al.*, 2003). In cell cultures, overexpression of DJ-1 protects cells from oxidative stress, and knockdown of DJ-1 increases susceptibility to oxidative stress, endoplasmic reticulum stress and proteasomal inhibition (Taira *et al.*, 2004; Yokota *et al.*, 2003). Further, mutations in DJ-1 reduce its ability to inhibit the aggregation of α-synuclein both *in vitro* and *in vivo* (Shendelman *et al.*, 2004). Interestingly, deletion of DJ-1 in transgenic mice does not induce neurodegeneration (Goldberg *et al.*, 2005), suggesting that other factors might be involved in the pathogenic process in PD. Thus, one may speculate that mutations in DJ-1 might lead to a loss of its putative anti-oxidant, chaperone and proteolytic activity.

PINK1

More than 20 homozygous or compound heterozygous mutations in the gene (1p35–p36, PARK 6) that codes for a 581 amino acid/62.8 kDa protein, designated PINK1 (PTEN (phosphatase and tensin homolog deleted on chromosome 10)-induced kinase 1), are known to cause autosomal recessive early-onset PD (Hatano *et al.*, 2004; Healy, Abou-Sleiman and Wood, 2004; Valente *et al.*, 2004; Valente *et al.*, 2001; Valente *et al.*, 2002). Clinically, this form of PD is characterized by early onset of symptoms (20–40 years), slow progression and a good response to levodopa (Healy, Abou-Sleiman and Wood, 2004; Valente *et al.*, 2001). Late-onset forms of the disease that resemble sporadic PD have also been described.

PINK1 is localized to mitochondria but additional studies are required to determine its precise cellular and anatomical distribution (Valente *et al.*, 2004). The normal function of PINK1 is unknown. It appears to be a serine/threonine protein kinase that phosphorylates proteins involved in signal transduction pathways. In cell culture studies, wild-type PINK1 prevents proteasome inhibitor-induced mitochondrial dysfunction and apoptosis, but this protection is lost with the mutations found in PD (Valente *et al.*, 2001). Interestingly, loss of function mutations in

PINK1 in *Drosophila* causes male sterility, muscle wasting, dopaminergic neuronal degeneration, and increased sensitivity to stressors (Clark *et al.*, 2006; Park *et al.*, 2006). These changes are associated with mitochondrial morphologic abnormalities, notably enlargement and fragmentation of christae. Thus, mitochondrial dysfunction appears to play a role in the pathogenesis of cell death associated with PINK1 mutations. Interestingly, defects in the parkin gene induced by knockout or by RNA interference also lead to alterations in mitochondrial morphology with dopamine neuronal degeneration, and enhance the degree of mitochondrial damage seen with PINK1 mutations (Park *et al.*, 2006; Yang, Gehrke and Imai, 2006). Further, overexpression of wild-type parkin restores mitochondrial morphology in the PINK1 mutant *Drosophila*, suggesting that PINK1 and parkin act in a common pathway that is critical for normal mitochondrial function (Yang, Gehrke and Imai, 2006). PINK-1 mutations have been found in normal control subjects who do not have clinical features of parkinsonism (Rogaeva *et al.*, 2004), again raising again the possibility that multiple factors may be necessary for the development of PD.

SPORADIC PD

Pathogenic Factors

The majority of PD cases occur sporadically, and are of unknown cause. It is thought that a combination of factors, acting sequentially or in parallel, and perhaps to varying degrees in each individual, might underlie the development of sporadic PD. The widely held view is that environmental toxins might cause PD in individuals who are susceptible due to their genetic profile, poor ability to metabolize toxins and/or advancing age. However, a specific infectious agent or toxin has not as yet been identified and the biological basis of possible vulnerabilities is unknown. Several pathogenic factors have been implicated in the disorder, including mitochondrial dysfunction, oxidative stress, excitotoxicity and inflammation (see reviews in reference Olanow, 2006). These defects may interact with each other and form a cascade or network of events that lead to apoptosis and cell death. It should be noted, however, that none of these pathogenetic factors have been established to be the primary source of neurodegeneration or for that matter to actually be involved in the cell death process (Olanow, 2007). It is certainly possible that as yet undiscovered pathogenic factors play a more critical role, and further that the pathogenic factors involved in cell death in an individual patient may differ.

Oxidative stress has been implicated in PD (Jenner, 2003) based on findings in the SNc of reduced levels of the major brain antioxidant reduced glutathione (GSH) (Sian *et al.*, 1994), increased levels of the pro-oxidant iron

(Dexter *et al.*, 1991; Hirsch *et al.*, 1991; Sofic *et al.*, 1988), and evidence of oxidative damage to proteins, lipids and DNA (Alam *et al.*, 1997; Dexter *et al.*, 1989; Dexter *et al.*, 1994; Zhang *et al.*, 1999). It is noteworthy that oxidative stress can be linked to the various gene mutations associated with PD, and that oxidative stress can lead to mitochondrial damage and cause proteasome dysfunction (Ding and Keller, 2001; Jha *et al.*, 2002; Okada *et al.*, 1999). However, clinical trials of anti-oxidants have failed to provide benefit in PD patients (Parkinson Study Group, 1993). Mitochondrial dysfunction has been implicated in PD based on findings of reduced activity and decreased staining for complex I of the mitochondrial respiratory chain (Schapira *et al.*, 1990). Further, toxins that specifically damage complex I such as rotenone and MPTP selectively damage dopamine neurons and induce a model of PD (Langston *et al.*, 1983; Betarbet *et al.*, 2000). As mentioned above, it is also noteworthy that mutations in DJ-1 and parkin are associated with mitochondrial abnormalities. However, whether mitochondrial defects found in PD are primary or secondary is not known, and bioenergetic agents have not yet been established to have disease-modifying effects in PD. Recent interest has also focused on the possibility that calcium cytotoxicity might contribute to neurodegeneration in PD. Recent studies have also demonstrated that with maturation, SNc dopamine neurons convert from using sodium channels to 1.3 L-type calcium channels in order to maintain their pacemaker activities which could make these cells vulnerable to calcium cytotoxicity. It is noteworthy that blockage of these channels in cultured dopamine neurons causes them to revert to using sodium channels and is protective (Chan *et al.*, 2007).

Proteolytic Stress

Much of our own interest has focused on the possibility that cell death in PD results from proteolytic stress due to increased formation and/or a failure to clear misfolded proteins (McNaught *et al.*, 2001). There is abundant evidence for protein accumulation in areas that undergo neurodegeneration in PD. Quantitative western blot analyses demonstrate a marked increase in the levels of truncated, full-length, oligomeric and aggregates (of high and various molecular weights) of α-synuclein and other proteins in the SNc (Baba *et al.*, 1998; Tofaris *et al.*, 2003). These α-synuclein species have various post-translation modifications, including phosphorylation, glycosylation, nitration and ubiquitination (Tofaris *et al.*, 2003; Giasson *et al.*, 2000; Hasegawa *et al.*, 2002; Sampathu *et al.*, 2003). Accumulated α-synuclein can exist in a fibrillar form and cross-link with other proteins (e.g., by advanced glycation endproducts) and with neuromelanin (Fasano *et al.*, 2003; Munch *et al.*, 2000; Spillantini *et al.*, 1998). In addition to α-synuclein, many other proteins accumulate and are post-translationally modified in the SNc and other brain regions in PD. There is a several-fold increase in levels of ubiquitin–protein conjugates and phosphorylated proteins in the SNc (McNaught *et al.*, 2002; Zhu *et al.*, 2002). There is also an increase in the content of oxidatively damaged proteins, as indicated by an elevation in the levels of protein carbonyls and protein adducts of 4-hydroxy-2-nonenal (derived from lipid peroxidation) (Alam *et al.*, 1997; Yoritaka *et al.*, 1996). Nuclear magnetic relaxation field-cycling relaxometry, which measures water solubility in tissues, has also been used to demonstrate a generalized increase in protein aggregates in the SNc in PD (Shimura *et al.*, 1999).

Lewy Bodies

The most striking evidence for protein dysfunction in PD is the presence of Lewy bodies, Lewy neurites and small protein aggregates in the SNc and other sites of neurodegeneration (McNaught *et al.*, 2002). The Lewy body is usually 8–30 μm in diameter, and in the SNc in PD it demonstrates an intensely stained central core with a lightly staining surrounding halo with the protein-binding dye eosin. Electron microscopy demonstrates a core comprised of dense granular material, which may contain punctate aggregates of ubiquitinated proteins, while the outer region is an arrangement of radiating filaments (7–20 nm in diameter) comprised of fibrillar α-synuclein and neurofilaments (Spillantini *et al.*, 1998; McNaught *et al.*, 2002). Immuno-histochemical staining shows that Lewy bodies contain a wide range of proteins, the most prominent being α-synuclein (Spillantini *et al.*, 1998; McNaught *et al.*, 2002; Spillantini *et al.*, 1997), neurofilaments (Schmidt *et al.*, 1991), and ubiquitin/ubiquitinated proteins (McNaught *et al.*, 2002; Lennox *et al.*, 1989). Lewy bodies also contain components of the UPS (e.g., ubiquitination/de-ubiquitination enzymes, proteasomal subunits, and proteasome activators) (McNaught *et al.*, 2002; Ii *et al.*, 1997; Lowe *et al.*, 1990; Schlossmacher *et al.*, 2002), and heat shock proteins (e.g., HSP70 and HSP90) (McNaught *et al.*, 2002), but it is not known if the proteasome subunits unite to form a functioning proteasomal complex. Within Lewy bodies, proteins may be oxidized (Castellani *et al.*, 2002), nitrated (Giasson *et al.*, 2000; Good *et al.*, 1998), ubiquitinated and/or phosphorylated (Fujiwara *et al.*, 2002). It is noteworthy that not all proteins are found in Lewy bodies (e.g., synaptophysin, β-tubulin, and tau).

The consistent organization and composition of Lewy bodies suggests that they are unlikely to be formed in a random manner by the non-specific passive diffusion and coalescing of cellular proteins. Recent studies have led to the speculation that Lewy bodies could be formed and function in an aggresome-like manner (McNaught *et al.*, 2002; Ardley *et al.*, 2003; Kopito, 2000; Olanow *et al.*, 2004). Aggresomes are inclusion bodies that form at the

centrosome in response to proteolytic stress. They serve to sequester, segregate and degrade excess levels of abnormal and potentially toxic proteins when these products cannot be cleared by other proteolytic systems (Kopito, 2000; Olanow *et al.*, 2004; Taylor *et al.*, 2003). In this respect, we and others have postulated that aggresomes appear to have a cytoprotective role (Olanow *et al.*, 2004; Taylor *et al.*, 2003; Kawaguchi *et al.*, 2003; Tanaka *et al.*, 2003). In support of this concept, inhibition of aggresome formation in cells undergoing proteolytic stress impairs the clearance of abnormal proteins and enhances cellular toxicity (Taylor *et al.*, 2003; Johnston, Illing and Kopito, 2002; Johnston, Ward and Kopito, 1998; Junn *et al.*, 2002). Lewy bodies resemble aggresomes and stain positively for γ-tubulin and pericentrin, specific markers of the centrosome/aggresome. These observations have led to the suggestion that Lewy bodies might be aggresome-related inclusions that are cytoprotective, and slow or halt the demise of some neurons in PD (McNaught *et al.*, 2002; Olanow *et al.*, 2004; Chen and Feany, 2005). This hypothesis is consistent with other lines of evidence indicating that Lewy bodies are not deleterious to cells (Gertz, Siegers and Kuchinke, 1994; Tompkins and Hill, 1997). Indeed, neurodegeneration can occur in the SNc without Lewy bodies in both sporadic and familial forms of PD (Mori *et al.*, 1998; Wakabayashi *et al.*, 1999), and Lewy bodies can be present without neurodegeneration (van Duinen *et al.*, 1999). Indeed, degeneration in disorders such as parkin, which lack Lewy bodies, appear to have an aggressive form of dopamine cell loss such that patients present at a very early age, perhaps because they are incapable of manufacturing these protective structures.

The ultimate fate of Lewy bodies and their host cell in PD seems to vary. Some Lewy bodies are observed in the cytoplasm of remaining neurons, while others are extruded into the extracellular space following destruction of the host neuron (Katsuse *et al.*, 2003). In addition, Lewy bodies may be internalized and destroyed by the lysosomal/autophagic system, as has been reported for aggresomes (Taylor *et al.*, 2003; Fortun *et al.*, 2003). Finally, Lewy bodies could be engulfed along with the host cell by activated microglia cells, which are observed at pathological sites in PD (Iseki *et al.*, 2000). Thus, while excess levels of abnormal proteins and aggregates can interfere with intracellular processes and alter cell viability, the formation of Lewy body inclusions might be a cytoprotective response aimed at segregating unwanted proteins to preserve cell viability.

While protein accumulation might occur as a result of increased production in genetic cases (e.g., mutant or excess production of wild-type α-synuclein), there is evidence that protein aggregation in sporadic PD might result from impaired clearance of unwanted proteins due to proteasomal dysfunction (McNaught *et al.*, 2001).

Altered Proteasomal Fuction

Proteasomes are multicatalytic enzymes primarily responsible for the degradation and clearance of unwanted proteins within eukaryocytic cells. Several studies have examined the structure and function of proteasomes in the PD. In one study comparing PD patients to controls, all three proteolytic activities of the 20S proteasome in the SNc were reduced by approximately 45%, but not in other unaffected brain areas (McNaught et al., 2003; McNaught and Jenner, 2001). This defect was accompanied by a marked reduction in the levels of the 20S proteasome α-, but not β-, subunits in dopaminergic neurons of the SNc in PD. In addition, while levels of the PA700 proteasome activator are reduced in the SNc in PD, PA700 expression is increased in other brain regions, such as the frontal cortex and striatum, possibly as a compensation to a proteasomal toxin. This finding raised the possibility that the compensatory capacity of the 26S proteasome is also altered in PD. Further, levels of the PA28 proteasome activator are very low to almost undetectable in the SNc, compared to other brain areas, in both PD and normal subjects. Another study reported a 55% decrease in 20S proteasomal enzyme activity in the SNc, but not elsewhere in the brain of PD subjects (Tofaris et al., 2003). Interestingly, this investigation used PD cases with relatively mild neuropathology, suggesting that proteasomal dysfunction occurs early in the pathogenic process. An additional study also demonstrated that proteasomal activity is not inhibited in extranigral areas in the brain of patients with sporadic PD (Furukawa et al., 2002). Indeed, there was marked upregulation of proteasomal enzymatic activity in the striatum and cerebral cortex in PD patients compared to control subjects, consistent with our demonstration of increased expression of PA700 in these brain areas (McNaught et al., 2003).

The basis of proteasomal dysfunction in sporadic PD is presently unknown, but could relate to encoding changes, oxidative damage, ATP depletion, and toxic modifications. Recently, DNA microarray analyses in the SNc in PD demonstrated a reduction in the mRNA levels of 20S proteasome α-subunits (PSAM2, PSMA3 and PSMA5), a non-ATPase subunit (PSMD8/Rpn12) and an ATPase subunit (PSMC4/Rpt3) of PA700 (Grunblatt et al., 2004). Proteasomal subunits are susceptible to free radical-mediated injury and to mitochondrial damage, and this could account for secondary proteasomal damage in PD (Ding and Keller, 2001; Jha et al., 2002; Okada et al., 1999; Hoglinger et al., 2003; Shamoto-Nagai et al., 2003). Assembly/re-assembly of proteasomal components and their subsequent proteolytic activity require ATP (Hoglinger et al., 2003; Eytan et al., 1989; Hendil, Hartmann-Petersen and Tanaka, 2002; Imai et al., 2003). Thus, primary or secondary inhibition of complex I activity could contribute to proteasomal dysfunction in PD. Interestingly, continuous administration of low doses of MPTP, which inhibits complex I through its active metabolite MPP+, was recently shown to impair proteasomal function and to cause neurodegeneration with inclusion body formation in mice (Fornai et al., 2005). Abnormal proteins themselves may also interfere with proteasomal function in PD (Snyder et al., 2003; Tanaka et al., 2001; Bennett et al., 2005; Hyun et al., 2002; Lindersson et al., 2004). Consistent with this possibility, recent studies have shown that incompletely or partially degraded α-synuclein directly inhibits proteasomal function (Liu et al., 2005). Finally, naturally occurring environmental toxins could play a role in proteasomal dysfunction in PD (McNaught et al., 2001).

The stage at which proteasomal dysfunction first occurs is not known. If this occurs early it might play a role in the initiation of the neurodegenerative processes, or if it occurs late it could contribute to the progression of the disease process. Either way, proteasomal dysfunction could be a central feature of cell death in PD and underlie the protein accumulation/aggregation and Lewy body formation that characterize PD. In support of this concept, we (McNaught et al., 2002; McNaught et al., 2002) and others (Fornai et al., 2003; Rideout et al., 2005; Rideout et al., 2001; Miwa et al., 2005) showed that proteasome inhibitors induced selective degeneration of dopaminergic cells in culture and nigrostriatal degeneration with motor dysfunction when injected directly into the SNc or striatum of rats. Importantly, neuronal death was associated with the accumulation of α-synuclein and ubiquitin, and the formation of intracytoplasmic Lewy body-like inclusions containing these and other proteins. Further, several studies have shown that lactacystin, PSI and other proteasome inhibitors can also induce degeneration of non-dopaminergic cells with inclusion body formation (Kisselev and Goldberg, 2001; Rideout and Stefanis, 2002). This observation has important implications for a role of proteasomal dysfunction in PD, since brain regions containing non-dopaminergic neurons also degenerate in the illness. Indeed, we and others recently demonstrated that systemic administration of proteasome inhibitors to rats induces degeneration of nigral dopaminergic neurons (McNaught et al., 2004; Nair et al., 2006; Schapira et al., 2006; Zeng et al., 2006). However, these results are somewhat controversial, as several groups have not been able to confirm these findings (Kordower et al., 2006; Manning-Bog et al., 2006). In addition, inhibition of proteasomal function can induce cellular, biochemical and molecular changes that are similar to those that occur in PD (Hoglinger et al., 2003; Kikuchi et al., 2003; Sullivan et al., 2004). Further, there is a strong theoretical basis for considering that mutations in α-synuclein, UCH-L1 and parkin genes could theoretically lead to interference with UPS function and protein accumulation (Olanow and McNaught, 2006). Therefore, it is reasonable to suggest that proteolytic stress could play a key role in the pathogenesis of PD, and that therapies designed to prevent the formation or enhance the clearance of misfolded proteins might have neuroprotective effects in PD.

Recent attention has also focused on the role of autophagy in clearing misfolded and unwanted proteins, raising the possibility that defects in this lysosomal system could also lead to protein accumulation and Lewy body formation (Martinez-Vicente and Cueve, 2007). No studies have as yet examined the status of the autophage system in PD.

Apoptosis

Regardless of the precise pathogenic mechanism, there is considerable evidence indicating that cell death in PD occurs by way of a signal-mediated apoptotic process. Numerous studies have found increased numbers of apoptotic nuclei in the SNc of PD patients in comparison to controls (Hirsch *et al.*, 1999). Further, Tatton and colleagues showed evidence of both chromatin clumping and DNA fragmentation in the same nigral neurons, virtually eliminating the possibility of false positive results (Tatton *et al.*, 1998). In addition, there is increased expression of pro-apoptotic signals such as caspase 3 and Bax and nuclear translocation of GAPDH in SNc neurons in PD (Tatton, 2000), supporting the concept that these cells have been injured and are in a pro-apoptotic state. Recent studies also demonstrate increased levels of p-p53 in PD nigral neurons compared to controls (Nair *et al.*, 2006). As a non-transcriptional increase in p53 is a key signal mediating cell death following proteasome inhibition, this may be a particularly relevant finding (Nair *et al.*, 2006).

CONCLUSIONS

The mechanism of cell death in PD remains unknown, despite many promising and even tantalizing clues. Small numbers of familial cases of PD are known to be caused by gene mutations, and mutations have now been identified in some cases with sporadic forms of PD. However, it is not at all clear that genetic factors cause the majority of sporadic cases. Environmental toxins have been implicated, but none has as yet been established to cause PD. It is possible that there are many different forms of PD, and many different causes. Post mortem studies have implicated oxidative stress, mitochondrial dysfunction, inflammation and exictotoxicity, but what role each of these play remains uncertain, and it is possible that some or even all are epiphenomena and do not directly contribute to cell death. More recently, attention has focused on the possibility that proteolytic stress due to impaired clearance of unwanted proteins is at the heart of cell death in PD. This is supported by the almost universal finding of protein accumulation and inclusion body formation in areas that undergo neurodegeneration. This concept is also supported by the observation that increased production of both mutant and wild-type α-synuclein can cause PD in humans and dopamine degeneration in animal models. Similarly, proteasome dysfunction is found in sporadic PD and proteasome inhibitors induce dopamine cell death with inclusion bodies in animal models. It is possible that many or all of these various pathogenic factors might interact in a cascade of events leading to cell death and that the precipitating factor may be different in different individuals. Many candidate targets for developing possible neuroprotective therapies have been identified, but to date no agent has been shown to have disease-modifying effects in PD. The identification of gene mutations that cause PD provide additional opportunities for identifying mechanisms that lead to cell death that hopefully will also be relevant to sporadic PD. Already, transgenic models that carry these mutations have begun to shed light on how cells might die in PD, although it is disturbing that no animal model to date fully replicates the dopaminergic and non-dopaminergic pathology of PD. Still, there is enthusiasm that with further research we will better understand why cells die in PD, develop animal models that replicate all of the features of the disease, and ultimately produce a drug which slows or stops disease progression.

ACKNOWLEDGEMENT

This study was supported by grants from the NIH/NINDS (1 RO1 NS045999-01), the Bendheim Parkinson's Disease Center, and the Morris and Alma Schapiro Foundation.

References

Alam, Z.I., Daniel, S.E., Lees, A.J., Marsden, D.C., Jenner, P. and Halliwell, B. (1997) A generalised increase in protein carbonyls in the brain in Parkinson's but not incidental Lewy body disease. *Journal of Neurochemistry*, **69** (3), 1326–1329.

Alam, Z.I., Daniel, S.E., Lees, A.J., Marsden, D.C., Jenner, P. and Halliwell, B.(Sep 1997) A generalised increase in protein carbonyls in the brain in Parkinson's but not incidental Lewy body disease. *Journal of Neurochemistry*, **69** (3), 1326–1329.

Ardley, H.C., Scott, G.B., Rose, S.A., Tan, N.G., Markham, A.F. and Robinson, P.A. (2003) Inhibition of proteasomal activity causes inclusion formation in neuronal and non-neuronal cells overexpressing parkin. *Molecular Biology of the Cell*, **14** (11), 4541–4556.

Auberger, G., Kessker, K., Kang, J.-S., Gispert, S., Stoltenburg, G. and Braak, H. (2005) Is the PARK5 I93M mutation a cause of Parkinson's disease with cognitive deficits and cortical Lewy pathology? 16th International Congress on Parkinson's Disease and Related Disorders Berlin (2), pp. PT042.

Auluck, P.K. and Bonini, N.M. (2002) Pharmacological prevention of Parkinson's disease in Drosophila. *Nature Medicine*, **8**, 1185–1186.

Auluck, P.K., Chan, H.Y., Trojanowski, J.Q. *et al.* (2002) Chaperone suppression of alpha-synuclein toxicity in a Drosophila model for Parkinson's disease. *Science*, **295**, 865–868.

Baba, M., Nakajo, S., Tu, P.H., Tomita, T., Nakaya, K., Lee, V.M., Trojanowski, J.Q. and Iwatsubo, T. (1998) Aggregation of alpha-synuclein in Lewy bodies of sporadic Parkinson's disease and dementia with Lewy bodies. *The American Journal of Pathology*, **152** (4), 879–884.

Bandopadhyay, R., Kingsbury, A.E., Cookson, M.R., Reid, A.R., Evans, I.M., Hope, A.D., Pittman, A.M., Lashley, T., Canet-Aviles, R., Miller, D.W., McLendon, C., Strand, C., Leonard, A.J., Abou-Sleiman, P.M., Healy, D.G., Ariga, H., Wood, N.W., de Silva, R., Revesz, T., Hardy, J.A. and Lees, A.J. (2004) The expression of DJ-1 (PARK7) in normal human CNS and idiopathic Parkinson's disease. *Brain: A Journal of Neurology*, **127** (Pt 2), 420–430.

Bence, N.F., Sampat, R.M. and Kopito, R.R. (2001) Impairment of the ubiquitin-proteasome system by protein aggregation. *Science*, **292** (5521), 1552–1555.

Bennett, M.C., Bishop, J.F., Leng, Y., Chock, P.B., Chase, T.N. and Mouradian, M.M. (1999) Degradation of alpha-synuclein by proteasome. *The Journal of Biological Chemistry*, **274** (48), 33855–33858.

Bennett, E.J., Bence, N.F., Jayakumar, R. and Kopito, R.R. (2005) Global impairment of the ubiquitin-proteasome system by nuclear or cytoplasmic protein aggregates precedes inclusion body formation. *Molecular Cell*, **17** (3), 351–365.

Betarbet, R., Sherer, T.B., MacKenzie, G., Garcia-Osuna, M., Panov, A.V. and Greenamyre, J.T. (2000) Chronic systemic pesticide exposure reproduces features of Parkinson's disease. *Nature Neuroscience*, **3**, 1301–1306.

Bonifati, V., Rizzu, P., van Baren, M.J., Schaap, O., Breedveld, G.J., Krieger, E., Dekker, M.C., Squitieri, F., Ibanez, P., Joosse, M., van Dongen, J.W., Vanacore, N., van Swieten, J.C., Brice, A., Meco, G., van Duijn, C.M., Oostra, B.A. and Heutink, P. (2003) Mutations in the DJ-1 gene associated with autosomal recessive early-onset parkinsonism. *Science*, **299** (5604), 256–259.

Bonifati, V., Oostra, B.A. and Heutink, P. (2004) Linking DJ-1 to neurodegeneration offers novel insights for understanding the pathogenesis of Parkinson's disease. *Journal of Molecular Medicine*, **82** (3), 163–174.

Braak, H., Tredici, K.D., Rub, U., de Vos, R.A., Jansen Steur, E.N. and Braak, E. (2003) Staging of brain pathology related to sporadic Parkinson's disease. *Neurobiology of Aging*, **24** (2), 197–211.

Castellani, R.J., Perry, G., Siedlak, S.L., Nunomura, A., Shimohama, S., Zhang, J., Montine, T., Sayre, L.M. and Smith, M.A. (2002) Hydroxynonenal adducts indicate a role for lipid peroxidation in neocortical and brainstem Lewy bodies in humans. *Neuroscience Letters*, **319** (1), 25–28.

Caughey, B. and Lansbury, P.T. (2003) Protofibrils, pores, fibrils, and neurodegeneration: separating the responsible protein aggregates from the innocent bystanders. *Annual Review of Neuroscience*, **26**, 267–298.

Chan, C.S., Guzman, J.N., Ilijic, E. *et al.* (2007) "Rejuvenation" protects neurons in mouse models of Parkinson's disease. *Nature*, **447**, 1081–1086.

Chartier-Harlin, M.C., Kachergus, J., Roumier, C., Mouroux, V., Douay, X., Lincoln, S., Levecque, C., Larvor, L., Andrieux, J., Hulihan, M., Waucquier, N., Defebvre, L., Amouyel, P., Farrer, M. and Destee, A. (2004) Alpha-synuclein locus duplication as a cause of familial Parkinson's disease. *Lancet*, **364** (9440), 1167–1169.

Chen, L. and Feany, M.B. (2005) alpha-Synuclein phosphorylation controls neurotoxicity and inclusion formation in a Drosophila model of Parkinson's disease. *Nature Neuroscience*, **8** (5), 657–663.

Clark, I.E., Dodson, M.W., Jiang, C., Cao, J.H., Huh, J.R., Seol, J.H., Yoo, S.J., Hay, B.A. and Guo, M. (2006) Drosophila pink1 is required for mitochondrial function and interacts genetically with parkin. *Nature*, **441** (7097), 1162–1166.

Conway, K.A., Harper, J.D. and Lansbury, P.T. (1998) Accelerated in vitro fibril formation by a mutant alpha-synuclein linked to early-onset Parkinson's disease. *Nature Medicine*, **4** (11), 1318–1320.

Conway, K.A., Lee, S.J., Rochet, J.C., Ding, T.T., Williamson, R.E. and Lansbury, P.T., Jr (2000) Acceleration of oligomerization, not fibrillization, is a shared property of both alpha-synuclein mutations linked to early-onset Parkinson's disease: implications for pathogenesis and therapy. *Proceedings of the National Academy of Sciences, of the United States of America*, **97** (2), 571–576.

Cuervo, A.M., Stefanis, L., Fredenburg, R., Lansbury, P.T. and Sulzer, D. (2004) Impaired degradation of mutant alpha-synuclein by chaperone-mediated autophagy. *Science*, **305** (5688), 1292–1295.

Cyr, D.M., Hohfeld, J. and Patterson, C. (2002) Protein quality control: U-box-containing E3 ubiquitin ligases join the fold. *Trends in Biochemical Sciences*, **27** (7), 368–375.

Dachsel, J.C., Lucking, C.B., Deeg, S., Schultz, E., Lalowski, M., Casademunt, E., Corti, O., Hampe, C., Patenge, N., Vaupel, K., Yamamoto, A., Dichgans, M., Brice, A., Wanker, E.E., Kahle, P.J. and Gasser, T. (2005) Parkin interacts with the proteasome subunit alpha4. *FEBS Letters*, **579** (18), 3913–3919.

Dauer, W., Kholodilov, N., Vila, M. *et al.* (2002) Resistance of alpha-synuclein null mice to the parkinsonian neurotoxin MPTP. *Proceedings of the National Academy of Sciences, of the United States of America*, **99**, 14524–14529.

Dexter, D.T., Carter, C.J., Wells, F.R., Javoy-Agid, F., Agid, Y., Lees, A., Jenner, P. and Marsden, C.D. (1989) Basal lipid peroxidation in substantia nigra is increased in Parkinson's disease. *Journal of Neurochemistry*, **52** (2), 381–389.

Dexter, D.T., Carayon, A., Javoy-Agid, F., Agid, Y., Wells, F.R., Daniel, S.E., Lees, A.J., Jenner, P. and Marsden, C.D. (1991) Alterations in the levels of iron, ferritin and other trace metals in Parkinson's disease and other neurodegenerative diseases affecting the basal ganglia. *Brain: A Journal of Neurology*, **114** (Pt 4), 1953–1975.

Dexter, D.T., Holley, A.E., Flitter, W.D., Slater, T.F., Wells, F.R., Daniel, S.E., Lees, A.J., Jenner, P. and Marsden, C.D. (1994) Increased levels of lipid hydroperoxides in the parkinsonian substantia nigra: an HPLC and ESR study. *Movement Disorders*, **9** (1), 92–97.

Di Fonzo, A., Rohe, C.F., Ferreira, J., Chien, H.F., Vacca, L., Stocchi, F., Guedes, L., Fabrizio, E., Manfredi, M., Vanacore, N., Goldwurm, S., Breedveld, G., Sampaio, C., Meco, G., Barbosa, E., Oostra, B.A. and Bonifati, V. (2005) A frequent LRRK2 gene mutation associated with autosomal dominant Parkinson's disease. *Lancet*, **365** (9457), 412–415.

Ding, Q. and Keller, J.N. (2001) Proteasome inhibition in oxidative stress neurotoxicity: implications for heat shock proteins. *Journal of Neurochemistry*, **77**, 1010–1017.

Dorsey, E.R., Constantinescu, R., Thompson, J.P., Biglan, K.M., Holloway, R.G., Kieburtz, K., Marshall, F.J., Ravina, B.M., Schifitto, G., Siderowf, A. and Tanner, C.M. (2007) Projected number of people with Parkinson's disease in the most populous nations, 2005 through 2030. *Neurology*, **68** (5), 384–386.

Duda, J.E., Giasson, B.I., Mabon, M.E., Miller, D.C., Golbe, L.I., Lee, V.M. and Trojanowski, J.Q. (2002) Concurrence of alpha-synuclein and tau brain pathology in the Contursi kindred. *Acta Neuropathologica*, **104** (1), 7–11.

Elbaz, A., Nelson, L.M., Payami, H. *et al.* (2006) Lack of replication of thirteen single-nucleotide polymorphisms implicated in Parkinson's disease: a large-scale international study. *Lancet Neurology*, **5**, 917–923.

Eytan, E., Ganoth, D., Armon, T. and Hershko, A. (1989) ATP-dependent incorporation of 20S protease into the 26S complex that degrades proteins conjugated to ubiquitin. *Proceedings of the National Academy of Sciences, of the United States of America*, **86** (20), 7751–7755.

Farrer, M.J. (2006) Genetics of Parkinson's disease: paradigm shifts and future prospects. *Nature Reviews Genetics*, **7** (4), 306–318.

Farrer, M., Chan, P., Chen, R., Tan, L., Lincoln, S., Hernandez, D., Forno, L., Gwinn-Hardy, K., Petrucelli, L., Hussey, J., Singleton, A., Tanner, C., Hardy, J. and Langston, J.W. (2001) Lewy bodies and parkinsonism in families with parkin mutations. *Annals of Neurology*, **50** (3), 293–300.

Farrer, M., Kachergus, J., Forno, L., Lincoln, S., Wang, D.S., Hulihan, M., Maraganore, D., Gwinn-Hardy, K., Wszolek, Z., Dickson, D. and Langston, J.W. (2004) Comparison of kindreds with parkinsonism and alpha-synuclein genomic multiplications. *Annals of Neurology*, **55** (2), 174–179.

Fasano, M., Giraudo, S., Coha, S., Bergamasco, B. and Lopiano, L. (2003) Residual substantia nigra neuromelanin in Parkinson's disease is cross-linked to alpha-synuclein. *Neurochemistry International*, **42** (7), 603–606.

Feany, M.B. and Bender, W.W. (2000) A Drosophila model of Parkinson's disease. *Nature*, **404** (6776), 394–398.

Fernagut, P.O. and Chesselet, M.F. (2004) Alpha-synuclein and transgenic mouse models. *Neurobiology of Disease*, **17** (2), 123–130.

Fornai, F., Lenzi, P., Gesi, M., Ferrucci, M., Lazzeri, G., Busceti, C.L., Ruffoli, R., Soldani, P., Ruggieri, S., Alessandri, M.G. and Paparelli, A. (2003) Fine structure and biochemical mechanisms underlying nigrostriatal inclusions and cell death after proteasome inhibition. *The Journal of Neuroscience*, **23** (26), 8955–8966.

Fornai, F., Schluter, O.M., Lenzi, P., Gesi, M., Ruffoli, R., Ferrucci, M., Lazzeri, G., Busceti, C.L., Pontarelli, F., Battaglia, G., Pellegrini, A., Nicoletti, F., Ruggieri, S., Paparelli, A. and Sudhof, T.C. (2005) Parkinson-like syndrome induced by continuous MPTP infusion: Convergent roles of the ubiquitin-proteasome system and {alpha}-synuclein. *Proceedings of the National Academy of Sciences, of the United States of America*, **102**, 3413–3418.

Forno, L.S. (1996) Neuropathology of Parkinson's disease. *Journal of Neuropathology and Experimental, Neurology*, **55** (3), 259–272.

Foroud, T., Uniacke, S.K., Liu, L., Pankratz, N., Rudolph, A., Halter, C., Shults, C., Marder, K., Conneally, P.M. and Nichols, W.C. (2003) Heterozygosity for a mutation in the parkin gene leads to later onset Parkinson's disease. *Neurology*, **60** (5), 796–801.

Fortun, J., Dunn, W.A., Jr, Joy, S., Li, J. and Notterpek, L. (2003) Emerging role for autophagy in the removal of aggresomes in Schwann cells. *The Journal of Neuroscience*, **23** (33), 10672–10680.

Fujiwara, H., Hasegawa, M., Dohmae, N., Kawashima, A., Masliah, E., Goldberg, M.S., Shen, J., Takio, K. and Iwatsubo, T. (2002) alpha-Synuclein is phosphorylated in synucleinopathy lesions. *Nature Cell Biology*, **4** (2), 160–164.

Funayama, M., Hasegawa, K., Kowa, H., Saito, M., Tsuji, S. and Obata, F. (2002) A new locus for Parkinson's disease (PARK8) maps to chromosome 12p11.2-q13.1. *Annals of Neurology*, **51** (3), 296–301.

Fung, H..-C., Scholz, S., Matarin, M. *et al.* (2006) Genome-wide genotyping in Parkinson's disease and neurologically normal controls: first stage analysis and public release of data. *Lancet Neurology*, **5**, 911–916.

Furukawa, Y., Vigouroux, S., Wong, H., Guttman, M., Rajput, A.H., Ang, L., Briand, M., Kish, S.J. and Briand, Y. (2002) Brain proteasomal function in sporadic Parkinson's disease and related disorders. *Annals of Neurology*, **51**, 779–782.

Gertz, H.J., Siegers, A. and Kuchinke, J. (1994) Stability of cell size and nucleolar size in Lewy body containing neurons of substantia nigra in Parkinson's disease. *Brain Research*, **637** (1–2), 339–341.

Giasson, B.I., Duda, J.E., Murray, I.V., Chen, Q., Souza, J.M., Hurtig, H.I., Ischiropoulos, H., Trojanowski, J.Q. and Lee, V.M. (2000) Oxidative damage linked to neurodegeneration by selective alpha-synuclein nitration in synucleinopathy lesions. *Science*, **290** (5493), 985–989.

Gilks, W.P., Abou-Sleiman, P.M., Gandhi, S. *et al.* (2005) A common LRRK2 mutation in idiopathic Parkinson's disease. *Lancet*, **365**, 415–416.

Gilks, W.P., Abou-Sleiman, P.M., Gandhi, S., Jain, S., Singleton, A., Lees, A.J., Shaw, K., Bhatia, K.P., Bonifati, V., Quinn, N.P., Lynch, J., Healy, D.G., Holton, J.L., Revesz, T. and Wood, N.W. (2005) A common LRRK2 mutation in idiopathic Parkinson's disease. *Lancet*, **365** (9457), 415–416.

Goedert, M. (2001) Alpha-synuclein and neurodegenerative diseases. *Nature Reviews. Neuroscience*, **2** (7), 492–501.

Goldberg, M.S., Fleming, S.M., Palacino, J.J., Cepeda, C., Lam, H.A., Bhatnagar, A., Meloni, E.G., Wu, N., Ackerson, L.C., Klapstein, G.J., Gajendiran, M., Roth, B.L., Chesselet, M.F., Maidment, N.T., Levine, M.S. and Shen, J. (2003) Parkin-deficient mice exhibit nigrostriatal deficits but not loss of dopaminergic neurons. *The Journal of Biological Chemistry*, **278** (44), 43628–43635.

Goldberg, M.S., Pisani, A., Haburcak, M., Vortherms, T.A., Kitada, T., Costa, C., Tong, Y., Martella, G., Tscherter, A., Martins, A., Bernardi, G., Roth, B.L., Pothos, E.N., Calabresi, P. and Shen, J. (2005) Nigrostriatal dopaminergic deficits and hypokinesia caused by inactivation of the familial parkinsonism-linked gene DJ-1. *Neuron*, **45**, 489–496.

Good, P.F., Hsu, A., Werner, P., Perl, D.P. and Olanow, C.W. (1998) Protein nitration in Parkinson's disease. *Journal of Neuropathology and Experimental, Neurology*, **57** (4), 338–342.

Greggio, E., Jain, S., Kingsbury, A. *et al.* (2006) Kinase activity is required for the toxic effects of mutant LRRK2/dardarin. *Neurobiology of Disease*, **23**, 329–341.

Grunblatt, E., Mandel, S., Jacob-Hirsch, J., Zeligson, S., Amariglo, N., Rechavi, G., Li, J., Ravid, R., Roggendorf, W., Riederer, P. and Youdim, M.B. (2004) Gene expression profiling of parkinsonian substantia nigra pars compacta; alterations in ubiquitin-proteasome, heat shock protein, iron and oxidative stress regulated proteins, cell adhesion/cellular matrix and vesicle trafficking genes. *Journal of Neural Transmission*, **111**, 1543–1573.

Hardy, J., Cai, H., Cookson, M.R., Gwinn-Hardy, K. and Singleton, A. (2006) Genetics of Parkinson's disease and parkinsonism. *Annals of Neurology*, **60**, 389–398.

Hasegawa, M., Fujiwara, H., Nonaka, T., Wakabayashi, K., Takahashi, H., Lee, V.M., Trojanowski, J.Q., Mann, D. and Iwatsubo, T. (2002) Phosphorylated alpha-synuclein is ubiquitinated in alpha-synucleinopathy lesions. *The Journal of Biological Chemistry*, **277** (50), 49071–49076.

Hashimoto, M., Rockenstein, E., Mante, M. *et al.* (2004) An antiaggregation gene therapy strategy for Lewy body disease utilizing beta-synuclein lentivirus in a transgenic model. *Gene Therapy*, **11**, 1713–1723.

Hatano, Y., Li, Y., Sato, K., Asakawa, S., Yamamura, Y., Tomiyama, H., Yoshino, H., Asahina, M., Kobayashi, S., Hassin-Baer, S., Lu, C.S., Ng, A.R., Rosales, R.L., Shimizu, N., Toda, T., Mizuno, Y. and Hattori, N. (2004) Novel PINK1 mutations in early-onset parkinsonism. *Annals of Neurology*, **56** (3), 424–427.

Hattori, N. and Mizuno, Y. (2004) Pathogenetic mechanisms of parkin in Parkinson's disease. *Lancet*, **364** (9435), 722–724.

Hawkes, C.H., Del Tredici, K. and Braak, H. (2007) Parkinson's disease: a dual-hit hypothesis. *Neuropathology and Applied Neurobiology*, **33** (6), 599–614.

Healy, D.G., Abou-Sleiman, P.M. and Wood, N.W. (2004) PINK, PANK, or PARK? A clinicians' guide to familial parkinsonism. *Lancet Neurology*, **3** (11), 652–662.

Healy, D.G., Abou-Sleiman, P.M., Casas, J.P., Ahmadi, K.R., Lynch, T., Gandhi, S., Muqit, M.M., Foltynie, T., Barker, R., Bhatia, K.P., Quinn, N.P., Lees, A.J., Gibson, J.M., Holton, J.L., Revesz, T., Goldstein, D.B. and Wood, N.W. (2006) UCHL-1 is not a Parkinson's disease susceptibility gene. *Annals of Neurology*, **59** (4), 627–633.

Hendil, K.B., Hartmann-Petersen, R. and Tanaka, K. (2002) 26S Proteasomes Function as Stable Entities. *Journal of Molecular Biology*, **315** (4), 627–636.

Hirsch, E.C., Brandel, J.P., Galle, P., Javoy-Agid, F. and Agid, Y. (1991) Iron and aluminum increase in the substantia nigra of patients with Parkinson's disease: an X-ray microanalysis. *Journal of Neurochemistry*, **56** (2), 446–451.

Hirsch, E.C., Hunot, S., Faucheux, B., Agid, Y., Mizuno, Y., Mochizuki, H., Tatton, W.G., Tatton, N. and Olanow, C.W. (1999) Dopaminergic neurons degenerate by apoptosis in Parkinson's disease. *Movement Disorders*, **14**, 383–385.

Hoglinger, G.U., Carrard, G., Michel, P.P. *et al.* (2003) Dysfunction of mitochondrial complex I and the proteasome: interactions between two biochemical deficits in a cellular model of Parkinson's disease. *Journal of Neurochemistry*, **86**, 1297–1307.

Horowitz, J.M., Vernace, V.A., Myers, J., Stachowiak, M.K., Hanlon, D.W., Fraley, G.S. and Torres, G. (2001) Immunodetection of Parkin protein in vertebrate and invertebrate brains: a comparative study using specific antibodies. *Journal of Chemical Neuroanatomy*, **21** (1), 75–93.

Hyun, D.H., Lee, M.H., Halliwell, B. and Jenner, P. (2002) Proteasomal dysfunction induced by 4-hydroxy-2,3-trans-nonenal, an end-product of lipid peroxidation: a mechanism contributing to neurodegeneration? *Journal of Neurochemistry*, **83** (2), 360–370.

Ibanez, P., Bonnet, A.M., Debarges, B., Lohmann, E., Tison, F., Pollak, P., Agid, Y., Durr, A. and Brice, A. (2004) Causal relation between alpha-synuclein gene duplication and familial Parkinson's disease. *Lancet*, **364** (9440), 1169–1171.

Ii, K., Ito, H., Tanaka, K. and Hirano, A. (1997) Immunocytochemical co-localization of the proteasome in ubiquitinated structures in neurodegenerative diseases and the elderly. *Journal of Neuropathology and Experimental, Neurology*, **56** (2), 125–131.

Imai, Y., Soda, M. and Takahashi, R. (2000) Parkin suppresses unfolded protein stress-induced cell death through its E3 ubiquitin-protein ligase activity. *The Journal of Biological Chemistry*, **275** (46), 35661–35664.

Imai, Y., Soda, M., Inoue, H., Hattori, N., Mizuno, Y. and Takahashi, R. (2001) An Unfolded Putative Transmembrane Polypeptide, which Can Lead to Endoplasmic Reticulum Stress, Is a Substrate of Parkin. *Cell*, **105** (7), 891–902.

Imai, J., Maruya, M., Yashiroda, H., Yahara, I. and Tanaka, K. (2003) The molecular chaperone Hsp90 plays a role in the assembly and maintenance of the 26S proteasome. *EMBO Journal*, **22** (14), 3557–3567.

Iseki, E., Marui, W., Akiyama, H., Ueda, K. and Kosaka, K. (2000) Degeneration process of Lewy bodies in the brains of patients with dementia with Lewy bodies using alpha-synuclein-immunohistochemistry. *Neuroscience Letters*, **286** (1), 69–73.

Itier, J.M., Ibanez, P., Mena, M.A., Abbas, N., Cohen-Salmon, C., Bohme, G.A., Laville, M., Pratt, J., Corti, O., Pradier, L., Ret, G., Joubert, C., Periquet, M., Araujo, F., Negroni, J., Casarejos, M. J., Canals, S., Solano, R., Serrano, A., Gallego, E., Sanchez, M., Denefle, P., Benavides, J., Tremp, G., Rooney, T.A., Brice, A. and Garcia de Yebenes, J. (2003) Parkin gene inactivation alters behaviour and dopamine neurotransmission in the mouse. *Human Molecular Genetics*, **12** (18), 2277–2291.

Jakes, R., Spillantini, M.G. and Goedert, M. (1994) Identification of two distinct synucleins from human brain. *FEBS Letters*, **345** (1), 27–32.

Jenner, P. (2003) Oxidative stress in Parkinson's disease. *Annals of Neurology*, **53** (Suppl 3), S26–S36 discussion S36–28.

Jha, N., Kumar, M.J., Boonplueang, R. and Andersen, J.K. (2002) Glutathione decreases in dopaminergic PC12 cells interfere with the ubiquitin protein degradation pathway: relevance for Parkinson's disease? *Journal of Neurochemistry*, **80**, 555–561.

Johnston, J.A., Ward, C.L. and Kopito, R.R. (1998) Aggresomes: a cellular response to misfolded proteins. *The Journal of Cell Biology*, **143** (7), 1883–1898.

Johnston, J.A., Illing, M.E. and Kopito, R.R. (2002) Cytoplasmic dynein/dynactin mediates the assembly of aggresomes. *Cell Motility and the Cytoskeleton*, **53** (1), 26–38.

Junn, E., Lee, S.S., Suhr, U.T. and Mouradian, M.M. (2002) Parkin accumulation in aggresomes due to proteasome impairment. *The Journal of Biological Chemistry*, **277** (49), 47870–47877.

Katsuse, O., Iseki, E., Marui, W. and Kosaka, K. (2003) Developmental stages of cortical Lewy bodies and their relation to axonal transport blockage in brains of patients with dementia with Lewy bodies. *Journal of the Neurological Sciences*, **211** (1–2), 29–35.

Kawaguchi, Y., Kovacs, J.J., McLaurin, A., Vance, J.M., Ito, A. and Yao, T.P. (2003) The deacetylase HDAC6 regulates aggresome formation and cell viability in response to misfolded protein stress. *Cell*, **115** (6), 727–738.

Kikuchi, S., Shinpo, K.,Tsuji, S. *et al.* (2003) Effect of proteasome inhibitor on cultured mesencephalic dopaminergic neurons. *Brain Research*, **964**, 228–236.

Kirik, D., Annett, L.E., Burger, C., Muzyczka, N., Mandel, R.J. and Bjorklund, A. (2003) Nigrostriatal alpha-synucleinopathy induced by viral vector-mediated overexpression of human alpha-synuclein: a new primate model of Parkinson's disease. *Proceedings of the National Academy of Sciences, of the United States of America*, **100** (5), 2884–2889.

Kisselev, A.F. and Goldberg, A.L. (2001) Proteasome inhibitors: from research tools to drug candidates. *Chemistry & Biology*, **8** (8), 739–758.

Kitada, T., Asakawa, S., Hattori, N., Matsumine, H., Yamamura, Y., Minoshima, S., Yokochi, M., Mizuno, Y. and Shimizu, N. (1998) Mutations in the parkin gene cause autosomal recessive juvenile parkinsonism. *Nature*, **392** (6676), 605–608.

Kopito, R.R. (2000) Aggresomes, inclusion bodies and protein aggregation. *Trends in Cell Biology*, **10** (12), 524–530.

Kordower, J.H., Kanaan, N.M., Chu, Y., Suresh Babu, R., Stansell, J., 3rd, Terpstra, B.T., Sortwell, C.E., Steece-Collier, K. and Collier, T.J. (2006) Failure of proteasome inhibitor administration to provide a model of Parkinson's disease in rats and monkeys. *Annals of Neurology*, **60** (2), 264–268.

Kotzbauer, P.T., Giasson, B.I., Kravitz, A.V., Golbe, L.I., Mark, M.H., Trojanowski, J.Q. and Lee, V.M. (2004) Fibrillization of alpha-synuclein and tau in familial Parkinson's disease caused by the A53T alpha-synuclein mutation. *Experimental Neurology*, **187** (2), 279–288.

Lang, A.E. and Lozano, A.M. (1998) Parkinson's disease. First of two parts. *The New England Journal of Medicine*, **339** (15), 1044–1053.

Lang, A.E. and Lozano, A.M. (1998) Parkinson's disease. Second of two parts. *The New England Journal of Medicine*, **339** (16), 1130–1143.

Langston, J.W., Ballard, P., Tetrud, J.W. and Irwin, I. (1983) Chronic parkinsonism in humans due to a product of meperidine-analog synthesis. *Science*, **219**, 979–980.

Lashuel, H.A., Petre, B.M., Wall, J., Simon, M., Nowak, R.J., Walz, T. and Lansbury, P.T., Jr (2002) Alpha-synuclein, especially the Parkinson's disease-associated mutants, forms pore-like annular and tubular protofibrils. *Journal of Molecular Biology*, **322** (5), 1089–1102.

Lee, S.J., Kim, S.J., Kim, I.K., Ko, J., Jeong, C.S., Kim, G.H., Park, C., Kang, S.O., Suh, P.G., Lee, H.S. and Cha, S.S. (2003) Crystal structures of human DJ-1 and Escherichia coli Hsp31, which share an evolutionarily conserved domain. *The Journal of Biological Chemistry*, **278** (45), 44552–44559.

Lee, H.J., Khoshaghideh, F., Patel, S. and Lee, S.J. (2004) Clearance of alpha-synuclein oligomeric intermediates via the lysosomal degradation pathway. *The Journal of Neuroscience*, **24** (8), 1888–1896.

Lennox, G., Lowe, J., Morrell, K., Landon, M. and Mayer, R.J. (1989) Anti-ubiquitin immunocytochemistry is more sensitive than conventional techniques in the detection of diffuse Lewy body disease. *Journal of Neurology, Neurosurgery, and, Psychiatry*, **52** (1), 67–71.

Leroy, E., Boyer, R., Auburger, G., Leube, B., Ulm, G., Mezey, E., Harta, G., Brownstein, M.J., Jonnalagada, S., Chernova, T., Dehejia, A., Lavedan, C., Gasser, T., Steinbach, P.J., Wilkinson, K.D. and Polymeropoulos, M.H. (1998) The ubiquitin pathway in Parkinson's disease. *Nature*, **395** (6701), 451–452.

Lesage, S., Dürr, A., Tazir, M. *et al.* (2006) LRRK2 G2019S as a cause of Parkinson's disease in North African Arabs. *The New England Journal of Medicine*, **354**, 422–423.

Lesage, S., Dürr, A., Tazir, M. *et al.* (2006) LRRK2 G2019S as a cause of Parkinson's disease in North African Arabs. *The New England Journal of Medicine*, **354**, 422–423.

Li, J., Uversky, V.N. and Fink, A.L. (2001) Effect of familial Parkinson's disease point mutations A30P and A53T on the structural properties, aggregation, and fibrillation of human alpha-synuclein. *Biochemistry*, **40** (38), 11604–11613.

Li, X., Tan, Y.C., Poulose, S., Olanow, C.W., Huang, X.Y. and Yue, Z. (2007) Leucine-rich repeat kinase 2 (LRRK2)/PARK8 possesses GTPase activity that is altered in familial Parkinson's disease R1441C/G mutants. *Journal of Neurochemistry*, **103**, 238–247.

Lim, K.L., Chew, K.C., Tan, J.M., Wang, C., Chung, K.K., Zhang, Y., Tanaka, Y., Smith, W., Engelender, S., Ross, C.A., Dawson, V.L. and Dawson, T.M. (2005) Parkin mediates nonclassical, proteasomal-independent ubiquitination of synphilin-1: implications for Lewy body formation. *The Journal of Neuroscience*, **25** (8), 2002–2009.

Lincoln, S.J., Maraganore, D.M., Lesnick, T.G., Bounds, R., de Andrade, M., Bower, J.H., Hardy, J.A. and Farrer, M.J. (2003) Parkin variants in North American Parkinson's disease: cases and controls. *Movement Disorders*, **18** (11), 1306–1311.

Lindersson, E., Beedholm, R., Hojrup, P., Moos, T., Gai, W., Hendil, K.B. and Jensen, P.H. (2004) Proteasomal inhibition by alpha-synuclein filaments and oligomers. *The Journal of Biological Chemistry*, **279** (13), 12924–12934.

Liu, Y., Fallon, L., Lashuel, H.A., Liu, Z. and Lansbury, P.T., Jr (2002) The UCH-L1 gene encodes two opposing enzymatic activities that affect alpha-synuclein degradation and Parkinson's disease susceptibility. *Cell*, **111** (2), 209–218.

Liu, C.W., Corboy, M.J., DeMartino, G.N. and Thomas, P.J. (2003) Endoproteolytic Activity of the Proteasome. *Science*, **299**, 408–411.

Liu, C.W., Giasson, B.I., Lewis, K.A., Lee, V.M., Demartino, G.N. and Thomas, P.J. (2005) A precipitating role for truncated alpha-synuclein and the proteasome in alpha-synuclein aggregation: implications for pathogenesis of Parkinson's disease. *The Journal of Biological Chemistry*, **280** (24), 22670–22678.

Lockhart, P.J., Lincoln, S., Hulihan, M., Kachergus, J., Wilkes, K., Bisceglio, G., Mash, D.C. and Farrer, M.J. (2004) DJ-1 mutations are a rare cause of recessively inherited early onset parkinsonism mediated by loss of protein function. *Journal of Medical Genetics*, **41** (3), e22.

Lopiano, L., Fasano, M., Giraudo, S., Digilio, G., Koenig, S.H., Torre, E., Bergamasco, B. and Aime, S. (2000) Nuclear magnetic relaxation dispersion profiles of substantia nigra pars compacta in Parkinson's disease patients are consistent with protein aggregation. *Neurochemistry International*, **37** (4), 331–336.

Lowe, J., McDermott, H., Landon, M., Mayer, R.J. and Wilkinson, K.D. (1990) Ubiquitin carboxyl-terminal hydrolase (PGP 9.5) is selectively present in ubiquitinated inclusion bodies characteristic of human neurodegenerative diseases. *The Journal of Pathology*, **161** (2), 153–160.

Lucking, C.B., Durr, A., Bonifati, V., Vaughan, J., De Michele, G., Gasser, T., Harhangi, B.S., Meco, G., Denefle, P., Wood, N.W., Agid, Y. and Brice, A. (2000) Association between early-onset Parkinson's disease and mutations in the parkin gene. French Parkinson's Disease Genetics Study Group. *The New England Journal of Medicine*, **342** (21), 1560–1567.

Manning-Bog, A.B., Reaney, S.H., Chou, V.P., Johnston, L.C., McCormack, A.L., Johnston, J., Langston, J.W. and Di Monte, D.A. (2006) Lack of nigrostriatal pathology in a rat model of proteasome inhibition. *Annals of Neurology*, **60** (2), 256–260.

Maraganore, D.M., Lesnick, T.G., Elbaz, A., Chartier-Harlin, M.-C., Gasser, T., Krüger, R., Hattori, N., Mellick, G.D., Quattrone, A., Satoh, J.-I., Toda, T., Wang, J., Ioannidis, J.P.A., de Andrade, M., Rocca, W.A. and Consortium, U.G.G. (2004) UCHL1 is a Parkinson's disease susceptibility gene. *Annals of Neurology*, **55**, 512–521.

Maroteaux, L., Campanelli, J.T. and Scheller, R.H. (1988) Synuclein: a neuron-specific protein localized to the nucleus and presynaptic nerve terminal. *The Journal of Neuroscience*, **8** (8), 2804–2815.

Martinez-Vicente, A. and Cuevo, A.M. (2007) Autophagy and neurodegeneration: when the cleaning crew goes on strike. *Lancet Neurology*, **6**, 352–359.

Masliah, E., Rockenstein, E., Adame, A. *et al.* (2005) Effects of alpha-synuclein immunization in a mouse model of Parkinson's disease. *Neuron*, **46**, 857–868.

Matsumine, H., Saito, M., Shimoda-Matsubayashi, S., Tanaka, H., Ishikawa, A., Nakagawa-Hattori, Y., Yokochi, M., Kobayashi, T., Igarashi, S., Takano, H., Sanpei, K., Koike, R., Mori, H., Kondo, T., Mizutani, Y., Schaffer, A.A., Yamamura, Y., Nakamura, S., Kuzuhara, S., Tsuji, S. and Mizuno, Y. (1997) Localization of a gene for an autosomal recessive form of juvenile Parkinsonism to chromosome 6q25.2–27. *American Journal of Human Genetics*, **60** (3), 588–596.

McNaught, K.S. and Jenner, P. (2001) Proteasomal function is impaired in substantia nigra in Parkinson's disease. *Neuroscience Letters*, **297** (3), 191–194.

McNaught, K.St.P., Olanow, C.W., Halliwell, B., Isacson, O. and Jenner, P. (2001) Failure of the ubiquitin-proteasome system in Parkinson's disease. *Nature Reviews/Neuroscience*, **2**, 589–594.

McNaught, K.S.P., Mytilineou, C., JnoBaptiste, R., Jabut, J., Shashidharan, P., Jenner, P. and Olanow, C.W. (2002) Impairment of the ubiquitin-proteasome system causes dopaminergic cell death and inclusion body formation in ventral mesencephalic cultures. *Journal of Neurochemistry*, **81** (301–6), 301–306.

McNaught, K.S., Shashidharan, P., Perl, D.P., Jenner, P. and Olanow, C.W. (2002) Aggresome-related biogenesis of Lewy bodies. *The European Journal of Neuroscience*, **16** (11), 2136–2148.

McNaught, K.S.P., Bjorklund, L.M., Belizaire, R., Jenner, P. and Olanow, C.W. (2002) Proteasome Inhibition Causes Nigral Degeneration with Inclusion Bodies in Rats. *NeuroReport*, **13** (1437–1441), 1437–1441.

McNaught, K.S., Belizaire, R., Isacson, O., Jenner, P. and Olanow, C.W. (2003) Altered Proteasomal Function in Sporadic Parkinson's Disease. *Experimental Neurology*, **179** (38–46), 38–45.

McNaught, K.S.P., Perl, D.P., Brownell, A.L. and Olanow, C.W. (2004) Systemic exposure to proteasome inhibitors causes a progressive model of Parkinson's disease. *Annals of Neurology*, **56** (1), 149–162.

Miller, D.W., Hague, S.M., Clarimon, J., Baptista, M., Gwinn-Hardy, K., Cookson, M.R. and Singleton, A.B. (2004) Alpha-synuclein in blood and brain from familial Parkinson's disease with SNCA locus triplication. *Neurology*, **62** (10), 1835–1838.

Miwa, H., Kubo, T., Suzuki, A., Nishi, K. and Kondo, T. (2005) Retrograde dopaminergic neuron degeneration following intrastriatal proteasome inhibition. *Neuroscience Letters*, **380** (1–2), 93–98.

Moore, D.J., Zhang, L., Dawson, T.M. and Dawson, V.L. (2003) A missense mutation (L166P) in DJ-1, linked to familial Parkinson's disease, confers reduced protein stability and impairs homo-oligomerization. *Journal of Neurochemistry*, **87** (6), 1558–1567.

Moore, D.J., Zhang, L., Troncoso, J., Lee, M.K., Hattori, N., Mizuno, Y., Dawson, T.M. and Dawson, V.L. (2005) Association of DJ-1 and parkin mediated by pathogenic DJ-1 mutations and oxidative stress. *Human Molecular Genetics*, **14** (1), 71–84.

Mori, H., Kondo, T., Yokochi, M., Matsumine, H., Nakagawa-Hattori, Y., Miyake, T., Suda, K. and Mizuno, Y. (1998) Pathologic and biochemical studies of juvenile parkinsonism linked to chromosome 6q. *Neurology*, **51** (3), 890–892.

Munch, G., Luth, H.J., Wong, A., Arendt, T., Hirsch, E., Ravid, R. and Riederer, P. (2000) Crosslinking of alpha-synuclein by advanced glycation endproducts – an early pathophysiological step in Lewy body formation? *Journal of Chemical Neuroanatomy*, **20** (3–4), 253–257.

Nagakubo, D., Taira, T., Kitaura, H., Ikeda, M., Tamai, K., Iguchi-Ariga, S.M. and Ariga, H. (1997) DJ-1, a novel oncogene which transforms mouse NIH3T3 cells in cooperation with ras. *Biochemical and Biophysical Research, Communications*, **231** (2), 509–513.

Nair, V.D., McNaught, K.S., Gonzalez-Maeso, J., Sealfon, S.C. and Olanow, C.W. (2006) p53 Mediates non-transcriptional cell death in dopaminergic cells in response to proteasome inhibition. *The Journal of Biological Chemistry*, **281**, (51), 39550–39560.

Nair, V.D., McNaught, K.St.P., Gonzalez-Maeso, J., Sealfon, S. and Olanow, C.W. (2006) P53 mediates non-transcriptional cell death in dopaminergic cells in response to proteasome inhibitors. *The Journal of Biological Chemistry*, **281**, 39550–39560.

Nichols, W.C., Pankratz, N., Hernandez, D., Paisan-Ruiz, C., Jain, S., Halter, C.A., Michaels, V.E., Reed, T., Rudolph, A., Shults, C.W., Singleton, A. and Foroud, T. (2005) Genetic screening for a single common LRRK2 mutation in familial Parkinson's disease. *Lancet*, **365** (9457), 410–412.

Nishikawa, K., Li, H., Kawamura, R., Osaka, H., Wang, Y.L., Hara, Y., Hirokawa, T., Manago, Y., Amano, T., Noda, M., Aoki, S. and Wada, K. (2003) Alterations of structure and hydrolase activity of parkinsonism-associated human ubiquitin carboxyl-terminal hydrolase L1 variants. *Biochemical and Biophysical Research, Communications*, **304** (1), 176–183.

Okada, K., Wangpoengtrakul, C., Osawa, T., Toyokuni, S., Tanaka, K. and Uchida, K. (1999) 4-Hydroxy-2-nonenal-mediated impairment of intracellular proteolysis during oxidative stress. Identification of proteasomes as target molecules. *The Journal of Biological Chemistry*, **274**, 23787–23793.

Olanow, C.W. and Schapira , A.H.V. (2008) New Can we obtain neuroprotection in Parkinson's Disease?, *Annals of Neurology*, (in press).

Olanow, C.W. (2007) Pathogenesis of cell death in Parkinson's disease – 2007. *Movement Disorders*, **22**, S335–S342.

Olanow, C.W. and McNaught, K. (2006) The Ubiquitin-Proteasome System in Parkinson's Disease. *Movement Disorders*, **21**, 1806–1823.

Olanow, C.W., Perl, D.P., DeMartino, G.N. and McNaught, K. (2004) Lewy-body formation is an aggresome-related process: a hypothesis. *Lancet Neurology*, **3**, 496–503.

Olzmann, J.A., Brown, K., Wilkinson, K.D., Rees, H.D., Huai, Q., Ke, H., Levey, A.I., Li, L. and Chin, L.S. (2004) Familial Parkinson's disease-associated L166P mutation disrupts DJ-1 protein folding and function. *The Journal of Biological Chemistry*, **279** (9), 8506–8515.

Osaka, H., Wang, Y.L., Takada, K., Takizawa, S., Setsuie, R., Li, H., Sato, Y., Nishikawa, K., Sun, Y.J., Sakurai, M., Harada, T., Hara, Y., Kimura, I., Chiba, S., Namikawa, K., Kiyama, H., Noda, M., Aoki, S. and Wada, K. (2003) Ubiquitin carboxy-terminal hydrolase L1 binds to and stabilizes monoubiquitin in neuron. *Human Molecular Genetics*, **12** (16), 1945–1958.

Ozelius, L.J., Senthil, G., Saunders-Pullman, R. *et al.* (2006) LRRK2 G2019S as a cause of Parkinson's disease in Ashkenazi Jews. *The New England Journal of Medicine*, **354**, 424–425.

Ozelius, L.J., Senthil, G., Saunders-Pullman, R. *et al.* (2006) LRRK2 G2019S as a cause of Parkinson's disease in Ashkenazi Jews. *The New England Journal of Medicine*, **354**, 424–425.

Paisan-Ruiz, C., Jain, S., Evans, E.W., Gilks, W.P., Simon, J., van der Brug, M., de Munain, A.L., Aparicio, S., Gil, A.M., Khan, N., Johnson, J., Martinez, J.R., Nicholl, D., Carrera, I.M., Pena, A.S., de Silva, R., Lees, A., Marti-Masso, J.F., Perez-Tur, J., Wood, N.W. and Singleton, A.B. (2004) Cloning of the gene containing mutations that cause PARK8-linked Parkinson's disease. *Neuron*, **44** (4), 595–600.

Pandey, N., Schmidt, R.E. and Galvin, J.E. (2006) The alpha-synuclein mutation E46K promotes aggregation in cultured cells. *Experimental Neurology*, **197** (2), 515–520.

Park, J., Lee, S.B., Lee, S., Kim, Y., Song, S., Kim, S., Bae, E., Kim, J., Shong, M., Kim, J.M. and Chung, J. (2006) Mitochondrial dysfunction in Drosophila PINK1 mutants is complemented by parkin. *Nature*, **441** (7097), 1157–1161.

Parkinson Study Group (1993) Effects of tocopherol and deprenyl on the progression of disability in early Parkinson's disease. *The New England Journal of Medicine*, **328**, 176–183.

Perez, F.A. and Palmiter, R.D. (2005) Parkin-deficient mice are not a robust model of parkinsonism. *Proceedings of the National Academy of Sciences, of the United States of America*, **102**, 2174–2179.

Pickart, C.M. and Cohen, R.E. (2004) Proteasomes and their kin: proteases in the machine age. *Nature Reviews. Molecular Cell Biology*, **5** (3), 177–187.

Polymeropoulos, M.H., Higgins, J.J., Golbe, L.I., Johnson, W. G., Ide, S.E., Di Iorio, G., Sanges, G., Stenroos, E.S., Pho, L. T., Schaffer, A.A., Lazzarini, A.M., Nussbaum, R.L. and Duvoisin, R.C. (1996) Mapping of a gene for Parkinson's disease to chromosome 4q21-q23. *Science*, **274** (5290), 1197–1199.

Polymeropoulos, M.H., Lavedan, C., Leroy, E., Ide, S.E., Dehejia, A., Dutra, A., Pike, B., Root, H., Rubenstein, J., Boyer, R., Stenroos, E.S., Chandrasekharappa, S., Athanassiadou, A., Papapetropoulos, T., Johnson, W.G., Lazzarini, A.M., Duvoisin, R.C., Di Iorio, G., Golbe, L.I. and Nussbaum, R.L. (1997) Mutation in the alpha-synuclein gene identified in families with Parkinson's disease. *Science*, **276** (5321), 2045–2047.

Pramstaller, P.P., Schlossmacher, M.G., Jacques, T.S., Scaravilli, F., Eskelson, C., Pepivani, I., Hedrich, K., Adel, S., Gonzales-McNeal, M., Hilker, R., Kramer, P.L., and Klein, C. (2005) Lewy body Parkinson's disease in a large pedigree with 77 Parkin mutation carriers. *Annals of Neurology*, **58** (3), 411–422.

Rideout, H.J. and Stefanis, L. (2002) Proteasomal inhibition-induced inclusion formation and death in cortical neurons require transcription and ubiquitination. *Molecular and Cellular Neurosciences*, **21** (2), 223–238.

Rideout, H.J., Larsen, K.E., Sulzer, D. and Stefanis, L. (2001) Proteasomal inhibition leads to formation of ubiquitin/alpha-synuclein-immunoreactive inclusions in PC12 cells. *Journal of Neurochemistry*, **78** (4), 899–908.

Rideout, H.J., Lang-Rollin, I.C.J., Savalle, M. and Stefanis, L. (2005) Dopaminergic neurons in rat ventral midbrain cultures undergo selective apoptosis and form inclusions, but do not up-regulate iHSP, following proteasomal inhibition. *Journal of Neurochemistry*, **93** (2), 1304–1313.

Rogaeva, E., Johnson, J., Lang, A.E., Gulick, C., Gwinn-Hardy, K., Kawarai, T., Sato, C., Morgan, A., Werner, J., Nussbaum, R., Petit, A., Okun, M.S., McInerney, A., Mandel, R., Groen, J.L., Fernandez, H.H., Postuma, R., Foote, K.D., Salehi-Rad, S., Liang, Y., Reimsnider, S., Tandon, A., Hardy, J., St George-Hyslop, P. and Singleton, A.B. (2004) Analysis of the PINK1 gene in a large cohort of cases with Parkinson's disease. *Archives of Neurology*, **61** (12), 1898–1904.

Sakata, E., Yamaguchi, Y., Kurimoto, E., Kikuchi, J., Yokoyama, S., Yamada, S., Kawahara, H., Yokosawa, H., Hattori, N., Mizuno, Y., Tanaka, K. and Kato, K. (2003) Parkin binds the Rpn10 subunit of 26S proteasomes through its ubiquitin-like domain. *EMBO Reports*, **4** (3), 301–306.

Sampathu, D.M., Giasson, B.I., Pawlyk, A.C., Trojanowski, J.Q. and Lee, V.M. (2003) Ubiquitination of alpha-synuclein is not required for formation of pathological inclusions in alpha-synucleinopathies. *The American Journal of Pathology*, **163** (1), 91–100.

Schapira, A.H. and Olanow, C.W. (2004) Neuroprotection in Parkinson's disease: mysteries, myths, and misconceptions. *Jama*, **291** (3), 358–364.

Schapira, A.H., Mann, V.M., Cooper, J.M., Dexter, D., Daniel, S.E., Jenner, P., Clark, J.B. and Marsden, C.D. (1990) Anatomic and disease specificity of NADH CoQ1 reductase (complex I) deficiency in Parkinson's disease. *Journal of Neurochemistry*, **55** (6), 2142–2145.

Schapira, A.H., Cleeter, M.W., Muddle, J.R., Workman, J.M., Cooper, J.M. and King, R.H. (2006) Proteasomal inhibition causes loss of nigral tyrosine hydroxylase neurons. *Annals of Neurology*, **60** (2), 253–255.

Schlossmacher, M.G., Frosch, M.P., Gai, W.P., Medina, M., Sharma, N., Forno, L., Ochiishi, T., Shimura, H., Sharon, R., Hattori, N., Langston, J.W., Mizuno, Y., Hyman, B.T., Selkoe, D.J. and Kosik, K.S. (2002) Parkin localizes to the lewy bodies of Parkinson's disease and dementia with lewy bodies. *The American Journal of Pathology*, **160** (5), 1655–1667.

Schmidt, M.L., Murray, J., Lee, V.M., Hill, W.D., Wertkin, A. and Trojanowski, J.Q. (1991) Epitope map of neurofilament protein domains in cortical and peripheral nervous system Lewy bodies. *The American Journal of Pathology*, **139** (1), 53–65.

Shamoto-Nagai, M., Maruyama, W., Kato, Y. *et al.* (2003) An inhibitor of mitochondrial complex I, rotenone, inactivates proteasome by oxidative modification and induces aggregation of oxidized proteins in SH-SY5Y cells. *Journal of Neuroscience Research*, **74**, 589–597.

Shang, H., Lang, D., Jean-Marc, B. and Kaelin-Lang, A. (2004) Localization of DJ-1 mRNA in the mouse brain. *Neuroscience Letters*, **367** (3), 273–277.

Shendelman, S., Jonason, A., Martinat, C., Leete, T. and Abeliovich, A. (2004) DJ-1 is a redox-dependent molecular chaperone that inhibits alpha-synuclein aggregate formation. *PLoS Biol*, **2** (11), e362.

Shimura, H., Hattori, N., Kubo, S., Yoshikawa, M., Kitada, T., Matsumine, H., Asakawa, S., Minoshima, S., Yamamura, Y., Shimizu, N. and Mizuno, Y. (1999) Immunohistochemical and subcellular localization of Parkin protein: absence of protein in autosomal recessive juvenile parkinsonism patients. *Annals of Neurology*, **45** (5), 668–672.

Shimura, H., Hattori, N., Kubo, S., Mizuno, Y., Asakawa, S., Minoshima, S., Shimizu, N., Iwai, K., Chiba, T., Tanaka, K. and Suzuki, T. (2000) Familial Parkinson's disease gene product, parkin, is a ubiquitin-protein ligase. *Nature Genetics*, **25** (3), 302–305.

Shimura, H., Schlossmacher, M.G., Hattori, N., Frosch, M.P., Trockenbacher, A., Schneider, R., Mizuno, Y., Kosik, K.S. and Selkoe, D.J. (2001) Ubiquitination of a New Form of {alpha}-Synuclein by Parkin from Human Brain: Implications for Parkinson's Disease. *Science*, **293**, 263–269.

Sian, J., Dexter, D.T., Lees, A.J., Daniel, S., Agid, Y., Javoy-Agid, F., Jenner, P., Marsden, C.D. (1994) Alterations in glutathione levels in Parkinson's disease and other neurodegenerative disorders affecting basal ganglia. *Annals of Neurology*, **36** (3), 348–355.

Simon-Sanchez, J., Herranz-Perez, V., Olucha-Bordonau, F. and Perez-Tur, J. (2006) LRRK2 is expressed in areas affected by Parkinson's disease in the adult mouse brain. *The European Journal of Neuroscience*, **23** (3), 659–666.

Singleton, A.B., Farrer, M., Johnson, J., Singleton, A., Hague, S., Kachergus, J., Hulihan, M., Peuralinna, T., Dutra, A., Nussbaum, R., Lincoln, S., Crawley, A., Hanson, M., Maraganore, D., Adler, C., Cookson, M.R., Muenter, M., Baptista, M., Miller, D., Blancato, J., Hardy, J. and Gwinn-Hardy, K. (2003) alpha-Synuclein locus triplication causes Parkinson's disease. *Science*, **302** (5646), 841.

Smith, W.W., Pei, Z., Jiang, H. *et al.* (2006) Kinase activity of mutant LRRK2 mediates neuronal toxicity. *Nature Neuroscience*, **9**, 1231–1233.

Snyder, H., Mensah, K., Theisler, C., Lee, J.M., Matouschek, A. and Wolozin, B. (2003) Aggregated and monomeric alpha-synuclein bind to the S6' proteasomal protein and inhibit proteasomal function. *The Journal of Biological Chemistry*, **278**, 11753–11759.

Sofic, E., Riederer, P., Heinsen, H., Beckmann, H., Reynolds, G.P., Hebenstreit, G. and Youdim, M.B. (1988) Increased iron (III) and total iron content in post mortem substantia nigra of parkinsonian brain. *Journal of Neural Transmission*, **74** (3), 199–205.

Solano, S.M., Miller, D.W., Augood, S.J., Young, A.B. and Penney, J.B., Jr (2000) Expression of alpha-synuclein, parkin, and ubiquitin carboxy-terminal hydrolase L1 mRNA in human brain: genes associated with familial Parkinson's disease. *Annals of Neurology*, **47** (2), 201–210.

Spillantini, M.G., Schmidt, M.L., Lee, V.M., Trojanowski, J.Q., Jakes, R. and Goedert, M. (1997) Alpha-synuclein in Lewy bodies. *Nature*, **388** (6645), 839–840.

Spillantini, M.G., Crowther, R.A., Jakes, R., Hasegawa, M. and Goedert, M. (1998) alpha-Synuclein in filamentous inclusions of Lewy bodies from Parkinson's disease and dementia with lewy bodies. *Proceedings of the National Academy of Sciences, of the United States of America*, **95** (11), 6469–6473.

Stefanis, L., Larsen, K.E., Rideout, H.J., Sulzer, D. and Greene, L.A. (2001) Expression of A53T Mutant But Not Wild-Type alpha -Synuclein in PC12 Cells Induces Alterations of the Ubiquitin-Dependent Degradation System, Loss of Dopamine Release, and Autophagic Cell Death. *The Journal of Neuroscience*, **21** (24), 9549–9560.

Sullivan, P.G., Dragicevic, N.B., Deng, J.H. *et al.* (2004) Proteasome inhibition alters neural mitochondrial homeostasis and mitochondria turnover. *The Journal of Biological Chemistry*, **279**, 20699–20707.

Taira, T., Saito, Y., Niki, T., Iguchi-Ariga, S.M., Takahashi, K. and Ariga, H. (2004) DJ-1 has a role in antioxidative stress to prevent cell death. *EMBO Reports*, **5** (2), 213–218.

Tanaka, Y., Engelender, S., Igarashi, S., Rao, R.K., Wanner, T., Tanzi, R.E., Sawa, A., Dawson, V.L., Dawson, T.M. and Ross, C.A. (2001) Inducible expression of mutant alpha-synuclein decreases proteasome activity and increases sensitivity to mitochondria-dependent apoptosis. *Human Molecular Genetics*, **10** (9), 919–926.

Tanaka, M., Kim, Y.M., Lee, G., Junn, E., Iwatsubo, T. and Mouradian, M.M. (2003) Aggresomes formed by alpha -synuclein and synphilin-1 are cytoprotective. *The Journal of Biological Chemistry*, **279**, 4625–4631.

Tanner, C.M. (2003) Is the cause of Parkinson's disease environmental or hereditary? Evidence from twin studies. *Advances in Neurology*, **91**, 133–142.

Tatton, N.A. (2000) Increased caspase 3 and Bax immunoreactivity accompany nuclear GAPDH translocation and neuronal apoptosis in Parkinson's disease. *Experimental Neurology*, **166**, 29–43.

Tatton, N.A., Maclean-Fraser, A., Tatton, W.G., Perl, D.F. and Olanow, C.W. (1998) A Fluorescent Double-Labeling Method to Detect and Confirm Apoptotic Nuclei in Parkinson's Disease. *Annals of Neurology*, **44** (suppl 1), 142–148.

Taylor, J.P., Tanaka, F., Robitschek, J., Sandoval, C.M., Taye, A., Markovic-Plese, S. and Fischbeck, K.H. (2003) Aggresomes protect cells by enhancing the degradation of toxic polyglutamine-containing protein. *Human Molecular Genetics*, **12** (7), 749–757.

Tofaris, G.K., Layfield, R. and Spillantini, M.G. (2001) alpha-Synuclein metabolism and aggregation is linged to ubiquitin-independent degradation by the proteasome. *FEBS Letters*, **25504**, 1–5.

Tofaris, G.K., Razzaq, A., Ghetti, B., Lilley, K. and Spillantini, M.G. (2003) Ubiquitination of alpha-synuclein in Lewy bodies is a pathological event not associated with impairment of proteasome function. *The Journal of Biological Chemistry*, **278**, 44405–44411.

Tompkins, M.M. and Hill, W.D. (1997) Contribution of somal Lewy bodies to neuronal death. *Brain Research*, **775** (1-2), 24–29.

Valente, E.M., Bentivoglio, A.R., Dixon, P.H., Ferraris, A., Ialongo, T., Frontali, M., Albanese, A. and Wood, N.W. (2001) Localization of a novel locus for autosomal recessive early-onset parkinsonism, PARK6, on human chromosome 1p35-p36. *American Journal of Human Genetics*, **68** (4), 895–900.

Valente, E.M., Brancati, F., Ferraris, A., Graham, E.A., Davis, M. B., Breteler, M.M., Gasser, T., Bonifati, V., Bentivoglio, A.R., De Michele, G., Durr, A., Cortelli, P., Wassilowsky, D., Harhangi, B.S., Rawal, N., Caputo, V., Filla, A., Meco, G., Oostra, B.A., Brice, A., Albanese, A., Dallapiccola, B. and Wood, N.W. (2002) PARK6-linked parkinsonism occurs in several European families. *Annals of Neurology*, **51** (1), 14–18.

Valente, E.M., Abou-Sleiman, P.M., Caputo, V., Muqit, M.M., Harvey, K., Gispert, S., Ali, Z., Del Turco, D., Bentivoglio, A.R., Healy, D.G., Albanese, A., Nussbaum, R., Gonzalez-Maldonado, R., Deller, T., Salvi, S., Cortelli, P., Gilks, W.P., Latchman, D.S., Harvey, R.J., Dallapiccola, B., Auburger, G. and Wood, N.W. (2004) Hereditary early-onset Parkinson's disease caused by mutations in PINK1. *Science*, **304** (5674), 1158–1160.

van Duijn, C.M., Dekker, M.C., Bonifati, V., Galjaard, R.J., Houwing-Duistermaat, J.J., Snijders, P.J., Testers, L., Breedveld, G.J., Horstink, M., Sandkuijl, L.A., van Swieten, J.C., Oostra, B.A. and Heutink, P. (2001) Park7, a novel locus for autosomal recessive early-onset parkinsonism, on chromosome 1p36. *American Journal of Human Genetics*, **69** (3), 629–634.

van Duinen, S.G., Lammers, G.J., Maat-Schieman, M.L. and Roos, R.A. (1999) Numerous and widespread alpha-synuclein-negative Lewy bodies in an asymptomatic patient. *Acta Neuropathologica*, **97** (5), 533–539.

Von Coelln, R., Thomas, B., Savitt, J.M., Lim, K.L., Sasaki, M., Hess, E.J., Dawson, V.L. and Dawson, T.M. (2004) Loss of locus coeruleus neurons and reduced startle in parkin null mice. *Proceedings of the National Academy of Sciences, of the United States of America*, **101** (29), 10744–10749.

Wakabayashi, K., Toyoshima, Y., Awamori, K., Anezaki, T., Yoshimoto, M., Tsuji, S. and Takahashi, H. (1999) Restricted occurrence of Lewy bodies in the dorsal vagal nucleus in a patient with late-onset parkinsonism. *Journal of the Neurological Sciences*, **165** (2), 188–191.

Weinreb, P.H., Zhen, W., Poon, A.W., Conway, K.A. and Lansbury, P.T., Jr (1996) NACP, a protein implicated in Alzheimer's disease and learning, is natively unfolded. *Biochemistry*, **35** (43), 13709–13715.

West, A.B., Moore, D.J. and Biskup, S. (2005) Parkinson's disease-associated mutations in leucine-rich repeat kinase 2 augment kinase activity. *Proceedings of the National Academy of Sciences, of the United States of America*, **102**, 16842–16847.

West, A.B., Moore, D.J., Biskup, S., Bugayenko, A., Smith, W.W., Ross, C.A., Dawson, V.L. and Dawson, T.M. (2005) Parkinson's disease-associated mutations in leucine-rich repeat kinase 2 augment kinase activity. *Proceedings of the National Academy of Sciences, of the United States of America*, **102** (46), 16842–16847.

West, A.B., Moore, D.J., Choi, C. *et al.* (2007) Parkinson's disease-associated mutations in LRRK2 link enhanced GTP-binding and kinase activities to neuronal toxicity. *Human Molecular Genetics*, **16**, 223–232.

Whitesell, L., Mimnaugh, E.G., De Costa, B., Myers, C.E. and Neckers, L.M. (1994) Inhibition of heat shock protein HSP90-pp60v-src heteroprotein complex formation by benzoquinone ansamycins: essential role for stress proteins in oncogenic transformation. *Proceedings of the National Academy of Sciences of the United States of America*, **91**, 8324–8328.

Wilkinson, K.D., Lee, K.M., Deshpande, S., Duerksen-Hughes, P., Boss, J.M. and Pohl, J. (1989) The neuron-specific protein PGP

9.5 is a ubiquitin carboxyl-terminal hydrolase. *Science*, **246** (4930), 670–673.

Wilkinson, K.D., Deshpande, S. and Larsen, C.N. (1992) Comparisons of neuronal (PGP 9.5) and non-neuronal ubiquitin C-terminal hydrolases. *Biochemical Society Transactions*, **20** (3), 631–637.

Wilson, M.A., St Amour, C.V., Collins, J.L., Ringe, D. and Petsko, G.A. (2004) The 1.8-A resolution crystal structure of YDR533Cp from Saccharomyces cerevisiae: a member of the DJ-1/ThiJ/PfpI superfamily. *Proceedings of the National Academy of Sciences, of the United States of America*, **101** (6), 1531–1536.

Wintermeyer, P., Kruger, R., Kuhn, W., Muller, T., Woitalla, D., Berg, D., Becker, G., Leroy, E., Polymeropoulos, M., Berger, K., Przuntek, H., Schols, L., Epplen, J.T. and Riess, O. (2000) Mutation analysis and association studies of the UCHL1 gene in German Parkinson's disease patients. *Neuroreport*, **11** (10), 2079–2082.

Wood-Kaczmar, A., Gandhi, S. and Wood, N.W. (2006) Understanding the molecular causes of Parkinson's disease. *Trends in Molecular Medicine*, **12** (11), 521–528.

Wszolek, Z.K., Pfeiffer, R.F., Tsuboi, Y., Uitti, R.J., McComb, R.D., Stoessl, A.J., Strongosky, A.J., Zimprich, A., Muller-Myhsok, B., Farrer, M.J., Gasser, T., Calne, D.B. and Dickson, D.W. (2004) Autosomal dominant parkinsonism associated with variable synuclein and tau pathology. *Neurology*, **62** (9), 1619–1622.

Yang, Y., Nishimura, I., Imai, Y., Takahashi, R. and Lu, B. (2003) Parkin suppresses dopaminergic neuron-selective neurotoxicity induced by Pael-R in Drosophila. *Neuron*, **37** (6), 911–924.

Yang, Y., Gehrke, S. and Imai, Y. (2006) Mitochondrial pathology and muscle and dopaminergic neuron degeneration caused by inactivation of Drosophila Pink1 is rescued by Parkin. *Proceedings of the National Academy of Sciences, of the United States of America*, **103**, 10793–10798.

Yokota, T., Sugawara, K., Ito, K., Takahashi, R., Ariga, H. and Mizusawa, H. (2003) Down regulation of DJ-1 enhances cell death by oxidative stress, ER stress, and proteasome inhibition. *Biochemical and Biophysical Research, Communications*, **312** (4), 1342–1348.

Yoritaka, A., Hattori, N., Uchida, K., Tanaka, M., Stadtman, E.R. and Mizuno, Y. (1996) Immunohistochemical detection of 4-hydroxynonenal protein adducts in Parkinson's disease. *Proceedings of the National Academy of Sciences, of the United States of America*, **93** (7), 2696–2701.

Zarow, C., Lyness, S.A., Mortimer, J.A. and Chui, H.C. (2003) Neuronal loss is greater in the locus coeruleus than nucleus basalis and substantia nigra in Alzheimer and Parkinson's diseases. *Archives of Neurology*, **60** (3), 337–341.

Zarranz, J.J., Alegre, J., Gomez-Esteban, J.C., Lezcano, E., Ros, R., Ampuero, I., Vidal, L., Hoenicka, J., Rodriguez, O., Atares, B., Llorens, V., Gomez Tortosa, E., del Ser, T., Munoz, D.G. and de Yebenes, J.G. (2004) The new mutation, E46K, of alpha-synuclein causes Parkinson and Lewy body dementia. *Annals of Neurology*, **55** (2), 164–173.

Zeng, B.Y., Bukhatwa, S., Hikima, A., Rose, S. and Jenner, P. (2006) Reproducible nigral cell loss after systemic proteasomal inhibitor administration to rats. *Annals of Neurology*, **60** (2), 248–252.

Zhang, J., Perry, G., Smith, M.A., Robertson, D., Olson, S.J., Graham, D.G. and Montine, T.J. (1999) Parkinson's disease is associated with oxidative damage to cytoplasmic DNA and RNA in substantia nigra neurons. *The American Journal of Pathology*, **154** (5), 1423–1429.

Zhang, Y., Gao, J., Chung, K.K., Huang, H., Dawson, V.L. and Dawson, T.M. (2000) Parkin functions as an E2-dependent ubiquitin- protein ligase and promotes the degradation of the synaptic vesicle-associated protein, CDCrel-1. *Proceedings of the National Academy of Sciences, of the United States of America*, **97** (24), 13354–13359.

Zhu, J.H., Kulich, S.M., Oury, T.D. and Chu, C.T. (2002) Cytoplasmic aggregates of phosphorylated extracellular signal-regulated protein kinases in lewy body diseases. *The American Journal of Pathology*, **161** (6), 2087–2098.

Zimprich, A., Biskup, S., Leitner, P., Lichtner, P., Farrer, M., Lincoln, S., Kachergus, J., Hulihan, M., Uitti, R.J., Calne, D.B., Stoessl, A.J., Pfeiffer, R.F., Patenge, N., Carbajal, I.C., Vieregge, P., Asmus, F., Muller-Myhsok, B., Dickson, D.W., Meitinger, T., Strom, T.M., Wszolek, Z.K. and Gasser, T. (2004) Mutations in LRRK2 cause autosomal-dominant parkinsonism with pleomorphic pathology. *Neuron*, **44** (4), 601–607.

2

Physiology of Parkinson's Disease

Shlomo Elias[1], Zvi Israel[2] and Hagai Bergman[1,3,4]

[1] Department of Physiology, The Hebrew University—Hadassah Medical School, Jerusalem, Israel
[2] Department of Neurosurgery, Hadassah—Hebrew University Medical Center, Jerusalem, Israel
[3] The Interdisciplinary Center for Neural Computation, The Hebrew University—Hadassah Medical School, Jerusalem, Israel
[4] The Eric Roland Center for Neurodegenerative Diseases, The Hebrew University—Hadassah Medical School, Jerusalem, Israel

INTRODUCTION

Parkinson's disease (PD) is a common and disabling disorder of movement in humans. The main symptoms of PD are poverty and slowing of voluntary movements (akinesia and bradykinesia), muscle rigidity and low-frequency rest tremor. These clinical symptoms are due to dopaminergic denervation of the striatum—the input nucleus of the basal ganglia. However, how this striatal dopamine depletion perverts normal functioning to cause the clinical symptoms of PD has remained unclear. Recent work in tissue slice preparations, animal models and in humans with PD has demonstrated abnormally synchronized oscillatory activity at multiple levels of the basal ganglia-cortical loop. These excessive oscillations correlate with the motor deficits and their suppression by dopaminergic therapies; ablative surgery or deep brain stimulation ameliorate the motor symptoms of PD. Nevertheless, persistent and robust correlation between the basal ganglia oscillations and the Parkinsonian tremor has not been established in the minute-to-minute time scale.

In this chapter we will discuss the clinical physiology of PD symptoms, and will outline the hypothesis that abnormal basal ganglia oscillations and synchronization disrupt motor cortex and brain stem activity leading to akinesia and bradykinesia (core negative symptoms of the disease). The positive motor symptoms of Parkinsonism—rigidity and tremor—are probably generated by compensatory mechanisms downstream to the basal ganglia.

PARKINSON'S DISEASE: CLINICAL SYMPTOMS

In 1817 the English physician James Parkinson wrote an "Essay on the Shaking Palsy" providing the first clinical description of the motor symptoms of the disease now bearing his name (Parkinson, 1817). Today, PD is the most common basal ganglia movement disorder, and affects from 1% to as many as 5% of those in the 65 and 85 year age brackets, respectively (Van Den Eeden et al., 2003).

Only 5% of PD cases can be attributed to specific genetic causes (Farrer, 2006; Benmoyal-Segal and Soreq, 2006). Most of the remaining cases cannot be attributed to metabolic or toxic causes either, and are therefore classified as idiopathic PD. The clinical manifestations of PD are the result of a neurodegenerative process that causes damage to multiple neuronal circuits (Braak et al., 2003). The dopaminergic system is the most seriously damaged (Sulzer, 2007), but the noradrenergic, serotonergic and the cholinergic systems are also affected ((Jellinger, 1991), and see also Chapter 1: The Etiopathogenesis of Parkinson's Disease: Basic Mechanisms of Neurodegeneration, this volume).

Based on a very small number of clinical observations (six patients, including two whom he met on the street and a third he observed at a distance) James Parkinson pinpointed two of the most important and paradoxically related symptoms of PD—shaking and palsy. PD shaking is now characterized as a low frequency (4–7 Hz) tremor at rest. However, other non-harmonically related forms (e.g., postural/kinetic 7–12 Hz tremor) are very common in PD (Elble and Koller, 1990; Deuschl et al., 2000). Palsy (or akinesia in modern terminology) is a hypokinetic disorder characterized by a poverty of voluntary goal-directed movements. Automatic (involuntary) movements, such as emotional facial expression are more severely reduced than instructed (voluntary) movements. Bradykinesia (slowness of voluntary movements) and related hypokinetic PD clinical features are also considered as akinetic symptoms. The other cardinal motor symptoms of PD include rigidity (increased muscular tone), and postural abnormalities,

Therapeutics of Parkinson's Disease and Other Movement Disorders   Edited by Mark Hallett and Werner Poewe
© 2008 John Wiley & Sons, Ltd.

characteristically loss of postural reflexes. Cognitive and mood (emotional) deficits frequently (Ravina *et al.*, 2007) accompany the motor symptoms (see Chapter 6, Managing the Non-Motor Symptoms of Parkinson's Disease, this volume). However, in this review we focus on the pathophysiology of the three main motor symptoms of PD: akinesia, tremor and rigidity.

PD is not a homogenous disease, either across patients or even during the natural progression of a single patient. Unlike rigidity and akinesia, there is no correlation between the clinical severity of PD tremor and the severity of the dopaminergic deficit in the striatum or the clinical progression of the disease (Deuschl *et al.*, 2000). Temporally, tremor is a more episodic phenomenon, as opposed to other PD symptoms. The classic PD tremor is a rest tremor, since its amplitude decreases during voluntary action. PD tremor increases during mental and emotional stress and is absent during sleep (Elble and Koller, 1990; Deuschl *et al.*, 2000). Although our clinical impression is that akinesia and rigidity fluctuate less in the daily course of a PD patient, quantitative data is still missing. The heterogeneous nature of PD between patients is revealed by its broad spectrum and clinical sub-types. PD can present as a predominant resting tremor (T-sub-type) or primarily as marked akinesia and rigidity (AR-sub-type), sometime defined as the "postural instability gait difficulty (PIGD) sub-type" (Jankovic *et al.*, 1990; Burn *et al.*, 2006). As early as the nineteenth century, the great French neurologist Jean-Martin Charcot noted that tremor is not always present in human PD patients, and therefore suggested changing the name of the disease from *paralysis agitans* (Latin for shaking palsy) to *la maladie de Parkinson* (French for Parkinson's disease). T-sub-type PD patients have a better prognosis and slower disease progression than AR-sub-type patients (Jankovic *et al.*, 1990). Interestingly, most forms of non-idiopathic PD (as most animal models of the disease, see below) display akinesia and rigidity but not rest tremor (Rajput, 1995). Anti-cholinergic agents, which were the first drugs available for the symptomatic treatment of PD, tend to have better effects on tremor than on akinetic-rigid symptoms, whereas akinesia may show better and earlier response to dopamine replacement therapy (Tolosa and Marin, 1995). Several studies have indicated that the pathology of human T-type PD differs from the AR-type PD, with the retrorubral area (A8) more severely affected than the substantia nigra pars compacta (A9) in the tremor dominant form (Paulus and Jellinger, 1991). Taken together, it therefore seems logical to conclude that PD akinesia and tremor are not caused by a single pathophysiological process.

Physiology of PD Tremor

The frequency of tremor in a given PD patient is often remarkably similar in different muscles of the extremities and trunk (Hunker and Abbs, 1990). These observations led to the assumption that a common single central oscillator controls all tremulous muscles. Coherence analysis, however, has shown that although the *muscles* within one body part (e.g., a limb) are mostly coherent, the tremor in *different extremities*, even on the same body side, is almost never coherent (Raethjen *et al.*, 2000; Ben-Pazi *et al.*, 2001), indicating that different oscillators underlie PD tremor in the different extremities. This lack of tremor coherence may hint at mechanical or spinal reflex mechanisms rather than a single central oscillator. However, several studies have failed to demonstrate any frequency reduction of PD tremor after loading of the trembling limb (Elble and Koller, 1990; Deuschl *et al.*, 2000). Resetting experiments have been less conclusive. Initial studies indicated that resetting of tremor by mechanical perturbation is much more easily achieved in essential tremor than in PD tremor (Lee and Stein, 1981). However, later studies have shown that the resetting index varies significantly with the magnitude of the mechanical perturbation and with the tremor amplitude (Britton *et al.*, 1992). No significant difference was found in mean resetting indexes between PD tremor, essential tremor and normal subjects mimicking tremor when these mechanical factors were equalized. Resetting experiments with electrical stimulation of the median nerve or transcranial magnetic stimulation of the motor cortex did not show consistent resetting of the tremor rhythm when the periphery (median nerve) was stimulated, but depicted complete tremor resetting when the cortex was stimulated (see review in (Deuschl *et al.*, 2000)). Thus, PD tremor seems to be generated in the central nervous system (CNS) by more than one single (coupled) oscillator; however, the central oscillators and the tremor can be modulated by peripheral inputs.

In line with the CNS hypothesis on the origin of PD tremor, it has long been known that different lesions within the CNS can suppress PD tremor. Early attempts to remove parts of the motor cortex or its downstream projections were successful in suppressing tremor, but produced unacceptable side effects. The cerebellar receiving nuclei of the thalamus (e.g., the ventralis-intermedius, Vim) have traditionally been considered the optimal target for stereotaxic procedures for amelioration of PD and other tremors. Recently it has been demonstrated that chronic high-frequency stimulation of these same thalamic targets, as well as the subthalamic nucleus and the pallidum are all able to efficiently suppress Parkinsonian tremor and other motor symptoms ((Machado *et al.*, 2006), and see Chapter 7: Surgery for Parkinson's Disease, this volume).

Physiology of PD Rigidity

PD rigidity is often characterized as a uniform resistance to passive movements, but it may also have a cogwheel intermittency due to superposition of tremor on the rigidity. Rigidity is evident throughout the full amplitude velocity and range of movements, in both flexor and extensor muscles (although more evident in flexor muscles). Early in the disease, rigidity is more evident in the axial (trunk) muscles, and later it extends to the distal limb muscles.

Increased passive mechanical stiffness of the muscles may play some role in PD rigidity (Dietz, 1987; Watts, Wiegner and Young, 1986), but its contribution to PD rigidity is probably minimal. Early studies (Pollock and Davis, 1930) showing that PD rigidity can be abolished by section of the dorsal root indicate that PD rigidity is maintained by spinal reflexes. Muscle spindle afferent activity of PD patients seems to be normally correlated with the degree of their muscular activation (Hagbarth *et al.*, 1975). Similarly, many spinal cord reflexes, including the tendon jerk, H-reflex and the tonic vibration reflex, and the excitability of the alpha motor neurons appear normal in Parkinsonian patients (Delwaide, Sabbatino and Delwaide, 1986). Thus, spinal cord responses to stretch seem to be close to normal in PD patients. However, passive stretch of muscle can evoke long-latency reflexes (Lee and Tatton, 1975; Tatton *et al.*, 1975), which are exaggerated in PD patients (Tatton *et al.*, 1984). Several studies indicate that the tonic muscle responses, initiated by slow and sustained stretch, and probably involving secondary muscle afferents, contribute more to PD rigidity than muscle reflexes triggered by brisk stretches. The long-latency reflexes are in many cases due to activation of long, for example, transcranial loops; although, as for the secondary muscle afferent reflex, they might be dependent on spinal loops.

In summary, most clinical human studies indicate that PD tremor, rigidity and akinesia, although sharing many common origins and similarities, have significantly distinct characteristics. The role of striatal dopamine depletion and the central generators seem to be much more important in akinesia. PD tremor and rigidity may be modulated by peripheral manipulation and by the activity of other central neuronal systems. It is highly possible that transmitter systems other than dopamine (e.g., cholinergic, serotonergic) or neural circuits other than the basal ganglia (e.g., cerebellum, red nucleus) play a critical additive role in these positive symptoms of PD.

ANIMAL MODELS OF PARKINSON'S DISEASE AND PARKINSONISM

Early animal models of PD were based on lesions of midbrain areas in monkeys (Poirier *et al.*, 1975). These anatomical lesions mainly produce akinesia and rigidity, but only rarely result in a spontaneous sustained tremor. Careful analysis of the correlation between the clinical symptoms and the extent of the lesion led to the conclusion

that experimental rest tremor is the result of damage to the nigro-striatal dopaminergic projections as well as to the cerebellar outflow (to the red nucleus and thalamus). Damage to only one of these neuronal systems was not sufficient for reliable generation of tremor (Jenner and Marsden, 1984).

More modern animal models of PD have shifted from anatomical to chemical lesions. Early chemical—for example, the 6-hydroxydopamine (6-OHDA)—rodent models of PD were limited to dopaminergic damage, and mainly reproduced the main negative symptoms of PD; namely, akinesia (Wilms, Sievers and Deuschl, 1999). The more recently introduced primate 1-methyl-4-phenyl-1,2,3,6-tetrahydropyridine (MPTP) model of PD (Burns *et al.*, 1983; Langston, Irwin and Langston, 1984) better mimics the clinical and the pathological picture of PD. Post-mortem examination of the brains of MPTP-treated primates reveals that the primary damage is to the dopaminergic system. However, as in human PD, other neuromodulators are also affected (Pifl, Schingnitz and Hornykiewicz, 1991). Rhesus monkeys treated with MPTP mainly exhibit the akinetic-rigid symptoms of PD (Burns *et al.*, 1983). Low-frequency (4–7 Hz) resting tremor is not readily replicated in MPTP-treated macaque monkeys; but some primate species, notably the vervet (African green) monkey often develop a prominent low-frequency tremor following MPTP injections (Bergman *et al.*, 1994; Raz, Vaadia and Bergman, 2000). It is important to note that the tremor usually appears several days after the development of clinical akinesia and rigidity (Bergman *et al.*, 1994; Heimer *et al.*, 2006). This order of presentation of clinical symptoms is reversed compared to human reports. It may be due to the fast induction of dopamine depletion in the MPTP model that impedes the development of compensatory processes found in the slowly evolving human disease. On the other hand, tremor is a much more overt phenomenon than akinesia and rigidity. A human patient or his/her family may first be aware of the slow development of PD by the more easily recognizable tremor. As in human studies there is a low coherence level between the tremor of the limbs of MPTP-treated vervet monkeys following dopamine replacement therapy (Heimer *et al.*, 2006).

THE CLINICAL ANATOMY OF THE BASAL GANGLIA AND THEIR CONNECTIONS

The major pathological event leading to the motor symptoms of PD, and especially to akinesia, is the death of midbrain dopaminergic neurons and their striatal projections. The striatum (composed of caudate, putamen and ventral striatum) is the main input stage of the basal ganglia, receiving inputs from all cortical areas as well as from many thalamic nuclei and even from the cerebellum (Hoshi *et al.*, 2005). Therefore, a good grasp of the pathophysiology of

PD depends on understanding the anatomy and physiology of the basal ganglia and dopamine networks.

The motor system has been classically described as consisting of two parts: the pyramidal and the extra-pyramidal sub-systems. The pyramidal system starts at the motor cortices, and, through the brain-stem pyramids, projects to spinal interneurons and alpha-motoneurons, innervating the distal parts of the limbs, and controls the execution of accurate, voluntary movements. In contrast, it was assumed that the extra-pyramidal system originates at the basal ganglia and the cerebellum, descends parallel to the pyramidal system, and innervates the spinal circuits involved with more axial (postural), automatic non-voluntary movements.

The revolution in anatomical methods during the second half of the twentieth century led to the conclusion that the basal ganglia are the feed-forward part of a closed loop connecting all cortical areas sequentially through the striatum, pallidum and thalamus with the frontal cortex. The frontal cortex projects downstream to the spinal level. This view of the basal ganglia networks assumes that there are two segregated internal pathways that start in the striatum and converge on the output structures of the basal ganglia (the internal segment of the globus pallidus (GPi), and the substantia nigra pars reticulata (SNr)). The "direct pathway" is a direct GABAeregic inhibitory pathway, whereas the "indirect pathway" is a polysynaptic disinhibitory pathway through the external segment of the globus pallidus (GPe) and the subthalamic nucleus (STN). The projection striatal neurons in the direct pathway express D1 dopamine receptors, whereas those in the indirect pathway express D2 dopamine receptors (Gerfen et al., 1990). Dopamine has differential effects on the two striato-pallidal pathways: it facilitates transmission along the direct pathway via the D1 receptors and inhibits transmission along the indirect pathway via the D2 receptors (Gerfen et al., 1990; Albin, Young and Penney, 1989). Since the output structures of the basal ganglia inhibit their thalamic targets, the direct pathway (cortex, striatum, GPi, thalamus, frontal cortex) contain two inhibitory paths (striatum to GPi and GPi to thalamus) and can be regarded as a positive feedback—facilitatory—loop and the indirect pathway, containing three inhibitory paths (striatum to GPe, GPe to STN and GPi to thalamus) connected by an excitatory path from the STN to the GPi is regarded as a negative feedback—inhibitory—loop. The dopamine facilitation of movements is therefore the combined results of its excitatory effects on the direct positive feedback loop and the inhibition of the indirect negative feedback loops.

Recently, single axon tracing anatomical studies have revealed an even more complex map of basal ganglia connectivity. Striatal neurons projecting to the GPi and SNr have been shown to send collaterals to the GPe (Levesque and Parent, 2005). The physiological evidence for the

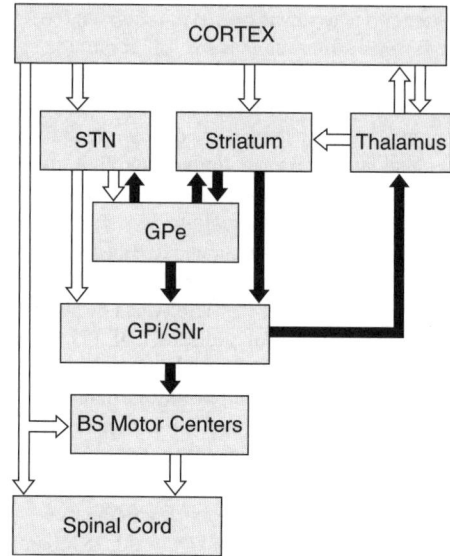

Figure 2.1 Schematic view of the connectivity of the cortex–basal ganglia–muscle networks. White arrows indicate excitatory connections, and black arrows denote inhibitory connections. The dopamine projections to the striatum are not shown. Abbreviations: STN, subthalamic nucleus; GPe, GPi, external, internal segment of the globus pallidus; SNc, SNr, substantia nigra pars compacta and reticulata; BS motor centers, brain stem motor centers, for example, superior colliculus and the pedunculopontine nucleus.

importance of the direct projections from the motor cortex to the STN (the "hyper-direct" pathway, (Nambu, 2004)) indicates that, like the striatum, the STN is an input stage of the basal ganglia. Moreover, the recently described feedback projections from the GPe to the striatum, as well as the GPe to GPi projection (Bolam et al., 2000), strongly suggest that the GPe is a central nucleus in the basal ganglia circuitry rather than a simple relay station in the indirect pathway. The last twist in our understanding of the basal ganglia anatomy came with the re-discovery of basal ganglia outputs to brain-stem motor centers, such as the pedunculopontine nucleus and the superior colliculus (Delwaide et al., 2000). Figure 2.1 summarizes the current view of the complex connectivity among the basal ganglia nuclei.

PHYSIOLOGICAL STUDIES OF THE BASAL GANGLIA IN NORMAL PRIMATES

Analysis of neuronal activity at the level of single spikes of single cells is probably the best way to study the computational physiology of a neuronal network. The background (during a quiet awake state) spiking activity of the basal ganglia nuclei is very characteristic. The low-frequency discharge of striatal neurons (<1 spikes/s by the projection neurons and 4–10 spikes/s by the tonically active neurons (TANs), the cholinergic interneurons of the striatum resembles cortical discharge rates. However, this slow discharge contrasts strikingly with the high frequency (50–80 spikes/s) discharge of GPe, GPi and SNr neurons. In all these structures the firing rate is irregular (Poisson-like). Furthermore, neuronal oscillations are seldom observed in normal awake subjects (DeLong, 1971; Elias et al., 2007).

Studies exploring the relationship between the spiking activity of basal ganglia neurons and movements have found even more unexpected results. The akinesia associated with PD suggests that the basal ganglia may play a critical role in movement initiation. Nevertheless, most basal ganglia neurons change their firing rate after initiation of stereotyped, over-learned, stimulus-triggered movements (Putamen: (Crutcher and DeLong, 1984; Alexander and Crutcher, 1990); GP: (DeLong, 1971; Anderson and Horak, 1985; Mink and Thach, 1991); SNr: (Schultz, 1986)), and do not have any exclusive or consistent relationships to movement parameters such as start/end, velocity or amplitude (Mink and Thach, 1991). The data regarding basal ganglia discharge related to voluntary, self-initiated movements (Romo, Scarnati and Schultz, 1992; Schultz and Romo, 1992) are still scarce and under debate. Together with the inconclusive findings of lesion studies of the output structures of the primate basal ganglia (Horak and Anderson, 1984; Mink and Thach, 1991; Kato and Kimura, 1992) the physiological results revealing late timing of basal ganglia discharge has led to the surprising conclusion that the basal ganglia do not initiate movements (Mink, 1996). Rather, basal ganglia inhibitory control of the thalamic-cortical network probably enables and facilitates the execution of learned and semi-automatic movements. Recent advances of our understanding of the role of striatal dopamine (Schultz, 2007; Calabresi et al., 2007; Arbuthnott and Wickens, 2007) and acetylcholine (Morris et al., 2004; Cragg, 2006; Wang et al., 2006) indicate that these movements are those acquired and shaped by implicit learning (Bar-Gad, Morris and Bergman, 2003; Daw and Doya, 2006).

PHYSIOLOGICAL STUDIES IN THE BASAL GANGLIA NETWORKS OF MPTP-TREATED PRIMATES AND HUMAN PATIENTS WITH PARKINSON'S DISEASE

Early physiological studies of Parkinsonian MPTP-treated monkeys reported increases in the discharge rate within the GPi (Miller and DeLong, 1987; Filion and Tremblay, 1991) and the STN (Bergman et al., 1994) as opposed to a decrease in discharge rate in the GPe (Miller and DeLong, 1987; Filion and Tremblay, 1991). Reversed trends of pallidal discharge rates in response to dopamine replacement therapy have been reported in both human patients (Hutchinson et al., 1997; Merello et al., 1999) and primates (Heimer et al., 2006; Filion, Tremblay and Bedard, 1991; Papa et al., 1999). The possible role of these rate changes in the pathophysiology of PD has been verified by the subsequent findings showing that inactivation of STN and GPi could improve the motor symptoms in Parkinsonian animals (Bergman, Wichmann and DeLong, 1990; Aziz et al., 1991) and human patients (Machado et al., 2006).

These findings contributed to the formulation and the popularity of the direct/indirect model of the basal ganglia (see above). Nevertheless, several studies have failed to find the expected significant changes of firing rates in the pallidum (Boraud et al., 2002), thalamus (Pessiglione et al., 2005) or motor cortical areas (Goldberg et al., 2002) of MPTP monkeys. This and other inconsistencies with the assumptions and the predictions of the direct/indirect rate model have attracted more attention to the potential role of other aspects of neuronal activity, such as firing patterns and neuronal synchronization in the pathophysiology of PD. MPTP monkeys show an increase in the fraction of basal ganglia neurons that discharge in bursts. These bursts are either irregular or oscillatory and have been found in the STN, GPe, GPi and also in the primary motor cortex (Bergman et al., 1994; Raz, Vaadia and Bergman, 2000; Miller and DeLong, 1987; Filion and Tremblay, 1991; Goldberg et al., 2002; Boraud et al., 2001; Wichmann and Soares, 2006). In most cases the cells tend to oscillate at the tremor frequency as well as at double or even triple the tremor frequency (Bergman et al., 1994; Raz, Vaadia and Bergman, 2000; Heimer et al., 2006). Nevertheless, these studies have failed to reveal a significant fraction of neurons whose oscillations are consistently coherent with the simultaneous recorded tremor (Raz, Vaadia and Bergman, 2000; Heimer et al., 2006). Both STN inactivation (Wichmann, Bergman and DeLong, 1994) and dopamine replacement therapy (Heimer et al., 2006) significantly ameliorate the 4–7 Hz tremor and reduce the GPi 8–20 Hz oscillations, indicating the critical role of beta range, higher frequency oscillations, rather than the tremor frequency oscillations, in tremor generation.

Physiological studies of simultaneously recorded neurons in the pallidum (Raz, Vaadia and Bergman, 2000; Heimer et al., 2006; Nini et al., 1995; Heimer et al., 2002), as well as in the primary motor cortex (Goldberg et al., 2002), among striatal TANs and between TANs and pallidal neurons (Raz et al., 1996; Raz et al., 2001) in MPTP-treated monkeys demonstrate that their pair-wise cross-correlograms become peaked and oscillatory. The abnormal pallidal synchronization decreases in response to dopamine replacement therapy (Heimer et al., 2006). In most cases, the maximal power of the synchronous oscillations was found to be at double the tremor frequency (Raz, Vaadia and Bergman, 2000; Heimer *et al.*, 2006; Raz *et al.*, 1996; Raz *et al.*, 2001). Similar, double tremor frequencies were observed also in the STN of both akinetic-rigid- and tremor-dominant human PD patients undergoing DBS procedures (Moran, Bergman, Israel, Bar-Gad, unpublished results). These correlation studies therefore suggest that striatal dopamine depletion induces abnormal coupling of basal ganglia loops, but mainly in a higher, beta frequency range.

As in the MPTP primate, single unit studies of the basal ganglia of human PD patients (performed during electrophysiological mapping of the target area for therapeutic implantation of stimulating electrodes) have reported a high fraction of GPi and STN cells oscillating at the tremor frequency (Hutchison *et al.*, 1997; Weinberger *et al.*, 2006; Levy *et al.*, 2002). However as in the primate, the human studies (Lemstra *et al.*, 1999; Hurtado *et al.*, 1999; Hurtado *et al.*, 2005) show that these oscillations are not fully coherent with the simultaneously recorded tremor. Advanced time-dependent phase correlation techniques have been applied to pairs of tremor-related GPi single units and EMG of PD patients undergoing stereotactic neurosurgery. Analysis using short sliding windows shows that oscillatory activity in both GPi oscillatory units and muscles occurs intermittently over time. There is partial overlap in the times of oscillatory activity but, in most cases, no correlation has been found between the times of oscillatory episodes in the two signals. Phase-locking analysis reveals that pallidal oscillations and tremor are punctuated by phase slips, which have been classified as synchronizing or desynchronizing. The results of this high-level quantitative characterization of PD tremor and pallidal oscillations can be explained by either a very dynamic connectivity from the basal ganglia to the periphery, or by tremor generators downstream of the basal ganglia. The sharp contrast between this transient and inconsistent pallidal-tremor synchronization and the high synchronicity found between thalamic Vim neurons and the tremor (Lenz *et al.*, 1988) suggest that pallidal neurons cannot be viewed as the tremor generators, or as simple encoders of the proprioceptive feedback of the tremor.

PHYSIOLOGICAL STUDIES OF POPULATION ACTIVITY IN THE BASAL GANGLIA NETWORKS OF DOPAMINE-DEPLETED ANIMAL MODELS AND HUMAN PATIENTS WITH PARKINSON'S DISEASE

Synchronization of basal ganglia neuronal activity is also evident in the local field potentials (LFP) recorded in the basal ganglia of PD patients through macro-electrodes used for high-frequency stimulation of these structures. These oscillations occur mainly in the high beta range (15–30 Hz) and following treatment with levodopa shift to higher frequencies (40–70 Hz) in the gamma range (Kuhn *et al.*, 2006; Hammond, Bergman and Brown, 2007). In line with both the single unit and the LFP studies, magnetoencephalographic (MEG) studies (Timmermann *et al.*, 2003) of tremor-type PD patients have revealed a strong coherence between the tremor and activity in the motor and sensory cortices and the cerebellum at tremor frequency, and an even stronger coherency at double tremor frequency. Spectra of coherence between thalamic activity and cerebellum as well as several other brain areas have revealed additional broad peaks at around 20 Hz.

Studies of LFPs recorded from the frontal cortex and STN of rats following 6-OHDA lesions of midbrain dopamine neurons (Sharott *et al.*, 2005) have revealed significant increases in the power and coherence of beta-frequency oscillatory activity. Administration of the dopamine receptor agonist apomorphine to these dopamine-depleted animals suppressed the beta-frequency oscillations, and increased coherent activity at gamma frequencies in the cortex and STN. Thus, the pattern of synchronization between population activity in the STN and cortex in the 6-OHDA-lesioned rodent model of PD is closely paralleled to that seen in PD human patients and the primate MPTP model.

Recordings of both LFPs and multi-neuronal activity from microelectrodes inserted into the STN in PD patients during functional neurosurgery suggests that the discharges of some of the neurons in the STN are locked to beta oscillations in the LFP (Kuhn *et al.*, 2005). LFPs probably represent the synaptic input to a neural structure and its sub-threshold slow activity. The discrepancies between LFP oscillatory activity as compared to neuronal activity (both in their frequency domains, prevalence and power) may be due to the fact that even quite strong synchronized inputs (as reflected in the LFP) may lead to weak correlations in the neuronal discharge. On the other hand, correlations can be very low at the neuronal pair-wise level, but still summate and become substantial at the population (LFP) level (Goldberg *et al.*, 2004; Schneidman *et al.*, 2006). We therefore conclude that the hallmark of the dopamine-depleted basal ganglia network is its abnormally strong synchronized state.

ADVANCED NEUROSURGICAL TREATMENTS OF PARKINSON'S DISEASE: WHAT THEY TELL US ABOUT PD PHYSIOLOGY

The most important prediction of the dual pathway model of the basal ganglia (see above) and the finding of abnormal tonic firing rate in the basal ganglia of MPTP monkeys was that ablation or inactivation of the GPi or STN should lead to the alleviation of parkinsonian symptoms. Inactivation of the GPi would remove the excessive inhibitory drive to the frontal cortex (via the thalamus) and the resulting suppression of voluntary movements. Similarly, destroying the STN would remove the excessive excitatory drive to the GPi. This would normalize GPi output, thereby reducing the inhibition of the frontal cortex.

These predictions were in fact supported by early pallidal ablation therapy of PD. Pallidotomy, which had been largely abandoned since the advent of levodopa therapy, was shown to be very successful at alleviating akinesia and rigidity of human patients (Laitinen, Bergenheim and Hariz, 1992; Lozano et al., 1995; Vitek and Bakay, 1997). Injection of excitatory amino acid antagonists into the GPi of MPTP-treated monkeys was shown to reverse the motor symptoms of parkinsonism (Graham et al., 1990). STN permanent lesions and temporal inactivation (by injection of the GABA agonist, muscimol) were shown by several groups to reverse parkinsonian symptoms in MPTP primates (Bergman, Wichmann and DeLong, 1990; Wichmann, Bergman and DeLong, 1994; Aziz et al., 1991; Guridi et al., 1993; Guridi et al., 1996). The primate results set the stage for the introduction of subthalamotomy as a treatment for PD patients (Obeso et al., 1997; Gill and Heywood, 1997) and for the development of deep brain stimulation (DBS) of the STN as an alternative treatment for PD. DBS of the STN and the GPi have been successful at alleviating parkinsonism both in PD patients (Limousin et al., 1995; Pollak et al., 1996; Kumar et al., 1998) and in MPTP primates (Benazzouz et al., 1996). Today DBS is preferred by neurosurgeons over ablative surgery due to its reversibility and parameter tuning capabilities (Lang and Lozano, 1998; Gross et al., 1999). There are indications that GPi stimulation is best suited to treat levodopa-induced dyskinesia (LID) and rigidity, whereas STN stimulation is best fit for treatment of akinesia, rigidity and tremor (Limousin et al., 1995; Pollak et al., 1996; Kumar et al., 1998; Benabid et al., 1994). However, significant reduction of the dopamine replacement therapy is better achieved with STN DBS, and therefore this is the procedure of choice in most centers. An updated description of surgical techniques and patient management during DBS surgery for advanced PD has been published as Supplement 14 to Volume 21 of *Movement Disorders*, 2006 (see also Chapter 7: Surgery for Parkinson's Disease, this volume).

The mechanism of DBS on neuronal discharge is still debated. Early studies (Ranck, 1975; Stoney, Thompson and Asanuma, 1968) showed that when metal microelectrodes are used, the susceptibility of nerve fibers is much higher than that of the cell bodies, suggesting that microstimulation activates bypassing fibers. In any case, the classical interpretation of the effect of micro-stimulation on the motor cortices has been that the stimulation induces excitation of the cortex or cortico-spinal axonal pathways and thus evokes movement of different body parts. Since the effect of DBS in PD is paradoxically similar to the effect of lesions (e.g., neuronal inactivation) the question of the actual effect of DBS has been recently addressed both in the MPTP primate model and in human PD patients. In the MPTP primate, DBS in the GPi has been shown to reduce the discharge rates to within the normal range (Boraud et al., 1996). Similar results have been described in rodent studies (Benazzouz et al., 2000) and in human PD patients (Dostrovsky et al., 2000; Maltete et al., 2007). There are several possible mechanisms to explain these results: depolarization block of the stimulated neurons, stimulation of bypassing inhibitory pathways, and/or induction of GABA release from the terminals of the GPe projection neurons, thereby inhibiting the target GPi neurons. A major difference between human DBS and primate or human microstimulation is that the former uses macro-electrodes (with impedances in the ranges of a few kΩ). The current densities around the stimulating macro-electrodes are much smaller than with micro-stimulation, and therefore the mechanisms of clinical macro deep brain high-frequency stimulation are still debated.

Application of DBS to the STN of MPTP primates has also generated conflicting results. In one early study, DBS was found to differentially affect the mean discharge rates in the GPe and GPi for several hours after the DBS: it caused an increase in the former and a decrease in the latter (Hayase et al., 1996). In a more recent study the mean firing rates increased in both pallidal segments during STN DBS (Hashimoto et al., 2003) and GPi DBS lead to suppression of thalamic discharge (Anderson, Postupna and Ruffo, 2003). DBS with macro-electrodes has been recently shown in rats *in vivo* to directly depolarize the membrane potential of the STN neurons (Garcia et al., 2003). Thus, DBS may enforce high-frequency homogenous (in time and space) discharge in the basal ganglia and "jamming" of their abnormal output rather than inhibition (Benabid, 2003; Bar-Gad et al., 2004; Miocinovic et al., 2006).

In summary, the precise neuronal mechanism of DBS (e.g., effects on neurons or fibers in the area of electrode, effect of the stimulated area or remote structures, etc.) is still an open issue. In any case, the similar effects of thalamic and STN/GPi DBS, despite the GABAergic connectivity between these two structures, supports the hypothesis that the main effect of DBS is mediated by enforcing a constant spatio-temporal firing pattern, rather than modulation of discharge rate, on pallidal or thalamic neurons. This enables the cortical network to ignore the pathological synchronized oscillatory "noisy" drive of the basal ganglia, and to provide a compensation for their missing gating signal.

SUMMARY AND CONCLUSIONS

In this review we have explored the possible relationships between basal ganglia neuronal activity and PD clinical symptoms. PD is the result of dopamine depletion in the striatum—the input stage of the basal ganglia. Akinesia, rigidity and rest tremor are the major motor symptoms of PD. Nevertheless, cumulative clinical and experimental evidence support the view that they are not generated by identical neuronal mechanisms. Following striatal dopamine depletion, many basal ganglia neurons develop synchronous oscillations at the tremor frequency and at their higher harmonics, as well as in the beta range. However, the PD tremor does not strictly follow the basal ganglia oscillatory activity. The recent demonstration of anatomical connections between the cerebellum and the basal ganglia, both at the cortical, striatal and brain stem level may suggest that the cerebellum is associated with the movement disorders classically described as pure basal ganglia disorders. The critical role of the cerebellar output in the generation of PD tremor has been demonstrated by primate lesion studies and the efficacy of Vim intervention in treatment of PD tremor. These findings, along with the physiological studies of the normal basal ganglia indicating that the basal ganglia do not initiate movements, strengthen the supposition that the abnormal synchronous beta-range (higher than tremor frequency) oscillations in the basal ganglia provide noisy input to the frontal cortex. The abnormal driven activity of the frontal cortex hinders the normal functioning of the motor cortices and hence leads to PD akinesia. We further suggest that rigidity and tremor are generated by basal ganglia downstream mechanisms struggling to compensate for PD akinesia. The stronger association between akinesia and rigidity as opposed to the more independent nature of PD tremor may indicate that rigidity and tremor are generated by different mechanisms.

ACKNOWLEDGMENTS

This research was supported in part by the "Fighting against Parkinson" Foundation of the Hebrew University Netherlands Association (HUNA).

References

Albin, R.L., Young, A.B. and Penney, J.B. (1989) The functional anatomy of basal ganglia disorders. *Trends in Neurosciences*, **12**, 366–375.

Alexander, G.E. and Crutcher, M.D. (1990) Preparation for movement: neural representations of intended direction in three motor areas of the monkey. *Journal of Neurophysiology*, **64**, 133–150.

Anderson, M.E. and Horak, F.B. (1985) Influence of the globus pallidus on arm movements in monkeys. III. Timing of movement-related information. *Journal of Neurophysiology*, **54**, 433–448.

Anderson, M.E., Postupna, N. and Ruffo, M. (2003) Effects of high-frequency stimulation in the internal globus pallidus on the activity of thalamic neurons in the awake monkey. *Journal of Neurophysiology*, **89**, 1150–1160.

Arbuthnott, G.W. and Wickens, J. (2007) Space, time and dopamine. *Trends in Neurosciences*, **30**, 62–69.

Aziz, T.Z., Peggs, D., Sambrook, M.A. and Crossman, A.R. (1991) Lesion of the subthalamic nucleus for the alleviation of 1-methyl-4-phenyl-1,2,3,6-tetrahydropyridine (MPTP)-induced parkinsonism in the primate. *Movement Disorders*, **6**, 288–292.

Aziz, T.Z., Peggs, D., Sambrook, M.A. and Crossman, A.R. (1991) Lesion of the subthalamic nucleus for the alleviation of 1-methyl-4-phenyl-1,2,3,6-tetrahydropyridine (MPTP)-induced parkinsonism in the primate. *Movement Disorders*, **6**, 288–293.

Bar-Gad, I., Morris, G. and Bergman, H. (2003) Information processing, dimensionality reduction and reinforcement learning in the basal ganglia. *Progress in Neurobiology*, **71**, 439–473.

Bar-Gad, I., Elias, S., Vaadia, E. and Bergman, H. (2004) Complex locking rather than complete cessation of neuronal activity in the globus pallidus of a 1-methyl-4-phenyl-1,2,3,6-tetrahydropyridine-treated primate in response to pallidal microstimulation. *The Journal of Neuroscience*, **24**, 9410–9419.

Benabid, A.L. (2003) Deep brain stimulation for Parkinson's disease. *Current Opinion in Neurobiology*, **13**, 696–706.

Benabid, A.L., Pollak, P., Gross, C., Hoffmann, D., Benazzouz, A., Gao, D.M., Laurent, A., Gentil, M. and Perret, J. (1994) Acute and long-term effects of subthalamic nucleus stimulation in Parkinson's disease. *Stereotactic and Functional Neurosurgery*, **62**, 76–84.

Benazzouz, A., Boraud, T., Feger, J., Burbaud, P., Bioulac, B. and Gross, C. (1996) Alleviation of experimental hemiparkinsonism by high-frequency stimulation of the subthalamic nucleus in primates: a comparison with L-Dopa treatment. *Movement Disorders*, **11**, 627–632.

Benazzouz, A., Gao, D.M., Ni, Z.G., Piallat, B., Bouali, B.R. and Benabid, A.L. (2000) Effect of high-frequency stimulation of the subthalamic nucleus on the neuronal activities of the substantia nigra pars reticulata and ventrolateral nucleus of the thalamus in the rat. *Neuroscience*, **99**, 289–295.

Benmoyal-Segal, L. and Soreq, H. (2006) Gene-environment interactions in sporadic Parkinson's disease. *Journal of Neurochemistry*, **97**, 1740–1755.

Ben-Pazi, H., Bergman, H., Goldber, J.A., Giladi, N., Hansel, D., Reches, A. and Simon, E.S. (2001) Synchrony of rest tremor in multiple limbs in parkinson's disease: evidence for multiple oscillators. *Journal of Neural Transmission*, **108**, 287–296.

Bergman, H., Wichmann, T. and DeLong, M.R. (1990) Reversal of experimental parkinsonism by lesions of the subthalamic nucleus. *Science*, **249**, 1436–1438.

Bergman, H., Wichmann, T., Karmon, B. and DeLong, M.R. (1994) The primate subthalamic nucleus. II. Neuronal activity in the MPTP model of parkinsonism. *Journal of Neurophysiology*, **72**, 507–520.

Bolam, J.P., Hanley, J.J., Booth, P.A. and Bevan, M.D. (2000) Synaptic organisation of the basal ganglia. *Journal of Anatomy*, **196**Pt (4), 527–542.

Boraud, T., Bezard, E., Bioulac, B. and Gross, C. (1996) High frequency stimulation of the internal Globus Pallidus (GPi) simultaneously improves parkinsonian symptoms and reduces the firing frequency of GPi neurons in the MPTP-treated monkey. *Neuroscience Letters*, **215**, 17–20.

Boraud, T., Bezard, E., Bioulac, B. and Gross, C.E. (2001) Dopamine agonist-induced dyskinesias are correlated to both firing pattern and frequency alterations of pallidal neurones in the

MPTP-treated monkey. *Brain: A Journal of Neurology*, **124**, 546–557.

Boraud, T., Bezard, E., Bioulac, B. and Gross, C.E. (2002) From single extracellular unit recording in experimental and human Parkinsonism to the development of a functional concept of the role played by the basal ganglia in motor control. *Progress in Neurobiology*, **66**, 265–283.

Braak, H., Del, T.K., Rub, U., de Vos, R.A., Jansen Steur, E.N. and Braak, E. (2003) Staging of brain pathology related to sporadic Parkinson's disease. *Neurobiology of Aging*, **24**, 197–211.

Britton, T.C., Thompson, P.D., Day, B.L., Rothwell, J.C., Findley, L.J. and Marsden, C.D. (1992) "Resetting" of postural tremors at the wrist with mechanical stretches in Parkinson's disease, essential tremor, and normal subjects mimicking tremor. *Annals of Neurology*, **31**, 507–514.

Burn, D.J., Rowan, E.N., Allan, L.M., Molloy, S., O'Brien, J.T. and McKeith, I.G. (2006) Motor subtype and cognitive decline in Parkinson's disease, Parkinson's disease with dementia, and dementia with Lewy bodies. *Journal of Neurology, Neurosurgery, and Psychiatry*, **77**, 585–589.

Burns, R.S., Chiueh, C.C., Markey, S.P., Ebert, M.H., Jacobowitz, D.M. and Kopin, I.J. (1983) A primate model of parkinsonism: selective destruction of dopaminergic neurons in the pars compacta of the substantia nigra by N-methyl-4-phenyl-1,2,3,6-tetrahydropyridine. *Proceedings of the National Academy of Sciences of the United States of America*, **80**, 4546–4550.

Calabresi, P., Picconi, B., Tozzi, A. and Di, F.M. (2007) Dopamine-mediated regulation of corticostriatal synaptic plasticity. *Trends in Neurosciences*, **30**, 211–219.

Cragg, S.J. (2006) Meaningful silences: how dopamine listens to the ACh pause. *Trends in Neurosciences*, **29**, 125–131.

Crutcher, M.D. and DeLong, M.R. (1984) Single cell studies of the primate putamen. II. Relations to direction of movement and pattern of muscular activity. *Experimental Brain Research*, **53**, 244–258.

Daw, N.D. and Doya, K. (2006) The computational neurobiology of learning and reward. *Current Opinion in Neurobiology*, **16**, 199–204.

DeLong, M.R. (1971) Activity of pallidal neurons during movement. *Journal of Neurophysiology*, **34**, 414–427.

Delwaide, P.J., Sabbatino, M. and Delwaide, C. (1986) Some pathophysiological aspects of the parkinsonian rigidity. *Journal of Neural Transmission Supplementum*, **22**, 129–139.

Delwaide, P.J., Pepin, J.L., De, P.V. and de Noordhout, A.M. (2000) Projections from basal ganglia to tegmentum: a subcortical route for explaining the pathophysiology of Parkinson's disease signs? *Journal of Neurology*, **247** (Suppl 2), II75–II81.

Deuschl, G., Raethjen, J., Baron, R., Lindemann, M., Wilms, H. and Krack, P. (2000) The pathophysiology of parkinsonian tremor: a review. *Journal of Neurology*, **247** (Suppl 5), V33–V48.

Dietz, V. (1987) Changes of inherent muscle stiffness in Parkinson's disease. *Journal of Neurology, Neurosurgery, and Psychiatry*, **50**, 944.

Dostrovsky, J.O., Levy, R., Wu, J.P., Hutchison, W.D., Tasker, R.R. and Lozano, A.M. (2000) Microstimulation-induced inhibition of neuronal firing in human globus pallidus. *Journal of Neurophysiology*, **84**, 570–574.

Elble, R.J. and Koller, W.C. (1990) *Tremor*, The Johns Hopkins University Press; Baltimore and London.

Elias, S., Joshua, M., Goldberg, J.A., Heimer, G., Arkadir, D., Morris, G. and Bergman, H. (2007) Statistical properties of pauses of the high-frequency discharge neurons in the external segment of the globus pallidus. *The Journal of Neuroscience*, **27**, 2525–2538.

Farrer, M.J. (2006) Genetics of Parkinson's disease: paradigm shifts and future prospects. *Nature Reviews Genetics*, **7**, 306–318.

Filion, M. and Tremblay, L. (1991) Abnormal spontaneous activity of globus pallidus neurons in monkeys with MPTP-induced parkinsonism. *Brain Research*, **547**, 142–151.

Filion, M., Tremblay, L. and Bedard, P.J. (1991) Effects of dopamine agonists on the spontaneous activity of globus pallidus neurons in monkeys with MPTP-induced parkinsonism. *Brain Research*, **547**, 152–161.

Garcia, L., Audin, J., D'Alessandro, G., Bioulac, B. and Hammond, C. (2003) Dual effect of high-frequency stimulation on subthalamic neuron activity. *The Journal of Neuroscience*, **23**, 8743–8751.

Gerfen, C.R., Engber, T.M., Mahan, L.C., Susel, Z., Chase, T.N., Monsma, F.,J. Jr and Sibley, D.R. (1990) D1 and D2 dopamine receptor-regulated gene expression of striatonigral and striatopallidal neurons. *Science*, **250**, 1429–1432.

Gill, S.S. and Heywood, P. (1997) Bilateral dorsolateral subthalamotomy for advanced Parkinson's disease. *Lancet*, **350**, 1224.

Goldberg, J.A., Boraud, T., Maraton, S., Haber, S.N., Vaadia, E. and Bergman, H. (2002) Enhanced synchrony among primary motor cortex neurons in the 1-methyl-4-phenyl-1,2,3,6-tetrahydropyridine primate model of Parkinson's disease. *The Journal of Neuroscience*, **22**, 4639–4653.

Goldberg, J.A., Rokni, U., Boraud, T., Vaadia, E. and Bergman, H. (2004) Spike synchronization in the cortex-Basal Ganglia networks of parkinsonian primates reflects global dynamics of the local field potentials. *The Journal of Neuroscience*, **24**, 6003–6010.

Graham, W.C., Robertson, R.G., Sambrook, M.A. and Crossman, A.R. (1990) Injection of excitatory amino acid antagonists into the medial pallidal segment of a 1-methyl-4-phenyl-1,2,3,6-tetrahydropyridine (MPTP) treated primate reverses motor symptoms of parkinsonism. *Life Sciences*, **47**, PL91–PL97.

Gross, C.E., Boraud, T., Guehl, D., Bioulac, B. and Bezard, E. (1999) From experimentation to the surgical treatment of Parkinson's disease: prelude or suite in basal ganglia research? *Progress in Neurobiology*, **59**, 509–532.

Guridi, J., Luguin, M.R., Herrero, M.T., Guillen, J. and Obeso, J.A. (1993) Antiparkinsonian effect of subthalmotomy in MPTP-exposed monkeys. *Movement Disorders*, **8**, 415.

Guridi, J., Herrero, M.T., Luquin, M.R., Guillen, J., Ruberg, M., Laguna, J., Vila, M., Javoy, A.F., Agid, Y., Hirsch, E. and Obeso, J.A. (1996) Subthalamotomy in parkinsonian monkeys. Behavioural and biochemical analysis. *Brain: A Journal of Neurology*, **119**, 1717–1727.

Hagbarth, K.E., Wallin, G., Lofstedt, L. and Aquilonius, S.M. (1975) Muscle spindle activity in alternating tremor of Parkinsonism and in clonus. *Journal of Neurology, Neurosurgery, and Psychiatry*, **38**, 636–641.

Hammond, C., Bergman, H. and Brown, P. (2007) Pathological synchronization in Parkinson's disease: networks, models and treatments. *Trends Neuroscience*, **70**, 357–364.

Hashimoto, T., Elder, C.M., Okun, M.S., Patrick, S.K. and Vitek, J.L. (2003) Stimulation of the subthalamic nucleus changes the firing pattern of pallidal neurons. *The Journal of Neuroscience*, **23**, 1916–1923.

Hayase, N., Filion, M., Richard, H. and Boraud, T. (1996) Electrical stimulation of the subthalamic nucleus in fully parkinsonian (MPTP) monkeys: effect on clinical signs and pallidal activity, in *The Basal Ganglia V.* (eds C. Ohye, M. Kimura and J.S. McKenzie), Plenum, pp. 241–248.

Heimer, G., Bar-Gad, I., Goldberg, J.A. and Bergman, H. (2002) Dopamine replacement therapy reverses abnormal synchronization of pallidal neurons in the 1-methyl-4-phenyl-1,2,3,6-tetrahydropyridine primate model of parkinsonism. *The Journal of Neuroscience*, **22**, 7850–7855.

Heimer, G., Rivlin-Etzion, M., Bar-Gad, I., Goldberg, J.A., Haber, S.N. and Bergman, H. (2006) Dopamine replacement therapy does not restore the full spectrum of normal pallidal activity in the 1-methyl-4-phenyl-1,2,3,6-tetra-hydropyridine primate model of Parkinsonism. *The Journal of Neuroscience*, **26**, 8101–8114.

Horak, F.B. and Anderson, M.E. (1984) Influence of globus pallidus on arm movements in monkeys. I. Effects of kainic acid-induced lesions. *Journal of Neurophysiology*, **52**, 290–304.

Hoshi, E., Tremblay, L., Feger, J., Carras, P.L. and Strick, P.L. (2005) The cerebellum communicates with the basal ganglia. *Nature Neuroscience*, **8**, 1491–1493.

Hunker, C.J. and Abbs, J.H. (1990) Uniform frequency of parkinsonian resting tremor in the lips, jaw, tongue, and index finger. *Movement Disorders*, **5**, 71–77.

Hurtado, J.M., Gray, C.M., Tamas, L.B. and Sigvardt, K.A. (1999) Dynamics of tremor-related oscillations in the human globus pallidus: a single case study. *Proceedings of the National Academy of Sciences of the United States of America*, **96**, 1674–1679.

Hurtado, J.M., Rubchinsky, L.L., Sigvardt, K.A., Wheelock, V.L. and Pappas, C.T. (2005) Temporal evolution of oscillations and synchrony in GPi/muscle pairs in Parkinson's disease. *Journal of Neurophysiology*, **93**, 1569–1584.

Hutchinson, W.D., Levy, R., Dostrovsky, J.O., Lozano, A.M. and Lang, A.E. (1997) Effects of apomorphine on globus pallidus neurons in parkinsonian patients. *Annals of Neurology*, **42**, 767–775.

Hutchinson, W.D., Lozano, A.M., Tasker, R.R., Lang, A.E. and Dostrovsky, J.O. (1997) Identification and characterization of neurons with tremor-frequency activity in human globus pallidus. *Experimental Brain Research*, **113**, 557–563.

Jankovic, J., McDermott, M., Carter, J., Gauthier, S., Goetz, C., Golbe, L., Huber, S., Koller, W., Olanow, C., Shoulson, I. *et al.* (1990) Variable expression of Parkinson's disease: a base-line analysis of the DATATOP cohort. The Parkinson Study Group. *Neurology*, **40**, 1529–1534.

Jellinger, K.A. (1991) Pathology of Parkinson's disease. Changes other than the nigrostriatal pathway. *Molecular and Chemical Neuropathology*, **14**, 153–197.

Jenner, P. and Marsden, C.D. (1984) Neurochemical basis of parkinsonian tremor, in *Movement disorders: tremor* (eds L.J. Findley and R. Capildeo), Oxford University Press, New York, pp. 305–319.

Kato, M. and Kimura, M. (1992) Effects of reversible blockade of basal ganglia on voluntary arm movement. *Journal of Neurophysiology*, **68**, 1516–1534.

Kuhn, A.A., Trottenberg, T., Kivi, A., Kupsch, A., Schneider, G.H. and Brown, P. (2005) The relationship between local field potential and neuronal discharge in the subthalamic nucleus of patients with Parkinson's disease. *Experimental Neurology*, **194**, 212–220.

Kuhn, A.A., Kupsch, A., Schneider, G.H. and Brown, P. (2006) Reduction in subthalamic 8–35 Hz oscillatory activity correlates with clinical improvement in Parkinson's disease. *The European Journal of Neuroscience*, **23**, 1956–1960.

Kumar, R., Lozano, A.M., Montgomery, E. and Lang, A.E. (1998) Pallidotomy and deep brain stimulation of the pallidum and subthalamic nucleus in advanced Parkinson's disease. *Movement Disorders*, **13** (Suppl 1), 73–82.

Laitinen, L.V., Bergenheim, A.T. and Hariz, M.I. (1992) Leksell's posteroventral pallidotomy in the treatment of Parkinson's disease. *Journal of Neurosurgery*, **76**, 53.

Lang, A.E. and Lozano, A.M. (1998) Parkinson's disease. Second of two parts. *The New England Journal of Medicine*, **339**, 1130–1143.

Langston, J.W., Irwin, I. and Langston, E.B. (1984) A comparison of the acute and chronic effects of 1-methyl-4-phenyl-1,2,5,6-tetrahydropyridine (MPTP)-induced parkinsonism in humans and the squirrel monkey. *Neurology*, **34** (Suppl 1), 268.

Lee, R.G. and Stein, R.B. (1981) Resetting of tremor by mechanical pertubation: a comparison of essential tremor and parkinsonian tremor. *Annals of Neurology*, **10**, 523–531.

Lee, R.G. and Tatton, W.G. (1975) Motor responses to sudden limb displacements in primates with specific CNS lesions and in human patients with motor system disorders. *The Canadian Journal of Neurological Sciences*, **2**, 285–293.

Lemstra, A.W., Verhagen, M.L., Lee, J.I., Dougherty, P.M. and Lenz, F.A. (1999) Tremor-frequency (3–6 Hz) activity in the sensorimotor arm representation of the internal segment of the globus pallidus in patients with Parkinson's disease. *Neuroscience Letters*, **267**, 129–132.

Lenz, F.A., Tasker, R.R., Kwan, H.C., Schnider, S., Kwong, R., Murayama, Y., Dostrovsky, J.O. and Murphy, J.T. (1988) Single unit analysis of the human ventral thalamic nuclear group: correlation of thalamic "tremor cells" with the 3–6\component of parkinsonian tremor. *The Journal of Neuroscience*, **8**, 754–764.

Levesque, M. and Parent, A. (2005) The striatofugal fiber system in primates: a reevaluation of its organization based on single-axon tracing studies. *Proceedings of the National Academy of Sciences of the United States of America*, **102**, 11888–11893.

Levy, R., Hutchison, W.D., Lozano, A.M. and Dostrovsky, J.O. (2002) Synchronized neuronal discharge in the basal ganglia of parkinsonian patients is limited to oscillatory activity. *The Journal of Neuroscience*, **22**, 2855–2861.

Limousin, P., Pollak, P., Benazzouz, A., Hoffmann, D., Broussolle, E., Perret, J.E. and Benabid, A.L. (1995) Bilateral subthalamic nucleus stimulation for severe Parkinson's disease. *Movement Disorders*, **10**, 672–674.

Lozano, A.M., Lang, A.E., Galvez Jimenez, N., Miyasaki, J., Duff, J., Hutchinson, W.D. and Dostrovsky, J.O. (1995) Effect of GPi pallidotomy on motor function in Parkinson's disease. *Lancet*, **346**, 1383–1387.

Machado, A., Rezai, A.R., Kopell, B.H., Gross, R.E., Sharan, A.D. and Benabid, A.L. (2006) Deep brain stimulation for Parkinson's disease: Surgical technique and perioperative management. *Movement Disorders*, **21**, S247–S258.

Maltete, D., Jodoin, N., Karachi, C., Houeto, J.L., Navarro, S., Cornu, P., Agid, Y. and Welter, M.L. (2007) Subthalamic stimulation and neuronal activity in the substantia nigra in Parkinson's disease. *Journal of Neurophysiology*, **97**, 4017–4022.

Merello, M., Balej, J., Delfino, M., Cammarota, A., Betti, O. and Leiguarda, R. (1999) Apomorphine induces changes in GPi spontaneous outflow in patients with Parkinson's disease. *Movement Disorders*, **14**, 45–49.

Miller, W.C. and DeLong, M.R. (1987) Altered tonic activity of neurons in the globus pallidus and subthalamic nucleus in the primate MPTP model of parkinsonism, in *The Basal Ganglia II* (eds M.B. Carpenter and A. Jayaraman), Plenum Press, New York, pp. 415–427.

Mink, J.W. (1996) The basal ganglia: focused selection and inhibition of competing motor programs. *Progress in Neurobiology*, **50**, 381–425.

Mink, J.W. and Thach, W.T. (1991) Basal ganglia motor control. II. Late pallidal timing relative to movement onset and inconsistent pallidal coding of movement parameters. *Journal of Neurophysiology*, **65**, 301–329.

Mink, J.W. and Thach, W.T. (1991) Basal ganglia motor control. I. Nonexclusive relation of pallidal discharge to five movement modes. *Journal of Neurophysiology*, **65**, 273–300.

Mink, J.W. and Thach, W.T. (1991) Basal ganglia motor control. III. Pallidal ablation: normal reaction time, muscle cocontraction, and slow movement. *Journal of Neurophysiology*, **65**, 330–351.

Miocinovic, S., Parent, M., Butson, C.R., Hahn, P.J., Russo, G.S., Vitek, J.L. and McIntyre, C.C. (2006) Computational analysis of subthalamic nucleus and lenticular fasciculus activation during therapeutic deep brain stimulation. *Journal of Neurophysiology*, **96**, 1569–1580.

Morris, G., Arkadir, D., Nevet, A., Vaadia, E. and Bergman, H. (2004) Coincident but distinct messages of midbrain dopamine and striatal tonically active neurons. *Neuron*, **43**, 133–143.

Nambu, A. (2004) A new dynamic model of the cortico-basal ganglia loop. *Progress in Brain Research*, **143**, 461–466.

Nini, A., Feingold, A., Slovin, H. and Bergman, H. (1995) Neurons in the globus pallidus do not show correlated activity in the normal monkey, but phase-locked oscillations appear in the MPTP model of parkinsonism. *Journal of Neurophysiology*, **74**, 1800–1805.

Obeso, J.A., Alvarez, L.M., Macias, R.J., Guridi, J., Teijeiro, J., Juncos, J.L., Rodriguez, M.C., Ramos, E., Linazasoro, G.J., Gorospe, A. and DeLong, M.R. (1997) Lesion of the subthalamic nucleus is Parkinson's disease. *Neurology*, **48**, A138.

Papa, S.M., DeSimone, R., Fiorani, M. and Oldfield, E.H. (1999) Internal globus pallidus discharge is nearly suppressed during levodopa-induced dyskinesias. *Annals of Neurology*, **46**, 732–738.

Parkinson, J. (1817) *An essay on the shaking palsy*, Sherwood, Neely and Jones, London.

Paulus, W. and Jellinger, K. (1991) The neuropathologic basis of different clinical subgroups of Parkinson's disease. *Journal of Neuropathology and Experimental Neurology*, **50**, 743–755.

Pessiglione, M., Guehl, D., Rolland, A.S., Francois, C., Hirsch, E.C., Feger, J. and Tremblay, L. (2005) Thalamic neuronal activity in dopamine-depleted primates: evidence for a loss of functional segregation within basal ganglia circuits. *The Journal of Neuroscience*, **25**, 1523–1531.

Pifl, C., Schingnitz, G. and Hornykiewicz, O. (1991) Effect of 1-methyl-4-phenyl-1,2,3,6-tetrahydropyridine on the regional distribution of brain monoamines in the rhesus monkey. *Neuroscience*, **44**, 591–605.

Poirier, L.J., Filion, M., LaRochelle, L. and Pechadre, J.C. (1975) Physiopathology of experimental Parkinsonism in the monkey. *The Canadian Journal of Neurological Sciences*, **2**, 255–263.

Pollak, P., Benabid, A.L., Limousin, P., Benazzouz, A., Hoffmann, D., Le Bas, J.F. and Perret, J. (1996) Subthalamic nucleus stimulation alleviates akinesia and rigidity in parkinsonian patients. *Advances in Neurology*, **69**, 591–594.

Pollock, L.J. and Davis, L. (1930) Muscle tone in parkinsonan states. *Archives of Neurology: Psychiatry*, **23**, 303–319.

Raethjen, J., Lindemann, M., Schmaljohann, H., Wenzelburger, R., Pfister, G. and Deuschl, G. (2000) Multiple oscillators are causing parkinsonian and essential tremor. *Movement Disorders*, **15**, 84–94.

Rajput, A.H. (1995) Clinical features of tremor in extrapyramidal syndromes, in *Handbook of Tremor Disorders* (eds L.J. Findley and W.C. Koller), Marcel Dekker, Inc., New York.

Ranck, J.B. (1975) Which elements are excited in electrical stimulation of mammalian central nervous system: A review. *Brain Research*, **98**, 417–440.

Ravina, B., Camicioli, R., Como, P.G., Marsh, L., Jankovic, J., Weintraub, D. and Elm, J. (2007) The impact of depressive symptoms in early Parkinson's disease. *Neurology*, **69**, 342–347.

Raz, A., Feingold, A., Zelanskaya, V., Vaadia, E. and Bergman, H. (1996) Neuronal synchronization of tonically active neurons in the striatum of normal and parkinsonian primates. *Journal of Neurophysiology*, **76**, 2083–2088.

Raz, A., Vaadia, E. and Bergman, H. (2000) Firing patterns and correlations of spontaneous discharge of pallidal neurons in the normal and the tremulous 1-methyl-4-phenyl-1,2,3,6-tetrahydropyridine vervet model of parkinsonism. *The Journal of Neuroscience*, **20**, 8559–8571.

Raz, A., Frechter-Mazar, V., Feingold, A., Abeles, M., Vaadia, E. and Bergman, H. (2001) Activity of pallidal and striatal tonically active neurons is correlated in mptp-treated monkeys but not in normal monkeys. *The Journal of Neuroscience*, **21**, RC128.

Romo, R., Scarnati, E. and Schultz, W. (1992) Role of primate basal ganglia and frontal cortex in the internal generation of movements. II. Movement-related activity in the anterior striatum. *Experimental Brain Research*, **91**, 385–395.

Schneidman, E., Berry, M.J., Segev, R. and Bialek, W. (2006) Weak pairwise correlations imply strongly correlated network states in a neural population. *Nature*, **440**, 1007–1012.

Schultz, W. (1986) Activity of pars reticulata neurons of monkey substantia nigra in relation to motor, sensory, and complex events. *Journal of Neurophysiology*, **55**, 660–677.

Schultz, W. (2007) Behavioral dopamine signals. *Trends in Neurosciences*, **30**, 203–210.

Schultz, W. and Romo, R. (1992) Role of primate basal ganglia and frontal cortex in the internal generation of movements. I. Preparatory activity in the anterior striatum. *Experimental Brain Research*, **91**, 363–384.

Sharott, A., Magill, P.J., Harnack, D., Kupsch, A., Meissner, W. and Brown, P. (2005) Dopamine depletion increases the power and coherence of beta-oscillations in the cerebral cortex and subthalamic nucleus of the awake rat. *The European Journal of Neuroscience*, **21**, 1413–1422.

Stoney, S.D., Jr, Thompson, W.D. and Asanuma, H. (1968) Excitation of pyramidal tract cells by intracortical microstimulation: effective treatment of stimulating current. *Journal of Neurophysiology*, **31**, 659–669.

Sulzer, D. (2007) Multiple hit hypotheses for dopamine neuron loss in Parkinson's disease. *Trends in Neurosciences*, **30**, 244–250.

Tatton, W.G., Forner, S.D., Gerstein, G.L., Chambers, W.W. and Liu, C.N. (1975) The effect of postcentral cortical lesions on motor responses to sudden upper limb displacements in monkeys. *Brain Research*, **96**, 108–113.

Tatton, W.G., Eastman, M.J., Bedingham, W., Verrier, M.C. and Bruce, I.C. (1984) Defective utilization of sensory input as the basis for bradykinesia, rigidity and decreased movement repertoire in Parkinson's disease: a hypothesis. *The Canadian Journal of Neurological Sciences*, **11**, 136–143.

Timmermann, L., Gross, J., Dirks, M., Volkmann, J., Freund, H.J. and Schnitzler, A. (2003) The cerebral oscillatory network of parkinsonian resting tremor. *Brain: A Journal of Neurology*, **126**, 199–212.

Tolosa, E.S. and Marin, C. (1995) Medical Management of Parkinsonian Tremor, in *Handbook of Tremor Disorders* (eds L.J. Findley and W.C. Koller Marcel Dekker, Inc., New York, pp. 333–350.

Van Den Eeden, S.K., Tanner, C.M., Bernstein, A.L., Fross, R. D., Leimpeter, A., Bloch, D.A. and Nelson, L.M. (2003) Incidence of Parkinson's disease: variation by age, gender, and race/ethnicity. *American Journal of Epidemiology*, **157**, 1015–1022.

Vitek, J.L. and Bakay, R.A. (1997) The role of pallidotomy in Parkinson's disease and dystonia. *Current Opinion in Neurology*, **10**, 332–339.

Wang, Z., Kai, L., Day, M., Ronesi, J., Yin, H.H., Ding, J., Tkatch, T., Lovinger, D.M. and Surmeier, D.J. (2006) Dopaminergic control of corticostriatal long-term synaptic depression in medium spiny neurons is mediated by cholinergic interneurons. *Neuron*, **50**, 443–452.

Watts, R.L., Wiegner, A.W. and Young, R.R. (1986) Elastic properties of muscles measured at the elbow in man: II. Patients with parkinsonian rigidity. *Journal of Neurology, Neurosurgery, and Psychiatry*, **49**, 1177–1181.

Weinberger, M., Mahant, N., Hutchison, W.D., Lozano, A.M., Moro, E., Hodaie, M., Lang, A.E. and Dostrovsky, J.O. (2006) Beta oscillatory activity in the subthalamic nucleus and its relation to dopaminergic response in Parkinson's disease. *Journal of Neurophysiology*, **96**, 3248–3255.

Wichmann, T. and Soares, J. (2006) Neuronal firing before and after burst discharges in the monkey Basal Ganglia is predictably patterned in the normal state and altered in parkinsonism. *Journal of Neurophysiology*, **95**, 2120–2133.

Wichmann, T., Bergman, H. and DeLong, M.R. (1994) The primate subthalamic nucleus. III. Changes in motor behavior and neuronal activity in the internal pallidum induced by subthalamic inactivation in the MPTP model of parkinsonism. *Journal of Neurophysiology*, **72**, 521–530.

Wilms, H., Sievers, J. and Deuschl, G. (1999) Animal models of tremor. *Movement Disorders*, **14**, 557–571.

3

Pharmacology of Parkinson's Disease

Jonathan M. Brotchie

Toronto Western Research Institute, Toronto Western Hospital, Toronto, Canada

OVERVIEW

Over the last decade, significant advances in understanding the neural mechanisms underlying Parkinson's disease have been driven by, and led to, a paradigm shift in our understanding of the pharmacology of this disorder. This chapter will review how our understanding of the pharmacology of Parkinson's disease now combines an increasing appreciation of:

1. The manner in which the functioning of different parts of the basal ganglia circuitry must be integrated to understand the pharmacological processes underlying the pathophysiology of both parkinsonism per se and the motor complications of dopamine replacement therapy in Parkinson's disease,
2. Interactions between dopamine and many non-dopaminergic transmitters,
3. The means by which various sub-types of dopaminergic and non-dopaminergic receptors, each with anatomically distinct distribution and different downstream signaling cascades, mediate their effects.

A CIRCUIT-BASED MODEL OF BASAL GANGLIA PHARMACOLOGY

Thirty years ago, explanations of the pharmacology of Parkinson's disease were often reduced to a model whereby the basal ganglia were represented as a single black box whose pharmacology could be described by a simple, "see-saw"-like mechanism balancing the effects of dopamine and acetylcholine transmission. It was seen as something of an advance when, in the early 1980s, this model was refined to highlight instead the balance between dopaminergic and glutamatergic systems. In these simple models, parkinsonism was characterized by a reduction in dopaminergic transmission and an increase in cholinergic or glutamatergic signaling. Hyperkinetic syndromes such as

L-DOPA-induced dyskinesia were seen simply as the direct opposite, with the balance reversed. These explanations of basal ganglia pharmacology were generally devoid of any anatomical detail; it was usually assumed, if not made explicit, that they referred to the pharmacology of the striatum. Furthermore, they did not explain the roles of the many other transmitter systems found within the basal ganglia, sub-types of receptors or second messenger signaling systems. The models provided no explanation as to how, or why, the proposed imbalances might effect pathophysiological processes, such as changes in firing rate or pattern or indeed motor control overall. However, while capturing little of the complexity of our current understanding of basal ganglia pharmacology, these ideas did at least open the door for the concept that non-dopaminergic mechanisms might be involved in a spectrum of movement disorders.

Today, an understanding of the pharmacology of movement disorders requires a multi-dimensional perspective, where the effects of a panoply of transmitters, each acting at several sub-types of receptors, regulate distinct neuronal populations and the activity of discrete anatomical pathways within the basal ganglia. The path to this understanding was trail-blazed in the mid-1980s by a small number of research groups worldwide, who built the idea that the pharmacology of movement disorders could not be understood unless the models were expanded to include a representation of circuits combined with an involvement of several non-dopaminergic transmitter systems (Penney and Young, 1986; Mitchell et al., 1989; Mitchell et al., 1986; Bergman et al., 1990). This required an appreciation of how dopaminergic and non-dopaminergic transmitter systems interact to regulate the activity of the different component nuclei of the basal ganglia with most importance to the control of movement. The power of this approach to conceptualizing basal ganglia pharmacology derives from the fact that it incorporates sufficient, but not too much, anatomical detail, to enable it to provide apparently

Therapeutics of Parkinson's Disease and Other Movement Disorders   Edited by Mark Hallett and Werner Poewe
© 2008 John Wiley & Sons, Ltd.

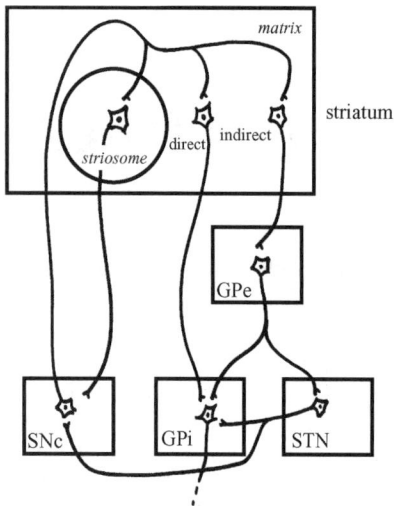

Figure 3.1 Basal ganglia circuitry. Dopaminergic neurons of the substantia nigra pars compacta (SNc) provide a dense innervation of the striatum. The striatum projects to other regions of the basal ganglia via medium-sized spiny neurons (MSNs). Two major classes of MSNs can be defined on both anatomical and pharmacological bases, the first project the output regions of the basal ganglia, internal globus pallidus (GPi) and the substantia nigra pars reticulata, the so-called "direct pathway" neurons. The second class of MSN project to the external globus pallidus (GPe), as this projection influences the basal ganglia outputs via the intermediary of the GPi and subthalamic nucleus (STN), they are described as components of the indirect pathway. MSNs projecting to the dopaminergic neurons of the SNC can be considered, in terms of their pharmacology, to be similar to direct pathway MSNs.

meaningful explanations as to how transmitters interact and how such interactions would impact on behavior. Although many circuits likely work in parallel to subserve multiple functions (Alexander *et al.*, 1990), the core components of this circuitry are illustrated in Figure 3.1. At its most simple, the model places the striatum as the major input region of the basal ganglia and the internal globus pallidus (GPi) and the substantia nigra pars reticulata (SNr) as the source of outputs to non-basal ganglia regions of the brain. The inputs to the striatum are primarily glutamatergic and dopaminergic. Striatal output neurons are medium sized with many dendritic spines and are termed medium spiny neurons (MSNs). MSNs are GABAergic but utilize a range of peptides as co-transmitters. MSNs do not function in isolation, but communicate with each other via a rich network of recurrent collaterals and are integrated with several classes of interneurons, including those employing acetylcholine, GABA and nitric oxide as transmitters.

Two major routes by which the striatum can influence the GPi/SNr are identified, a "direct" monosynaptic pathway and an "indirect" pathway, or network. The indirect pathway involves poly-synaptic connections through the intermediary of the external globus pallidus (GPe) and the subthalamic nucleus. In addition to their involvement in the direct and indirect pathways, MSNs project from the striatum to the dopaminergic neurons of the substantia nigra pars compacta (SNc) and ventral tegmental area (VTA). These projections are localized within specific patches in the striatum, "striosomes," which are surrounded by a "matrix" containing neurons projecting to the GPi, SNr and GPe.

This core circuitry is used as the basis for models to describe the functioning pharmacology of the basal ganglia in health and disease. Thus, the impact of dopamine depletion, with progressive death of dopamine neurons in Parkinson's disease, is to generate an imbalance in the activities of the direct and indirect pathways. The details of these imbalances and their causation can be debated, but it is generally considered that the generation of parkinsonian symptoms is associated with:

1. Overactivity of MSNs of the indirect pathway,
2. Overactivity of the subthalamic nucleus and,
3. Overactivity of basal ganglia outputs from GPi and SNr.

In contrast, in situations where the treatment of Parkinson's disease is compromised by motor complications, such as L-DOPA-induced dyskinesia, "on–off" or "wearing-off" fluctuations, the situation is almost the mirror of parkinsonism (Brotchie, 2005; Bezard *et al.*, 2001; Cenci, 2007). Thus, the expression of motor complications is associated primarily with:

1. Overactivity of MSNs of the direct pathway,
2. Underactivity of the subthalamic nucleus and,
3. Underactivity of basal ganglia outputs from the GPi and SNr.

In accepting the above-described descriptions of functional pharmacology, it is important to realize that there has been much debate about the ability of the model to capture the complexity of basal ganglia anatomy and its apparent inability to explain how firing patterns, and not just rates, change in pathological conditions (Obeso *et al.*, 2000; Wichmann and DeLong, 1999; Obeso *et al.*, 1997). Indeed, while these parameters are not explicitly modeled, in interpreting the model we must consider that terms such as overactivity reflect both average firing rate, over minutes, and changes in firing pattern such as increased incidence of burst, and over single firing, that might impact on average rate. Furthermore, these changes are reflected in, and likely result from, changes in the synchronization of neuronal ensembles within and across regions of the basal ganglia.

It can be argued that the advances it provides are minimal in that the earlier single black box models are just replaced by a model that has five, or more, functionally dependent black boxes. These cannot explain basal ganglia function in detail and at best can only be regarded as a metaphor for basal ganglia function. However, it is remarkable that such a simple framework can accurately predict how specific manipulations of transmitter systems within the basal ganglia circuitry will impact on motor function and also define efficacy of potential pharmacological approaches. In this latter respect, the model is particularly predictive in defining the pharmacology of parkinsonism and dyskinesia.

CELLULAR AND MOLECULAR PHARMACOLOGY OF THE BASAL GANGLIA

The, now classic, framework of the functional anatomy of the basal ganglia circuits, described above, has, in the last decade, been enriched by an evolving understanding of its molecular and cellular pharmacology. In particular the understanding of the functions of, and interactions between, dopamine, glutamate and acetylcholine are much better appreciated. The differences between the roles played by these transmitters in neurons of the direct and indirect pathway have become clearer, with an evolving understanding of the differential distribution of dopamine, acetylcholine and glutamate receptors; this is summarized in Figure 3.2.

Dopamine

Dopaminergic afferents to the striatum are provided by the substantia nigra pars compacta (SNc) and the ventral tegmental area (VTA). These inputs impact on medium-sized spiny neurons (MSNs), which represent the output neurons of the striatum, and on a variety of interneurons. Dopamine has differential effects on MSNs of the direct and indirect pathway. Thus, at least when considered at the level of intact circuits, dopamine has an inhibitory effect on the indirect pathway and an excitatory effect on the direct pathway. Over recent years, there has been much debate as to the cellular and molecular basis of these functional properties. It is now accepted that neurons of the direct pathway preferentially express the D1 sub-type of dopamine receptors while those of the indirect pathway express predominantly D2 dopamine receptors. The respective excitatory and inhibitory actions of dopamine on neurons of the direct and indirect pathway could thus be explained by D1 and D2 receptors having different second-messenger signal-transduction pathways, the former being via an activation of adenylyl cylcase and increase in cAMP levels, the latter by inhibiting adenylyl cyclase. However, it is likely not as simple as D1 receptors being excitatory and D2 receptors being inhibitory. In fact, dopamine is invariably inhibitory on all MSNs if applied to striatal slices in standard electrophysiological experiments. The difference in dopaminergic regulation of the functioning of the direct and indirect pathways probably results from a combination of the D1–D2 split, the functioning of the circuit as a whole and interactions with other transmitter systems.

Dopamine also provides powerful regulation of interneuron function in the striatum. D1 receptor stimulation drives acetylcholine release. D2 receptor stimulation reduces acetylcholine release (Maurice et al., 2004). As will be described below, acetylcholine has multiple actions in the striatum and this dichotomy of D1 and D2 effects provides a further way in which the functional outcome of D1 and D2 receptor stimulation, on the activity of the direct and indirect pathways, is determined by mechanisms in addition to their actions on MSNs.

Striatal D2 receptors are also localized pre-synaptically on dopamine terminals and their activation can reduce dopamine release. In this way, D2 receptor activation can further modulate D1 receptor activity indirectly.

In addition to D1 and D2 receptors, the striatum also expresses D3 (which are D2-like in terms of pharmacology) and D5 (D1-like) receptors. D3 receptors appear to be expressed primarily in MSNs of the direct pathway. The role of D3 receptors in many ways appears to oppose that of D1 receptors with which they are co-expressed, though their levels of expression in the normal situation are relatively low, at least in the sensorimotor and associative regions of the striatum. D5 receptors are expressed in MSNs and cholinergic interneurons. In MSNs, D5 receptors work in concert with D2 receptors to regulate GABA$_A$ channel signalling, D5 receptor stimulation reduces the expression of GABA$_A$ channel sub-units, and thus inhibits GABA signalling in MSNs.

Outside the striatum, dopamine has a multitude of actions, which are often overlooked. The GPe has high levels of D2 receptors; these are localized pre-synaptically on terminals of inputs from the striatum. Activation of pallidal D2 receptors reduces GABA release from these indirect pathway neurons. In a similar way, D1 receptors are localized on terminals of direct pathway neurons in the GPi and SNr, activation of these receptors enhances GABA release. In the subthalamic nucleus, both D1 and D2-like receptors regulate neuronal excitability, enhancing and reducing activity respectively. While D1 and D2 receptors mediate these effects in part, there is increasing evidence of an involvement of D4 (inhibitory) and D5 (excitatory) receptors in these actions.

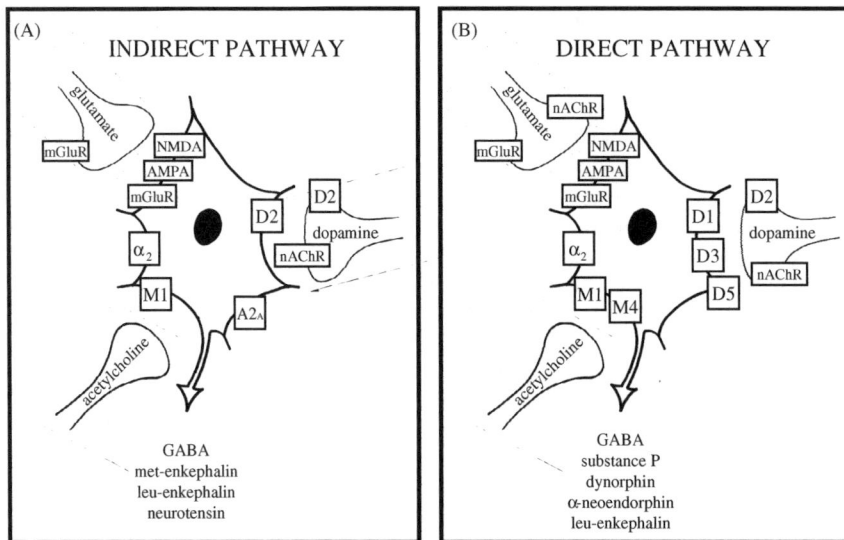

Figure 3.2 Relative distribution of sub-types of receptors between direct and indirect pathway neurons of the striatum. Medium spiny neurons (MSNs) of the striatum are GABAergic but use a range of peptides as co-transmitters. In addition, MSNs receive glutamatergic, dopaminergic and cholinergic afferent connections. The nature of receptors mediating signaling by these transmitters differs between MSNs of the indirect (A) and direct (B) pathways. This figure does not attempt to illustrate the sub-cellular distribution of receptors, which varies significantly between dendritic spine or soma depending on the case.

Glutamate

Excitatory glutamatergic inputs to the basal ganglia derive from diverse regions of the cerebral cortex and the centromedian and parafascicular nuclei (CM/Pf) of the thalamus. These are targeted mainly on the striatum and the subthalamic nucleus. In terms of the sub-cellular organization the glutamatergic afferents to the striatum, the corticostriatal inputs impinge upon the spines of MSNs while those of the thalamostriatal pathways synapse more proximally on dendrites close to cell bodies. The functional relevance of this is reflected in potential modulation of cortical afferents by dopaminergic afferents, which synapse on the base of dendritic spines. This localization allows dopamine to gate the spreading of glutamatergic excitation by the corticostriatal pathway to a much greater extent than the thalamocortical projection. Glutamatergic excitation of striatal neurons appears to involve all major classes of glutamate receptor, namely the ionotropic receptors (NMDA, AMPA and kainate receptors) and metabotropic receptors (mGluRs).

A single glutamatergic nucleus, the subthalamic nucleus, is intrinsic to the basal ganglia and provides substantial excitatory influence on the output regions of the basal ganglia, GPi and SNr, as well as on functionally important projection to the SNc, GPe and CM/Pf thalamus.

NMDA receptors are composed of heteromeric complexes of, most likely four, sub-units, from two families

termed NR1 and NR2. Two NR1 sub-units are required for the formation of functional channels activated by glutamate. The NR2 composition, in particular, defines the pharmacology of an NMDA receptor, and to some extent also its function, particularly with respect to channel opening kinetics and involvement in synaptic plasticity. In striatal MSNs, NMDA receptors are composed of the ubiquitous NR1 sub-units, and express NR2A and NR2B sub-units. The precise molecular composition of these receptors is not clear, be they binary, that is, containing two sub-units each of NR1 and NR2A, or two each of NR1 and NR2B, or ternary, containing two NR1 sub-units and one each of NR2A and NR2B. Furthermore, at present, it is not clear whether the nature of NMDA receptors differs in MSNs of the direct pathway and the indirect pathway.

AMPA receptors mediate fast excitatory transmission by glutamate in the striatum. All MSNs and interneurons appear to express AMPA receptors. However, there appears to be differences in the sub-units expressed, which suggests functional differences in AMPA transmission in different neuronal types.

In addition to effects in the striatum, NMDA and AMPA receptors also mediate excitation by the subthalamic nucleus. In the subthalamic nucleus, activation of NMDA, but not AMPA, receptors is thought to be responsible for switching from single spike to burst firing modes.

Metabotropic glutamate receptors (mGluRs) are classified in three groups, I, II and III. Group I mGluRs (mGlu$_1$ and mGlu$_5$) are typically post-synaptic and excitatory. Group II (mGlu$_2$ and mGlu$_3$) and Group III (mGlu$_4$, mGlu$_6$, mGlu$_7$ and mGlu$_8$) are typically pre-synaptic, their activation leading to reduced release of neurotransmitter.

In the striatum, Group I mGluRs excite MSNs of both the direct and indirect pathways. However, the effects of Group I mGluR activation are complex and an initial excitatory response is often followed by an inhibitory response, this latter effect involving mGlu$_5$ and release of endogenous cannabinoids (see below). In addition, mGlu$_5$ also plays a role in integrating signals between glutamate, adenosine and dopamine; mGlu$_5$, A$_{2A}$ and D$_2$ receptors, being closely co-localized on spines of MSNs on the indirect pathway (Diaz-Cabiale *et al.*, 2002; Fuxe *et al.*, 2003). Group II mGluRs in the striatum reduce NMDA receptor-mediated release of acetylcholine from cholinergic interneurons, by a mechanism dependent on dopamine.

Outside the striatum, other actions of mGluRs are seen. Thus, Group I mGluRs mediate long-lasting excitation, and may support burst firing, in the GPe, GPi and substantia nigra. Group II mGluRs can reduce glutamate release from the subthalamic efferents to the globus pallidus. Activation of group III mGluRs pre-synaptically reduces both GABAergic and glutamatergic transmission in the rat globus pallidus and substantia nigra.

Acetylcholine

Large spiny interneurons provide an intrinsic cholinergic innervation of the striatum. These cholinergic neurons are tonically active and play a critical role in learning and memory, reducing their activity immediately prior to learning components of motor tasks and providing encoding of contextual information that is important in selection of appropriate motor functions (Apicella, 2007; Cragg, 2006; Pisani *et al.*, 2001).

Cholinergic receptors of both muscarinic (mAChR) and nicotinic (nAChR) families are important mediators of cholinergic regulation of signalling within the striatum. Two sub-types of mAChRs are found in high levels on striatal MSNs, M1 and M4. Although not complete, there is a differential expression of these receptors such that the MSNs of the direct pathway express M4 receptors at much higher levels than those of the indirect pathway (Ince *et al.*, 1997). M1 receptors couple to the G protein G$_{q/11}$ and are generally excitatory, whereas M4 receptors couple to Go and are generally inhibitory. In the direct pathway, there is a functional balance between D1 receptors and both M1, which enhance, and M4, which reduce D1 signalling (Sanchez-Lemus and Arias-Montano, 2006).

Nicotinic receptors regulate pre-synaptic function in the striatum, acetylcholine stimulation of striatal nAChRs

enhances the release of dopamine. Interestingly, selective activation of a sub-type nAChRs, termed $\alpha_4\beta_2$, leads to dopamine release that is preferentially targeted to stimulate D2 receptors of the indirect pathway, whereas stimulation of both $\alpha_4\beta_2$ and α_7 receptors leads to stimulation of D1 receptors on the direct pathway, via a mechanism involving α_7-induced release of glutamate (Hamada *et al.*, 2004).

Peptides

A characteristic of striatal MSNs is that they utilize neuropeptides as co-transmitters with GABA. In fact, the use of neuropeptide transmitters by neurons equivalent to MSNs is highly conserved across a range of vertebrate species. MSNs of both the direct and indirect pathways utilize opioid peptides as co-transmitters with GABA. These are released within the striatum, and in the target regions of these pathways, that is, the GPe/GPi and SNr. However, there is a qualitative difference between the opioid employed by the two classes of MSN (Figure 3.2).

MSNs of the indirect pathway utilize opioid peptides produced from a high molecular weight precursor termed pre-proenkephalin-A (PPE-A). This precursor produces peptides, leu- and met-encephalin, which are relatively selective ligands for δ-opioid receptors. In contrast, neurons of the direct pathway produce opioid peptides derived from pre-proenkephalin-B (PPE-B). While PPE-B is often termed pro-dynorphin, and indeed is a precursor of several dynorphins, in MSNs it is, in addition, processed to produce other opioid peptides, including leu-enkephalin and α-neoendorphin. These peptides can be released from collaterals in the striatum as well as in the output regions of the basal ganglia and the SNc and VTA. Opioid peptides produced from PPE-B show some promiscuity between opioid receptors, but, in general terms, dynorphins, leu-enkephalin and α-neoendorphin show some selectivity for κ-, δ- and μ-opioid receptors respectively. κ-opioid receptors are distributed throughout the striatum and mediate pre-synaptic regulation of afferent inputs to the striatum. By virtue of being localized pre-synaptically on dopaminergic and glutamatergic terminals κ receptors can reduce the release of both these transmitters. Within the striatum, μ-opioid receptors, are localized pre-synaptically on dopamine terminals; stimulation of these receptors enhances dopamergic transmission. μ-receptors are more concentrated in striosomes, where, presumably, they play a role in the regulation, by dopamine, of striosomal MSNs that project back onto dopaminergic neurons in the mesencephalon.

In GPe, the terminals of the indirect pathway MSNs release enkephalins, which acting via δ-opioid receptors, reduce GABA release. In GPi/SNr, release of peptides produced from PPE-B, from terminals of the direct pathway, have potential to reduce glutamate release from subthalamic efferents, via κ-opioid receptors, and inhibit output neurons, via μ-opioids.

In addition to opioid peptides, MSNs use additional peptides as co-transmitters. Thus, neurons of the direct pathway synthesise tachykinins, especially substance P, from pro-tachykinin. Release of tachykinins by the direct pathway may contribute to D1 receptor-mediated actions to produce movements; these actions involve NK1 and NK3 tachykinin receptors in the substantia nigra and NK1 receptors in the striatum. On the other hand, MSNs of the indirect pathway do not produce tachykinins but do utilize neurotensin. The NTR-1 sub-type of neurotensin receptors are located in the GPe and their stimulation provides excitation of these neurons. This action is mediated via both a post-synaptic action and a facilitation of glutamate release (Chen et al., 2006; Martorana et al., 2006). Neurotensin is also released in the striatum, presumably from recurrent collateral of indirect pathway neurons. In the striatum, neurotensin increases dopamine, glutamate and acetylcholine release, this latter action being unmasked only in the absence of D2 receptor stimulation.

Two other opioid-related peptides have been described as having relevance to striatal function. Firstly, the striatum contains high levels of endomorphin-1. Endomorphin-1 is a potent and selective endogenous ligand for μ-opioid receptors and thus offers an alternative to PPE-B-derived α-neoendorphin as a means to stimulate μ- opioid receptors and regulate striatal dopamine release. However, it is not clear whether endomorphin-1 is synthesized within the striatum or released from one of the striatal afferents.

Other Transmitters

In addition to the transmitters discussed above, over 40 additional neurotransmitters and neuromodulators have been described as having functions within the basal ganglia. A brief review of those for which there is most evidence of an involvement in the pathophysiology of movement disorders is given here.

5-Hydroxytryptamine (5-HT, serotonin) provides a dense and widespread innervation of the basal ganglia, involving a range of 5-HT receptors. In the striatum, $5HT_{1A}$ receptors located pre-synaptically can reduce the synthesis of dopamine and reduce the release of glutamate. In contrast, $5\text{-}HT_{2A}$ receptors are located on MSNs, mainly on dendrites. Stimulation of $5HT_{2A}$ receptors enhances motor behaviors elicited by D1 receptor stimulation. Outside the striatum, the globus pallidus and substantia nigra contain high levels of $5HT_{2C}$ receptors. Stimulation of these receptors excites GABAergic neurons, output neurons of GPi and SNr.

Although α_2 adrenergic receptors are found in high levels in the basal ganglia, there has been some debate as to the functional relevance of any noradrenergic innerva-

tion of these regions. The endogenous activator of basal ganglia α_2 receptors may be dopamine as well as noradrenaline. α_2 adrenergic receptors are localized post-synaptically on striatal MSNs. It has been proposed that they enhance behaviors mediated via the direct pathway. The interplay between sub-types of α_2 adrenergic receptors is of importance. In general terms, it can be assumed that stimulation of pre-synaptic α_{2A} receptors reduces release of noradrenaline and thus reduces stimulation of α_{2C} receptors, which might either be post-synaptic, for example, on MSNs in the striatum, or pre-synaptic, for example, heteroreceptors on GABAergic terminals of MSN projections to the SNr. Thus, in the striatum, noradrenaline release is reduced by stimulation of α_2 receptors, particularly α_{2A} receptors, and this can lead to reduced stimulation of post-synaptic α_{2C} receptors. In the SNr, GABA release is increased by α_2 stimulation, because stimulation of α_{2A} receptors reduces noradrenaline release, which leads to decreased inhibition of GABA release by α_{2C} receptors.

The striatum and GPi contain amongst the highest concentration of adenosine A_{2A} receptors in the CNS (Schwarzschild et al., 2006). A_{2A} receptors are coupled to the G-protein Gs and stimulate adenylyl cyclase and cAMP synthesis. As such they work to balance the effects of D2 dopamine receptors, with which they are intimately linked. A_{2A} and D_2 receptors form functional integrative units, along with Group I mGluRs, in the dendritic spines of MSNs. Indeed, A_{2A} and D_2 receptors may be so closely linked as to be physically associated in heteromeric complex (Fuxe et al., 2003). There is also some evidence that CB1 cannabinoid receptors might also contribute to these complexes. Adenosine release and A_{2A} stimulation are driven, in part at least, via NMDA receptor stimulation, and thus A_{2A} receptors contribute indirectly to glutamatergic excitatory processes in the striatum. In the GPe, A_{2A} receptors on the terminals of MSN projections from the striatum, stimulate the release of GABA.

Endogenous cannabinoids (endocannabinoids) are neurotransmitters capable of stimulating cannabinoid receptors. Within the basal ganglia, the principal endocannabinoids are anandamide and 2-AG, their cannabinoid-like actions are mediated via the CB1 cannabinoid receptor. These endocannabinoids are small lipophilic molecules and share an important property of being able to move freely from the neuron in which they are synthesized to an adjacent neuron without requiring the molecular machinery typical of synaptic transmission. Their synthesis can thus be triggered by a classical neurotransmitter and their release mediates signaling across a synapse in a retrograde manner. Endocannabinoids are released from post-synaptic neurons by strong depolarization and resultant Ca^{2+} elevation or activation of $G_{q/11}$-coupled receptors such as Group I mGluRs or M1 muscarinic acetylcholine receptors. In the striatum, the actions of endocannabinoids, once released, are to reduce glutamate, dopamine and GABA transmission (Narushima *et al.*, 2006; Narushima *et al.*, 2007). Outside the striatum, endocannabinoids and CB1 receptors modulate GABA and glutamate transmission, predominately via pre-synaptic actions. Actions on GABA re-uptake and GABA release, both acting to enhance GABAergic signaling are seen in the GPe, GPi, and SNr. Cannabinoids also depress the excitation of the globus pallidus by the subthalamic nucleus.

The growth factor sonic hedgehog (Shh), acting at its receptor Patched, has been suggested as an inhibitory transmitter in the pallido-subthalamic pathway (Bezard *et al.*, 2003a).

PHARMACOLOGY OF THERAPEUTICS IN PARKINSON'S DISEASE: CURRENT STATUS AND EMERGING OPPORTUNITIES

The above discussion highlights the range of neurotransmitters and receptors that might be targeted as therapy for parkinsonism or treatment-related motor complications in Parkinson's disease. This section discusses currently available treatments for parkinsonism (Tables 3.1 and 3.2) and motor complications (Table 3.4) and highlights therapies in development for these indications (Tables 3.3 and 3.5 respectively).

Parkinsonism

In considering the changes in basal ganglia circuit activity that underlie parkinsonism and the detailed pharmacology

regulating the activity of these circuits, several principles emerge for treating Parkinson's disease.

In parkinsonism, the principal abnormality in the functioning of the circuitry is overactivity of MSNs of the indirect pathway. Thus, targeting receptors present on MSNs of the indirect pathway (see Figure 3.2a) to reduce activity of this pathway could provide multiple means to alleviate parkinsonism.

Overactivity of MSNs of the indirect pathway leads to enhanced GABAergic transmission in the GPe, and decreased inhibition of the subthalamic nucleus by the pallido-subthalamic pathway. Along with overactivity of cortico-subthalamic projections, this leads to overactivity of the subthalamic nucleus. Together, these processes drive overactivity of GPi/SNr. Pharmacological manipulation at any point in this circuitry downstream of the striatum appears able to alleviate parkinsonism.

Additionally, though probably of lesser importance, underactivity of the direct pathway contributes to the generation of parkinsonian symptoms. As with overactivity of the indirect pathway, this leads to overactivity of the GPi/SNr. Reversal of this overactivity could have anti-parkinsonian actions and/or could enhance the anti-parkinsonian actions of therapeutics primarily targeting overactivity of the indirect pathway.

The immediate cause of overactivity of the indirect pathway in parkinsonism is loss of inhibition by D2 dopamine receptors. This provides a rationale for employing dopamine-replacing drugs, in particular those stimulating D2 receptors. All currently available classes of dopaminergic therapy have, by one means or another,

Table 3.1 Currently available approaches to the pharmacological treatment of parkinsonism.

Class of drug	Example	Proposed mechanism of action
Dopamine precursor	L-DOPA	Increases dopamine levels, anti-parkinsonian action provided by stimulation of D1-like and D2-like dopamine receptors on direct and indirect striatal output pathways respectively
Non-selective dopamine receptor agonist	Apomorphine	Directly stimulates D1 and D2-like dopamine receptors on direct and indirect striatal output pathways to provide anti-parkinsonian action
D2/D3 selective dopamine receptor agonist	Ropinirole	Directly stimulates D2-like dopamine receptors on indirect pathway to provide anti-parkinsonian action
MAO-B inhibitors	Rasagiline	As monotherapy, enhances levels of endogenous dopamine to stimulate D1-like and D2-like dopamine receptors on direct and indirect striatal output pathways respectively and thus provide anti-parkinsonian benefit
Muscarinic cholinergic antagonist	Biperiden	Blockade of M1 mAChRs provides anti-parkinsonian action by reducing activity of overactive indirect striatal output pathway
NMDA antagonist	Amantadine	Reduces excitation of MSNs of indirect striatal output pathway and thereby provides anti-parkinsonian benefit

Table 3.2 Pharmacology of currently available dopamine receptor agonists.

Treatments	Receptor selectivity			$t_{1/2}$	Structural class
	D1-like	D2-like	Other		
Ropinirole	0	+ + +	Negligible	6 h	Non-ergoline
Pramipexole	0	+ + +	Negligible	8 h	Non-ergoline
Cabergoline	0	+ + +	5-HT$_{2A}$ and 5-HT$_{2B}$ agonist	60 + h	Ergoline
Bromocriptine	−	+ + +	5-HT$_{2A}$ and 5-HT$_{2B}$ agonist	8–14 h	Ergoline (ergopeptine)
Apomorphine	+ + +	+ + +	5-HT$_{2A}$ and 5-HT$_{2B}$ agonist	0.5–1 h	Ergoline
Pergolide	+	+ + +	5-HT$_{2A}$ and 5-HT$_{2B}$ agonist	16–30 h	Ergoline
Lisuride	+	+ + +	α_2 agonist	2–5 h	Ergoline
Piribedil	0	+ + +	α_2 and 5-HT$_{2B}$ antagonist	20 h	Non-ergoline
Rotigotine	+ + +	+ + +	α_2 antagonist and 5-HT$_{1A}$ agonist	7–8 h	Non-ergoline

D2 receptor-stimulating properties (Table 3.1). In considering the use of these approaches, it is worth considering actions of individual therapies in addition to D2 receptor stimulation (Table 3.2). These actions could modify anti-parkinsonian efficacy. Thus, D1 receptor activation can enhance D2 actions, perhaps due to correcting the underactivity of the direct pathway. This may, in part, underlie the perceived ability of L-DOPA, which, by increasing

Table 3.3 Emerging non-dopaminergic approaches to the pharmacological treatment of parkinsonism.

Class of drug	Proposed mechanism of action
Sub-type-selective NMDA antagonist	Reduced excitation of MSNs of indirect striatal output pathway. Fewer off-target actions and thus improved efficacy over non-selective agents such as amantadine
A$_{2A}$ adenosine antagonist	Reduced excitation of MSNs of indirect striatal output pathway
FAAH inhibitor	Elevated levels of endogenous cannabinoids and enhanced inhibition of MSNs of indirect striatal output pathway
mGluR Group I antagonist	Reduced excitation of MSNs of indirect striatal output pathway
mGluR Group III agonist	Reduced release of GABA in GPe
CB1 antagonist	Increased re-uptake and reduced release of GABA in GPe
Sonic hedgehog agonist	Increased inhibition of subthalamic nucleus

dopamine levels, stimulates both D1 and D2-like receptors, to provide more efficacious anti-parkinsonian benefit than dopamine receptor agonists selective for D2-like receptors. Similarly, L-DOPA has potential to lead to the formation of noradrenaline as well as dopamine, this may afford additional benefits to those of dopamine receptor stimulation alone. On the other hand, non-D2 receptor actions could compromise anti-parkinsonian benefit by facilitating the emergence of motor complications. This is discussed in more detail below.

In parkinsonism, loss of D2 dopamine receptor stimulation also causes a loss of dopaminergic inhibition of acetylcholine release from cholinergic interneurons. Enhanced acetylcholine release leads, via M1 muscarinic receptor activation, to excitation of indirect pathway medium spiny neurons. The long-appreciated anti-parkinsonian actions of muscarinic antagonists may result from blockade of this mechanism. The lack of profound anti-parkinsonian efficacy may be a reflection of the inability of available muscarinic antagonists to target M1 receptors over other sub-types of muscarinic receptor, or to selectively target the M1 receptors of the indirect over the M1 receptors on the direct pathway.

Furthermore, the loss of D2 receptor stimulation has impact on transmitter systems other than acetylcholine. These cause effects at least as important in rendering the indirect pathway overactive and are amenable to pharmacological intervention by novel means (Table 3.3). Firstly, after loss of dopamine, the glutamatergic drive to indirect pathway MSNs can act unimpeded by D2 dopaminergic inhibition. This leads to enhanced glutamatergic excitation and ultimately underlies overactivity of indirect pathway MSNs in parkinsonism. Glutamate antagonists, acting at NMDA, AMPA or Group I mGluRs have potential to reduce the activity of the indirect pathway. However, given that both direct and indirect pathway MSNs express all

Table 3.4 Currently available approaches to the pharmacological treatment of treatment-related motor complications.

Class of drug	Example	Proposed mechanism of action
MAO-B inhibitors	Rasagiline	As adjuncts to L-DOPA can reduce metabolism of dopamine, increase its half life and thus extend duration of L-DOPA action and thus provide enhanced benefit in advanced disease
COMT inhibitors	Entacapone	As adjuncts to L-DOPA can increase brain availability and extend half life of L-DOPA action, provide enhanced benefit in advanced disease
NMDA antagonist	Amantadine	As adjuncts to L-DOPA may reduce excitation of direct striatal output pathway and thereby reduce expression of motor complications

these classes of glutamate receptor, the therapeutic window where benefit can be attained may be narrow, that is, while an action to reduce excitation of the indirect pathway may attenuate parkinsonism, an action to reduce excitation of the direct pathway may exacerbate it. Amantadine, an NMDA antagonist that is available for use clinically, does have anti-parkinsonian actions though these are only of moderate efficacy and exhibit tachyphylaxis. However, targeting sub-types of glutamate receptor may have potential as an approach to developing novel therapeutics with greater efficacy (Nash and Brotchie, 2002). Antagonists selective for NMDA receptors containing NR2B sub-units alleviate symptoms, with efficacy equivalent to L-DOPA, in parkinsonian monkeys (Steece-Collier et al., 2000; Nash et al., 2000; Nash et al., 1999; Loschmann et al., 2004). However, this approach has not yet been translated into successful clinical application.

Loss of D2 transmission, and enhanced NMDA and M1 signaling, contribute to enhanced signaling by A_{2A} adenosine receptors. A_{2A} antagonists offer an opportunity to reverse the impact of these changes of the activity of the indirect pathway (Jenner, 2003; Kanda et al., 1998). The possibility is especially attractive given the discrete

localization of A_{2A} receptors to MSNs of the indirect pathway (Schwarzschild et al., 2006).

Outside the striatum, the effects of the indirect pathway could also be reversed by manipulation of the processes responsible for the release of GABA in the GPe. Antagonism of CB1 cannabinoid receptors can reduce GABAergic transmission in the GPe, and has some anti-parkinsonian action in animal models of Parkinson's disease. Similarly, stimulation of Group III mGluRs reduces GABA release in the GPe and has potential to offer anti-parkinsonian benefit.

Endogenous cannabinoid levels are elevated in the CSF of Parkinson's disease patients (Pisani et al., 2005) and CB1 antagonists can have mild anti-parkinsonian actions in monkeys, suggesting an involvement in the pathophysiology of parkinsonism (van der Stelt et al., 2005). It is suggested that enhanced levels of endocannabinoids in the GPe lead to increased CB1 cannabinoid receptor stimulation in the GPe and enhances GABAergic signaling in the GPe by the indirect pathway. On the other hand, reduced levels of endocannabinoids in the striatum contribute to the generation of parkinsonian symptoms, by decreasing synaptic plasticity on MSNs of the indirect pathway (Kreitzer and Malenka, 2007). In this case, enhancing striatal endocannabinoid levels, for example, by inhibiting the enzyme degrading them, FAAH, is a potential anti-parkinsonian approach (Maccarrone et al., 2003). These findings further

Table 3.5 Emerging approaches to the pharmacological treatment of treatment-related motor complications.

Class of drug	Proposed mechanism of action
Dopamine re-uptake inhibitor	Increased availability of synaptic dopamine, may combat wearing-off
α_2 adrenergic antagonist	Decreased sensitivity of direct pathway to dopaminergic stimulation
5-HT$_{1A}$ agonist	Decreased glutamatergic transmission in striatum leading to decreased excitation of direct pathway
5-HT$_{2A}$ antagonist	Decreased sensitivity of direct pathway to dopaminergic stimulation
CB1 cannabinoid antagonist	Increased re-uptake and reduced release of GABA in GPi/SNr
A_{2A} adenosine antagonist	Prevent development of motor complications if given with dopamine replacement de novo
H3 histamine agonist	Reduced release of GABA in GPi/SNr

illustrate the concept that in developing novel pharmaco-logical strategies for Parkinson's disease it may be necessary to have drugs act selectively in different components of the basal ganglia circuitry, or even act in different ways in different regions, in order to maximize anti-parkinsonian efficacy.

Motor Complications

With respect to motor complications of treatment in Parkinson's disease, few effective treatments are available today (Table 3.4). However, enhancement of L-DOPA and/ or dopamine availability by inhibition of MAO-B or COMT can offer some benefit with respect to reducing the problem of wearing-off, that is, it can extend on-time. The principal abnormality of the neural circuitry generating side effects is overactivity of the direct striatal output pathway and resul-tant overinhibition of the GPi and SNc (Cenci, 2007). Thus, targeting receptors on MSNs of the direct pathway, see Figure 3.2b, offers opportunities for treating motor com-plications. Blockade of excitatory NMDA receptors on the direct pathway may underlie the ability of amantadine to reduce L-DOPA-induced dyskinesia (see below).

In considering the cause of overactivity of the direct pathway in motor complications, two processes need to be understood:

1. The mechanisms by which repeated dopamine replace-ment therapy leads to the development of the state associated with motor complications, and,
2. The mechanisms by which, once the "complicated" state has developed, motor complications are ex-pressed on subsequent treatments with dopamine-replacing drugs.

Our increased understanding of these processes has led to the pre-clinical validation of many novel approaches to treating motor complications, several of which are now in development (Table 3.5).

With respect to the development of motor complications, the propensity of a dopaminergic treatment to cause such problems is determined by a combination of its dopamine receptor selectivity and the nature of stimulation of those receptors, be it intermittent or continuous throughout the day. Those drugs selective for D2-like dopamine receptors have less propensity to lead to the development of motor complications (Pearce et al., 1998). On the other hand, treatments with long half-lives or those administered in such a way as to provide continuous dopaminergic stimu-lation, even if they are not receptor sub-type-selective, have lower propensity to lead to the development of motor complications (Smith et al., 2003). The receptor selectivity and half-lives of currently available dopamine agonists are illustrated in Table 3.2. This understanding has led to

D2-like selective agonists becoming an option for first line therapy in Parkinson's disease, with aim to delay the initiation of L-DOPA therapy and development of motor complications. More recently, alternative means to provide continuous dopaminergic stimulation have attracted atten-tion, for instance by patch delivery of agonists or by combining L-DOPA with COMT inhibitors to increase effective half-life.

In animal models, the development of motor complica-tions appears to be dependant on, or at least facilitated by, stimulation of NMDA and A_{2A} receptors. Attenuation of these systems thus provides attractive possibilities for developing therapies to be used as adjuncts to dopamine replacement, though to date, despite proof of principle in animal models (Wessell et al., 2004; Hadj Tahar et al., 2004), these have not entered clinical practice.

Once motor complications have developed, it appears that all dopaminergic treatments, whether D2-like selective or not, elicit dyskinesia and are associated with motor fluctuations. The mechanisms by which dopaminergic stimulation leads to overactivity of the direct pathway have yet to be fully unraveled, though it is likely that they involve an increase in signaling downstream of D1 receptors and altered sub-cellular localization of D1 receptors, and not simply an increase in receptor number (Guigoni et al., 2007; Bezard et al., 2005; Aubert et al., 2005). Even if it is difficult to avoid motor complications once they have developed, studies in parkinsonian monkeys suggest that switching from L-DOPA to a D2-like receptor-selective dopamine agonist may reduce the severity of motor com-plications (Smith et al., 2006; Jackson et al., 2007). It has been suggested that once motor complications are estab-lished, stimulation of the D3 receptor may be one mecha-nism that is responsible for their expression. This remains controversial though there is evidence that D3 stimulation may contribute to dyskinesia (Bezard et al., 2003b) and wearing-off (Silverdale et al., 2004). Dopaminergic thera-pies that stimulate D2 receptors, to provide anti-parkinso-nian benefit, but not D3 receptors, to avoid motor complications, are thus of interest, though have not, to date, been developed.

Many non-dopaminergic mechanisms downstream of dopamine receptor stimulation contribute to overactivity of the direct pathway. NMDA, AMPA and Group I mGluRs provide excitation of the direct pathway (Hallett et al., 2005; Calon et al., 2003; Dunah et al., 2000). Antagonists of these receptors reduce dyskinesia and motor fluctuations in animal models and are thus attractive adjuncts to reduce motor complications of treatment in Parkinson's disease (Blanchet et al., 1999; Silverdale et al., 2005). The use of amantadine to attenuate NMDA transmission is the first successful clinical application of this approach. In contrast to their use as monotherapy to alleviate parkinsonism, the off-target actions of non-sub-type selective glutamate antagonists may be beneficial and not only reduce side effects but also enhance the anti-parkinsonian benefit of a dopaminergic therapy. Thus, within the striatum, an action on indirect pathway MSNs or cholinergic interneurons may enhance anti-parkinsonian actions. The challenge with such anti-glutamate therapies is likely avoiding actions outside the basal ganglia that might reduce benefit in other ways, for example, by interfering with learning and memory processes, causing ataxia or sedation.

Alternative means to reduce the excitability of the direct pathway, and thus reduce motor complication, include the use of $5HT_{1A}$ agonists, $5HT_{2A}$ antagonists and α_2 adrenergic receptor antagonists (Savola *et al.*, 2003). All three of these approaches are validated in animal models and have been the subject of several clinical studies. It is of interest that many of the available dopamine agonists, particularly the ergoline derivatives, have actions at these non-dopaminergic receptors (Table 3.2). Theoretically, such actions could reduce, for example, α_2 adrenergic receptor antagonist properties of piribedil, or exacerbate, for example, 5-HT (Cenci, 2007) agonist properties of pergolide, the motor complications associated with the anti-parkinsonian benefits of an agonist. While still experimental, additional approaches with some promise, and a strong theoretical basis, are to employ CB1 antagonists or H3 histamine receptor agonists to reduce GABAergic transmission in the GPi/SNr (van der Stelt *et al.*, 2005) and thereby reduce the expression of dyskinesia.

The challenge with all the above-discussed potential approaches to motor complications is to develop drugs that are selective for the receptors being targeted and define approaches that will not be compromised by actions outside the target structure.

CONCLUSIONS

The problem of parkinsonism and motor complications of dopamine-replacement therapy are issues of abnormal circuitry rather than a simple loss, or inefficient replacement of dopamine. Indeed, an understanding of the pharmacology of these disorders requires an appreciation of the role of multiple transmitters and their interactions at several levels of the basal ganglia circuitry. While this adds complexity to the process of understanding the pharmacology of Parkinson's disease, it does offer many opportunities for therapeutic intervention that had not been considered until recently and are likely to revolutionize clinical practice in years to come.

References

Alexander, G.E., Crutcher, M.D. and DeLong, M.R. (1990) *Progress in Brain Research*, **85**, 119–146.

Apicella, P. (2007) *Trends in Neurosciences*, **30**, 299–306.

Aubert, I., Guigoni, C., Hakansson, K., Li, Q., Dovero, S., Barthe, N., Bioulac, B.H., Gross, C.E., Fisone, G., Bloch, B. and Bezard, E. (2005) *Annals of Neurology*, **57**, 17–26.

Bergman, H., Wichmann, T. and DeLong, M.R. (1990) *Science*, **249**, 1436–1438.

Bezard, E., Brotchie, J.M. and Gross, C.E. (2001) *Nature Reviews. Neuroscience*, **2**, 577–588.

Bezard, E., Baufreton, J., Owens, G., Crossman, A.R., Dudek, H., Taupignon, A. and Brotchie, J.M. (2003a) *The FASEB Journal*, **17**, 2337–2338.

Bezard, E., Ferry, S., Mach, U., Stark, H., Leriche, L., Boraud, T., Gross, C. and Sokoloff, P. (2003b) *Nature Medicine*, **9**, 762–767.

Bezard, E., Gross, C.E., Qin, L., Gurevich, V.V., Benovic, J.L. and Gurevich, E.V. (2005) *Neurobiology of Disease*, **18**, 323–335.

Blanchet, P.J., Konitsiotis, S., Whittemore, E.R., Zhou, Z.L., Woodward, R.M. and Chase, T.N. (1999) *The Journal of Pharmacology and Experimental, Therapeutics* **290**, 1034–1040.

Brotchie, J.M. (2005) *Movement Disorders*, **20**, 919–931.

Calon, F., Rajput, A.H., Hornykiewicz, O., Bedard, P.J. and Di Paolo, T. (2003) *Neurobiology of Disease*, **14**, 404–416.

Cenci, M.A. (2007) *Trends in Neurosciences*, **30**, 236–243.

Chen, L., Yung, K.K. and Yung, W.H. (2006) *Neuroscience*, **141**, 1871–1878.

Cragg, S.J. (2006) *Trends in Neurosciences*, **29**, 125–131.

Diaz-Cabiale, Z., Vivo, M., Del Arco, A., O'Connor, W.T., Harte, M.K., Muller, C.E., Martinez, E., Popoli, P., Fuxe, K. and Ferre, S. (2002) *Neuroscience Letters*, **324**, 154–158.

Dunah, A.W., Wang, Y., Yasuda, R.P., Kameyama, K., Huganir, R.L., Wolfe, B.B. and Standaert, D.G. (2000) *Molecular Pharmacology*, **57**, 342–352.

Fuxe, K., Agnati, L.F., Jacobsen, K., Hillion, J., Canals, M., Torvinen, M., Tinner-Staines, B., Staines, W., Rosin, D., Terasmaa, A., Popoli, P., Leo, G., Vergoni, V., Lluis, C., Ciruela, F., Franco, R. and Ferre, S. (2003) *Neurology*, **61**, S19–S23.

Guigoni, C., Doudnikoff, E., Li, Q., Bloch, B. and Bezard, E. (2007) *Neurobiology of Disease*, **26**, 452–463.

Hadj Tahar, A., Gregoire, L., Darre, A., Belanger, N., Meltzer, L. and Bedard, P.J. (2004) *Neurobiology of Disease*, **15**, 171–176.

Hallett, P.J., Dunah, A.W., Ravenscroft, P., Zhou, S., Bezard, E., Crossman, A.R., Brotchie, J.M. and Standaert, D.G. (2005) *Neuropharmacology*, **48**, 503–516.

Hamada, M., Higashi, H., Nairn, A.C., Greengard, P. and Nishi, A. (2004) *Journal of Neurochemistry*, **90**, 1094–1103.

Ince, E., Ciliax, B.J. and Levey, A.I. (1997) *Synapse*, **27**, 357–366.

Jackson, M.J., Smith, L.A., Al-Barghouthy, G., Rose, S. and Jenner, P. (2007) *Experimental Neurology*, **204**, 162–170.

Jenner, P. (2003) *Neurology*, **61**, S32–S38.

Kanda, T., Jackson, M.J., Smith, L.A., Pearce, R.K., Nakamura, J., Kase, H., Kuwana, Y. and Jenner, P. (1998) *Annals of Neurology*, **43**, 507–513.

Kreitzer, A.C. and Malenka, R.C. (2007) *Nature*, **445**, 643–647.

Loschmann, P.A., De Groote, C., Smith, L., Wullner, U., Fischer, G., Kemp, J.A., Jenner, P. and Klockgether, T. (2004) *Experimental Neurology*, **187**, 86–93.

Maccarrone, M., Gubellini, P., Bari, M., Picconi, B., Battista, N., Centonze, D., Bernardi, G., Finazzi-Agro, A. and Calabresi, P. (2003) *Journal of Neurochemistry*, **85**, 1018–1025.

Martorana, A., Martella, G., D'Angelo, V., Fusco, F.R., Spadoni, F., Bernardi, G. and Stefani, A. (2006) *Synapse*, **60**, 371–383.

Maurice, N., Mercer, J., Chan, C.S., Hernandez-Lopez, S., Held, J., Tkatch, T. and Surmeier, D.J. (2004) *The Journal of Neuroscience*, **24**, 10289–10301.

Mitchell, I.J., Cross, A.J., Sambrook, M.A. and Crossman, A.R. (1986) *Neuroscience Letters*, **63**, 61–65.

Mitchell, I.J., Clarke, C.E., Boyce, S., Robertson, R.G., Peggs, D., Sambrook, M.A. and Crossman, A.R. (1989) *Neuroscience*, **32**, 213–226.

Narushima, M., Hashimoto, K. and Kano, M. (2006) *Neuroscience Research*, **54**, 159–164.

Narushima, M., Uchigashima, M., Fukaya, M., Matsui, M., Manabe, T., Hashimoto, K., Watanabe, M. and Kano, M. (2007) *The Journal of Neuroscience*, **27**, 496–506.

Nash, J.E. and Brotchie, J.M. (2002) *Movement Disorders*, **17**, 455–466.

Nash, J.E., Hill, M.P. and Brotchie, J.M. (1999) *Experimental Neurology*, **155**, 42–48.

Nash, J.E., Fox, S.H., Henry, B., Hill, M.P., Peggs, D., McGuire, S., Maneuf, Y., Hille, C., Brotchie, J.M. and Crossman, A.R. (2000) *Experimental Neurology*, **165**, 136–142.

Obeso, J.A., Rodriguez, M.C. and DeLong, M.R. (1997) *Advances in Neurology*, **74**, 3–18.

Obeso, J.A., Rodriguez-Oroz, M.C., Rodriguez, M., DeLong, M.R. and Olanow, C.W. (2000) *Annals of Neurology*, **47**, S22–S32; discussion S32–4.

Pearce, R.K., Banerji, T., Jenner, P. and Marsden, C.D. (1998) *Movement Disorders*, **13**, 234–241.

Penney, J.B. Jr and Young, A.B. (1986) *Movement Disorders*, **1**, 3–15.

Pisani, A., Bonsi, P., Picconi, B., Tolu, M., Giacomini, P. and Scarnati, E. (2001) Progress in Neuro-Psychopharmacology & Biological Psychiatry **25**, 211–230.

Pisani, A., Fezza, F., Galati, S., Battista, N., Napolitano, S., Finazzi-Agro, A., Bernardi, G., Brusa, L., Pierantozzi, M.,

Stanzione, P. and Maccarrone, M. (2005) *Annals of Neurology*, **57**, 777–779.

Sanchez-Lemus, E. and Arias-Montano, J.A. (2006) *Neurochemical Research*, **31**, 555–561.

Savola, J.M., Hill, M., Engstrom, M., Merivuori, H., Wurster, S., McGuire, S.G., Fox, S.H., Crossman, A.R. and Brotchie, J.M. (2003) *Movement Disorders*, **18**, 872–883.

Schwarzschild, M.A., Agnati, L., Fuxe, K., Chen, J.F. and Morelli, M. (2006) *Trends in Neurosciences*, **29**, 647–654.

Silverdale, M.A., Nicholson, S.L., Ravenscroft, P., Crossman, A.R., Millan, M.J. and Brotchie, J.M. (2004) *Experimental Neurology*, **188**, 128–138.

Silverdale, M.A., Nicholson, S.L., Crossman, A.R. and Brotchie, J.M. (2005) *Movement Disorders*, **20**, 403–409.

Smith, L.A., Jackson, M.J., Hansard, M.J., Maratos, E. and Jenner, P. (2003) *Movement Disorders*, **18**, 487–495.

Smith, L.A., Jackson, M.J., Johnston, L., Kuoppamaki, M., Rose, S., Al-Barghouthy, G., Del Signore, S. and Jenner, P. (2006) *Clinical Neuropharmacology*, **29**, 112–125.

Steece-Collier, K., Chambers, L.K., Jaw-Tsai, S.S., Menniti, F.S. and Greenamyre, J.T. (2000) *Experimental Neurology*, **163**, 239–243.

van der Stelt, M., Fox, S.H., Hill, M., Crossman, A.R., Petrosino, S., Di Marzo, V. and Brotchie, J.M. (2005) *The FASEB Journal*, **19**, 1140–1142.

Wessell, R.H., Ahmed, S.M., Menniti, F.S., Dunbar, G.L., Chase, T.N. and Oh, J.D. (2004) *Neuropharmacology*, **47**, 184–194.

Wichmann, T. and DeLong, M.R. (1999) *Nature*, **400**, 621–622.

The Treatment of Early Parkinson's Disease

Olivier Rascol[1] and Regina Katzenschlager[2]

[1] Department of Clinical Pharmacology and Neurosciences, Clinical Investigation Center and INSERM U825,
Toulouse University Hospital, France
[2] Department of Neurology, Danube Hospital/SMZ-Ost, Vienna, Austria

At the beginning of the twentieth century, anticholinergic drugs were the only available efficacious medications for the treatment of early and advanced Parkinson's disease (PD). When levodopa was discovered (Birkmayer and Hornykiewics, 1961; Cotzias, 1968) in the 1960s, the number of alternative pharmacological options was still limited, and decisions on how to treat PD remained relatively simple, regardless of the stage of the disease. Nowadays, at the beginning of the twenty-first century, the situation has markedly changed, because levodopa monotherapy is not the sole option to treat PD any more, and this is especially the case when patients are not severely disabled, in the early stages of the disease.

More than a dozen anti-parkinsonian medications have been developed and approved during the levodopa era. This is mainly due to the fact that levodopa has a number of limitations beside its spectacular efficacy. It does not cure the disorder and there is no convincing evidence that it improves the progression of the underlying pathological process. It may induce side effects such as nausea, vomiting, orthostatic hypotension and psychosis and its long-term use is frequently associated with the emergence of motor complications. Seeking solutions for these problems drove the development of other pharmacological approaches, including dopamine agonists (e.g., bromocriptine, lisuride, pergolide, piribedil, cabergoline, pramipexole, ropinirole), MAO-B inhibitors (selegiline, rasagiline) and COMT inhibitors (entacapone, tolcapone). Unfortunately, none of these turned out to be good enough to replace levodopa. They can, at best, complement its effect when used before it, as initial therapy, or when added as a second line strategy. Hence, doctors must choose among numerous therapeutic strategies, combining different drugs in a variety of ways and sequences. Making the most appropriate choice at each stage of the disease and for each patient is a difficult exercise, and must be based on various parameters, such as pathophysiological concepts, clinical evidence regarding efficacy and safety, but also empirical experience, economical environment, and patients' preferences, expectations and needs.

We shall summarize in the first part of this chapter the clinical evidence supporting the efficacy and safety of anti-parkinsonian medications as assessed by randomized controlled trials (RCTs) conducted in untreated patients with early PD. In the second part of this chapter, we will provide a pragmatic approach for routine clinical practice.

OVERVIEW OF THE CLINICAL EVIDENCE FOR ANTI-PARKINSONIAN MEDICATIONS IN THE TREATMENT OF EARLY PD: THE MOVEMENT DISORDER SOCIETY (MDS) EVIDENCE-BASED MEDICINE (EBM) ASSESSMENT OF ANTI-PARKINSONIAN INTERVENTIONS

The Movement Disorder Society (MDS) is an international professional society of clinicians, scientists, and other healthcare professionals who are interested in PD and related disorders of motor control. In the late 1990s MDS established and funded a taskforce to review the different available anti-parkinsonian therapeutic interventions according to the robustness of the published clinical evidence. The approach followed was to develop an evidence-based medicine (EBM) systematic review where therapeutic interventions were classified according to specified criteria regarding efficacy, clinical usefulness and safety

Table 4.1 Standard definitions of the terms used to qualify efficacy, clinical usefulness and safety of therapeutic interventions.

Efficacious	Evidence shows that the intervention has a positive effect on studied outcomes (at least one good quality RCT).
Efficacy likely	Evidence suggests, but is not sufficient to show that the intervention has a positive effect on studied outcomes.
Efficacy unlikely	Evidence suggests that the intervention does not have a positive effect on studied outcomes.
Non-efficacious	Evidence shows that the intervention does not have a positive effect on studied outcomes.
Insufficient evidence	There are no data available or available data do not provide enough evidence either for or against the use of the intervention in treatment of Parkinson's disease.
Clinical usefulness	
Clinically useful	For a given situation, evidence available is sufficient to conclude that the intervention provides clinical benefit.
Possibly useful	For a given situation, evidence available suggests, but insufficient to conclude that the intervention provides clinical benefit.
Investigational	Available evidence is insufficient to support the use of the intervention in clinical practice, but further study is warranted.
Not useful	For a given situation, available evidence is sufficient to say that the intervention provides no clinical benefit.
Safety	
Acceptable risk without specialized monitoring.	
Acceptable risk, with specialized monitoring.	
Unacceptable risk.	
Insufficient evidence to make conclusions on the safety of the intervention.	

(see Table 4.1). The scientific basis for that classification was defined as all identified original articles (Medline and Cochrane Library, English peer-reviewed literature) reporting RCTs that enrolled a minimum of 20 patients with an established diagnosis of PD, used objective scales for measuring target symptoms, and had a minimum of four-weeks' treatment.

It was acknowledged that this basis was most appropriate to establish efficacy, but much less so for safety, because RCTs are not designed to identify rare adverse reactions. Therefore, additional sources were used for safety, such as post-marketing surveillance and regulatory publications.

We shall focus in the present chapter on three efficacy issues of special importance for the management of untreated patients with early PD, namely (i) impact on disease progression, (ii) symptomatic efficacy on motor symptoms as monotherapy and (iii) prevention of motor complications. A brief description of the main RCTs will be presented, as well as summaries of adverse drug

reactions to be expected with medications used at this stage of the disease. An extensive report of the MDS EBM systematic review was published as a supplement of the *Movement Disorder Journal* in 2002. This document was updated in 2005 (Goetz *et al.*, 2005) and is currently in its third updating process. Readers interested in a detailed description and a complete list of all relevant RCTs are invited to refer to these MDS documents (MDS Evidence based medicine taskforce, 2002; Rascol *et al.*, 2002; Goetz *et al.*, 2005) and to forthcoming ones.

Drug Efficacy on Disease Progression

Over time, symptoms of PD progressively worsen. The need for symptomatic medications increases, the quality of their effects deteriorates and non-motor symptoms as well as motor problems unresponsive to dopaminergic treatment, such as balance problems and freezing during on-periods, develop. A major theoretical therapeutic goal is therefore to limit the progression of PD as early as possible, ideally before the occurrence of symptoms. Etiologic mechanisms including free radical-mediated damage, excitotoxicity, mitochondrial dysfunction, or inflammation-mediated cell damage are supposed to contribute to the pathogenesis. In addition, the recent interest in apoptosis, protein misfolding and aggregation, and proteasomal activity has provided new insights into pathogenetic pathways in PD. This has increased efforts to develop drugs that might modify such biochemical abnormalities in order to alter the course of the disease, either by retarding the rate of cell death, or by restoring function to neurons that are likely to be damaged, but not irremediably dead.

We have chosen to briefly describe in this section eight large RCTs conducted to test various disease-modifying hypotheses in PD. These RCTs illustrate the huge efforts invested since the "decade of the brain" to identify drugs that could reduce PD progression. Unfortunately, to this date, no "neuroprotective" or "disease-modifying" agent with robust positive clinical findings has been identified.

- Selegiline (DATATOP study; Parkinson Study Group, 1993): Selegiline is a propargylamine with MAO-B inhibiting properties. The symptomatic anti-parkinsonian efficacy of selegiline is believed to be related to MAO-B inhibition. *In vivo*, MAO-B inhibition reduces the toxicity of MPTP in animal models of PD. Moreover, *in vitro*, propargylamines increase neuronal survival independently of MAO-B inhibition by interfering with apoptosis signaling pathways.

  DATATOP was the first prospective, randomized, controlled trial to test the impact of a drug on PD progression. It was a double-blind placebo-controlled parallel 2×2 factorial design study, comparing selegiline (10 mg/d) and α-tocopherol (vitamine E, 2000 units/d) in 800 untreated patients with early PD. The development of disability requiring levodopa therapy was the primary endpoint to measure disease progression. Tocopherol had no effect on this endpoint. Conversely, selegiline significantly delayed "time to levodopa therapy" during an average 12-month follow-up. However, the interpretation of this encouraging result was soon challenged when it was realized that UPDRS motor scores improved after initiation of selegiline (wash-in effect) and deteriorated after drug withdrawal (wash-out effect), suggesting that the response was not sustained. These observations strongly suggest that the beneficial effect of the drug may be related, at least in part, to a symptomatic improvement of parkinsonism, precluding conclusions on an effect on disease progression.

- Bromocriptine (SINDEPAR trial; Olanow *et al.*, 1995): Bromocriptine is a dopamine agonist with putative "neuroprotective" properties including direct scavenging of free radicals, increasing the activities of radical-scavenging enzymes, and enhancing neurotrophic activity in *in vitro* and *in vivo* animal models.

  SINDEPAR was a prospective parallel-group double-blind placebo-controlled 14-month RCT to compare the effects of selegiline with or without either bromocriptine or SINEMET in 101 untreated patients with early PD. Deterioration of UPDRS total score between baseline and final visit was used as an index of PD progression, patients being assessed seven days after withdrawal of bromocriptine or SINEMET (to avoid potential confounding symptomatic effects) and after two months of selegiline wash-out. There was no difference in deterioration in UPDRS scores between the bromocriptine and SINEMET groups, suggesting that PD progressed at the same rate on both treatments. Conclusions were hampered by the absence of a placebo group and the short duration of the wash-out period, which may have been insufficient to completely clear symptomatic drug effects.

- Pramipexole (CALM-PD trial; Parkinson Study Group, 2002): The D2/D3 dopamine agonist pramipexole may have neuroprotective activity that is, at least in part, unrelated to its dopamine agonist action. Protection in cell and animal models against a variety of toxins, including MPTP and 6-hydroxydopamine, suggests neuroprotective effects that might be mediated by antioxidant properties, direct action on mitochondrial membrane potential or the inhibition of apoptosis.

  CALM-PD allowed a four-year sub-analysis of a double-blind prospective parallel-group RCT comparing pramipexole and levodopa in 84 untreated patients with early PD. The primary endpoint of this sub-study was the percentage change measured with single photon emission tomography (SPECT) at month 46 from baseline in striatal [^{123}I]β-CIT (2 β-carboxymethoxy-3 β-[4-iodophenyl]tropane) uptake. This dopamine transporter ligand was chosen as a putative biomarker of dopamine innervation. A significant difference in mean percentage decline of approximately 40% was identified in favor of pramipexole ($p = 0.01$). However, the lack of a clinical correlate, the absence of a placebo control and the potentially different regulatory effects of levodopa or dopamine agonists on the imaging biomarker preclude conclusions on any modifying effects of pramipexole on the progression of PD.

- Ropinirole (REAL-PET trial; Whone *et al.*, 2003): Ropinirole scavenges free radicals and suppresses lipid peroxidation *in vitro*. It protects striatal dopaminergic neurons against 6-hydroxydopamine (6-OHDA) in *in vivo* animal models.

  REAL-PET was a parallel-group prospective levodopa-controlled two-year RCT to assess the effect of ropinirole in 186 untreated patients with early PD. The primary endpoint to measure disease progression was the percentage decrease of the putaminal Ki value of [^{18}F]dopa uptake from baseline, as measured with positron emission tomography (PET). There was a statistically significant reduction in putaminal Ki values in the ropinirole group compared with the levodopa group (-13% on ropinirole vs -20% on levodopa, $p < 0.05$), but the same limits as discussed for the CALM-PD study preclude any firm conclusions on the effect of ropinirole on PD progression.

- Levodopa (ELLDOPA trial; Fahn *et al.*, 2004): Levodopa therapy has been claimed to be toxic for the remaining dopaminergic neurons because, in theory, it could enhance free radical generation from dopamine metabolism. Conversely, chronic levodopa treatment has been reported to promote the recovery of striatal innervation in rats with partial dopaminergic lesions (Murer *et al.*, 1998).

    ELLDOPA was a parallel-group double-blind placebo-controlled 40-week RCT conducted in 361 untreated patients with early PD to assess the effects of different doses (150, 300, and 600 mg/d) of levodopa on PD progression. The primary endpoint was the change in UPDRS score from baseline, after two weeks of levodopa wash-out at the end of the 40-week follow-up. A sub-group of 142 subjects also had striatal [^{123}I] β-CIT SPECT imaging, as a biomarker for disease progression. The mean UPDRS change between baseline and endpoint was larger in the placebo group than in all levodopa groups (differences >5 UPDRS units, $p < 0.0001$). Conversely, the decline in [^{123}I] β-CIT signal was significantly greater with levodopa than placebo. These results are inconsistent and do not allow one to conclude definitely on the impact of levodopa on PD progression: the clinical data suggested that the drug either slowed the progression of PD or had a prolonged effect (>2 weeks) on the symptoms, while the neuroimaging data suggested that either levodopa accelerated the loss of nigrostriatal dopamine nerve terminals or that its pharmacologic effects modified the dopamine transporter signal.

- Rasagiline (TEMPO delayed-start trial; Parkinson Study Group, 2004): Rasagiline is a MAO-B inhibitor and a propargylamine. As a propargylamine, it binds to glyceraldehyde-3-phosphate dehydrogenase (GAPDH). GAPDH binding is associated with decreased synthesis of pro-apoptotic proteins like BAX, c-JUN and GAPDH, but increased synthesis of anti-apoptotic proteins like BCL-2, Cu-Zn superoxide dismutase and heat shock protein 70.

    TEMPO was a double-blind parallel-group randomized delayed-start clinical trial, a six-month extension of a six-month placebo-controlled RCT (Parkinson Study Group, 2004), which compared the effects of early vs later initiation of rasagiline (1 or 2 mg/d) on progression of disability in 404 untreated patients with early PD. Change in total UPDRS from baseline was the primary endpoint. Subjects who were on rasagiline 2 mg/d for one year had a significantly smaller increase in UPDRS than those who received placebo for six months followed by rasagiline 2 mg/d for six months (< 2 UPDRS units difference between the two groups, $p <$ 0.05). These pilot results showed that patients treated late with rasagiline did not "catch-up" compared with those who started early. This difference cannot be explained by a pure symptomatic effect of the drug and suggests that some disease-modifying effect may have occurred. A larger study, using a comparable design, known as the ADAGIO trial, is presently ongoing to try to replicate these results. Nevertheless, the design of these studies will not allow one to determine if the different reduction in functional decline between the groups is related to a true "neuroprotective" effect or to an enhancement of yet unknown brain "compensatory" mechanisms.

- Pergolide (Grosset *et al.*, 2005): As other dopamine agonists, pergolide exhibits neuroprotective properties *in vitro* and *in vivo* in animal models of PD. This trial tested the effects of a sub-therapeutic dose of pergolide (50 mcg/d) in a prospective placebo-controlled parallel-group RCT conducted in 106 untreated patients with early PD. Levodopa initiation was used as the primary endpoint to assess PD progression. There was a non-significant trend in favor of pergolide in "time to levodopa therapy", but recruitment problems compromised the power of the trial and the wash-in effect of pergolide measured at six weeks indicated a mild symptomatic benefit at a dose normally considered sub-therapeutic. These results therefore do not allow any firm conclusion on an effect of pergolide on PD progression.

- TCH 346 (Olanow, Obeso and Stocchi, 2006): TCH 346 incorporates a propargyl ring within its molecular structure. The drug resembles selegiline, but does not inhibit MAO-B. Like other propargylamines, it is a glyceraldehyde-3-phosphate (GAPDH) ligand and a potent anti-apoptotic drug that protects against loss of dopaminergic neurons in laboratory animals. In this study, 301 patients with early, untreated PD were assessed in a placebo-controlled parallel-group double-blind 12–18-month RCT testing three doses of TCH 346 (0.5 mg/d, 2.5 mg/d and 10 mg/d). The primary outcome was time to development of disability requiring dopaminergic treatment. TCH 346 did not differ from placebo at any dose for any of the study outcomes, suggesting that the drug did not modify the course of the disease under the experimental conditions used.

Other drugs have also been tested in untreated patients with early PD in large RCTs for putative disease-modifying properties. The results of these trials have not yet all been published in detail, but are known to be negative. This is the case for the anti-glutamate agent riluzole (Rascol *et al.*, 2002) and the anti-apoptotic mixed lineage kinase inhibitor CEP-1347 (Parkinson Study Group, 2007). Other compounds have been prioritized for testing in Phase II proof-of-concept trials, including CoEnzyme Q10, GPI-1458, creatine and minocycline. Encouraging pilot results from small placebo-controlled trials (Shults *et al.*, 2002) or futility trials (The NINDS NET-PD investigators, 2006, 2007) have been reported. These results deserve further confirmation in larger trials before any conclusions can be drawn.

In summary, based on the MDS EBM Taskforce methods, there is presently no sufficiently robust clinical evidence to conclude that any drug is "efficacious" for improving PD progression. Any intervention to achieve this goal remains at this stage, at best, "investigational". The reasons for these negative conclusions are numerous, including incomplete understanding of cell death mechanisms, inadequate targets for drug action, poorly predictive animal models, imperfect RCT design, absence of validated surrogate endpoints, and lack of simple and reliable clinical outcomes. Future developments of novel drugs will need to improve such shortcomings.

Drugs with Symptomatic Efficacy as Monotherapy

Based on our current understanding of the pathophysiology of PD, the striatal dopaminergic deficit caused by the degeneration of the nigro-striatal dopamine neurons represents the most widely accepted factor to explain the occurrence of motor symptoms in PD, especially in the early stages of the disease. However, it is possible that non-dopaminergic mechanisms are involved, even at the early disease stages, possibly related to an indirect functional imbalance secondary to the initial dopaminergic deficit within the basal ganglia circuitry.

Whatever these mechanisms are, several dopaminergic and non-dopaminergic drugs can be used to improve the symptoms of patients with early PD. A universally accepted manner to demonstrate that a drug is efficacious in controlling motor symptoms in patients with early PD consists in measuring the changes from baseline to endpoint in the scores of the Motor Examination Section (Part III) and/or of the Activity of Daily Living (Part II) of the UPDRS (Fahn *et al.*, 1987). This is best achieved in prospective parallel-group, double-blind placebo-controlled RCTs lasting from three to six months. Unfortunately, such RCTs became standard practice at times when the "oldest" anti-parkinsonian medications, like anticholinergics and amantadine had already been used for many years. Such trials to assess the efficacy of these compounds are therefore lacking.

According to current methodological standards and following the methods recommended by the MDS EBM Taskforce, there is enough clinical evidence (at least one good quality RCT and sometimes several consistent ones) to conclude that nine anti-parkinsonian medications are efficacious when used as monotherapy in early PD drugs, namely levodopa, six dopamine agonists (dihydroergocryptine (DHEK), pergolide, piribedil, pramipexole, ropinirole and rotigotine) and two MAO-B inhibitors (selegiline, rasagiline) (Table 4.2). Some anti-parkinsonian drugs have been compared with others using an active comparator—in most cases levodopa—instead of placebo. The most relevant trials are discussed below. For a complete list of all RCTs, readers should refer to the original MDS publications.

Table 4.2 Symptomatic interventions for the treatment of parkinsonism (motor features) as monotherapies in early PD patients.

	Efficacious	Likely efficacious	Insufficient evidence
Medications	Standard levodopa	Bromocriptine	Apomorphine
	CR levodopa	Lisuride	Cabergoline
	Dihydroergocriptine	Anticholinergics	Entacapone[a]
	Pergolide	Amantadine	Tolcapone[a]
	Piribedil		
	Pramipexole		
	Ropinirole		
	Rotigotine		
	Selegiline		
	Rasagiline		
Surgery			All interventions
Rehabilitation			All interventions

[a] Based on their mechanism of action, COMT-inhibitors are not considered as efficacious when used as monotherapy in PD, but no published clinical trial was identified.

RCTs Using Placebo as a Comparator

- *Levodopa*: Standard levodopa has been tested in a recent placebo-controlled RCT, which confirmed its long-established anti-parkinsonian efficacy in early PD (ELLDOPA Study, Fahn *et al.*, 2004).
- *Dopamine agonists*: Several dopamine agonists improved UPDRS scores better than placebo in good quality RCTs: pergolide (Barone *et al.*, 1999), dihydroergocriptine (DHEK) (Bergamasco *et al.*, 2000), piribedil (Rascol *et al.*, 2006b), pramipexole (Shannon *et al.*, 1997), ropinirole (Adler *et al.*, 1997) and rotigotine (Watts *et al.*, 2007; Giladi *et al.*, 2007a). These agonists are considered efficacious as monotherapy in the treatment of early PD, according to the methods of the MDS EBM review.

  There is less convincing, but still supportive, evidence for bromocriptine. This conclusion is mainly based on levodopa-controlled RCTs showing that the efficacy of the drug was comparable to levodopa (Riopelle 1987; Montastruc *et al.*, 1994) (these studies were not powered to demonstrate non-inferiority), or slightly less efficacious (Parkinson's Disease Research Group of the UK, 1993). Similarly, cabergoline was never compared with placebo in early PD but results comparable to levodopa in two double-blind RCTs suggest efficacy (Rinne *et al.*, 1997, 1998). There are only open-label studies to support the effect of lisuride (Rinne, 1989) in early PD. Therefore, these latter three agonists are considered likely efficacious in this indication according to the MDS EBM methods. Apomorphine, being only used sub-cutaneously, has never been tested as monotherapy for the treatment of PD at this early stage.
- *MAO-B inhibitors*: Selegiline (Parkinson Study Group, 1996) and rasagiline (Parkinson Study Group, 2002) have both been compared with placebo in good quality RCTs and improved parkinsonism better than placebo. They can therefore be considered efficacious.
- *COMT inhibitors*: These drugs are only active when combined with levodopa and are therefore not efficacious as monotherapy in the treatment of untreated patients with early PD.
- *Other anti-parkinsonian medications*: Amantadine and anticholinergics are considered *likely efficacious* as monotherapy in PD, because they have been tested in ancient RCTs of lower quality or in studies without placebo control, but consistently showing improvement compared to baseline. Data on other monotherapy treatments are insufficient for conclusions.

RCTs Using an Active Comparator

- *Controlled-released (CR) levodopa* vs *standard levodopa*: CR levodopa was compared to standard levodopa in different studies with equivalent improvement in

parkinsonism at short-term and long-term evaluations (Koller *et al.*, 1999).
- *Agonist monotherapy* vs *levodopa in untreated patients with early PD*: Levodopa proved to be more efficacious than any orally active dopamine agonist monotherapy in most available RCTs. This common clinical practice observation is documented in RCTs assessing agonists like cabergoline (Rinne *et al.*, 1997), pramipexole (Parkinson Study Group, 2000), ropinirole (Rascol *et al.*, 1998) and bromocriptine (Parkinson's Disease Research Group of the UK, 1993; Olanow *et al.*, 1995). There are no published levodopa-controlled head-to-head RCTs with the other agonists.

  The proportion of patients with early PD remaining on an agonist monotherapy falls progressively over years to less than 20% after five years of treatment with bromocriptine (Montastruc *et al.*, 1994; Parkinson's Disease Research Group of the UK, 1993), cabergoline (Rinne *et al.*, 1998), pramipexole (Parkinson Study Group, 2000), ropinirole (Rascol *et al.*, 2000). For this reason, after some years of treatment, most patients who start on an agonist will receive levodopa as a replacment or an adjunct treatment to maintain control of the parkinsonian motor syndrome. The optimal timing of when best to combine both drugs has never been assessed. In the last decade, the most frequently tested strategy has been to start with an agonist and to postpone the adjunction of levodopa for as long as possible as a second step of the therapeutic strategy. However, previously it had been common practice to combine an agonist (bromocriptine or lisuride) with levodopa within the first months of treatment ("early combination strategy") (Przuntek *et al.*, 1996; Allain *et al.*, 2000). There are no data to assess if one strategy is better than the other.
- *Agonist monotherapy* vs *another agonist*: There are only few trials comparing the efficacy of a dopamine agonist vs that of another as monotherapy. When such data are available (bromocriptine vs ropinirole [Korczyn *et al.*, 1998, 1999] and vs pergolide [Mizuno, Kondo and Narabayashi, 1995]), the clinical relevancy of the reported difference, if any, remains questionable, especially since the exact dose equivalence between the different agonists remains unknown. No published systematic reviews, such as by the Cochrane Collaboration, have investigated any differences in efficacy among various agonists in early PD. A recent, large, placebo-controlled, randomised trial compared the transdermally administered dopamine agonist rotigotine vs ropinirole as an active comparator. Non-inferiority of rotigotine could not be demonstrated. However, a potential bias in terms of predefined dose equivalence prevented definite conclusions, the maximum daily doses permitted in this trial being 24 mg for ropinirole but only 8 mg for

rotigotine. In a post hoc sub-group analysis, rotigotine ≤ 8 mg/24 hours had a similar efficacy to ropinirole at doses ≤ 12 mg/day, and in studies in advanced PD, a rotigotine dose of 16 mg was used. Therefore the fact that UPDRS scores and other measures showed more improvement on ropinirole in this study does not allow the conclusion of an inferior efficacy of rotigotine as such (Giladi et al., 2007a).

In summary, there is no convincing evidence of clinically relevant differences in the efficacy of the currently available dopamine agonists when used for the treatment of early PD.

- *Other anti-parkinsonian medications*: There are no published direct head-to-head comparisons between other drugs as monotherapy in early PD (e.g., MAO-B inhibitors, amantadine, anticholinergics). The changes in UPDRS scores reported in placebo-controlled RCTs are usually greater on agonists than on MAO-B inhibitors. This could be interpreted as an indirect indication of a greater symptomatic efficacy of the agonists, but one cannot firmly establish if this putative difference is of clinical importance.

Prevention of Motor Complications

Motor complications, such as fluctuations of the wearing-off or on–off types and dyskinesias are frequent, difficult to treat, disabling and they may be partly irreversible. An appealing pathophysiological concept that is currently put forward to explain the occurrence of motor complications in PD patients on levodopa is known as the "continuous dopamine stimulation" or "CDS" hypothesis (Olanow, Obeso and Stocchi, 2006). This theory proposes that dopaminergic agents that provide continuous stimulation of striatal dopamine receptors will delay or prevent the onset of levodopa-related motor complications. Nigro-striatal dopaminergic neurons normally fire in a random, but continuous, manner, and striatal dopamine concentrations are therefore supposed to remain at a relatively constant level. Pre-clinical data obtained in 6-OH-treated rats and MPTP-intoxicated monkeys have shown that a parkinsonian brain cannot adequately buffer the peaks of dopamine concentrations elicited by the intermittent administration of short-acting drugs like oral levodopa. Intermittent oral doses of levodopa may therefore induce discontinuous stimulation of striatal dopamine receptors. Such pulsatile stimulation could drive a cascade of molecular and physiologic changes at the level of basal ganglia relays and outputs, including dysregulation of striatal dopamine and non-dopamine receptors, abnormal intracellular signaling of striatal neurones, and abnormal output of the basal ganglia motor loop, resulting in abnormal motor programs and behaviors such as motor fluctuations and dyskinesias. According to this concept, these effects should be reduced

or avoided when dopaminergic therapies are delivered in a more continuous and physiologic manner. Several observations in primate models support the CDS hypothesis, showing that continuous or long-acting dopaminergic agents are associated with a decreased risk of motor complications compared with short-acting dopamine agonists or levodopa (Pearce et al., 1998; Smith et al., 2005). However, other observations have challenged the CDS hypothesis, which requires further validation (Nutt, 2007).

On this basis, investigations have been performed to assess the impact of initial treatment using drugs with longer elimination half-life than levodopa, in order to reduce or delay the incidence of motor complications. Several prospective long-term, double-blind levodopa-controlled RCTs compared the probability of developing motor complications within up to five years in previously untreated patients. Such trials did not use standardized methods to define the onset of motor complications. Each trial used its own definition, with consequent variable numbers from one study to another.

CR levodopa: The CDS hypothesis would predict that the early use of CR levodopa formulations should reduce the risk of long-term motor complications. However, two large (several hundred patients), prospective, double-blind, five-year, standard levodopa-controlled RCTs tested the impact of the early use of CR-levodopa on the occurrence of long-term motor complications (Dupont et al., 1996; Block et al., 1997). Both studies found no difference between the two groups. CR levodopa is therefore considered not efficacious in preventing the long-term occurrence of motor complications, according to the methods of the MDS EBM Taskforce.

Dopamine agonists: The only medications considered to be efficacious therapies in reducing the risk of motor complication when used early in the treatment of PD are three dopamine agonists: cabergoline (Rinne et al., 1998), ropinirole (Rascol et al., 2000) and pramipexole (Parkinson Study Group, 2000) (Table 4.3). Pergolide and bromocriptine are considered likely efficacious. The design of the RCTs of the first three agonists was quite comparable. They were prospective, parallel-group, levodopa-controlled, large (several hundreds of patients), two- to five-year, double-blind RCTs, using the time when the first motor complication (fluctuations or dyskinesias) occurred as the primary endpoint. In these trials, levodopa could be added early or late to the agonist, in order to keep control on parkinsonism if the anti-parkinsonian effect of agonist monotherapy was waning. In the cabergoline RCT, motor fluctuations occurred in 34% of the patients allocated to early levodopa vs 22% of those randomized to the agonist ($p < 0.02$). In the pramipexole RCT, motor complications occurred in 55% of the patients randomized to receive levodopa as initial therapy vs 28% of those allocated to the agonist first ($p < 0.0001$). In the ropinirole RCT, dyskinesias were

Table 4.3 Preventive interventions for motor complications in levodopa-naive PD patient.

	Efficacious	Likely efficacious	Non efficacious	Insufficient data
Medications	Cabergoline Pramipexole Ropinirole	Bromocriptine Pergolide	Standard levodopa CR levodopa	Apomorphine Dihydroergocriptine Lisuride Piribedil Selegiline Rasagiline Entacapone Tolcapone Amantadine Anticholinergics
Surgery				All interventions
Rehabilitation				All interventions

observed in 45% of the patients randomized to early levodopa vs 20% in those randomized to early agonist ($p < 0.001$) (Figure 4.1). A post hoc analysis of this study suggests that the risk of developing dyskinesias during maintained initial agonist monotherapy is very low. Only once levodopa is added to the agonist does the risk increase substantially. Early use of agonists postpones the onset of dyskinesia, but these benefits decline when levodopa therapy is started, with no evidence of a subsequent rapid "catch-up" or persisting preventive effect (Rascol et al., 2006b). Open-label five-year data from another ropinirole trial (Whone et al., 2003) are limited by a relatively small residual sample, but support these findings by showing significantly less dyskinesia in the ropinirole arm compared with levodopa, and similar motor control (Poewe et al., 2005). A new, prolonged-release formulation

of ropinirole already available in some countries has been shown to be non-inferior to immediate-release ropinirole as monotherapy in early PD (Stocchi and Giorgi, 2006), although no published studies are available investigating the effect of this new formulation on the emergence of motor complications when used as the initial treatment.

A fourth, large, three-year RCT using a comparable design compared pergolide to levodopa as initial therapy in untreated patients with early PD (Oertel et al., 2006). However, levodopa supplementation was not allowed during the trial. The primary outcome of this trial (time to onset of motor complications) was not different between the two groups after three years, although the severity of motor complications was significantly lower and time to onset of dyskinesia was significantly delayed in the agonist group. It was therefore concluded, according to the MDS EBM

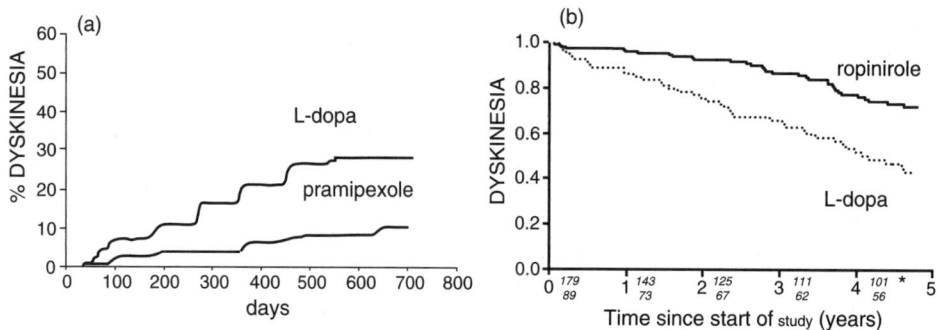

Figure 4.1 Rates of dyskinesias in studies comparing initial levodopa and agonist treatment. [(a) Reproduced from Parkinson Study Group (2000) *J. Am. Med. Assoc.*; **284**: 1931–1938, with permission from the American Medical Association (b) reproduced with permission from Rascol et al., *N. Engl. J. Med.* 2000; **342**: 1484–1491, Copyright © 2000, Massachusetts Medical Society].

definitions, that pergolide is likely efficacious in reducing the risk of motor complication over three years as compared with initial levodopa monotherapy.

Similar conclusions were reported in trials with bromocriptine (Parkinson Study group of the UK 1993; Hely *et al.*, 1994; Montastruc *et al.*, 1994) although these were designed at a time when trial methodology was less standardised and rigorous than current standards.

The fact that five different agonists proved to be efficacious or likely efficacious suggests that this property might be a "class effect". However, conflicting results have been reported with lisuride (Rinne, 1989; Allain *et al.*, 2000), and published controlled data are lacking for other orally active agonists (dihydroergocryptine, piribedil), apomorphine not being used and tested in this situation. In the absence of adequate published RCTs or because of conflicting results, there is insufficient data to conclude on the effect of using these agonists as initial therapy for patients with early PD on the development of motor complications.

There is no indication that one agonist might be more efficacious than another in preventing or delaying "time to motor complication". The only published head-to-head RCT comparing two agonists in this situation (ropinirole vs bromocriptine) (Korczyn *et al.*, 1999) did not show any difference at three years in the incidence of dyskinesias.

It is important to note that these trials covered the first few (up to five) years following the initiation of therapy, but data on longer follow-up periods are important to consider. Until recently, little was known on whether the initial choice of drug still had effects 10 years or more into the course of the disease. No studies have maintained blinding for more than five years, but data are now emerging on the subsequent development in patients who were initially randomized to one of the dopamine agonists vs levodopa. Ten-year data for the original double-blind five-year ropinirole study (Hauser *et al.*, 2007) showed that dyskinesias— but not disabling dyskinesias—continued to occur less frequently ($p = 0.046$) in the original ropinirole arm, while motor scores had converged. However, only 69 of 268 patients entered the extension part of this study. In the randomized but open-label study of the PD Research Group of the UK, patients initially randomized to bromocriptine had a significantly lower incidence of dyskinesias than those randomized to levodopa at 10 years (rate ratio 0.73 [95% CI 0.57, 0.93]) (Lees *et al.*, 2001). This difference was not significant when only moderate to severe forms were considered, and the incidence of fluctuations was similar in both arms. At 14 years of follow-up, frequencies of motor complications had converged (Katzenschlager *et al.*, 2008). A smaller 15-year study of bromocriptine vs levodopa (Hely *et al.*, 2005) reported that 94% of patients had experienced dyskinesias, but this was severe in only 12%. The mean duration of treatment before the onset of dyskinesia was 4.2 years for the levodopa group and 6.9 years for the

bromocriptine group ($p = 0.009$). Fluctuations were reported by 96% of patients, but there were no significant differences between the arms in the time to onset of fluctuations, or in the duration of off-periods.

In summary, evidence from these trials shows lower frequencies of both dyskinesias and motor fluctuations during the first years of treatment in patients randomized to a dopamine agonist as compared to levodopa, but open-label long-term observations suggest that these differences tend to diminish as the disease progresses.

While trials reporting on agonists vs levodopa as initial treatment for up to five years found that initial agonist treatment led to fewer dyskinesias and usually fewer motor fluctuations compared with levodopa, this occurred at the expense of smaller UPDRS score improvements (Figure 4.2). It has been argued that these UPDRS differences in favor of levodopa may or may not be clinically relevant. It is not possible at this stage to conclude definitely on this issue because of methodological differences from one trial to another: Levodopa supplementation was allowed during the course of some trials (cabergoline, ropinirole, pramipexole), but not in others (pergolide), agonists were used at fixed doses in some studies (pramipexole) while continuous up-titration was permitted over years in others (ropinirole). One study suggested that a difference of 5 points on the UPDRS motor score represents a clinically meaningful difference (Schrag *et al.*, 2006), and the differences between the levodopa and agonist arms in the early treatment trials were sometimes of that magnitude. However, it must be acknowledged that a minimally clinically meaningful UPDRS difference has never been clearly established (Schrag *et al.*, 2006; Rascol 2006a) and that global assessments, such as clinical global impression scales, did not differ between agonist and levodopa arms in some trials. Another possible cause of this persisting modest advantage of levodopa might partly be artefactual due to patients' and physicians' expectations being influenced by the degree of initial improvement (Parkinson Study Group, 2000). Another explanation is the possibility that early symptomatic treatment—or early treatment with more efficacious drugs, such as levodopa, compared with agonists–might enable compensatory mechanisms within the basal ganglia, which may delay sustained damage (see below). It has also been suggested that early levodopa might have greater potential to sensitize a long-lasting motor response (Nutt, 2007).

In levodopa-controlled trials, adverse drug reactions such as somnolence, leg oedema or hallucinations were more common with agonists (see safety section below). Finally, after a disease duration of 15 years and more, no differences between treatment arms were detected in other clinically important factors such as disability, falls, independent living and dementia. Therefore, other factors besides the induction of motor complications during the first years of treatment

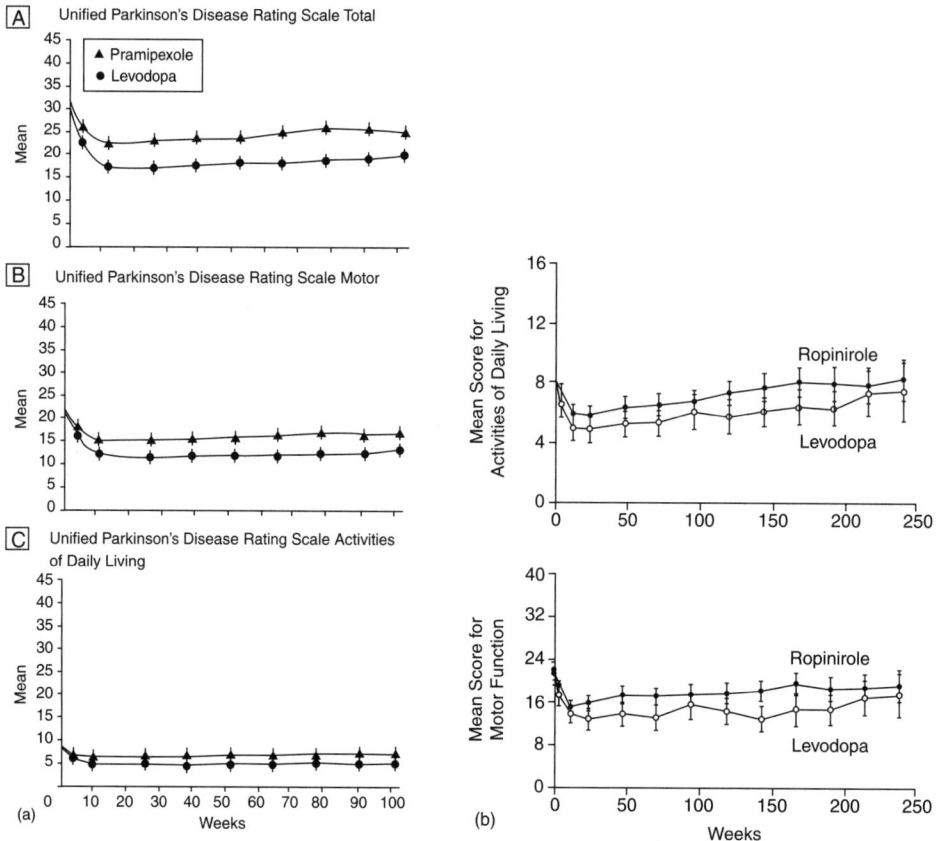

Figure 4.2 UPDRS scores in studies comparing initial levodopa and agonist treatment. [(a) Reproduced from Parkinson Study Group (2000) *J. Am. Med. Assoc.*; **284**: 1931–1938, with permission from the American Medical Association (b) reproduced with permission from Rascol *et al.*, *N. Engl. J. Med.* 2000; **342**: 1484–1491, Copyright © 2000, Massachusetts Medical Society].

need to be taken into account when choosing the initial treatment for a given patient (see below).

MAO-B inhibitors: According to the published literature and MDS EBM methods, the early use of selegiline is non-efficacious for the prevention of dyskinesias. This conclusion is based on the negative results of a large (473 patients), three-year RCT comparing the effect of early therapy with levodopa, a dopamine agonist (bromocriptine or lisuride) or selegiline on the occurrence of motor complications (primary endpoint) (Caraceni and Musicco, 2001) and on the analysis after two years of follow-up of a second independent randomization of 368 patients from the original DATATOP cohort, which showed that the frequency of new occurrence of any of the pre-specified primary outcome events (wearing-off, dyskinesias, or on–off fluctuations) was not different between the two arms (Shoulson *et al.*, 2002).

COMT inhibitors: According to the "CDS" hypothesis, the early combination of a COMT inhibitor with levodopa therapy should be desirable, in order to reduce the

development of motor complications. Indeed entacapone prolongs levodopa elimination half-life without increasing its C_{max} and this should help in reducing the inadequate pulsatility of levodopa stimulation. Because of liver toxicity, tolcapone is not recommended as first-line therapy in PD patients, so it should not be considered in early PD. Preliminary results in MPTP-intoxicated monkeys show that, indeed, when entacapone is combined with levodopa in untreated animals, the incidence of dyskinesias over the next few weeks is reduced as compared with animals on levodopa monotherapy (Smith *et al.*, 2005). A large, prospective, double-blind two-year, levodopa-controlled double-blind RCT, known as STRIDE-PD, is presently underway to test this hypothesis in untreated patients with early PD. Until the results of this trial are available, there is still insufficient data to conclude on the benefit of adding entacapone to levodopa early, in order to reduce the incidence of long-term motor complications.

Other anti-parkinsonian medications: It is now known that neurotransmitters other than dopamine contribute to the generation of motor complications (Brotchie, 2005). It is therefore conceivable that the early use of drugs with effects on such transmitters could have a positive impact on the later development of motor complications. This might be of particular interest in the case of amantadine, which has proven to be efficacious in symptomatically treating dyskinesias, once present, in levodopa-treated patients with advanced PD. Unfortunately, at present, no controlled data are available and there is therefore insufficient evidence to conclude on the use of amantadine in early PD.

SAFETY ISSUES

It is beyond the scope of this article to review in detail all known side effects of all anti-parkinsonian medications. This is, however, an important issue to consider when deciding which drug to introduce in a patient with early PD, who has not been previously exposed to such therapies. As already pointed out, the scientific data to base conclusions on for safety cannot be restricted to RCTs, especially because such trials are never powered to identify rare and/or idiosyncratic adverse reactions that are nevertheless clinically meaningful. Therefore, for the safety part of a risk/benefit assessment, other sources must be reviewed, including post-marketing surveillance, case reports, pharmacovigilance studies and regulatory publications, like those issued by the Committee of Proprietary Medicinal Product (CPMP) in Europe and the Food and Drug Administration (FDA) in the USA.

Adverse drug reactions (ADRs) are defined as any appreciably harmful or unpleasant reaction, resulting from an intervention related to the use of a medicinal product, which predicts hazard from future administration and warrants prevention or specific treatment, or alteration of the dosage regime, or withdrawal of the product (Edwards and Aronson, 2000). They can be classified as type A or type B reactions (Rawlins and Thompson, 1977). Type A reactions are generally expected and predictable, since they are frequently related to the known pharmacological properties of the drug. Their prevalence is relatively high. They are usually non-serious, non-lethal, dose dependent and can be managed with dose adjustment. Conversely, type B reactions are unexpected, unpredictable, rare, often serious reactions and most of the time they lead to drug withdrawal.

Many dopaminergic medications share a similar qualitative safety profile. Their adverse drug reactions can be divided into peripheral and central ADRs.

Peripheral Adverse Drug Reactions of Dopaminergic Medications

- *Gastro-intestinal and cardiovascular type A adverse reactions* are common at the onset of therapy with any dopamine agent, and usually diminish over time. They are explained by the agonistic effect of the drugs on dopamine receptors in the gut and in the area postrema (gastrointestinal effects) and at the pre-synaptic level of the sympathetic system (orthostatic hypotension). They can be managed by slow titration. Anti-emetics like domperidone, a dopamine blocker agent that does not cross the blood–brain barrier, help to treat nausea. In large, levodopa- controlled double-blind RCTs, gastrointestinal and cardiovascular ADRs are not necessarily reported to be more frequent with agonists than with levodopa (Rascol et al., 2000), while it is frequently empirically believed that this is the case in clinical practice.

- *Leg oedema* is known to be associated with dopamine agonists (ergot and non-ergot derivatives). It is also observed with amantadine (which can also induce livedo reticularis). Reported incidences vary widely and this reaction is more frequent with agonists than with levodopa. For example, the incidence of leg oedema reported in levodopa-controlled trials was 14% for ropinirole vs 6% for levodopa (Rascol et al., 2000), 42% for pramipexole vs 15% for levodopa (Holloway et al., 2004) and 16% for cabergoline vs 3% for levodopa (Bracco et al., 2004). The mechanism of this side effect is unknown. This adverse drug reaction is sometimes reported as dose-dependent, but can also be idiosyncratic. It is reversible, with discontinuation of the agonist, while the use of diuretics should be discouraged, because these agents are not efficacious and can induce or aggravate other problems, such as orthostatic hypotension.

- *Fibrosis* has been detected in post-marketing surveillance studies with all ergot-derivative dopamine agonists including bromocriptine, lisuride, cabergoline and pergolide. Classically, such fibrotic reactions have been reported as pleuropulmonary, pericardiac and/or retroperitoneal syndromes (Bhatt et al., 1991; Ling et al., 1999; Shaunak et al., 1999; Mondal and Suri, 2000). These adverse reactions are usually considered rare events, although their exact prevalence is unknown. Their mechanism is possibly related to the dose and duration of exposure to the ergot compounds. Erythrocyte-sedimentation and protein-C-reactive inflammatory markers are usually increased and may be helpful for an early diagnosis. The risk of developing such a fibrosis on non-ergot agonists is much lower, if it exists. These reactions are sometimes life-threatening, although they can be at least partially reversible after drug withdrawal. In general, when a patient develops this kind of adverse reaction on an ergot agonist, the strategy is to switch to a non-ergot one.

Recently, several cases of another type of fibrotic adverse reaction, severe multi-valvular heart disease, have been reported with pergolide and other ergot derivative agonists, namely bromocriptine and cabergoline (Horvath et al., 2004; Agarwal, Fahn and Frucht, 2004; Vergeret et al., 1984). For the moment, the risk is best documented with pergolide and cabergoline (Van Camp *et al.*, 2004; Peralta *et al.*, 2006; Yamamoto, Uesugi and Nakayama, 2006; Junghanns *et al.*, 2007; Dewey *et al.*, 2007; Zanettini *et al.*, 2007; Gentile *et al.*, 2007) and a recent review of the literature showed that moderate to severe regurgitation in at least one heart valve was present in 34% of patients on cabergoline and in 22% on pergolide, compared to 4% on non-ergot agonists and 6% in controls (Antonini and Poewe, 2007), while the prevalence on bromocriptine is less well known. The most likely mechanism is considered to be via the $5HT_{2B}$ receptor, rather than a direct effect of a drug's ergoline structure. A dose effect seems likely, but it is not known whether the restrictive heart valve changes are reversible on discontinuation of the drug involved. Pergolide has been withdrawn from the market in some countries and both pergolide and cabergoline are now only recommended as second-line alternative options, when other agonists have not provided a satisfying response. In many countries, specific guidelines on the frequency of echocardiography follow-ups have been issued (usually before initiating therapy and then yearly, and discontinuation of the drug is recommended in cases of any relevant changes).

- *Other peripheral ADRs:* Examples of type B reactions due to agonists are alopecia, which has been reported with bromocriptine (Fabre, Montastruc and Rascol, 1993), visual cortical disturbances with bromocriptine (Lane and Routledge, 1983), loss of color vision with pramipexole (Müller, Przuntek and Kuhlmann, 2003) and hypersensitivity (allergic reactions) to many agonists (Martindale, 2005). These adverse reactions are rare, but their real prevalence and mechanisms often remain unknown.

Central Adverse Drug Reactions of Dopaminergic Drugs

- *Psychiatric symptoms* are among the most disabling dopaminergic medication-related ADRs. These may occur with any efficacious dopaminergic medication. The prevalence of these symptoms on agonists varies according to the reports, and usually ranges between 5 and 20%. In most levodopa-controlled double-blind trials, psychiatric adverse reactions are reported to be more common with agonists than with levodopa (Rascol *et al.*, 2000; Parkinson Study Group, 2000), and this is also empirically observed in clinical practice. Such psychotic symptoms can present as delusions, usually paranoid, or hallucinations, predominantly visual, though an auditory component is common.

  Abnormal behaviors linked to the role of dopamine in natural reward mechanisms, such as hypersexuality, pathological gambling and other related syndromes, are now recognized to be associated with the use of dopamine agonists, although no association with one particular agonist has been demonstrated (Lawrence, Evans and Lees, 2003; Weintraub *et al.*, 2006; Voon *et al.*, 2007; Gallagher *et al.*, 2007). These problems occur in 3–8% of PD patients seen in specialized clinics (Voon *et al.*, 2006; Weintraub *et al.*, 2006). There is some dose-relationship, but it is important to be aware of the fact that these abnormal behaviors may occur on regular doses, including on the small doses of dopamine agonist monotherapy often used in the initial management of early PD. This possibility is highlighted by the observation of impulse control problems brought on by the small doses used in the treatment of restless legs syndrome (Driver-Dunckley *et al.*, 2007). Factors that have been found to increase the risk of developing these behaviors in PD patients include younger age, male gender, impulse control issues in the past (such as alcohol or substance dependence), socially accepted gambling, and high scores for novelty-seeking personality traits (Giladi *et al.*, 2007b; Weintraub *et al.*, 2006; Voon and Fox, 2007). Depression and irritability have been found to often co-occur with impulse control disorders (Pontone *et al.*, 2006).

  The usual management of impulse control disorders, if occurring in patients with early PD, is to reduce the dose or to stop the drug and to replace it with other anti-parkinsonian medications, especially levodopa. It may take weeks before the effect clears, but the response to reducing dopamine agonists (and partially switching to levodopa) has recently been shown to be sustained in many cases (Mamikonyan *et al.*, 2008). Other measures, such as the use of atypical neuroleptics or, in the case of extreme hypersexuality, anti-androgens, are occasionally helpful, although there is no evidence from controlled studies to support any particular treatment. DBS has occasionally been reported to improve impulse control disorders, although the opposite effect has also been observed.

  In contrast, the dopamine dysregulation syndrome is less often a problem in the management of early PD, as it tends to occur after a period of treatment (Evans *et al.*, 2006). This disorder involves the use of increasing doses of any dopaminergic drug, often levodopa, which is associated with the subsequent development of emotional and behavioral changes similar to those in various forms of substance abuse (Evans *et al.*, 2005). Predisposing factors are similar to those for impulse control disorders, and both disorders may occur separately or in combination (Evans *et al.*, 2005). All attempts should be made to reduce the overall dopaminergic drug dose.

- *Abnormal daytime somnolence* was not listed among common type A adverse reactions of anti-parkinsonian medications until the publication in 1999 of cases of "sleep attacks" at the wheel, in patients with PD treated with ropinirole or pramipexole (Frucht et al., 1999). It was thereafter realized that such problems are common with any dopamine agonist, including ergot and non-ergot ones. This is based on post-marketing surveillance case reports with apomorphine (Homann et al., 2000), bromocriptine (Ferreira et al., 2000), cabergoline (Ebersbach, Norden and Tracik, 2000), lisuride (Ferreira et al., 2000), pergolide (Scharpira, 2000; Ferreira et al., 2000), piribedil (Ferreira et al., 2000; Tan, 2003), pramipexole (Frucht et al., 1999; Ryan, Slevin and Wells, 2000), ropinirole (Frucht et al., 1999), but also with other anti-parkinsonian medications, such as entacapone (Ebersbach, Norden and Tracik, 2000) and levodopa (Ferreira et al., 2001). Pharmaco-epidemiological surveys confirmed that all agonists share the risk of daytime somnolence (Hobson et al., 2002; Paus et al., 2003). In levodopa-controlled double-blind RCTs, the agonists usually induce greater somnolence than levodopa (Etiman et al., 2001). The prevalence of abnormal daytime somnolence varies greatly according to the studies (6% according to Paus et al., 2003; 16% Tandberg, Larsen and Karlsen, 1999; 18% Razmy, Lang and Shapiro, 2004; 27% Ferreira et al., 2006; 30% Montastruc et al., 2001b; 32% Manni et al., 2004; 34% Schlesinger and Ravin, 2003; 76% Brodsky et al., 2003). This is probably mainly due to different definitions ("sleep attacks", "sudden onset of sleep", "unintended sleep episodes", "irresistible sleep episodes", "abnormal daytime sleepiness", "excessive daytime sleepiness"), different populations (non-demented patients, patients on agonists only, patients who drive vehicles, or normal population) and different methods of assessment (questionnaires, scales like the Epworth scale, electro-physiological techniques like the Multiple Sleep Latency Test etc.). In placebo-controlled RCTs conducted in healthy volunteers, ropinirole induced somnolence (Ferreira et al., 2002). This was also true for levodopa (Andreu et al., 1999). Risk factors are poorly known and might be related to the patient (age, gender, genetic susceptibility), the disease (severity, duration, associated symptoms such as dysautonomia, dementia, depression) or the drug (dose, duration of exposure, co-medications). One must now recognize that somnolence is a frequent dopaminergic type A adverse reaction, shared by most, if not all, dopaminergic medications (Homann et al., 2002), although dopamine agonists appear to pose a greater risk than levodopa (Etiman et al., 2001). Patients should be informed of this potential effect, and be advised not to drive if present. The practical management of agonist-induced, inappropriate daytime sleepiness is poorly known and remains empirical. In some instances, dose reduction is efficacious. Switching from one agonist to another is an option, but the same reaction can occur with another agonist. Relatively small placebo-controlled RCTs do not support the prescription of "specific" therapies, such as modafinil (Ondo et al., 2005).

Adverse Drug Reactions Caused by Anticholinergics

With anti-muscarinic agents, the most frequent adverse reactions are urinary retention, constipation, dry mouth, increase in intraocular pressure and central effects such as confusion and cognitive deterioration, which may occur even in non-demented persons (Sadeh, Braham and Modan, 1982). Such a safety profile is obviously crucial to consider when initiating treatment. Cognitively impaired or aged patients are unlikely to tolerate anticholinergics, and are better managed with other drugs, mainly standard levodopa. Even in cognitively intact patients, anti-cholinergics should only be prescribed in selected cases and with great caution, and patients need to be monitored for the emergence of anticholinergic side effects (Katzenschlager et al., 2003).

Adverse Drug Reactions Caused by MAO-B Inhibitors

MAO-B inhibitors are generally well tolerated. A possible, but rare, adverse effect is the serotonergic syndrome: MAO-B inhibitors may increase central serotonergic tone when taken together with serotonergic drugs such as selective serotonine re-uptake inhibitors (SSRIs) and other drugs including opiates, lithium and St John's wort. This may result in confusional states, myoclonus, nausea and fever. No safety concerns were observed in those patients from the large rasagiline trials who had been on concomitant SSRIs, but the combination of MAO-B inhibitors and the SSRIs fluvoxamine and fluoxetine (which block CYP oxidase) is not recommended.

Although both selegiline and rasagiline are relatively selective MAO-B inhibitors, some effect on MAO-A cannot entirely be ruled out, particularly at higher doses. However, interactions of rasagiline with food intake have been investigated and no effect on blood pressure suggestive of a tyramine effect (as observed with older MAO-A inhibiting anti-depressants) was found (deMarcaida et al., 2006).

Mortality and the Early Use of Dopaminergic Drugs

In the few available long-term trials conducted in patients with PD, the mortality rate of patients randomized early to a dopamine agonist like bromocriptine was not different from that of patients randomized to levodopa (Hely et al., 1999; Katzenschlager et al., 2008; Montastruc et al., 2001).

A few years ago, concerns on selegiline safety were raised because of increased mortality in the levodopa + selegiline arm of a large levodopa-controlled RCT conducted in early patients with PD (Lees 1995). A subsequent meta-analysis and smaller RCTs failed to reproduce or to support this finding (Macleod *et al.*, 2005). In the absence of clear confirmatory reports, there is still insufficient data for definite conclusions. However, despite some small studies reporting increased cardiovascular risk due to orthostatic hypotension and autonomic nerve system dysfunction on selegiline (Churchyard, Mathias and Lees, 1999), most prescribers now consider an impact on mortality unlikely.

PRAGMATIC APPROACH IN ROUTINE CLINICAL PRACTICE

The management of patients with early PD involves different steps. The first is to establish the diagnosis of "idiopathic" PD. Then, the patient and their family should be adequately informed and receive appropriate answers to their questions about PD, including causes, symptoms, progression, prognosis, genetic transmission, treatments, on-going research and future perspectives. It is also important, at this stage, to evaluate the individual and specific needs and expectations of each patient, because these can be markedly different depending on age, profession, culture, hobbies, mood, cognition, and co-morbidity. On this basis, the next step is to choose the most adequate therapeutic option and finally to start follow-up.

Two issues are important to consider in this context (refer to Figure 4.3):

1. When to start treatment: It is currently an unresolved issue whether treating patients as early as possible, that is, as soon as the diagnosis has been made, is preferable to treating as late as possible and waiting until symptoms impair the patient's functioning.

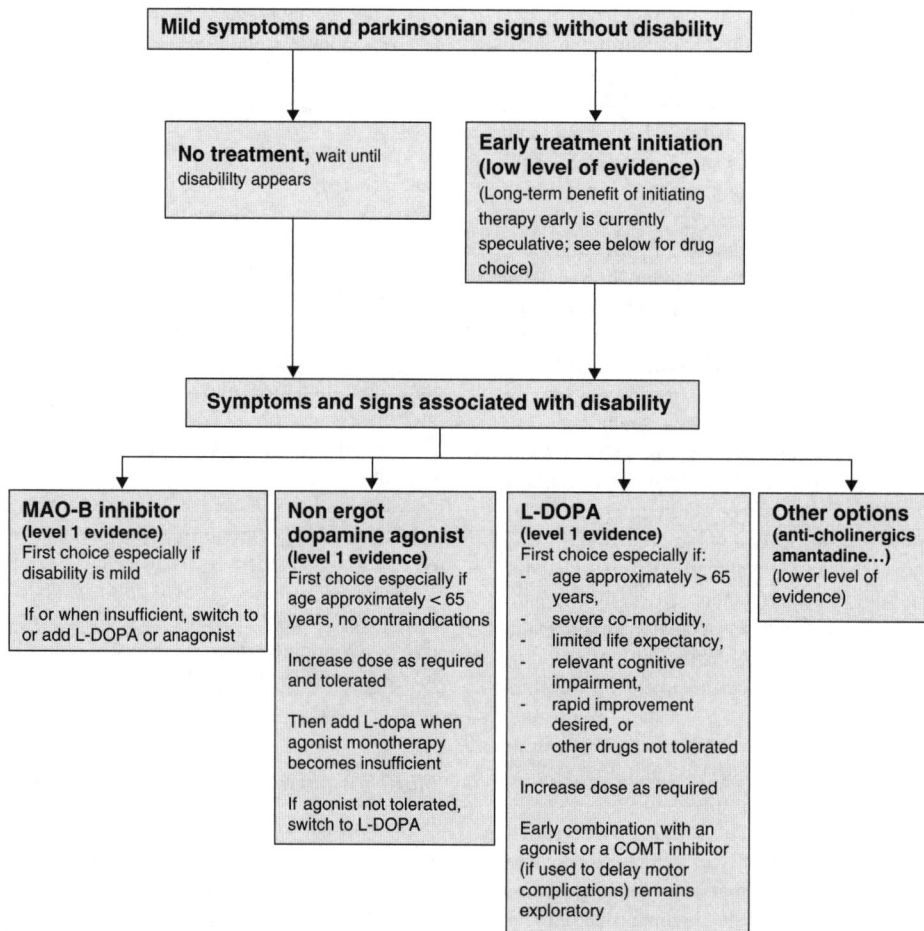

Figure 4.3 Summary of the different treatment options.

If a drug had proven to positively influence the progression of PD, one would expect that it should be prescribed as early as possible (even at pre-symptomatic stages of the disease, if detectable), provided short-term and long-term tolerability and safety are acceptable. However, up to now, no intervention has demonstrated definite efficacy in this indication (see above). Results from a recent trial of the MAO-B inhibitor rasagiline in early PD (the TEMPO study) have been interpreted as showing a sustained clinical benefit to initiating drug treatment early (Parkinson Study Group, 2002). The trial used a "delayed-start" design, where patients received the active drug either from the beginning of the study, or with a six-month delay. Over the following six months, patients who had started with a delay improved, but not to the same degree as those who had received initial active drug treatment. An on-going larger study is currently attempting to replicate these findings with rasagiline. A similar effect has been found in a study of the transdermal dopamine agonist rotigotine, although these results have not yet been fully published (Poewe, personal communication), and a delayed-start trial is currently ongoing with another dopamine agonist, pramipexole.

Similarly, it is conceivable that not just early initiation but initiating treatment with a more powerful drug or higher doses may have some long-term benefit. The only existing placebo-controlled trial of levodopa (ELLDOPA Fahn *et al.*, 2004) showed that following a two-week wash-out period, UPDRS motor scores remained better in the levodopa arms than with placebo and patients on higher doses of levodopa did better than on lower doses. These findings are broadly in keeping with a general perception that has emerged over the past few years, that starting treatment early may convey some sustained benefit to patients in terms of motor function. It has been speculated that this may be, at least partly, due to compensatory mechanisms within the basal ganglia which are enabled by alleviating the dopamine deficiency early (Schapira and Obeso, 2006).

However, it remains to be confirmed in larger and long-term studies whether these observed differences are clinically relevant or not and whether they correspond to a subsequent long-lasting and sustained effect.

The different side-effect profiles of drugs used in the treatment of early PD also need to be considered when deliberating on the best time to start any symptomatic treatment. As long as a definite benefit of treating early has not been established, it remains important to consider that in very mildly affected patients, the induction of drug-related adverse events may outweigh any improvement of motor symptoms.

2. Which drug to prefer as first line when initiating therapy: Once the decision has been made to start symptomatic treatment, the best choice for each individual patient must be identified. It is important to remember that very few of the various possible strategies have been directly compared in randomized trials. Ideally, any treatment should be simple, efficacious, safe in the long and the short term, and cost effective (Table 4.4). None of the available drugs for the treatment of early PD meets all these criteria and each of the options has advantages and disadvantages (Table 4.5):

- Levodopa: This is clinically useful in the early management of PD because it has the strongest efficacy among the anti-parkinsonian drugs. It also has a long background of clinical use and is not expensive. Due to its marked symptomatic efficacy, levodopa remains the "gold standard" for the treatment of PD, but in the early stages of the disease, when symptoms are not severe, less efficacious drugs can be sufficient to control mild symptoms. Like any dopaminergic medication, levodopa can induce dopaminergic peripheral and central ADRs, but it is generally better tolerated than other dopaminergic agents, such as agonists. The emergence of motor complications on chronic therapy represents an important disadvantage of levodopa. Up to now, levodopa CR formulations or an early combination with entacapone have not demonstrated convincing clinical advantages vs standard formulations with respect to motor complications. Some years ago, the question of a

Table 4.4 Issues to consider in the early management of Parkinson's disease.

Objectives
  1. Efficacy
  2. Safety (long/short term)
  3. Simplicity
  4. Cost
  5. Patient's circumstances/preferences

Pathophysiological basis
  1. Symptomatic therapy:
     Non-dopaminergic agents? for example, amantadine, (anticholinergics)
     Dopamine replacement: MAO-B inhibitors, dopamine agonists, L-dopa
  2. Continuous dopaminergic stimulation
  3. Neuroprotection
  4. Compensatory mechanisms/lasting benefit by initiating treatment early?

Table 4.5 Characteristics of drugs used in the treatment of early PD.

	Neuro-protection	Efficacy	Motor complications	Practicality	Cost	Psychiatric ADRs
Amantadine	?	+	?	+	Low	+ +
Anticholinergics	?	+	?	+	Low	+ + +
COMT inhibitors (Entacapone[a])	?	?	?	+ +	Expensive	+
Dopamine agonists	?	+ +	+	− (titration)	Expensive	+ +
Levodopa	?	+ + +	−	+ +	Low	+
MAO-B inhibitors	?	+	?	+ + +	Low[b]/expensive[c]	+

[a] Not licensed for the indication early PD.
[b] Selegiline.
[c] Rasagiline.

putative negative impact of levodopa therapy on PD progression was put forward, because dopamine metabolism produces free radicals. Based on *in vitro* data, and according to the pathophysiological concept that oxidative stress causes neurodegeneration, many physicians became reluctant to prescribe levodopa early. They rather delayed its use as much as possible, in order to "protect" the remaining neurones from this potential toxicity. The concept of levodopa "toxicity" has no clinical data to support the hypothesis (Olanow *et al.*, 2004) and it is not good clinical practice to delay levodopa therapy for this purpose, when it is required to adequately control motor symptoms.

- MAO-B inhibitors represent a possible option as a first-line treatment in early PD for patients with mild symptoms, because the regimen is simple for the patients (once daily, no titration, one dose). They are efficacious—although their symptomatic efficacy is relatively modest—and they generally have a favorable tolerability profile, although food and drug interactions (tyramine cheese effect,

serotonergic syndrome) are rare, but possible. However, the long-term impact of using MAO-B inhibitors as the initial choice is not known, nor is the impact of subsequent supplementation with a dopamine agonist or with levodopa. These issues are due to be assessed in the future in the course of the development program of drugs like safinamide. The daily dosages are listed in Table 4.6.

- Anticholinergics and amantadine are likely useful, because they have moderate symptomatic efficacy, and because they are cheap (an important issue in countries where the social security system does not pay for medical care in all patients). Data from trials are insufficient for specific recommendations regarding these drugs in early PD, but their side-effect profiles, as outlined above, should be kept in mind, especially when considering anticholinergics.

- Dopamine agonists: Dopamine agonists are clinically useful in the early management of PD patients because they have demonstrated symptomatic efficacy and because they induce fewer

Table 4.6 Licensed maximum dosages of selected drugs used in early PD.

Dopamine agonists		MAO inhibitors	
Ropinirole	24 mg/d	Selegiline	Oral: 10 mg/d
Pramipexole	3.3 mg/d (base)		Buccal: 1.25 mg/d
Rotigotine	16 mg/d	Rasagiline	1 mg/d
Cabergoline[a]	4 mg/d		
Pergolide[a]	5 mg/d		

[a] Not recommended as first-line options.

motor complications than levodopa, at least during the first years of follow-up. Non-ergot compounds should be preferred to ergot derivatives because of fibrotic adverse reactions, and the risk of restrictive heart valve changes with some agonists must be kept in mind. The most controversial issue in the early management of PD patients remains, after years of debate, whether a dopamine agonist or levodopa should be chosen first. The disadvantages of the agonists are that they are less efficacious (the clinical relevancy of this difference remains controversial) and that they can induce more adverse drug reactions, such as daytime somnolence, leg oedema, hallucinations and impulse control disorders, than levodopa (see above). Moreover, the long-term benefit of the early use of dopamine agonists (>10 years) in terms of motor complications remains questionable, while they offer no benefit over levodopa on other relevant long-term issues, such as balance and gait problems, dementia and mortality. The maximum daily dosages for dopamine agonists are listed in Table 4.6. No universally accepted conversion factor exists for one dopamine agonist to another.

In summary, the question of which treatment to use as first line in early PD remains unresolved, and at this stage, no recommendations can be given that would suit every situation: for each patient it remains important to consider the patient's preferences, age, co-morbidity including cognitive function, and occupation. In patients with mild symptoms, the use of an MAO-B inhibitor can be considered, due to the simplicity of its use and its good tolerability profile. If or when symptoms require more "potent" medications, levodopa or an agonist are usually considered, with their respective advantages and disadvantages (see above). Quality of life data are currently unavailable to help with this decision, as the difference favoring levodopa at two years (in two separate measures) in the pramipexole study was no longer significant after four years of follow-up (CALM-PD, Holloway *et al.*, 2004). As nearly all patients require levodopa after a few years, it is important to be aware that prolonged under-treatment with agonist monotherapy may lead to increased disability, social withdrawal and diminished professional prospects in some patients. Similarly, it is important to adjust the dose of a dopamine agonist according to the patient's needs during the first months and years of treatment, when dopamine agonist monotherapy is still an option, using high enough doses, depending on tolerability, and to add levodopa when it becomes necessary.

It is generally recommended in young patients (below around 60–65 years), where the risk of motor complications is relatively high, to start with a dopamine agonist and to monitor the patients for potential adverse reactions. Levodopa should then be added as a second line when the efficacy of the agonist wanes and requires complementing. Conversely, in aged patients (> around 65 years), it is usually preferable to start with levodopa, because the risk of motor complications is lower in this group. As long as the agonist is maintained as monotherapy, the risk of motor complications is extremely low. However, as all currently available oral dopamine agonists are less symptomatically efficacious than levodopa, low doses of levodopa are needed after months to years in nearly all patients to maintain sufficient symptom control. Patients should then receive the combination of the agonist and levodopa rather than switching to levodopa. This is supported by the conclusions of the post hoc 056 trial (Rascol *et al.*, 2006b) and of the CALM-PD trial (Constantinescu *et al.*, 2007) showing that when levodopa is added on top of an agonist after some years of initial monotherapy, the risk of dyskinesia is not precipitated, but simply reappears, whereas if the patient is switched to levodopa, the incidence of dyskinesias can be expected to catch up rapidly, as if levodopa had been used from the beginning. This is suggestive of a levodopa sparing effect as a mechanism to delay and reduce the risk of dyskinesia.

From a pharmacokinetic perspective, different options can theoretically be discussed in order to achieve more continuous receptor stimulation. This includes using levodopa controlled-release (CR) formulations (because they reduce peak plasma concentrations (C_{max}) and prolong elimination half-life), agonists with very long half-life, or entacapone (because it prolongs levodopa elimination half-life without increasing its C_{max}). It could be speculated that these drugs should be used early. However, while the hypothesis is attractive, proof of these concepts from clinical data is currently lacking. As already mentioned in the case of CR levodopa, two large RCTs showed no effect on the incidence of motor complications. Moreover, although we lack head-to head comparisons, it is a challenging observation that cabergoline, with its long elimination half-life of 70 hours, does not seem to reduce the risk of long-term motor complications much more than lisuride, with its short half-life (three hours). The addition of entacapone to levodopa from the initiation of treatment is based on promising *in vitro* and animal data, but this strategy cannot be generally recommended before the data become available from the on-going study investigating this concept in PD patients (STRIDE-PD). Attempts by some physicians to prescribe levodopa divided into six or more daily doses from the initiation of treatment to avoid pulsatile plasma concentration changes, may cause inconvenience to patients and might impair compliance. Therefore, strategies that reflect pathophysiological concepts should be subjected to clinical trials before adopting them into clinical practice.

SUMMARY

In conclusion, it is clear that any practitioner will base his/her own therapeutic decision to initiate treatment in a given patient with PD on a combination of several considerations. The weight of these different factors varies markedly from one patient to another, from one physician to another and from one country to another. In regions with a low economical level and poor social-security system, for example, theoretical hypotheses such as "continuous dopamine stimulation" and long-term concerns about motor complications might not be seen realistically as crucial factors when initiating therapy. The most affordable and efficacious treatments allow treatment of the largest numbers of patients and will be the most appropriate pragmatic choices. In richer countries, there is more space for long-term concerns and attractive, but speculative, theories, and marketing pressure have a stronger impact.

We believe that an evidence-based approach should be promoted and favored as much as possible, to help make the best decisions. This is often a difficult task, because it is not easy to have access to the appropriate data, to analyze them and to draw clear conclusions, and this is where working groups such as the Cochrane and the MDS EBR one are valuable in interpreting the data from clinical trials. Armed with this knowledge, it is then the task of each physician to weigh the benefits and drawbacks of each therapeutic strategy and make the right choice, taking into account the patient's level of disability, personal and professional circumstances, and expectations. These deliberations must be continued as the patient is followed up further, and changes in circumstances, individual response and tolerability, and the relentless progression of the disease make it necessary to adapt each patient's medication on an individualized basis.

References

Adler, C.H., Sethi, K.D., Hauser, R.A., Davis, T.L., Hammerstad, J. P., Bertoni, J., Taylor, R.L., Sanchez-Ramos, J., O'Brien, C.F., for the Ropinirole Study Group (1997) Ropinirole for the treatment of early Parkinson's disease. *Neurology*, **49**, 393–399.

Agarwal, P., Fahn, S. and Frucht, S.J. (2004) Diagnosis and management of pergolide-induced fibrosis. *Movement Disorders*, **19**, 699–704.

Allain, H., Destée, A., Petit, H., Patay, M., Schück, S., Bentué-Ferrer, D. and Le Cavorzin, P. (2000) Five-year follow-up of early lisuride and levodopa combination therapy versus levodopa monotherapy in de novo Parkinson's disease. The French Lisuride Study Group. *European Neurology*, **44**, 22–30.

Andreu, N., Chalé, J.J., Senard, J.M., Thalamas, C., Montastruc, J. L. and Rascol, O. (1999) L-Dopa-induced sedation: a double-blind cross-over controlled study versus triazolam and placebo in healthy volunteers. *Clinical Neuropharmacology*, **22**, 15–23.

Antonini, A. and Poewe, W. (2007) Fibrotic heart-valve reactions to dopamine-agonist treatment in Parkinson's disease. *Lancet Neurology*, **6**, 826–829.

Barone, P., Bravi, D., Bermejo-Pareja, F., Marconi, R., Kulisevsky, J., Malagú, S., Weiser, R., Rost, N., the Pergolide Monotherapy Study Group (1999) Pergolide monotherapy in the treatment of early Parkinson's disease: A randomized, controlled study. *Neurology*, **53**, 573–579.

Bergamasco, B., Frattola, L., Muratorio, A., Piccoli, F., Mailland, F. and Parnetti, L. (2000) Alpha-dihydroergocryptine in the treatment of de novo parkinsonian patients: results of a multicentre, randomised, double-blind, placebo-controlled study. *Acta Neurologica Scandinavica*, **101**, 372–380.

Bhatt, M.H., Keenan, S.P., Fleetham, J.A. and Calne, D.B. (1991) Pleuropulmonary disease associated with dopamine agonist therapy. *Annals of Neurology*, **30**, 613–616.

Birkmayer W., Hornykiewicz, O. (1961) The L-3,4-dioxyphenylalanine (DOPA)-effect in Parkinson-akinesia. *Wiener Klinische Wochenschrift*, **73**, 787–788.

Block, G., Liss, C., Scott, R., Irr, J. and Nibbelink, D. (1997) Comparison of immediate-release and controlled release carbidopa/levodopa in Parkinson's disease. A multicenter 5-year study. *European Neurology*, **37**, 23–27.

Bracco, F., Battaglia, A., Chouza, C. *et al.*, the PKDS009 Study Group (2004) The long-acting dopamine receptor agonist cabergoline in early Parkinson's disease: final results of a 5-year, double-blind, levodopa-controlled study. *CNS Drugs*, **18**, 733–746.

Brodsky, M.A., Godbold, J., Roth, T. and Olanow, C.W. (2003) Sleepiness in Parkinson's disease: a controlled study. *Movement Disorders*, **18**, 668–672.

Brotchie, J.M. (2005) Nondopaminergic mechanisms in levodopa-induced dyskinesia. *Movement Disorders*, **20**, 919–931.

Caraceni, T. and Musicco, M. (2001) Levodopa or dopamine agonists, or deprenyl as initial treatment for Parkinson's disease. A randomized multicenter study. *Parkinsonism & Related Disorders*, **7**, 107–114.

Churchyard, A., Mathias, C.J. and Lees, A.J. (1999) Selegiline-induced postural hypotension in Parkinson's disease: a longitudinal study on the effects of drug withdrawal. *Movement Disorders*, **14**, 246–251.

Constantinescu, R., Romer, M., McDermott, M.P., Kamp, C., Kieburtz, K., CALM-PD Investigators of the Parkinson Study Group (2007) Impact of pramipexole on the onset of levodopa-related dyskinesias. *Movement Disorders*, **22**, 1317–1319.

Cotzias, G.C. (1968) L-Dopa for Parkinsonism. *The New England Journal of Medicine*, **278**, 630.

deMarcaida, J.A., Schwid, S.R., White, W.B., Blindauer, K., Fahn, S., Kieburtz, K., Stern, M., Shoulson, I., Parkinson Study Group TEMPO (2006) PRESTO Tyramine Substudy Investigators and Coordinators. Effects of tyramine administration in Parkinson's disease patients treated with selective MAO-B inhibitor rasagiline. *Movement Disorders*, **21**, 1716–1721.

Dewey, R.B., Reimold, S.C. and O'Suilleabhain, P.E. (2007) Cardiac valve regurgitation with pergolide compared with non-ergot agonists in Parkinson disease. *Archives of Neurology*, **64**, 377–380.

Driver-Dunckley, E.D., Noble, B.N., Hentz, J.G., Evidente, V.G., Caviness, J.N., Parish, J., Krahn, L. and Adler, C.H. (2007) Gambling and increased sexual desire with dopaminergic medications in restless legs syndrome. *Clinical Neuropharmacology*, **30**, 249–255.

Dupont, E., Anderson, A., Boqs, J., Boisen, E., Borgmann, R., Helgetveit, A.C., Kjaer, A.C., Kristensen, T.N., Mikkelsen, B., Pakkenberg, H., Presthus, J., Stien, R., Worm-Petersen, J. and Buch, D. (1996) Sustained-release Madopar HBS compared with standard Madopar in the long-term treatment of de novo parkinsonian patients. *Acta Neurologica Scandinavica*, **93**, 14–20.

Ebersbach, G., Norden, J. and Tracik, F. (2000) Sleep attacks in Parkinson's disease: polysomnographic recordings. *Movement Disorders*, **15** (Suppl. 3), 89.

Edwards, I.R. and Aronson, J.K. (2000) Adverse drug reactions: definitions, diagnosis, and management. *Lancet*, **356**, 1255–1259.

Etiman, M., Samii, A., Takkouche, B. and Rochon, P.A. (2001) Increased risk of somnolence with the new dopamine agonists in patients with Parkinson's disease: a meta-analysis of randomised controlled trials. *Drug Safety*, **24**, 863–868.

Evans, A.H., Lawrence, A.D., Potts, J., Appel, S. and Lees, A.J. (2005) Factors influencing susceptibility to compulsive dopaminergic drug use in Parkinson disease. *Neurology*, **65**, 1570–1574.

Evans, A.H., Pavese, N., Lawrence, A.D., Tai, Y.F., Appel, S., Doder, M., Brooks, D.J., Lees, A.J. and Piccini, P. (2006) Compulsive drug use linked to sensitized ventral striatal dopamine transmission. *Annals of Neurology*, **59**, 852–858.

Fabre, N., Montastruc, J.L. and Rascol, O. (1993) Alopecia: an adverse effect of bromocriptine. *Clinical Neuropharmacology*, **16**, 266–268.

Fahn, S., Elton, R.L., Members of the UPDRS development committee (1987) Unified Parkinson's Disease rating scale, in Recent Development in Parkinson's Disease, **Vol. 2** (eds S. Fahn, C.D. Marsden, D.B. Calne and M. Goldstein) MacMillan Healthcare Information, Florham Park, NJ, pp. 153–163.

Fahn, S., Oakes, D., Shoulson, I., Kieburtz, K., Rudolph, A., Lang, A., Olanow, C.W., Tanner, C., Marek, K., Parkinson Study Group (2004) Levodopa and the progression of Parkinson's disease. *The New England Journal of Medicine* **351**, 2498–2508.

Ferreira, J.J., Galitzky, M., Montastruc, J.L. and Rascol, O. (2000) Sleep attacks and Parkinson's disease treatment. *Lancet*, **355**, 1333–1334.

Ferreira, J.J., Thalamas, C., Montastruc, J.L., Castro-Caldas, A. and Rascol, O. (2001) Levodopa monotherapy can induce "sleep attacks" in Parkinson's disease patients. *Journal of Neurology*, **248**, 426–427.

Ferreira, J.J., Galitzky, M., Thalamas, C., Tiberge, M., Montastruc, J.L., Sampaio, C. and Rascol, O. (2002) Effect of ropinirole on sleep onset: a randomized, placebo-controlled study in healthy volunteers. *Neurology*, **58**, 460–462.

Ferreira, J.J., Desboeuf, K., Galitzky, M., Thalamas, C., Brefel-Courbon, C., Fabre, N., Senard, J.M., Montastruc, J.L., Sampaio, C. and Rascol, O. (2006) Sleep disruption, daytime somnolence and 'sleep attacks' in Parkinson's disease: a clinical survey in PD patients and age-matched healthy volunteers. *European Journal of Neurology*, **13**, 209–214.

Frucht, S., Rogers, J.D., Greene, P.E., Gordon, M.F. and Fahn, S. (1999) Falling asleep at the wheel: motor vehicle mishaps in persons taking pramipexole and ropinirole. *Neurology*, **52**, 1908–1910.

Giladi, N., Boroojerdi, B., Korczyn, A.D., Burn, D.J., Clarke, C.E., Schapira, A.H., SP513 Investigators (2007a) Rotigotine transdermal patch in early Parkinson's disease: A randomized, double-blind, controlled study versus placebo and ropinirole. *Movement Disorders*, **22**, 2398–2404.

Giladi, N., Weitzman, N., Schreiber, S., Shabtai, H. and Peretz, C. (2007b) New onset heightened interest or drive for gambling, shopping, eating or sexual activity in patients with Parkinson's disease: the role of dopamine agonist treatment and age at motor symptoms onset. *Journal of Psychopharmacology*, **21**, 501–506.

Goetz, C.G., Poewe, W., Rascol, O. and Sampaio, C. (2005) Evidence-based medical review update: Pharmacological and surgical treatments of Parkinson's disease: 2001 to 2004. *Movement Disorders*, **20**, 523–539.

Grosset, K., Grosset, D., Lees, A., Parkinson's Disease Research Group of the United Kingdom (2005) Trial of subtherapeutic pergolide in de novo Parkinson's disease. *Movement Disorders*, **20**, 363–366.

Hauser, R.A., Rascol, O., Korczyn, A.D., Stoessl, J.A., Watts, R.L., Poewe, W., De Deyn, P.P. and Lang, A.E. (2007) Ten-year follow-up of Parkinson's disease patients randomized to initial therapy with ropinirole or levodopa. *Movement Disorders*, **22**, 2409–2417.

Hely, M.A., Morris, J.G., Reid, W.G., O'Sullivan, D.J., Williamson, P.M., Rail, D., Broe, G.A. and Margrie, S. (1994) The Sydney Multicentre Study of Parkinson's disease: a randomised, prospective five year study comparing low dose bromocriptine with low dose levodopa-carbidopa. *Journal of Neurology, Neurosurgery, and Psychiatry*, **57**, 903–910.

Hely, M.A., Morris, J.G., Traficante, R., Reid, W.G., O'Sullivan, D.J. and Williamson, P.M. (1999) The sydney multicentre study of Parkinson's disease: progression and mortality at 10 years. *Journal of Neurology, Neurosurgery, and Psychiatry*, **67**, 300–307.

Hely, M.A., Morris, J.G.L., Reid, W.G.J. and Trafficante, R. (2005) Sydney multicenter study of Parkinson's disease: Non-L-dopaLevodopa-responsive problems dominate at 15 years. *Movement Disorders*, **20**, 190–199.

Hobson, D.E., Lang, A.E., Martin, W.R., Razmy, A., Rivest, J. and Fleming, J. (2002) Excessive daytime sleepiness and sudden-onset sleep in Parkinson disease: a survey by the Canadian Movement Disorders Group. *The Journal of the American Medical Association*, **287**, 455–463.

Holloway, R.G., Shoulson, I., Fahn, S., Kieburtz, K., Lang, A., Marek, K., McDermott, M., Seibyl, J., Weiner, W., Musch, B., Kamp, C., Welsh, M., Shinaman, A., Pahwa, R., Barclay, L., Hubble, J., LeWitt, P., Miyasaki, J., Suchowersky, O., Stacy, M., Russell, D.S., Ford, B., Hammerstad, J., Riley, D., Standaert, D., Wooten, F., Factor, S., Jankovic, J., Atassi, F., Kurlan, R., Panisset, M., Rajput, A., Rodnitzky, R., Shults, C., Petsinger, G., Waters, C., Pfeiffer, R., Biglan, K., Borchert, L., Montgomery, A., Sutherland, L., Weeks, C., DeAngelis, M., Sime, E., Wood, S., Pantella, C., Harrigan, M., Fussell, B., Dillon, S., Alexander-Brown, B., Rainey, P., Tennis, M., Rost-Ruffner, E., Brown, D., Evans, S., Berry, D., Hall, J., Shirley, T., Dobson, J., Fontaine, D., Pfeiffer, B., Brocht, A., Bennett, S., Daigneault, S., Hodgeman, K., O'Connell, C., Ross, T., Richard, K., Watts, A., Parkinson Study Group (2004) Pramipexole vs levodopa as initial treatment for Parkinson disease: a 4-year randomized controlled trial. *Archives of Neurology*, **61**, 1044–1053.

Homann, C.N., Wenzel, K., Suppan, K., Feichtinger, M., Ivanic, G., Kriechbaum, N. and Ott, E. (2000) Sleep attacks after acute administration of apomorphine. *Movement Disorders*, **15**, 585.

Homann, C.N., Suppan, K., Wenzel, K., Ivanic, G., Kriechbaum, N. and Ott, E. (2002) Sleep attacks with apomorphine. *Wiener Klinische Wochenschrift*, **114**, 430–431.

Horvath, J., Fross, R.D., Kleiner-Fisman, G., Lerch, R., Stalder, H., Liaudat, S., Raskoff, W.J., Flachsbart, K.D., Rakowski, H., Pache, J.C., Burkhard, P.R. and Lang, A.E. (2004) Severe multivalvular heart disease: a new complication of the ergot derivative dopamine agonists. *Movement Disorders*, **19**, 656–662.

Junghanns, S., Fuhrmann, J.T., Simonis, G., Oelwein, C., Koch, R., Strasser, R.H., Reichmann, H. and Storch, A. (2007) Valvular heart disease in Parkinson's disease patients treated with dopamine agonists: a reader-blinded monocenter echocardiography study. *Movement Disorders*, **22**, 234–238.

Katzenschlager, R., Head, J., Schrag, A., Ben-Shlomo, Y., Evans, A. and Lees, A.J., on behalf of the Parkinson's Disease Research Group of the United Kingdom (2008) 14-year final report of the randomized PDRG-UK trial comparing three initial treatments in PD. *Neurology*, **71**, 474–480.

Katzenschlager, R., Sampaio, C., Costa, J. and Lees, A. (2003) Anticholinergics for symptomatic management of Parkinson's disease. *Cochrane Database of Systematic Reviews*, (2), CD003735.

Koller, W.C., Hutton, J.T., Tolosa, E., Capildeo, R., Carbidopa/Levodopa Study Group (1999) Immediate-release and controlled-release carbidopa/levodopa in PD: a 5-year randomized multicenter study. *Neurology*, **53**, 1012–1019.

Korczyn, A.D., Brooks, D.J., Brunt, E.R., Poewe, W.H., Rascol, O., Stocchi, F., on behalf of the 053 Study Group (1998) Ropinirole versus bromocriptine in the treatment of early Parkinson's disease: 6-month interim report of a 3-year study. *Movement Disorders*, **13**, 46–51.

Korczyn, A.D., Brunt, E.R., Larsen, J.P., Nagy, Z., Poewe, W.H. and Ruggieri, S. (1999) A 3-year randomized trial of ropinirole and bromocriptine in early Parkinson's disease. The 053 Study Group. *Neurology*, **53**, 364–370.

Lane, R.J.M. and Rontledge, P.A. (1983) Drug-induced neurological disorders. *Drugs*, **26**, 124–147.

Lawrence, A.D., Evans, A.H. and Lees, A.J. (2003) Compulsive use of dopamine replacement therapy in Parkinson's disease: reward systems gone awry? *Lancet Neurology*, **2**, 595–604.

Lees, A.J., Katzenschlager, R., Head, J., Ben-Shlomo, Y., on behalf of the Parkinson's Disease Research Group of the United Kingdom (2001) Ten-year follow-up of three different initial treatments in de-novo PD. *Neurology*, **57**, 1687–1694.

Lees, A.J. (1995) Comparison of therapeutic effects and mortality data of levodopa and levodopa combined with selegiline in patients with early, mild Parkinson's disease. Parkinson's Disease Research Group of the United Kingdom. *BMJ*, **311**, 1602–1607.

Ling, L.H., Ahlskog, J.E., Munger, T.M., Limper, A.H. and Oh, J. K. (1999) Constrictive pericarditis and pleuropulmonary disease linked to ergot dopamine agonist therapy (cabergoline) for Parkinson's disease. *Mayo Clinic Proceedings*, **74**, 371–375.

Mamikonyan, E., Siderowf, A.D., Duda, J.E., Potenza, M.N., Horn, S., Stern, M.B. and Weintraub, D. (2008) Long-term follow-up of impulse control disorders in Parkinson's disease. *Movement Disorders*, **23**, 75–80.

Manni, R., Terzaghi, M., Sartori, I., Mancini, F. and Pacchetti, C. (2004) Dopamine agonists and sleepiness in PD: review of the literature and personal findings. *Sleep Medicine*, **5**, 189–193.

Martindale (2005) The Complete Drug Reference. 34th edn London Pharmaceutical Press.

Mizuno, Y., Kondo, T. and Narabayashi, H. Pergolide in the treatment of Parkinson's disease. *Neurology* 1995; **45** (3 Suppl 3), S13–S21.

Mondal, B.K. and Suri, S. (2000) Pergolide-induced retroperitoneal fibrosis. *International Journal of Clinical Practice*, **54**, 403.

Montastruc, J.L., Desboeuf, K., Lapeyre-Mestre, M., Senard, J.M., Rascol, O. and Brefel-Courbon, C. (2001) Long-term mortality results of the randomized controlled study comparing bromocriptine to which levodopa was later added with levodopa alone in previously untreated patients with Parkinson's disease. *Movement Disorders*, **16**, 511–514.

Montastruc, J.L., Brefel-Courbon, C., Senard, J.M., Bagheri, H., Ferreira, J., Rascol, O. and Lapeyre-Mestre, M. (2001b) Sleep attacks and antiparkinsonian drugs: a pilot prospective pharmacoepidemiologic study. *Clinical Neuropharmacology*, **24**, 181–183.

Montastruc, J.L., Rascol, O., Senard, J.M. and Rascol, A. (1994) A randomised controlled study comparing bromocriptine to which levodopa was later added, with levodopa alone in previously untreated patients with Parkinson's disease:a five year follow-up. *Journal of Neurology, Neurosurgery, and Psychiatry*, **57**, 1034–1038.

Movement Disorder Society (2002) Management of Parkinson's Disease: An Evidence-Based Review; Supplement **4**, S1–S166.

Müller, T., Przuntek, H. and Kuhlmann, A. (2003) Loss of color vision during long-term treatment with pramipexole. *Journal of Neurology*, **250**, 101–102.

Murer, M.G., Dziewczapolski, G., Menalled, L.B., García, M.C., Agid, Y., Gershanik, O. and Raisman-Vozari, R. (1998) Chronic levodopa is not toxic for remaining dopamine neurons, but instead promotes their recovery, in rats with moderate nigrostriatal lesions. *Annals of Neurology*, **43**, 561–575.

Nutt, J.G. (2007) Continuous dopaminergic stimulation: Is it the answer to the motor complications of Levodopa? *Movement Disorders*, **22**, 1–9.

Oertel, W.H., Wolters, E., Sampaio, C., Gimenez-Roldan, S., Bergamasco, B., Dujardin, M., Grosset, D.G., Arnold, G., Leenders, K.L., Hundemer, H.P., Lledo, A., Wood, A., Frewer, P. and Schwarz, J. (2006) Pergolide versus levodopa monotherapy in early Parkinson's disease patients: The PELMOPET study. *Movement Disorders*, **21**, 343–353.

Olanow, C.W., Hauser, R.A., Gauger, L., Malapira, T., Koller, W., Hubble, J., Bushenbark, K., Lilienfeld, D. and Esterlitz, J. (1995) The effect of deprenyl and levodopa on the pro- gression of Parkinson's disease. *Annals of Neurology*, **38** (5), 771–777.

Olanow, C.W., Agid, Y., Mizuno, Y., Albanese, A., Bonuccelli, U., Damier, P., De Yebenes, J., Gershanik, O., Guttman, M., Grandas, F., Hallett, M., Hornykiewicz, O., Jenner, P., Katzenschlager, R., Langston, W.J., LeWitt, P., Melamed, E., Mena, M.A., Michel, P.P., Mytilineou, C., Obeso, J.A., Poewe, W., Quinn, N., Raisman-Vozari, R., Rajput, A.H., Rascol, O., Sampaio, C. and Stocchi, F. (2004) Levodopa in the treatment of Parkinson's disease: current controversies. *Movement Disorders*, **19**, 997–1005.

Olanow, C.W., Obeso, J.A. and Stocchi, F. (2006) Drug insight: Continuous dopaminergic stimulation in the treatment of Parkinson's disease. *Nature Clinical Practice Neurology*, **2**, 382–392.

Ondo, W.G., Fayle, R., Atassi, F. and Jankovic, J. (2005) Modafinil for daytime somnolence in Parkinson's disease: double blind, placebo controlled parallel trial. *Journal of Neurology, Neurosurgery, and Psychiatry*, **76**, 1636–1639.

Parkinson Study Group PRECEPT Investigators (2007) Mixed lineage kinase inhibitor CEP-1347 fails to delay disability in early Parkinson disease. *Neurology*, **69**, 1480–1490.

Parkinson Study Group (1993) Effects of tocopherol and deprenyl on the progression of disability in early Parkinson's disease. *N Engl J Med* **328**, 176–183.

Parkinson Study Group (2002) A controlled trial of rasagiline in early Parkinson disease: the TEMPO Study. *Archives of Neurology*, **59**, 1937–1943.

Parkinson Study Group (2004) A controlled, randomized, delayed-start study of rasagiline in early Parkinson disease. *Archives of Neurology*, **61**, 561–566.

Parkinson Study Group (2002b) Dopamine transporter brain imaging to assess the effects of pramipexole vs levodopa on Parkinson disease progression. *The Journal of the American Medical Association*, **287**, 1653–1661.

Parkinson Study Group (1996) Impact of deprenyl and tocopherol treatment of Parkinson's disease in DATATOP subjects not requiring levodopa. *Annals of Neurology*, **39**, 29–36.

Parkinson Study Group (2000) Pramipexole versus levodopa as initial treatment for Parkinson's disease: a randomized controlled trial. *The Journal of the American Medical Association*, **284**, 1931–1938.

Parkinson's Disease Research Group in the United Kingdom (1993) Comparisons of therapeutic effects of levodopa, levodopa and selegiline, and bromocriptine in patients with early, mild Parkinson's disease: three year interim report. *British Medical Journal*, **307**, 469–472.

Paus, S., Brecht, H.M., Köster, J., Seeger, G., Klockgether, T. and Wüllner, U. (2003) Sleep attacks, daytime sleepiness, and dopamine agonists in Parkinson's disease. *Movement Disorders*, **18**, 659–667.

Pearce, R.K., Banerji, T., Jenner, P. and Marsden, C.D. (1998) *De novo* administration of ropinirole and bromocriptine induces less dyskinesia than L-dopa in the MPTP-treated marmoset. *Movement Disorders*, **13**, 234–241.

Peralta, C., Wolf, E., Alber, H., Seppi, K., Müller, S., Bösch, S., Wenning, G.K., Pachinger, O. and Poewe, W. (2006) Valvular heart disease in Parkinson's disease vs. controls: An echocardiographic study. *Movement Disorders*, **21**, 1109–1113.

Poewe, W., Rascol, O., Watts, R., Lang, A., Stoessl, J. and Hauser, R. (2005) 5-year follow-up of patients with early Parkinson's disease (PD) initially receiving ropinirole compared with L-dopa in the REAL-PET study. *Parkinsonism & Related Disorders*, **11** (Suppl. 2), 215.

Pontone, G., Williams, J.R., Bassett, S.S. and Marsh, L. (2006) Clinical features associated with impulse control disorders in Parkinson disease. *Neurology*, **67**, 1258–1261.

Przuntek, H., Welzel, D., Gerlach, M., Blumner, E., Danielczyk, W., Kaiser, H.J., Krauss, P.H., Letzel, H., Riederer, P. and Uberla, K. (1996) Early institution of bromocriptine in Parkinson's disease inhibits the emergence of levodopa-associated motor side effects. Long-term results of the PRADO study. *Journal of Neural Transmission*, **103**, 699–715.

Rascol, O., Olanow, W., Brooks, D., Koch, G., Truffinet, P. and Bejuit, R. (2002) A 2-year multicenter placebo-controlled double-blind parallel group study of the effect of riluzole on Parkinson's disease progression. *Movement Disorders*, **17** (Suppl. 5), 39.

Rascol, O. (2006a) Defining a minimal clinically relevant difference for the unified Parkinson's rating scale: An important but still unmet need. *Movement Disorders*, **21**, 1059–1061.

Rascol, O., Brooks, D.J., Brunt, E.R., Korczyn, A.D., Poewe, W.H., Stocchi, F., on behalf of the 056 Study Group (1998) Ropinirole in the treatment of early Parkinson's disease: a 6-month interim report of a 5-year levodopa-controlled study. *Movement Disorders*, **13**, 39–45.

Rascol, O., Brooks, D.J., Korczyn, A.D., De Deyn, P.P., Clarke, C.E. and Lang, A.E. for the 056 Study Group (2000) A five-year study of the incidence of dyskinesia in patients with early Parkinson's disease who were treated with ropinirole or levodopa. *The New England Journal of Medicine*, **342**, 1484–1491.

Rascol, O., Brooks, D.J., Korczyn, A.D., De Deyn, P.P., Clarke, C.E., Lang, A.E., Abdalla, M., 056 Study Group (2006b) Development of dyskinesias in a 5-year trial of ropinirole and L-dopa. *Movement Disorders*, **21**, 1844–1850(b).

Rascol, O., Dubois, B., Caldas, A.C., Senn, S., Del Signore, S., Lees, A., Parkinson REGAIN Study Group (2006b) Early piribedil monotherapy of Parkinson's disease: A planned seven-month report of the REGAIN study. *Movement Disorders*, **21**, 2110–2115.

Rawlins, M.D. and Thompson, G.W. (1977) Pathogenesis of adverse drug reactions, in Textbook of Adverse Drug Reactions (ed. D.M. Davies), Oxford University Press, p. 44.

Razmy, A., Lang, A.E. and Shapiro, C.M. (2004) Predictors of impaired daytime sleep and wakefulness in patients with Parkinson disease treated with older (ergot) vs newer (nonergot) dopamine agonists. *Archives of Neurology*, **61**, 97–102.

Rinne, U.K., Bracco, F., Chouza, C., Dupont, E., Gershanik, O., Marti masso, J.F., Montastruc, J.L., Marsden, C.D., the PKDS009 Study Group (1998) Early treatment of Parkinson's disease with cabergoline delays the onset of motor complications. *Drugs*, **55** (Suppl. 1), 23–30.

Rinne, U.K., Bracco, F., Chouza, C., Dupont, E., Gershanik, O., Marti Masso, J.F., Montastruc, J.L., Marsden, C.D., Dubini, A., Orlando, N. and Grimaldi, R. (1997) Cabergoline in the treatment of early Parkinson's disease: results of the first year of treatment in a double-blind comparison of cabergoline and levodopa. The PKDS009 Collaborative Study Group. *Neurology*, **48**, 363–368.

Rinne, U.K. (1989) Lisuride, a dopamine agonist in the treatment of early Parkinson's disease. *Neurology*, **39**, 336–339.

Riopelle, R.J. (1987) Bromocriptine and the clinical spectrum of Parkinson's disease. *The Canadian Journal of Neurological Sciences*, **14** (Suppl), 455–459.

Ryan, M., Slevin, J.T. and Wells, A. (2000) Non-ergot dopamine agonist-induced sleep attacks. *Pharmacotherapy*, **20**, 724–726.

Sadeh, M., Braham, J. and Modan, M. (1982) Effects of anticholinergic drugs on memory in Parkinson's disease. *Archives of Neurology*, **39**, 666–667.

Schapira, A.H. and Obeso, J. (2006) Timing of treatment initiation in Parkinson's disease: a need for reappraisal? *Annals of Neurology*, **59**, 559–562.

Scharpira, A.H.V. (2000) Sleep attacks (sleep episodes) with pergolide [letter]. *Lancet*, **355**, 1332.

Schlesinger, I. and Ravin, P.D. (2003) Dopamine agonists induce episodes of irresistible daytime sleepiness. *European Neurology*, **49**, 30–33.

Schrag, A., Sampaio, C., Counsell, N. and Poewe, W. (2006) Minimal clinically important change on the unified Parkinson's disease rating scale. *Movement Disorders*, **21**, 1200–1207.

Shannon, K.M., Bennett, J.P., Friedman, J.H., for the Pramipexole Study Group (1997) Efficacy of pramipexole, a novel dopamine agonist, as monotherapy in mild to moderate Parkinson's disease. *Neurology*, **49**, 724–728.

Shaunak, S., Wilkins, A., Pilling, J.B. and Dick, D.J. (1999) Pericardial, retroperitoneal, and pleural fibrosis induced by pergolide. *Journal of Neurology, Neurosurgery, and Psychiatry*, **66**, 79–81.

Shoulson, I., Oakes, D., Fahn, S., Lang, A., Langston, J.W., LeWitt, P., Olanow, C.W., Penney, J.B., Tanner, C., Kieburtz, K., Rudolph, A., Parkinson Study Group (2002) Impact of sustained deprenyl (selegiline) in levodopa-treated Parkinson's disease: a randomized placebo-controlled extension of the deprenyl and tocopherol antioxidative therapy of parkinsonism trial. *Annals of Neurology*, **51**, 604–612.

Shults, C.W., Oakes, D., Kieburtz, K., Beal, M.F., Haas, R., Plumb, S., Juncos, J.L., Nutt, J., Shoulson, I., Carter, J., Kompoliti, K., Perlmutter, J.S., Reich, S., Stern, M., Watts, R.L., Kurlan, R., Molho, E., Harrison, M., Lew, M., Parkinson Study Group (2002) Effects of coenzyme Q10 in early Parkinson disease: evidence of slowing of the functional decline. *Archives of Neurology*, **59**, 1541–1550.

Smith, L.A., Jackson, M.J., Al-Barghouthy, G., Rose, S., Kuoppamaki, M., Olanow, W. and Jenner, P. (2005) Multiple small doses of levodopa plus entacapone produce continuous dopaminergic stimulation and reduce dyskinesia induction in MPTP-treated drug-naive primates. *Movement Disorders*, **20**, 306–314.

Stocchi, F. and Giorgi, L. (2006) Efficacy of ropinirole 24-hour prolonged release compared with ropinirole immediate release in early Parkinson's disease: the EASE-PD Monotherapy Study. *European Journal of Neurology*, **13** (suppl 2), 205.

Tan, E.K. (2003) Piribedil-induced sleep attacks in Parkinson's disease. *Fundamental & Clinical Pharmacology*, **17**, 117–119.

Tandberg, E., Larsen, J.P. and Karlsen, K. (1999) Excessive daytime sleepiness and sleep benefit in Parkinson's disease: a community-based study. *Movement Disorders*, **14**, 922–927.

The NINDS NET-PD investigators (2007) A randomized clinical trial of coenzyme Q10 and GPI-1485 in early Parkinson disease. *Neurology*, **68**, 20–28.

The NINDS NET-PD Investigators (2006) A randomized, double-blind, futility clinical trial of creatine and minocycline in early Parkinson disease. *Neurology*, **66**, 664–671.

Van Camp, G., Flamez, A., Cosyns, B., *et al.* (2004) Treatment of Parkinson's disease with pergolide and relation to restrictive valvular heart disease. *Lancet*, **363**, 1179–1183.

Vergeret, J., Barat, M., Taytard, A., Bellvert, P., Domblides, P., Douvier, J.J. and Fréour, P. (1984) Pleuropulmonary fibrosis and bromocriptine. *Semaine des Hôpitaux*, **60**, 741–744.

Voon, V., Hassan, K., Zurowski, M., de Souza, M., Thomsen, T., Fox, S., Lang, A.E. and Miyasaki, J. (2006) Prevalence of repetitive and reward-seeking behaviors in Parkinson's disease. *Neurology*, **67**, 1254–1257.

Voon, V. and Fox, S.H. (2007) Medication-related impulse control and repetitive behaviors in Parkinson disease. *Archives of Neurology*, **64**, 1089–1096.

Watts, R.L., Jankovic, J., Waters, C., Rajput, A., Boroojerdi, B. and Rao, J. (2007) Randomized, blind, controlled trial of transdermal rotigotine in early Parkinson disease. *Neurology*, **68**, 272–276.

Weintraub, D., Siderowf, A.D., Potenza, M.N., Goveas, J., Morales, K.H., Duda, J.E., Moberg, P.J. and Stern, M.B. (2006) Association of dopamine agonist use with impulse control disorders in Parkinson disease. *Archives of Neurology*, **63**, 969–973.

Whone, A.L., Watts, R.L., Stoessl, A.J., Davis, M., Reske, S., Nahmias, C., Lang, A.E., Rascol, O., Ribeiro, M.J., Remy, P., Poewe, W.H., Hauser, R.A., Brooks, D.J., REAL-PET Study Group (2003) Slower progression of Parkinson's disease with ropinirole versus levodopa: The REAL-PET study. *Annals of Neurology*, **54**, 93–101.

Yamamoto, M., Uesugi, T. and Nakayama, T. (2006) Dopamine agonists and cardiac valvulopathy in Parkinson disease: a case-control study. *Neurology*, **67**, 1225–1229.

Zanettini, R., Antonini, A., Gatto, G., Gentile, R., Tesei, S. and Pezzoli, G. (2007) Valvular heart disease and the use of dopamine agonists for Parkinson's disease. *The New England Journal of Medicine*, **356**, 39–46.

5

Treatment of Motor Complications in Advanced Parkinson's Disease

Susan H. Fox and Anthony E. Lang

Toronto Western Hospital, Movement Disorders Clinic, Division
of Neurology, University of Toronto, Toronto, Canada

INTRODUCTION

Early treatment of Parkinson's disease (PD) with dopaminergic drugs, including dopamine agonists and levodopa, results in effective and sustained control of motor symptoms which may last for several years. With progression of the disease and the requirement for higher doses of levodopa, the vast majority of patients start to experience a variety of problems, including a reduced and variable benefit from medication, with a range of motor and non-motor symptoms. These motor problems can be divided into those that are drug-responsive, including motor fluctuations and dyskinesia and those that are either less or non-drug-responsive, including speech, swallowing, drooling problems, gait and balance, and drug resistant tremor (Tables 5.1 and 5.2). Treatment of associated non-motor symptoms is further discussed in Chapter 6.

DRUG-RESPONSIVE MOTOR COMPLICATIONS

Motor Fluctuations

A PD patient exhibiting parkinsonian symptoms when medication benefit wanes is described as being "OFF" (in the text indicated as OFF) and an improvement in symptoms in response to dopaminergic medication is termed "on" (ON). Thus, the emergence of motor fluctuations is apparent when a patient starts to notice these two states and reports variable responses to levodopa. At the same time, patients often experience involuntary movements, dyskinesia. Levodopa-induced dyskinesia can occur at variable times in the levodopa cycle. A careful history of the patient's problems in relation to the timing of a dose of

levodopa is critical to management and treatment of motor fluctuations (Table 5.3).

Predictable Fluctuations: Wearing-Off

Clinical Features

In early PD, the clinical response to a single dose of levodopa is stable and lasts for several hours, despite the half-life of levodopa being only 60–90 minutes (Muenter and Tyce, 1971). The first motor fluctuation that is usually appreciated by the patient is a predictable shortening in the duration of response to levodopa with gradual emergence of parkinsonian symptoms, called "wearing-off" or end-of-dose deterioration (Shoulson, Glaubiger and Chase, 1975; Fahn, 1982). The earliest manifestation of this is usually "morning akinesia" since the time between doses is generally longest overnight before the morning dose or alternatively, symptoms emerge if the patient forgets or is delayed in taking a dose during the day. As a result they become more reliant on the timing of the doses of levodopa and begin to shorten the time intervals between doses to usually less than four hours. Some PD patients also experience a predictable loss of benefit, or further shortening of the duration of action, in response to exercise.

Mechanisms

Wearing-off symptoms are probably due to a progressive loss of presynaptic dopaminergic terminals with a loss of dopamine storage (Verhagen Metman, Konitsiotis and Chase, 2000). Loss of dopaminergic terminals means levodopa is converted to dopamine in other aromatic acid-decarboxylase containing cells, such as serotonergic and endothelial cells (Ng, Colburn and Kopin, 1971; Melamed, Hefti and Wurtman, 1980). These cells lack the ability to

Therapeutics of Parkinson's Disease and Other Movement Disorders   Edited by Mark Hallett and Werner Poewe
© 2008 John Wiley & Sons, Ltd.

Table 5.1 Levodopa-responsive motor complications Motor Fluctuations.

Motor Fluctuations
   Predictable
      End of dose deterioration/wearing-off
   Unpredictable
      Unpredictable OFF or sudden OFF
      Delayed ON or partial ON or dose failure
      Beginning or end-of-dose worsening
      ON–OFF fluctuations
   Dyskinesia
      Peak-dose dyskinesia
      Diphasic dyskinesia (Beginning and
        end-of-dose dyskinesia)
      OFF period and wearing-off dystonia

store dopamine and thus non-regulated release of dopamine into the synaptic space may cause fluctuations. In addition, post-synaptic mechanisms may also play a role (see Chapter 1).

Treatment (Figure 5.1)

- *Alter Dose Interval or Preparation of Levodopa*: end-of-dose or wearing-off phenomenon, if mild, can be initially treated by decreasing the time interval between each dose of levodopa to give the next dose just before the beneficial effects have worn off. Alternatively or in addition, if the patient is not experiencing dyskinesia and OFF periods predominate, then individual doses of levodopa can be increased. In advanced PD, increasing individual doses of levodopa will not improve the quality of the ON period, but will simply increase the duration (Nutt and Woodward 1986; Marsden, 1994).

    Longer-acting levodopa preparations such as levodopa/carbidopa (Sinemet) CR or levodopa/benserazide (Madopar) CR may help improve ON time by 1–1.5 hours (Ahlskog *et al.*, 1988; MacMahon *et al.*, 1990). However, double-blind randomized controlled trials

Table 5.2 Levodopa non-responsive motor complications.

Speech problems
Dysphagia
Drooling
Freezing of gait
Postural instability/falls
Drug-resistant tremor

Table 5.3 Definitions of ON and OFF periods in response to levodopa.

ON	Patient experiences improved PD symptoms after taking levodopa
Beginning of dose	Onset of effect of levodopa; usually within 15–30 min post dose
Peak dose	Time of maximal improvement in PD symptoms
End of dose	Time when effects of levodopa start to wane.
OFF	Patient experiences PD symptoms

(RCTs) have shown no significant difference with standard levodopa preparations in reducing OFF time (Jankovic *et al.*, 1989; Lieberman *et al.*, 1990) and, as such, are not recommended to reduce OFF time by the American Academy of Neurology Practice Parameter (level C recommendation); for definitions see Pahwa *et al.*, 2006). The bioavailability of these longer-acting preparations is 20–30% less than standard release preparations and patients usually end up on higher overall daily doses of levodopa, with a risk of exacerbating dyskinesia, particularly later in the day (Lieberman *et al.*, 1990). In addition, these preparations also typically have a longer latency to benefit so patients may experience "delayed-on" problems; especially if doses are not overlapping (i.e., the patient wears OFF before the next dose). The commonest use for these long-lasting preparations is as a last dose of the day to reduce nocturnal or early morning OFF period symptoms.

- *Add a catechol-O-methytransferease (COMT) inhibitor*: COMT is an enzyme involved in the breakdown of levodopa and dopamine to methylated derivatives. Inhibition of this enzyme therefore increases the elimination half-life of levodopa, thus increasing bioavailability (Ruottinen and Rinne, 1996a). There are currently two COMT inhibitors available, entacapone and tolcapone. Tolcapone is administered three times daily, usually in 100 mg doses, irrespective of levodopa dosing. The shorter half life of entacapone, (one hour) means that each 200 mg dose has to be co-administered with levodopa, up to 9–10 times per day, as necessary. A combined preparation of levodopa/carbidopa and entacapone (Stalevo) in a single tablet is now available (Koller *et al.*, 2005). There is no difference in efficacy between standard levodopa/carbidopa with entacapone compared to Stalevo, but rather increased patient preference for the combined rather than the separate tablets (Brooks *et al.*, 2005).

    Many clinical trials have demonstrated improved ON time with the addition of entacapone (Ruottinen

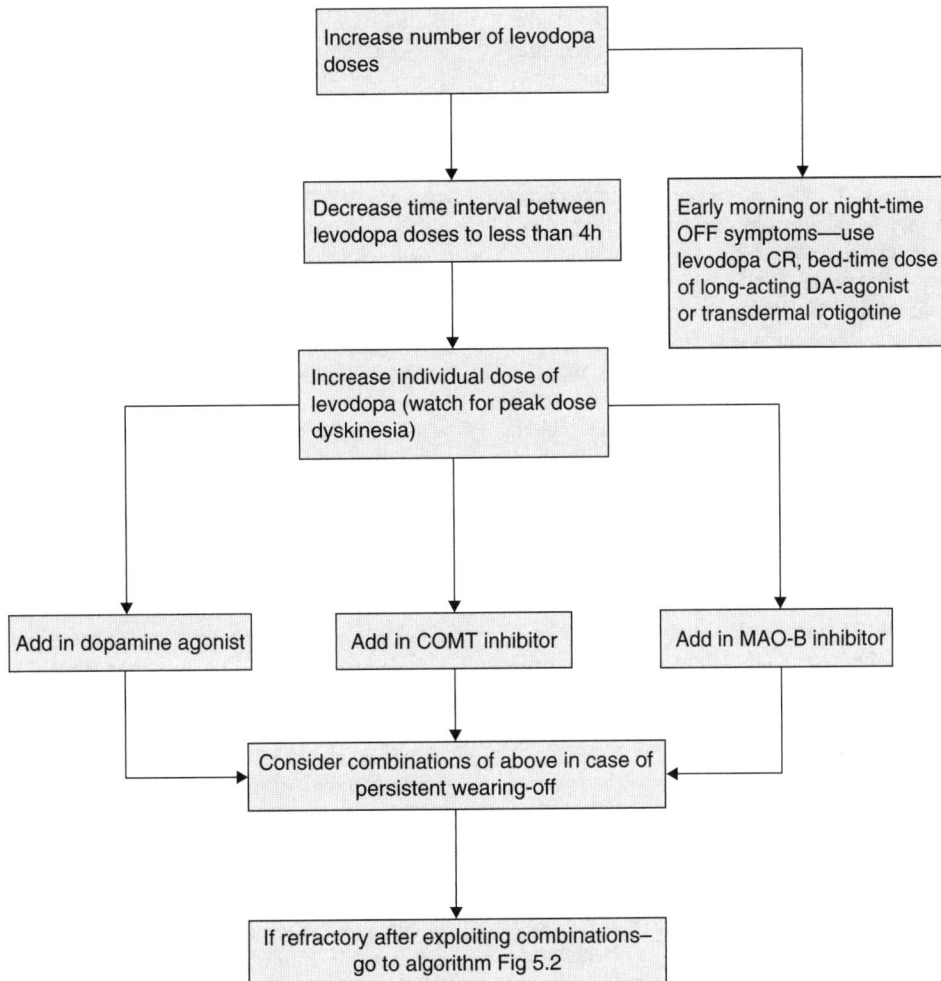

Figure 5.1 Algorithm of practical approach to management of predictable wearing off.

and Rinne, 1996b; Parkinson Study Group, 1997) or tolcapone (Rajput *et al.*, 1997; Kurth *et al.*, 1997) to levodopa; on average by 1–2 hours. In open-label extension studies, three-year follow up of the six-month double-blind RCT (NOMECOMT trial) (Rinne *et al.*, 1998) showed on-going benefit, with 64% of patients reporting benefit (Larsen *et al.*, 2003). There are no differences in the responses obtained using levodopa/carbidopa, levodopa/benserazide preparations or with controlled release preparations of levodopa (Poewe *et al.*, 2002). However, the clinical benefit of entacapone in PD patients with fluctuations may be rather modest. A three-year follow-up study of 222 patients found that 122 (56%) had discontinued entacapone, 46% due to lack of efficacy (Parashos, Wielinski and Kern, 2004).

Early side effects of COMT inhibitors include prolongation of existing ON period dyskinesia. In addition, as the level of levodopa may accumulate following repeated dosing, severity of dyskinesia may also increase (Ruottinen and Rinne, 1996a; Kurth *et al.*, 1997; Muller *et al.*, 2000). Dyskinesia can be improved by reducing the dose of levodopa, usually by 20% (Myllyla *et al.*, 2001). Later side effects include abdominal pain and severe, explosive diarrhoea that can occur after a few weeks of treatment and may lead to discontinuation in 5% patients (Rajput *et al.*, 1997; Myllyla *et al.*, 2001). A recent study has also shown that entacapone 100 mg is equally efficacious to the usual 200 mg, in Japanese PD patients with wearing-off and with improved tolerability (Mizuno *et al.*, 2007).

Tolcapone can cause significant elevation of transa-minases, which occurs in about 3% of patients and three unmonitored patients died of acute hepatic failure before this complication was recognized (Rajput et al., 1997; Assal et al., 1998). This led to the prior withdrawal of tolcapone; it has now been re-introduced into many countries with a liver enzyme monitoring requirement and restricted use only in those failing other therapies. Entacapone does not cause elevation of liver enzymes (Myllyla et al., 2001).

Although randomized comparative studies have not been performed, it is a common clinical impression that tolcapone may be more efficacious than entacapone in controlling motor fluctuations (Factor et al., 2001; Entacapone to Tolcapone Switch Investigators, 2007). This may relate to the purely peripheral effects of entacapone on degradation of levodopa, as compared to the additional central effects of tolcapone on dopamine metabolism (Kaakkola, Gordin and Mannisto, 1994; Forsberg et al., 2003). The American Academy of Neurology Practice Parameter recommends entacapone to reduce OFF times (level A) (Pahwa et al., 2006). The Movement Disorder Society Evidence-Based Medicine (EBM) Review Task Force recommends entacapone as clinically useful and tolcapone as possibly useful (for definitions of specific recommendations see Goetz et al., 2005)).

- *Add a monoamine oxidase B inhibitor*: Monoamine oxidase B (MAO-B) inhibition can extend the duration of action of levodopa by inhibiting the metabolism of dopamine and increasing dopamine levels by up to 70% in the brain (Riederer and Youdim, 1986). Several early clinical studies demonstrated that the MAO-B inhibitor, selegiline, (Eldepryl), (5–10 mg/d) had a mild effect on PD patients with wearing-off motor fluctuations (Lees et al., 1977; Golbe et al., 1988). There was no benefit in patients with marked, disabling ON–OFF fluctuations and the main side effects related to increased dopamine levels, such as nausea, postural hypotension, hallucinations and dyskinesia, which improved on reduction of the levodopa dose. The earlier concerns of higher risk of death in PD patients taking selegiline combined with levodopa by the UK study (Lees, 1995) have not been confirmed in subsequent meta-analysis (Ives et al., 2004), although these involved studies of patients using selegiline in early PD and similar meta-analysis of the risks of selegiline as add-on in PD patients with motor fluctuations have not been performed.

A new transmucosal preparation of selegiline (Zydis selegiline) is now available. This is placed on the tongue and is rapidly absorbed directly into the systemic circulation (Seager, 1997). This bypasses first pass hepatic metabolism and reduces production of theoretically toxic amphetamine-like metabolites (Clarke et al., 2003). A single double-blind, RCT has shown that Zydis selegiline (2.5 mg/d) significantly reduced total daily OFF time in PD patients with predictable wearing-off, by 2.2 h compared to 0.6 h for placebo (Waters et al., 2004). The main side effects were dizziness, hallucinations, headache and dyskinesia. To date, no comparisons have been made with conventional selegiline in terms of improving wearing-off symptoms.

Rasagiline (Azilcet), a newly developed irreversible MAO-B inhibitor, is 10–15 times more potent than selegiline and is not associated with amphetamine metabolites (Finberg et al., 1999). In a double-blind RCT over 26 weeks, rasagiline 0.5 mg/d and 1 mg/d reduced total daily OFF time by 1.41 and 1.85 hours compared to 0.9 h with placebo, respectively (Parkinson Study Group, 2005). Another RCT using rasagline 1 mg/d showed similar efficacy to entacapone (200 mg/dose of levodopa) in reducing OFF time (−1.18 h for rasagiline; −1.2 h for entacapone compared to −0.4 h for placebo) with the one potential advantage of improved morning akinesia, possibly due to its longer duration of action (Rascol et al., 2005). Side effects with rasagiline were similar to those seen with selegiline.

On a practical basis, the use of MAO-B inhibitors as a treatment for wearing-off in advanced PD patients can be limited due to potential perceived drug interactions. Thus the manufacturers of both selegiline and rasagiline advise concomitant use of selective serotonin reuptake inhibitors (SSRIs) and tricyclic anti-depressants is contraindicated due to the potential risk of the serotonin syndrome. The serotonin syndrome has been reported with use of serotonergic drugs in combination with non-selective MAO inhibitors and consists of mental changes such as confusion and agitation with myoclonus, tremor, hyperreflexia and diaphoresis. However, up to 40% of PD patients have depression and frequently use anti-depressants. A review of experts in treatment of PD, published case reports and adverse experiences reported to the FDA revealed out of 4568 PD patients using selegiline combined with an anti-depressant, 11 patients (0.2%) had symptoms suggestive of serotonin syndrome, with only 2 patients having serious symptoms and no deaths (Richard et al., 1997). This suggests that in clinical practice, serotonin syndrome is extremely rare. The incidence of serotonin syndrome with rasagline is as yet unknown. However, low doses of anti-depressants were allowed in the phase III trials of rasagline, without any reported problems.

The American Academy of Neurology Practice Parameter recommends rasagiline to reduce OFF times (level A), while selegiline has level C recommendation (Pahwa et al., 2006). The Movement Disorder Society EBM Review Task Force reports insufficient data for selegiline as a treatment for motor complications and at the time of the report, rasagiline was undergoing investigation

(Goetz *et al.*, 2005). To date, there are no direct comparison studies of selegiline vs rasagiline as add-on therapy for the treatment of wearing-off.

• *Add a Dopamine Receptor Agonist*: Adding an oral dopamine receptor agonist may be a better option due to the longer duration of action, as well as bypassing erratic gastric absorption, which may be a factor in motor fluctuations (see below), and also may allow a reduction in levodopa. All dopamine agonists in clinical practice, bromocriptine, ropinirole, pergolide, pramipexole, and cabergoline reduce OFF time and improve the duration of ON time when combined with levodopa (Hoehn and Elton, 1985; Lieberman *et al.*, 1993; Olanow *et al.*, 1994; Rascol *et al.*, 1996; Pinter, Pogarell and Oertel, 1999). Systematic review and analysis of clinical trials comparing bromocriptine with ropinirole, cabergoline and pramipexole as add-on therapy have shown no significant differences in efficacy (Clarke and Deane, 2001a; Clarke and Deane, 2001b; Clarke *et al.*, 2000; Goetz, 2003). In two trials, pergolide was more efficacious at reducing motor impairment and disability compared to bromocripine (Clarke and Speller, 2000). To date, there are no comparisons of efficacy between ropinirole and pramipexole as treatment for wearing-off.

A transdermal (patch) formulation of the non-ergot dopamine agonist, rotigotine (Neupro) is approved for use in advanced PD in Europe and has recently received FDA approval. Transdermal therapy has an additional advantage over oral dopamine agonists in patients unable to swallow or take medication by mouth, for example, post-operatively and by reducing the number of drugs a patient takes. The side effects of rotigotine are similar to other dopamine agonists with the addition of application site reactions. A recent phase III RCT investigated rotigotine, 8 mg and 12 mg/24 h in 351 PD patients with wearing-off and demonstrated a significant reduction in OFF time of 1.8 h and 1.2 h, respectively, without increasing bothersome dyskinesia (LeWitt *et al.*, 2007).

Side effects of dopamine agonists are frequently the limiting factor in use or escalation of dose in advanced PD. The commonest problems include nausea, symptomatic postural hypotension, somnolence, hallucinations and oedema, with no difference between drugs (Pahwa *et al.*, 2006) (see also Chapter 3). Other rarer issues include the recently highlighted impulse control disorders such as problem gambling, compulsive shopping and hypersexuality, with a prevalence of about 6% (Voon *et al.*, 2006; Weintraub *et al.*, 2006). Recent concerns regarding valvular fibrosis with the ergot dopamine agonists, pergolide and cabergoline, may also limit use of these particular drugs (Schade *et al.*, 2007; Zanettini *et al.*, 2007). The FDA has recently announced that pergolide is being voluntarily withdrawn from the market. The evidence of similar valvular problems with bromocriptine is unknown and to date lisuride has not shown any problems, possibly due to $5HT_{2B}$ antagonist properties of the drug. Pleuropulmonary and retroperitoneal fibrosis seems to be a complication of all ergot-derived agonists.

The American Academy of Neurology Practice Parameter recommends pergolide, pramipexole and ropinirole for treatment of wearing-off (level B) (Pahwa *et al.*, 2006). The Movement Disorder Society EBM Review Task Force recommends pergolide, pramipexole, and ropinirole as "clinically useful" and bromocriptine and cabergoline as "possibly useful" for treatment of wearing-off (Goetz *et al.*, 2005).

Practical Approach to Managing Predictable Wearing-Off

PD patients with predictable wearing-off will usually respond well to increased frequency or dose of levodopa. The key to managing such patients is not to be afraid of using levodopa. The last two decades has seen a swing in prescribing habits from use of levodopa early to avoidance at all costs, or under-use, due to the "fear" of long-term levodopa-induced motor fluctuations. Frequently, patients are now seen struggling on low doses of levodopa (300–400 mg/d) with many hours OFF time in the day. Remember to strike a balance between the long-term risks of motor fluctuations and present quality of life.

Unpredictable Fluctuations: Unpredictable OFFs, Sudden OFFs and ON–OFF Fluctuations

Clinical Features

Patients can also experience wearing-off that is fast, random and unrelated to the timing of the last dose of levodopa, called "unpredictable OFFs." Such patients can suffer OFF periods that come on over a few seconds with resultant severe akineisa called a "sudden-OFF" (Fahn, 1974). Such problems are more resistant to treatment than predictable wearing-off. Patients may experience predictable or unpredictable switching from being ON and mobile with dyskinesia to being OFF and immobile, known as "ON–OFF fluctuations" (Duvoisin, 1974; Fahn, 1974). The term "ON–OFF" implies a transition from one state to the other akin to switching on and off a light. Patients with advanced PD can develop a "yo-yoing" effect where they rapidly, unpredictably and repeatedly switch from being ON with dyskinesia to OFF and then ON again (Fahn, 1974; Fahn, 1982; Marsden and Parkes, 1976). Such fluctuations are typically difficult to manage using pharmacological means and such patients often require functional surgical intervention, to reduce the motor fluctuations and improve quality of life (see Chapter 7).

Mechanism

Unpredictable motor fluctuations occur with further disease progression. Thus such problems arise due to ongoing loss of pre-synaptic dopaminergic terminals, as well as post-synaptic changes in the striatal medium spiny neurons and resultant altered neurotransmitter activity within basal ganglia circuitry (see Chapter 1). Peripheral pharmacokinetics of levodopa also play a role (see below), resulting in variable levodopa absorption in the small intestine and transport across the blood–brain barrier. In addition, PD patients often report sudden OFFs in response to anxiety, being in a crowd, suggesting cortical influences on basal ganglia motor circuits.

Treatment (Figure 5.2)

- *Increase oral dopaminergic agents (as for predictable wearing-off):* Increasing dopaminergic stimulation with increased frequency and or dosing of levodopa may reduce sudden ON–OFF fluctuations by smoothing out dopamine levels. However, these unpredictable ON– OFF fluctuations do not appear to correlate with levodopa timing or levels. Patients often have associated ON period choreiform dyskinesia and so this regime can exacerbate involuntary movements. Increasing the dose of a dopamine agonist is a better option, as this may permit a reduction in the levodopa dose. Several studies have shown that dopamine agonists are efficacious in alleviating motor fluctuations using higher than normally recommended dosing, for example, ropinirole average daily dose 34 mg (Cristina *et al.*, 2003); pergolide 8.2 mg/d (Storch *et al.*, 2005) and cabergoline 6.4 mg/d (Odin *et al.*, 2006). In all cases, levodopa doses were significantly reduced and the commonest side effects were hallucinations. Since the discovery of cardiac valvulopathy complicating pergolide and cabergoline use and the suggestion that it may be, at least partially, dose-related, this high-dose approach with these agents is not recommended. The addition of entacapone is less helpful for unpredictable sudden OFFs compared to predictable wearing-off (Gordin, Kaakkola and Teravainen, 2003).
- *Use liquid/soluble oral levodopa preparations:* Soluble levodopa pro-drug preparations are rapidly hydrolyzed to levodopa and thus more rapidly and reliably absorbed, compared to conventional levodopa. Such preparations may be helpful for rapid reversal of OFF periods (Steiger *et al.*, 1991; Stocchi, Nordera and Marsden, 1997). Preparations that exist include levodopa/benserazide (Madopar dispersible), levodopa methylester, levodopa ethylester and orally disintegrating tablets of levodopa/carbidopa (Parcopa). Although these preparations are more reliably absorbed than conventional tablets, the duration of action may be shorter at 1–1.5 hours. Thus, in clinical practice, such preparations are only useful for intermittent use as rescue treatment for OFF periods or more often, as treatments for dose failures or for rapid switching-on required in the early morning (see below).

  Alternatively, patients can crush oral levodopa preparations and take them with a carbonated beverage. This may result in more rapid absorption for rescuing OFF periods. Patients requiring frequent smaller doses to control complicated fluctuations and disabling dyskinesias can take liquid levodopa preparations by crushing tablets in water combined with ascorbic acid, however, the solutions are unstable after 24 hours (Kurth *et al.*, 1993a). In our experience, the inconvenience of liquid levodopa therapy (e.g., taking hourly doses, having to carry a supply whenever the patient leaves home, preparations every 1–2 days), usually results in patients and families abandoning this approach after a relatively short period of time.
- *Enteral levodopa:* There have been several attempts at delivering levodopa directly into the duodenum as a way of circumventing the stomach to improve absorption and reduce ON–OFF fluctuations. To date, however, only open-label studies have been performed in small numbers of advanced PD patients with ON–OFF motor fluctuations. These studies have demonstrated efficacy in improved daily OFF times, with a reduction in dyskinesia (e.g., Kurlan *et al.*, 1986; Kurth *et al.*, 1993b; Stocchi *et al.*, 2005). To aid solubility of the levodopa methyl ester, however, large volumes of water are required (Nyholm and Aquilonius, 2004). An alternative stable suspension of levodopa and carbidopa in methylcellulose (Duodopa) has been recently developed, with improved solubility for enteral administration (Nyholm, 2006). To date, clinical studies have been performed in small numbers of patients and have not been double blind or placebo controlled so the true efficacy is unclear. However, Duodopa infusions have shown improved ON time without an increase in dyskinesia, in advanced PD patients (Nyholm *et al.*, 2005). This treatment, which combines a gastrostomy with placement of the tube into the duodenum and a specially designed pump carried in a "holster" has now been marketed in Scandinavia, Europe, the UK and approval is pending in North America.

  In all cases of enteral infusion of levodopa, the cost, as well as technical and mechanical issues may limit widespread use. For PD patients with disabling fluctuations who are not suitable for functional neurosurgery (DBS) however, such an approach is a potential alternative. The more continuous dopaminergic stimulation and ability to reduce intermittent oral levodopa provided with this treatment may also be associated with a reduction in dyskinesia.

```
┌─────────────────────────────────────────────┐
│  Revise L-Dopa regimen (consider less        │
│  frequent higher doses, convert CR levodopa  │
│  to standard levodopa)                       │
└─────────────────────────────────────────────┘
                      │
                      ▼
┌─────────────────────────────────────────────┐
│  Consider dose increase of DA-agonists       │
└─────────────────────────────────────────────┘
                      │
                      ▼
┌─────────────────────────────────────────────┐
│  Consider parenteral DA-agonists             │
│  (transdermal rotigotine, intermittent       │
│  s.c. apomorphine)                           │
└─────────────────────────────────────────────┘
                      │
                      ▼
┌─────────────────────────────────────────────┐
│  If refractory consider invasive             │
│  therapies (if available)                    │
└─────────────────────────────────────────────┘
           ┌──────────┼──────────┐
           ▼          ▼          ▼
┌───────────────┐ ┌──────────┐ ┌───────────┐
│  Continuous   │ │ Enteral  │ │ Bilateral │
│  s.c.         │ │ levodopa │ │ STN-DBS   │
│  apomorphine  │ │ infusions│ │           │
│  infusions    │ │          │ │           │
└───────────────┘ └──────────┘ └───────────┘
```

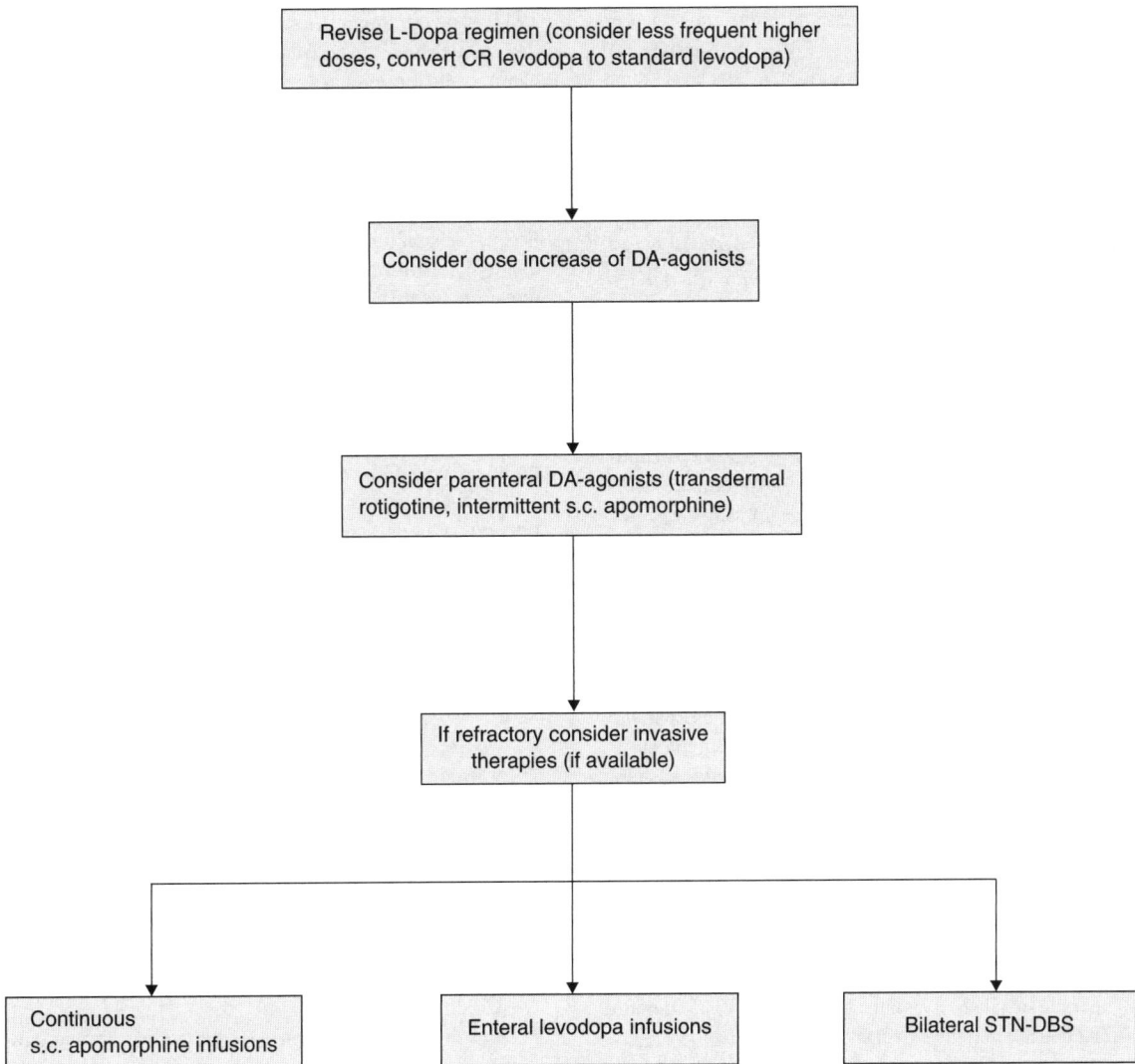

Figure 5.2 Algorithm of practical approach to management of unpredictable motor fluctuations.

• *Parenteral dopamine agonist: apomorphine*: The injectable mixed dopamine D_1/D_2 receptor agonist, apomorphine, has been used in Europe for many years as a treatment for ON–OFF motor fluctuations, particularly as rescue therapy for OFF periods and sudden or unpredictable OFF periods (Stibe *et al.*, 1988; Frankel *et al.*, 1990) and has recently been approved for use in the USA. Due to the pro-emetic action of apomorphine, prior treatment for 2–3 days and continued treatment using the oral anti-emetics, domperidone (20 mg t.i.d.) or trimethobenzamide hydrochloride (300 mg t.i.d) is required. Some patients can discontinue the anti-emetic after a few weeks.

A single s.c. injection of apomorphine alleviates parkinsonian symptoms within 5–15 min for 60–90 minutes and so can be used as a "rescue" for OFF-period disability (Chaudhuri *et al.*, 1988; Dewey *et al.*, 2001). Apomorphine can be used either as intermittent s.c injections (2–8 mg per injection, average daily total dose approximately 100 mg/d) and/or as an infusion (20–160 mg) ranging over 10–24 hours (Manson, Turner and Lees, 2002; Tyne *et al.*, 2004). The anti-parkinsonian actions of apomorphine and levodopa are equivalent (Cotzias *et al.*, 1970). Long-term use of apomorphine does not result in loss of benefit (Hughes *et al.*, 1993; Gancher, Nutt and Woodward, 1995). For patients with frequent OFF periods requiring several injections per day, s.c infusion of apomorphine (using specially designed pumps) is useful and more practical. Continuous infusion of apomorphine not only markedly reduces OFF time but also reduces ON period dyskinesia. This reduction in dyskinesia is only partly due to a concomitant reduction in levodopa dose (Colzi, Turner and Lees, 1998; Manson, Turner and Lees, 2002). However, despite the potential advantages, there has been a general under-usage of apomorphine (Chaudhuri and Clough, 1998). In many countries, this has been because of a lack of a peripheral dopamine receptor antagonist, such as domperidone. Another common reason also relates to practicalities of using apomorphine, as most patients will need support from family and specialist PD nurses (Manson, Turner and Lees, 2002; Tyne *et al.*, 2004).

The main side effect of apomorphine is formation of skin nodules. These can occur in 20–78% of patients (Colzi, Turner and Lees, 1998; Tyne *et al.*, 2004), but are only bothersome in about a third of these patients (Manson, Turner and Lees, 2002). Management includes rotating the injection site, ensuring strict aseptic technique; diluting the apomorphine 1:1 with normal saline, massage or local skin ultrasound. Neuropsychiatric side effects appear to be less common than with oral dopamine agonists, but hallucinations and confusion can occur at high doses. New methods of administering apomorphine are being developed in an attempt to reduce the problems associated with injections. These include sub-lingual (Montastruc *et al.*, 1991), intranasal (Kapoor *et al.*, 1990), rectal (Hughes *et al.*, 1991) and transdermal (Priano *et al.*, 2004), which have all been tried, but with sub-optimal absorption and tolerability.

Both apomorphine and enteral levodopa (as discussed above) are viable options for use in elderly patients with motor fluctuations where the risks of functional neurosurgery (STN DBS) are thought too great. The relative safety, efficacy and patient satisfaction of these treatment compared to STN DBS in younger patients who are good surgical candidates is under active assessment at present (e.g., De Gaspari *et al.*, 2006).

Dose Failure "No-ON"; Delayed or Partial "ON" Response

Clinical Features

PD patients may experience delay in benefit ("delayed ON") or absence of benefit from a dose of levodopa called "dose-failure" or "no-ON" response (Melamed and Bitton,

1984). The commonest times include the first dose of the day or after meals. The delay in a PD patient switching-on can account for a significant proportion of the total daily OFF time (Merims, Djaldetti and Melamed, 2003).

Mechanism

Such problems may occur due to impaired levodopa absorption in the small intestine or across the blood–brain barrier due to competition with large neutral amino acids found in dietary protein (peripheral pharmacokinetics of levodopa) (Nutt and Fellman, 1984; Leenders *et al.*, 1986; Alexander *et al.*, 1994). Absorption of levodopa in the small intestine may also be impaired by delay in gastric emptying secondary to the presence of food per se (Fahn, 1977; Baruzzi *et al.*, 1987). Gastric emptying is also erratic and slow in PD due to the underlying disease, as well as secondary to dopaminergic and anti-cholinergic medications (Evans *et al.*, 1981; Edwards, Quigley and Pfeiffer, 1992). In addition, constipation via a cologastric reflex, leads to delayed gastric emptying (Bojo and Cassuto, 1992). A slower speed of gastric emptying has been demonstrated to correlate with the presence of motor fluctuations (Djaldetti *et al.*, 1996).

Treatment (Figure 5.2)

- *Modify dietary protein*: Either reducing protein intake, or leaving large protein meals to the end of the day may improve motor fluctuations (Pincus and Barry, 1987; Karstaedt and Pincus, 1992).
- *Take levodopa on an empty stomach*: Initially patients are advised to take levodopa with food to prevent nausea, but with time this requirement diminishes. Thus advising a patient to take levodopa on an empty stomach will improve absorption and reduce dose failures (Contin *et al.*, 1998).
- *Improve gastric emptying*: Reducing or stopping anticholinergics may help improve gastic emptying and thus levodopa absorption. In addition, treatment of constipation may also help.
- *Treat* H. pylori *infection*: A recent study has suggested an important role for *Helicobacter pylori* infection in altering levodopa absorption and contributing to motor fluctuations. Eradication of the *H. pylori* infection improved levodopa pharmacokinetic profiles and clinical response (Pierantozzi *et al.*, 2006).
- *Soluble oral levodopa preparations*: The more rapidly absorbed, fast-acting soluble levodopa pro-drug preparations may be helpful for improving dose failures (see above). A small study demonstrated that equivalent doses of oral levodopa methyl ester and dispersible Madopar (levodopa/benserazide) improved latency to switching ON in 13 PD patients in the fasting state after overnight drug withdrawal and were significantly faster compared to standard levodopa/carbidopa (Steiger

et al., 1992). A recent RCT study of levodopa methyl ester (melevodopa)/carbidopa, as the first dose of the afternoon, in 74 fluctuating PD patients showed a significant reduction in latency to switch-on from 66.7 to 47.4 min compared to 68.5 to 58 min with an equivalent dose of standard levodopa/carbidopa (Stocchi et al., 2007). A small open-label study comparing patient preference and benefit in 61 PD patients, when switched from conventional to the orally disintegrating tablets (ODT) of levodopa/carbidopa showed significantly more patients (45%) preferred ODTs compared with 20% who preferred the conventional tablets, in terms of ease of use, although there was no difference in daily OFF times between the two groups (Nausieda et al., 2005).

A study using levodopa ethyl ester (etilevodopa)/carbidopa as a replacement for the first dose of the day and first dose after lunch demonstrated a reduction in mean latency to switching ON by 21% (morning dose) and 17% (post-lunch dose) compared to conventional levodopa/carbidopa and a decrease in percentage of no-ON episodes after the post-lunch dose by 21% compared to conventional levodopa/carbidopa (Djaldetti et al., 2002). However, a recent double-blind RCT in 327 PD patients with motor fluctuations comparing etilevodopa/carbidopa (as the only levodopa preparation) vs standard levodopa/carbidopa, failed to show any significant benefit in total daily time to turn-on or dose failures (Blindauer et al., 2006). This suggests that such soluble preparations are probably only useful for intermittent use in reducing motor fluctuations.

- *Apomorphine*: Apomorphine s.c. injections can also be used to switch on when there is a delay or dose failure (see above).

Beginning-of-Dose Worsening, End-of-Dose Rebound

Some patients can experience a transient worsening of symptoms at the beginning of a dose, often as an increase in tremor ("beginning-of-dose worsening") (Merello and Lees, 1992). Patients may experience an exacerbation or rebound in their symptoms at the end of dose ("end-of-dose rebound") (Nutt, Gancher and Woodward, 1988). In some cases, the OFF state may be considerably worse than in the untreated state or after longer periods of drug withdrawal ("super-OFF").

Take Levodopa When Still in ON State

Occasionally patients with advanced PD experiencing motor fluctuations may report that the first dose of the day is less effective (Melamed and Bitton, 1984) (in general, however, PD patients tend to notice that their response to medication is usually better in the morning

and deteriorates over the course of the day). Some patients need a larger dose to "kick in;" or if they become very parkinsonian or experience a "super-OFF", then a usually effective dose of levodopa does not switch them ON.

Practical Approach to Treating Unpredictable Motor Fluctuations

Whatever approach is taken, PD patients with advanced disease often cannot tolerate even small increases in dopaminergic stimulation because of a disabling increase in dyskinesia or the development of behavioral and psychiatric problems. At this stage, the response to intermittent oral medication becomes brittle and unpredictable. More frequent, smaller doses attempting to address the shortening response without aggravating dyskinesias sometimes result in a more unpredictable response pattern with a greater number of dose failures. At this stage many patients seem to have an "all-or-none" response to levodopa that requires a threshold level of dopaminergic stimulation. Frequent, small doses may under-shoot this threshold. In such patients with very complicated, unpredictable fluctuations, simplifying the dosage schedule using fewer, but larger, doses will often result in a return to a more predictable response pattern.

Counseling and educating patients and families as to the nature of the fluctuations is vital in management, and for some symptoms, may be as effective as changing drugs. Resist the pressure to change medication just because the patient is with you in the clinic; sometimes doing nothing is the best course of action. Warn patients and relatives that changes to drugs may take time (weeks rather than days) to be effective. Make changes to one drug at a time so you know what has caused the improvement or change. (Watch out when stopping selegiline or anti-cholinergics for rebound symptoms, especially tremor).

Dyskinesia

Clinical Features

Dyskinesia varies in phenomenology and management according to the timing in response to levodopa. Dyskinesia most commonly occurs at the time of best ON response to levodopa ("peak-dose dyskinesia") or throughout the duration of the ON period ("square-wave dyskinesia") and can be a mixture of chorea, ballism and dystonia and to a lesser extent myoclonus (Nutt, 1990). Choreiform movements in the limbs are most common, but dystonic posturing in the limbs and craniocervical dystonia and chorea are also common (Luquin et al., 1992).

Dyskinesia also occurs when the levels of levodopa are low. This occurs during OFF periods or wearing-off and is predominantly dystonic, affecting the lower limbs (Poewe, Lees and Stern, 1988; Bravi *et al.*, 1993). Patients often experience a more fixed posture (e.g., ankle intorsion with toe flexion or extension), especially early morning, often associated with pain ("early morning dystonia") (Melamed, 1979). Less common is dyskinesia occurring at the beginning and end-of-dose, when the levels of levodopa are rising and falling, respectively, known as "diphasic dyskinesia," or "beginning and end-of-dose" dyskinesia (Muenter *et al.*, 1977). Diphasic dyskinesia also tends to affect the legs predominantly and can involve stereotypic rapid alternating leg movements, as well as unusual ballistic kicking or dystonia (Luquin *et al.*, 1992).

Mechanism

Levodopa-induced dyskinesia is due to a combination of pre- and post-synaptic changes in the nigrostriatal dopaminergic system and possibly other dopamine pathways, for example, the nigropallidal pathway (this is further discussed in Chapter 1).

Peak-Dose Dyskinesia

Treatment (Figure 5.3)

The need to treat dyskinesia has to be carefully evaluated since symptoms are often non-bothersome and many patients prefer this to the disability associated with OFF periods. A recent population-based study from the Mayo Clinic found that although dyskinesia developed in nearly 60% of patients after 10 years, the dyskinesia was severe enough to require medication adjustments in only 43% of patients and nearly 90% of the patients were spared dyskinesia that could not be controlled by drug adjustments (Van Gerpen *et al.*, 2006).

- *Reduce levodopa lose*: Management of peak-dose dyskinesia is based on reducing the level of dopaminergic stimulation without increasing parkinsonian disability. Frequently, however, small reductions in levodopa will result in unacceptable worsening of parkinsonism. This can be counteracted by increasing the dose of dopamine agonists, which have a lower propensity to cause dyskinesia (although in practice, advanced PD patients may find higher doses of dopamine agonists difficult to tolerate).
- *Reduce mildly active dopaminergic drugs; MAO-B inhibitors and COMT inhibitors*: At the stage when PD patients are experiencing brittle ON–OFF fluctuations with unpredictable motor fluctuations and peak-dose dyskinesia, the benefit of MAO-B inhibitors and COMT inhibitors may be less. Thus discontinuing or

reducing the dose of these drugs may reduce peak-dose dyskinesia.

- *Amantadine*: To date, the most effective drug in alleviating peak-dose dyskinesia is the non-sub-type-selective NMDA receptor antagonist, amantadine. Several lines of evidence have demonstrated abnormal glutamatergic activity within the striatum in dyskinesia, involving both NMDA and AMPA subtypes of glutamate receptors (see Chapter 1). Amantadine, significantly reduces dyskinesia, between 24 and 60%, without exacerbating parkinsonism (Verhagen Metman *et al.*, 1998; Snow *et al.*, 2000). However, amantadine can induce side effects such as psychosis, confusion, livido reticularis and oedema that can limit tolerability. In addition, clinical practice has shown that only a proportion of PD patients appear to respond well and benefit may only last a few months (Thomas *et al.*, 2004). For the treatment of dyskinesia, the American Academy of Neurology Practice Parameter recommends amantadine as possibly effective (level C), (Pahwa *et al.*, 2006). The Movement Disorder Society EBM Review Task Force advises that amantadine is efficacious and clinically useful (Goetz *et al.*, 2005).
- *Clozapine*: Clozapine has been suggested as a possible treatment for peak-dose dyskinesia in PD, as clinical experience in schizophrenia has shown a lower propensity to induce extra pyramidal side effects, including tardive dyskinesia, when used in the treatment of psychosis. This "atypical" antipsychotic effect has been suggested to be due to changes in the distribution and affinity of dopamine D_2 receptor binding as well as affinity for non-dopaminergic receptors, including $5HT_{2A/2C}$, amongst others (Kapur and Seeman, 2001). A double blind RCT in PD patients with dyskinesia using low-dose clozapine (39.4 ± 4.5 mg/day) reduced ON time with dyskinesias as well as the severity of dyskinesia in response to a single dose of levodopa in a 10-week placebo-controlled trial (Durif *et al.*, 2004). However, on clinical evaluation, only dyskinesia at rest, but not activated dyskinesia (as with talking, performing various activities) were reduced and so it is not clear whether this effect will translate into a meaningful improvement in disability caused by dyskinesia in practice. The American Academy of Neurology Practice Parameter states there is insufficient data to recommend clozapine (Pahwa *et al.*, 2006).

The atypical anti-psychotic drug, quetiapine has also been evaluated, but low-dose treatment (25 mg) was found to be ineffective (Katzenschlager *et al.*, 2004), however, animal studies suggest that higher

```
┌─────────────────────────────────────────────────────┐
│  Revise levodopa regimen (reduce individual dose     │
│  size, convert levodopa CR to standard levodopa)     │
└─────────────────────────────────────────────────────┘
```

No improvement

```
┌──────────────────────────────┐        ┌──────────────────────────────────┐
│  Dyskinesias improve,         │ ◄───── │  Discontinue mildly active drugs  │
│  parkinsonism worsens         │        │  like MAO-B-inhibitors,           │
│                               │        │  COMT-inhibitors                  │
└──────────────────────────────┘        └──────────────────────────────────┘
```

```
┌──────────────────────────────┐
│  Increase dose of DA-agonist  │
└──────────────────────────────┘
```

Re-emergence of dyskinesias

```
┌──────────────────────────────┐
│  Add Amantadine               │
└──────────────────────────────┘
```

Insufficient response

```
┌──────────────────────────────┐
│  Consider invasive            │
│  therapies (if available)     │
└──────────────────────────────┘
```

```
┌──────────────────────────────┐        ┌──────────────────────────────────┐
│  Continuous s.c. apomorphine  │        │  Surgery – bilateral STN-DBS      │
│  or enteral levodopa          │        │  unilateral pallidotomy for       │
│  infusions                    │        │  selected patients                │
└──────────────────────────────┘        └──────────────────────────────────┘
```

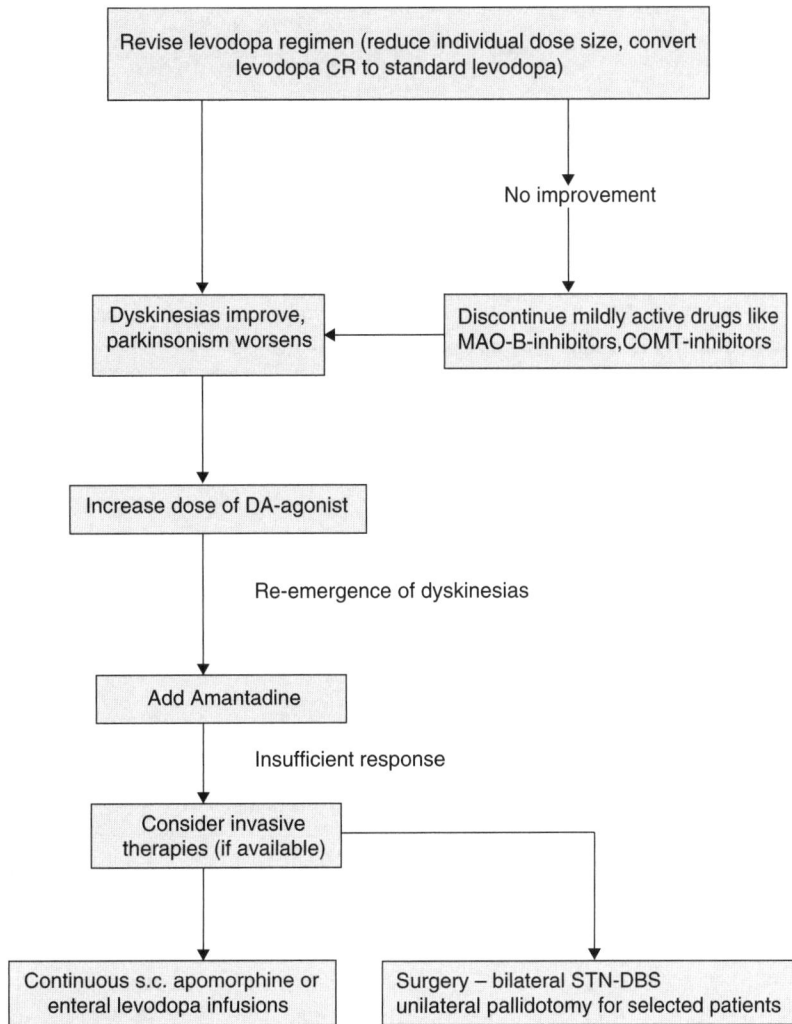

Figure 5.3 Algorithm of practical management of peak-dose (*high-dose*) dyskinesia.

doses might be beneficial (Oh, Bibbiani and Chase, 2002). The other atypical anti-psychotics, olanzapine and risperidone have been shown to significantly worsen parkinsonism (Goetz *et al.*, 2000; van de Vijver *et al.*, 2002) and are not recommended in PD for the treatment of dyskinesia.

- *Enteral levodopa/parenteral dopaminergic drugs*: Many studies have demonstrated an improvement in peak-dose dyskinesia with administration of continuous dopaminergic stimulation (e.g., Sage *et al.*, 1988; Kurth *et al.*, 1993b; Nutt, Obeso and Stocchi, 2000). Thus Duodopa and apomorphine infusions (Katslanger *et al.*, 2005) (as discussed above) can also reduce levodopa-induced dyskinesia, by reducing the oral levodopa dose and also possibly by a "de-priming" effect within the basal ganglia circuitry (see Chapter 1). A study in 40 PD patients with an infusion of the dopamine agonist, lisuride over a four-year period also showed a significant reduction in dyskinesia, as well as OFF time compared to oral levodopa (Stocchi *et al.*, 2002). The same was reported in a small pharmacokinetic study using duodenal infusions of levodopa methyl ester (Stocchi *et al.*, 2005). To date, it is not clear if similar effects on reducing peak-dose dyskinesia will be seen with transdermal patches of dopamine agonists.

Diphasic Dyskinesia

Treatment (Figure 5.4)

- *Improve OFF periods; use of dopamine agonists*: The problem of OFF-period and diphasic dyskinesia is due to low levels of dopaminergic stimulation. Thus, treatments designed to reduce OFF periods, as discussed above, will reduce OFF period dystonia. In particular dopamine agonists, due to the long duration of action, are useful in the treatment of diphasic dyskinesia.
- *Amantadine*: Amantadine may also improve diphasic dyskinesia. (Paci, Thomas and Onofrj, 2001).

Early Morning OFF Dystonia

Treatment (Figure 5.4)

- *Early morning dose of levodopa*: Painful OFF-period morning foot dystonia is often helped by taking the first daily dose of levodopa early on awakening or using an extra early morning dose, especially crushed (e.g., setting an alarm clock and taking a dose left out at the bedside before returning to sleep for 1–2 h). Other alternatives include using s.c. apomorphine or one of the fast-acting levodopa preparations for quicker onset (Lees, 1993; Factor, Brown and Molho, 2000). The other option is the use of long-acting dopamine agonists or controlled-release levodopa prior to bedtime (Lees, 1987).

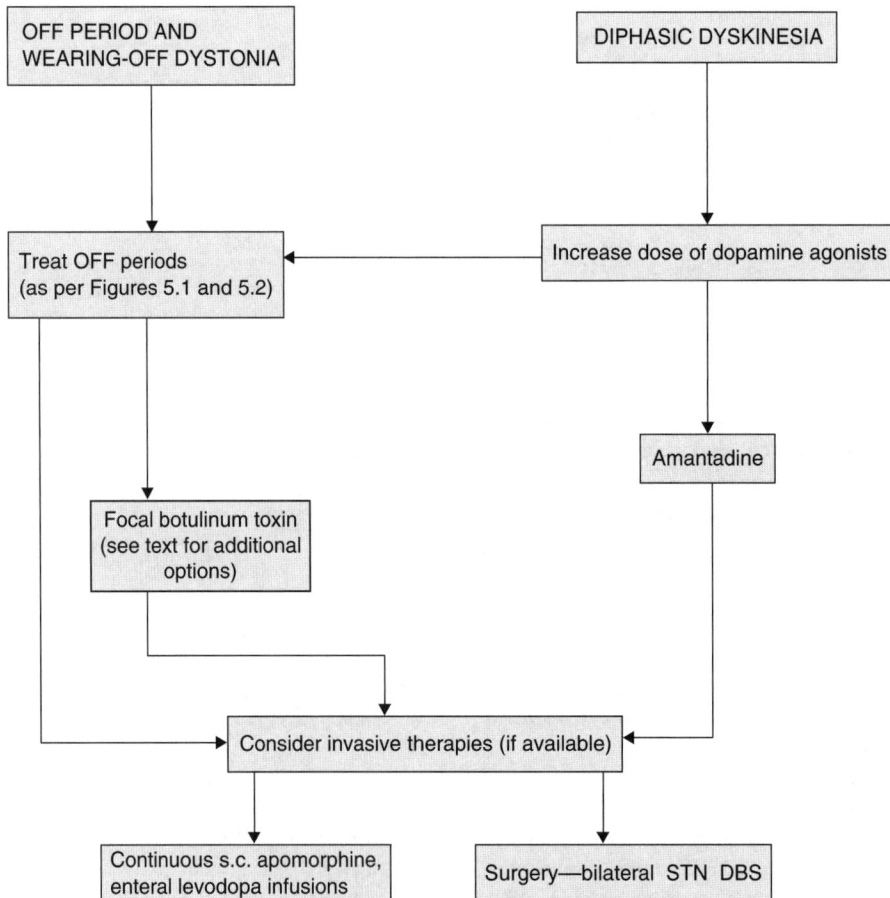

Figure 5.4 Algorithm of practical management of OFF-period dystonia and diphasic dyskinesia (*low-dose*) dyskinesia.

- *Botulinum toxin*: Focal injection of botulinum toxin frequently helps, especially extension of the big toe and foot inversion. (Pacchetti *et al.*, 1995).

Drug-Resistant Motor Complications

Advanced PD patients experience a range of symptoms that may not respond, or only partially respond, to dopaminergic drugs. These comprise predominantly "midline" or axial symptoms associated with bulbar function, gait and balance (Table 5.2). The underlying pathophysiology is probably outside the dopaminergic system and involves neurodegeneration within other brainstem structures and connections. This explains the overall poor response obtained from dopaminergic therapy. The neuropharmacology of many of these functions is complex, involving cholinergic, noradrenergic and serotonergic systems and is unlikely to derive from dysfunction of one neurotransmitter system. Thus, to date, no effective drug treatments exist for the majority of these problems. The management of these drug-resistant motor symptoms therefore relies primarily on non-pharmacological means.

Speech Problems

Clinical Features

Speech problems are a common source of disability in advanced PD patients. Patients can develop reduced volume (hypophonia), monotony of pitch, breathy phonation and imprecise articulation, amongst other problems, resulting in unintelligible speech (often termed hypokinetic dysarthria).

Mechanism

The cause of these speech problems is not clearly defined, but probably results from a combination of impaired vocal cord, laryngeal and respiratory muscle movement combined with altered basal ganglia drive and cortical dysfunction (reviewed in Pinto *et al.*, 2004).

Treatment of Speech Problems See Table 5.4

Dysphagia

Clinical Features

Swallowing difficulties can be a common and important problem in advanced PD. Patients may complain of food or tablets sticking in the throat or coughing after fluids.

Table 5.4 Treatment of speech problems.

Treatment	Randomized Clinical trials (RCT) and Evidence based recommendations	Practical approach and comments
Increase dopaminergic medications	None	May help in early disease
		Care – can worsen speech (peak-dose dysphonia) (Critchley, 1974). Tachyphemia (fast, low-volume speech) can be an ON phenomena
Speech therapy	Possibly effective (Level C) (Suchowersky *et al.*, 2006). Unknown relative benefits of different techniques (Deane *et al.*, 2001).	Main approach to treatment
Various techniques, for example, Lee Silverman Voice Treatment (LSVT) (Ramig, Fox and Sapir, 2004)		
Collagen vocal cord augmentation	None	Usually temporary benefit (Kim, Kearney and Atkins, 2002; Hill *et al.*, 2003
Technological means of improving communication, for example, voice amplification systems and electronic communicators	None	

Mechanism

On examination of PD patients with dysphagia, abnormalities in the oral and pharyngeal phases of swallowing (including the facial, tongue and palatal muscles) are common, with hypokinetic lingual transfer movements and palatal elevation (Ertekin *et al.*, 2002; Alfonsi *et al.*, 2007). Investigation with videofluoroscopy helps determine the severity (Stroudley and Walsh, 1991).

Treatment of Dysphagia See Table 5.5

Drooling of Saliva

Clinical Features

PD patients often report drooling of saliva (sialorrhea) which can range from mild, nocturnal only or intermittent daytime between the sides of the mouth, to severe drooling with constantly wet face and clothes (Bateson, Gibberd and Wilson, 1973).

Mechanism

Sialorrhea is probably due to associated dysphagia as absolute saliva production is normal or even reduced in PD (Bagheri *et al.*, 1999; Proulx *et al.*, 2005). In addition,

the open-mouth and flexed neck postures will exacerbate the problem.

Treatment of Sialorrhea – See Table 5.6

Gait Disturbances

Problems with gait and balance, resulting in falls are frequent, dopamine-resistant symptoms in advanced PD. This topic is discussed in Chapter 28.

Drug-Resistant Tremor

Certain PD patients can experience marked tremor that is apparently resistant to dopaminergic drugs. In such patients, tremor may respond to much higher doses of levodopa, but often at the expense of development of other dopaminergic side effects. Alternatives may include clozapine (Friedman *et al.*, 1997); the exact mechanism of action of clozapine in reducing tremor is unknown. The option of surgery, either bilateral STN DBS, or now less frequently, thalamic VIM nucleus stimulation is often the best means of managing the tremor in such patients (see Chapter 7).

Table 5.5 Treatment of dysphagia.

Treatment	Randomized Clinical trial (RCT) and Evidence based recommendations	Practical approach and comments
Increase dopaminergic medications	None	May help if dysphagia is an OFF period symptom (Bushmann *et al.*, 1989; Witjas *et al.*, 2002). Usually is unhelpful
Speech therapy and nutritionist	None (Deane *et al.*, 2002)	A multi-disciplinary team including a speech therapist for swallow assessments and advice on safe eating and drinking, and nutritionist/dietician with regard to dietary advice such as change in food consistency and so on, is main approach to treatment required
Percutaneous endoscopic gastrostomy (PEG) feeding tube		May be considered if patient is unable to maintain adequate nutrition or has frequent aspiration pneumonia. Only consider following counseling with patient and family.

Table 5.6 Treatment of sialorrhea.

Treatment	Randomized Clinical trial (RCT) and Evidence based recommendations	Practical approach and comments
Increased dopaminergic drugs	None	Fluctuations in salivation can occur with worsening in the OFF periods (Raudino, 2001; Gunal *et al.*, 2002). In advanced disease rarely helpful
Oral anti-cholinergic or transdermal anti-choloinergic preparations.	None	All can be effective but side effects (confusion, memory loss, hallucinations, urinary hesitancy) limit use
Sub-lingual anti-cholinergic	Open label use of atropine drops (5 mg in 1%w/v bid) effective (Hyson, Johnson and Jog, 2002)	Systemic side effects still occur, including delirium and hallucinations
	RCT ipratropium bromide spray was in effective (Fox *et al.*, 2006)	No systemic side effects encountered; maybe helpful in some PD patients
Botulinum toxin	RCT of Botulinum toxin type A (Mancini *et al.*, 2003; Lagalla *et al.*, 2006 and type B (Ondo, Hunter and Moore, 2004) have shown significant reduction in sialorrhoea	No major side effects
	The relative efficacy of type A over B, or different sources of botulinum is unknown (Benson and Daugherty, 2007)	Botulinum toxin should not be used in patients with significant dysphagia.
		Effect of use of ultrasound to aid localization is not clear (Dogu *et al.*, 2004)
Surgery; salivary gland transposition, salivary gland excision or ligation. Denervation of the salivary glands	None in PD. Several studies in other neurological diseases showing benefit (Crysdale *et al.*, 2001; Hockstein *et al.*, 2004)	May be helpful in advanced PD with intractable sialorrhea where botulinum toxin may be unsafe due to dysphagia
Irradiation of the parotid glands	None; benefit in other neurological diseases (Borg and Hirst, 1996)	Alternative in elderly, advanced PD patients unsuitable for surgery

References

Ahlskog, J.E., Muenter, M.D., McManis, P.G. *et al.* (1988) Controlled-release Sinemet (CR-4): a double-blind crossover study in patients with fluctuating Parkinson's disease. *Mayo Clinic Proceedings*, **63**, 876–886.

Alexander, G.M., Schwartzman, R.J., Grothusen, J.R. and Gordon, S.W. (1994) Effect of plasma levels of large neutral amino acids and degree of parkinsonism on the blood-to-brain transport of levodopa in naive and MPTP parkinsonian monkeys. *Neurology*, **44**, 1491–1499.

Alfonsi, E., Versino, M., Merlo, I.M. *et al.* (2007) Electrophysiologic patterns of oral-pharyngeal swallowing in parkinsonian syndromes. *Neurology*, **20** (68), 583–589.

Assal, F., Spahr, L., Hadengue, A., Rubbia-Brandt, L. and Burkhard, P.R. (1998) Tolcapone and fulminant hepatitis. *Lancet*, **352**, 958.

Bagheri, H., Damase-Michel, C., Lapeyre-Mestre, M. *et al.* (1999) A study of salivary secretion in Parkinson's disease. *Clinical Neuropharmacology*, **22** (4), 213–215.

Baruzzi, A., Contin, M., Riva, R. *et al.* (1987) Influence of meal ingestion time on pharmacokinetics of orally administered levodopa in parkinsonian patients. *Clinical Neuropharmacology*, **10**, 527–537.

Bateson, M.C., Gibberd, F.B. and Wilson, R.S. (1973) Salivary symptoms in Parkinson's disease. *Archives of Neurology*, **29**, 274–275.

Benson, J. and Daugherty, K.K. (2007) Botulinum toxin A in the treatment of sialorrhea. *The Annals of Pharmacotherapy*, **41** (1), 79–85.

Blindauer, K., Shoulson, I., Oakes, D. *et al.*, Parkinson Study Group (2006) A randomized controlled trial of etilevodopa in patients with Parkinson's disease who have motor fluctuations. *Archives of Neurology*, **63** (2), 210–216.

Bojo, L. and Cassuto, J. (1992) Gastric reflex relaxation by colonic distension. *Journal of the Autonomic Nervous System*, **38**, 57–64.

Borg, M. and Hirst, F. (1998) The role of radiation therapy in the management of sialorrhea. *International Journal of Radiation Oncology, Biology, Physics*, **41** (5), 1113–1119.

Bravi, D., Mouradian, M.M., Roberts, J.W. *et al.* (1993) End-of-dose dystonia in Parkinson's disease. *Neurology*, **43**, 2130–2131.

Brooks, D.J., Agid, Y., Eggert, K. *et al.*, TC-INIT Study Group (2005) Treatment of end-of-dose wearing-off in parkinson's disease: stalevo (levodopa/carbidopa/entacapone) and levodopa/DDCI given in combination with Comtess/Comtan (entacapone) provide equivalent improvements in symptom control superior to that of traditional levodopa/DDCI treatment. *European Neurology*, **53** (4), 197–202.

Bushmann, M., Dobmeyer, S.M., Leeker, L. and Perlmutter, J.S. (1989) Swallowing abnormalities and their response to treatment in Parkinson's disease. *Neurology*, **39**, 1309–1312.

Chaudhuri, K.R. and Clough, C. (1998) Subcutaneous apomorphine in Parkinson's disease. *BMJ*, **316**, 641.

Chaudhuri, K.R., Critchley, P., Abbott, R.J. *et al.* (1988) Subcutaneous apomorphine for on–off oscillations in Parkinson's disease. *Lancet*, **26**, 1260.

Clarke, A., Brewer, F., Johnson, E.S. *et al.* (2003) A new formulation of selegiline: improved bioavailability and selectivity for MAO-B inhibition. *Journal of Neural Transmission*, **110**, 1241–1255.

Clarke, C.E. and Speller, J.M. (2000) Pergolide versus bromocriptine for levodopa-induced motor complications in Parkinson's disease. *Cochrane Database of Systematic Reviews*, (2), CD000236.

Clarke, C.E., Speller, J.M. and Clarke, J.A. (2000) Pramipexole versus bromocriptine for levodopa-induced complications in Parkinson's disease. *Cochrane Database of Systematic Reviews*, (2), CD002259.

Clarke, C.E. and Deane, K. (2001) Ropinirole versus bromocriptine for levodopa-induced complications in Parkinson's disease. *Cochrane Database of Systematic Reviews*, (1), CD001517.

Clarke, C.E. and Deane, K. (2001) Cabergoline versus bromocriptine for levodopa-induced complications in Parkinson's disease. *Cochrane Database of Systematic Reviews*, (1), CD001519.

Colzi, A., Turner, K. and Lees, A.J. (1998) Continuous subcutaneous waking day apomorphine in the long term treatment of levodopa induced interdose dyskinesias in Parkinson's disease. *Journal of Neurology, Neurosurgery, and Psychiatry*, **64**, 573–576.

Contin, M., Riva, R., Martinelli, P. *et al.* (1998) Effect of meal timing on the kinetic-dynamic profile of levodopa/carbidopa controlled release in parkinsonian patients. *European Journal of Clinical Pharmacology*, **54**, 303–308.

Cotzias, G.C., Papavasiliou, P.S., Fehling, C. *et al.* (1970) Similarities between neurologic effects of L-dipa and of apomorphine. *The New England Journal of Medicine*, **282**, 31–33.

Cristina, S., Zangaglia, R., Mancini, F. *et al.* (2003) High-dose ropinirole in advanced Parkinson's disease with severe dyskinesias. *Clinical Neuropharmacology*, **26** (3), 146–1450.

Critchley, E.M. (1976) Peak-dose dysphonia in parkinsonism. *Lancet*, **6** (7958), 544.

Crysdale, W.S., Raveh, E., McCann, C. *et al.* (2001) Management of drooling in individuals with neurodisability: a surgical experience. *Developmental Medicine and Child Neurology*, **43** (6), 379–383.

Deane, K.H., Whurr, R., Playford, E.D. *et al.* (2001) A comparison of speech and language therapy techniques for dysarthria in Parkinson's disease. *Cochrane Database of Systematic Reviews*, (2), CD002814.

Deane, K.H., Ellis-Hill, C., Jones, D. *et al.* (2002) Systematic review of paramedical therapies for Parkinson's disease. *Movement Disorders*, **17**, 984–991.

De Gaspari, D., Siri, C., Landi, A. *et al.* (2006) Clinical and neuropsychological follow up at 12 months in patients with complicated Parkinson's disease treated with subcutaneous apomorphine infusion or deep brain stimulation of the subthalamic nucleus. *Journal of Neurology, Neurosurgery, and Psychiatry*, **77**, 450–453.

Dewey, R.B., Jr, Hutton, J.T., LeWitt, P.A. and Factor, S.A. (2001) A randomized, double-blind, placebo-controlled trial of subcutaneously injected apomorphine for parkinsonian off-state events. *Archives of Neurology*, **58**, 1385–1392.

Djaldetti, R., Baron, J., Ziv, I. and Melamed, E. (1996) Gastric emptying in Parkinson's disease: patients with and without response fluctuations. *Neurology*, **46**, 1051–1054.

Djaldetti, R., Inzelberg, R., Giladi, N. *et al.* (2002) Oral solution of levodopa ethylester for treatment of response fluctuations in patients with advanced Parkinson's disease. *Movement Disorders*, **17**, 297–302.

Dogu, O., Apaydin, D., Sevim, S. *et al.* (2004) Ultrasound-guided versus 'blind' intraparotid injections of botulinum toxin-A for the treatment of sialorrhoea in patients with Parkinson's disease. *Clinical Neurology and Neurosurgery*, **106**, 93–936.

Durif, F., Debilly, B., Galitzky, M. *et al.* (2004) Clozapine improves dyskinesias in Parkinson's disease – A double-blind, placebo-controlled study. *Neurology*, **62**, 381–388.

Duvoisin, R.C. (1974) Variations in the "on–off" phenomena. *Advances in Neurology*, **5**, 339–340.

Edwards, L.L., Quigley, E.M. and Pfeiffer, R.F. (1992) Gastrointestinal dysfunction in Parkinson's disease: frequency and pathophysiology. *Neurology*, **42**, 726–732.

Entacapone to Tolcapone Switch Study Investigators (2007) Entacapone to tolcapone switch: Multicenter double-blind, randomized, active-controlled trial in advanced Parkinson's disease. *Movement Disorders*, **22**, 14–19.

Ertekin, C., Tarlaci, S., Aydogdu, I. *et al.* (2002) Electrophysiological evaluation of pharyngeal phase of swallowing in patients with Parkinson's disease. *Movement Disorders*, **17**, 942–949.

Evans, M.A., Broe, G.A., Triggs, E.J. *et al.* (1981) Gastric emptying rate and the systemic availability of levodopa in the elderly parkinsonian patient. *Neurology*, **31**, 1288–1294.

Factor, S.A., Molho, E.S., Feustel, P.J. *et al.* (2001) Long-term comparative experience with tolcapone and entacapone in advanced Parkinson's disease. *Clinical Neuropharmacology*, **24**, 295–299.

Factor, S.A., Brown, D.L. and Molho, E.S. (2000) Subcutaneous apomorphine injections as a treatment for intractable pain in Parkinson's disease. *Movement Disorders*, **15**, 167–169.

Fahn, S. (1974) "On–off" phenomenon with levodopa therapy in parkinsonism: Clinical and pharmacological correlations and the effects of intramuscular pyridoxine. *Neurology*, **24**, 431–444.

Fahn, S. (1977) Episodic failure of absorption of levodopa: a factor in the control of clinical fluctuations in the treatment of parkinsonism. *Neurology*, **27**, 390.

Fahn, S. (1982) Fluctuations of disability in Parkinson's disease: pathophysiological aspects, in *Movement Disorders* (eds C.D. Marsden and S. Fahn) Butterworth Scientific, London, pp. 123–145.

Finberg, J.P., Lamensdorf, I., Weinstock, M. *et al.* (1999) Pharmacology of rasagiline (N-propargyl-1R-aminoindan). *Advances in Neurology*, **80**, 495–499.

Forsberg, M., Lehtonen, M., Heikkinen, M. *et al.* (2003) Pharmacokinetics and pharmacodynamics of entacapone and tolcapone after acute and repeated administration: a comparative study in the rat. *The Journal of Pharmacology and Experimental Therapeutics*, **304**, 498–506.

Fox, S.H., Thomsen, T., Asante, A. and Galpern, W. (2006) Ipratropium bromide spray as a treatment for sialorrhea in Parkinson's disease. *Movement Disorders*, **21** (Suppl. 15), 900.

Frankel, J.P., Lees, A.J., Kempster, P.A. and Stern, G.M. (1990) Subcutaneous apomorphine in the treatment of Parkinson's disease. *Journal of Neurology, Neurosurgery, and Psychiatry*, **53**, 96–101.

Friedman, J.H., Koller, W.C., Lannon, M.C. *et al.* (1997) Benztropine versus clozapine for the treatment of tremor in Parkinson's disease. *Neurology*, **48**, 1077–1081.

Gancher, S.T., Nutt, J.G. and Woodward, W.R. (1995) Apomorphine infusional therapy in Parkinson's disease: clinical utility and lack of tolerance. *Movement Disorders*, **10**, 37–43.

Goetz, C.G. (2003) Treatment of advanced Parkinson's disease: an evidence-based analysis. *Advances in Neurology*, **91**, 213–228.

Goetz, C.G., Blasucci, L.M., Leurgans, S. and Pappert, E.J. (2000) Olanzapine and clozapine: comparative effects on motor function in hallucinating PD patients. *Neurology*, **26**, 789–794.

Goetz, C.G., Poewe, W., Rascol, O. and Sampaio, C. (2005) Evidence-based medical review update: pharmacological and surgical treatments of Parkinson's disease: 2001 to 2004. *Movement Disorders*, **20**, 523–539.

Golbe, L.I., Lieberman, A.N., Muenter, M.D. *et al.* (1988) Deprenyl in the treatment of symptom fluctuations in advanced Parkinson's disease. *Clinical Neuropharmacology*, **11**, 45–55.

Gordin, A., Kaakkola, S. and Teravainen, H. (2003) Position of COMT inhibition in the treatment of Parkson's disease, in Parkinson's Disease (eds A. Gordin, S. Kaakkola and H. Teravainen) Lippincott Williams and Williams, USA, **Vol. 91**, pp. 237–250.

Gunal, D.I., Nurichalichi, K., Tuncer, N. *et al.* (2002) The clinical profile of nonmotor fluctuations in Parkinson's disease patients. *The Canadian Journal of Neurological Sciences*, **29**, 61–64.

Hill, A.N., Jankovic, J., Vuong, K.D. and Donovan, D. (2003) Treatment of hypophonia with collagen vocal cord augmentation in patients with parkinsonism. *Movement Disorders*, **18**, 1190–1192.

Hockstein, N.G., Samadi, D.S., Gendron, K. and Handler, S.D. (2004) Sialorrhea: a management challenge. *American Family Physician*, **69**, 2628–2634.

Hoehn, M.M. and Elton, R.L. (1985) Low dosages of bromocriptine added to levodopa in Parkinson's disease. *Neurology*, **35**, 199–206.

Hughes, A.J., Bishop, S., Lees, A.J. *et al.* (1991) Rectal apomorphine in Parkinson's disease. *Lancet*, **337**, 118.

Hughes, A.J., Bishop, S., Kleedorfer, B. *et al.* (1993) Subcutaneous apomorphine in Parkinson's disease: response to chronic administration for up to five years. *Movement Disorders*, **8**, 165–170.

Hyson, H.C., Johnson, A.M. and Jog, M.S. (2002) Sublingual atropine for sialorrhea secondary to parkinsonism: a pilot study. *Movement Disorders*, **17**, 1318–1320.

Ives, N.J., Stowe, R.L., Marro, J. *et al.* (2004) Monoamine oxidase type B inhibitors in early Parkinson's disease: meta-analysis of 17 randomised trials involving 3525 patients. *BMJ*, **329**, 593.

Jankovic, J., Schwartz, K. and Vander Linden, C. (1989) Comparison of Sinemet CR4 and standard Sinemet: double blind and long-term open trial in parkinsonian patients with fluctuations. *Movement Disorders*, **4**, 303–309.

Kaakkola, S., Gordin, A. and Mannisto, P.T. (1994) General properties and clinical possibilities of new selective inhibitors of catechol O-methyltransferase. *General Pharmacology*, **25**, 813–824.

Kapoor, R., Turjanski, N., Frankel, J. *et al.* (1990) Intranasal apomorphine: a new treatment in Parkinson's disease. *Journal of Neurology, Neurosurgery, and Psychiatry*, **53**, 1015.

Kapur, S. and Seeman, P. (2001) Does fast dissociation from the dopamine d(2) receptor explain the action of atypical antipsychotics?: A new hypothesis. *The American Journal of Psychiatry*, **158**, 360–369.

Karstaedt, P.J. and Pincus, J.H. (1992) Protein redistribution diet remains effective in patients with fluctuating parkinsonism. *Archives of Neurology*, **49**, 149–151.

Katzenschlager, R., Manson, A.J., Evans, A. *et al.* (2004) Low dose quetiapine for drug induced dyskinesias in Parkinson's disease: a double blind cross over study. *Journal of Neurology, Neurosurgery, and Psychiatry*, **75**, 295–297.

Katzenschlager, R., Hughes, A., Evans, A. *et al.* (2005) Continuous subcutaneous apomorphine therapy improves dyskinesias in Parkinson's disease: a prospective study using single-dose challenges. *Movement Disorders*, **20**, 151–157.

Kim, S.H., Kearney, J.J. and Atkins, J.P. (2002) Percutaneous laryngeal collagen augmentation for treatment of parkinsonian hypophonia. *Otolaryngology and Head and Neck Surgery*, **126**, 653–656.

Koller, W., Guarnieri, M., Hubble, J. *et al.* (2005) An open-label evaluation of the tolerability and safety of Stalevo(R) (carbidopa, levodopa and entacapone) in Parkinson's disease patients experiencing wearing-off. *Journal of Neural Transmission*, **112**, 221–230.

Kurlan, R., Rubin, A.J., Miller, C. *et al.* (1986) Duodenal delivery of levodopa for on-off fluctuations in parkinsonism: preliminary observations. *Annals of Neurology*, **20**, 262–265.

Kurth, M.C., Tetrud, J.W., Irwin, I. *et al.* (1993) Oral levodopa/carbidopa solution versus tablets in Parkinson's patients with severe fluctuations: a pilot study. *Neurology*, **43**, 1036–1039.

Kurth, M.C., Tetrud, J.W., Tanner, C.M. *et al.* (1993) Double-blind, placebo-controlled, crossover study of duodenal infusion of levodopa/carbidopa in Parkinson's disease patients with 'on-off' fluctuations. *Neurology*, **43**, 1698–1703.

Kurth, M.C., Adler, C.H., Hilaire, M.S. *et al.* (1997) Tolcapone improves motor function and reduces levodopa requirement in patients with Parkinson's disease experiencing motor fluctuations: a multicenter, double-blind, randomized, placebo-controlled trial. Tolcapone Fluctuator Study Group I. *Neurology*, **48**, 81–87.

Lagalla, G., Millevolte, M., Capecci, M. *et al.* (2006) Botulinum toxin type A for drooling in Parkinson's disease: a double-blind, randomized, placebo-controlled study. *Movement Disorders*, **21**, 704–707.

Larsen, J.P., Worm-Petersen, J., Siden, A. *et al.*, NOMESAFE Study Group (2003) The tolerability and efficacy of entacapone over 3 years in patients with Parkinson's disease. *European Journal of Neurology*, **10** (2), 137–146.

Leenders, K.L., Poewe, W.H., Palmer, A.J. *et al.* (1986) Inhibition of L-[18F]fluorodopa uptake into human brain by amino acids demonstrated by positron emission tomography. *Annals of Neurology*, **20**, 258–262.

Lees, A.J. (1987) A sustained-release formulation of L-dopa (Madopar HBS) in the treatment of nocturnal and early-morning disabilities in Parkinson's disease. *European Neurology*, **27** (Suppl. 1), 126–134.

Lees, A.J. (1993) Dopamine agonists in Parkinson's disease: a look at apomorphine. *Fundamental & Clinical Pharmacology*, **7** (3–4), 121–128.

Lees, A.J. (1995) Comparison of therapeutic effects and mortality data of levodopa and levodopa combined with selegiline in patients with early, mild Parkinson's disease Parkinson's Disease Research Group of the United Kingdom. *BMJ*, **311**, 1602–1607.

Lees, A.J., Shaw, K.M., Kohout, L.J. *et al.* (1977) Deprenyl in Parkinson's disease. *Lancet*, **15**, 791–795.

LeWitt, P.A., Lyons, K.E., and Pahwa, R., SP 650 Study Group (2007) Advanced Parkinson's disease treated with rotigotine transdermal system: PREFER Study. *Neurology*, **268** (16), 1262–1267.

Lieberman, A., Gopinathan, G., Miller, E. *et al.* (1990) Randomized double-blind cross-over study of Sinemet-controlled release (CR4 50/200) versus Sinemet 25/100 in Parkinson's disease. *European Neurology*, **30**, 75–78.

Lieberman, A., Imke, S., Muenter, M. *et al.* (1993) Multicenter study of cabergoline, a long-acting dopamine receptor agonist, in Parkinson's disease patients with fluctuating responses to levodopa/carbidopa. *Neurology*, **43**, 1981–1984.

Luquin, M.R., Scipioni, O., Vaamonde, J. *et al.* (1992) Levodopa-induced dyskinesias in Parkinson's disease: clinical and pharmacological classification. *Movement Disorders*, **7**, 117–124.

MacMahon, D.G., Sachdev, D., Boddie, H.G. *et al.* (1990) A comparison of the effects of controlled-release levodopa (Madopar CR) with conventional levodopa in late Parkinson's disease. *Journal of Neurology, Neurosurgery, and Psychiatry*, **53**, 220–223.

Mancini, F., Zangaglia, R., Cristina, S. *et al.* (2003) Double-blind placebo controlled study to evaluate the efficacy and safety of botulinum toxin type A in the treatment of drooling in parkinsonism. *Movement Disorders*, **18**, 685–688.

Manson, A.J., Turner, K. and Lees, A.J. (2002) Apomorphine monotherapy in the treatment of refractory motor complications of Parkinson's disease: long-term follow-up study of 64 patients. *Movement Disorders*, **17**, 1235–1241.

Marsden, C.D. (1994) Parkinson's disease. *Journal of Neurology, Neurosurgery, and Psychiatry*, **57**, 672–681.

Marsden, C.D. and Parkes, J.D. (1976) "On-off" effects in patients with Parkinson's disease on chronic levodopa therapy. *Lancet*, **1**, 292–296.

Melamed, E. (1979) Early morning dystonia: A late side effect of long-term levodopa therapy in Parkinson's disease. *Archives of Neurology*, **36**, 308–310.

Melamed, E. and Bitton, V. (1984) Delayed onset of responses to individual doses of L-dopa in parkinsonian fluctuators: an additional side effect of long-term L-dopa therapy. *Neurology*, **34** (Suppl. 2), 270.

Melamed, E., Hefti, F. and Wurtman, R.J. (1980) Nonaminergic striatal neurons convert exogenous L-dopa to dopamine in parkinsonism. *Annals of Neurology*, **8**, 558–563.

Merello, M. and Lees, A.J. (1992) Beginning-of-dose motor deterioration following the acute administration of levodopa and apomorphine in Parkinson's disease. *Journal of Neurology, Neurosurgery, and Psychiatry*, **55**, 1024–1026.

Merims, D., Djaldetti, R. and Melamed, E. (2003) Waiting for ON: a major problem in patients with Parkinson's disease and ON/OFF motor fluctuations. *Clinical Neuropharmacology*, **26**, 196–198.

Mizuno, Y., Kanazawa, I., Kuno, S. *et al.* (2007) Placebo-controlled, double-blind dose-finding study of entacapone in fluctuating parkinsonian patients. *Movement Disorders*, **22**, 75–80.

Montastruc, J.L., Rascol, O., Senard, J.M. *et al.* (1991) Sublingual apomorphine in Parkinson's disease: a clinical and pharmacokinetic study. *Clinical Neuropharmacology*, **14**, 432–437.

Muenter, M.D. and Tyce, G.M. (1971) L-dopa therapy of Parkinson's disease: plasma L-dopa concentration, therapeutic response, and side effects. *Mayo Clinic Proceedings*, **46**, 231–239.

Muenter, M.D., Sharpless, N.S., Tyce, G.M. and Darley, F.L. (1977) Patterns of dystonia (I-D-I and D-I-D) in response to L-dopa therapy in Parkinson's disease. *Mayo Clinic Proceedings*, **52**, 163–174.

Muller, T., Woitalla, D., Schulz, D. *et al.* (2000) Tolcapone increases maximum concentration of levodopa. *Journal of Neural Transmission*, **107**, 113–119.

Myllyla, V.V., Kultalahti, E.R., Haapaniemi, H., and Leinonen, M., FILOMEN Study Group (2001) Twelve-month safety of entacapone in patients with Parkinson's disease. *European Journal of Neurology*, **8**, 53–60.

Nausieda, P.A., Pfeiffer, R.F., Tagliati, M. *et al.* (2005) A multi-center, open-label, sequential study comparing preferences for carbidopa-levodopa orally disintegrating tablets and conventional tablets in subjects with Parkinson's disease. *Clinical Therapeutics*, **27**, 58–63.

Ng, K.Y., Colburn, R.W. and Kopin, I.J. (1971) Effects of L-dopa on efflux of cerebral monoamines from synaptosomes. *Nature*, **230**, 331–332.

Nutt, J.G. (1990) Pharmacokinetics of Levodopa-induced dyskinesia: review, observations, and speculations. *Neurology*, **40**, 340–345.

Nutt, J.G. and Fellman, J.H. (1984) Pharmacokinetics of levodopa. *Clinical Neuropharmacology*, **7**, 35–49.

Nutt, J.G. and Woodward, W.R. (1986) Levodopa pharmacokinetics and pharmacodynamics in fluctuating parkinsonian patients. *Neurology*, **36** (6), 739–744.

Nutt, J.G., Gancher, S.T. and Woodward, W.R. (1988) Does an inhibitory action of levodopa contribute to motor fluctuations? *Neurology*, **38**, 1553–1557.

Nutt, J.G., Obeso, J.A. and Stocchi, F. (2000) Continuous dopamine-receptor stimulation in advanced Parkinson's disease. *Trends in Neurosciences*, **23** (Suppl), S109–S115.

Nyholm, D. and Aquilonius, S.M. (2004) Levodopa infusion therapy in Parkinson's disease: state of the art in 2004. *Clinical Neuropharmacology*, **27**, 245–256.

Nyholm, D., Nilsson Remahl, A.I., Dizdar, N. *et al.* (2005) Duodenal levodopa infusion monotherapy vs oral polypharmacy in advanced Parkinson's disease. *Neurology*, **64**, 216–223.

Nyholm, D. (2006) Enteral levodopa/carbidopa gel infusion for the treatment of motor fluctuations and dyskinesias in advanced Parkinson's disease. *Expert Review of Neurotherapeutics*, **6**, 1403–1411.

Odin, P., Oehlwein, C., Storch, A. *et al.* (2006) Efficacy and safety of high-dose cabergoline in Parkinson's disease. *Acta Neurologica Scandinavica*, **113**, 18–24.

Oh, J.D., Bibbiani, F. and Chase, T.N. (2002) Quetiapine attenuates levodopa-induced motor complications in rodent and primate parkinsonian models. *Experimental Neurology*, **177**, 557–564.

Olanow, C.W., Fahn, S., Muenter, M. *et al.* (1994) A multicenter double-blind placebo-controlled trial of pergolide as an adjunct to Sinemet in Parkinson's disease. *Movement Disorders*, **9**, 40–47.

Ondo, W.G., Hunter, C. and Moore, W. (2004) A double-blind placebo-controlled trial of botulinum toxin B for sialorrhea in Parkinson's disease. *Neurology*, **62**, 37–40.

Paci, C., Thomas, A. and Onofrj, M. (2001) Amantadine for dyskinesia in patients affected by severe Parkinson's disease. *Neurological Sciences*, **22**, 75–76.

Pacchetti, C., Albani, G., Martignoni, E. *et al.* (1995) "Off" painful dystonia in Parkinson's disease treated with botulinum toxin. *Movement Disorders*, **10**, 333–336.

Pahwa, R., Factor, S.A., Lyons, K.E. *et al.*, Quality Standards Subcommittee of the American Academy of Neurology (2006) Practice Parameter: treatment of Parkinson's disease with motor fluctuations and dyskinesia (an evidence-based review): report of the Quality Standards Subcommittee of the American Academy of Neurology. *Neurology*, **66**, 983–995.

Parashos, S.A., Wielinski, C.L. and Kern, J.A. (2004) Frequency, reasons, and risk factors of entacapone discontinuation in Parkinson's disease. *Clinical Neuropharmacology*, **27**, 119–123.

Parkinson Study Group (1997) Entacapone improves motor fluctuations in levodopa-treated Parkinson's disease patients. *Annals of Neurology*, **42** 747–755.

Parkinson Study Group (2005) A randomized placebo-controlled trial of rasagiline in levodopa-treated patients with Parkinson's disease and motor fluctuations: the PRESTO study. *Archives of Neurology*, **62** 241–248.

Pierantozzi, M., Pietroiusti, A., Brusa, L. *et al.* (2006) Helicobacter pylori eradication and l-dopa absorption in patients with PD and motor fluctuations. *Neurology*, **66**, 1824–1829.

Pincus, J.H. and Barry, K. (1987) Influence of dietary protein on motor fluctuations in Parkinson's disease. *Archives of Neurology*, **44**, 270–272.

Pinter, M.M., Pogarell, O. and Oertel, W.H. (1999) Efficacy, safety, and tolerance of the non-ergoline dopamine agonist pramipexole in the treatment of advanced Parkinson's disease: a double blind, placebo controlled, randomised, multicentre study. *Journal of Neurology, Neurosurgery, and Psychiatry*, **66**, 436–441.

Pinto, S., Ozsancak, C., Tripoliti, E. *et al.* (2004) Treatments for dysarthria in Parkinson's disease. *Lancet Neurology*, **3**, 547–556.

Poewe, W.H., Lees, A.J. and Stern, G.M. (1988) Dystonia in Parkinson's disease: clinical and pharmacological features. *Annals of Neurology*, **23**, 73–78.

Poewe, W.H., Deuschl, G., Gordin, A. *et al.*, Celomen Study Group (2002) Efficacy and safety of entacapone in Parkinson's disease patients with suboptimal levodopa response: a 6-month randomized placebo-controlled double-blind study in Germany and Austria (Celomen study). *Acta Neurologica Scandinavica*, **105**, 245–255.

Priano, L., Albani, G., Brioschi, A. *et al.* (2004) Transdermal apomorphine permeation from microemulsions: a new treatment in Parkinson's disease. *Movement Disorders*, **19**, 937–942.

Proulx, M., de Courval, F.P., Wiseman, M.A. and Panisset, M. (2005) Salivary production in Parkinson's disease. *Movement Disorders*, **20**, 204–207.

Rajput, A.H., Martin, W., Saint-Hilaire, M.H. *et al.* (1997) Tolcapone improves motor function in parkinsonian patients with the "wearing-off" phenomenon: a double-blind, placebo-controlled, multicenter trial. *Neurology*, **49**, 1066–1071.

Ramig, L.O., Fox, C. and Sapir, S. (2004) Parkinson's disease: speech and voice disorders and their treatment with the Lee Silverman Voice Treatment. *Seminars in Speech and Language*, **25**, 169–180.

Rascol, O., Lees, A.J., Senard, J.M. *et al.* (1996) Ropinirole in the treatment of levodopa-induced motor fluctuations in patients with Parkinson's disease. *Clinical Neuropharmacology*, **19**, 234–245.

Rascol, O., Brooks, D.J., Melamed, E. *et al.*, LARGO Study Group (2005) Rasagiline as an adjunct to levodopa in patients with Parkinson's disease and motor fluctuations (LARGO, Lasting effect in Adjunct therapy with Rasagiline Given Once daily, study): a randomised, double-blind, parallel-group trial. *Lancet*, **365**, 947–954.

Raudino, F. (2001) Non motor off in Parkinson's disease. *Acta Neurologica Scandinavica*, **104**, 312–315.

Richard, I.H., Kurlan, R., Tanner, C. *et al.* (1997) Serotonin syndrome and the combined use of deprenyl and an antidepressant in Parkinson's disease. Parkinson Study Group. *Neurology*, **48**, 1070–1077.

Riederer, P. and Youdim, M.B. (1986) Monoamine oxidase activity and monoamine metabolism in brains of parkinsonian patients treated with l-deprenyl. *Journal of Neurochemistry*, **46**, 1359–1365.

Rinne, U.K., Larsen, J.P., Siden, A. and Worm-Petersen, J. (1998) Entacapone enhances the response to levodopa in parkinsonian patients with motor fluctuations. Nomecomt Study Group. *Neurology*, **51** (5), 1309–1314.

Ruottinen, H.M. and Rinne, U.K. (1996) Effect of one month's treatment with peripherally acting catechol-O-methyltransferase inhibitor, entacapone, on pharmacokinetics and motor response to levodopa in advanced parkinsonian patients. *Clinical Neuropharmacology*, **19**, 222–233.

Ruottinen, H.M. and Rinne, U.K. (1996) Entacapone prolongs levodopa response in a one month double blind study in parkinsonian patients with levodopa related fluctuations. *Journal of Neurology, Neurosurgery, and Psychiatry*, **60**, 36–40.

Sage, J.I., Trooskin, S., Sonsalla, P.K. *et al.* (1988) Long-term duodenal infusion of levodopa for motor fluctuations in parkinsonism. *Annals of Neurology*, **24**, 87–89.

Schade, R., Andersohn, F., Suissa, S. *et al.* (2007) Dopamine agonists and the risk of cardiac-valve regurgitation. *The New England Journal of Medicine*, **356**, 29–38.

Scott, S. and Caird, F.I. (1983) Speech therapy for Parkinson's disease. *Journal of Neurology, Neurosurgery, and Psychiatry*, **46**, 140–144.

Seager, H. (1997) Drug delivery products and the Zydis fast-dissolving dosage form. *Journal of Pharmacy and Pharmacology*, **50**, 375–382.

Shoulson, I., Glaubiger, G.A. and Chase, T.N. (1975) On-off response. Clinical and biochemical correlations during oral and intravenous levodopa administration in parkinsonian patients. *Neurology*, **25**, 1144–1148.

Snow, B.J., Macdonald, L., McAuley, D. and Wallis, W. (2000) The effect of amantadine on levodopa-induced dyskinesias in Parkinson's disease: a double-blind, placebo-controlled study. *Clinical Neuropharmacology*, **23**, 82–85.

Steiger, M.J., Stocchi, F., Carta, A. *et al.* (1991) The clinical efficacy of oral levodopa methyl ester solution in reversing afternoon "off" periods in Parkinson's disease. *Clinical Neuropharmacology*, **14**, 241–244.

Steiger, M.J., Stocchi, F., Bramante, L. *et al.* (1992) The clinical efficacy of single morning doses of levodopa methyl ester: dispersible Madopar and Sinemet plus in Parkinson's disease. *Clinical Neuropharmacology*, **15**, 501–504.

Stibe, C.M., Lees, A.J., Kempster, P.A. and Stern, G.M. (1988) Subcutaneous apomorphine in parkinsonian on-off oscillations. *Lancet*, **20**, 403–406.

Stocchi, F., Nordera, G. and Marsden, C.D. (1997) Strategies for treating patients with advanced Parkinson's disease with disastrous fluctuations and dyskinesias. *Clinical Neuropharmacology*, **20**, 95–115.

Stocchi, F., Ruggieri, S., Vacca, L. and Olanow, C.W. (2002) Prospective randomized trial of lisuride infusion versus oral levodopa in patients with Parkinson's disease. *Brain*, **125**, 2058–2066.

Stocchi, F., Vacca, L., Ruggieri, S. and Olanow, C.W. (2005) Intermittent vs continuous levodopa administration in patients with advanced Parkinson's disease: a clinical and pharmacokinetic study. *Archives of Neurology*, **62**, 905–910.

Stocchi, F., Fabbri, L., Vecsei, L. *et al.* (2007) Clinical efficacy of a single afternoon dose of effervescent levodopa-carbidopa preparation (CHF 1512) in fluctuating Parkinson's disease. *Clinical Neuropharmacology*, **30**, 18–24.

Storch, A., Trenkwalder, C., Oehlwein, C. *et al.* (2005) High-dose treatment with pergolide in Parkinson's disease patients with motor fluctuations and dyskinesias. *Parkinsonism & Related Disorders*, **11**, 393–398.

Stroudley, J. and Walsh, M. (1991) Radiological assessment of dysphagia in Parkinson's disease. *British Journal of Radiology*, **64**, 890–893.

Suchowersky, O., Gronseth, G., Perlmutter, J. *et al.*, Quality Standards Subcommittee of the American Academy of Neurology (2006) Practice Parameter: neuroprotective strategies and alternative therapies for Parkinson's disease (an evidence-based review): report of the Quality Standards Subcommittee of the American Academy of Neurology. *Neurology*, **66**, 976–982.

Thomas, A., Iacono, D., Luciano, A.L. *et al.* (2004) Duration of amantadine benefit on dyskinesia of severe Parkinson's disease. *Journal of Neurology, Neurosurgery, and Psychiatry*, **75**, 141–143.

Tyne, H.L., Parsons, J., Sinnott, A. *et al.* (2004) A 10 year retrospective audit of long-term apomorphine use in Parkinson's disease. *Journal of Neurology*, **251**, 1370–1374.

van de Vijver, D.A., Roos, R.A., Jansen, P.A. *et al.* (2002) Antipsychotics and Parkinson's disease: association with disease and drug choice during the first 5 years of antiparkinsonian drug treatment. *European Journal of Clinical Pharmacology*, **58**, 157–161.

Van Gerpen, J.A., Kumar, N., Bower, J.H. *et al.* (2006) Levodopa-associated dyskinesia risk among Parkinson's disease patients in Olmsted County, Minnesota, 1976–1990. *Archives of Neurology*, **63**, 205–209.

Verhagen Metman, L., Del Dotto, P., van den Munckhof, P. *et al.* (1998) Amantadine as treatment for dyskinesias and motor fluctuations in Parkinson's disease. *Neurology*, **50**, 1323–1326.

Verhagen Metman, L., Konitsiotis, S. and Chase, T.N. (2000) Pathophysiology of motor response complications in Parkinson's disease: hypotheses on the why, where, and what. *Movement Disorders*, **15**, 3–8.

Voon, V., Hassan, K., Zurowski, M. *et al.* (2006) Prevalence of reward-seeking and repetitive behaviors in Parkinson's disease. *Neurology*, **67**, 1254–1257.

Waters, C.H., Sethi, K.D., Hauser, R.A. *et al.*, Zydis Selegiline Study Group (2004) Zydis selegiline reduces off time in Parkinson's disease patients with motor fluctuations: a 3-month, randomized, placebo-controlled study. *Movement Disorders*, **19**, 426–432.

Weintraub, D., Siderowf, A.D., Potenza, M.N. *et al.* (2006) Association of dopamine agonist use with impulse control disorders in Parkinson's disease. *Archives of Neurology*, **63**, 969–973.

Witjas, T., Kaphan, E., Azulay, J.P. *et al.* (2002) Nonmotor fluctuations in Parkinson's disease: frequent and disabling. *Neurology*, **59**, 408–413.

Zanettini, R., Antonini, A., Gatto, G. *et al.* (2007) Valvular heart disease and the use of dopamine agonists for Parkinson's disease. *The New England Journal of Medicine*, **356** (1), 39–46.

6

Managing the Non-Motor Symptoms of Parkinson's Disease

Werner Poewe and Klaus Seppi

Department of Neurology, Medical University of Innsbruck, Innsbruck, Austria

CLASSIFICATION AND CLINICAL SPECTRUM

Although idiopathic Parkinson's disease (PD) is generally considered a paradigmatic movement disorder, it has long been recognized that the neuropathology underlying PD involves many brain areas that are not directly involved in motor control, like the locus coeruleus, dorsal vagal nucleus, raphe nuclei of the brainstem, the hypothalamus, the olfactory tubercle and large parts of the limbic cortex and neocortex (Braak *et al.*, 2003). Pathology also extends into the peripheral autonomic nervous system involving sympathetic ganglia, cardiac sympathetic efferents and the myenteric plexus of the gut (Braak *et al.*, 2003; Braak *et al.*, 2006a). It is therefore not surprising that a majority, if not all PD patients, also suffer from non-motor symptoms (Poewe, 2006), adding to the overall burden of parkinsonian morbidity. Non-motor symptoms in PD involve a multitude of functions, including disorders of sleep–wake cycle regulation, cognitive dysfunction, disorders of mood and affect, autonomic dysfunction as well as sensory symptoms and pain. They become increasingly prevalent and obvious over the course of the illness and are a major determinant of quality of life, progression of overall disability and of nursing-home placement in PD (Hely *et al.*, 2005). In their various combinations, non-motor symptoms may become the chief therapeutic challenge in advanced stages of PD.

NEUROPSYCHIATRIC FEATURES (TABLE 6.1)

Depression

Clinical Features

Apathy, or some degree of loss of initiative and decisiveness, are almost universal, even in the early stages of PD, and some decline in the capacity to derive pleasure from enjoyable activities is also reported by many patients or their partners. The majority, however, do not complain about depressed mood, and there is some ambiguity regarding the exact clinical definition of PD-associated depression vs PD-specific alterations of psychomotor drive and hedonistic tone (Barone *et al.*, 2006). Loss of interest and anhedonia are core features of the depressive syndrome in PD. Anxiety and panic attacks are also common in PD and may antedate the first manifestation of the parkinsonian motor syndrome. Insomnia, loss of appetite and fatigue are also frequently present, while other depressive features common in major depression in non-PD patients, like feelings of self-blame, guilt, sense of failure and self-destructive thoughts, are much less common in PD, as are suicides or suicidal ideation (Mayeux 1990).

Prevalence

According to published reports, the prevalence of major depression in PD ranges from a low of 4% to a high of 70% (Poewe 2006; Tandberg *et al.*, 1996; Starkstein *et al.*, 1990; Cummings, 1992; Meara, Mitchelmore and Hobson, 1999). Recent studies suggest the presence of depressive symptoms in 36–50% of patients with PD (Shulman *et al.*, 2001), but less than half of these will actually meet DSM IV criteria for major depression (Tandberg *et al.*, 1996).

Pathophysiology and Clinico-Pathological Correlations

While some of the depressive symptoms in Parkinson's disease may actually occur as a reaction at the time of first diagnosis, there is general consensus that PD-specific pathology, with multiple transmitter deficiencies in mesocortical monoaminergic systems, plays a major role—including the mesocorticolimbic dopaminergic projection, as well as the

Therapeutics of Parkinson's Disease and Other Movement Disorders   Edited by Mark Hallett and Werner Poewe
© 2008 John Wiley & Sons, Ltd.

Table 6.1 Neuropsychiatric features in PD.

Mood disorder
- anhedonia, apathy
- anxiety
- depression

Cognitive dysfunction
- dysexecutive syndrome
- visuospatial dysfunction
- dementia
- psychosis

Complex behavioral disorders
- dopamine dysregulation syndrome (hedonistic homeostatic dysregulation)
- punding
- impulse control disorders

mesocortical noradrenergic and serotonergic projections. Specifically dopaminergic cell-loss in the ventral tegmental area (VTA) with subsequent orbitofrontal dopaminergic denervation may contribute to apathy and anhedonia, which are typical of parkinsonian depression (Damier et al., 1999). In addition, corticolimbic noradrenergic denervation through cell-loss in the locus coeruleus and serotonergic denervation via serotonergic cell-loss in the raphe nucleus likely play a role. Recent functional imaging studies have confirmed dopaminergic and noradrenergic denervation in limbic areas and have also demonstrated reduction of 5-HT$_{1A}$ receptor binding in the limbic cortex and frontal and temporal cortical areas in depressed PD-patients (Remy et al., 2005).

Principles of Management

Psychosocial support, counseling and various forms of psychotherapy all have a role in the management of patients with PD and depression, particularly in relation to reactive depressive episodes around the time of diagnosis. The mainstay of treatment for most patients, however, is pharmacological therapy.

Available Studies

In contrast to the frequency and clinical impact of depression of PD, there are very limited data from controlled clinical trials to guide treatment decisions (Goetz et al., 2002). In those therapeutic trials available, placebo effects have generally been large (Weintraub et al., 2005) and virtually no study to date has unequivocally demonstrated anti-depressive efficacy of any intervention targeting PD-related depression in a placebo-controlled design—the only

exception relating to an old trial of nortriptiline using an unconventional outcome measure (Wermuth, Sorensen and Timm, 1998; Andersen et al., 1980).

Available open-label and controlled drug trials in PD depression have assessed both classical anti-depressants, as well as the anti-depressive potential of dopaminergic drugs used to treat the motor symptoms of PD. In addition, some studies have assessed the efficacy of electroconvulsive therapy or transcranial magnetic stimulation.

Dopaminergic Agents

The role of dopaminergic deficiency in PD depression is illustrated by the common clinical occurrence of OFF-period-related depressive symptoms in fluctuating PD (Witjas et al., 2002). Consistent with this, Maricle and co-workers (Maricle et al., 1995) have shown anti-anxiolytic and mood brightening short-term effects of L-Dopa infusions in a double-blind, single-dose placebo-controlled study of eight patients with fluctuating Parkinson's disease. There have also been claims of anti-depressant efficacy of the dopamine (DA) agonist bromocriptine in a small open-label study (Jouvent et al., 1983). More recently, the non-ergot dopamine agonist pramipexole was shown to exert anti-depressant effects in two randomized open-label studies in PD patients with depression (Barone et al., 2006; Rektorova et al., 2003). Both studies showed significant improvements on the Hamilton Depression Rating scale (HAM-D), but are limited by the lack of a placebo-control arm (see Table 6.2). Two randomized studies have assessed the anti-depressant effects of monoamine oxidase (MAO) inhibitors in PD (Lees et al., 1977; Mann et al., 1989). Results were inconsistent and both studies were confounded by motor improvement and also lacked placebo controls.

Anti-depressant Drugs

Tricyclic anti-depressants (TCAs) were identified as the second most commonly used drug class to treat PD depression in a large North American survey involving 49 investigators of the Parkinson Study Group (Richard and Kurlan, 1997), but there are only very limited data from clinical trials in PD to support this use.

The only randomized placebo-controlled study with this class of agents in PD depression dates back more than 20 years and is related to nortriptyline (titrated from 25 mg/day to a maximum of 150 mg/day) (Andersen et al., 1980), which showed a significant improvement over placebo, on a depression rating scale designed by the author. The now more commonly used anti-muscarinic anti-depressants clomipramine, imipramine or amitryptiline have never been tested in a placebo-controlled trial in PD depression, although amitryptiline was more efficacious than fluoxetine in one randomized comparator trial (Serrano-Duenas, 2002) and received a level C recommendation for treating

Table 6.2 Treatment of depression in PD: randomized controlled trials.

	Study	Intervention	Daily dose	Design	Duration	Patients included (n)	Outcome
Anti-depressants	Andersen et al. (1980)	Nortriptyline vs placebo	25–150 mg	Randomized, double-blind, cross-over	16 wk with 8 wk cross-over period	22	Significantly greater improvement of depression in the nortriptyline group compared to placebo
	Wermuth, Sorensen and Timm (1998)	Citalopram vs placebo	10–40 mg	Randomized, double-blind, parallel group	6 wk acute phase, additional 46 wk continuation phase	37	Significant decrease of HAM-D scores within both treatment groups at 6 wk; no difference between groups at week 6 or 52. Withdrawal rate of 19% in the acute phase and of 73% in the continuation phase
	Leentjens et al. (2003)	Sertraline vs placebo	25–100 mg	Randomized, double-blind, parallel group	10 wk	12	Significant decrease of MADRS scores within both treatment groups at 10 wk; no difference between groups.
	Serrano-Duenas (2002)	Amitriptyline vs fluoxetine	Amitriptyline: 25–75 mg; Fluoxetine: 20–40 mg	Randomized, parallel group	12 mo	77	Patients randomized to amitriptyline significantly improved on the HAM-D, while those treated with fluoxetine did not.
	Avila et al. (2003)	Nefazodone vs fluoxetine	Nefazodone: 100–300 mg; Fluoxetine: 20–40 mg	Randomized, single-blind, parallel group	90 d	16	Significant decrease of BDI scores within both treatment groups without difference between groups. Significant improvement on the UPDRS II + III in the nefazodone group, no change on UPDRS II + III in the fluoxetine group

(continued)

Table 6.2 (*Continued*)

	Study	Intervention	Daily dose	Design	Duration	Patients included (*n*)	Outcome
Dopaminergic drugs	Rektorova *et al.* (2003)	Pramipexole *vs* pergolide	Pramipexole: 2.7 mg; pergolide 3 mg	Randomized, parallel group, open label	6 and 12 mo	41	Patients in both arms had significant improvements in Zung scores over baseline while only patients on pramipexole also significantly improved on the MADRS.
	Barone *et al.* (2006)	Pramipexole *vs* sertraline	Pramipexole: 3 mg; sertraline: 48 mg	Randomized, parallel group, open label	12 wk	67	Significant decrease of HAM-D scores within both treatment groups at 12 wk; no difference between groups. 61% of patients on pramipexole *vs* 27% on sertraline had HAM-D scores of ≤7 at week 12
rTMS	Okabe, Ugawa and Kanazawa (2003)	Motor cortical, occipital and sham rTMS	0.2 Hz	Randomized, double-blind, parallel group	8 wk	85	Significant decrease of HAM-D and UPDRS scores motor cortical and sham group with no difference between groups.
	Fregni *et al.* (2004)	active rTMS and placebo drug treatment *vs* sham rTMS and fluoxetine	15 Hz rTMS for 10 d; fluoxetine: 20 mg	Randomized, double-blind, parallel group	8 wk	42	Significant decrease of HAM-D and BDI scores within both groups without any difference between groups at week 2. No change at week 8 in either group. No effects on UPDRS III.

wk: week; mo: month; d: day; BDI: Beck Depression Inventory; HAM-D: Hamilton Rating Scale for Depression; MADRS: Montgomery-Asberg Depression Rating Scale; UPDRS: Unified PD Rating Scale.

PD depression in a recent AAN practice parameter (Miyasaki *et al.*, 2006).

Serotonine Reuptake Inhibitors (SSRIs)

SSRIs were the most commonly used class of drugs to treat depression in PD, considered the first-line option in 63% of their patients by the North American Parkinson Study Group (PSG) investigators (Richard and Kurlan, 1997). The efficacy of SSRIs in PD-associated depression has been suggested by numerous open-label studies covering a variety of agents (fluoxetine, sertraline, paroxetine) (Goetz *et al.*, 2002; Weintraub *et al.*, 2005). To date, only two small double-blind placebo-controlled studies have assessed this approach. When Leentjens and colleagues randomized 12 patients to treatment with sertraline or placebo for 10 weeks no statistically significant differences in the change of Montgomery-Asberg Depression Rating Scale (MADRS) scores was detected (Leentjens *et al.*, 2003), and Wermuth and co-workers also failed to detect statistically significant differences in treatment response between citalopram and placebo in a larger trial involving 37 patients treated for 52 weeks (Wermuth, Sorensen and Timm, 1998).

Newer Anti-depressants

Reboxetine (Lemke, 2002) is a selective noradrenergic re-uptake inhibitor devoid of serotonergic activity, while nefazodone (Avila *et al.*, 2003) and venlafaxine (Cunningham, 1994) are both serotonergic and noradrenergic re-uptake inhibitors. Mirtazapine is a potent pre-synaptic α_2-adrenergic autoreceptor antagonist, and in addition has antagonistic activity at both 5-HT_2 and 5-HT_3 serotonin receptors enhancing 5-HT_1-mediated neurotransmission. The only available randomized trial with this class of drugs has compared nefazodone with fluoxetine (see Table 6.2) and found similar anti-depressant activity, in a small group of patients with PD (Avila *et al.*, 2003).

Non-Pharmacological Treatment

A recent review identified 21 articles, covering a total of 71 patients with PD receiving electroconvulsive therapy (ECT) to treat concomitant depression (Goetz *et al.*, 2002). These data are insufficient to conclude about the efficacy and safety of ECT to treat depression in PD. Two double-blind studies have assessed repetitive transcranial magnetic stimulation (rTMS) in PD depression. There was no difference between sham and effective stimulation with respect to depression and PD measures (Okabe, Ugawa and Kanazawa, 2003). Another study (Fregni *et al.*, 2004) found rTMS as effective as fluoxetine in improving depression at week 2—an effect maintained to week 8. However, interpretation of this study is hampered by lack of a placebo arm (see Table 6.2).

Pragmatic Management of PD Depression

In the absence of controlled-trial data on drug-treatment of depression in PD, routine clinical management has to rely on extrapolation from data obtained in trials in non-PD populations with major depression and open-label observations in PD depression, taking into account current knowledge on the pathogenesis of depressive symptoms in PD (see Figure 6.1). In general, patients should be receiving sufficient dopamine-substitution for optimal control of motor symptoms, including attempts to smooth out motor response oscillations that can go along with profound mood swings. In cases with advanced PD this will usually be based on combinations of L-Dopa with or without catechol-O-methyltransferase (COMT)-inhibitors and dopamine agonists. Currently there is insufficient evidence to support the use of dopamine agonists as primary anti-depressants in PD patients with optimized motor control.

Add-on anti-depressant drug treatment is often needed, and the choice between anti-muscarinic agents, SSRIs or the newer combined serotonergic-adrenergic agents depends on the patient profile and individual safety and tolerability (see Figure 6.1). The anti-cholinergic profile of anti-muscarinic anti-depressants may help to further improve PD symptoms, such as tremor or rigidity, and their sedating properties may make them suitable options for patients with agitated depression and insomnia. Their main safety risks are related to a potential to induce cardiac arrhythmias, orthostatic hypotension, cognitive dysfunction or delirium when used in patients with PD dementia. Concomitant treatment of PD patients with TCAs can contribute to psychosis, sedation and daytime sleepiness and abrupt withdrawal has been associated with dysautonomia, anxiety and panic.

SSRIs may help to improve anhedonia and loss of interest and relieve anxiety and panic attacks. SSRIs, when studied in psychiatric populations, have been found to exhibit an improved safety profile over TCAs with lower incidences of anti-cholinergic side effects or cardiac arrhythmias. They may, however, worsen PD tremor in some 4 to 5% of patients (Ceravolo *et al.*, 2000) and there are concerns about the induction of the serotonin syndrome when used in conjunction with MAOB inhibitors. This somewhat loosely defined condition involves hyperpyrexia, tremor, agitation and other mental status changes and has been found to occur in severe form in 0.24% of PD cases exposed to SSRIs in the presence of the MAOB inhibitor selegeline, in one large survey (Richard *et al.*, 1997).

The class of newer anti-depressant agents targeting both the noradrenergic and serotonergic systems may be useful in PD depression, given that both systems are involved in its pathogenesis, but so far there are very limited data to actually support their efficacy or safety. Venlafaxine has activating effects that can be useful in apathic patients and

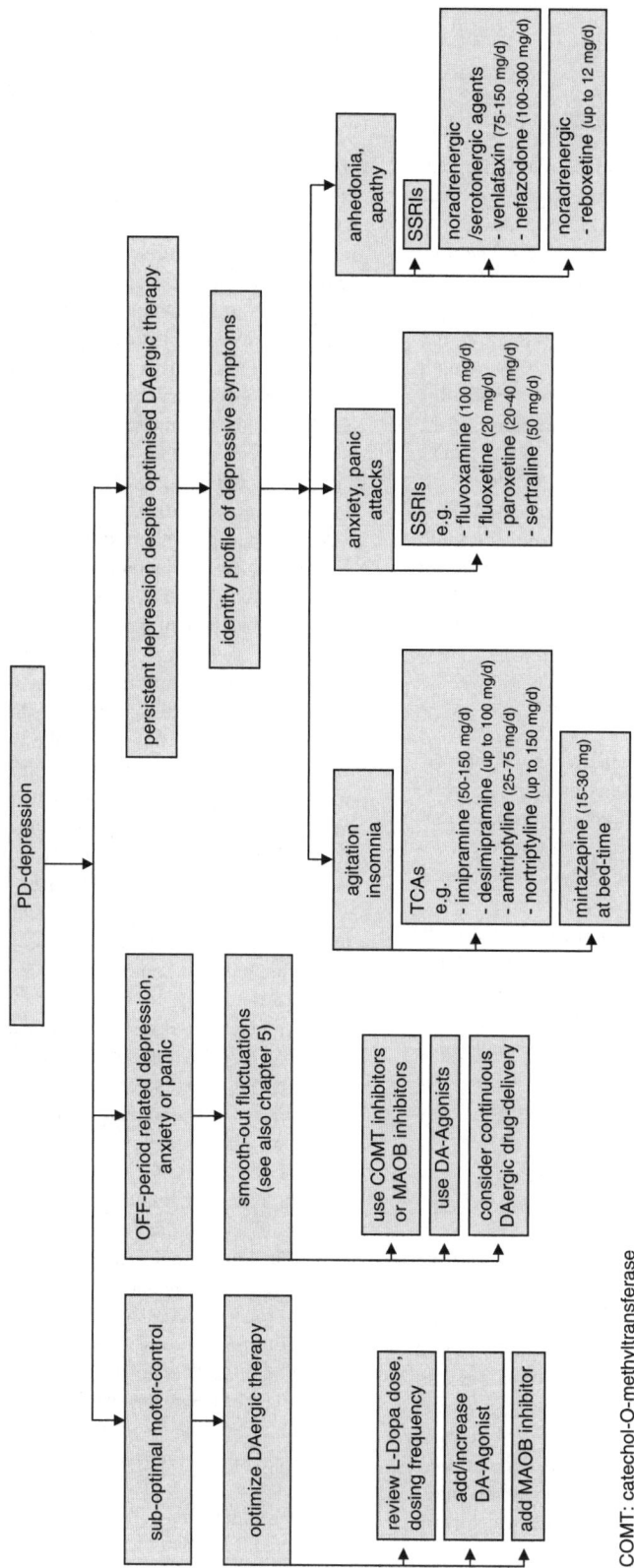

COMT: catechol-O-methyltransferase
DA: dopamine
MAOB: monoamine oxidase B
TCAs: tricyclic antidepressants
Tx: therapy
SSRIs: selective serotonin reuptake inhibitors
PD: Parkinson's disease

Figure 6.1 Pragmatic management of PD-associated depression.

withdrawn patients with PD depression, but needs to be avoided in agitated subjects (Okun and Watts, 2002). Because of its anti-histaminic activity mirtazapine can induce some sedation and should be given at bedtime. It has been claimed to reduce anxiety and insomnia in depressed PD patients (Okun and Watts, 2002).

Currently available evidence does not support the use of ECT or rTMS to treat depression in PD.

Cognitive Dysfunction and Dementia

The development of dementia has significant impact on the natural history of Parkinson's disease and has been shown to be associated with more rapid progression of disability, increased risk for nursing-home placement and increased mortality (Goetz and Stebbins, 1993; Biggins *et al.*, 1992; Marder *et al.*, 1995).

Definition and Clinical Features

The clinical profile of PD dementia (PD-D) is identical to that of dementia with Lewy Bodies (DLB) except for later development of the dementia syndrome (more than 12 months after onset of parkinsonism in PD-D and before that in DLB) (McKeith *et al.*, 2005). The dementia syndrome of PD-D includes aspects of psychomotor slowing, apathy and bradyphrenia, but the core cognitive dysfunction in PD-D is characterized by deficits in memory, attention, visuospatial and visuoconstructive capabilities and executive function. The memory deficit in PD predominantly affects retrieval, but there is also impairment of cued recall and recognition, both in the verbal and visual domains (Emre *et al.*, 2007). Attentional deficits in PD-D may show similar fluctuations as reported for DLB (Ballard *et al.*, 2002), and executive dysfunction includes impaired verbal fluency tests, concept formation, set shifting and problem solving. In addition, affected patients may show prominent mood and behavioral disorders, including anxiety and depression, as well as hallucinations, delusions and confusional states, while language and praxis remain largely intact (Emre, 2003). Cognitive dysfunction in PD-D is progressive at an average annual rate of decline of Mini-Mental State Examination (MMSE)-scores in the order of two to three points (Emre 2003; Aarsland *et al.*, 2004).

Prevalence

Subtle cognitive deficits are almost universally identified even in early Parkinson's disease upon detailed neuropsychological testing (Lees and Smith, 1983). A recent meta-analysis of prevalence studies on dementia in Parkinson's disease has estimated that 31% of PD patients fulfill diagnostic criteria for dementia and that PD-D accounts for around 4% of degenerative dementias with a population-based prevalence of between 0.2 and 0.5% in those aged older than 65 (Aarsland, Zaccai and Brayne, 2005a).

Pathophysiology and Clinico-Pathological Correlations

The pathophysiology of cognitive decline and dementia in PD is complex and includes multiple pathologies in multiple brain areas. Neocortical Alzheimer-type changes, limbic and neocortical Lewy Body degeneration as well as subcortical vascular lesions are often present in combination, but cortical Lewy Body degeneration has been suggested to be the major driving factor for the development of dementia in PD (Aarsland *et al.*, 2005b; Apaydin *et al.*, 2002). Similar to DLB, dementia in PD has been correlated with cortical cholinergic denervation (Whitehouse *et al.*, 1983; Perry *et al.*, 1993; Bohnen *et al.*, 2003).

Principles of Management

In trying to improve cognitive function and erratic behavior in patients with PD-D, it is important to control or eliminate potential aggravators (see Figure 6.2) and in the majority of patients additional treatment with anti-dementia agents will deserve a trial.

Available Studies

Based on the role of cortical cholinergic denervation in the pathogenesis of PD-D, cholinesterase inhibitors (ChE-Is) are the most widely studied class of agents for this condition. Small open-label series with usually less than 10 patients were initially performed with tacrine (Hutchinson and Fazzini, 1996), subsequently with rivastigmine and donepezil (Werber and Rabey, 2001; Reading, Luce and McKeith, 2001; Linazasoro *et al.*, 2005), and have claimed efficacy in improving cognition and reducing erratic behavior. More recently, efficacy and safety of donepezil and rivastigmine have been evaluated in placebo-controlled randomized trials (see Table 6.3).

Donepezil

Aarsland and colleagues performed the first randomized placebo-controlled study using donepezil in a crossover design of two 10-week treatment periods (Aarsland *et al.*, 2002). In this small study of 14 patients with PD and mild to moderate dementia, MMSE scores significantly improved with 10 mg of donepezil vs placebo (see Table 6.3). However, two subsequent studies using a similar design in equally small patient numbers have not been able to demonstrate consistent benefits of donepezil on a variety of measures including the MMSE, Alzheimer's Disease Assessment Scale Cognitive Subscale (ADAScog) and Mattis Dementia Rating Scale (Leroi *et al.*, 2004; Ravina *et al.*, 2005). Studies were consistent, however, in showing good tolerability of donepezil in PD-D, without worsening of

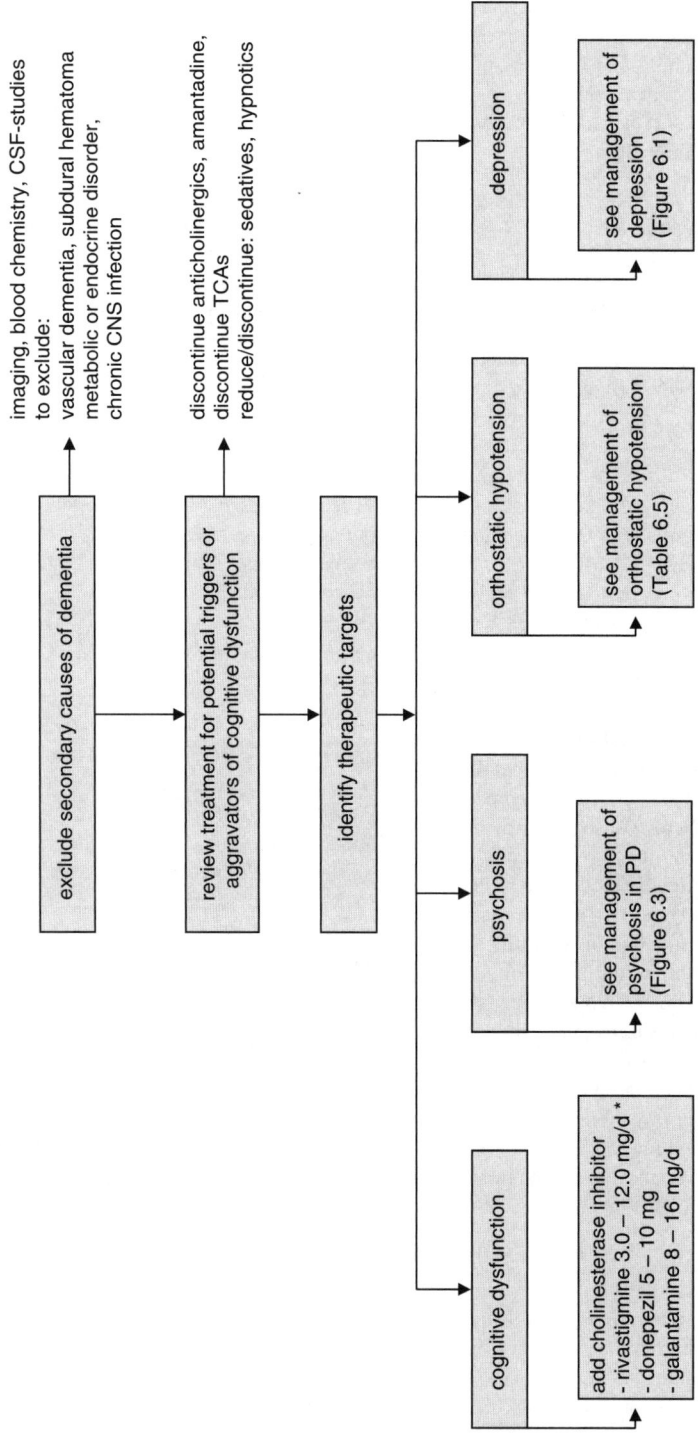

Figure 6.2 Pragmatic management of PD-dementia.

imaging, blood chemistry, CSF-studies
to exclude:
vascular dementia, subdural hematoma
metabolic or endocrine disorder,
chronic CNS infection

discontinue anticholinergics, amantadine,
discontinue TCAs
reduce/discontinue: sedatives, hypnotics

exclude secondary causes of dementia

review treatment for potential triggers or
aggravators of cognitive dysfunction

identify therapeutic targets

cognitive dysfunction

add cholinesterase inhibitor
- rivastigmine 3.0 – 12.0 mg/d *
- donepezil 5 – 10 mg
- galantamine 8 – 16 mg/d

psychosis

see management of
psychosis in PD
(Figure 6.3)

orthostatic hypotension

see management of
orthostatic hypotension
(Table 6.5)

depression

see management of
depression
(Figure 6.1)

CNS: central nervous system
CSF: cerebrospinal fluid
PD: Parkinson's disease
TCAs: tricyclic antidepressants

Table 6.3 Treatment of dementia in PD: randomized controlled trials.

Study	Intervention	Dosage (range/day or mean/day)	Design	Duration	Patients included (n)	Outcome
Aarsland et al. (2002)	donepezil vs placebo	10 mg	Randomized, double-blind, cross-over	20 wk with 10 wk cross-over point	14	Significant effect of donepezil vs placebo on MMSE (2.1 vs 0.3) and CIBIC + (42% vs 17% improved on donepezil vs placebo). No motor deterioration.
Leroi et al. (2004)	donepezil vs placebo	10 mg	Randomized, double-blind, parallel group	18 wk	16	No significant differences within and between groups on MMSE and MDRS (primary outcome). Significant group difference on MDRS memory sub-scale in favor of donepezil group. No motor deterioration.
Ravina et al. (2005)	donepezil vs placebo	5–10 mg	Randomized, double-blind, cross-over	10 wk treatment periods with a washout period of 6 wk between treatment periods	22	Trend toward better scores on the ADAScog (primary outcome) on donepezil compared with placebo. Significant effect of donepezil vs placebo on MMSE and CGI. No change on the MDRS. No motor deterioration.
Emre (2004)	rivastigmine vs placebo	8.7 mg (3–12 mg)	Randomized, double-blind, parallel group 2 : 1 randomization ratio	6 mo	541	Significant improvement on primary outcomes (ADAScog and ADCS-CGIC) and secondary outcomes including the NPI on patients treated with rivastigmine vs those who received placebo. 2.8 points improvement on ADAScog on rivastigmine vs placebo. Clinically meaningful improvements in the scores for the ADCS-CGIC in 19.8% of patients in the rivastigmine group and 14.5% of those in the placebo group. No significant difference between treatment groups on Unified Parkinson's Disease Rating Scale (UPDRS part III), although rivastigmine was associated with higher rates of tremor (10.2% vs 3.9%).

MMSE: Mini-Mental State Examination; NPI: Neuro-Psychiatric Inventory; MDRS: Mattis Dementia Rating Scale; CGI: Clinical Global Impression of Change; CIBIC + : Clinician's Interview Based Impression of Change plus Caregiver Input; ADAScog: Alzheimer's Disease Assessment Scale Cognitive Subscale; ADCS-CGIC: Alzheimer's Disease Cooperative Study-Clinician's Global Impression of Change.

Unified PD Rating Scale (UPDRS) motor scores. A large placebo-controlled randomized trial of donepezil in patients with PD-D has recently been completed, and results have been published in abstract form only. They include statistically significant improvement of ADAScog scores after 24 weeks of treatment with donepezil compared to placebo (Dubois *et al.*, 2007).

Rivastigmine

A recent randomized placebo-controlled trial assessing the efficacy and safety of rivastigmine to treat PD-D included a total of 541 patients and found that rivastigmine at a mean dose of 8.7 mg/day, was associated with a significant improvement of ADAScog and Alzheimer's Disease Cooperative Study-Clinician's Global Impression of Change (ADCS-CGIC) scores (see Table 6.3) (Emre *et al.*, 2004). Nausea and vomiting were the most common side effects observed with rivastigmine, affecting between 17 and 29% of patients. Although there were no statistically significant differences in UPDRS motor scores between rivastigmine and placebo-treated patients, more patients on rivastigmine reported tremor as an adverse event. A sub-analysis of this study has shown greater response in patients experiencing visual hallucinations at baseline, compared to those without these phenomena (Burn *et al.*, 2006) and an open-label extension of the trial has shown sustained efficacy over 12 months (Poewe *et al.*, 2006).

Other Agents

Galantamine, a cholinesterase inhibitor with some additional effects on nicotonic cholinergic transmission, has only been assessed in a small open-label study reporting global clinical improvement, increases in MMSE scores and improvement of selected items of the Neuropsychiatric Inventory (NPI) (Aarsland, Hutchinson and Larsen, 2003). Worsening of tremor occurred in some patients.

Pragmatic Management of PD Dementia

Treatment of cognitive decline and dementia in PD should always start with careful assessment of potential differential diagnoses or alternate causes of dementia other than PD (see Figure 6.2). This process may involve brain imaging to exclude new-onset structural brain pathology, like sub-dural hematomas, as a consequence of recurrent PD-related falls or, rarely, CSF studies to exclude encephalitis, chronic meningitis, or other CNS inflammation. Next, it is mandatory to review current PD and other CNS-active treatments for their potential to induce or aggravate cognitive dysfunction. Anti-cholinergics or amantadine should be discontinued in any cognitively impaired PD patient, co-treatment with anti-depressants should not use agents like TCAs or others with prominent anti-muscarinic activity. Sedatives or hypnotics may also add to cognitive dysfunction and should only be used when absolutely necessary.

In *bona fide* PD dementia, orthostatic hypotension can be a contributor to fluctuations in attention and alertness and should be treated accordingly (Peralta *et al.*, 2007).

Cholinesterase inhibitor therapy should be initiated in all patients with a MMSE score of less than 24. The best-studied drug in PD-D is rivastigmine and, to date, is the only member of this class approved in this indication in the US and EU. Donepezil may also be efficacious, but data from controlled trials currently do not unequivocally support its use. Data on galantamine and memantine are few and these agents are considered investigational in PD-D. Results to be expected from treatment of PD-D with ChE-Is include improvement in memory, attention, concentration and alertness, reduced fluctuations in cognitive performance, as well as improved hallucinosis and erratic behavior. There can be substantial gains in independence of activities of daily living, and reduced caregiver burden, but responses may be disappointing in a fair proportion of patients. Declining response over time may reflect ongoing cortical Lewy Body degeneration, but stopping therapy in such instances may still be associated with further worsening of cognitive performance.

Psychosis

Definition and Clinical Features

Hallucinosis and psychotic episodes are among the most challenging of the parkinsonian non-motor symptoms. Psychosis is often used as an umbrella term encompassing a spectrum of disordered thought and perception including illusions, delusions, hallucinations, confusion and paranoid ideation (Ravina *et al.*, 2007). Illusions and hallucinations are the predominant psychotic manifestations in PD and most commonly are visual in nature, while acoustic and tactile hallucinations are less frequent and, if present, usually occur in association with visual hallucinations (Poewe, 2003). Visual hallucinations in PD can be minor, such as fleeting sensations of presence or passage, but when fully expressed they are usually well formed, colorful and rich in detail (Ebersbach, 2003). In milder forms, insight into the hallucinatory nature of these perceptions is at least partially maintained, while in severe forms there is loss of insight with or without paranoid interpretation.

Psychosis has been identified as a major risk factor for nursing-home placement in PD (Goetz and Stebbins, 1993) and early psychotic reactions to dopaminergic replacement in PD have been correlated with subsequent development of cognitive decline and dementia (Goetz *et al.*, 1998).

Prevalence

Although there are few systematic and prospective studies of incidence and risk factors for psychosis in PD, recent drug trials in early PD have found incidences of hallucinosis and psychosis in up to 17% of patients (Poewe, 2003) and cross-sectional surveys in outpatient clinic populations have reported a 40% prevalence of hallucinations in PD during the previous three months when "minor forms" of psychosis, like illusions or transient sensations of the presence of a person were included (Fenelon *et al.*, 2000). The total lifetime prevalence of hallucinations occurring at any time period of the disease course was close to 50% in this cohort.

Pathophysiology and Clinicopathological Correlations

While psychosis in PD is commonly triggered by drug exposure, it can also occur spontaneously as a genuine feature of PD. Visual hallucinations in patients with PD are thought to be related to Lewy body pathology in the visuoperceptual systems including the basolateral nucleus of the amygdala and parahippocampus (Williams and Lees, 2005; Harding, Broe and Halliday, 2002). A recent clinicopathological study has found a high positive predictive value of visual hallucinations in life for a pathological diagnosis of Lewy body (PD and DLB) vs non-Lewy body parkinsonism (MSA, PSP or vascular parkinsonism) (Williams and Lees, 2005). In addition, psychosis can be induced or triggered by all major classes of anti-parkinsonian agents, including dopamine agonists, L-Dopa, monoamine oxidase-B (MAOB) inhibitors, catechol-O-methyl-transferase (COMT)-inhibitors, anti-cholinergics, and amantadine (Poewe, 2003; Poewe and Seppi, 2001). The frequency of psychosis is higher with dopamine agonist treatment compared to L-Dopa monotherapy (Poewe, 2003; Weintraub *et al.*, 2006). Additional risk factors include older age, cognitive decline and dementia.

Principles of Management

Management of psychosis in PD is based on careful assessment of triggering or contributing factors, including a rigorous review of the current anti-parkinsonian treatment schedule, and frequently will include the addition of an anti-psychotic agent.

Available Studies

In recent years a number of atypical anti-psychotic drugs with low potential for causing extrapyramidal adverse reactions have been tested in the setting of psychosis in patients with PD, in order to control psychiatric symptoms without reducing motor function (see Table 6.4). As a group, atypical anti-psychotics have a greater affinity for serotonin 5-HT_2 than dopamine D_2 receptors compared to typical anti-psychotics. Cholinesterase inhibitors may be another treatment option for psychotic behavior specifically in patients with PD and dementia (see above).

Anti-psychotics

Clozapine

Clozapine remains the only atypical anti-psychotic agent with consistent evidence for efficacy from open-label and randomized controlled studies (Goetz *et al.*, 2002). Two randomized placebo-controlled trials have documented anti-psychotic efficacy without worsening of UPDRS motor scores after four weeks of double-blind treatment (FCPSG, 1999; The Parkinson Study Group, 1999) (see Table 6.4). Open-label extensions of these studies provided evidence for maintained efficacy of clozapine over an additional 12 weeks (Pollak *et al.*, 2004; Factor *et al.*, 2001). Consistently reported side effects, even with low-dose clozapine, in these studies include sedation, dizziness, increased drooling, orthostatic hypotension and weight gain (Poewe and Seppi, 2001). In addition, clozapine is associated with the rare (0.38% according to Honigfeld *et al.* 1998), but serious and potentially life-threatening occurrence of agranulocytosis.

Olanzapine

Olanzapine has consistently failed to show anti-psychotic efficacy in several randomized controlled trials (Breier *et al.*, 2002; Ondo *et al.*, 2002a; Goetz *et al.*, 2000), but was associated with significant motor worsening in all trials (see Table 6.4).

Quetiapine

Four randomized controlled trials have assessed the efficacy of quetiapine to treat psychosis in PD (Ondo *et al.*, 2005a; Rabey *et al.*, 2007; Morgante *et al.*, 2004; Merims *et al.*, 2006). Two of these failed to show superiority of quetiapine over placebo on the primary outcome measures (see Table 6.4) (Ondo *et al.*, 2005a; Rabey *et al.*, 2007), while the other two trials (Morgante *et al.*, 2004; Merims *et al.*, 2006) found similar efficacy of quetiapine and clozapine (see Table 6.4). In open-label trials, quetiapine was generally associated with improvement in some 70 to 80% of patients (Poewe, 2003; Chou and Fernandez, 2006; Fernandez *et al.*, 2003) and some motor worsening was reported at one point during prolonged treatment in up to one third of patients (Fernandez *et al.*, 2003). One study compared efficacy and safety of quetiapine between parkinsonian patients with and without dementia and found demented patients to have a higher propensity for worsening of motor symptoms (Reddy *et al.*, 2002).

Other Anti-psychotics

Studies with risperidone to treat PD psychosis have generally been open-label with very small patient numbers and one small double-blind study (Goetz *et al.*, 2002; Ellis *et al.*,

Table 6.4 Treatment of psychosis in PD: randomized controlled trials.[a]

Study	Intervention	Dosage (range/ day or mean/ day)	Design	Duration	Patients included (n)	Outcome
FCPSG (1999)	Clozapine vs placebo	35.8 mg (12.5–50 mg)	Randomized, double-blind, parallel group	4 wk	60	Significant improvement in the clozapine vs placebo group in the psychosis rating scores (CGI and PANSS positive sub-score). No evidence of motor decline as assessed by the UPDRS.
PSG (1999)	Clozapine vs placebo	24.7 mg (6.25–50 mg)	Randomized, double-blind, parallel group	4 wk	60	Significant improvement in the clozapine vs placebo group in all psychosis rating scores (CGI, primary outcome; SAPS, BPRS-M). No evidence of motor decline as assessed by the UPDRS, significant improvement on the tremor item of the UPDRS III in the clozapine group.
Ondo et al. (2005a)	Quetiapine vs placebo	169.1 mg (75–200 mg)	Randomized, double-blind, parallel group	12 wk	31	No significant difference in psychosis rating scores (BPRS and Baylor PD Hallucination Questionnaire) between quetiapine and placebo group at week 12. No evidence of motor decline as assessed by the UPDRS.
Rabey et al. (2007)	Quetiapine vs placebo	123.3 mg	Randomized, double-blind, parallel group	12 wk	58	No significant difference in psychosis rating scales (BPRS and CGI) within and between groups. No evidence of motor decline as assessed by the UPDRS. Drop-out rate of 45% due to dosing guidelines in the protocol.
Morgante et al. (2004)	Quetiapine vs clozapine		Randomized, rater-blinded, parallel group	12 wk	40	No significant differences between clozapine- and quetiapine- treated patients concerning psychosis outcome measures (CGI and BPRS). Significant improvements on CGI and BPRS within both treatment groups. Parkinsonism did not deteriorate in either of the groups.

Study	Comparison	Dose	Design	Duration	N	Results
Merims *et al.* (2006)	Quetiapine vs clozapine		Randomized, rater-blinded, parallel group	22 wk	27	No significant differences between clozapine- and quetiapine- treated patients concerning psychosis outcome measures (CGI, hallucination frequency and severity as well as delusion severity as assessed by the NPI). Significant reduction of delusion frequency in favor of clozapine as assessed by the NPI. Significant improvements on most of the psychosis rating scores with both treatment groups. Parkinsonism did not deteriorate in either of the groups.
Goetz *et al.* (2002)	Olanzapine vs clozapine	Olanzapine: 11.4 mg (2.5–15 mg); clozapine: 25.8 mg (6.25–50 mg)	Randomized, double-blind, parallel group	9 wk	15	28 patients were originally planned for inclusion, but the study was prematurely stopped after only 15 patients had completed the study because of unacceptable deterioration of parkinsonism in the olanzapine arm. Significant improvement on psychosis outcome variables (SAPS, BPRS) in the clozapine arm only. Significant negative effect of olanzapine on motor function.
Breier *et al.* (2002)[a]	Olanzapine vs placebo	4.2 mg (2.5–15 mg)	Randomized, double-blind, parallel group	4 wk	158	Significant improvements within both groups on most psychosis efficacy measures (BPRS, CGI, NPI) without any difference between groups. Significant motor worsening (UPDRS) with olanzapine.
Ellis *et al.* (2000)	Risperidone vs clozapine	Risperidone: 1.2 mg (1–1.5 mg); clozapine: 62.5 mg (25–100 mg)	Randomized, double-blind, parallel group	3 mo	10	Significant improvement on BPRS in the risperidone group only without any differences between groups. No significant change on UPDRS within and between groups, although UPDRS motor score worsened in one subject in the clozapine group and in three subjects in the risperidone group.

[a] Single publication covering two seperate trails with identical design performed in the US and the EU. Pooled results are shown here.
CGI: Clinical Global Impression Scale; BPRS: Brief Psychiatric Rating Scale; NPI: Neuro-Psychiatric Inventory; SAPS: Schedule for Assessment of Positive Symptoms; PANSS: Positive and Negative Syndrome Scale; UPDRS: Unified PD Rating Scale; BPRS-M: modified BPRS

2000). Motor worsening has been reported in most of the studies (Goetz *et al.*, 2002) so that risperidone does not rank as a first-line therapeutic option for psychosis in PD. Both ziprasidone (Connemann and Schonfeldt-Lecuona, 2004; Gomez-Esteban *et al.*, 2005) and aripiprazole (Friedman *et al.*, 2006;Wickremaratchi, Morris and Ali, 2006) have been studied in small-scale open-label trials including less than 15 patients each. Overall, both agents were associated with improvement in a majority of cases, but close to one third also had some worsening of motor symptoms leading to discontinuation in some. Further controlled trials are needed to establish the usefulness of these agents in the treatment of psychosis in PD.

Cholinesterase Inhibitors

More recently, several open-label studies have reported anti-psychotic efficacy of rivastigmine (Reading, Luce and McKeith, 2001; Bullock and Cameron, 2002), donepezil (Fabbrini *et al.*, 2002; Bergman and Lerner, 2002) or galantamine (Aarsland, Hutchinson and Larsen, 2003) in demented and non-demented PD patients. In addition, post hoc analysis of a large placebo-controlled study of rivastigmine in PD dementia showed improvement of hallucinations on rivastigmine (Emre *et al.*, 2004).

Pragmatic Management of Psychosis in PD

Identification and removal of aggravating or triggering factors is paramount in the management of PD psychosis. This includes control of medical conditions like infections, dehydration, and electrolyte disturbances, or reductions of polypharmacy with anti-parkinsonian and other centrally active drugs like anti-muscarinic anti-depressants, anxiolytics, and sedatives (see Figure 6.3) (Poewe and Seppi, 2001). In cases of new-onset confusion and delirium not readily explained by any of these triggers or medication changes, brain imaging should be used liberally to exclude new structural brain pathology like sub-dural hematomas or stroke. When reducing and simplifying anti-parkinsonian combination therapy, drugs with high-risk benefit ratios regarding cognitive side effects vs anti-parkinsonian efficacy should be tapered first, that is, anti-cholinergics, amantadine, but also MAOB inhibitors before reducing dopamine agonists and L-Dopa. Similarly, dopamine agonists, by virtue of their greater potential to induce psychosis, should be tapered before L-Dopa (Poewe, 2003).

Dose reductions of anti-parkinsonian drugs to a level that will lead to a resolution of psychotic symptoms, while maintaining sufficient symptomatic motor control is not always feasible and start of anti-psychotic therapy becomes necessary. Quetiapine, although not formally established as efficacious in RCTs, should be a pragmatic first choice due to its improved safety profile as compared to clozapine.

Treatment should start with 25–50 mg at bedtime, increasing to 200 mg/d if needed. Clozapine is the only anti-psychotic agent with proven efficacy based on RCTs and should be used in all cases failing treatment with quetiapine, but can also be considered as a first-line option, despite of onerous weekly blood-count monitoring. It should be started with 6.25 mg/d at bedtime and increased by the same amount every other day until psychosis remits or adverse events occur. Rivastigmine and donepezil may be another treatment option for psychotic behavior, specifically in patients with PD and dementia.

Medication-Related Impulse Dyscontrol and Abnormal Repetitive Behaviors

A sub-group of patients with PD develop behavioral abnormalities in response to dopaminergic medication, which include medication overuse, abnormal repetitive non-goal oriented behaviors and reward or incentive-based compulsive actions. Collectively they are not uncommon and can have major and sometimes devastating psychosocial consequences.

Definition and Clinical Features

Impulse control disorders (ICDs) are characterized by a failure to resist an impulse, drive or temptation to perform an act that is harmful to the person or to others (Potenza, Voon and Weintraub, 2007). In PD, such behaviors include pathological gambling, hypersexuality, pathological shopping and binge eating (Potenza, Voon and Weintraub, 2007; Voon and Fox, 2007). Compulsive medication-overuse in PD is the hallmark of what has been termed "dopamine dysregulation syndrome" (DDS) or "hedonistic homeostatic dysregulation" (Giovannoni *et al.*, 2000). Affected patients increase their dopaminergic medication in excess of the amount needed to control motor symptoms and inspite of marked degrees of drug-induced dyskinesia. They often perform drug hoarding, become severely irritated by attempts to reduce their drug intake and show marked neglect of occupational and social responsibilities and relations.

"Punding" refers to purposeless, non-goal oriented repetitive behaviors, which are frequently related to a patient's pre-morbid occupational habits or interests and hobbies (Evans *et al.*, 2004). Behaviors include sorting objects or papers, dismantling devices like computers, radios or household equipment, or hobbyism, occupy the greater part of the day and may be continued through the night leading to severly disordered sleep–wake regulation.

Risk factors for the development of impulse dyscontrol and the other abnormal behaviors described above include younger age at onset, a previous history of alcohol or substance abuse and exposure to dopaminergic medication. Impulse dyscontrol is mainly associated with dopamine

check for and eliminate non-drug triggering factors::
(e.g. : infections, dehydration and electrolyte disturbances)

review current treatment regime.
reduce polypharmacy / reduce antiparkinsonian drugs:
stop drugs with high risk-benefit ratio in combination regimes, maintain sufficient symptomatic motor control:
1. stop anti-cholinergics, deprenyl, amantadine first
2. reduce or stop dopamine agonists next
3. reduce levodopa dose as last measure (stop COMT-inhibitors first)

persistent psychosis?

add anti-psychotics:
1. quetiapine start with 25 mg at bed time, then increase (up to 200 mg/d) as needed
2. clozapine (6.25 mg/d at bed time and increase in 6.25 mg steps until pschosis remits or adverse events occur)—weekly blood count monitoring

PD-dementia

add cholinesterase inhibitors

persistent psychosis?

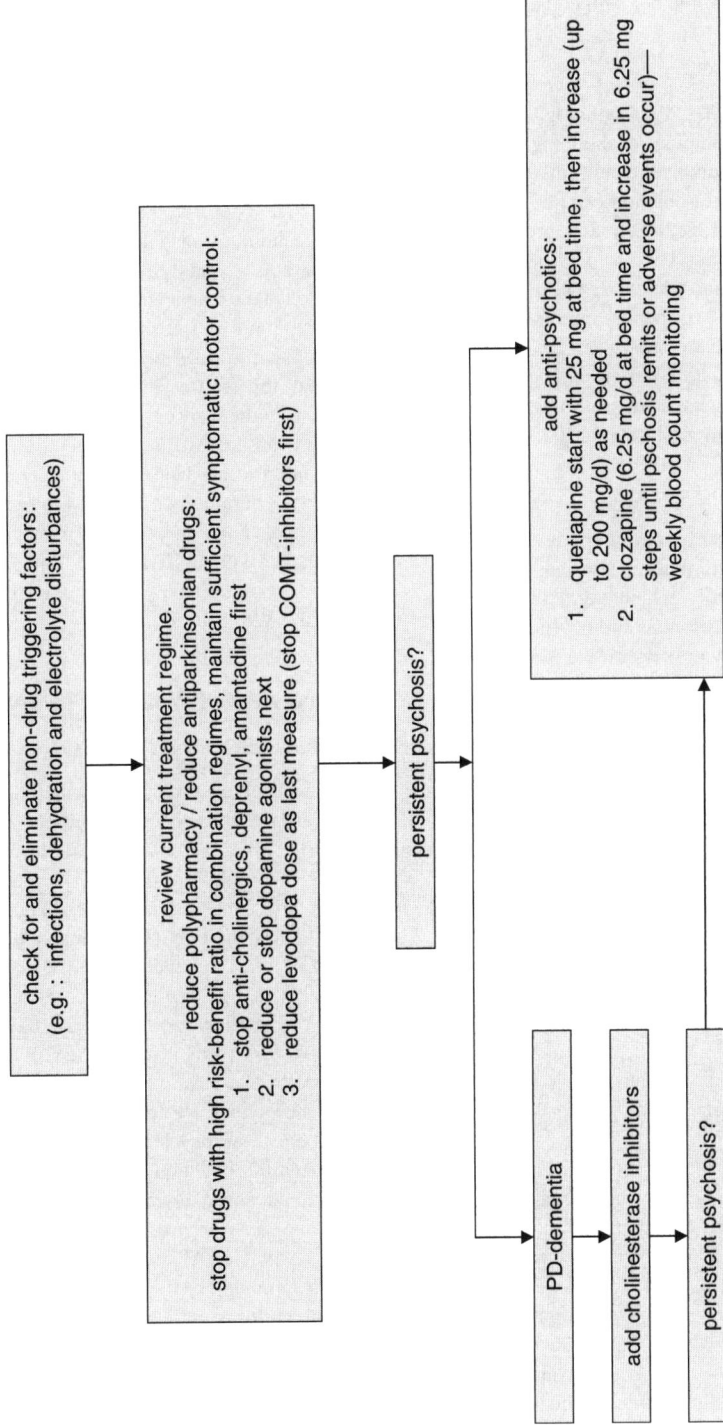

COMT: catechol-O-methyltransferase
PD: Parkinson's disease

Figure 6.3 Pragmatic management of psychosis in PD.

agonists as a class, while dopamine dysregulation and punding appear to mainly correlate with total dopaminergic dose, implicating both L-Dopa and dopamine agonists.

Prevalence

The overall prevalence of ICDs, like pathological gambling, hypersexuality and compulsive shopping, in PD appears to be around 6%, according to recent surveys, with point prevalences around 4% (Voon and Fox, 2007). For patients treated with dopamine agonists, overall prevalence figures for these behaviors have been as high as 13.7% (Voon and Fox, 2007). The prevalence of the dopamine dysregulation syndrome has been reported to be around 4% in one study of patients in a tertiary referral centre (Giovannoni et al., 2000), while punding was identified in 1.5% of patients in a movement disorder clinic with community-based referrals (Miyasaki et al., 2007).

Pathophysiology and Clinico-Pathological Correlations

The exact pathophysiology and brain regions involved in these different behavioral abnormalities are only incompletely understood. It is generally held that they are linked to dysfunction of brain-reward systems and neuroanatomical structures involved may include dopamine projections from the midbrain ventral tegmental area to the ventral striatum as well as limbic and pre-frontal cortical areas (Voon and Fox, 2007). One ^{11}C-raclopide PET study in PD patients with the dopamine dysregulation syndrome has indeed shown increased release of dopamine in the ventral striatum in response to L-dopa challenges (Evans et al., 2006).

Management

Management of ICDs and other behavioral abnormalities in PD is largely based on pragmatic recommendations without firm evidence for efficacy from controlled clinical trials. Based on few empirical data on treatment approaches for ICDs in PD, the management of each patient must be tailored according to the particular clinical setting (Potenza, Voon and Weintraub, 2007).

A first step will often be to decrease the dopamine agonist dosage with concomitant careful increase in L-Dopa dosage as necessary to maintain motor control (Potenza, Voon and Weintraub, 2007; Dodd et al., 2005; Drapier et al., 2006; Evans et al., 2005). In subjects with compulsive medication use, management comprises decreasing total dopaminergic dosage including external controls of doses, keeping the lowest medication dose required to overcome motor disabilities (Potenza, Voon and Weintraub, 2007; Evans et al., 2005). There may need to be a period of in-patient admission whilst tapering the medication. Disabling dyskinesias and distressing OFF-

period depression and dysphoria in patients with compulsive medication use may respond to continuous dopaminergic stimulation via subcutaneous apomorphine infusion (Evans et al., 2005; Katzenschlager et al., 2005).

If dose reduction of dopamine agonist or of total dopaminergic therapy to a level that will lead to resolution of behavioral abnormalities is not possible, a trial of a SSRI or of low-dose clozapine or quetiapine has to be considered (Voon and Fox, 2007; Kessel, 2006; Kurlan, 2004; Voon, Potenza and Thomsen, 2007). In addition, behavioral therapy techniques may be useful (Voon, Potenza and Thomsen, 2007). Ideally, specialized psychiatrists should be included in the management of PD patients with ICDs or other behavioral abnormalities. Functional neurosurgery with subthalamic deep brain stimulation (DBS) may be considered for well-selected patients refractory to the above management recognizing that history of an ICD is a potential risk factor for post-operative suicide attempts and that intermittent worsening of ICDs may occur postoperatively. Therefore, caution has to be applied in selection of patients and peri-operative management of a selected PD patient with an ICD (Voon, Potenza and Thomsen, 2007; Ardouin et al., 2006; Grimsby et al., 1997; Smeding et al., 2007; Witjas et al., 2005).

AUTONOMIC DYSFUNCTION

Definition and Clinical Features

Orthostatic hypotension (OH), urogenital and bowel dysfunction are the commonest autonomic problems in PD.

Clinically, OH is defined as a decrease of at least 20 mmHg in systolic or 10 mmHg in diastolic blood pressure or both within 3 min in an upright position, without or with postural symptoms (Lahrmann et al., 2006). Symptoms of OH in PD include blurred vision, postural instability, dizziness, lightheadedness, coat-hanger pain (pain in the back of the neck and shoulders) and syncope (Pathak and Senard, 2006). OH is one of the risk factors for falls in PD (Michalowska et al., 2005; Martignoni, Tassorelli and Nappi, 2006), which are among the most common reasons for emergency hospital admissions in this illness (Woodford and Walker, 2005). Although troublesome OH is thought to complicate advanced disease, up to 14% of de novo PD patients may have asymptomatic OH (Bonuccelli et al., 2003) and, rarely, OH may precede the onset of motor symptoms in bona fide PD (Kaufmann et al., 2004).

Urinary dysfunction is a common feature of advanced PD and includes urinary frequency and urgency, incomplete bladder emptying, double micturition and urge incontinence (Fowler and O'Malley, 2003; Winge and Fowler, 2006). Urodynamic studies in series of patients with PD have found that the commonest urodynamic abnormality is detrusor hyperreflexia while detrusor hypoactivity seems to be less prominent (Fowler and O'Malley, 2003; Winge and Fowler, 2006).

Sexual dysfunction in male patients with PD includes erectile (ED) and ejaculatory dysfunction (Basson, 2001; Brown *et al.*, 1990). ED typically affects men several years after a diagnosis of PD has been established, and the risk increases with advanced disease stage (Papatsoris *et al.*, 2006).

Constipation is another common autonomic symptom of PD and has been reported prior to onset of overt motor symptoms in about half of the patients in one series (Korczyn, 1990). In severe cases it may cause intestinal pseudo-obstruction and toxic mega-colon (Kaufmann and Biaggioni, 2003). Constipation in healthy male individuals has been associated with an increased risk to develop PD (Abbott *et al.*, 2001).

Prevalence

Retrospective chart reviews in a large series of 135 cases of pathologically proven PD found evidence for symptomatic OH in life in 30% of cases, bladder dysfunction in 32%, and constipation in 36% (Magalhaes *et al.*, 1995). Several studies—most of them case control studies—have reported even greater prevalences of up to 60% or approximately twofold above the prevalence of OH, constipation or urogenital dysfunction in non-PD elderly controls (Hely *et al.*, 2005; Winge and Fowler, 2006; Papatsoris *et al.*, 2006; Kaufmann and Biaggioni, 2003; Allcock *et al.*, 2004; Clara, De Macedo and Pego, 2007; Edwards, Quigley and Pfeiffer, 1992; Feldman *et al.*, 1994; Hobson *et al.*, 2003; Lemack *et al.*, 2000; Magerkurth, Schnitzer and Braune, 2005; Sakakibara *et al.*, 2001; Senard *et al.*, 1997; Visser *et al.*, 2004).

Pathophysiology and Clinicopathological Correlations

The pathophysiology and clinicopathological correlations of dysautonomia in PD are not entirely understood. Lewy body-type neurodegeneration in PD affects lower brainstem nuclei mediating autonomic functions such as the dorsal vagal nucleus, the nucleus ambiguous, and other medullary centers (rostral ventrolateral medulla, ventromedial medulla, and caudal raphe nuclei), as well as peripheral sympathetic ganglia and efferents of the gastrointestinal and cardiovascular systems (Braak *et al.*, 2003; Forno, 1996; Braak *et al.*, 2006b). The pontine micturition and defecation centre, as well as the amygdala and the paraventricular hypothalamic nucleus, which are involved in sexual function, may also be affected in PD (Braak *et al.*, 2003; Braak *et al.*, 2006b; Braak *et al.*, 1994; Wakabayashi and Takahashi, 1997).

Principles of Management (see Table 6.5)

Management of autonomic failure in PD is largely based on pragmatic recommendations without firm evidence for efficacy from controlled clinical trials (Goetz *et al.*, 2002; Horstink *et al.*, 2006).

Orthostatic Hypotension

Available Studies

Controlled-trial data on the treatment of OH in PD derive mostly from studies performed in mixed populations of patients with neurogenic hypotension. Two randomized placebo-controlled trials of midodrine—a pro-drug with the post-synaptic α_1-adrenergic metabolite desglymidodrine—have included patients with PD (Low *et al.*, 1997; Jankovic *et al.*, 1993). Both showed efficacy of midodrine in improving orthostatic hypotension. Small open-label studies have shown beneficial effects of etilefrine hydrochloride, dihydroergotamine and fludrocortisone on OH in patients with PD (Goetz *et al.*, 2002; Pathak and Senard, 2006). A recent multi-center, placebo-controlled trial of L-Dihydroxyphenyl Scrine (L-DOPS) to treat OH in patients with PD and multiple system atrophy (MSA) only found a marginal decrease in blood pressure fall during orthostatism without any change in postural symptoms (Pathak and Senard, 2006).

Pragmatic Management of Orthostatic Hypotension in PD

If a PD patient presents with symptoms suggestive for OH, OH should be confirmed on active standing test or passive head-up tilt (60°) testing. The current drug regimen should be reviewed for possible drug-induced OH. Before initiating adjunct treatment with anti-hypotensive agents, it is usually worthwhile to try a variety of non-pharmacological measures (see Table 6.5).

Fludrocortisone and midodrine are the two most commonly used agents to treat OH in PD. The full benefit of fludrocortisone requires high dietary salt and adequate fluid intake. The development or aggravation of supine hypertension can complicate treatment with both drugs, such that supine blood pressure tests, especially in the evening, are recommended.

Bladder Dysfunction

Available Studies

Therapeutic trials to treat detrusor overactivity-related urgency, frequency and urge incontinence have been performed in non-PD patients with neurogenic bladder syndromes and have shown efficacy of anti-cholinergics agents like oxybutinin, tolterodine and trospium chloride (Goetz *et al.*, 2002; Winge and Fowler, 2006; Horstink *et al.*, 2006).

Table 6.5 Practical management of autonomic dysfunction in PD.

Orthostatic Hypotension:
- *Non-pharmacological measures*
  o Sleeping in head-up position
  o Fragmentation of meals
  o Physical counter manoeuvres such as squatting, bending over forward or leg crossing with tension of the thigh, bottom and calf muscles (party position) at the onset of pre-syncopal symptoms
  o Avoidance of low-sodium and carbohydrate rich meals
  o Increased water (2–2.5 l/day) and salt intake (>8 g or 150 mmol/day)
  o Elastic stockings
- *Pharmacological treatment*
  o Fludrocortisone 0.1–0.4 mg/d
  o Midodrine 2.5–10 mg/d
  o Etilefrine 7.5–15 mg/d

Neurogenic Bladder Symptoms (nocturia, urgency, frequency, urge incontinence):
Nocturnal polyuria:
- Reduced fluid intake or avoiding coffee in the evening
- Desmopressin Spray (10–40 mcg/night)

Detrusor overactivity
- Check for bladder infections, antibiotic treatment if positive
- Add Anti-cholinergics
  o Oxybutynine 5–15 mg/d
  o Tolterodine 2–4 mg/d
  o Trospiumchloride 20–40 mg/d
- Clean intermittent self-catheterization if post-micturitional residual volume is increased in several measurements (>100 ml)
- Long-term urethral catheter when neurogenic bladder symptoms become unmanageable

Erectile Dysfunction:
- Oral PDE-5 inhibitor
  o 50 mg Sildenafil (CAVE: OH)
  o 10 mg Vardenafil
  o 20 mg Tadalafil
- 3 mg Apomorphine sub-lingual

Constipation:
- *Stop anti-cholinergics*
- *Non-pharmacological measures*
  o Sufficient or additional fluid intake
  o Use of stool softener
  o Adequate fibre (e.g., bran, unprocessed foods and fibre additives)
- *Pharmacological treatment*
  o Lactulose (20–60 g/d) and laxatives such as sodiumpicosulfate (5–10 mg/d) or macrogol (13.125–39.375 g/d)
  o Prokinetic agents such as domperidone (30–60 mg/d), tegaserod (6–12 mg/d) or mosapride (15–45 mg/d)
  o Botulinum toxin A injections into the puborectalis for muscle outlet-obstruction constipation

In one study, apomorphine and L-Dopa improved detrusor overactivity in PD (Aranda and Cramer, 1993), while results were inconsistent in another study in patients with motor fluctuations (Fitzmaurice *et al.*, 1985). Several reports of the effect of subthalamic nucleus (STN) deep brain stimulation on bladder function in patients with PD suggest improvement of bladder capacity and increase of the volume at first desire to void (Herzog *et al.*, 2006; Winge *et al.*, 2007). In a small open-label study, desmopressin, given intranasaly, has shown reductions in the frequency of nocturnal voids in five out of eight patients with PD and nocturia (Suchowersky, Furtado and Rohs, 1995).

Novel approaches to manage neurogenic detrusor over-activity include intravesical instillation of anti-cholinergic agents, vanilloids, and botulinum toxin, and have shown promising effects in non-parkinsonian patients (Sahai *et al.*, 2006).

Pragmatic Management of Bladder Dysfunction in PD

Obtaining a detailed history, including drug history, is a prerequisite for planning further investigation and treatment of urinary dysfunction in PD. The approach in PD is similar to that for non-PD elderly patients with urinary dysfunction and should exclude underlying treatable causes, such as drug side effects, infection, diabetes, gender-specific causes, such as prostate or gynecological causes. In addition, measurement of post-micturition residual volume and urodynamic studies provide critical information.

If nocturia is the major complaint, it may be improved by reducing fluid intake or avoiding coffee in the evening. Distressing nocturia which is refractory to these non-pharmacological measures may respond to night-time doses of intranasal desmopressin. This approach requires electrolyte monitoring in blood and urine.

Based on findings in therapeutic trials in other types of neurogenic bladder symptoms, anti-cholinergic agents should be tried to treat detrusor hyperreflexia. While oxybutinine and tolterodine may worsen cognitive dysfunction in PD, this is not the case for trospium chloride, which may be preferable in PD dementia (Fowler and O'Malley, 2003). Adverse effects of anti-cholinergic agents include dry mouth, constipation and, possibly, urinary retention that may complicate treatment. In the latter instance, combination with clean intermittent self-catheterization may become necessary. A long-term urethral catheter may be required and restore a degree of independence when urge incontinence and frequency are unmanageable. If infections are frequent, a suprapubic catheter is preferable to a urethral catheter for chronic use (Fowler and O'Malley, 2003; Winge and Fowler, 2006).

Erectile Dysfunction

Available Studies

Sildenafil has been found efficacious in several clinical trials for the treatment of ED in patients with PD, including one small randomized placebo-controlled study (Zesiewicz, Helal and Hauser, 2000; Raffaele *et al.*, 2002; Hussain *et al.*, 2001). The latter trial found a significant improvement in the ability to achieve and maintain an erection, as assessed by the International Index of Erectile Function (IIEF), and in quality of sex life on 50 mg sildenafil in 12 patients with PD (Hussain *et al.*, 2001). Sildenafil was well tolerated; minor transient adverse effects included headache and flushing.

No data are available on the use of other phosphodiesterase-5 (PDE-5) inhibitors in patients with PD, but in non-parkinsonian populations, efficacy and safety profiles of all PDE-5 inhibitors seem to be similar (Briganti *et al.*, 2005). Cautious use is advised in parkinsonian patients with OH and PDE-5 inhibitors are contraindicated in patients on nitrate medications for coronary heart disease (Briganti *et al.*, 2005).

Open-label reports have claimed efficacy of the dopamine agonists pergolide and s.c. apomorphine for ED in patients with PD (O'Sullivan and Hughes, 1998; Pohanka *et al.*, 2005), while randomized studies with sub-lingual apomorphine have shown efficacy in non-parkinsonian patients with ED.

Pragmatic Management of ED in PD

Management of ED in men with PD should first exclude alternative underlying causes such as drug side effects, depression, prostate disorders or diabetes. SSRIs and other anti-depressants may interfere with sexual function on both men and women (Taylor, 2006), and affected patients should be switched to anti-depressant agents with lower risks for sexual dysfunction such as reboxetine and bupropion (Taylor, 2006), When drug treatment is indicated for ED in men with PD, oral PDE-5 inhibitors (sildenafil, tadalafil and vardenafil) should be considered (see Table 6.5) (Briganti *et al.*, 2005). Sub-lingual apomorphine may represent an alternative, but has been less effective in studies in non-parkinsonian populations (Porst *et al.*, 2007). Second-line options include vacuum devices, intraurethral, and intracavernosal administration of vasoactive drugs alone, or combined with a PDE-5 inhibitor. Penile prosthesis implantation can be considered as a last resort (Kendirci *et al.*, 2006).

Generally, treatment of ED should follow the model of proceeding from the least to most invasive procedure (process of care), taking into account patient and partner satisfaction (Kendirci *et al.*, 2006).

Constipation

Available Studies

Different pro-kinetic agents including cisapride (which has been withdrawn from the market in several countries worldwide due to the risk of fatal arrhythmia), tegaserod and mosapride have been reported as beneficial in small-scale trials in PD (Liu *et al.*, 2005; Morgan and Sethi, 2007; Jost and Schimrigk, 1993). The only double-blind, placebo-controlled trial found a trend for improvement of constipation measures with tegaserod over a four week period, in 15 patients with PD (Sullivan *et al.*, 2006). Open-label trials with macrogol, a polyethylene glycol electrolyte solution working on an osmotic basis, and dietary herb extracts have also reported improvement of constipation in small PD cohorts (Eichhorn and Oertel, 2001; Sakakibara *et al.*, 2005). Botulinum toxin A injections into the puborectalis muscle have been efficacious for outlet-obstruction constipation in PD (Albanese *et al.*, 2003; Maria *et al.*, 2000).

Pragmatic Management of Constipation in PD

Sufficient fluid intake and the use of stool softener are simple ways to help maintain soft bowel movements. Adequate fibre (e.g., bran, unprocessed foods and fibre additives) intake is important to keep bowel movements of sufficient calibre and consistency to be propelled through the intestinal tract (Maria *et al.*, 2000; Lembo and Camilleri, 2003). Treatment of constipation in PD should also include increased exercise. In general, patients should be receiving sufficient dopamine-substitution for optimal control of motor symptoms, since difficulties with defecation may be worsened during OFF periods (Witjas *et al.*, 2002).

Drug treatment should start with lactulose and laxatives such as sodium picosulfate, bisacodyl or macrogol, followed by pro-kinetic agents such as domperidone, tegaserod or mosapride, if needed.

In cases of outlet-obstruction constipation, botulinum toxin injections into the puborectalis muscle can be tried, but this requires some expertise regarding correct targeting of the injection. Fecal incontinence may represent a potentially troublesome side effect of such a strategy.

DISORDERS OF SLEEP AND WAKEFULNESS

Clinical Manifestations

Sleep disorders are among the most frequent non-motor problems of PD (Tandberg, Larsen and Karlsen, 1998). They include insomnia, with difficulties falling asleep, frequent awakenings and overall reduced sleep efficiency, as well as excessive daytime sleepiness. Sleep problems in PD are due to a multitude of factors, including primary dysfunction of sleep–wake-cycle regulation, Rapid Eye Movement (REM) Sleep Behavior Disorder (RBD) and secondary effects of parkinsonian motor and non-motor symptoms on sleep onset and maintenance. In addition PD medications, as well as the impact of co-morbid conditions like RLS/PLMS or sleep disordered breathing, may affect sleep and wakefulness. (see Table 6.6) (Boeve *et al.*, 2007).

Prevalence

Sleep problems are almost universal in PD, but prevalence data differ widely between studies depending on definitions and types of assessment used. Lees and colleagues, using a mailed questionnaire, found some type of sleep disturbance in more than 90% of cases, while Tandberg *et al.* reported a somewhat lower figure of 67% in a community-based study

Table 6.6 Disturbances of sleep and wakefulness in PD.

Primary sleep–wake dysregulation
- altered sleep microstructure
- sleep fragmentation
- REM Sleep Behavior Disorder (RBD)
- excessive daytime sleepiness ("narcoleptic phenotype")

Secondary effects of PD symptoms
- nocturnal akinesia, tremor and rigidity
- nocturnal off-period dystonia and pain
- nocturia and incontinence
- nighttime confusion and hallucinosis
- depression

Effects of PD medications
- medication-induced insomnia (L-dopa, DA-Agonists, Selegiline)
- medication induced daytime sleepiness (L-dopa, DA-Agonists)
- drug-induced delirium

Effects of co-morbid conditions
- sleep-disordered breathing
- RLS/PLMS

(Tandberg, Larsen and Karlsen, 1998; Lees, Blackburn and Campbell, 1988). RBD and excessive daytime somnolence can affect up to 50% of patients with PD (Comella, 2003; Gagnon *et al.*, 2002; Hobson *et al.*, 2002). Several studies have also reported increased prevalence rates of RLS affecting around 20% of individuals with PD (Ondo, Vuong and Jankovic, 2002b) and others have found sleep disordered breathing in 20% of their patients (Arnulf *et al.*, 2002).

Clinicopathological Correlations

Disturbances of sleep architecture found in PD include sleep fragmentation, reduced sleep efficiency, reduced slow-wave sleep, reduced REM sleep, and RBD. The mechanisms underlying these are only partially understood, but are likely related to brainstem Lewy-body degeneration. Of those disturbances of sleep architecture described in PD patients, RBD may be the most closely related to Lewy body neurodegeneration in lower brainstem nuclei (Boeve *et al.*, 2007; Boeve *et al.*, 1998).

Principles of Management

Due to the multiple causative factors involved, treatment of PD-related sleep problems and daytime somnolence is usually complex. Careful history taking—often including information from a spouse or caregiver—is essential, to identify the most likely and relevant underlying causes. Treatment options include optimizing PD therapies to improve nocturnal symptom control or reduce daytime somnolence, treatment of non-motor symptoms, like nocturia or mental dysfunction, counseling about sleep hygiene, as well as the addition of drugs promoting sleep or wakefulness. In most instances therapeutic decisions are pragmatic without formal evidence from controlled clinical trials.

REM Sleep Behavior Disorder (RBD)

RBD is a parasomnia characterized by lack of atonia during REM sleep, resulting in dream-enacting behaviors, occasionally associated with violent motor activity (Mahowald, Schenck and Bornemann, 2007). Symptomatic RBD has been found in one-third of patients in polysomnographic studies (Hobson *et al.*, 2002) and several reports have drawn attention to the fact that idiopathic RBD may precede the onset of PD, MSA or dementia with Lewy bodies by years (Olson, Boeve and Silber, 2000; Iranzo *et al.*, 2006; Schenck, Bundlie and Mahowald, 1996). RBD is frequently associated with sleep related injuries (either self injuries or injuries of bed partners) and can contribute to poor sleep quality and daytime somnolence in PD.

Available Studies

There are no controlled trials of any medication used to treat RBD. Clonazepam has been found to completely suppress dream-enacting behaviors in several open-label case series, where responder rates have been as high as 90% (Ozekmekci, Apaydin and Kilic, 2005; Schenck *et al.*, 1987; Schenck and Mahowald, 1996). Treatment with the dopamine agonist pramipexole was described as beneficial in two small studies (Fantini *et al.*, 2003; Schmidt, Koshal and Schmidt, 2006), but was found ineffective in another report (Iranzo *et al.*, 2005). There is also a single anecdotal report of beneficial effects of L-dopa in three patients with PD and RBD (Tan, Salgado and Fahn, 1996). Melatonin, either as the sole agent or in combination with clonazepam, has consistently been reported as beneficial for observation periods of up to two years in three open-label studies involving between 6 and 25 patients with RBD occurring in the context of PD, DLB, MSA and a variety of other conditions (Boeve, Silber and Ferman, 2003; Kunz and Bes, 1999; Takeuchi *et al.*, 2001).

Pragmatic Management of RBD in PD

Before initiating pharmacotherapy for RBD, potential aggravators should be identified and, if possible, removed. In PD the most common of these are TCAs and SSRIs (Mahowald, Schenck and Bornemann, 2007). Clonazepam,

given as a single dose of 0.5 to 1.0 mg about two hours before bed-time is considered first-line treatment for RBD in PD. It is generally effective in some 90% of cases, suppressing abnormal motor activity and injurious behavior, as well as nightmares, often within a few days. There is little concern about tolerance or loss of effect over time and most patients can stay on the drug long-term.

Melatonin at doses between 3 and 12 mg at night may also be effective and can be considered a second-line option in patients in whom clonazepam is found poorly tolerated or ineffective. Third-line options may include additional bedtime doses of L-dopa or non-ergot dopamine agonists.

Sleep Fragmentation and Insomnia

Available Studies

There is a paucity of trials specifically assessing the effect of anti-parkinsonian therapies on sleep quality and nocturnal disability in PD. The U.K. Madopar CR study group (1989) performed a double-blind crossover study of bedtime doses of either standard or controlled-release madopar in 103 patients with PD and a variety of nocturnal and early morning motor disabilities. Nocturnal or early morning disability scores did not differ between the two treatment periods (The U.K. Madopar CR Study Group, 1989). Chauduri and colleagues (Chaudhuri *et al.*, 2001) found bedtime doses of the long-acting ergot agonist cabergoline superior to slow-release Levodopa in patients with nocturnal akinesia and painful dystonia. On the other hand, Comella and colleagues failed to detect beneficial effects of pergolide 1 mg at night-time on sleep fragmentation and sleep efficiency in a small placebo-controlled actigraphic study in 22 patients (Comella, Morrissey and Janko, 2005). Likewise, when Hoegl and colleagues compared polysomnographic variables of total sleep time and sleep efficiency before and after adding cabergoline, there was no significant difference, although patients scored their sleep quality as subjectively improved (Hogl *et al.*, 2003).

Recent controlled trials of the transdermal DA agonist rotigotine in patients with fluctuating PD have included PD specific sleep scales and reported improvement on the Parkinson's Disease Sleep Scale (PDSS) which were largely related to the motor benefit derived from the drug, and were similar to those seen with the oral agonist pramipexole (Poewe *et al.*, 2007).

No studies have formally assessed the efficacy of COMT inhibitors, MAOB inhibitors, amantadine or anticholinergics on sleep function and nocturnal disability in PD.

Deep Brain Stimulation (DBS) of the subthalamic nucleus (STN) has been found to improve total sleep time in a cohort of 89 patients followed for six months, with persistent effects in those followed further, for up to two years (Lyons and Pahwa, 2006). Self-reported sleep problems and early-morning dystonia were also improved, and improvements in total sleep time correlated with improvements in bradykinesia.

A single double-blind placebo controlled cross-over study has reported modest but statistically significant beneficial effects of 50 mg of melatonin on total sleep time in 40 PD patients, as well as subjective improvements on several items of the General Sleep Disturbance Scale (GSDS) (Dowling *et al.*, 2005).

A small open-label study found improvement on the Pittsburgh Sleep Quality Index (PSQI) following bedtime doses of the atypical anti-psychotic quetiapine in non-psychotic PD patients with insomnia (Juri *et al.*, 2005).

Pragmatic Management of Sleep Fragmentation and Insomnia

Management of sleep fragmentation and insomnia in PD has to target the main underlying mechanisms, which differ from patient to patient (see Figure 6.4). A first step should always be a careful review of the patient's drug history, with an aim to identify drug-induced insomnia, which can occur following the introduction or dose increase of dopamine agonists or, rarely, even of L-dopa.

If, on the other hand, difficulties falling asleep or sleep fragmentation are due to nocturnal akinesia, painful OFF-period dystonic foot cramps or nocturnal tremor episodes, bedtime doses of long-acting dopamine agonists may improve sleep. Because of a risk of inducing cardiac vavulopathy associated with cabergoline and pergolide, non-ergot drugs like ropinirole, pramipexole or transdermal rotigotine will be the preferred choices. Slow-release L-dopa preparations given at bedtime usually do not provide sufficient duration of action to prevent problems in the second half of the night. Exceptional cases with prolonged and severe nocturnal OFF-periods may require more invasive drug-delivery approaches like jejunal infusions of L-dopa or s.c. infusions of apomorphine (see also Chapter 4).

When difficulties falling asleep or sleep fragmentation are mainly caused by co-morbid RLS/PLMS, bedtime doses of ropinirol (2–4 mg) or pramipexole (0.125–0.5 mg) may be sufficient. The addition of a once daily patch of rotigotine (2–6 mg), when given two hours before bedtime, will also improve RLS/PLMS, with an additional effect on parkinsonism throughout a 24 hour cycle, if that is needed.

Clonazepam (0.5 mg at bed-time) is the treatment of choice in cases of RBD-related sleep fragmentation, and atypical neuroleptics or cholinesterase inhibitors may improve sleep in patients with nocturnal episodes of confusion or hallucinosis (see above sections on dementia and psychosis).

Sleep disruption due to urinary urge and incontinence should be treated according to the principles outlined above for neurogenic bladder disturbances, and suspicion of co-morbid sleep disordered breathing requires poly-somnographic verification to decide on a need for continuous positive airway pressure (CPAP) therapy.

Daytime Sleepiness and Sudden Onset Sleep

Excessive daytime sleepiness (EDS) has been found in up to 50% of non-demented, fully functioning PD patients (Hobson *et al.*, 2002). Sudden-onset sleep (SOS) episodes were reported by 4 to 6% of subjects in two large questionnaire-based surveys (Hobson *et al.*, 2002; Paus *et al.*, 2003). Dopaminergic drugs can exacerbate sleepiness in PD, but potential causes are many and include co-morbid primary sleep disorders, like sleep apnea or RBD, sleep fragmentation and insomnia caused by PD itself (see above), as well as risk factors like older age, cognitive impairment and orthostatic hypotension (Rye, 2006).

Available Studies

Following the original alert by Frucht and colleagues about dopamine agonist-induced episodes of irresistible sleep in patients taking pramipexole or ropinirole (Frucht *et al.*, 1999), a number of studies have confirmed that EDS and SOS in PD are related to dopaminergic therapy and can be caused both by L-dopa and, more commonly, by DA-agonists (Paus *et al.*, 2003; Hobson *et al.*, 2002; Brodsky *et al.*, 2003). Findings have consistently included significant correlations between total dopaminergic drug dose and Epworth Sleepiness Scale (ESS) scores, as well as prevalence of EDS and SOS (Rye, 2006; Arnulf, 2005). One study assessed relative frequencies of SOS with different types of dopaminergic treatments and found ESS in 2.9% of those on L-dopa monotherapy as compared to 5.3% on dopamine agonist monotherapy vs 7.3% on combined treatments with L-Dopa and dopamine agonists (Paus *et al.*, 2003). In summary, studies on EDS and SOS in PD have failed to detect significant differences between patients on ergot dopamine agonists as compared to non-ergot dopamine agonists (Paus *et al.*, 2003; Brodsky *et al.*, 2003; Hobson *et al.*, 2002).

Few studies have assessed the efficacy of wake-promoting agents to treat EDS in PD. Following an initial open-label study of modafinil (maximum of 400 mg/d, average 172 mg/d), showing clear benefit on the ESS in 10 patients (Nieves and Lang, 2002), three randomized, placebo-controlled trials (two cross-over and one parallel group study including a total of 15, 21 and 40 patients, respectively) have tested this approach to reduce daytime sleepiness (Adler *et al.*, 2003; Hogl *et al.*, 2002; Ondo *et al.*, 2005b). Overall, at doses of modafinil of around 200 mg/d, there were modest, but significant, positive effects in the two cross-over trials on the ESS, but not on the Maintenance of Wakefulness Test (MWT), while the larger parallel group study failed to detect significant differences vs identify causal factors

nocturnal motor-symptoms (immobility, tremor, off-period dystonia)

optimise nocturnal motor-control

- add/increase evening dose DA-Agonist
- use 24 hr transdermal agonist delivery
- add evening or nocturnal dose of L-Dopa (Std. or CR ± COMT-inhibitor)
- add MAOB-inhibitor (morning dose for 24 hr efficacy)
- consider semi-invasive/invasive continuous drug delivery signs (s.c. jejunal/L-Dopa infusions)
- consider DBS if also indicated for daytime motor control

nocturia

treat detrusor overactivity

see table 6.5

nocturnal confusion, hallucinosis

treat PD-psychosis

bed time antipsychotic
- clozapine 0.25 – 5 mg
- quetiapine 75 – 250 mg

start cholinesterase inhibitor

RBD

add bedtime dose of clonazepam 0.5 mg

co-morbidities

RLS

sleep-apnea

perform PSG

consider CPAP

evening dose of DA-Agonist
- pramipexole 0,125 – 0,5 mg
- ropinirole 1.0 – 4.0 mg

evening dose of L-Dopa (100 mg Std. + 100 mg CR)

depression

add sleep promoting anti-depressants
- amitriptyline 25-75 mg
- mirtazapine 15-30 mg

COMT: catechol-O-methyltransferase
CPAP: continuous positive airway pressure
RLS: restless legs syndrome
CR: controlled release
DA: dopamine
DBS: deep brain stimulation

MAOB: monoamine oxidase B
PD: Parkinson's disease
PSG: polysomonography
RBD: REM sleep behavior disorder
Std.: standard

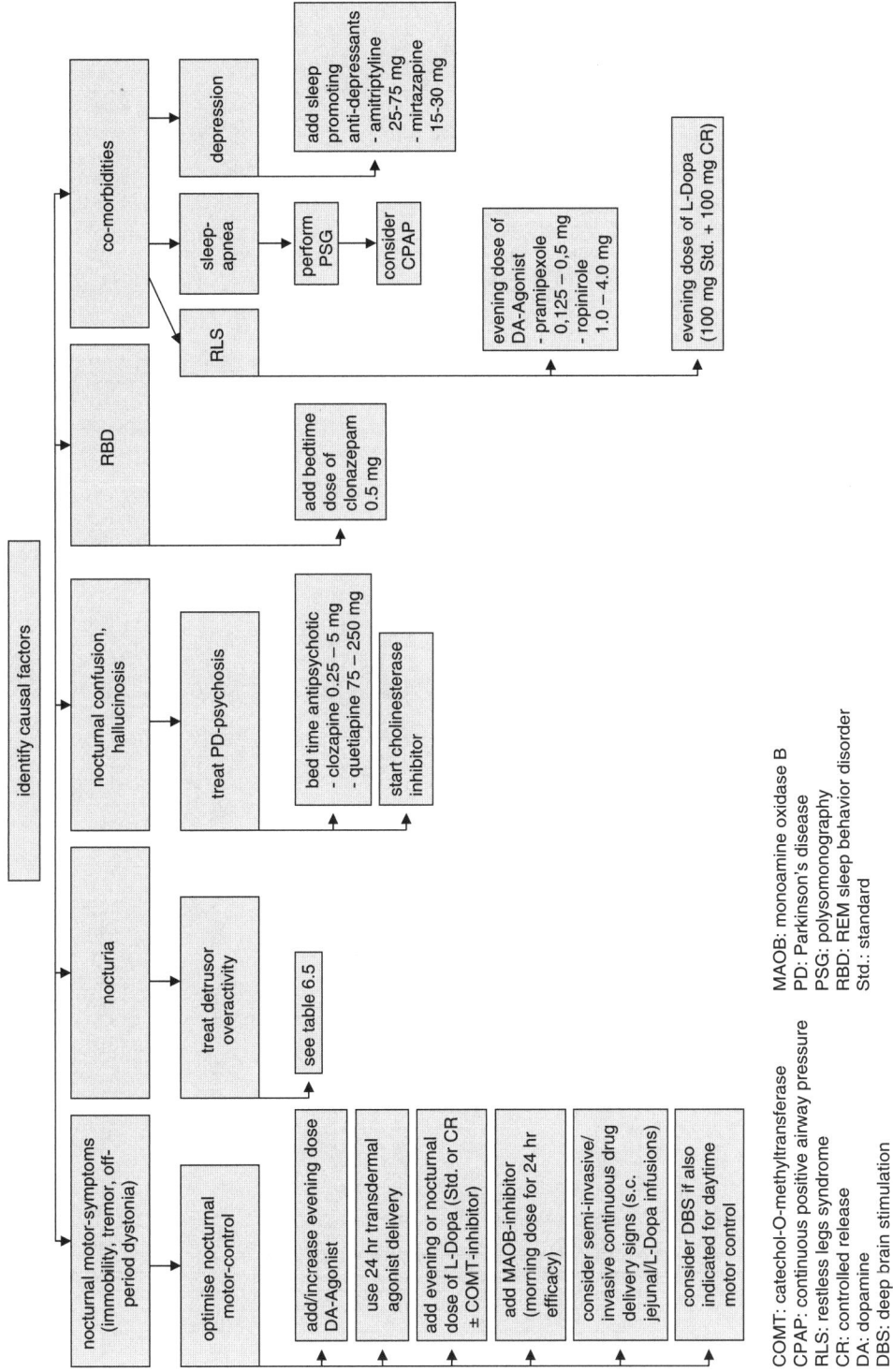

Figure 6.4 Pragmatic management of insomnia in PD.

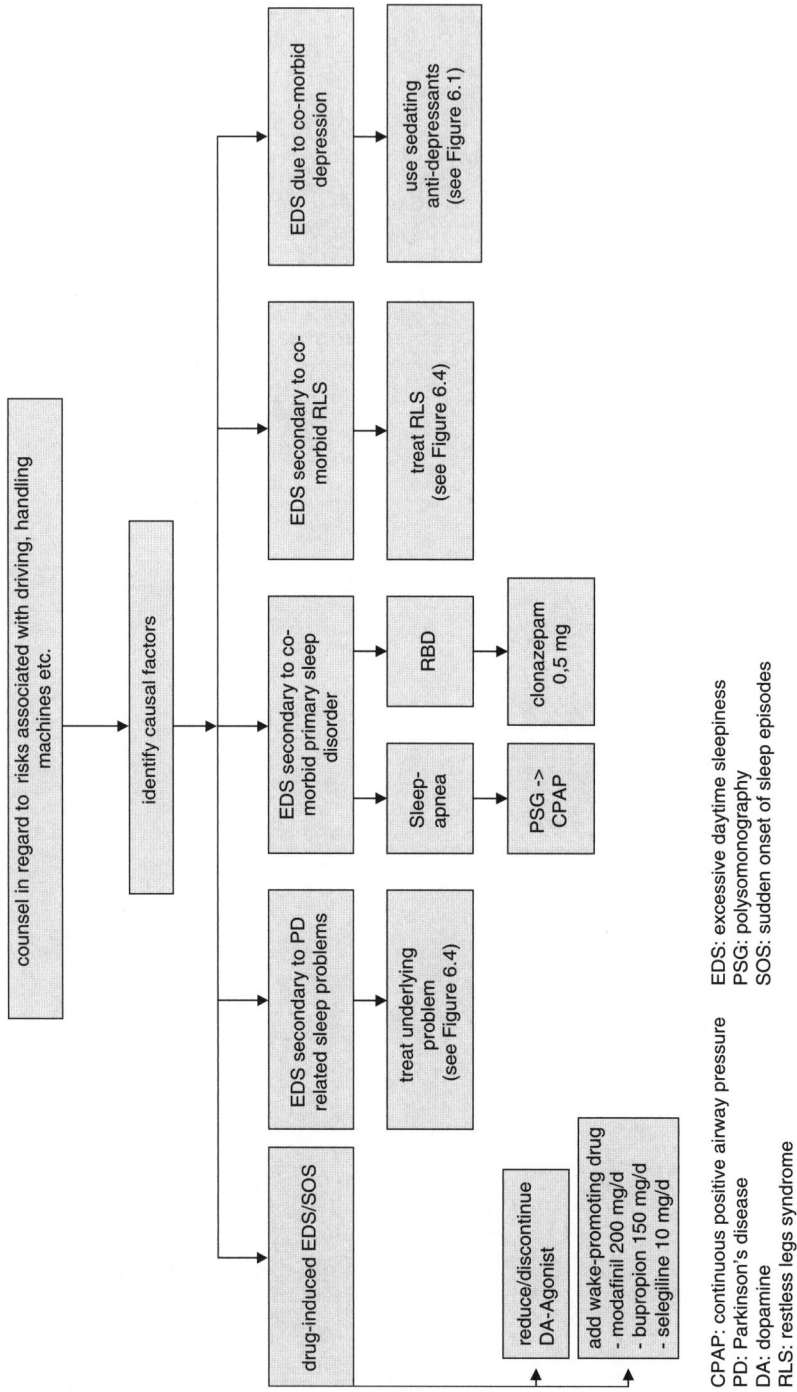

Figure 6.5 Pragmatic management of EDS/SOS in PD.

counsel in regard to risks associated with driving, handling machines etc.

identify causal factors

drug-induced EDS/SOS

EDS secondary to PD related sleep problems

EDS secondary to co-morbid primary sleep disorder

EDS secondary to co-morbid RLS

EDS due to co-morbid depression

reduce/discontinue DA-Agonist

add wake-promoting drug
- modafinil 200 mg/d
- bupropion 150 mg/d
- selegiline 10 mg/d

treat underlying problem
(see Figure 6.4)

Sleep-apnea

RBD

PSG -> CPAP

clonazepam 0,5 mg

treat RLS
(see Figure 6.4)

use sedating anti-depressants
(see Figure 6.1)

CPAP: continuous positive airway pressure
PD: Parkinson's disease
DA: dopamine
RLS: restless legs syndrome

EDS: excessive daytime sleepiness
PSG: polysomonography
SOS: sudden onset of sleep episodes

placebo on the ESS or the MSLT (Adler *et al.*, 2003; Hogl *et al.*, 2002; Ondo *et al.*, 2005b).

Pragmatic Management

As for the treatment of sleep fragmentation and insomnia, managing PD patients with daytime sleepiness and SOS requires careful assessment of causative factors, including drug history, co-morbid conditions affecting sleep–wake regulation and PD-related contributors to reduced wakefulness (see Figure 6.5). New-onset EDS or SOS, following changes in dopaminergic drug type and dose should raise a suspicion of drug-induced EDS leading to trials of dose reduction or other medication change. If that is not feasible, the addition of a wake-promoting drug like modafinil should be considered. If EDS appears to be caused by insomnia due to PD or co-morbid conditions like sleep apnea, RLS or depression these should be treated accordingly (see algorithm Figures 6.1 and 6.4). Often times, treating EDS in PD will involve combinations of these measures.

References

Aarsland, D., Laake, K., Larsen, J.P. *et al.* (2002) Donepezil for cognitive impairment in Parkinson's disease: a randomised controlled study. *Journal of Neurology, Neurosurgery, and Psychiatry*, **72**, 708–712.

Aarsland, D., Hutchinson, M. and Larsen, J.P. (2003) Cognitive, psychiatric and motor response to galantamine in Parkinson's disease with dementia. *International Journal of Geriatric Psychiatry*, **18**, 937–941.

Aarsland, D., Andersen, K., Larsen, J.P. *et al.* (2004) The rate of cognitive decline in Parkinson's disease. *Archives of Neurology*, **61**, 1906–1911.

Aarsland, D., Zaccai, J. and Brayne, C. (2005a) A systematic review of prevalence studies of dementia in Parkinson's disease. *Movement Disorders*, **20**, 1255–1263.

Aarsland, D., Perry, R., Brown, A. *et al.* (2005b) Neuropathology of dementia in Parkinson's disease: a prospective, community-based study. *Annals of Neurology*, **58**, 773–776.

Abbott, R.D., Petrovitch, H., White, L.R. *et al.* (2001) Frequency of bowel movements and the future risk of Parkinson's disease. *Neurology*, **57**, 456–462.

Adler, C.H., Caviness, J.N., Hentz, J.G. *et al.* (2003) Randomized trial of modafinil for treating subjective daytime sleepiness in patients with Parkinson's disease. *Movement Disorders*, **18**, 287–293.

Albanese, A., Brisinda, G., Bentivoglio, A.R. *et al.* (2003) Treatment of outlet obstruction constipation in Parkinson's disease with botulinum neurotoxin A. *The American Journal of Gastroenterology*, **98**, 1439–1440.

Allcock, L.M., Ullyart, K., Kenny, R.A. *et al.* (2004) Frequency of orthostatic hypotension in a community based cohort of patients with Parkinson's disease. *Journal of Neurology, Neurosurgery, and Psychiatry*, **75**, 1470–1471.

Andersen, J., Aabro, E., Gulmann, N. *et al.* (1980) Anti-depressive treatment in Parkinson's disease. A controlled trial of the effect of nortriptyline in patients with Parkinson's disease treated with L-DOPA. *Acta Neurologica Scandinavica*, **62**, 210–219.

Apaydin, H., Ahlskog, J.E., Parisi, J.E. *et al.* (2002) Parkinson's disease neuropathology: later-developing dementia and loss of the L-Dopa response. *Archives of Neurology*, **59**, 102–112.

Aranda, B. and Cramer, P. (1993) Effects of apomorphine and L-dopa on the parkinsonian bladder. *Neurourology and Urodynamics*, **12**, 203–209.

Ardouin, C., Voon, V., Worbe, Y. *et al.* (2006) Pathological gambling in Parkinson's disease improves on chronic subthalamic nucleus stimulation. *Movement Disorders*, **21**, 1941–1946.

Arnulf, I. (2005) Excessive daytime sleepiness in parkinsonism. *Sleep Medicine Reviews*, **9**, 185–200.

Arnulf, I., Konofal, E., Merino-Andreu, M. *et al.* (2002) Parkinson's disease and sleepiness: an integral part of PD. *Neurology*, **58**, 1019–1024.

Avila, A., Cardona, X., Martin-Baranera, M. *et al.* (2003) Does nefazodone improve both depression and Parkinson's disease? A pilot randomized trial. *Journal of Clinical Psychopharmacology*, **23**, 509–513.

Ballard, C.G., Aarsland, D., McKeith, I. *et al.* (2002) Fluctuations in attention: PD dementia vs DLB with parkinsonism. *Neurology*, **59**, 1714–1720.

Barone, P., Scarzella, L., Marconi, R. *et al.* (2006) Pramipexole vs sertraline in the treatment of depression in Parkinson's disease: a national multicenter parallel-group randomized study. *Journal of Neurology*, **253**, 601–607.

Basson, R. (2001) Sex and idiopathic Parkinson's disease. *Advances in Neurology*, **86**, 295–300.

Bergman, J. and Lerner, V. (2002) Successful use of donepezil for the treatment of psychotic symptoms in patients with Parkinson's disease. *Clinical Neuropharmacology*, **25**, 107–110.

Biggins, C.A., Boyd, J.L., Harrop, F.M. *et al.* (1992) A controlled, longitudinal study of dementia in Parkinson's disease. *Journal of Neurology, Neurosurgery, and Psychiatry*, **55**, 566–571.

Boeve, B.F., Silber, M.H., Ferman, T.J. *et al.* (1998) REM sleep behavior disorder and degenerative dementia: an association likely reflecting Lewy body disease 81. *Neurology*, **51**, 363–370.

Boeve, B.F., Silber, M.H. and Ferman, T.J. (2003) Melatonin for treatment of REM sleep behavior disorder in neurologic disorders: results in 14 patients. *Sleep Medicine*, **4**, 281–284.

Boeve, B.F., Silber, M.H., Saper, C.B. *et al.* (2007) Pathophysiology of REM sleep behaviour disorder and relevance to neurodegenerative disease. *Brain*, **130**, 2770–2788.

Bohnen, N.I., Kaufer, D.I., Ivanco, L.S. *et al.* (2003) Cortical cholinergic function is more severely affected in parkinsonian dementia than in Alzheimer disease: an in vivo positron emission tomographic study. *Archives of Neurology*, **60**, 1745–1748.

Bonuccelli, U., Lucetti, C., Del Dotto, P. *et al.* (2003) Orthostatic hypotension in de novo Parkinson's disease. *Archives of Neurology*, **60**, 1400–1404.

Braak, H., Braak, E., Yilmazer, D. *et al.* (1994) Amygdala pathology in Parkinson's disease. *Acta Neuropathologica*, **88**, 493–500.

Braak, H., Del Tredici, K., Rub, U. *et al.* (2003) Staging of brain pathology related to sporadic Parkinson's disease. *Neurobiology of Aging*, **24**, 197–211.

Braak, H., de Vos, R.A., Bohl, J. *et al.* (2006a) Gastric alpha-synuclein immunoreactive inclusions in Meissner's and Auerbach's plexuses in cases staged for Parkinson's disease-related brain pathology. *Neuroscience Letters*, **396**, 67–72.

Braak, H., Muller, C.M., Rub, U. *et al.* (2006b) Pathology associated with sporadic Parkinson's disease–where does it end? *Journal of Neural Transmission. Supplementa*, **70**, 89–97.

Breier, A., Sutton, V.K., Feldman, P.D. *et al.* (2002) Olanzapine in the treatment of dopamimetic-induced psychosis in patients with Parkinson's disease. *Biological Psychiatry*, **52**, 438–445.

Briganti, A., Salonia, A., Gallina, A. *et al.* (2005) Drug Insight: oral phosphodiesterase type 5 inhibitors for erectile dysfunction. *Nature Clinical Practice Urology*, **2**, 239–247.

Brodsky, M.A., Godbold, J., Roth, T. *et al.* (2003) Sleepiness in Parkinson's disease: a controlled study. *Movement Disorders*, **18**, 668–672.

Brown, R.G., Jahanshahi, M., Quinn, N. *et al.* (1990) Sexual function in patients with Parkinson's disease and their partners. *Journal of Neurology, Neurosurgery, and Psychiatry*, **53**, 480–486.

Bullock, R. and Cameron, A. (2002) Rivastigmine for the treatment of dementia and visual hallucinations associated with Parkinson's disease: a case series. *Current Medical Research and Opinion*, **18**, 258–264.

Burn, D., Emre, M., McKeith, I. *et al.* (2006) Effects of rivastigmine in patients with and without visual hallucinations in dementia associated with Parkinson's disease. *Movement Disorders*, **21**, 1899–1907.

Ceravolo, R., Nuti, A., Piccinni, A. *et al.* (2000) Paroxetine in Parkinson's disease: effects on motor and depressive symptoms. *Neurology*, **55**, 1216–1218.

Chaudhuri, K.R., Pal, S., Bridgman, K. *et al.* (2001) Achieving 24-hour control of Parkinson's disease symptoms: use of objective measures to improve nocturnal disability. *European Neurology*, **46** (Suppl 1), 3–10.

Chou, K.L. and Fernandez, H.H. (2006) Combating psychosis in Parkinson's disease patients: the use of antipsychotic drugs. *Expert Opinion on Investigational Drugs*, **15**, 339–349.

Clara, J.G., De Macedo, M.E. and Pego, M. (2007) Prevalence of isolated systolic hypertension in the population over 55 years old. Results from a national study. *Revista Portuguesa de Cardiologia (Lisboa)*, **26**, 11–18.

Comella, C.L. (2003) Sleep disturbances in Parkinson's disease. *Current Neurology and Neuroscience Reports*, **3**, 173–180.

Comella, C.L., Morrissey, M. and Janko, K. (2005) Nocturnal activity with nighttime pergolide in Parkinson's disease: a controlled study using actigraphy. *Neurology*, **64**, 1450–1451.

Connemann, B.J. and Schonfeldt-Lecuona, C. (2004) Ziprasidone in Parkinson's disease psychosis. *Canadian Journal of Psychiatry*, **49**, 73.

Cummings, J.L. (1992) Depression and Parkinson's disease: a review. *The American Journal of Psychiatry*, **149**, 443–454.

Cunningham, L.A. (1994) Depression in the medically ill: choosing an antidepressant. *Journal of Clinical Psychiatry*, **55** (Suppl A), 90–97.

Damier, P., Hirsch, E.C., Agid, Y. *et al.* (1999) The substantia nigra of the human brain. II. Patterns of loss of dopamine-containing neurons in Parkinson's disease. *Brain*, **122** (Pt 8), 1437–1448.

Dodd, M.L., Klos, K.J., Bower, J.H. *et al.* (2005) Pathological gambling caused by drugs used to treat Parkinson's disease. *Archives of Neurology*, **62**, 1377–1381.

Dowling, G.A., Mastick, J., Colling, E. *et al.* (2005) Melatonin for sleep disturbances in Parkinson's disease. *Sleep Medicine*, **6**, 459–466.

Drapier, D., Drapier, S., Sauleau, P. *et al.* (2006) Pathological gambling secondary to dopaminergic therapy in Parkinson's disease. *Psychiatry Research*, **144**, 241–244.

Dubois, B., Tolosa, E., Kulisevsky, J., Reichmann, H., Jones, R.W., Burn, D.J., Harre, M., Thomas, G., Harris, R., Moline, M., Silver, G., Swartz, J.E., Schindler, R. and Gray, J. (2007) Efficacy and safety of donepezil in the treatment of Parkinson's disease patients with dementia. *Neurodegenerative Dis*, **4** (Suppl 1), 86.

Ebersbach, G. (2003) An artist's view of drug-induced hallucinosis. *Movement Disorders*, **18**, 833–834.

Edwards, L.L., Quigley, E.M. and Pfeiffer, R.F. (1992) Gastrointestinal dysfunction in Parkinson's disease: frequency and pathophysiology. *Neurology*, **42**, 726–732.

Eichhorn, T.E. and Oertel, W.H. (2001) Macrogol 3350/electrolyte improves constipation in Parkinson's disease and multiple system atrophy. *Movement Disorders*, **16**, 1176–1177.

Ellis, T., Cudkowicz, M.E., Sexton, P.M. *et al.* (2000) Clozapine and risperidone treatment of psychosis in Parkinson's disease. *Journal of Neuropsychiatry and Clinical Neurosciences*, **12**, 364–369.

Emre, M. (2003) Dementia associated with Parkinson's disease. *Lancet Neurology*, **2**, 229–237.

Emre, M., Aarsland, D., Albanese, A. *et al.* (2004) Rivastigmine for dementia associated with Parkinson's disease. *The New England Journal of Medicine*, **351**, 2509–2518.

Emre, M., Aarsland, D., Brown, R. *et al.* (2007) Clinical diagnostic criteria for dementia associated with Parkinson's disease. Movement Disorder Society Task Force. *Movement Disorders*, **22**, 1689–1707.

Evans, A.H., Costa, D.C., Gacinovic, S. *et al.* (2004) L-Dopa-responsive Parkinson's syndrome in association with phenylketonuria: In vivo dopamine transporter and D2 receptor findings. *Movement Disorders*, **19**, 1232–1236.

Evans, A.H., Lawrence, A.D., Potts, J. *et al.* (2005) Factors influencing susceptibility to compulsive dopaminergic drug use in Parkinson's disease. *Neurology*, **65**, 1570–1574.

Evans, A.H., Pavese, N., Lawrence, A.D. *et al.* (2006) Compulsive drug use linked to sensitized ventral striatal dopamine transmission. *Annals of Neurology*, **59**, 852–858.

Fabbrini, G., Barbanti, P., Aurilia, C. *et al.* (2002) Donepezil in the treatment of hallucinations and delusions in Parkinson's disease. *Neurological Sciences*, **23**, 41–43.

Factor, S.A., Friedman, J.H., Lannon, M.C. *et al.* (2001) Clozapine for the treatment of drug-induced psychosis in Parkinson's disease: results of the 12 week open label extension in the PSYCLOPS trial. *Movement Disorders*, **16**, 135–139.

Fantini, M.L., Gagnon, J.F., Filipini, D. *et al.* (2003) The effects of pramipexole in REM sleep behavior disorder. *Neurology*, **61**, 1418–1420.

FCPSG (The French Clozapine Parkinson Study Group) (1999) Clozapine in drug-induced psychosis in Parkinson's disease. *Lancet*, **353**, 2041–2042.

Feldman, H.A., Goldstein, I., Hatzichristou, D.G. *et al.* (1994) Impotence and its medical and psychosocial correlates: results of the Massachusetts Male Aging Study. *The Journal of Urology*, **151**, 54–61.

Fenelon, G., Mahieux, F., Huon, R. *et al.* (2000) Hallucinations in Parkinson's disease: prevalence, phenomenology and risk factors. *Brain*, **123** (Pt 4), 733–745.

Fernandez, H.H., Trieschmann, M.E., Burke, M.A. *et al.* (2003) Long-term outcome of quetiapine use for psychosis among Parkinsonian patients. *Movement Disorders*, **18**, 510–514.

Fitzmaurice, H., Fowler, C.J., Rickards, D. *et al.* (1985) Micturition disturbance in Parkinson's disease. *British Journal of Urology*, **57**, 652–656.

Forno, L.S. (1996) Neuropathology of Parkinson's disease. *Journal of Neuropathology and Experimental Neurology*, **55**, 259–272.

Fowler, C.J. and O'Malley, K.J. (2003) Investigation and management of neurogenic bladder dysfunction. *Journal of Neurology, Neurosurgery, and Psychiatry*, **74** (Suppl 4), iv27–iv31.

Fregni, F., Santos, C.M., Myczkowski, M.L. *et al.* (2004) Repetitive transcranial magnetic stimulation is as effective as fluoxetine in the treatment of depression in patients with Parkinson's disease. *Journal of Neurology, Neurosurgery, and Psychiatry*, **75**, 1171–1174.

Friedman, J.H., Berman, R.M., Goetz, C.G. *et al.* (2006) Open-label flexible-dose pilot study to evaluate the safety and tolerability of aripiprazole in patients with psychosis associated with Parkinson's disease. *Movement Disorders*, **21**, 2078–2081.

Frucht, S., Rogers, J.D., Greene, P.E. *et al.* (1999) Falling asleep at the wheel: motor vehicle mishaps in persons taking pramipexole and ropinirole. *Neurology*, **52**, 1908–1910.

Gagnon, J.F., Bedard, M.A., Fantini, M.L. *et al.* (2002) REM sleep behavior disorder and REM sleep without atonia in Parkinson's disease. *Neurology*, **59**, 585–589.

Giovannoni, G., O'Sullivan, J.D., Turner, K. *et al.* (2000) Hedonistic homeostatic dysregulation in patients with Parkinson's disease on dopamine replacement therapies. *Journal of Neurology, Neurosurgery, and Psychiatry*, **68**, 423–428.

Goetz, C.G. and Stebbins, G.T. (1993) Risk factors for nursing home placement in advanced Parkinson's disease. *Neurology*, **43**, 2227–2229.

Goetz, C.G., Vogel, C., Tanner, C.M. *et al.* (1998) Early dopaminergic drug-induced hallucinations in parkinsonian patients. *Neurology*, **51**, 811–814.

Goetz, C.G., Blasucci, L.M., Leurgans, S. *et al.* (2000) Olanzapine and clozapine: comparative effects on motor function in hallucinating PD patients. *Neurology*, **55**, 789–794.

Goetz, C.G., Koller, W.C., Poewe, W. *et al.* (2002) Management of Parkinson's disease: an evidence-based review. *Movement Disorders*, **17** (Suppl 4), S1–166.

Gomez-Esteban, J.C., Zarranz, J.J., Velasco, F. *et al.* (2005) Use of ziprasidone in parkinsonian patients with psychosis. *Clinical Neuropharmacology*, **28**, 111–114.

Grimsby, J., Toth, M., Chen, K. *et al.* (1997) Increased stress response and beta-phenylethylamine in MAOB-deficient mice. *Nature Genetics*, **17**, 206–210.

Harding, A.J., Broe, G.A. and Halliday, G.M. (2002) Visual hallucinations in Lewy body disease relate to Lewy bodies in the temporal lobe. *Brain*, **125**, 391–403.

Hely, M.A., Morris, J.G., Reid, W.G. *et al.* (2005) Sydney Multicenter Study of Parkinson's disease: non-L-dopa-responsive problems dominate at 15 years. *Movement Disorders*, **20**, 190–199.

Herzog, J., Weiss, P.H., Assmus, A. *et al.* (2006) Subthalamic stimulation modulates cortical control of urinary bladder in Parkinson's disease. *Brain*, **129**, 3366–3375.

Hobson, D.E., Lang, A.E., Martin, W.R. *et al.* (2002) Excessive daytime sleepiness and sudden-onset sleep in Parkinson's disease: a survey by the Canadian Movement Disorders Group. *The Journal of the American Medical Association*, **287**, 455–463.

Hobson, P., Islam, W., Roberts, S. *et al.* (2003) The risk of bladder and autonomic dysfunction in a community cohort of Parkinson's disease patients and normal controls. *Parkinsonism & Related Disorders*, **10**, 67–71.

Hogl, B., Saletu, M., Brandauer, E. *et al.* (2002) Modafinil for the treatment of daytime sleepiness in Parkinson's disease: a double-blind, randomized, crossover, placebo-controlled polygraphic trial. *Sleep*, **25**, 905–909.

Hogl, B., Rothdach, A., Wetter, T.C. *et al.* (2003) The effect of cabergoline on sleep, periodic leg movements in sleep, and early morning motor function in patients with Parkinson's disease. *Neuropsychopharmacology*, **28**, 1866–1870.

Honigfeld, G., Arellano, F., Sethi, J. *et al.* (1998) Reducing clozapine-related morbidity and mortality: 5 years of experience with the Clozaril National Registry. *Journal of Clinical Psychiatry*, **59** (Suppl 3), 3–7.

Horstink, M., Tolosa, E., Bonuccelli, U. *et al.* (2006) Review of the therapeutic management of Parkinson's disease. Report of a joint task force of the European Federation of Neurological Societies (EFNS) and the Movement Disorder Society-European Section (MDS-ES). Part II: late (complicated) Parkinson's disease. *European Journal of Neurology*, **13**, 1186–1202.

Hussain, I.F., Brady, C.M., Swinn, M.J. *et al.* (2001) Treatment of erectile dysfunction with sildenafil citrate (Viagra) in parkinsonism due to Parkinson's disease or multiple system atrophy with observations on orthostatic hypotension. *Journal of Neurology, Neurosurgery, and Psychiatry*, **71**, 371–374.

Hutchinson, M. and Fazzini, E. (1996) Cholinesterase inhibition in Parkinson's disease. *Journal of Neurology, Neurosurgery, and Psychiatry*, **61**, 324–325.

Iranzo, A., Santamaria, J., Kumru, H., Valldeoriola, F., Marti, M.J. and Tolosa, E. (2005) Lack of effect of pramipexole on REM sleep behavior disorder in subjects with Parkinson's Disease. *Sleep*, **28** (Suppl), 266; Ref Type: Abstract.

Iranzo, A., Molinuevo, J.L., Santamaria, J. *et al.* (2006) Rapid-eye-movement sleep behaviour disorder as an early marker for a neurodegenerative disorder: a descriptive study. *Lancet Neurology*, **5**, 572–577.

Jankovic, J., Gilden, J.L., Hiner, B.C. *et al.* (1993) Neurogenic orthostatic hypotension: a double-blind, placebo-controlled study with midodrine. *The American Journal of Medicine*, **95**, 38–48.

Jost, W.H. and Schimrigk, K. (1993) Cisapride treatment of constipation in Parkinson's disease. *Movement Disorders*, **8**, 339–343.

Jouvent, R., Abensour, P., Bonnet, A.M. *et al.* (1983) Antiparkinsonian and antidepressant effects of high doses of bromocriptine. An independent comparison. *Journal of Affective Disorders*, **5**, 141–145.

Juri, C., Chana, P., Tapia, J. *et al.* (2005) Quetiapine for insomnia in Parkinson's disease: results from an open-label trial. *Clinical Neuropharmacology*, **28**, 185–187.

Katzenschlager, R., Hughes, A., Evans, A. *et al.* (2005) Continuous subcutaneous apomorphine therapy improves dyskinesias in Parkinson's disease: a prospective study using single-dose challenges. *Movement Disorders*, **20**, 151–157.

Kaufmann, H. and Biaggioni, I. (2003) Autonomic failure in neurodegenerative disorders. *Seminars in Neurology*, **23**, 351–363.

Kaufmann, H., Nahm, K., Purohit, D. *et al.* (2004) Autonomic failure as the initial presentation of Parkinson's disease and dementia with Lewy bodies. *Neurology*, **63**, 1093–1095.

Kendirci, M., Tanriverdi, O., Trost, L. *et al.* (2006) Management of sildenafil treatment failures. *Current Opinion in Urology*, **16**, 449–459.

Kessel, B.L. (2006) A case of hedonistic homeostatic dysregulation. *Age Ageing*, **35**, 540–541.

Korczyn, A.D. (1990) Autonomic nervous system disturbances in Parkinson's disease. *Advances in Neurology*, **53**, 463–468.

Kunz, D. and Bes, F. (1999) Melatonin as a therapy in REM sleep behavior disorder patients: an open-labeled pilot study on the possible influence of melatonin on REM-sleep regulation. *Movement Disorders*, **14**, 507–511.

Kurlan, R. (2004) Disabling repetitive behaviors in Parkinson's disease. *Movement Disorders*, **19**, 433–437.

Lahrmann, H., Cortelli, P., Hilz, M. *et al.* (2006) EFNS guidelines on the diagnosis and management of orthostatic hypotension. *European Journal of Neurology*, **13**, 930–936.

Leentjens, A.F., Vreeling, F.W., Luijckx, G.J. *et al.* (2003) SSRIs in the treatment of depression in Parkinson's disease. *International Journal of Geriatric Psychiatry*, **18**, 552–554.

Lees, A.J. and Smith, E. (1983) Cognitive deficits in the early stages of Parkinson's disease. *Brain*, **106** (Pt 2), 257–270.

Lees, A.J., Shaw, K.M., Kohout, L.J. *et al.* (1977) Deprenyl in Parkinson's disease. *Lancet*, **2**, 791–795.

Lees, A.J., Blackburn, N.A. and Campbell, V.L. (1988) The nighttime problems of Parkinson's disease. *Clinical Neuropharmacology*, **11**, 512–519.

Lemack, G.E., Dewey, R.B., Jr, Roehrborn, C.G. *et al.* (2000) Questionnaire-based assessment of bladder dysfunction in patients with mild to moderate Parkinson's disease. *Urology*, **56**, 250–254.

Lembo, A. and Camilleri, M. (2003) Chronic constipation. *The New England Journal of Medicine*, **349**, 1360–1368.

Lemke, M.R. (2002) Effect of reboxetine on depression in Parkinson's disease patients. *Journal of Clinical Psychiatry*, **63**, 300–304.

Leroi, I., Brandt, J., Reich, S.G. *et al.* (2004) Randomized placebo-controlled trial of donepezil in cognitive impairment in Parkinson's disease. *International Journal of Geriatric Psychiatry*, **19**, 1–8.

Linazasoro, G., Lasa, A. and Van Blercom, N. (2005) Efficacy and safety of donepezil in the treatment of executive dysfunction in Parkinson's disease: a pilot study. *Clinical Neuropharmacology*, **28**, 176–178.

Liu, Z., Sakakibara, R., Odaka, T. *et al.* (2005) Mosapride citrate, a novel 5-HT4 agonist and partial 5-HT3 antagonist, ameliorates constipation in parkinsonian patients. *Movement Disorders*, **20**, 680–686.

Low, P.A., Gilden, J.L., Freeman, R. *et al.* (1997) Efficacy of midodrine vs placebo in neurogenic orthostatic hypotension. A randomized, double-blind multicenter study. Midodrine Study Group. *The Journal of the American Medical Association*, **277**, 1046–1051.

Lyons, K.E. and Pahwa, R. (2006) Effects of bilateral subthalamic nucleus stimulation on sleep, daytime sleepiness, and early morning dystonia in patients with Parkinson's disease. *Journal of Neurosurgery*, **104**, 502–505.

Magalhaes, M., Wenning, G.K., Daniel, S.E. *et al.* (1995) Autonomic dysfunction in pathologically confirmed multiple system atrophy and idiopathic Parkinson's disease – a retrospective comparison. *Acta Neurologica Scandinavica*, **91**, 98–102.

Magerkurth, C., Schnitzer, R. and Braune, S. (2005) Symptoms of autonomic failure in Parkinson's disease: prevalence and impact on daily life. *Clinical Autonomic Research*, **15**, 76–82.

Mahowald, M.W., Schenck, C.H. and Bornemann, M.A. (2007) Pathophysiologic mechanisms in REM sleep behavior disorder. *Current Neurology and Neuroscience Reports*, **7**, 167–172.

Mann, J.J., Aarons, S.F., Wilner, P.J. *et al.* (1989) A controlled study of the antidepressant efficacy and side effects of (-)-deprenyl. A selective monoamine oxidase inhibitor. *Archives of General Psychiatry*, **46**, 45–50.

Marder, K., Tang, M.X., Cote, L. *et al.* (1995) The frequency and associated risk factors for dementia in patients with Parkinson's disease. *Archives of Neurology*, **52**, 695–701.

Maria, G., Brisinda, G., Bentivoglio, A.R. *et al.* (2000) Botulinum toxin in the treatment of outlet obstruction constipation caused by puborectalis syndrome. *Diseases of the Colon and Rectum*, **43**, 376–380.

Maricle, R.A., Nutt, J.G., Valentine, R.J. *et al.* (1995) Dose-response relationship of L-Dopa with mood and anxiety in fluctuating Parkinson's disease: a double-blind, placebo-controlled study. *Neurology*, **45**, 1757–1760.

Martignoni, E., Tassorelli, C. and Nappi, G. (2006) Cardiovascular dysautonomia as a cause of falls in Parkinson's disease. *Parkinsonism & Related Disorders*, **12**, 195–204.

Mayeux, R. (1990) Depression in the patient with Parkinson's disease. *Journal of Clinical Psychiatry*, **51** (Suppl), 20–23.

McKeith, I.G., Dickson, D.W., Lowe, J. *et al.* (2005) Diagnosis and management of dementia with Lewy bodies: third report of the DLB Consortium. *Neurology*, **65**, 1863–1872.

Meara, J., Mitchelmore, E. and Hobson, P. (1999) Use of the GDS-15 geriatric depression scale as a screening instrument for depressive symptomatology in patients with Parkinson's disease and their carers in the community. *Age Ageing*, **28**, 35–38.

Merims, D., Balas, M., Peretz, C. *et al.* (2006) Rater-blinded, prospective comparison: quetiapine vs clozapine for Parkinson's disease psychosis. *Clinical Neuropharmacology*, **29**, 331–337.

Michalowska, M., Fiszer, U., Krygowska-Wajs, A. *et al.* (2005) Falls in Parkinson's disease. Causes and impact on patients' quality of life. *Functional Neurology*, **20**, 163–168.

Miyasaki, J.M., Shannon, K., Voon, V. *et al.* (2006) Practice Parameter: evaluation and treatment of depression, psychosis, and dementia in Parkinson's disease (an evidence-based review): report of the Quality Standards Subcommittee of the American Academy of Neurology. *Neurology*, **66**, 996–1002.

Miyasaki, J.M., Al, H.K., Lang, A.E. *et al.* (2007) Punding prevalence in Parkinson's disease. *Movement Disorders*, **22**, 1179–1181.

Morgan, J.C. and Sethi, K.D. (2007) Tegaserod in constipation associated with Parkinson's disease. *Clinical Neuropharmacology*, **30**, 52–54.

Morgante, L., Epifanio, A., Spina, E. *et al.* (2004) Quetiapine and clozapine in parkinsonian patients with dopaminergic psychosis. *Clinical Neuropharmacology*, **27**, 153–156.

Nieves, A.V. and Lang, A.E. (2002) Treatment of excessive daytime sleepiness in patients with Parkinson's disease with modafinil. *Clinical Neuropharmacology*, **25**, 111–114.

O'Sullivan, J.D. and Hughes, A.J. (1998) Apomorphine-induced penile erections in Parkinson's disease. *Movement Disorders*, **13**, 536–539.

Okabe, S., Ugawa, Y. and Kanazawa, I. (2003) 0.2-Hz repetitive transcranial magnetic stimulation has no add-on effects as compared to a realistic sham stimulation in Parkinson's disease. *Movement Disorders*, **18**, 382–388.

Okun, M.S. and Watts, R.L. (2002) Depression associated with Parkinson's disease: clinical features and treatment. *Neurology*, **58**, S63–S70.

Olson, E.J., Boeve, B.F. and Silber, M.H. (2000) Rapid eye movement sleep behaviour disorder: demographic, clinical and laboratory findings in 93 cases. *Brain*, **123** (Pt 2), 331–339.

Ondo, W.G., Levy, J.K., Vuong, K.D. *et al.* (2002a) Olanzapine treatment for dopaminergic-induced hallucinations. *Movement Disorders*, **17**, 1031–1035.

Ondo, W.G., Vuong, K.D. and Jankovic, J. (2002b) Exploring the relationship between Parkinson's disease and restless legs syndrome. *Archives of Neurology*, **59**, 421–424.

Ondo, W.G., Tintner, R., Voung, K.D. *et al.* (2005a) Double-blind, placebo-controlled, unforced titration parallel trial of quetiapine for dopaminergic-induced hallucinations in Parkinson's disease. *Movement Disorders*, **20**, 958–963.

Ondo, W.G., Fayle, R., Atassi, F. *et al.* (2005b) Modafinil for daytime somnolence in Parkinson's disease: double blind, placebo controlled parallel trial. *Journal of Neurology, Neurosurgery, and Psychiatry*, **76**, 1636–1639.

Ozekmekci, S., Apaydin, H. and Kilic, E. (2005) Clinical features of 35 patients with Parkinson's disease displaying REM behavior disorder. *Clinical Neurology and Neurosurgery*, **107**, 306–309.

Papatsoris, A.G., Deliveliotis, C., Singer, C. *et al.* (2006) Erectile dysfunction in Parkinson's disease. *Urology*, **67**, 447–451.

Pathak, A. and Senard, J.M. (2006) Blood pressure disorders during Parkinson's disease: epidemiology, pathophysiology and management. *Expert Review of Neurotherapeutics*, **6**, 1173–1180.

Paus, S., Brecht, H.M., Koster, J. *et al.* (2003) Sleep attacks, daytime sleepiness, and dopamine agonists in Parkinson's disease. *Movement Disorders*, **18**, 659–667.

Peralta, C., Stampfer-Kountchev, M., Karner, E. *et al.* (2007) Orthostatic hypotension and attention in Parkinson's disease with and without dementia. *Journal of Neural Transmission*, **114**, 585–588.

Perry, E.K., Irving, D., Kerwin, J.M. *et al.* (1993) Cholinergic transmitter and neurotrophic activities in Lewy body dementia: similarity to Parkinson's and distinction from Alzheimer disease. *Alzheimer Disease & Associated Disorders*, **7**, 69–79.

Poewe, W. (2003) Psychosis in Parkinson's disease. *Movement Disorders*, **18** (Suppl 6), S80–S87.

Poewe, W. (2006) The natural history of Parkinson's disease. *Journal of Neurology*, **253** (Suppl 7), vii2–vii6.

Poewe, W. and Seppi, K. (2001) Treatment options for depression and psychosis in Parkinson's disease. *Journal of Neurology*, **248** (Suppl 3), III12–III21.

Poewe, W., Wolters, E., Emre, M. *et al.* (2006) Long-term benefits of rivastigmine in dementia associated with Parkinson's disease: an active treatment extension study. *Movement Disorders*, **21**, 456–461.

Poewe, W.H., Rascol, O., Quinn, N. *et al.* (2007) Efficacy of pramipexole and transdermal rotigotine in advanced Parkinson's disease: a double-blind, double-dummy, randomised controlled trial. *Lancet Neurology*, **6**, 513–520.

Pohanka, M., Kanovsky, P., Bares, M. *et al.* (2005) The long-lasting improvement of sexual dysfunction in patients with advanced, fluctuating Parkinson's disease induced by pergolide: evidence from the results of an open, prospective, one-year trial. *Parkinsonism & Related Disorders*, **11**, 509–512.

Pollak, P., Tison, F., Rascol, O. *et al.* (2004) Clozapine in drug induced psychosis in Parkinson's disease: a randomised, placebo controlled study with open follow up. *Journal of Neurology, Neurosurgery, and Psychiatry*, **75**, 689–695.

Porst, H., Behre, H.M., Jungwirth, A. *et al.* (2007) Comparative trial of treatment satisfaction, efficacy and tolerability of sildenafil vs apomorphine in erectile dysfunction–an open, randomized cross-over study with flexible dosing. *European Journal of Medical Research*, **12**, 61–67.

Potenza, M.N., Voon, V. and Weintraub, D. (2007) Drug insight: impulse control disorders and dopamine therapies in Parkinson's disease. *Nature Clinical Practice Neurology*, **3**, 664–672.

Rabey, J.M., Prokhorov, T., Miniovitz, A. *et al.* (2007) Effect of quetiapine in psychotic Parkinson's disease patients: a double-blind labeled study of 3 months' duration. *Movement Disorders*, **22**, 313–318.

Raffaele, R., Vecchio, I., Giammusso, B. *et al.* (2002) Efficacy and safety of fixed-dose oral sildenafil in the treatment of sexual dysfunction in depressed patients with idiopathic Parkinson's disease. *European Urology*, **41**, 382–386.

Ravina, B., Putt, M., Siderowf, A. *et al.* (2005) Donepezil for dementia in Parkinson's disease: a randomised, double blind, placebo controlled, crossover study. *Journal of Neurology, Neurosurgery, and Psychiatry*, **76**, 934–939.

Ravina, B., Marder, K., Fernandez, H.H. *et al.* (2007) Diagnostic criteria for psychosis in Parkinson's disease: Report of an NINDS, NIMH work group. *Movement Disorders*, **22**, 1061–1068.

Reading, P.J., Luce, A.K. and McKeith, I.G. (2001) Rivastigmine in the treatment of parkinsonian psychosis and cognitive impairment: preliminary findings from an open trial. *Movement Disorders*, **16**, 1171–1174.

Reddy, S., Factor, S.A., Molho, E.S. *et al.* (2002) The effect of quetiapine on psychosis and motor function in parkinsonian patients with and without dementia. *Movement Disorders*, **17**, 676–681.

Rektorova, I., Rektor, I., Bares, M. *et al.* (2003) Pramipexole and pergolide in the treatment of depression in Parkinson's disease: a national multicentre prospective randomized study. *European Journal of Neurology*, **10**, 399–406.

Remy, P., Doder, M., Lees, A. *et al.* (2005) Depression in Parkinson's disease: loss of dopamine and noradrenaline innervation in the limbic system. *Brain*, **128**, 1314–1322.

Richard, I.H. and Kurlan, R. (1997) A survey of antidepressant drug use in Parkinson's disease. Parkinson Study Group. *Neurology*, **49**, 1168–1170.

Richard, I.H., Kurlan, R., Tanner, C. *et al.* (1997) Serotonin syndrome and the combined use of deprenyl and an antidepressant in Parkinson's disease. Parkinson Study Group. *Neurology*, **48**, 1070–1077.

Rye, D.B. (2006) Excessive daytime sleepiness and unintended sleep in Parkinson's disease. *Current Neurology and Neuroscience Reports*, **6**, 169–176.

Sahai, A., Khan, M.S., Arya, M. *et al.* (2006) The overactive bladder: review of current pharmacotherapy in adults. Part 2: treatment options in cases refractory to anticholinergics. *Expert Opinion in Pharmacotherapy*, **7**, 529–538.

Sakakibara, R., Shinotoh, H., Uchiyama, T. *et al.* (2001) Questionnaire-based assessment of pelvic organ dysfunction in Parkinson's disease. *Autonomic Neuroscience: Basic & Clinical*, **92**, 76–85.

Sakakibara, R., Odaka, T., Lui, Z. *et al.* (2005) Dietary herb extract dai-kenchu-to ameliorates constipation in parkinsonian patients (Parkinson's disease and multiple system atrophy). *Movement Disorders*, **20**, 261–262.

Schenck, C.H. and Mahowald, M.W. (1996) Long-term nightly benzodiazepine treatment of injurious parasomnias and other disorders of disrupted nocturnal sleep in 170 adults. *The American Journal of Medicine*, **100**, 333–337.

Schenck, C.H., Bundlie, S.R., Patterson, A.L. *et al.* (1987) Rapid eye movement sleep behavior disorder. A treatable parasomnia affecting older adults. *The Journal of the American Medical Association*, **257**, 1786–1789.

Schenck, C.H., Bundlie, S.R. and Mahowald, M.W. (1996) Delayed emergence of a parkinsonian disorder in 38% of 29 older men initially diagnosed with idiopathic rapid eye movement sleep behaviour disorder. *Neurology*, **46**, 388–393.

Schmidt, M.H., Koshal, V.B. and Schmidt, H.S. (2006) Use of pramipexole in REM sleep behavior disorder: results from a case series. *Sleep Medicine*, **7**, 418–423.

Senard, J.M., Rai, S., Lapeyre-Mestre, M. *et al.* (1997) Prevalence of orthostatic hypotension in Parkinson's disease. *Journal of Neurology, Neurosurgery, and Psychiatry*, **63**, 584–589.

Serrano-Duenas, M. (2002) A comparison between low doses of amitriptyline and low doses of fluoxetin used in the control of depression in patients suffering from Parkinson's disease. *Rev Neurol*, **35**, 1010–1014.

Shulman, L.M., Taback, R.L., Bean, J. *et al.* (2001) Comorbidity of the nonmotor symptoms of Parkinson's disease. *Movement Disorders*, **16**, 507–510.

Smeding, H.M., Goudriaan, A.E., Foncke, E.M. *et al.* (2007) Pathological gambling after bilateral subthalamic nucleus stimulation in Parkinson's disease. *Journal of Neurology, Neurosurgery, and Psychiatry*, **78**, 517–519.

Starkstein, S.E., Preziosi, T.J., Bolduc, P.L. *et al.* (1990) Depression in Parkinson's disease. *The Journal of Nervous and Mental Disease*, **178**, 27–31.

Suchowersky, O., Furtado, S. and Rohs, G. (1995) Beneficial effect of intranasal desmopressin for nocturnal polyuria in Parkinson's disease. *Movement Disorders*, **10**, 337–340.

Sullivan, K.L., Staffetti, J.F., Hauser, R.A. *et al.* (2006) Tegaserod (Zelnorm) for the treatment of constipation in Parkinson's disease. *Movement Disorders*, **21**, 115–116.

Takeuchi, N., Uchimura, N., Hashizume, Y. *et al.* (2001) Melatonin therapy for REM sleep behavior disorder. *Psychiatry and Clinical Neurosciences*, **55**, 267–269.

Tan, A., Salgado, M. and Fahn, S. (1996) Rapid eye movement sleep behavior disorder preceding Parkinson's disease with therapeutic response to L-Dopa. *Movement Disorders*, **11**, 214–216.

Tandberg, E., Larsen, J.P., Aarsland, D. *et al.* (1996) The occurrence of depression in Parkinson's disease. A community-based study. *Archives of Neurology*, **53**, 175–179.

Tandberg, E., Larsen, J.P. and Karlsen, K. (1998) A community-based study of sleep disorders in patients with Parkinson's disease. *Movement Disorders*, **13**, 895–899.

Taylor, M.J. (2006) Strategies for managing antidepressant-induced sexual dysfunction: a review. *Current Psychiatry Reports*, **8**, 431–436.

The Parkinson Study Group, (1999) Low-dose clozapine for the treatment of drug-induced psychosis in Parkinson's disease. *The New England Journal of Medicine*, **340**, 757–763.

The U.K. Madopar CR Study Group (1989) A comparison of Madopar CR and standard Madopar in the treatment of nocturnal and early-morning disability in Parkinson's disease. *Clinical Neuropharmacology*, **12**, 498–505.

Visser, M., Marinus, J., Stiggelbout, A.M. *et al.* (2004) Assessment of autonomic dysfunction in Parkinson's disease: the SCOPA-AUT. *Movement Disorders*, **19**, 1306–1312.

Voon, V. and Fox, S.H. (2007) Medication-related impulse control and repetitive behaviors in Parkinson's disease. *Archives of Neurology*, **64**, 1089–1096.

Voon, V., Potenza, M.N. and Thomsen, T. (2007) Medication-related impulse control and repetitive behaviors in Parkinson's disease. *Current Opinion in Neurology*, **20**, 484–492.

Wakabayashi, K. and Takahashi, H. (1997) Neuropathology of autonomic nervous system in Parkinson's disease. *European Neurology*, **38** (Suppl 2), 2–7.

Weintraub, D., Morales, K.H., Moberg, P.J. *et al.* (2005) Antidepressant studies in Parkinson's disease: a review and meta-analysis. *Movement Disorders*, **20**, 1161–1169.

Weintraub, D., Morales, K.H., Duda, J.E. *et al.* (2006) Frequency and correlates of co-morbid psychosis and depression in Parkinson's disease. *Parkinsonism & Related Disorders*, **12**, 427–431.

Werber, E.A. and Rabey, J.M. (2001) The beneficial effect of cholinesterase inhibitors on patients suffering from Parkinson's disease and dementia. *Journal of Neural Transmission*, **108**, 1319–1325.

Wermuth, L., Sorensen, P. and Timm, S. (1998) Depression in diopathic Parkinson's disease treated with citalopram. A placebo-controlled trial. *Nord J Psychiatry*, **52**, 163–169.

Whitehouse, P.J., Hedreen, J.C., White, C.L. III, *et al.* (1983) Basal forebrain neurons in the dementia of Parkinson's disease. *Annals of Neurology*, **13**, 243–248.

Wickremaratchi, M., Morris, H.R. and Ali, I.M. (2006) Aripiprazole associated with severe exacerbation of Parkinson's disease. *Movement Disorders*, **21**, 1538–1539.

Williams, D.R. and Lees, A.J. (2005) Visual hallucinations in the diagnosis of idiopathic Parkinson's disease: a retrospective autopsy study. *Lancet Neurology*, **4**, 605–610.

Winge, K. and Fowler, C.J. (2006) Bladder dysfunction in Parkinsonism: mechanisms, prevalence, symptoms, and management. *Movement Disorders*, **21**, 737–745.

Winge, K., Nielsen, K.K., Stimpel, H. *et al.* (2007) Lower urinary tract symptoms and bladder control in advanced Parkinson's disease: effects of deep brain stimulation in the subthalamic nucleus. *Movement Disorders*, **22**, 220–225.

Witjas, T., Kaphan, E., Azulay, J.P. *et al.* (2002) Nonmotor fluctuations in Parkinson's disease: frequent and disabling. *Neurology*, **59**, 408–413.

Witjas, T., Baunez, C., Henry, J.M. *et al.* (2005) Addiction in Parkinson's disease: impact of subthalamic nucleus deep brain stimulation. *Movement Disorders*, **20**, 1052–1055.

Woodford, H. and Walker, R. (2005) Emergency hospital admissions in idiopathic Parkinson's disease. *Movement Disorders*, **20**, 1104–1108.

Zesiewicz, T.A., Helal, M. and Hauser, R.A. (2000) Sildenafil citrate (Viagra) for the treatment of erectile dysfunction in men with Parkinson's disease. *Movement Disorders*, **15**, 305–308.

7

Surgery for Parkinson's Disease

Jens Volkmann

Department of Neurology, Christian-Albrechts-University, Germany

INTRODUCTION

Over the last two decades surgical therapies have established a firm place in the treatment of movement disorders. The recent progress in functional neurosurgery probably marks the second most important therapeutic advance in Parkinson's disease (PD) after the introduction of levodopa. Deep brain stimulation of the subthalamic nucleus (STN-DBS) is now considered an evidence-based, routine therapy for patients with severe tremor or motor complications of long-term levodopa therapy. A recent controlled trial confirmed the superiority of this surgical therapy over best medical treatment alone in improving quality of life of patients with advanced Parkinson's disease. Optimal "palliative" care is the best we can currently provide to patients with PD in the absence of effective disease-modifying strategies. This conceptual change has prompted a re-evaluation of different symptomatic treatments in PD within the multi-dimensional physical-psychosocial framework of disability and health-related quality of life. As a result, the role of surgery within the treatment algorithm of PD may even need to be redefined in the near future, because the goal of maintaining quality of life and preventing the psychosocial decline associated with PD may be better achieved in younger patients operated on at an earlier stage of disease.

Not every patient suffering from parkinsonism is a good candidate for surgery. In fact, the majority of patients are not, and inappropriate neurological patient selection is the most common reason for failed deep brain stimulation, besides poor surgical lead placement or inadequate programming (Okun *et al.*, 2005). Therefore, the discussion of predictive factors and patient selection criteria will be a special emphasis of this chapter, after summarizing the historical evolution of surgical therapies for PD and evaluating their clinical efficacy and safety.

HISTORICAL ASPECTS

Functional neurosurgery for Parkinson's disease has a long history dating back to the late nineteenth century. Before the basal ganglia became recognized as a target for the surgical treatment of movement disorders, various operations on the peripheral and central nervous system were performed. In general, only the positive symptoms of Parkinson's disease, tremor and rigidity, were considered to be treatable by surgery at that time, not akinesia, as a "negative symptom" resulting from loss of function. Lesions in the sensory system including posterior rhizotomy, cordotomy and sympathetic ramisectomy improved rigidity somewhat, but were unsuccessful in treating Parkinsonian tremor and therefore rapidly abandoned. Other procedures directly targeted the motor system, involving excisions of the motor and pre-motor cortex or sectioning of the pyramidal tract at the level of the internal capsule, cerebral peduncle or spinal cord. Tremor could be successfully reduced by these interventions, but at the cost of a variable degree of paralysis, which was soon considered unacceptable.

Basal ganglia surgery was pioneered by Russel Meyers, who performed open resections of the head of the caudate and lesions within the putamen, ansa lenticularis or pallidum in a series of 58 patients with various movement disorders, including parkinsonism, choreoathetosis, hemiballism and dystonia, between 1939 and 1949 (Meyers, 1951; Meyers, 1968). His first patient was a 26-year-old woman suffering from Parkinsonian tremor. After unsuccessfully undercutting the pre-motor cortex, Meyers extirpated the head of the caudate via a transventricular approach. Post-operatively, the tremor had disappeared and the patient did not suffer from a hemiparesis. In his subsequent series, improvement was noted in approximately 60% of the patients, but the operative mortality and morbidity was high with this and other open approaches.

In 1952 Irving Cooper accidentally ligated the anterior choroidal artery while carrying out a pedunculotomy to treat tremor in a patient with Parkinson's disease. The tremor was much improved after surgery, which Cooper considered the result of an ischemic lesion of the pallidum. He used the technique in a series of Parkinsonian patients, but the mortality was 13% (Cooper, 1954), and he subsequently turned to chemopallidotomy by injecting alcohol into the pallidum (Cooper, 1961).

Lesional neurosurgery for movement disorders was revolutionized by the introduction of a stereotactic head frame for use in humans by Spiegel and colleagues in 1947 (Spiegel *et al.*, 1947). Stereotaxis allowed the targeting of deep brain areas on the basis of a three-dimensional coordinate system defined by internal landmarks, which were visible on plain X-ray or pneumencephalography, such as the pineal calcification or the foramen of Monro. By use of the stereotactic technique, more precise and confined lesions could be placed using chemical injections, implantation of radioactive isotopes or ultimately electrocoagulation, which markedly reduced the morbidity associated with any free-hand approach. During the subsequent years, stereotactic neurosurgery flourished. Several groups around the world developed their own frame systems stimulated by the work of Spiegel and Wycis, human brain atlases were published providing the stereotactic coordinates of basal ganglia and thalamic nuclei and imaging was improved by replacing pneumencephalography with positive contrast ventriculography.

In the 1950s the first pathophysiological models of Parkinsomism emerged. The pallidum was thought to be directly involved in the generation of rigidity, but tremor was explained as a result of a disturbance in the postural mechanism of the cerebellum and brainstem (Levy, 1967). Hassler pioneered thalamotomy (Hassler and Riechert, 1954) and subsequently reported that the procedure was more effective than pallidotomy in the treatment of tremor, which convinced neurosurgeons of his time to gradually replace pallidal by thalamic surgery. An important report of Svennilson and colleagues (Svennilson *et al.*, 1960) was published almost unnoticed. The authors had varied the pallidal lesion location and reported a better efficacy on rigidity, tremor, but most notably also on the speed, range and accuracy of contralateral movements with more posteriorly placed pallidotomies. The introduction of levodopa therapy (Birkmayer and Hornykiewicz, 1961; Cotzias, Van Woert and Schiffer, 1967) then rapidly brought surgical therapies for Parkinson's disease to a halt, except for few cases with intractable tremors.

Surgery for Parkinson's disease made a return in the early 1990s, when it became apparent that medical therapy was associated with intractable long-term complications, such as motor fluctuations and dyskinesia. In addition, a better understanding of the pathophysiology in Parkinson's

disease had derived from studies in the MPTP-primate model (Albin, Young and Penney, 1995; Delong, 1990b). Most importantly, akinesia was now no longer considered a "negative symptom" as a direct consequence of neurodegeneration within the basal ganglia, but rather as the result of neuronal overactivity within the internal globus pallidus and subthalamic nucleus. This allowed a testable hypothesis on the effect of lesions within the basal ganglia circuitry. The seminal work on the beneficial effect of lesioning the subthalamic nucleus in the MPTP monkey (Bergmann, Wichmann and Delong, 1990) was published around the same time that Laitinen and colleagues reported on a series of patients with Parkinson's disease treated by posteroventral pallidotomy (Laitinen, Bergenheim and Hariz, 1992) (refer to Figure 7.1). They found marked improvements in all cardinal symptoms of Parkinson's disease and levodopa-induced dyskinesias with a procedure that was thought to interrupt the excessive inhibitory output from the sensorimotor pallidum to the ventrolateral thalamus. The procedure was rapidly adopted by other groups in Europe, USA and Canada, because it was felt to be safer than subthalamic lesioning, which could cause hemiballism or hemichorea. In 1996 an initial survey among 28 centers practicing pallidotomy in North America reported on 1015 patients (Favre *et al.*, 1996), but it was estimated that at least twice as many centers were active in the USA and Canada, which underlines the rapid renaissance of pallidal surgery. A novelty in contemporary surgery for movement disorders was the strong involvement of neurologists in patient selection, post-operative management and often intraoperative assessment of clinical symptoms. This also provided more objective reports on the outcome after surgery, according to the same rigid criteria that were used to evaluate medical therapies for Parkinson's disease.

High-frequency deep brain stimulation (DBS) as an alternative to ablative stereotaxy, was first introduced for the treatment of movement disorders in the 1970s (Mundinger, 1977; Mundinger and Neumuller, 1982), but had not been routinely used until the pioneering work of Alim-Louis Benabid in Grenoble and Jean Siegfried in Zürich became public in the early 1990s (Benabid *et al.*, 1991; Siegfried and Lippitz, 1994b). Encouraged by the efficacy and safety of thalamic DBS for tremor, and previous animal experiments (Benazzouz *et al.*, 1993), Benabid soon extended the technique to the subthalamic nucleus. The first patient was implanted in Grenoble in February 1993 and post-operatively demonstrated a remarkable reduction of all Parkinsonian symptoms, including akinesia, but without any hyperkinetic adverse effects (Pollak *et al.*, 1993). The publication of the first series of STN-DBS in *Lancet* triggered a worldwide interest in this novel approach (Limousin *et al.*, 1995). The therapy was approved by the European Commision in 1998 and by the US Food and Drug administration in 2002, for treating

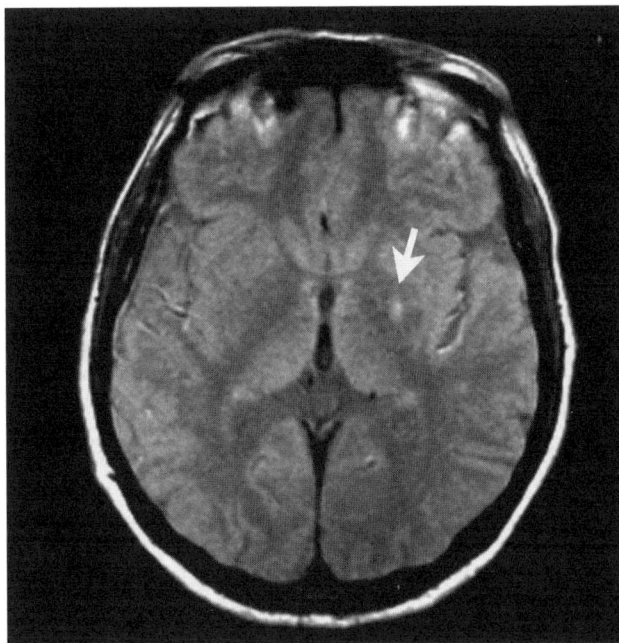

Figure 7.1 Pallidotomy lesion on magnetic resonance imaging.

advanced stages of Parkinson's disease. DBS has rapidly replaced ablative neurosurgery for Parkinson's disease during the past decade. It is currently by far the most frequent surgery for movement disorders with an estimated 40 000 patients treated worldwide.

PATHOPHYSIOLOGICAL MODELS OF PARKINSON'S DISEASE AND THE "PARADOX" OF BASAL GANGLIA SURGERY

Contemporary stereotactic neurosurgery for Parkinson's disease was built on advances in the understanding of PD pathophysiology, which derived from anatomical studies on the connectivity of the basal ganglia, and physiological recordings in the MPTP-primate model of parkinsonism. The popular models forwarded by Albin and colleagues (Albin, Young and Penney, 1995) and Delong (Delong, 1990) view the basal ganglia as part of several parallel negative-feedback loops linking them to specific thalamic nuclei and frontal cortical areas. These circuits within the basal ganglia thalamocortical system subserve motor, limbic, associative and cognitive functions. The motor territories are segregated from the other functional areas within each basal ganglia nucleus and lie, for example, within the posterolateral segment of the internal pallidum (GPi) and the dorsolateral portion of the subthalamic nucleus. Ablative therapies were developed from the observation that neuronal activity is abnormally increased in the subthalamic nucleus (STN) and GPi in animal models of Parkinson's disease. Lesioning or high-frequency stimulation to reduce the outflow from these overactive areas reversed symptoms of MPTP-induced parkinsonism (Bergmann, Wichmann and Delong, 1990; Benazzouz et al., 1993). Excitatory afferents from STN are driving GPi neurons to be overactive, according to the rate model (Delong, 1990b), which in turn provide excessive inhibitory outflow to the ventrolateral thalamus and motor cortical projection areas.

As predicted by the primate model, pallidotomy can restore a normal level of activity in the thalamocortical motor pathways of Parkinsonian patients, by decreasing the abnormal inhibitory output of the GPi. This was demonstrated by positron emission tomography (PET) studies after pallidotomy, which showed increased regional cerebral blood flow (rCBF) and metabolism in the ipsilateral supplementary motor area (SMA) and dorsolateral prefrontal cortex (DLPFC). These changes in cerebral blood flow were associated with improvements in motor functions (Samuel et al., 1997; Eidelberg et al., 1996; Ceballos-Baumann et al., 1994). Similar reversible changes of rCBF in the SMA and DLPFC were described after high-frequency stimulation of the internal pallidum (Davis et al., 1997) or subthalamic nucleus (Ceballos Baumann et al., 1999).

While these observations may explain the alleviation of akinesia, they provide little insight into the mechanisms by which tremor, rigidity or dyskinesias might be improved.

The simple "rate model" of abnormal neuronal activity in Parkinson's disease would predict reduced pallidal discharge rates in hyperkinetic states, and thus a further worsening with pallidal lesioning or DBS (Marsden and Obeso, 1994). Clinically, however, the most consistent effect of pallidal surgery is a marked reduction of contralateral hyperkinesias. Moreover, thalamotomy improves tremor and rigidity if pallidal receiving areas are included in the lesion, but does not aggravate akinesia as predicted by the rate model. These contradictions between clinical reality and predictions of the classical rate model of parkinsonism have been described as the "paradox of basal ganglia surgery" by Marsden and Obeso (Marsden and Obeso, 1994).

More recently, it has therefore been suggested that pallidal or subthalamic nucleus surgery, in more general terms, are effective by removing the disturbing influence of a "noisy" basal ganglia operator onto thalamocortical motor areas (Marsden and Obeso, 1994; Hammond, Bergman and Brown, 2007). "Noisy" or unphysiological basal ganglia activity could not only result from changes in discharge rate, but also from abnormal patterning, oscillation or synchronization of neuronal firing (Hammond, Bergman and Brown, 2007). Furthermore, descending projections from the basal ganglia to the brainstem nuclei and spinal cord are often neglected and may also play an important role in the pathophysiology of rigidity, postural instability and gait disorders in Parkinson's disease (Pahapill and Lozano, 2000; Nandi et al., 2002a; Nandi et al., 2002b; Delwaide et al., 2000; Potter et al., 2004).

LESIONAL STEREOTAXY

Lesion surgery, despite the undoutable success, has fallen out of favor with the advent of deep brain stimulation in most medical centers. The most eminent problem lies in adapting the lesion size to the volume and shape of the target structure using thermocoagulation. Larger lesions are often more effective, but have a greater risk of extending into adjacent structures, thus causing permanent neurological deficits. Multiple small lesions may be better shaped to the target, but with smaller lesions symptoms may recur over time and repeated surgery may be required. On the other hand, deep brain stimulation may be associated with a considerable proportion of hardware-associated problems, such as device infection, lead fracture, IPG (internal pulse generator) failure, skin erosions, pain and repeated battery replacements, which according to series from experienced centers lies somewhere around 15–25% in the long term (Seijo et al., 2007; Hamani and Lozano, 2006; Blomstedt and Hariz, 2005; Lyons et al., 2004; Oh et al., 2002). Moreover, deep brain stimulation is not accessible in all countries, due to political sanctions or cost issues. Few studies have directly compared ablative stereotaxy and

neuromodulation; in a double-blind randomized study Schuurman et al. demonstrated, after two years of follow-up, that thalamotomy and thalamic stimulation were equally effective in suppressing parkinsonian and other tremors, but that functional outcome according to the Frenchay activity index was significantly better in the DBS group (Schuurman et al., 2000a; Schuurman, Bosch and Speelman, 2001). The authors related this difference to permanent mild neurological sequelae of thalamotomy, such as impairment of fine motor skills due to lesions encroaching upon the internal capsule. Another small study showed no difference between pallidotomy and pallidal stimulation for Parkinson's disease (Merello et al., 1999). In summary, the current evidence is too scarce to entirely abandon lesional surgery and research in this field should continue (Okun and Vitek, 2004). Ablative neurosurgery may return to the stage with advances in lesioning techniques, that could overcome the current limitations of radiofrequency lesioning, such as fiber-sparing neurotoxins or immunological methods to selectively inactivate certain cell types.

Thalamotomy

In the thalamus, the ventrointermediate nucleus (VIM) is the primary target for the relief of Parkinsonian tremor. VIM-thalamotomy is highly effective with a success rate of over 85%, defined as complete or nearly complete suppression of contralateral tremor. If the lesions are extended anteriorly to include the pallidal receiving areas of the thalamus, rigidity and levodopa-induced dyskinesias also improve, but akinesia remains unchanged. The most frequent adverse effects include dysarthria and worsening of gait and balance. Bilateral procedures are not recommended, due to the high incidence of severe speech problems and cognitive deficits.

Pallidotomy

Two prospective, single-blinded studies have compared pallidotomy to best medical treatment. Vitek and colleagues (Vitek et al., 2003) randomized a total of 36 patients to either immediate surgery or optimal drug therapy for a period of six months. With the total Unified Parkinson's Disease Rating Scale (UPDRS) score as the primary outcome, they demonstrated that pallidotomy induced a 32% improvement, compared to a 5% decline in the control group. Baseline to six-month differences were statistically significant for the surgery group (mean baseline: 80.4 vs. 54.9; $P < 0.0001$), but not for the group receiving medical management (mean baseline: 76.8 vs 76.6). Dyskinesias, measured objectively, and motor fluctuations, assessed by the UPDRS, significantly improved only in the surgery group. A total of 20 patients were followed for two years to assess the effect of time on clinical outcome. These patients had sustained improvement in the total UPDRS ($p < 0.0001$), "off" motor ($p < 0.0001$) and complications of therapy sub-scores ($p < 0.0001$).

A Dutch multi-center trial (De Bie et al., 1999) with 37 patients found a reduction of the UPDRS motor score by 31% in the surgical arm at six months, whereas the medical group worsened by 7.6%. On-phase dyskinesias improved 50% in pallidotomy patients, compared with no change in controls.

From these studies and an estimated several hundred cases of pallidotomies reported in open-label trials over the past two decades, the most reliable effect of the procedure is a marked reduction or complete suppression of contralateral levodopa-induced dyskinesias. The amount of improvement of contralateral motor symptoms differs between studies, but is around 30% in most of them. Benefits in ipsilateral and midline symptoms of parkinsonism are usually lost after the first years, but some studies have found persistent improvements in gait and balance beyond two years. Patients followed up to 10 years after pallidotomy had sustained improvements in contralateral dyskinesia and tremor. Pallidotomy, however, did not alter the natural course of Parkinson's disease, as indicated by a progression of akinesia, axial motor symptoms and cognitive decline causing additional disability (Baron et al., 2000; Fine et al., 2000; Hariz and Bergenheim, 2001; Pal et al., 2000).

The risks of unilateral pallidotomy have been analyzed in a systematic review by de Bie and colleagues (Cooper, 1954) including 12 prospective studies with 334 patients. Permanent adverse effects were reported in 13.8% of the patients. A symptomatic infarction or hemorrhage occurred in 3.9% of patients, and the associated mortality rate was 1.2%. The most frequent adverse effects were problems with speech (11.1%) and facial paresis (8.4%).

Unilateral pallidotomy was found to be safe in terms of cognitive adverse effects in several clinical studies (Alegret et al., 2003; Rettig et al., 2000), if the lesions were confined to the sensorimotor region of the internal globus pallidus (Lombardi et al., 2000). More anteriorly placed lesions were associated with declines in memory and frontal-executive functions (Lombardi et al., 2000). Simultaneous or staged bilateral pallidotomies were only exceptionally performed in the past, because historical series had suggested a marked risk of dysarthria and cognitive decline. Although contemporary pallidotomy targets the ventroposterolateral GP_i and tries to avoid the associative and limbic anteromedial parts of the nucleus, several reports still found a significant proportion of speech and long-term memory problems (De Bie et al., 2002a, 2002b; York et al., 2007).

After pallidotomy, patients do usually not improve beyond their best pre-operative on-state. Therefore, a presurgical levodopa challenge is useful in predicting the best possible therapeutic benefit for a given patient. Patients with little or no response to dopaminergic treatment should be excluded from surgery. Ideal candidates for pallidotomy, in summary, would have a preserved, good levodopa response, but motor fluctuations and severe asymmetrical dyskinesias (Van Horn et al., 2001). More problematic may be patients with bilateral dyskinesias or severe gait and balance disturbance, which may not be sufficiently treated with a unilateral procedure.

Subthalamotomy

Only few groups have explored ablative surgery of the subthalamic nucleus for Parkinson's disease as a less expensive alternative to deep brain stimulation. The procedure carries a risk of permanent hemiballism or hemichorea (Chen et al., 2002) depending on the size and location of the lesion (Tseng, Su and Liu, 2003). Patel and colleagues argued that lesions extending dorsally to the STN into pallidofugal fiber tracts could combine a subthalamotomy and "pallidotomy" effect, thereby avoiding unmanageable dyskinesias (Patel et al., 2003).

Three open-label studies have shown a 15–50% reduction of the UPDRS motor score at 1–2 years follow-up after unilateral subthalamotomy (Alvarez et al., 2001; Patel et al., 2003; Su et al., 2003). The levodopa requirement was reduced by about half. Gait and postural stability improved up to one year after surgery, but showed a gradual decline thereafter (Su et al., 2003) treated by contralateral subthalamic deep brain stimulation in some patients (Patel et al., 2003). With bilateral subthalamotomy Alvarez and colleagues reported marked improvements in motor symptoms, on average 50% score reduction in the UPDRS after two years, including sustained benefits in axial symptoms. Interestingly, dyskinesia scores were reduced by about half after an average 50% reduction of the total daily levodopa dosage. Side effects of the procedure were transient chorea in 73% of the patients and severe dysarthria in 17%. No deterioration in cognitive functions was observed. The authors concluded that bilateral subthalamatomy could be an effective and relatively safe alternative to subthalamic deep brain stimulation, if the surgical procedure could be refined to assure precise lesioning of the dorsolateral STN. However, with the widespread use of deep brain stimulation, it seems unlikely that larger controlled studies on subthalamotomy will be available in the near future.

DEEP BRAIN STIMULATION

Deep brain stimulation (DBS) as an alternative to ablative stereotaxy, derived from the clinical observation during intraoperative neurophysiological testing, that high-frequency electrical stimulation of the target areas could mimic the effect of the subsequent lesion without the need for destroying brain tissue. DBS is accomplished by implanting an electrode with four contacts into the target area within the brain, and connecting it to an internal pulse generator, usually located in the chest region. The stimulator settings can be adjusted telemetrically with respect to electrode configuration, current amplitude, pulse width and pulse frequency. DBS has rapidly replaced ablative stereotactic surgery in movement disorders because of several advantages: (i) DBS does not require making a destructive lesion in the brain, (ii) it can be performed bilaterally with relative safety, in contrast to most lesioning procedures, (iii) stimulation parameters can be adjusted post-operatively to improve efficacy, to reduce adverse effects and to adapt DBS to the course of disease, and (iv) DBS is, in principle, reversible and does not preclude the use of possible future therapies in Parkinson's disease requiring integrity of the basal ganglia circuitry.

Physiological Mechanisms

DBS mimics the clinical effects of lesioning in all three target structures (ventrolateral thalamus, internal pallidum and subthalamic nucleus), when "high-frequency" (>100 Hz) stimulation is applied. Stimulation at lower frequencies has no beneficial effects or may even aggravate symptoms (Moro et al., 2002). The exact cellular mechanisms by which high-frequency DBS exerts a "lesioning-like" effect is still unknown, although several hypotheses have been postulated. In particular, it is strongly debated whether DBS effects result from "inhibition" or rather "excitation" of neural elements. Electrical stimulation of nervous tissue, in general, is more likely to activate large myelinated fibers before small axons or cell bodies, axons near the cathode before those near the anode and axons oriented parallel to the electrode before axons oriented transversely (Ranck, 1975). Chronaxy studies in DBS-treated patients also suggest that stimulation effects predominantly derive from excitation of myelinated fiber tracts (Holsheimer et al., 2000a; Holsheimer et al., 2000b). Given the short refractory period of myelinated axons, around 1–2 ms, a depolarization block at the cellular membrane is unlikely to occur at a stimulation rate around 100 Hz. Recent physiological experiments in animals, and intraoperatively in humans, instead propose the following possible mechanisms: (i) non-synaptic blocking of neuronal transmission through inactivation of voltage-dependant ion channels (Beurrier et al., 2001), (ii) antidromic excitation of inhibitory afferents to the target nucleus and local release of GABA (Dostrovsky et al., 2000), (iii) driving of efferents and masking (or jamming) of encoded information by superposition of an unphysiological, high-frequency pattern (Hashimoto et al., 2003), (iv) activation of local inhibitory circuits within the target structure (Strafella et al., 1997).

It is likely that some of the effects occur in combination, such as the blocking of intrinsic somatodendritic spike activity and excitation of the outgoing axon within the same neuron (Garcia et al., 2003). Which of these mechanisms is primarily responsible for the clinical benefit of DBS is unknown and may depend on the anatomy of the target structure (e.g., the thalamic target contains a local inhibitory circuitry of interneurons and projections from reticular thalamic nuclei, which does not exist in the pallidal and subthalamic target) and the exact location of the stimulating electrode. First clinical evidence in line with a predominantly axonal action of high-frequency stimulation, suggests that the optimal target point for DBS may not be within the target nuclei themselves, but rather at entry or exit sites of fiber tracts or adjacent crossings of large fiber bundles (Voges et al., 2002; Hamel et al., 2003; Herzog et al., 2007). These preliminary results, however, await further confirmation in larger series. For this reason, the exact documentation of the final electrode location post-operatively and the corresponding clinical effects does not only serve for internal quality control but is also essential to create a sufficiently large database to address the important controversy about DBS mechanisms and optimal target sites.

Thalamic Deep Brain Stimulation

Experience with DBS in the thalamus for the treatment of Parkinsonian tremor has been generally safe and effective. Clinical success is usually defined as a complete abolition or a reduction of contralateral tremor to grade 1 (mild and intermittent) on the tremor rating scale (Fahn, Tolosa and Marin, 1988) with chronic stimulation. The success rates of DBS in the following paragraph relate to this definition. For tremor in Parkinson's disease, Benabid et al. reported a success rate of 88% in 26 patients and very low morbidity, even after bilateral surgery (Benabid et al., 1991). These findings were confirmed in a European multi-center study with 74 patients and a follow-up of one year (Limousin et al., 1999). In another controlled, randomized trial, PD patients showed an 82% reduction ($p < 0.0001$) in contralateral tremor compared to baseline, and significant improvement in disability and global impressions. There was, however, no meaningful improvement in other motor aspects of the disease, and the total UPDRS part II (activities of daily living) score did not change (Ondo et al., 1998). Slightly less favorable results were reported in the first American multi-center trial of thalamic deep brain stimulation with "only" 58.3% of patients experiencing marked improvement.

Two long-term studies of up to six years have demonstrated persistent tremor reduction within this period (Hariz et al., 2008; Rehncrona et al., 2003). Axial motor sypmtoms (speech, gait and postural instability), however, worsened, and, in parallel, the initial improvement in activities of daily living scores at one year follow up had disappeared at six years, despite the sustained improvement of tremor.

Adverse events of thalamic deep brain stimulation are generally mild and can normally be eliminated by adjustment of the stimulation parameters. Transient tingling sensations when switching on the device, mild dysarthria or mild gait ataxia are the most common problems requiring changes in parameter settings.

Pallidal Deep Brain Stimulation

The majority of reports on pallidal deep brain stimulation refer to open-label observational studies (see Figure 7.2). The most consistent effect of pallidal stimulation in these studies is a marked and long-lasting reduction of contralateral levodopa-induced dyskinesias (Barcia-Salorio et al., 1999; Burchiel et al., 1999; Durif et al., 1999; Ghika et al., 1998; Gross et al., 1997; Krack et al., 1998b; Kumar et al., 1998; Lang and Group, 1998; Merello et al., 1999; Pahwa et al., 1997; Siegfried and Lippitz, 1994a; Tronnier et al., 1997; Volkmann et al., 1998; Volkmann et al., 2001; Volkmann et al., 2004; Anderson et al., 2005; Minguez-Castellanos et al., 2005). Improvement of "off-period" symptoms of parkinsonism is more variable, but significant in most studies and in the range of 20–30% for unilateral and 30–50% for bilateral stimulation. Patient diaries demonstrated a marked increase in "on-time without dyskinesias" with pallidal stimulation (Obeso et al., 2001).

In our own experience, bilateral GPi-stimulation ($n = 11$) led to a $54 \pm 33.1\%$ improvement of the "off"-period UPDRS motor score at one year follow up (Volkmann et al., 1998; Volkmann et al., 2001). In UPDRS sub-scores, we found significant improvements for bradykinesia, tremor and posture and gait, and a tendency towards improvement of rigidity. "On"-period motor symptoms did not significantly change after surgery, except for dyskinesias, which were reduced by 83% at one year follow-up.

Interestingly, one group reported a reduction of dyskinesias, but a worsening of motor function during the medication "on"-period (Tronnier et al., 1997) after bilateral pallidal stimulation, in contrast to all other available studies. Because the exact position of the stimulating electrodes is uncertain in this and most other studies, it is difficult to discern how far the variable effect of pallidal stimulation results from different target locations within GPi. Two studies (Bejjani et al., 1997; Krack et al., 1998a) claim, based on the observation of acute stimulation effects, that DBS of the ventral GPi may block dyskinesias, but aggravate akinesia, whereas dorsal GPi stimulation ameliorates akinesia on the account of being pro-dyskinetic.

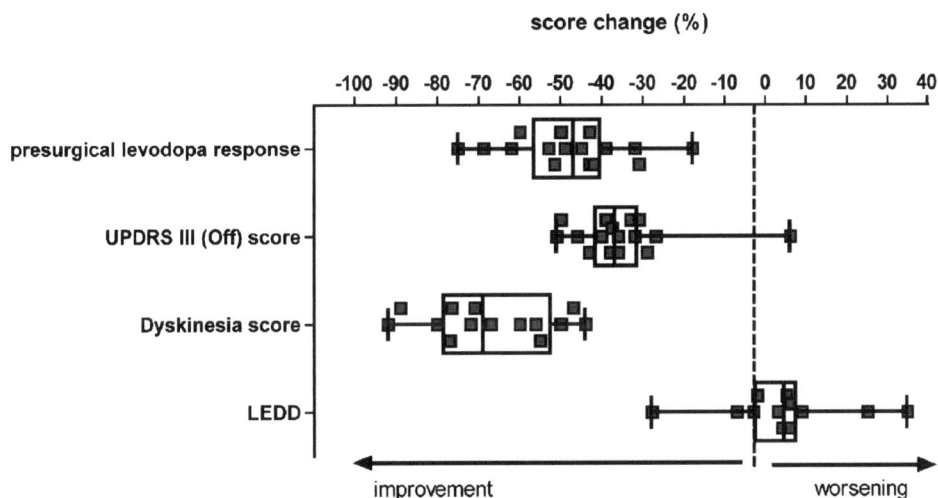

Figure 7.2 Summary of 16 publications on pallidal deep stimulation published between 1997 and 2005 including a total of 286 patients (54 unilateral treatments). For each study the average change in off-period motor symptoms by levodopa before surgery (levodopa response in %), by DBS at the final visit (UPDRS III Off score), the reduction of dyskinesias and the change in the LEDD (levodopa equivalent daily dose) compared to baseline are denoted by a symbol. The boxes represent the 25th–75th quartiles of the distribution of all studies with a line at the median. The whiskers represent the range. (Anderson et al., 2005; Burchiel et al., 1999; Durif et al., 2002; Ghika et al., 1998; Krack et al., 1998b; Kumar et al., 1998; Loher et al., 2002; Merello et al., 1999; Ogura et al., 2004; Pahwa et al., 1997; Peppe et al., 2004; The Deep-Brain Stimulation for Parkinson's Disease Study Group, 2001; Tronnier et al., 1997; Volkmann et al., 2001; Minguez-Castellanos et al., 2005).

The importance of these experimental observations for therapeutic long-term stimulation can only be determined in future studies carefully relating the efficacy of chronic pallidal stimulation to the exact target location within the GPi, determined by neuroimaging techniques and micro-electrode recordings.

Long-term assessments after pallidal deep brain stimulation are rare. Rodriguez and colleagues (Rodriguez-Oroz et al., 2005) reported on 20 patients from a multi-center study with 3–4 year follow-up after bilateral DBS of the GPi. They found a significant reduction of the off-period motor score, by 39% compared to baseline, and persistent benefits in dyskinesias, motor fluctuations and activites of daily living, Ghika et al. (Ghika et al., 1998) described persistent improvement in motor scores and activities of daily living two years after pallidal DBS, but noticed some decline in efficacy starting after 12 months in their patients. During the long-term follow-up (between two and four years), we also noted some decline in efficacy after 1–2 years of pallidal stimulation in three of our patients. In these patients, motor fluctuations returned and did not respond satisfactorily to changes in stimulation parameters or medication. Similar observations of secondary therapeutic failure after pallidal stimulation have been reported in small numbers of patients by other groups (Barcia-Salorio et al., 1999; Houeto et al., 2000a). Like in the two cases reported by Houeto et al. (Houeto et al., 2000a), we succesfully re-implanted our patients in the subthalamic nucleus. They had a similar benefit in terms of motor improvement and medication reduction as those patients primarily implanted within STN (Volkmann et al., 2004). These anecdotal reports underline the reversability of pallidal stimulation and suggest that the subthalamic target might be preferable to the pallidal target. They also emphasize that comparative trials of deep brain stimulation need a sufficiently long follow-up period to detect possible long-term differences.

Pallidal stimulation is adaptable and stimulation parameters can be set to achieve the optimal clinical efficacy in a given patient without inducing permanent stimulation-induced side effects. Therefore, visual field disturbances, facial weakness or dysarthria, which are characteristic side effects of pallidotomy, are rarely encountered after pallidal stimulation, unless deliberately accepted by the patient and physician on account of greater improvement in parkinsonian symptoms. Global scores of cognitive functions exhibit little changes after uni- or bilateral pallidal stimulation (Vingerhoets et al., 1999; Troster et al., 1997; Volkmann et al., 1998; Ghika et al., 1998). Subtle worsening of frontal scores, including verbal fluency, however, has been described by several authors (Vingerhoets et al., 1999; Troster et al., 1997; Volkmann et al., 1998). While most patients and relatives are unaware of these changes in daily life, behavioral alteration of a frontal nature has been reported in single cases after bilateral pallidal stimulation (Dujardin

et al., 2000; Volkmann et al., 1998). Old age and high pre-operative doses of levodopa were found to be predictive factors of post-operative cognitive worsening, in one study (Vingerhoets et al., 1999).

Subthalamic Deep Brain Stimulation

Deep brain stimulation of the subthalamic nucleus (STN-DBS) is the best established surgical treatment for Parkinson's disease. As of 2007 more than 25 000 patients were treated by subthalamic nucleus stimulation, world-wide. A recent systematic review of STN-DBS, commissioned by the Movement Disorder Society, identified a total of 34 articles using Medline and Ovid databases from 1993 until 2004, which reported on the outcome from 37 cohorts comprising of 921 patients (Kleiner-Fisman et al., 2006). STN-DBS significantly improved off-period motor symptoms and actvities of daily living, as indicated by an average reduction of the UPDRS II (activities of daily living) and III (motor) scores by 50 and 52%, respectively. The levodopa equivalent daily dosage of dopaminergic drugs could be reduced following surgery, by 55.9%. Dyskinesia scores decreased after surgery, on average by 69.1%, and the duration of daily off-periods by 68.2%. These outcome parameters underline the dramatic change in clinical status that well-selected patients can experience after successful STN-DBS. Patients with more severe off-period motor symptoms at baseline and a better responsiveness to levodopa, had the greatest benefit from STN-DBS, according to this review. The most common serious adverse event related to surgery was intracranial hemorrhage in 3.9% of patients. Psychiatric sequelae were common. The authors conclude, that the current literature suggests a consistent beneficial effect of STN-DBS on motor symptoms and activities of daily living (refer to Figure 7.3). The safety assessment, however, is limited by the small sample sizes and the uncontrolled nature of the open-label studies.

The open-label follow up of two large cohorts suggests that post-operative improvements in motor disability are sustained for up to five years after STN-DBS (Schupbach et al., 2005; Krack et al., 2003). Parkinson's disease, however, progresses, as reflected by a slight, but significant, worsening of the "on"-period motor score, in particular of axial symptoms, including dysarthria, gait freezing or postural imbalance. Cognitive decline, apathy and frontal dys-executive symptoms pose additional problems in the long-term management of DBS-treated patients (Rodriguez-Oroz et al., 2005; Lagrange et al., 2002). An important shortcoming of current long-term studies of STN-DBS is the lack of a medically treated control group. Without this control group one cannot discern whether STN-DBS has any positive or negative influence on the natural course of drug-treated PD. The neuropsychiatric problems reported after STN-DBS, for example, could be related to normal or accelerated

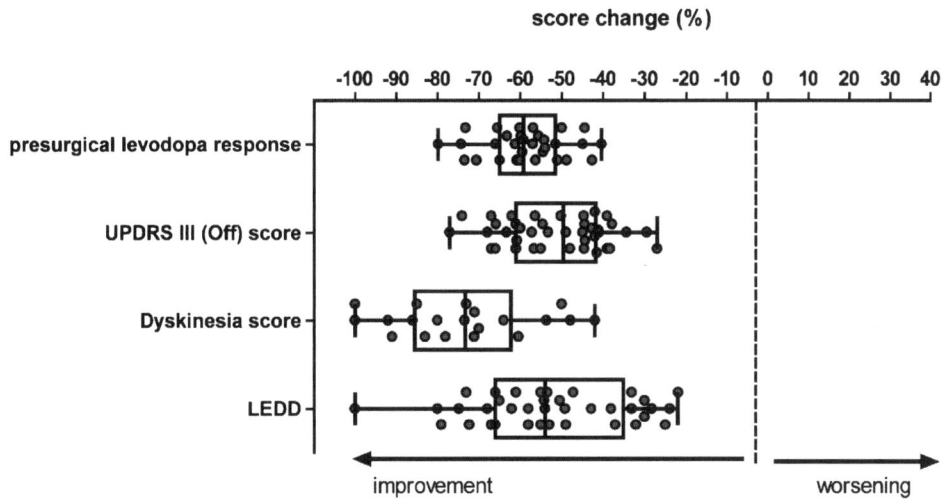

Figure 7.3 Summary of 40 publications on deep stimulation of the subthalamic nucleus published between 1999 and 2006 including a total of 1207 patients. For each study the average change in off-period motor symptoms by levodopa before surgery (levodopa response in %), by DBS at the final visit (UPDRS III Off score), the reduction of dyskinesias and the change in the LEDD (levodopa equivalent daily dose) are denoted by a symbol. The boxes represent the 25th–75th quartiles of the distribution of all studies with a line at the median. The whiskers represent the range. (Houeto *et al.*, 2000b; Molinuevo *et al.*, 2000; Pinter *et al.*, 1999; Broggi *et al.*, 2001; Rodriguez *et al.*, 1998; The Deep-Brain Stimulation for Parkinson's Disease Study Group, 2001; Katayama *et al.*, 2001; Krause *et al.*, 2001; Lopiano *et al.*, 2001; Martinez-Martin *et al.*, 2002; Ostergaard, Sunde and Dupont, 2002; Romito *et al.*, 2002b; Volkmann *et al.*, 2001; Lanotte *et al.*, 2002; Iansek, Rosenfeld and Huxham, 2002; Figueiras-Mendez *et al.*, 2002; Tavella *et al.*, 2002; Simuni *et al.*, 2002; Herzog *et al.*, 2003b; Thobois *et al.*, 2002; Valldeoriola *et al.*, 2002; Vesper *et al.*, 2002; Vingerhoets *et al.*, 2002; Doshi, Chhaya and Bhatt, 2002; Kleiner-Fisman *et al.*, 2002; Krack *et al.*, 2003; Lyons and Pahwa, 2005a; Landi *et al.*, 2003; Tamma *et al.*, 2003; Esselink *et al.*, 2004; Capecci *et al.*, 2005; Ford *et al.*, 2004; Jaggi *et al.*, 2004; Peppe *et al.*, 2004; Lyons and Pahwa, 2005b; Visser-Vandewalle *et al.*, 2005; Minguez-Castellanos *et al.*, 2005; Deuschl *et al.*, 2006; Varma *et al.*, 2003).

disease progression, post-operative medication changes, long-term stimulation effects or a combination of all.

STN-DBS is a non-curative therapy for Parkinson's disease, which will only be acceptable to patients if the burden of disease is more effectively reduced than optimal drug therapy. This fundamental question was addressed by a recent randomized, controlled multi-center study comparing neurostimulation to best medical management over a six-month period (Deuschl *et al.*, 2006). The study included 156 patients with severe motor symptoms of Parkinson's disease, who were randomly assigned in pairs to receive either bilateral DBS of the subthalamic nucleus in combination with medical treatment, or best medical therapy alone. The primary outcome of the trial was the change in health-related quality of life (PDQ-39 score) after six months. The Parkinson's Disease Questionnaire-39 summary index was 41.8 ± 13.9 out of 100 at baseline and 31.8 ± 16.3 at six months in the neurostimulation group, compared with 39.6 ± 16.0 and 40.2 ± 14.5 in the medication group. This corresponded to an improvement of about 25% in the neurostimulation group vs practically no change in the medication group. While serious adverse events were

more common with neurostimulation than with medication alone, and included a fatal intracerebral hematoma, and a suicide, the total number of adverse events was higher among medication-only patients. One patient in the medication-only group died from a car accident during a psychotic episode.

This study has set a new standard for surgical trials in movement disorders for several reasons: first, it has provided a realistic risk assessment of DBS in patients with advanced Parkinson's disease, whose natural course is already associated with major risks of disease or treatment-related complications, as evident in the medical control group. Second, it has proved the symptomatic benefits of DBS to outlast any adverse effects of the surgery on disability and quality of life. Previous open-label studies had raised concerns about the safety of STN-DBS on cognition (Saint-Cyr *et al.*, 2000b; Ardouin *et al.*, 1999b), mood (Berney *et al.*, 2002) or behaviour (Houeto *et al.*, 2002). Depression is known to have a higher impact on quality of life than motor symptoms in Parkinson's disease (Committee, 2002), such that neuropsychiatric adverse effects of neurostimulation could cancel out the motor benefits. This study (Deuschl *et al.*, 2006), however, found no evidence for an increased risk of cognitive or neuropsychiatric complications in the neurostimulation group, but confirmed a 25% improvement of quality of life with STN-DBS, which was within the range of the improvements previously found in uncontrolled case series (Drapier *et al.*, 2005; Erola *et al.*, 2005; Lezcano *et al.*, 2004; Lyons and Pahwa, 2005b; Martinez-Martin *et al.*, 2002; Ostergaard, Sunde and Dupont, 2002; Spottke *et al.*, 2002; Lagrange *et al.*, 2002).

A shortcoming of the study by Deuschl and colleagues (Deuschl *et al.*, 2006) is the limited follow-up period of only six months. As outlined before, some DBS effects may only become apparent in the long-term. The results of other ongoing trials with a longer parallel group comparison such as the UK PD SURG trial (http://www.pdsurg.bham.ac.uk) or the US Veterans Administration trial CSP#468 (CSP #468 Study Group Study Group #76 Study Group, 2006 #76) are awaited and may help to further clarify the role of STN-DBS in the treatment algorithm of PD.

Alternative Targets for Deep Brain Stimulation

A recent report suggested that the rostral zone of the zona incerta may be a better target for the cardinal motor symptoms of PD than the STN (Plaha *et al.*, 2006). The subthalamic area dorsomedial to the STN contains pallidofugal fiber tracts and the zona incerta, whose function within the basal ganglia-thalamocortical circuitry is still undetermined. The observation by Plaha and colleagues (Plaha *et al.*, 2006) underlines the necessity for a better delineation of the optimal "STN" target. Because the authors did not use intraoperative neurophysiology to confirm their anatomical targeting, one cannot decide whether the superior results of the "zona incerta" target in their series related to a sub-optimal placement of the STN electrodes. Due to the intraindividual variablity in the severity of motor symptoms and their responsiveness to levodopa, comparative trials of targets should rather use a relative score (e.g., percentage of the pre-operative levodopa response achieved by stimulation alone after surgery) than comparing average stimulation responses of two or more groups. Stimulation of optimally placed STN-electrodes is able to mimic the pre-operative levodopa response. Using this approach, in combination with intraoperative neurophysiology, (Herzog *et al.*, 2004) demonstrated earlier that stimulation of fiber tracts within the subthalamic area was clinically inferior to stimulation of the dorsal STN border or the STN proper.

More recently, a number of reports suggest an important role for the upper brainstem, and in particular, the pedunculopontine nucleus (PPN), in the genesis of PD motor symptoms, like akinesia, gait dysfunction and postural instability (Nandi *et al.*, 2002a; Munro-Davies *et al.*,

1999). The PPN is part of the mesencephalic locomotor reticular region (Jordan, 1998) and maintains dense interconnections with the basal ganglia and several other pontine and medullar areas (Delwaide, 2001; Pahapill and Lozano, 2000). Local injections of the GABA-antagonist bicuculine (Nandi *et al.*, 2002a) or low-frequency stimulation of the PPN (Jenkinson *et al.*, 2004; Jenkinson *et al.*, 2006) improved motor symptoms in the MPTP-primate model of parkinsonism. The feasibility of electrode implantations into the human PPN has been demonstrated in two recent case reports (Mazzone *et al.*, 2005; Plaha and Gill, 2005). The target is located lateral to the decussation of the superior cerebellar peduncle at the level of the inferior colliculus (Plaha and Gill, 2005). Low-frequency stimulation of the PPN resulted in up to 57% reduction of PD motor symptoms (Plaha and Gill, 2005). However, the first blinded comparison of STN and PPN stimulation in six patients with electrode implantations into both targets provided a less enthusiastic view (Stefani *et al.*, 2007): PPN stimulation alone was significantly inferior to STN-DBS (32% vs 54% motor score improvement). Combined stimulation of PPN and STN did not improve the overall motor score, but led to a significant additive effect on gait and balance symptoms and further improvement in the activities of daily living. A longer follow-up and larger sample size will be necessary to prove whether combined STN-PPN-DBS may overcome some of the limitations of STN-DBS alone, in particular the progression of levodopa-resistant axial symptoms.

Safety

Adverse events associated with DBS must be divided into those related to the surgical procedure, to the implanted device, to stimulation and to medication changes necessitated by DBS. Moreover, disappointed expectations, but also dramatic improvements of the motor handicap in patients that have been disabled for many years, may cause psychological difficulties in adapting to the new role after surgery. Social maladjustment may contribute to dissatisfaction or even psychiatric abnormalities after DBS.

Surgery- and Device-Related Adverse Effects

DBS requires a craniotomy and one or several needle passes through the brain carrying with it the risks of intracranial hemorrhage and damage to adjacent brain structures. The risk of unintended injury to adjacent brain structures, however, is much smaller than in ablative procedures, where the exact size of the final therapeutic lesion may be difficult to predict. A recent survey by Voges and others (Voges *et al.*, 2007) on the 30-day complication rate in 1183 patients operated on for various indications at five German DBS centers, provides a good estimation of the surgical risk of DBS in a sufficiently large patient group. According to this study, intracranial hemorrhages (2.2%) and pneumonia (0.6%) were the most common serious adverse effects of DBS surgery. The mortality rate was 0.4% and the permanent morbidity rate 1%. Skin infection occurred in 5 out of 1183 patients (0.4%). Older patients and patients with Parkinson's disease carried a slightly greater surgical risk.

The reported rate of hardware-related problems (e.g., lead dislocation, lead breakage, pulse generator dysfunction, skin erosion) varies greatly between different centers. Total rates between 3 and 50% (including scheduled pulse generator replacements) have been described in single center series with different follow-up periods. (Seijo et al., 2007; Hamani and Lozano, 2006; Blomstedt and Hariz, 2005; Lyons et al., 2004; Oh et al., 2002). The average lies somewhere in the range of 20–25%. Most hardware-related problems, however, occurred with the first patients of a series and were less frequent afterwards. This "learning curve"—even in experienced stereotactic centers—sheds light on the sophisticated nature of the procedure, which requires extensive neurosurgical skill before getting into a routine with DBS surgery.

The sudden failure of a DBS system is a medical emergency, because Parkinsonian symptoms return within minutes or hours and my lead to an akinetic crisis (Hariz and Johansson, 2001). Patients should be instructed to seek immediate medical attention if a sudden return of parkinsonian symptoms is experienced, and to take an emergency dose of levodopa to prevent a severe off-state. Electromagnetic interference (e.g., by household appliances, loadspeakers, etc.) was the most common cause of a sudden DBS failure before introduction of a new dual channel pulse generator (Kinetra, Medtronic Minneapolis, USA) that can be programmed to be insensitive to external magnetic sources. Recently, however, manufacturing problems caused sudden battery failures in several devices of certain production lots (Alesch, 2005). DBS is a complex therapy and despite continuous improvements in technology, hardware-associated problems must not be underestimated.

One must emphasize that the low morbidity and high efficacy of DBS reported here, was observed by multidisciplinary teams with extensive experience in movement disorder surgery. The increasing number of centers now offering DBS—sometimes with little previous experience in sterotactic and functional surgery and/or the neurological management of patients with advanced Parkinson's disease—increases the risk of poor outcomes and apparent DBS failures (Okun et al., 2005). Expert centers may be able to correct some of these treatment failures (Moro et al., 2006; Okun et al., 2005) by adjustments in medication, or programming or lead repositioning, but poor outcomes after surgery impose an unnecessary burden on patients

and threaten the general acceptance of DBS by the neurological community and patient advocacy groups.

Therapy-Related Adverse Effects

Stimulation induced adverse effects result from current leaking outside of the target structure into adjacent fiber tracts or nuclei. Optimal positioning of the stimulating electrode is therefore paramount for a large therapeutic window between beneficial effects of DBS and adverse effects caused by unintended co-stimulation of surrounding structures. Stimulation-induced adverse effects are easily recognized, because they are fully reversible when stimulation is stopped, and can be improved, in most cases, by changing stimulation parameters or electrode configuration. In some patients, in whom the suppression of motor symptoms is not achieved without side effects, patient and physician may deliberately accept a certain degree of stimulation-induced adverse effects.

In thalamic DBS, paraesthesias and dysarthria are among the most common stimulation-induced side effects. Especially with bilateral DBS, some dysarthria will have to be accepted in about 10% of cases, if optimal tremor control is desired. Less frequent are real dystonia or "pseudodystonia" resulting from co-stimulation of the pyramidal tract.

Stimulation-induced side effects in pallidal DBS are rare and mostly transient during the immediate post-operative adjustment of stimulation parameters. They include visual field disturbances from current spread to the optic tract, tetanic muscle contractions (pseudodystonia) from co-stimulation of the pyramidal tract and nausea or dizziness.

Possible therapeutic problems with deep brain stimulation of the subthalamic nucleus result from the complex interactions of drug therapy and electrical stimulation. Dopaminergic medication and STN-DBS act synergistically. In the immediate post-operative period, stimulation-induced dyskinesias are one of the most frequent and important specific side effects of STN stimulation. The appearance of dyskinesias indicates correct lead placement, but the necessity to downtitrate dopaminergic medication. To avoid severe dyskinetic states, initial programming should always be done early in the morning when the patient is in the medication off-state. Stimulation should be carefully increased over a period of days or weeks until a satisfactory effect on bradykinesia in the off-phase is achieved, and, at the same time, the levodopa dosage is downtitrated. The necessary withdrawal of levodopa, however, may be associated with adverse reactions, such as apathy, depression, hypophonia, postural imbalance or gait freezing, if the drugs are lowered too rapidly or extensively. The challenge of the post-operative neurological management in STN-DBS is to find the right balance between stimulation and medication and to distinguish clinically between "genuine" stimulation-induced side effects and pre-existing symptoms of the disease that are uncovered by a combination of reduced dopaminergic therapy and inadequate stimulation effects.

Either current diffusion due to excessive stimulation parameters, or incorrect lead placement may result in reversible stimulation-induced side effects, such as tonic muscle contractions, dysarthria, eyelid opening apraxia, ocular deviation, ipsilateral mydriasis, flushing, unilateral (ipsilateral) perspiration, (contralateral) paresthesias, worsening of akinesia and a reversal of the levodopa effect. These reversible side effects may help to define the optimal target intraoperatively or to track the deviation of a misplaced electrode after surgery (Volkmann, Fogel and Krack, 2000).

Effects On Cognition, Mood and Behavior

Despite the theoretical concern that pallidal or subthalamic nucleus stimulation could interfere with the functioning of cognitive basal ganglia loops, most studies found no, or clinically insignificant, changes in neuropsychological functioning after DBS (Ardouin *et al.*, 1999a; Jahanshahi *et al.*, 2000; Trepanier *et al.*, 2000; Alegret *et al.*, 2001; Pillon *et al.*, 2000). Some reports, however, have warned that STN-DBS has a risk of inducing cognitive decline with a frontal executive dysfunction similar to progressive supranuclear palsy in older patients (above 70 years) or those with minimal cognitive dysfunction prior to surgery (Saint-Cyr *et al.*, 2000a; Dujardin *et al.*, 2001).

An increasing number of reports on psychiatric and behavioral adverse effects of STN-DBS has raised concerns about the safety of this therapy and deserve special attention. Mood disorders are among the most frequently observed post-operative side effects in STN stimulation (Volkmann *et al.*, 2001; Limousin *et al.*, 1998), but the true prevalence is still difficult to estimate due to small sample sizes, uncontrolled study designs and possible biases in reporting on adverse events. The incidence of depression in the first post-operative months has been up to 25% in some reports (Volkmann *et al.*, 2001; Berney *et al.*, 2002) and suicidal ideation or completed suicides were reported in some patients (Berney *et al.*, 2002; Doshi, Chhaya and Bhatt, 2002; Deuschl *et al.*, 2006). Manic disorders seem to be less frequent, in the range of 5–10% (Daniele *et al.*, 2003; Romito *et al.*, 2002a; Kulisevsky *et al.*, 2002; Herzog *et al.*, 2003a). It is important to note that in most patients, psychiatric disturbances are mild and transient and do not require hospitalization.

The high incidence of psychiatric problems after STN-DBS is most likely multi-factorial, but the relevance of the individual factors still needs to be determined:

(1) Parkinson's disease is a neuro*psychiatric* disease most frequently associated with depression and anxiety, but also with behavioral abnormalities, such as impulse control disorders after long-term medical treatment. Mood and behavioral abnormalities after surgery often reflect a reactivation of a pre-existing psychiatric condition, as shown by Houeto and colleagues (Houeto *et al.*, 2002), underlining the necessity of careful neuropsychiatric assessment during the patient selection process (Voon *et al.*, 2005).

(2) Levodopa has psychotropic effects, in addition to the well-known motor effects. Patients describe the action of levodopa as pleasantly euphoria- and drive-enhancing. In extreme cases, mania, levodopa dysregulation syndrome or impulse control disorders (e.g., hypersexuality, gambling) can present as affective and behavioral side effects of dopaminergic therapy. The medication reduction after STN stimulation may, therefore, cause withdrawal phenomena, with an impact on mood and drive.

(3) The basal ganglia are integrated into associative-cognitive and limbic regulatory systems, such that psychiatric symptoms could also result as a direct side effect of stimulation. The acute emotional effect of STN-DBS is mood enhancing (Funkiewiez *et al.*, 2003; Schneider *et al.*, 2003). High stimulation amplitudes may cause laughing spells (Krack *et al.*, 2001). Stimulation of the medioventral, limbic part of the STN has been shown to evoke hypomanic states (Mallet *et al.*, 2007). There is currently no evidence that depression could result from stimulation inside the STN. The two spectacular cases of stimulation-induced depression rather resulted from high-frequency stimulation of the substantia nigra pars reticulata ventral to the STN (Bejjani *et al.*, 1999; Blomstedt *et al.*, 2008). Chronic stimulation within STN proper led to the intended improvements in motor symptoms in these patients without persistent side effects.

(4) Successful surgery allows a return to increased independence, which can affect partnership, social bonds, and profession, and at the same time, cause a loss of primary and secondary gains from the illness (Perozzo *et al.*, 2001). The process of adaptation to the new role after surgery is poorly understood in movement disorders, but is known to cause most of the psychological and behavioral problems after epilepsy surgery (Wilson, Bladin and Saling, 2001), and has also been identified as a reason for patient dissatisfaction after PD surgery, despite a good motor outcome (Schupbach *et al.*, 2006).

TRANSPLANTATION AND OTHER RESTORATIVE SURGERIES

The attempt to replace lost dopaminergic neurons in Parkinson's disease by transplantation pioneered the clinical application of restorative therapies in neurodegenerative disorders. Early attempts at autologous grafting using adrenal medullary cell transplants soon turned out to be ineffective and risky (Goetz *et al.*, 1989; Olanow *et al.*, 1990). Transplantation of human fetal cells, however, achieved early success in several unblinded case series. These series provided the proof of principle, that transplanted cells could survive and function for many years in the striatum of PD patients (Hauser *et al.*, 1999; Kordower *et al.*, 1995; Lindvall *et al.*, 1994). On the basis of these encouraging observations, two double blind, sham-surgery controlled trials were launched, which turned out to be more disappointing than expected (Olanow *et al.*, 2003; Freed *et al.*, 2001). Neither study found a significant improvement in off-period motor symptoms in the transplanted group, although graft survival could be demonstrated in PET imaging. Minor benefits were observed in sub-groups of patients under the age of 60 (Freed *et al.*, 2001) or with less severe disease (Olanow *et al.*, 2003). But a significant proportion of patients (15% in the Freed and 56% in the Olanow trial) with some initial benefit from transplantation, developed dyskinesia in the medication off-state (runaway dyskinesia) which could not be managed by medication adjustments. Despite some criticism about the transplant methodology in the two trials (storage of donor tissue, tissue preparation, immunosuppression), their results have definitively set back the field to an experimental stage. Alternative cell sources are now being explored including the use of neural stem cells, which could also solve the ethical problems associated with fetal transplants.

In the meantime, two small pilot trials evaluated the feasibility of non-neuronal cell therapy in Parkinson's disease. Autotransplantation of dopaminergic carotid body cell aggregates into the striatum resulted in modest clinical benefit (23% motor score reduction at six months) in 13 patients with advanced Parkinson's disease (Minguez-Castellanos *et al.*, 2007). None of the patients developed off-period dyskinesias. Based on the favorable results of a pilot study (Stover *et al.*, 2005) a double-blind, sham-controlled multi-center trial is currently investigating the safety and efficacy of intraputaminal implantation of human retinal pigment epithelial (RPE) cells. RPE cells produce levodopa and can be isolated from post-mortem human eye tissue, grown in culture, and implanted into the brain, attached to microcarriers. In the open-label pilot study, six patients with advanced Parkinson's disease were followed after unilateral implantation and had an average improvement of 48% in the motor score after 12 months (Stover *et al.*, 2005). This benefit was sustained at 24 months. No neurological side effects were observed.

Other restorative approaches include the use of growth factors and gene therapy (Kaplitt *et al.*, 2007), which are also in an experimental stage. Despite very favorable reports on the beneficial effects of intraputaminal infusion of glial cell line-derived neurotrophic factor (GDNF) in open studies (Gill *et al.*, 2003; Patel *et al.*, 2005), a recent randomized, controlled clinical trial failed to prove superiority of GDNF over placebo infusion in 34 PD patients (Lang *et al.*, 2006). Serious, device-related adverse events required surgical repositioning of catheters in two patients and removal of devices in another. Neutralizing antibodies were detected in three patients. Despite some issues on differences in methodology raised by the proponents of GDNF infusions, this study again demonstrates the need for a placebo control in surgical trials of PD. The magnitude of the placebo effect with any invasive therapy of PD must not be underestimated and may influence subjective patient ratings, such as quality of life, but also single-blinded physician ratings of motor symptoms, as demonstrated in a remarkable secondary analysis of a sham-controlled transplantation trial (Mcrae *et al.*, 2004).

COMPARISON OF SURGICAL THERAPIES

Lesional Stereotaxy vs Deep Brain Stimulation

Few studies have compared surgical therapies for Parkinson's disease in a controlled fashion. Thalamic deep brain stimulation is equally effective in symptomatic tremor control as thalamotomy, but offers a lower risk of permanent neurological deficits and better functional outcome (Schuurman *et al.*, 2000b). The same group later conducted a trial of pallidotomy vs subthalamic nucleus deep brain stimulation for advanced Parkinson's disease. Thirty-four patients with advanced PD were randomly assigned to have either unilateral pallidotomy or bilateral STN stimulation. STN-DBS was found to be more effective, at six months and one year, in reducing off-period motor symptoms, dyskinesias and anti-parkinsonian drugs (Esselink *et al.*, 2004; Esselink *et al.*, 2006). Secondary analysis of neuropsychological tests, however, suggested, that bilateral STN-DBS had slightly more negative effects on executive functioning than unilateral pallidotomy (Smeding *et al.*, 2005). A direct comparison between pallidotomy and the equivalent pallidal deep brain stimulation has been conducted in a single pilot trial. In a group of 13 patients randomized to either unilateral pallidal DBS or radiofrequency lesioning of the GPi, Merello and colleagues (Merello *et al.*, 1999) found about equal improvement of the UPDRS motor score after three months follow-up. There was greater reduction of contralateral dyskinesias after pallidotomy, whereas bilateral hand tapping scores improved more with DBS.

Comparison of DBS Targets

After the initial reports on the beneficial effects of STN-DBS, many groups worldwide quickly embraced the subthalamic nucleus as the overall best target for treating Parkinson's disease. Implantations into the thalamus or pallidum for Parkinson's disease rapidly decreased in number and the scientific evaluation of the two alternative targets almost came to a halt. This development, however, was driven by bias, not by sound clinical evidence.

In a retrospective analysis of their own series, Krack and colleagues described excellent control of marked to severe parkinsonian tremor by subthalamic nucleus stimulation (Krack et al., 1998a). The additional advantages of an anti-akinetic effect and savings in dopaminergic drugs, soon led to the suggestion that subthalamic nucleus stimulation should be preferred over thalamic stimulation for the treatment of tremor-dominant Parkinson's disease, especially in younger patients, who are likely to develop akinetic-rigid symptoms and treatment-related motor complications with disease progression. This common clinical practice has never been evaluated in a controlled clinical trial. Thalamic DBS is a reliable monosymptomatic treatment for parkinsonian tremor, which is easy to program, provides rapid and long-lasting benefit and has few adverse effects. In contrast, the temporal evolution of anti-tremor effects in STN-DBS is less predictable (Volkmann, Fogel and Krack, 2000; Volkmann et al., 2002). Some patients have an immediate benefit, while in others tremor may gradually decline over months. Therefore, we still consider thalamic DBS an option in tremor-dominant PD, especially for older patients with little akinesia and slow disease progression over the past years.

The preference of the subthalamic target over the pallidal target derives from an early open-label study, which found a slightly better efficacy of STN-DBS in reducing off-period motor symptoms (Obeso et al., 2001; Rodriguez-Oroz et al., 2005), but was never designed to compare both therapies. One single-center study supported this conclusion: Krack and colleagues (Krack et al., 1998b) reported a 71% improvement of the "off"-period UPDRS motor score with STN-stimulation, but only 39% with GPi-stimulation, in a group of 13 patients with young-onset Parkinson's disease. This significant difference resulted primarily from a greater reduction of bradykinesia in the STN-stimulated group, whereas other parkinsonian symptoms showed about equal improvement. Other open-label comparisons found little or no difference in the clinical efficacy of pallidal and subthalamic DBS (Minguez-Castellanos et al., 2005; Volkmann et al., 2001). In our own retrospective analysis of the initial 11 patients implanted within GPi and 16 patients implanted within STN, the main finding was a $54 \pm 33.1\%$ improvement of "off"-period motor symptoms in the first and $67 \pm 22.6\%$ improvement in the later group after one year of follow-up (Volkmann et al., 2001). The 10–15% difference between both groups was not significant and power analysis suggested that, based on the group variances, a much larger trial, including a minimum of 135 patients in each arm, would have been needed to prove significance of this possible small

difference in favor of STN-stimulation. A well-designed, but small, randomized-prospective trial described equal improvements in off-period symptoms and dyskinesia (Burchiel et al., 1999; Anderson et al., 2005) after STN- vs GPi-DBS.

The only consistent differences between pallidal and subthalamic nucleus stimulation reported so far concern medication requirements (Minguez-Castellanos et al., 2005) and stimulation parameters. Patients with pallidal stimulation continue to require pre-operative anti-PD medication doses and in some cases even higher doses are introduced post-operatively, whereas STN-stimulation allows an average reduction of dopaminergic medication in the range of 65% and equivalent improvement of "off"-period motor symptoms (Volkmann et al., 2001). The energy required for effective pallidal stimulation is about two- to threefold higher than values previously reported for subthalamic or thalamic stimulation (Benabid et al., 1996; Moro et al., 1999; Volkmann et al., 2001), which most probably reflects the larger anatomical size of the GPi target.

Better-powered, randomized studies of pallidal and subthalamic DBS are currently underway in the United States. The comparison should not only focus on the efficacy in reducing off-period motor symptoms, but needs to take into account aspects of safety and global treatment effects, such as improvements in quality of life. Hopefully, these studies will answer whether sub-groups of patients may be better suited for one or the other therapy.

PATIENT SELECTION

Despite the heterogeneity of surgical therapies for advanced Parkinson's disease, patient selection criteria are relatively uniform. Better results are obtained in patients with idiopathic Parkinson's disease, an excellent levodopa response, younger age and normal cognitive status.

DBS has not been evaluated for other forms of parkinsonism than idiopathic Parkinson's disease. From experience with a few patients with progressive supranuclear palsy, multiple system atrophy or other atypical parkinsonian syndroms, who underwent DBS, one can conclude that the overall progression of these disorders rapidly counteracts a possible transient benefit from surgery. Up to 10% of the therapeutic failures after DBS may result from an inappropriate diagnosis of Parkinson's disease (Okun et al., 2005), which underlines the importance of involving movement disorder specialists in the selection process.

The benefit of subthalamic DBS can be closely predicted by the "best motor on-state" of a patient after taking a suprathreshold dose of levodopa (Welter et al., 2002). Therefore, most centers routinely apply a levodopa challenge during the pre-surgical evaluation of surgical candidates. Symptoms that are not helped by levodopa, such as speech or postural problems, do not improve with long-term stimulation. The one exception to the rule is parkinsonian tremor, which may be refractory to anti-parkinsonian medication, but responds nicely to DBS. Another important factor is the age at surgery (Russmann *et al.*, 2004; Charles *et al.*, 2002). Patients over age 70 carry an increased risk of surgical complications (Voges *et al.*, 2007) including irreversible cognitive decline after surgery (Saint-Cyr *et al.*, 2000b). Moreover, their "stimulation-on" state after surgery does not reach the "best-medical-on" state, in contrast to younger patients (Russmann *et al.*, 2004). Russmann and colleagues (Russmann *et al.*, 2004) found in a retrospective analysis of their own series, that, in particular, gait and balance problems progressed after STN-DBS in the older patient group and became the primary reason for institutional care in 25%.

Cognitive decline is closely linked to advanced neuropathological stages of Parkinson's disease (Braak *et al.*, 2006). Because surgery may aggravate frontal dysexecutive scores or even global cognitive function in patients with pre-existing cognitive deficits, careful neuropsychological testing is mandatory during pre-surgical evaluation. The evolution of dementia correlates clinically with the progression of levodopa-resistant axial motor symptoms of PD (Alves *et al.*, 2006; Burn *et al.*, 2003). Particular attention must therefore be given to patients with a history of frequent falls in the on-state or a poor pull-test response after the levodopa challenge.

Currently surgery is performed in very advanced stages of Parkinson's disease after an average of 14 years of disease duration, when the psychosocial burden of the disease has been marked for many years. The majority of patients has retired from professional life, is dependent on help in their activities of daily living and has experienced marked changes in social participation due to the disease. Despite excellent motor improvements, these patients may have difficulties in returning to a "normal" life after STN-DBS. Schupbach and colleagues analyzed the factors contributing to psychosocial distress after DBS surgery in a group of 29 patients (Schupbach *et al.*, 2006). These patients experienced marked improvements in parkinsonian motor symptoms, activities of daily living and quality of life and had no signs of psychiatric disease. However, social adjustment, as measured by the social adjustment scale, did not improve after STN-DBS. Three types of maladjustment were observed: 19/29 patients expressed a feeling of strangeness and unfamiliarity with themselves. They had difficulties adopting to the new role after surgery and defining new goals in life after overcoming the burden of Parkinson's disease. Marital conflicts occurred in 17/24 patients living in couples before surgery and led to divorce in three couples. Only 9/16 patients, who were working before surgery, resumed their professional activity after surgery. Five of these patients preferred to engage in leisure activities instead of working, while others felt unable to work despite excellent motor improvement. This study underlines that deep brain stimulation is a therapy with profound impact on a patient's life, comparable to epilepsy surgery or organ transplantation (Wilson, Bladin and Saling, 2001). Maladjustment had previously been observed after these life-changing medical procedures and multi-disciplinary programs have been developed to help patients coping with re-integration (Wilson, Bladin and Saling, 2001).

The goal of improving quality of life and reducing the psychosocial burden of Parkinson's disease may be better achieved in younger patients operated on at an earlier stage of disease, once symptoms can no longer be managed optimally by medication. This time point is known among movement disorder specialists as the end of the "drug honeymoon period" in Parkinson's disease, when the first motor complications start to emerge. In patients with young-onset PD, mild fluctuations or dyskinesia may start as early as 3–5 years after disease onset. A small pilot study by the Paris group recently evaluated the impact of DBS at such an early stage. Twenty patients with a short duration of PD (6.8 ± 1 year) were randomized to either immediate STN-DBS surgery or best medical treatment for a period of 18 months (Schupbach *et al.*, 2007). Quality of life was significantly improved, by 24%, in the surgical group, but did not change in non-surgical patients. After 18 months, the severity of parkinsonian motor signs "off" medication, levodopa-induced motor complications, and the daily levodopa dose were reduced by 69, 83, and 57% in operated patients and increased by 29, 15, and 12% in the group with medical treatment only. Adverse events were mild or transient, and overall psychiatric morbidity and anxiety improved in the surgical group. After these encouraging results a large binational multi-center trial (EARLYSTIM) was initiated in France and Germany in 2006 to further evaluate the concept of early subthalamic nucleus deep brain stimulation in suitable patients with Parkinson's disease.

In the past years we have witnessed a paradigmatic change in movement disorder surgery from a "last resort treatment" for the most incapacitating motor symptoms to a routine therapy targeting quality of life and functional independence. The different levels of functioning of a patient within the multi-dimensional physical-psychosocial framework of health-related quality of life are best evaluated in a multi-disciplinary team of neurologists, neurosurgeons, psychologists, psychiatrists, specialized nurses and social workers. The symptomatic assessment of motor and cognitive function during the pre-surgical assessment is supplemented in our clinical practice by a psychiatric assessment to identify co-morbidities and disease- or treatment-related psychiatric complications. Moreover, areas of risk for social malad-justment are explored in one or several psychological interviews with the patient and a caregiver during the pre-surgical evaluation. The exploration should cover professional and leisure activities, social support, marital satisfaction, coping, future goals and expectations from surgery. Unrealistic expectations need to be corrected before advising surgery, to prevent disappointment with the outcome. The multi-faceted views are combined with an individual risk–benefit analysis, which is discussed with the patient and balanced against alternative treatment options.

PRAGMATIC MANAGEMENT

Surgical therapy is an option for patients with idiopathic Parkinson's disease suffering from hypokinetic fluctuations, dyskinesias or tremors that are no longer satisfactorily treated by medication. Deep brain stimulation is the best-established surgical therapy and can be applied in three different brain targets with a differential effect on parkinsonian motor symptoms. Patient selection criteria and guidelines for choosing the optimal target are summarized below:

Patients selection criteria:

- History of Parkinson's disease for at least five years (to exclude non-idiopathic parkinsonism)
- Disabling hypokinetic fluctuations, dyskinesia or tremor despite optimized drug therapy
- Excellent levodopa-responsiveness of akinetic-rigid symptoms
- Hoehn and Yahr stage $\leq$ III during best medical "on"
- Normal age-related cognitive status
- No major depression, acute psychosis or other unstable psychiatric conditions
- No structural brain abnormalities increasing surgical risk (MRI)
- General health condition allowing prolonged brain surgery.

Guidelines for selecting the brain target of deep brain stimulation in Parkinson' disease:

Thalamic (Vim) Deep Brain Stimulation

- Only effective on tremor, no improvement of akinesia, motor fluctuations or dyskinesia
- Usually well tolerated, risk of dysarthria or balance problems with bilateral procedures
- Benefit on tremor immediately obtained
- Simple adjustment of stimulation and medication after surgery

- Potentially useful in older patients with tremor-dominant PD, mild bradykinesia and little risk of developing motor fluctuations

Deep Brain Stimulaiton of theinternal globus pallidus(GPi)

- Effective on all cardinal symptoms of PD
- Effective in reducing hypokinetic fluctuations and dyskinesia
- Few therapy-related adverse effects
- Benefit on dyskinesia immediately obtained
- Simple adjustment of stimulation after surgery
- No savings in anti-parkinsonian medication
- Higher energy consumption

Deep Brain Stimulation of the subthalamic nucleus(STN)

- Effective on all cardinal symptoms of PD
- Effective in reducing hypokinetic fluctuations and dyskinesia
- Effective in improving health-related quality of life
- Risk of dysarthria
- Adjustment of stimulation and medication more complex and time consuming
- Significant savings in anti-parkinsonian medication
- Risk of (transient) psychiatric or behavioral adverse effects during the adjustment period
- Low energy consumption

CONCLUSION

Surgical therapies in Parkinson's disease have evolved from an empirical stage to treatment options with a sound scientific basis. Neurorestorative procedures are still in an experimental stage, but bear great potential for the future. In the meantime, deep brain stimulation will be the mainstay of surgery for Parkinson's disease. Sufficient evidence has accumulated to consider DBS of the subthalamic nucleus an effective and relatively safe therapy for all cardinal symptoms of Parkinson's disease and levodopa-induced motor complications. The improvements in motor symptoms are so profound, that quality of life is significantly improved by STN-DBS in well-selected patients. Research is ongoing and includes the exploration of alternative targets, improved definitions of candidacy and refinements in DBS technology with new electrode designs or improved stimulation protocols. The future looks bright, but the progress in surgical therapy will be critically dependent on support for this field, which has traditionally received far less attention than drug research.

References

Albin, R.L., Young, A.B. and Penney, J.B. (1995) The functional anatomy of disorders of the basal ganglia. _Trends in Neurosciences_, **18**, 63–64.

Alegret, M., Junque, C., Valldeoriola, F. *et al.* (2001) Effects of bilateral subthalamic stimulation on cognitive function in Parkinson's disease. *Archives of Neurology*, **58**, 1223–1227.

Alegret, M., Valldeoriola, F., Tolosa, E. *et al.* (2003) Cognitive effects of unilateral posteroventral pallidotomy: a 4-year follow-up study. *Movement Disorders*, **18**, 323–328.

Alesch, F. (2005) Sudden failure of dual channel pulse generators. *Movement Disorders*, **20**, 64–66.

Alvarez, L., Macias, R., Guridi, J. *et al.* (2001) Dorsal subthalamotomy for Parkinson's disease. *Movement Disorders*, **16**, 72–78.

Alves, G., Larsen, J.P., Emre, M. *et al.* (2006) Changes in motor subtype and risk for incident dementia in Parkinson's disease. *Movement Disorders*, **21**, 1123–1130.

Anderson, V.C., Burchiel, K.J., Hogarth, P. *et al.* (2005) Pallidal vs subthalamic nucleus deep brain stimulation in Parkinson's disease. *Archives of Neurology*, **62**, 554–560.

Ardouin, C., Klinger, H., Limousin, P. *et al.* (1999a) The effect of bilateral subthalamic nucleus stimulation on cognitive functions [abstract]. *Neurology*, **52**, A514.

Ardouin, C., Pillon, B., Peiffer, E. *et al.* (1999b) Bilateral subthalamic or pallidal stimulation for Parkinson's disease affects neither memory nor executive functions: a consecutive series of 62 patients. *Annals of Neurology*, **46**, 217–223.

Barcia-Salorio, J., Roldan, P., Talamantes, F. and Pascual-Leone, A. (1999) Electrical inhibition of basal ganglia nuclei in Parkinson's disease: long-term results. *Stereotact Funct Neurosurg*, **72**, 202–207.

Baron, M.S., Vitek, J.L., Bakay, R.A. *et al.* (2000) Treatment of advanced Parkinson's disease by unilateral posterior GPi pallidotomy: 4-year results of a pilot study. *Movement Disorders*, **15**, 230–237.

Bejjani, B., Damier, P., Arnulf, I. *et al.* (1997) Pallidal stimulation for Parkinson's disease: Two targets? *Neurology*, **49**, 1564–1569.

Bejjani, B.P., Damier, P., Arnulf, I. *et al.* (1999) Transient acute depression induced by high-frequency deep-brain stimulation. *The New England Journal of Medicine*, **340**, 1476–1480.

Benabid, A.L., Pollak, P., Gao, D. *et al.* (1996) Chronic electrical stimulation of the ventralis intermedius nucleus of the thalamus as a treatment of movement disorders. *Journal of Neurosurgery*, **84**, 203–214.

Benabid, A.L., Pollak, P., Gervason, C. *et al.* (1991) Long-term suppression of tremor by chronic stimulation of the ventral intermediate thalamic nucleus. *Lancet*, **337**, 403–406.

Benazzouz, A., Gross, C., Féger, J. *et al.* (1993) Reversal of rigidity and improvement in motor performance by subthalamic nucleus stimulation in MPTP-treated monkeys. *European Journal of Neuroscience*, **5**, 382–389.

Bergmann, H., Wichmann, T. and Delong, M.R. (1990) Reversal of experimental parkinsonism by lesions of the subthalamic nucleus. *Science (New York, NY)*, **249**, 1436–1438.

Berney, A., Vingerhoets, F., Perrin, A. *et al.* (2002) Effect on mood of subthalamic DBS for Parkinson's disease: a consecutive series of 24 patients. *Neurology*, **59**, 1427–1429.

Beurrier, C., Bioulac, B., Audin, J. and Hammond, C. (2001) High-frequency stimulation produces a transient blockade of voltage- gated currents in subthalamic neurons. *Journal of Neurophysiology*, **85**, 1351–1356.

Birkmayer, W. and Hornykiewicz, O. (1961) [The L-3,4-dioxyphenylalanine (DOPA)-effect in Parkinson-akinesia]. *Wiener Klinische Wochenschrift*, **73**, 787–788.

Blomstedt, P. and Hariz, M.I. (2005) Hardware-related complications of deep brain stimulation: a ten year experience. *Acta Neurochirurgica*, **147**, 1061–1064.

Blomstedt, P., Hariz, M.I., Lees, A. *et al.* (2008) Acute severe depression induced by intraoperative stimulation of the substantia nigra: A case report. *Parkinsonism & Related Disorders*, **14** (3), 253–256.

Braak, H., Rub, U. and Del Tredici, K. (2006) Cognitive decline correlates with neuropathological stage in Parkinson's disease. *Journal of the Neurological Sciences*, **248**, 255–258.

Broggi, G., Franzini, A., Ferroli, P. *et al.* (2001) Effect of bilateral subthalamic electrical stimulation in Parkinson's disease. *Surgical Neurology*, **56**, 89–94.

Burchiel, K.J., Anderson, V.C., Favre, J. and Hammerstad, J.P. (1999) Comparison of pallidal and subthalamic nucleus deep brain stimulation for advanced Parkinson's disease: results of a randomized, blinded pilot study. *Neurosurgery*, **45**, 1375–1382.

Burn, D.J., Rowan, E.N., Minett, T. *et al.* (2003) Extrapyramidal features in Parkinson's disease with and without dementia and dementia with Lewy bodies: A cross-sectional comparative study. *Movement Disorders*, **18**, 884–889.

Capecci, M., Ricciuti, R.A., Burini, D. *et al.* (2005) Functional improvement after subthalamic stimulation in Parkinson's disease: a non-equivalent controlled study with 12–24 month follow up. *Journal of Neurology, Neurosurgery, and Psychiatry*, **76**, 769–774.

Ceballos Baumann, A.O., Boecker, H., Bartenstein, P. *et al.* (1999) A positron emission tomographic study of subthalamic nucleus stimulation in Parkinson's disease: enhanced movement-related activity of motor-association cortex and decreased motor cortex resting activity. *Archives of Neurology*, **56**, 997–1003.

Ceballos-Baumann, A.O., Obeso, J.A., Vitek, J.L. *et al.* (1994) Restoration of thalamocortical activity after posteroventral pallidotomy in Parkinson's disease. *Lancet*, **344**, 814.

Charles, P.D., Van Blercom, N., Krack, P. *et al.* (2002) Predictors of effective bilateral subthalamic nucleus stimulation for PD. *Neurology*, **59**, 932–934.

Chen, C.C., Lee, S.T., Wu, T. *et al.* (2002) Hemiballism after subthalamotomy in patients with Parkinson's disease: report of 2 cases. *Movement Disorders*, **17**, 1367–1371.

Committee, G.P.S.D.S.S. (2002) Factors impacting on quality of life in Parkinson's disease: results from an international survey. *Movement Disorders*, **17**, 60–67.

Cooper, I.S. (1954) Surgical occlusion of the anterior choroidal artery in parkinsonism. *Surgery Gynecology & Obstetrics*, **92**, 207–219.

Cooper, I.S. (1961) Surgical treatment of parkinsonism. *British Medical Journal*, **1**, 1248–1249.

Cotzias, G.C., Van Woert, M.H. and Schiffer, L.M. (1967) Aromatic amino acids and modification of parkinsonism. *The New England Journal of Medicine*, **276**, 374–379.

Csp #468 Study Group (2006) Deep brain stimulation vs. best medical therapy for Parkinson's disease: patient outcomes from the VA CSP#468 prospective, randomized, multi-center trial. *Movement Disorders*, **21**, 1546–1547.

Daniele, A., Albanese, A., Contarino, M.F. *et al.* (2003) Cognitive and behavioural effects of chronic stimulation of the subthalamic nucleus in patients with Parkinson's disease. *Journal of Neurology, Neurosurgery, and Psychiatry*, **74**, 175–182.

Davis, K.D., Taub, E., Houle, S. *et al.* (1997) Globus pallidus stimulation activates the cortical motor system during alleviation of parkinsonian symptoms. *Nature Medicine*, **3**, 671–674.

De Bie, R.M., De Haan, R.J., Nijssen, P.C. *et al.* (1999) Unilateral pallidotomy in Parkinson's disease: a randomised, single-blind, multicentre trial. *Lancet*, **354**, 1665–1669.

De Bie, R.M., De Haan, R.J., Schuurman, P.R. *et al.* (2002a) Morbidity and mortality following pallidotomy in Parkinson's disease: a systematic review. *Neurology*, **58**, 1008–1012.

De Bie, R.M., Schuurman, P.R., Esselink, R.A. *et al.* (2002b) Bilateral pallidotomy in Parkinson's disease: a retrospective study. *Movement Disorders*, **17**, 533–538.

Delong, M.R. (1990) Primate models of movement disorders of basal ganglia origin. *Trends in Neurosciences*, **13**, 281–285.

Delwaide, P.J. (2001) Parkinsonian rigidity. *Functional Neurology*, **16**, 147–156.

Delwaide, P.J., Pepin, J.L., De Pasqua, V. and De Noordhout, A.M. (2000) Projections from basal ganglia to tegmentum: a subcortical route for explaining the pathophysiology of Parkinson's disease signs? *Journal of Neurology*, **247** (Suppl 2), II75–II81.

Deuschl, G., Schade-Brittinger, C., Krack, P. *et al.* (2006) A randomized trial of deep-brain stimulation for Parkinson's disease. *The New England Journal of Medicine*, **355**, 896–908.

Doshi, P.K., Chhaya, N. and Bhatt, M.H. (2002) Depression leading to attempted suicide after bilateral subthalamic nucleus stimulation for Parkinson's disease. *Movement Disorders*, **17**, 1084–1085.

Dostrovsky, J.O., Levy, R., Wu, J.P. *et al.* (2000) Microstimulation-induced inhibition of neuronal firing in human globus pallidus. *Journal of Neurophysiology*, **84**, 570–574.

Drapier, S., Raoul, S., Drapier, D. *et al.* (2005) Only physical aspects of quality of life are significantly improved by bilateral subthalamic stimulation in Parkinson's disease. *Journal of Neurology*, **252**, 583–588.

Dujardin, K., Defebvre, L., Krystkowiak, P. *et al.* (2001) Influence of chronic bilateral stimulation of the subthalamic nucleus on cognitive function in Parkinson's disease. *Journal of Neurology*, **248**, 603–611.

Dujardin, K., Krystkowiak, P., Defebvre, L. *et al.* (2000) A case of severe dysexecutive syndrome consecutive to chronic bilateral pallidal stimulation [In Process Citation]. *Neuropsychologia*, **38**, 1305–1315.

Durif, F., Lemaire, J.J., Debilly, B. and Dordain, G. (1999) Acute and chronic effects of anteromedial globus pallidus stimulation in Parkinson's disease. *Journal of Neurology, Neurosurgery, and Psychiatry*, **67**, 315–322.

Durif, F., Lemaire, J.J., Debilly, B. and Dordain, G. (2002) Long-term follow-up of globus pallidus chronic stimulation in advanced Parkinson's disease. *Movement Disorders*, **17**, 803–807.

Eidelberg, D., Moeller, J.R., Ishikawa, T. *et al.* (1996) Regional metabolic correlates of surgical outcome following unilateral pallidotomy for Parkinson's disease. *Annals of Neurology*, **39**, 450–459.

Erola, T., Karinen, P., Heikkinen, E. *et al.* (2005) Bilateral subthalamic nucleus stimulation improves health-related quality of life in Parkinsonian patients. *Parkinsonism & Related Disorders*, **11**, 89–94.

Esselink, R.A., De Bie, R.M., De Haan, R.J. *et al.* (2004) Unilateral pallidotomy versus bilateral subthalamic nucleus stimulation in PD: a randomized trial. *Neurology*, **62**, 201–207.

Esselink, R.A., De Bie, R.M., De Haan, R.J. *et al.* (2006) Unilateral pallidotomy versus bilateral subthalamic nucleus stimulation in Parkinson's disease: one year follow-up of a randomised observer-blind multi centre trial. *Acta Neurochirurgica*, **148**, 1247–1255, discussion 1255.

Fahn, S., Tolosa, E. and Marin, C. (1988) Clinical rating scale for tremor, in *Parkinson's Disease and Movement Disorders*

(eds J. Jankovic and E. Tolosa), Urban & Schwarzenberg, Baltimore.

Favre, J., Taha, J.M., Nguyen, T.T. *et al.* (1996) Pallidotomy: a survey of current practice in North America. *Neurosurgery*, **39**, 883–890, discussion 890-2.

Figueiras-Mendez, R., Regidor, I., Riva-Meana, C. and Magarinos-Ascone, C.M. (2002) Further supporting evidence of beneficial subthalamic stimulation in Parkinson's patients. *Neurology*, **58**, 469–470.

Fine, J., Duff, J., Chen, R. *et al.* (2000) Long-term follow-up of unilateral pallidotomy in advanced Parkinson's disease. *The New England Journal of Medicine*, **342**, 1708–1714.

Ford, B., Winfield, L., Pullman, S.L. *et al.* (2004) Subthalamic nucleus stimulation in advanced Parkinson's disease: blinded assessments at one year follow up. *Journal of Neurology, Neurosurgery, and Psychiatry*, **75**, 1255–1259.

Freed, C.R., Greene, P.E., Breeze, R.E. *et al.* (2001) Transplantation of embryonic dopamine neurons for severe Parkinson's disease. *The New England Journal of Medicine*, **344**, 710–719.

Funkiewiez, A., Ardouin, C., Krack, P. *et al.* (2003) Acute psychotropic effects of bilateral subthalamic nucleus stimulation and levodopa in Parkinson's disease. *Movement Disorders*, **18**, 524–530.

Garcia, L., Audin, J. and D'alessandro, G. *et al.* (2003) Dual effect of high-frequency stimulation on subthalamic neuron activity. *The Journal of Neuroscience*, **23**, 8743–8751.

Ghika, J., Villemure, J.G., Fankhauser, H. *et al.* (1998) Efficiency and safety of bilateral contemporaneous pallidal stimulation (deep brain stimulation) in levodopa-responsive patients with Parkinson's disease with severe motor fluctuations: a 2-year follow-up review. *Journal of Neurosurgery*, **89**, 713–718.

Gill, S.S., Patel, N.K., Hotton, G.R. *et al.* (2003) Direct brain infusion of glial cell line-derived neurotrophic factor in Parkinson's disease. *Nature Medicine*, **9**, 589–595.

Goetz, C.G., Olanow, C.W., Koller, W.C. *et al.* (1989) Multicenter study of autologous adrenal medullary transplantation to the corpus striatum in patients with advanced Parkinson's disease. *The New England Journal of Medicine*, **320**, 337–341.

Gross, C., Rougier, A., Guehl, D. *et al.* (1997) High-frequency stimulation of the globus pallidus internalis in Parkinson's disease: a study of seven cases. *Journal of Neurosurgery*, **87**, 491–498.

Hamani, C. and Lozano, A.M. (2006) Hardware-related complications of deep brain stimulation: a review of the published literature. *Stereotact Funct Neurosurg*, **84**, 248–251.

Hamel, W., Fietzek, U., Morsnowski, A. *et al.* (2003) Deep brain stimulation of the subthalamic nucleus in Parkinson's disease: evaluation of active electrode contacts. *Journal of Neurology, Neurosurgery and Psychiatry*, **74**, 1036–1046.

Hammond, C., Bergman, H. and Brown, P. (2007) Pathological synchronization in Parkinson's disease: networks, models and treatments. *Trends in Neurosciences*, **30**, 357–364.

Hariz, M.I. and Bergenheim, A.T. (2001) A 10-year follow-up review of patients who underwent Leksell's posteroventral pallidotomy for Parkinson's disease. *Journal of Neurosurgery*, **94**, 552–558.

Hariz, M.I. and Johansson, F. (2001) Hardware failure in parkinsonian patients with chronic subthalamic nucleus stimulation is a medical emergency. *Movement Disorders*, **16**, 166–168.

Hariz, M.I., Krack, P., Alesch, F. *et al.* (2008) Multicentre European study of thalamic stimulation for Parkinsonian tremor; a 6-year follow-up. *Journal of Neurology, Neurosurgery, and Psychiatry*, **79**, 694–699.

Hashimoto, T., Elder, C.M., Okun, M.S. *et al.* (2003) Stimulation of the subthalamic nucleus changes the firing pattern of pallidal neurons. *The Journal of Neuroscience*, **23**, 1916–1923.

Hassler, R. and Riechert, T. (1954) Indikationen und Lokalisationsmethode der gezielten Hirnoperationen. *Der Nervenarzt*, **25**, 441–447.

Hauser, R.A., Freeman, T.B., Snow, B.J. *et al.* (1999) Long-term evaluation of bilateral fetal nigral transplantation in Parkinson's disease. *Archives of Neurology*, **56**, 179–187.

Herzog, J., Fietzek, U., Hamel, W. *et al.* (2004) Most effective stimulation site in subthalamic deep brain stimulation for Parkinson's disease. *Movement Disorders*, **19**, 1050–1054.

Herzog, J., Hamel, W., Wenzelburger, R. *et al.* (2007) Kinematic analysis of thalamic versus subthalamic neurostimulation in postural and intention tremor. *Brain: A Journal of Neurology*, **130**, 1608–1625.

Herzog, J., Reiff, J., Krack, P. *et al.* (2003a) Manic episode with psychotic symptoms induced by subthalamic nucleus stimulation in a patient with Parkinson's disease. *Movement Disorders*, **18**, 1382–1384.

Herzog, J., Volkmann, J., Krack, P. *et al.* (2003b) Two year follow up of subthalamic deep brain stimulation in Parkinson's disease. *Movement Disorders*, **18**, 1332–1337.

Holsheimer, J., Demeulemeester, H., Nuttin, B. and De Sutter, P. (2000a) Identification of the target neuronal elements in electrical deep brain stimulation. *The European Journal of Neuroscience*, **12**, 4573–4577.

Holsheimer, J., Dijkstra, E.A., Demeulemeester, H. and Nuttin, B. (2000b) Chronaxie calculated from current-duration and voltage-duration data. *Journal of Neuroscience Methods*, **97**, 45–50.

Houeto, J.L., Bejjani, P.B., Damier, P. *et al.* (2000a) Failure of long-term pallidal stimulation corrected by subthalamic stimulation in PD. *Neurology*, **55**, 728–730.

Houeto, J.L., Damier, P., Bejjani, P.B. *et al.* (2000b) Subthalamic stimulation in Parkinson's disease: a multidisciplinary approach. *Archives of Neurology*, **57**, 461–465.

Houeto, J.L., Mesnage, V., Mallet, L. *et al.* (2002) Behavioural disorders, Parkinson's disease and subthalamic stimulation. *Journal of Neurology, Neurosurgery, and Psychiatry*, **72**, 701–707.

Iansek, R., Rosenfeld, J.V. and Huxham, F.E. (2002) Deep brain stimulation of the subthalamic nucleus in Parkinson's disease. *The Medical Journal of Australia*, **177**, 142–146.

Jaggi, J.L., Umemura, A., Hurtig, H.I. *et al.* (2004) Bilateral stimulation of the subthalamic nucleus in Parkinson's disease: surgical efficacy and prediction of outcome. *Stereotact Funct Neurosurg*, **82**, 104–114.

Jahanshahi, M., Ardouin, C.M., Brown, R.G. *et al.* (2000) The impact of deep brain stimulation on executive function in Parkinson's disease. *Brain: A Journal of Neurology*, **123** (Pt 6), 1142–1154.

Jenkinson, N., Nandi, D., Miall, R.C. *et al.* (2004) Pedunculopontine nucleus stimulation improves akinesia in a Parkinsonian monkey. *Neuroreport*, **15**, 2621–2624.

Jenkinson, N., Nandi, D., Oram, R. *et al.* (2006) Pedunculopontine nucleus electric stimulation alleviates akinesia independently of dopaminergic mechanisms. *Neuroreport*, **17**, 639–641.

Jordan, L.M. (1998) Initiation of locomotion in mammals. *Annals of the New York Academy of Sciences*, **860**, 83–93.

Just, H. and Ostergaard, K. (2002) Health-related quality of life in patients with advanced Parkinson's disease treated with deep brain stimulation of the subthalamic nuclei. *Movement Disorders*, **17**, 539–545.

Kaplitt, M.G., Feigin, A., Tang, C. *et al.* (2007) Safety and tolerability of gene therapy with an adeno-associated virus (AAV) borne GAD gene for Parkinson's disease: an open label, phase I trial. *Lancet*, **369**, 2097–2105.

Katayama, Y., Kasai, M., Oshima, H. *et al.* (2001) Subthalamic nucleus stimulation for Parkinson's disease: benefits observed in levodopa-intolerant patients. *Journal of Neurosurgery*, **95**, 213–221.

Kleiner-Fisman, G., Herzog, J., Fisman, D.N. *et al.* (2006) Subthalamic nucleus deep brain stimulation: summary and meta-analysis of outcomes. *Movement Disorders*, **21** (Suppl 14), S290–S304.

Kleiner-Fisman, G., Saint-Cyr, J.A., Miyasaki, J. *et al.* (2002) Subthalamic DBS replaces levodopa in Parkinson's disease. *Neurology*, **59**, 1293–1294.

Kordower, J.H., Freeman, T.B., Snow, B.J. *et al.* (1995) Neuropathological evidence of graft survival and striatal reinnervation after the transplantation of fetal mesencephalic tissue in a patient with Parkinson's disease. *The New England Journal of Medicine*, **332**, 1118–1124.

Krack, P., Batir, A., Van Blercom, N. *et al.* (2003) Five-year follow-up of bilateral stimulation of the subthalamic nucleus in advanced Parkinson's disease. *The New England Journal of Medicine*, **349**, 1925–1934.

Krack, P., Kumar, R., Ardouin, C. *et al.* (2001) Mirthful laughter induced by subthalamic nucleus stimulation. *Movement Disorders*, **16**, 867–875.

Krack, P., Pollak, P., Limousin, P. *et al.* (1998a) Opposite motor effects of pallidal stimulation in Parkinson's disease. *Annals of Neurology*, **43**, 180–192.

Krack, P., Pollak, P., Limousin, P. *et al.* (1998b) Subthalamic nucleus or internal pallidum stimulation in young onset Parkinson's disease. *Brain: A Journal of Neurology*, **121**, 451–457.

Krause, M., Fogel, W., Heck, A. *et al.* (2001) Deep brain stimulation for the treatment of Parkinson's disease: subthalamic nucleus versus globus pallidus internus. *Journal of Neurology, Neurosurgery, and Psychiatry*, **70**, 464–470.

Kulisevsky, J., Berthier, M.L., Gironell, A. *et al.* (2002) Mania following deep brain stimulation for Parkinson's disease. *Neurology*, **59**, 1421–1424.

Kumar, R., Lozano, A.M., Montgomery, E. and Lang, A.E. (1998) Pallidotomy and deep brain stimulation of the pallidum and subthalamic nucleus in advanced Parkinson's disease. *Movement Disorders*, **13**, 73–82.

Lagrange, E., Krack, P., Moro, E. *et al.* (2002) Bilateral subthalamic nucleus stimulation improves health-related quality of life in PD. *Neurology*, **59**, 1976–1978.

Laitinen, L.V., Bergenheim, A.T. and Hariz, M.I. (1992) Leksell's posteroventral pallidotomy in the treatment of Parkinson's disease. *Journal of Neurosurgery*, **76**, 53–61.

Landi, A., Antonini, A., Parolin, M. *et al.* (2003) Chronic subthalamus stimulation for the treatment of Parkinson's disease. Analysis of results by classes of symptoms and adverse effects. *Journal of Neurosurgical Sciences*, **47**, 24–27.

Lang, A.E., Gill, S., Patel, N.K. *et al.* (2006) Randomized controlled trial of intraputamenal glial cell line-derived neurotrophic factor infusion in Parkinson's disease. *Annals of Neurology*, **59**, 459–466.

Lang, A.E. and Group, for deep brain stimulation in advanced Parkinson's disease (1998) Deep brain stimulation (DBS) of the globus pallidus internus (GPi) in advanced Parkinson's disease (PD). *Movement Disorders*, **13** (Suppl 2), 264.

Lanotte, M.M., Rizzone, M., Bergamasco, B. *et al.* (2002) Deep brain stimulation of the subthalamic nucleus: anatomical, neurophysiological, and outcome correlations with the effects of stimulation. *Journal of Neurology, Neurosurgery, and Psychiatry*, **72**, 53–58.

Levy, A. (1967) Stereotaxic brain operations in Parkinson's syndrome and related motor disturbances. Comparison of lesions in the pallidum and thalamus with those in the internal capsule. *Confinia Neurologica*, **29** (Suppl), 1–70.

Lezcano, E., Gomez-Esteban, J.C., Zarranz, J.J. *et al.* (2004) Improvement in quality of life in patients with advanced Parkinson's disease following bilateral deep-brain stimulation in subthalamic nucleus. *European Journal of Neurology*, **11**, 451–454.

Limousin, P., Krack, P., Pollak, P. *et al.* (1998) Electrical stimulation of the subthalamic nucleus in advanced Parkinson's disease. *New England Journal of Medicine*, **339**, 1105–1111.

Limousin, P., Pollak, P., Benazzouz, A. *et al.* (1995) Effect of parkinsonian signs and symptoms of bilateral subthalamic nucleus stimulation. *Lancet*, **345**, 91–95.

Limousin, P., Speelman, J.D., Gielen, F. and Janssens, M. (1999) Multicentre European study of thalamic stimulation in parkinsonian and essential tremor. *Journal of Neurology, Neurosurgery, and Psychiatry*, **66**, 289–296.

Lindvall, O., Sawle, G., Widner, H. *et al.* (1994) Evidence for long-term survival and function of dopaminergic grafts in progressive Parkinson's disease. *Annals of Neurology*, **35**, 172–180.

Loher, T.J., Burgunder, J.M., Pohle, T. *et al.* (2002) Long-term pallidal deep brain stimulation in patients with advanced Parkinson's disease: 1-year follow-up study. *Journal of Neurosurgery*, **96**, 844–853.

Lombardi, W.J., Gross, R.E., Trepanier, L.L. *et al.* (2000) Relationship of lesion location to cognitive outcome following microelectrode-guided pallidotomy for Parkinson's disease: support for the existence of cognitive circuits in the human pallidum. *Brain: A Journal of Neurology*, **123** (Pt 4), 746–758.

Lopiano, L., Rizzone, M., Perozzo, P. *et al.* (2001) Deep brain stimulation of the subthalamic nucleus: selection of patients and clinical results. *Neurological Sciences*, **22**, 67–68.

Lyons, K.E. and Pahwa, R. (2005a) Long-term benefits in quality of life provided by bilateral subthalamic stimulation in patients with Parkinson's disease. *Journal of Neurosurgery*, **103**, 252–255.

Lyons, K.E., Wilkinson, S.B., Overman, J. and Pahwa, R. (2004) Surgical and hardware complications of subthalamic stimulation: a series of 160 procedures. *Neurology*, **63**, 612–616.

Mallet, L., Schupbach, M. and N'diaye, K. *et al.* (2007) Stimulation of subterritories of the subthalamic nucleus reveals its role in the integration of the emotional and motor aspects of behavior. *Proceedings of the National Academy of Sciences of the United States of America*, **104**, 10661–10666.

Marsden, C.D. and Obeso, J.A. (1994) The functions of the basal ganglia and the paradox of stereotaxic surgery in Parkinson's disease. *Brain: A Journal of Neurology*, **117**, 877–897.

Martinez-Martin, P., Valldeoriola, F., Tolosa, E. *et al.* (2002) Bilateral subthalamic nucleus stimulation and quality of life in advanced Parkinson's disease. *Movement Disorders*, **17**, 372–377.

Mazzone, P., Lozano, A., Stanzione, P. *et al.* (2005) Implantation of human pedunculopontine nucleus: a safe and clinically relevant target in Parkinson's disease. *Neuroreport*, **16**, 1877–1881.

Mcrae, C., Cherin, E., Yamazaki, T.G. *et al.* (2004) Effects of perceived treatment on quality of life and medical outcomes in a double-blind placebo surgery trial. *Archives of General Psychiatry*, **61**, 412–420.

Merello, M., Nouzeilles, M.I., Kuzis, G. *et al.* (1999) Unilateral radiofrequency lesion versus electrostimulation of posteroventral pallidum: a prospective randomized comparison. *Movement Disorders*, **14**, 50–56.

Meyers, R. (1951) Surgical experiments in the therapy of certain "extrapyramidal" diseases: a current evaluation. *Acta Psychiatrica et Neurologica Scandinavica Supplementum*, **67**, 1–42.

Meyers, R. (1968) The surgery of the hyperkinetic disorders, in *Handbook of Clinical Neurology* (eds P.J. Vinken and G.W. Bruyn), North Holland Publishers, Amsterdam.

Minguez-Castellanos, A., Escamilla-Sevilla, F., Hotton, G.R. *et al.* (2007) Carotid body autotransplantation in Parkinson's disease: A clinical and PET study. *Journal of Neurology, Neurosurgery, and Psychiatry*, **78**, 34–39.

Minguez-Castellanos, A., Escamilla-Sevilla, F., Katati, M.J. *et al.* (2005) Different patterns of medication change after subthalamic or pallidal stimulation for Parkinson's disease: target related effect or selection bias? *Journal of Neurology, Neurosurgery, and Psychiatry*, **76**, 34–39.

Molinuevo, J.L., Valldeoriola, F., Tolosa, E. *et al.* (2000) Levodopa withdrawal after bilateral subthalamic nucleus stimulation in advanced Parkinson's disease. *Archives of Neurology*, **57**, 983–988.

Moro, E., Esselink, R.J., Xie, J. *et al.* (2002) The impact on Parkinson's disease of electrical parameter settings in STN stimulation. *Neurology*, **59**, 706–713.

Moro, E., Poon, Y.Y., Lozano, A.M. *et al.* (2006) Subthalamic nucleus stimulation: improvements in outcome with reprogramming. *Archives of Neurology*, **63**, 1266–1272.

Moro, E., Scerrati, M., Romito, L.M. *et al.* (1999) Chronic subthalamic nucleus stimulation reduces medication requirements in Parkinson's disease. *Neurology*, **53**, 85–90.

Mundinger, F. (1977) [New stereotactic treatment of spasmodic torticollis with a brain stimulation system (author's transl)]. *Medizinische Klinik*, **72**, 1982–1986.

Mundinger, F. and Neumuller, H. (1982) Programmed stimulation for control of chronic pain and motor diseases. *Applied Neurophysiology*, **45**, 102–111.

Munro-Davies, L.E., Winter, J., Aziz, T.Z. and Stein, J.F. (1999) The role of the pedunculopontine region in basal-ganglia mechanisms of akinesia. *Experimental Brain Research*, **129**, 511–517.

Nandi, D., Aziz, T.Z., Giladi, N. *et al.* (2002a) Reversal of akinesia in experimental parkinsonism by GABA antagonist microinjections in the pedunculopontine nucleus. *Brain*, **125**, 2418–2430.

Nandi, D., Liu, X., Winter, J.L. *et al.* (2002b) Deep brain stimulation of the pedunculopontine region in the normal non-human primate. *Journal of Clinical Neuroscience*, **9**, 170–174.

Obeso, J.A., Guridi, J., Rodriguez-Oroz, M.C. *et al.* (2001) Deep-brain stimulation of the subthalamic nucleus or the pars interna of the globus pallidus in Parkinson's disease. *New England Journal of Medicine*, **345**, 956–963.

Ogura, M., Nakao, N., Nakai, E. *et al.* (2004) The mechanism and effect of chronic electrical stimulation of the globus pallidus for treatment of Parkinson's disease. *Journal of Neurosurgery*, **100**, 997–1001.

Oh, M.Y., Abosch, A., Kim, S.H. *et al.* (2002) Long-term hardware-related complications of deep brain stimulation. *Neurosurgery*, **50**, 1268–1274.

Okun, M.S., Tagliati, M., Pourfar, M. *et al.* (2005) Management of referred deep brain stimulation failures: a retrospective analysis from 2 movement disorders centers. *Archives of Neurology*, **62**, 1250–1255.

Okun, M.S. and Vitek, J.L. (2004) Lesion therapy for Parkinson's disease and other movement disorders: update and controversies. *Movement Disorders*, **19**, 375–389.

Olanow, C.W., Goetz, C.G., Kordower, J.H. *et al.* (2003) A double-blind controlled trial of bilateral fetal nigral transplantation in Parkinson's disease. *Annals of Neurology*, **54**, 403–414.

Olanow, C.W., Koller, W., Goetz, C.G. *et al.* (1990) Autologous transplantation of adrenal medulla in Parkinson's disease. 18-month results. *Archives of Neurology*, **47**, 1286–1289.

Ondo, W., Jankovic, J., Schwartz, K. *et al.* (1998) Unilateral thalamic deep brain stimulation for refractory essential tremor and Parkinson's disease tremor. *Neurology*, **51**, 1063–1069.

Ostergaard, K., Sunde, N. and Dupont, E. (2002) Effects of bilateral stimulation of the subthalamic nucleus in patients with severe Parkinson's disease and motor fluctuations. *Movement Disorders*, **17**, 693–700.

Pahapill, P.A. and Lozano, A.M. (2000) The pedunculopontine nucleus and Parkinson's disease. *Brain*, **123**, 1767–1783.

Pahwa, R., Wilkinson, S., Smith, D. *et al.* (1997) High-frequency stimulation of the globus pallidus for the treatment of Parkinson's disease. *Neurology*, **49**, 249–253.

Pal, P.K., Samii, A., Kishore, A. *et al.* (2000) Long term outcome of unilateral pallidotomy: follow up of 15 patients for 3 years. *Journal of Neurology, Neurosurgery, and Psychiatry*, **69**, 337–344.

Patel, N.K., Bunnage, M., Plaha, P. *et al.* (2005) Intraputamenal infusion of glial cell line-derived neurotrophic factor in PD: a two-year outcome study. *Annals of Neurology*, **57**, 298–302.

Patel, N.K., Heywood, P. and O'sullivan, K. *et al.* (2003) Unilateral subthalamotomy in the treatment of Parkinson's disease. *Brain*, **126**, 1136–1145.

Peppe, A., Pierantozzi, M., Bassi, A. *et al.* (2004) Stimulation of the subthalamic nucleus compared with the globus pallidus internus in patients with Parkinson's disease. *Journal of Neurosurgery*, **101**, 195–200.

Perozzo, P., Rizzone, M., Bergamasco, B. *et al.* (2001) Deep brain stimulation of subthalamic nucleus: behavioural modifications and familiar relations. *Neurological Sciences*, **22**, 81–82.

Pillon, B., Ardouin, C., Damier, P. *et al.* (2000) Neuropsychological changes between "off" and "on" STN or GPi stimulation in Parkinson's disease. *Neurology*, **55**, 411–418.

Pinter, M.M., Alesch, F., Murg, M. *et al.* (1999) Deep brain stimulation of the subthalamic nucleus for control of extrapyramidal features in advanced idiopathic parkinson's disease: one year follow-up. *Journal of Neural Transmission*, **106**, 693–709.

Plaha, P., Ben-Shlomo, Y., Patel, N.K. and Gill, S.S. (2006) Stimulation of the caudal zona incerta is superior to stimulation of the subthalamic nucleus in improving contralateral parkinsonism. *Brain*, **129**, 1732–1747.

Plaha, P. and Gill, S.S. (2005) Bilateral deep brain stimulation of the pedunculopontine nucleus for Parkinson's disease. *Neuroreport*, **16**, 1883–1887.

Pollak, P., Benabid, A.L., Gross, C. *et al.* (1993) [Effects of the stimulation of the subthalamic nucleus in Parkinson's disease]. *Revue Neurologique*, **149**, 175–176.

Potter, M., Illert, M., Wenzelburger, R. *et al.* (2004) The effect of subthalamic nucleus stimulation on autogenic inhibition in Parkinson's disease. *Neurology*, **63**, 1234–1239.

Ranck, J.B. (1975) Which elements are excited in electrical stimulation of mammalian central nervous system? A review. *Brain Research*, **98**, 417–440.

Rehncrona, S., Johnels, B., Widner, H. *et al.* (2003) Long-term efficacy of thalamic deep brain stimulation for tremor: double-blind assessments. *Movement Disorders*, **18**, 163–170.

Rettig, G.M., York, M.K., Lai, E.C. *et al.* (2000) Neuropsychological outcome after unilateral pallidotomy for the treatment of Parkinson's disease. *Journal of Neurology, Neurosurgery, and Psychiatry*, **69**, 326–336.

Rodriguez, M.C., Guridi, O.J., Alvarez, L. *et al.* (1998) The subthalamic nucleus and tremor in Parkinson's disease. *Movement Disorders*, **13** (Suppl 3), 111–118.

Rodriguez-Oroz, M.C., Obeso, J.A., Lang, A.E. *et al.* (2005) Bilateral deep brain stimulation in Parkinson's disease: a multicentre study with 4 years follow-up. *Brain*, **128**, 2240–2249.

Romito, L.M., Raja, M., Daniele, A. *et al.* (2002a) Transient mania with hypersexuality after surgery for high frequency stimulation of the subthalamic nucleus in Parkinson's disease. *Movement Disorders*, **17**, 1371–1374.

Romito, L.M., Scerrati, M., Contarino, M.F. *et al.* (2002b) Long-term follow up of subthalamic nucleus stimulation in Parkinson's disease. *Neurology*, **58**, 1546–1550.

Russmann, H., Ghika, J., Villemure, J.G. *et al.* (2004) Subthalamic nucleus deep brain stimulation in Parkinson's disease patients over age 70 years. *Neurology*, **63**, 1952–1954.

Saint-Cyr, J.A., Trepanier, L.L., Kumar, R. *et al.* (2000a) Neuropsychological consequences of chronic bilateral stimulation of the subthalamic nucleus in Parkinson's disease. *Brain*, **123** (Pt 10), 2091–2108.

Saint-Cyr, J.A., Trepanier, L.L., Kumar, R. *et al.* (2000b) Neuropsychological consequences of chronic bilateral stimulation of the subthalamic nucleus in Parkinson's disease. *Brain*, **123**, 2091–2108.

Samuel, M., Ceballos-Baumann, A.O., Turjanski, N. *et al.* (1997) Pallidotomy in Parkinson's disease increases supplementary motor area and prefrontal activation during performance of volitional movements an H2(15)O PET study. *Brain*, **120**, 1301–1313.

Schneider, F., Habel, U., Volkmann, J. *et al.* (2003) Deep brain stimulation of the subthalamic nucleus enhances emotional processing in Parkinson's disease. *Archives of General Psychiatry*, **60**, 296–302.

Schupbach, M., Gargiulo, M., Welter, M.L. *et al.* (2006) Neurosurgery in Parkinson's disease: a distressed mind in a repaired body? *Neurology*, **66**, 1811–1816.

Schupbach, W.M., Chastan, N., Welter, M.L. *et al.* (2005) Stimulation of the subthalamic nucleus in Parkinson's disease: a 5 year follow up. *Journal of Neurology, Neurosurgery, and Psychiatry*, **76**, 1640–1644.

Schupbach, W.M., Maltete, D., Houeto, J.L. *et al.* (2007) Neurosurgery at an earlier stage of Parkinson's disease: a randomized, controlled trial. *Neurology*, **68**, 267–271.

Schuurman, P., Bosch, D. and Speelman, J. (2001) Thalamic stimulation versus thalamotomy: long-term follow-up. *Parkinsonism & Related Disorders*, **7**, S85.

Schuurman, P.R., Bosch, D.A., Bossuyt, P.M. *et al.* (2000a) A comparison of continuous thalamic stimulation and thalamotomy for suppression of severe tremor. *New England Journal of Medicine*, **342**, 461–468.

Schuurman, P.R., Bosch, D.A., Bossuyt, P.M. *et al.* (2000b) A comparison of continuous thalamic stimulation and thalamotomy for suppression of severe tremor. *New England Journal of Medicine*, **342**, 461–468.

Seijo, F.J., Alvarez-Vega, M.A., Gutierrez, J.C. *et al.* (2007) Complications in subthalamic nucleus stimulation surgery for treatment of Parkinson's disease. Review of 272 procedures. *Acta Neurochirurgica*, **149**, 867–876.

Siegfried, J. and Lippitz, B. (1994a) Bilateral chronic electrostimulation of ventroposterolateral pallidum: a new therapeutic approach for alleviating all parkinsonian symptoms. *Neurosurgery*, **35**, 1126–1129.

Siegfried, J. and Lippitz, B. (1994b) Bilateral chronic electrostimulation of ventroposterolateral pallidum: a new therapeutic approach for alleviating all parkinsonian symptoms. *Neurosurgery*, **35**, 1126–1129.

Simuni, T., Jaggi, J.L., Mulholland, H. *et al.* (2002) Bilateral stimulation of the subthalamic nucleus in patients with Parkinson's disease: a study of efficacy and safety. *Journal of Neurosurgery*, **96**, 666–672.

Smeding, H.M., Esselink, R.A., Schmand, B. *et al.* (2005) Unilateral pallidotomy versus bilateral subthalamic nucleus stimulation in PD–a comparison of neuropsychological effects. *Journal of Neurology*, **252**, 176–182.

Spiegel, E.A., Wycis, H.T., Marks, M. and Lee, A.J. (1947) Stereotaxic Apparatus for Operations on the Human Brain. *Science (New York, NY)*, **106**, 349–350.

Spottke, E.A., Volkmann, J., Lorenz, D. *et al.* (2002) Evaluation of healthcare utilization and health status of patients with Parkinson's disease treated with deep brain stimulation of the subthalamic nucleus. *Journal of Neurology*, **249**, 759–766.

Stefani, A., Lozano, A.M., Peppe, A. *et al.* (2007) Bilateral deep brain stimulation of the pedunculopontine and subthalamic nuclei in severe Parkinson's disease. *Brain: A Journal of Neurology*, **130**, 1596–1607.

Stover, N.P., Bakay, R.A., Subramanian, T. *et al.* (2005) Intrastriatal implantation of human retinal pigment epithelial cells attached to microcarriers in advanced Parkinson's disease. *Archives of Neurology*, **62**, 1833–1837.

Strafella, A., Ashby, P., Munz, M. *et al.* (1997) Inhibition of voluntary activity by thalamic stimulation in humans: relevance for the control of tremor. *Movement Disorders*, **12**, 727–737.

Su, P.C., Tseng, H.M., Liu, H.M. *et al.* (2003) Treatment of advanced Parkinson's disease by subthalamotomy: one-year results. *Movement Disorders*, **18**, 531–538.

Svennilson, E., Torvik, A., Lowe, R. and Leksell, L. (1960) Treatment of parkinsonism by stereotatic thermolesions in the pallidal region. A clinical evaluation of 81 cases. *Acta Psychiatrica Scandinavica*, **35**, 358–377.

Tamma, F., Rampini, P., Egidi, M. *et al.* (2003) Deep brain stimulation for Parkinson's disease: the experience of the Policlinico-San Paolo Group in Milan. *Neurological Sciences*, **24** (Suppl 1), S41–S42.

Tavella, A., Bergamasco, B., Bosticco, E. *et al.* (2002) Deep brain stimulation of the subthalamic nucleus in Parkinson's disease: long-term follow-up. *Neurological Sciences*, **23** (Suppl 2), S111–S112.

The Deep-Brain Stimulation for Parkinson's Disease Study Group (2001) Deep-brain stimulation of the subthalamic nucleus or the pars interna of the globus pallidus in Parkinson's disease. *New England Journal of Medicine*, **345**, 956–963.

Thobois, S., Mertens, P., Guenot, M. *et al.* (2002) Subthalamic nucleus stimulation in Parkinson's disease: clinical evaluation of 18 patients. *Journal of Neurology*, **249**, 529–534.

Trepanier, L.L., Kumar, R., Lozano, A.M. *et al.* (2000) Neuropsychological outcome of GPi pallidotomy and GPi or STN deep brain stimulation in Parkinson's disease. *Brain and Cognition*, **42**, 324–347.

Tronnier, V.M., Fogel, W., Kronenbuerger, M. and Steinvorth, S. (1997) Pallidal stimulation: an alternative to pallidotomy? *Journal of Neurosurgery*, **87**, 700–705.

Troster, A.I., Fields, J.A., Wilkinson, S.B. *et al.* (1997) Unilateral pallidal stimulation for Parkinson's disease: neurobehavioral functioning before and 3 months after electrode implantation. *Neurology*, **49**, 1078–1083.

Tseng, H.M., Su, P.C. and Liu, H.M. (2003) Persistent hemiballism after subthalamotomy: the size of the lesion matters more than the location. *Movement Disorders*, **18**, 1209–1211.

Valldeoriola, F., Pilleri, M., Tolosa, E. *et al.* (2002) Bilateral subthalamic stimulation monotherapy in advanced Parkinson's disease: long-term follow-up of patients. *Movement Disorders*, **17**, 125–132.

Van Horn, G., Hassenbusch, S.J., Zouridakis, G. *et al.* (2001) Pallidotomy: a comparison of responders and nonresponders. *Neurosurgery*, **48**, 263–271.

Varma, T.R., Fox, S.H., Eldridge, P.R. *et al.* (2003) Deep brain stimulation of the subthalamic nucleus: effectiveness in advanced Parkinson's disease patients previously reliant on apomorphine. *Journal of Neurology, Neurosurgery, and Psychiatry*, **74**, 170–174.

Vesper, J., Klostermann, F., Stockhammer, F. *et al.* (2002) Results of chronic subthalamic nucleus stimulation for Parkinson's disease: a 1-year follow-up study. *Surgical Neurology*, **57**, 306–311.

Vingerhoets, F.J., Villemure, J.G., Temperli, P. *et al.* (2002) Subthalamic DBS replaces levodopa in Parkinson's disease: two-year follow-up. *Neurology*, **58**, 396–401.

Vingerhoets, G., Van Der Linden, C., Lannoo, E. *et al.* (1999) Cognitive outcome after unilateral pallidal stimulation in Parkinson's disease. *Journal of Neurology, Neurosurgery, and Psychiatry*, **66**, 297–304.

Visser-Vandewalle, V., Van Der Linden, C., Temel, Y. *et al.* (2005) Long-term effects of bilateral subthalamic nucleus stimulation in advanced Parkinson's disease: a four year follow-up study. *Parkinsonism & Related Disorders*, **11**, 157–165.

Vitek, J.L., Bakay, R.A., Freeman, A. *et al.* (2003) Randomized trial of pallidotomy versus medical therapy for Parkinson's disease. *Annals of Neurology*, **53**, 558–569.

Voges, J., Hilker, R., Botzel, K. *et al.* (2007) Thirty days complication rate following surgery performed for deep-brain-stimulation. *Movement Disorders*, **22**, 1486–1489.

Voges, J., Volkmann, J., Allert, N. *et al.* (2002) Bilateral high-frequency stimulation in the subthalamic nucleus for the treatment of Parkinson's disease: correlation of therapeutic effect with anatomical electrode position. *Journal of Neurosurgery*, **96**, 269–279.

Volkmann, J., Allert, N., Voges, J. *et al.* (2004) Long-term results of bilateral pallidal deep brain stimulation in Parkinson's disease. *Annals of Neurology*, **55**, 871–875.

Volkmann, J., Allert, N., Voges, J. *et al.* (2001) Safety and efficacy of pallidal or subthalamic nucleus stimulation in advanced PD. *Neurology*, **56**, 548–551.

Volkmann, J., Fogel, W. and Krack, P. (2000) Postoperatives neurologisches Management bei Stimulation des Nucleus subthalamicus. *Aktuelle Neurologie*, **27**, 23–39.

Volkmann, J., Herzog, J., Kopper, F. and Deuschl, G. (2002) Introduction to the programming of deep brain stimulators. *Movement Disorders*, **17** (Suppl 3), S181–S187.

Volkmann, J., Sturm, V., Weiss, P. *et al.* (1998) Bilateral high-frequency stimulation of the internal globus pallidus in advanced Parkinson's disease, *Annals of Neurology*, **44**, 953–961.

Voon, V., Saint-Cyr, J., Lozano, A.M. *et al.* (2005) Psychiatric symptoms in patients with Parkinson's disease presenting for deep brain stimulation surgery. *Journal of Neurosurgery*, **103**, 246–251.

Welter, M.L., Houeto, J.L., Tezenas Du Montcel, S. *et al.* (2002) Clinical predictive factors of subthalamic stimulation in Parkinson's disease. *Brain: A Journal of Neurology*, **125**, 575–583.

Wilson, S., Bladin, P. and Saling, M. (2001) The "burden of normality": concepts of adjustment after surgery for seizures. *Journal of Neurology, Neurosurgery, and Psychiatry*, **70**, 649–656.

York, M.K., Lai, E.C., Jankovic, J. *et al.* (2007) Short and long-term motor and cognitive outcome of staged bilateral pallidotomy: a retrospective analysis. *Acta Neurochirurgica*, **149**, 857–866.

Future Cell- and Gene-Based Therapies for Parkinson's Disease

Tomas Björklund[1], Asuka Morizane[2], Deniz Kirik[1] and Patrik Brundin[2]

[1] Brain Repair and Imaging in Neural Systems, Department
of Experimental Medical Science, Lund University, Sweden
[2] Neuronal Survival Unit, Wallenberg Neuroscience Center Department
of Experimental Medical Science, Lund University, Sweden

INTRODUCTION

In the 50 years since the discovery of dopamine (DA) as a neurotransmitter, and its involvement in Parkinson's disease (PD), pharmacologic DA replacement therapy has become the mainstay of PD treatment. Although, the introduction of long-lasting DA agonists and combined treatment with L-DOPA has improved the quality of life for the patients, it also dramatically increased the cost of treatment. However refined, these therapies still cannot modify the disease progression and the patients still face major adverse effects as the disease advances.

In this chapter, we will describe three major lines of experimental strategies, which hold great potential as future clinical therapies for PD patients (Figure 8.1). They differ significantly from each other in the way they interact with the host brain, but all aim at restoring basal ganglia function. The first section describes recent advances in cell replacement therapy, where the transplanted cells restore synaptic connectivity, DA synthesis and release in the parkinsonian striatum. The second section describes an alternative approach for neurotransmitter delivery. This strategy utilizes viral vector-mediated gene delivery and the cellular machinery of remaining neurons in the striatum to produce DA or its precursor. The final section covers advances in neuroprotective strategies to slow or even halt the disease progress.

CELL TRANSPLANTATION THERAPY

Historical Background

Cell transplantation has been considered a possible future therapy for PD for close to three decades. The first animal studies demonstrating that immature DA neurons grafted to the striatum could function in the adult mammalian nervous system surprised the neuroscience community. Earlier studies had already demonstrated that immature neurons could survive implantation into the anterior chamber of the eye (Olson and Malmfors, 1970; Olson and Seiger, 1972) and to a well-vascularized tissue bed adjacent to the hippocampus (Bjorklund, Stenevi and Svendgaard, 1976). Moreover, immature DA neurons could also survive *in vitro* culturing (Levitt, Moore and Garber, 1976). The fact that the neurons survived transplantation adjacent to the striatum was therefore not completely unexpected. Instead, the remarkable feature was that they could re-innervate the host brain, functionally "replace" the endogenous DA system and reverse behavioral abnormalities caused by a prior lesion of the nigrostriatal system. This dramatic functional plasticity of the adult brain, that is, that it could integrate a new set of neurons, went beyond all expectations. Immediately hopes were raised that the technique could be used to repair the brains of patients with PD. Several laboratories set out on a mission to characterize the grafted DA neurons morphologically and physiologically. The effects on the host brain neurons were studied in detail and the beneficial impact of the grafts on different lesion-induced deficits were described. In some studies the interaction between the recipient's immune system and the implants was monitored. A review of all the grafting studies in experimental animals is beyond the scope of this chapter; instead the reader may consult earlier publications that have focused on them (Brundin, Duan, and Sauer, 1994; Brundin and Hagell, 2001). The first clinical trials with transplantation in PD did not use immature DA neurons as donor tissue (Lindvall *et al.*, 1987). Instead the patients received

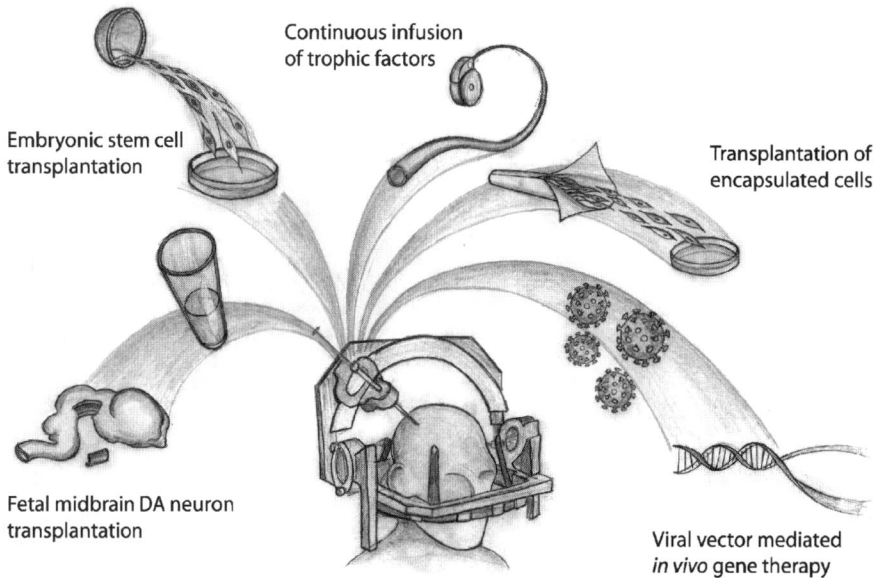

Figure 8.1 Schematic overview of novel therapeutic strategies in Parkinson's disease. *Fetal midbrain DA neuron transplantation*: Cells from the ventral mesencephalon are dissected from aborted embryos. They are then mechanically dissociated into a mixture of single cells and tissue aggregates before being stereotactically injected into the patients' putamen. *Embryonic stem cell transplantation*: Cells from the inner cell mass of early, *in vitro* fertilized embryos are collected, expanded and established as an embryonic stem cell line. Embryonic stem cells are cultured under controlled circumstances so that they differentiate into midbrain dopamine neurons before they are injected into the brain. *Continuous infusion of trophic factors*: A thin catheter is inserted either into the ventricle or the posterodorsal putamen and is connected to an infusion pump that delivers recombinant proteins, for example, glial cell line-derived neurotrophic factor (GDNF), at a continuous rate. *Transplantation of encapsulated cells*: The cells are genetically modified *in vitro* to stably express and secrete GDNF. They are then encapsulated in semi-permeable, hollow fibers before being inserted into the brain parenchyma. *Viral vector-mediated in vivo gene therapy*: Viral vectors such as recombinant adeno-associated viral (rAAV) vectors, coding for either neurotransmitter synthesizing enzymes or trophic factors, are injected into the brain parenchyma.

autografts of their own adrenal medulla. The supporting studies in experimental animals were fewer and the results less impressive than for immature DA neurons, but adrenal chromaffin cells were considered an ethically more acceptable source of catecholamine-producing tissue for clinical trials. Despite an initial optimism in the reports from Madrazo and co-workers (Madrazo *et al.*, 1987), the adrenal autografts were not successful in numerous follow-up trials and the approach was abandoned towards the end of the 1980s (Goetz *et al.*, 1991). In parallel, a number of clinical trials with transplants of human immature DA neurons in PD were initiated and actively pursued for about one decade. In the following section of this chapter we will briefly summarize the results of these trials and describe the problems the field has encountered. Subsequently we will discuss possible alternate sources of donor tissue, and in this context focus on different types of stem cells.

Fetal Neural Tissue Transplantation

From the initial clinical trials in 1987 to today, over 400 PD patients are estimated to have received transplants of human ventral mesencephalon from aborted embryos or fetuses. In several open-label trials, some of the grafted patients were reported to exhibit dramatic neurological improvement. Typically, the patients would display reductions in bradykinesia and rigidity, as well as a marked reduction in the time spent in the "off" phase. In the most impressive cases, it was possible to withdraw anti-parkinson medication. Positron emission tomography (PET) scans have shown increases in fluorodopa uptake such that in the best cases it has been normalized in the implanted putamen, even in cases where the expected level would be 10–20% of normal following numerous years of symptomatic PD. The graft's ability to release DA has been observed using PET with a DA D_2 receptor ligand (raclopride), where the level of DA receptor binding has been brought down to normal by the transplants (Piccini *et al.*, 1999). Using PET to measure cortical activation, the grafts have been found to normalize movement-related activity levels in the supplementary motor area and dorsolateral prefrontal cortex (Piccini *et al.*, 2000). In post-mortem studies of brains from grafted PD patients, sometimes in excess of 100 000 implanted DA neurons have been observed in each putamen (Kordower *et al.*, 1998; Mendez *et al.*, 2005). These cells have given rise to a dense network of dopaminergic axons and terminals in the host brain. Despite the apparent success of grafting in PD, it has, however, not become a standard therapy for PD.

Indeed, in recent years there have not been any additional transplantation surgeries as part of systematic clinical trials. This clinical field of research has virtually reached a standstill. There are several probable reasons for this. For example, it has been difficult to perform large series of surgeries due to difficulties in securing sufficient amounts of donor tissue from routine abortions. Moreover, the results in the open-label trials have varied markedly, with some patients showing no significant benefit whilst others have exhibited dramatic improvement (for review see (Lindvall *et al.*, 2000)). The reason for these variable results is not fully understood, and as a consequence, the reproducibility of the procedure has been question. Probably the most profound inhibitory effect on the clinical neural transplantation field was sparked by two NIH-sponsored, double-blind, placebo-controlled trials. The human mesencephalic transplants did not elicit any improvement in the respective primary endpoints of the studies (Freed *et al.*, 2001; Olanow *et al.*, 2003). The initial controlled trial also highlighted, for the first time, that some grafted patients can develop graft-induced dyskinesias, which persist in the absence of anti-parkinsonian medication (Freed *et al.*, 2001). Retrospective studies confirmed that the same type of dyskinesias had also been present in some of the patients from the open-label trials (Hagell *et al.*, 2002), and they were also seen in the second controlled trial (Olanow *et al.*, 2003). Taken together, the negative outcome of the controlled trials initiated a discussion on the future of neural transplantation (Bjorklund *et al.*, 2003). One conclusion is that more basic research is required to optimize the technique, so the chances of major benefit increase. Furthermore, it is necessary to understand, and create strategies to avoid, graft-induced dyskinesias.

What is the best way forward in order to maximize the chances of benefit and minimize the risk of side effects? First, the selection of patients has to be considered more carefully than before. Patients with PD are a heterogeneous group and aside from obvious variables, such as duration of disease, age of onset and genetics, other factors may influence suitability for transplantation therapy. Today it is not known which patients are most suited for transplanta-

tion therapy, although it has been suggested that mild disease or a good response to L-DOPA are predictors of a good response to grafting (Olanow *et al.*, 2003; Freed *et al.*, 2004). Second, the extent to which patient selection and surgical factors influence the risk of developing dyskinesias needs clarification. As mentioned above, it is necessary to design new animal experiments to examine when and why dyskinesias develop after transplantation (Hagell and Cenci, 2005). Graft-induced dyskinesias have so far not been possible to faithfully replicate in experimental rodents. Following administration of amphetamine, however, some grafted rats exhibit abnormal involuntary movements (Carlsson *et al.*, 2006; Lane *et al.*, 2006). These may be analogous to true graft-induced dyskinesias in PD patients. Interestingly, they only appear in rats that have previously displayed abnormal movements in response to prolonged L-DOPA treatment. Third, surgical factors, such as the numbers of cells implanted, the type of instrument used and the regions of the basal ganglia targeted, are definitely important for clinical outcome and need to be understood better. Fourth, the impact of the host immune system on the survival and function of neural grafts is not well understood. Without question, the brain constitutes an immunologically privileged transplantation site and incompatible grafts display prolonged survival compared to when they are placed in peripheral sites (Widner and Brundin, 1988). This does not mean, however, that immune rejection of grafted neurons cannot take place in the brain (Brevig, Holgersson and Widner, 2000). Finally, there is great need for a novel source of immature DA neurons that can replace the use of ventral mesencephalic tissue from aborted embryos. Ideally the cells should closely resemble the morphology and functions of human nigral DA neurons, should provide a minimal stimulus to the immune system and should be possible to produce in large numbers. The development of a reproducible supply of cells is necessary, if systematic, large-scale clinical trials are to be conducted in the future. In the following sections, we briefly review different types of stem cells and their potential suitability as starting material for the generation of DA neurons.

Stem-Cell Based Therapies

Stem cells have the capacity both to self-renew and to generate progeny that can differentiate into multiple types of specialized cells (Gage, 2000). Stem cells are classified based on the age of the tissue in which they are found (e.g., embryonic, fetal, adult). Those found in the adult are often called somatic stem cells. Stem cells are also grouped based on their level of plasticity, that is, potency to form different mature cell types. Thus, multipotent stem cells are capable of generating several types of mature cells (typically within one tissue type), whereas pluripotent stem cells can form all types of tissue, that is, from the three different germ layers. In the context of cell therapy for PD, stem cells from embryos, fetuses and adults have been explored as potential sources of DA neurons. Several studies have also addressed the capacity of stem cells found outside the brain, to form neurons. In this section we very briefly summarize the current state-of-the-art regarding stem cells as a source of transplantable neurons in PD.

Neural Stem Cells

Neural stem cells are multipotent and can differentiate into neurons, astrocytes and oligodendrocytes. They are found both in immature and adult central nervous system tissue. In human adult brain, neural stem cells are present in the subventricular zone and subgranular zone of the hippocampal dentate gyrus (Eriksson et al., 1998). Recently, the human equivalent of the rodents rostral migratory stream (RMS) was described, suggesting that newly born neurons migrate to the olfactory bulb from the subventricular zone (Curtis et al., 2007). Neural stem cells obtained from immature tissue of rodents readily prolifer-ate in culture medium that is supplemented with growth factors such as basic fibroblast growth factor (bFGF) and epidermal growth factor (EGF) (Gage, Ray and Fisher, 1995). Investigators often chose to proliferate these cells in small aggregates called neurospheres. Many groups have tried to induce DA neurons from embryonic/fetal neural stem cells by exposing them to a large variety of soluble growth factors, cytokines and substrates, or alter-natively by using gene-transfer techniques to express transcription factors involved in DA neuron development (Yang et al., 2004; Roybon, Brundin and Li, 2005; Christophersen et al., 2006; Park et al., 2006; Andersson et al., 2007; Kim et al., 2007). So far, no culture protocol has reliably and reproducibly generated large numbers of transplantable DA neurons from neural stem cells (Roybon et al., 2008). Why it is so difficult to drive neural stem cells to a dopaminergic fate is not well understood. Possibly, some of these so-called neural stem cells are already progenitors that are partially committed to another fate. Alternatively, the complex set of transcriptional and external signals needed to make a DA neuron from neural stem cells have simply not been possible to faithfully reproduce in the culture dish. Even if it were possible to obtain large numbers of DA neurons from rodent neural stem cells, it would not be always simple to transfer culture techniques from rodent to human neural stem cells. Typically, human neural stem cells display longer doubling time than those of rodents. Be-sides that, the telomeres of human neural stem cells are significantly shorter than their rodent counterparts, sug-gesting that they will senesce more rapidly (Ostenfeld et al., 2000).

Stem Cells Derived from Non-Neural Tissues

Stem cells are derived from tissues outside the nervous system have also been explored as potential sources of DA neurons. They include stem cells from bone marrow, skin, umbilical cord, and so on. A few years ago, several studies claimed that such stem cells can differentiate into neurons and thereby transcend classical tissue lineage boundaries (Priller et al., 2001; Cogle et al., 2004). This phenomenon has been named "transdifferentiation" and it is hotly debated to what extent it really exists (Rice and Scolding, 2004). For many studies claiming that transdifferentiation of non-neural stem cells into neurons can occur, it has subsequently been possible to explain it as an experimental artifact of the studied model system. For example, grafted bone marrow-derived stem cells carrying a cell-specific marker protein have been reported to differentiate into mature neurons that then express the same marker protein. Re-interpretation of these studies indicates that mature neurons expressing the marker protein do so because they have undergone fusion with the grafted stem cells (Alvarez-Dolado et al., 2003; Weimann et al., 2003). This fusion event is rare, but may explain all those (also rare) instances where transdiffer-entiation of a non-neural somatic stem cells into mature neurons has been suggested to take place. In short, trans-differentiation currently does not appear to be a viable approach to obtaining DA neurons for grafting in PD. A different, exciting, recent finding has rekindled the idea that adult somatic cells may one day be a source of DA neurons. By overexpressing four transcription factors (Oct3/4, Sox2, c-Myc and Klf4), it has been possible to induce mouse fibroblasts to become pluripotent stem cells (Takahashi and Yamanaka, 2006; Maherali et al., 2007; Okita, Ichisaka and Yamanaka, 2007; Wernig et al., 2007). Notably, it has been possible to obtain cells that can differentiate into DA neurons when applying the same strategy on human fibro-blasts cells (Takahashi et al., 2007). Consequently, "induced pluripotent stem cells", abbreviated iPS cells, have attracted great interest. They might become a powerful source of transplantable DA neurons and could even be derived from the PD patient's own fibroblasts.

Embryonic Stem Cells

Embryonic stem cells (ESCs) are a particularly interesting potential donor tissue source for transplantation in PD. They are highly proliferative and truly pluripotent. Taken together, they are eminently suited to generate large num-bers of DA neurons.

Several different cell culture protocols have been used to generate DA neurons or neural progenitors from mouse ESCs (Kawasaki et al., 2000; Lee et al., 2000). Some of these protocols for mouse ESCs have been adapted to suit human ESCs (Figure 8.2). This adaptation has not always

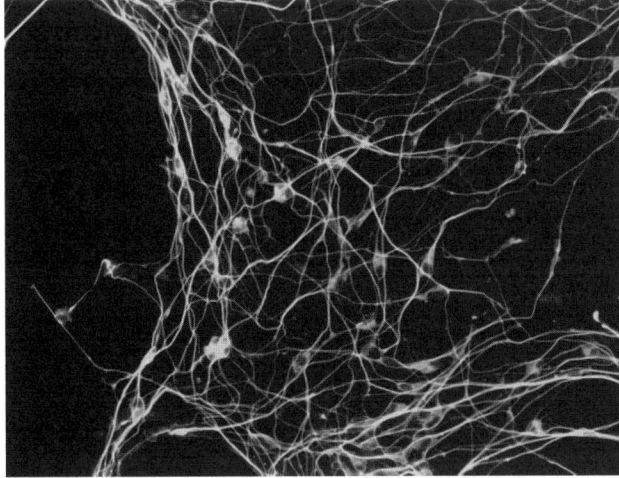

Figure 8.2 Neurons derived from human ESCs (HUES-3 cell line). Immunohisotochemical staining with TuJ1 antibody and their morphology show that human ESCs can differentiate into neurons after three weeks of culture.

been problem-free, in part because human cell development is much more protracted than murine. The main strategies have been co-culture with specific feeder cells (e.g., different forms of mesenchymal cells) and addition of defined soluble factors to the culture medium (e.g., sonic hedgehog and fibroblast growth factor 8) (Kim *et al.*, 2006). Regarding mouse ESCs, gene-transfer strategies have also been successfully employed. Genes encoding transcription factors that promote DA neurons development and survival (e.g., Lmx1a, Nurr1 and Pitx3) have been overexpressed (Kim *et al.*, 2002; Kanda *et al.*, 2004; Chung *et al.*, 2005; Andersson *et al.*, 2006). Using different combinations of these strategies, mouse ESC cultures containing around 50% TH-immunopositive neurons (Kim *et al.*, 2002) and human ESC cultures made up of approximately 25–30% TH-positive neurons have been obtained (Perrier *et al.*, 2004; Roy *et al.*, 2006). Despite the apparent success in obtaining TH- positive, dopaminergic neurons from ESCs in culture, there are at least three major obstacles facing clinical application of these cells in PD. First, many of the protocols use animal-derived products in the culture media or feeder cells. To eliminate the risk of transfer of zoonoses or molecules that stimulate immune rejection on the grafted cells, clinical grade ESCs must be completely xeno-free. Second, while the functional efficacy of grafted DA neurons derived from mouse ESCs has been well documented (Kim *et al.*, 2002), this is still not the case for human ESCs-derived DA neurons xenografted to immunosuppressed rats. For reasons that are not yet fully understood, it is more difficult to get good survival and function of TH-positive neurons derived from human than from mouse ESCs. Third, another major practical problem lies in the heterogeneity of the cultured cells. Somewhat unlike the

developing embryonic brain, neural differentiation from ESCs is not synchronous in the culture dish. Some ESCs can remain in an undifferentiated pluripotent state, even when most neighboring cells have initiated neural differentiation. Additionally, some cells escape neural commitment and differentiate into other cell types even under the currently best conditions for neural induction. The fact that some cells continue to proliferate, either as immature neuroepithelial progenitors or in the form of pluripotent stem cells, means that there is a risk for tumor or even teratoma formation after transplantation. Obviously, this risk has to be completely eliminated before clinical application can be considered. For these reason, methods that either purge the proliferating cells or positively select the DA neurons from the cultures—without jeopardizing their survival after grafting—need to be developed.

Keeping an Eye on Spheramine

Another cell type has been tested in transplantation studies in PD, namely human retinal pigment epithelial (hRPE) cells. In a commercially driven trial, cultured hRPE cells are attached to gelatin microcarriers (Spheramine) and injected stereotaxically into the putamen. An open-label pilot study in patients with advanced PD suggested that at least there were some short-term benefits (Bakay *et al.*, 2004). The mechanism of action of grafted hRPE cells on microcarriers is not well understood. Although hRPE cells do not form axons or synaptic connections with host tissue like fetal mesencephalic DA neurons, they can produce some DA and levodopa. They are also reported to secrete a number of growth factors, such as platelet-derived growth factor (PDGF), epidermal growth factor (EGF), fibroblast growth factor (FGF), insulin-like growth factor (IGF), transforming growth factor (TGF), vascular endothelial growth factor (VEGF), nitric oxide, pigment epithelial-derived factor (PEDF), and Fas-ligand.

The advantage of hRPE cells is their availability. Aside from the commercial development of Sphereamine, hRPE cells can be obtained from eye banks and be expanded easily in culture. Cells from single donor eyes could potentially treat several hundred patients. However, a recently completed Phase IIb clinical trial failed to reach neither it's primary nor key secondary endpoints for efficacy so the future of this strategy in the clinic is uncertain (Spheramine, 2008).

GENE THERAPY FOR PARKINSON'S DISEASE

The development of novel viral vector-based therapeutics has made considerable impact in pre-clinical studies during the last decade. Viral vectors have proven to be powerful tools to interfere with disease progress or restore normal function in slow, chronic, neurodegenerative diseases. Results obtained in models of PD have been particularly encouraging.

To date, the most-studied viral vectors for gene transfer to the brain are based on adeno-associated virus (AAV), lentivirus (LV), adenovirus, and to a lesser extent herpes simplex virus. The recombinant AAV (rAAV) vectors, in particular, have a functional and safety profile that makes them very well suited for CNS application in the clinic; Firstly, these vectors are not known to cause any pathology in humans (Chen et al., 2005; Schnepp et al., 2005). Secondly, 96% of the viral genome can be deleted without loss of the transduction ability. Thus, no viral genes are retained in the final therapeutic vector preparation. Thirdly, rAAV vectors can transduce non-dividing cells such as neurons, and, since the transgene does not integrate in the chromosomes, the risk of insertional mutagenesis is very low. Finally, transgene expression is very stable and long-lasting. Thus, genes transferred using rAAV vectors have been shown to be functional for over 12 months in rodents and up to six years in primates.

Due to their unique properties, rAAV vectors have been approved for the first pioneering clinical gene therapy trials in PD. There are currently three clinical trials for gene therapy in PD patients approved by the FDA (Clinical trial identifier numbers: NCT00195143, NCT00229736 and NCT00252850; see http://clinicaltrial.gov/ for more details). In this chapter we will review the rationale behind these gene therapy approaches and summarize the results obtained so far.

Continuous DOPA Delivery Strategy

The concept of continuous DOPA delivery to the brain using *in vivo* gene therapy is more attractive than oral L-DOPA administration. Continuous DOPA delivery might reverse DA-dependent motor deficits without generating the side effects seen with peripheral intermittent L-DOPA pharmacotherapy. Motor fluctuations and dyskinesias in PD are thought to develop, at least in part due to the intermittent and pulsatile nature of orally delivered L-DOPA acting on supersensitive DA receptors on striatal GABAergic neurons (Chase, 1998; Nutt, Obeso and Stocchi, 2000). This is directly supported by data obtained in patient trials, where continuous delivery of L-DOPA via duodenal or intravenous pumps, or subcutaneous infusion of the DA receptor agonist apomorphine can significantly reduce the severity and frequency of motor fluctuations and dyskinesias (Mouradian et al., 1990; Nutt, Obeso and Stocchi, 2000; Olanow, Obeso and Stocchi, 2006).

In line with these clinical data, it was recently shown that when rAAV vectors transduce striatal cells with human TH and GCH1 genes, continuous DOPA production can be reinstituted in the brain. The TH-cofactor tetrahydrobiopterin (BH_4) is important for proper functioning of the TH enzyme, and it is normally synthesized by the enzyme GCH1. This importance of GCH1 for DA neurons is evident from patients with hereditary progressive dystonia, who exhibit Parkinson-like symptoms due to mutations in the GCH1 gene (Ichinose et al., 1994). In rats previously rendered dyskinetic by chronic pulsatile L-DOPA injections, the severity of abnormal dyskinetic movements gradually declined by 85% after transduction of TH and GCH1 genes with rAAV vectors in the striatum (Carlsson et al., 2005). Moreover, efficient DOPA synthesis using these vectors also supported substantial improvements in both drug-induced and spontaneous motor tests in rodent models of PD (Kirik et al., 2002). These experimental data show that continuous DOPA delivery is a promising treatment strategy for PD. It is now being tested in MPTP-treated monkeys with the hope that the first clinical trials using this approach can be initiated, if the results are positive.

Continuous DA Delivery Strategy

Following degeneration of DA neurons in the substantia nigra, and their axon terminals in the striatum, not only TH but also AADC enzyme activity is reduced. Although oral L-DOPA medication provides symptomatic relief in PD patients, it has been argued that the residual, striatal AADC activity might be insufficient for optimal DA synthesis in the parkinsonian brain. Therefore, the effects of combining the TH gene transfer approach with supplementation of the AADC activity have been evaluated in rodents and primates (Fan et al., 1998; Shen et al., 2000; Muramatsu et al., 2002).

Muramatsu and colleagues successfully applied triple gene delivery of TH/GCH1/AADC in a primate brain, using a three-vector co-injection paradigm. Tremor and bradykinesia were ameliorated contralateral to the injected striatum in the monkeys (Muramatsu *et al.*, 2002). The animals improved on a primate parkinsonian rating scale by up to 64% after two weeks and this was stable for 10 months. Hand dexterity particularly improved and some of the treated monkeys could pick up raisins more quickly. Whether a single vector containing all three genes can provide functional improvement after injection into the brain of a parkinsonian primate remains to be studied. Although, all studies we have presented so far are based on rAAV vectors, rLV vectors are superior to rAAV vectors with regards to cloning capacity and would be required for a single vector delivery of the three genes TH/GCH1/AADC. These vectors have can also mediate long-term expression in terminally differentiated cells in the brain.

The striatal neurons targeted with the triple gene transfer protocol do not express any the vesicular monoamine transporter 2 (VMAT2), as they normally do not produce monoamines. Therefore they are unable to store the DA that is produced in the cytoplasm in vesicles. As a consequence, increased levels of cytoplasmic DA following gene therapy may inhibit the TH enzyme present in the same cell through a negative feedback mechanism. A truncated form of TH (tTH), which lacks 160 amino acids in the N-terminal regulatory domain, is less inhibited by DA (Moffat *et al.*, 1997). Using a non-human LV, the equine infectious anemia virus (EIAV), Azzouz and colleagues showed that a single transcript unit expressing tTH, GCH1 and AADC can successfully transduce these genes in rat striatal cells, forcing co-expression in each infected cell (Azzouz *et al.*, 2002). Using this construct, Oxford BioMedica conducted a pre-clinical study to show the efficacy of the treatment in non-human primates with MPTP lesions. The results publicly available at this date show increased motor performance in treated animals, compared to monkeys with lesions alone. The difference was already significant at two weeks and was maintained up to 15 months (ProSavin, 2007).

Enhanced DA Synthesis from Peripheral L-DOPA

An alternative strategy to transduction of the TH/GCH1/AADC genes is to express the AADC gene alone and provide L-DOPA by pharmacotherapy (Leff *et al.*, 1998). In this case, the transgene would have no effect until L-DOPA was given exogenously, thus providing a safety measure and the possibility to customize the dosing simply by adjusting the medication for each patient (Leff *et al.*, 1998; Bankiewicz *et al.*, 2000). Secondly, as AADC activity in the striatum is selectively enhanced, it is possible to reach to higher DA levels in the striatal target areas with a lower dose of systemic L-DOPA administration. This in turn may lead to fewer side effects that can occur with high doses of L-DOPA due to its actions in non-striatal brain regions.

High levels of AADC expression in circumscribed striatal regions may create unwanted large gradients in tissue DA concentrations. Bankiewicz and collaborators showed that such a focal striatal DA production can potentiate the dyskinetic side effects of L-DOPA. This problem was persistent at all doses of L-DOPA tested, even below the therapeutic doses (Bankiewicz *et al.*, 2006a). By contrast, in a study where more widespread transduction of the AADC gene was achieved, no serious side effects were observed. The response to acute L-DOPA was improved and stable after 12 months, and maintained up to six years (Bankiewicz *et al.*, 2006b). Interestingly, the first clinical trial combining AADC gene delivery with systemic L-DOPA has recently been completed (Eberling *et al.*, 2008) (http://clinicaltrial.gov/show/NCT00229736).

While the AADC-transduced striatal neurons decarboxylate L-DOPA very effectively, they cannot store and release DA. It is therefore unknown if and how the synthesized DA exits the cells and reaches striatal DA receptors. It is also unclear what the long-term consequences are of DA production in striatal neurons, and if high cytosolic DA levels, coupled with an inefficient release, will result in cellular dysfunction.

Targeting the Subthalamic Nucleus Through Gene Therapy

The loss of dopaminergic stimulation in the striatum of PD patients results in over-activity of the subthalamic nucleus (STN). This structure sends excitatory projections to both the substantia nigra pars reticulata and the internal segment of the globus pallidus. The net effect of this stimulation is an inhibition of the motor output pathways in the cortex, which is believed to underlie the motor symptoms in PD. Therefore, the STN is a therapeutic target in PD. The most widely used therapeutic intervention in STN is deep brain stimulation, (DBS, described in detail in Chapter 7). The success of DBS indicates that manipulation of STN activity is a valid approach to relieving motor problems in PD. Consequently a gene-therapy approach to reducing STN activity has been developed. This strategy is based on over-expression of the glutamic acid decarboxylase (GAD) in the glutamatergic cells of the STN, resulting in an increased production of the inhibitory neurotransmitter γ-aminobutyric acid (GABA) instead. Thereby, an intrinsic, inhibitory, signaling pathway in the overactive projection neurons of the STN would be created. If this hypothesis holds true, this intervention should alleviate PD symptoms. The first clinical trial testing the safety of rAAV vectors encoding the GAD gene, were recently reported (Kaplitt *et al.*, 2007) (http://clinicaltrial.gov/show/NCT00195143). Kaplitt *et al.* studied side effects from over-expression of GAD in the sub-thalamic nucleus in 12 patients with moderate or advanced PD, displaying motor complications with L-DOPA therapy. They were followed for 12 months after surgery and assessed for motor performance, complications of therapy, activities of daily living and metabolic changes in the brain, using positron emission tomography. They improved in both "on" and "off" motor scores by three months—an effect that was maintained in 10 out of 12 patients in "off" at 12 months. There was no improvement in activities of daily living, but a significant reduction of glucose metabolism of the thalamus ipsilateral to the injected STN at 12 months.

A major safety concern with clinical rAAV gene therapy is the risk of an immune reaction to the vector. This is based on the fact that up to 80% of the population is expected to have circulating antibodies against the capsid antigens of at least one wild-type AAV species. Thus, pre-existing neutralizing antibodies against the therapeutic rAAV vectors can be a potential complication and must be investigated carefully (Peden et al., 2004; Sanftner et al., 2004). In a phase I trial utilizing rAAV2 vectors for the treatment of Canavan's disease, neutralizing antibodies were detected in a subset (3 out of 10) of the treated patients (McPhee et al., 2006). In the study by Kaplitt and coworkers, two PD patients showed evidence of substantial anti-AAV2 immunity (the serotype of the injected rAAV-GAD) at baseline. Except for a small, transient spike in IgM concentration at six months, there were no changes in antibody titers recorded throughout the study.

This trial on GAD gene therapy is the first published study utilizing rAAV for in vivo gene delivery in adult patients. Therefore, it has wide-reaching implications for the whole field of gene therapy in PD. A positive outcome of this trial should pave the way for other rAAV-based clinical therapies in the brain, not only in PD (Stoessl,).

Growth Factor Therapy

In 1954, nerve growth factor was discovered by Rita Levi-Montalcini. It was the first known molecule with neurotrophic properties and marked the starting point for a novel area of research concerning growth factors for treatment of neurodegenerative disorders. Due to its potent actions on DA neurons, glial cell line-derived neurotrophic factor (GDNF), which was discovered in 1993, has attracted great interest in the last decade. GDNF therapy differs from some of the other novel therapeutic strategies we have discussed (e.g., DBS, GAD overexpression and DA replacement) in that it potentially is disease-modifying and does not only reduce symptoms. Thus, once patients are treated with GDNF, the course of the disease can be altered or even halted completely. In primate models of PD, GDNF has been shown to provide robust protection of the nigral dopaminergic neurons from toxin-induced (MPTP or 6-OHDA) degeneration, increase the DA levels in the striatum and improve the animals' motor function.

The first clinical trial utilizing GDNF was initiated in 1996. The study was based on infusion of recombinant GDNF protein into the intracerebroventricular space with mechanical pumps using a randomized, double-blind design (Nutt et al., 2003). Fifty subjects with moderate or advanced idiopathic PD were chosen for this study. Treated patients received bolus injections of 25–4000 µg GDNF into the ventricles once monthly over 28 months (the first eight months blinded). The results were disappointing, as patients did not improve in response to GDNF. Instead, several adverse events were observed. These included weight loss, nausea, vomiting, depression and paresthesias described as an electric shock (L'Hermitte's sign). In retrospect, the lack of symptomatic relief has been attributed to the limited penetration of GDNF from the cerebrospinal fluid into the brain parenchyma, as demonstrated by post-mortem analysis in one patient from this study (Kordower et al., 1999). The adverse events were probably the results of GDNF actions outside the basal ganglia; GDNF receptors are widely expressed in the central nervous system. This study illustrated that focal delivery of GDNF directly into the parenchyma of the basal ganglia may be a better strategy.

The second clinical GDNF trial had a phase I safety design. GDNF was infused using a pump (short pulses of delivery, several times a day) via an intraparenchymal catheter into the posterodorsal putamen on both sides of the brain (Gill et al., 2003). All five patients were L-DOPA responsive, idiopathic PD cases. The outcome was encouraging, with no serious adverse events and clear improvement in motor performance. At the one-year time point, the patients displayed about 40% improvement in the motor sub-score of UPDRS and about 60% improvement in the activities of daily living sub-score, coupled with a decrease in dyskinesias and increase in $[^{18}F]$-DOPA uptake in the putamen. One patient died 46 months after surgery and histological examination revealed an area of dense TH-immunoreactivity, presumed to be sprouting of nigrostriatal fibers, around an injection tract (Love et al., 2005). A second independent open-label trial by another group of investigators reported similar positive findings of motor improvement in 10 patients, as seen in the first trial (Slevin et al., 2005). After 12 months of GDNF infusion, these patients were shifted to saline infusion and monitored for an additional year. At 9–12 months after cessation of GDNF infusion, the UPDRS scores returned to baseline and the patients required increased pharmacotherapy (Slevin et al., 2007).

Based on these data, a multi-center, blinded, clinical trial of GDNF delivery into the putamen was conducted (Lang et al., 2006). The results from this trial differed from the open-label trials and there was no symptomatic relief. Some patients displayed adverse events due to the GDNF infusion, including paraesthesia and headache. Although there was an increase in $[^{18}F]$-DOPA uptake around the infusion cannula in the posterior putamen of the treated patients, they actually displayed a tendency towards a worsening of the UPDRS scores.

The discrepancies between the open-label and blinded GDNF trials remain unclear. The surgical protocol used in the blinded trial differed on several points to the one used in the open-label trials. Most notably, patient selection (milder disease in the open-label trials) and differences in the infusion protocol (cannula diameter and number of ports, etc.) could have played a role. In addition, it is also possible that placebo effects contributed to the positive outcome of the open-label trial (Sherer et al., 2006).

For continuous in vivo delivery of trophic factors, two alternatives to infusion of the growth factor have been developed. The first is based on an encapsulated cell bio-delivery platform, where genetically engineered cells that secrete GDNF have been used. Encapsulated cells can secrete significant amounts of GDNF for more than one year in the primate brain and have been placed both in the intracerebroventricular space and into the striatum (Kishima et al., 2004). Placement into the parenchyma has yielded the most promising results so far. The encapsulated cells are derived from well-characterized, immortalized cell lines that have been genetically modified in vitro to stably express and secrete GDNF. These cells are encapsulated in semi-permeable, polymeric, hollow fibers that are heat sealed after the loading of the cells to prevent migration out of the capsule. The clinical development of the encapsulated cell bio-delivery platform is being carried out by a Danish biotechnology company (see (ECB, 2007) for further information on this platform) (Ahn et al., 2005). A multi-center collaborative effort has now been initiated and plans to carry out the first clinical trials of encapsulated cells releasing GDNF in PD patients (LEAPS, 2005).

The second alternative strategy for continuous delivery of GDNF into the brains of PD patients uses viral vectors for in vivo genes encoding GDNF, or other members of the same family of trophic factors. Viral vector-mediated delivery of GDNF into the putamen is very efficient at protecting the DA system against MPTP-induced damage in monkeys. The neuroprotection is coupled to major behavioral benefits. Extensive efficacy data exists for both rLV and rAAV vectors encoding GDNF or related factors in rodent and primate models. These data form the basis for clinical applications. In fact, the first phase I safety trial was recently completed. The study tested the safety of rAAV-mediated delivery of neurturin, another member of the GDNF family that binds to the GDNF receptor with lower affinity (http://clinicaltrial.gov/show/NCT00252850). In this study, 12 patients received intraputaminal injections of rAAV coding for human neuturin gene driven by the NGF promoter. At nine months follow-up, the patients appear to tolerate the treatment well. In addition, they are reported to display a reduction of the UPDRS motor "off" score by 40%, shortening of "off" time by 50% and doubling of dyskinesias-free "on" time (Marks et al., 2008). Based on these data, a phase II trial comprising 51 patients has been initiated.

CONCLUDING REMARKS

Twenty years have passed since the first clinical cell transplantation trials in PD and 10 years since the first GDNF trial. In this chapter we have described some of the obstacles that need to be overcome for these novel therapies to be widely applicable in PD. In retrospect, the numerous clinical trials have led us to the conclusion that there are no "quick fixes" and no short cuts to a new effective treatment. We need to fully understand the mechanisms of cell differentiation to DA neurons and we need to master the delivery of cells and genes into the brain parenchyma in a safe and reliable way before we are likely to consistently succeed with these novel therapies in patients. A number of important pre-clinical discoveries and clinical trials have been made in recent years, both regarding cell- and gene-based therapy in PD. Hopefully they will pave the way for success with both these approaches in the not-too-distant future.

ACKNOWLEDGEMENTS

T.B. is supported by a National Institutes of Health R01 grant. A. M. is supported by Stiftelsen Olle Engkvist Byggmästare and the Swedish Institute. D.K. and P.B. are supported by the Swedish Research Council. All authors are members of NeuroFortis and of the Nordic Network of Excellence on Neurodegeneration.

References

Ahn, Y.H., Bensadoun, J.C., Aebischer, P. et al. (2005) Increased fiber outgrowth from xeno-transplanted human embryonic dopaminergic neurons with co-implants of polymer-encapsulated genetically modified cells releasing glial cell line-derived neurotrophic factor. Brain Research Bulletin, 66, 135–142.

Alvarez-Dolado, M., Pardal, R., Garcia-Verdugo, J.M. et al. (2003) Fusion of bone-marrow-derived cells with Purkinje neurons, cardiomyocytes and hepatocytes.e. Nature, 425, 968–973.

Andersson, E., Tryggvason, U., Deng, Q. et al. (2006) Identification of intrinsic determinants of midbrain dopamine neurons. Cell, 124, 393–405.

Andersson, E.K., Irvin, D.K., Ahlsio, J. and Parmar, M. (2007) Ngn2 and Nurr1 act in synergy to induce midbrain dopaminergic neurons from expanded neural stem and progenitor cells. Experimental Cell Research, 313, 1172–1180.

Azzouz, M., Martin-Rendon, E., Barber, R.D. et al. (2002) Multicistronic lentiviral vector-mediated striatal gene transfer of aromatic L-amino acid decarboxylase, tyrosine hydroxylase, and GTP cyclohydrolase I induces sustained transgene expression, dopamine production, and functional improvement in a rat model of Parkinson's disease. *The Journal of Neuroscience*, **22**, 10302–10312.

Bakay, R.A., Raiser, C.D., Stover, N.P. *et al.* (2004) Implantation of Spheramine in advanced Parkinson's disease (PD). *Frontiers in Bioscience: A Journal and Virtual Library*, **9**, 592–602.

Bankiewicz, K.S., Daadi, M., Pivirotto, P. *et al.* (2006a) Focal striatal dopamine may potentiate dyskinesias in parkinsonian monkeys. *Experimental Neurology*, **197**, 363–372.

Bankiewicz, K.S., Eberling, J.L., Kohutnicka, M. *et al.* (2000) Convection-enhanced delivery of AAV vector in parkinsonian monkeys; *in vivo* detection of gene expression and restoration of dopaminergic function using pro-drug approach. *Experimental Neurology*, **164**, 2–14.

Bankiewicz, K.S., Forsayeth, J., Eberling, J.L. *et al.* (2006b) Long-Term Clinical Improvement in MPTP-Lesioned Primates after Gene Therapy with AAV-hAADC. *Molecular Therapy: The Journal of the American Society of Gene Therapy*, **14**, 564–570.

Bjorklund, A., Stenevi, U. and Svendgaard, N. (1976) Growth of transplanted monoaminergic neurones into the adult hippocampus along the perforant path. *Nature*, **262**, 787–790.

Bjorklund, A., Dunnett, S.B., Brundin, P. *et al.* (2003) Neural transplantation for the treatment of Parkinson's disease. *Lancet Neurology*, **2**, 437–445.

Brevig, T., Holgersson, J. and Widner, H. (2000) Xenotransplantation for CNS repair: immunological barriers and strategies to overcome them. *Trends in Neurosciences*, **23**, 337–344.

Brundin, P. and Hagell, P. (2001) The neurobiology of cell transplantation in Parkinson's disease. *Clinical Neuroscience Research*, **1**, 507–520.

Brundin, P., Duan, W.-M. and Sauer, H. (1994) Functional effects of mesencephalic dopamine neurons and adrenal chromaffin cells grafted to the striatum, in Functional Neural Transplantation (eds S.B. Dunnett and A. Björklund), Raven Press, pp. 9–46.

Carlsson, T., Winkler, C., Lundblad, M. *et al.* (2006) Graft placement and uneven pattern of reinnervation in the striatum is important for development of graft-induced dyskinesia. *Neurobiology of Disease*, **21**, 657–668.

Carlsson, T., Winkler, C., Burger, C. *et al.* (2005) Reversal of dyskinesias in an animal model of Parkinson's disease by continuous L-DOPA delivery using rAAV vectors. *Brain: A Journal of Neurology*, **128**, 559–569.

Chase, T.N. (1998) Levodopa therapy: consequences of the non-physiologic replacement of dopamine. *Neurology*, **50**, S17–S25.

Chen, C.L., Jensen, R.L., Schnepp, B.C. *et al.* (2005) Molecular characterization of adeno-associated viruses infecting children. *Journal of Virology*, **79**, 14781–14792.

Christophersen, N.S., Meijer, X., Jorgensen, J.R. *et al.* (2006) Induction of dopaminergic neurons from growth factor expanded neural stem/progenitor cell cultures derived from human first trimester forebrain. *Brain Research Bulletin*, **70**, 457–466.

Chung, S., Hedlund, E., Hwang, M. *et al.* (2005) The homeodomain transcription factor Pitx3 facilitates differentiation of mouse embryonic stem cells into AHD2-expressing dopaminergic neurons. *Molecular and Cellular Neurosciences*, **28**, 241–252.

Cogle, C.R., Yachnis, A.T., Laywell, E.D. *et al.* (2004) Bone marrow transdifferentiation in brain after transplantation: a retrospective study. *Lancet*, **363**, 1432–1437.

Curtis, M.A., Kam, M., Nannmark, U. *et al.* (2007) Human neuroblasts migrate to the olfactory bulb via a lateral ventricular extension. *Science (New York, NY)*, **315**, 1243–1249.

ECB (2007) NsGene: EC-biodelivery Platform, http://www.nsgene.dk/Default.aspx?ID=26.

Eberling, J.L., Jagust, W.J., Christine, C.W. *et al.* (2008) Results from a phase I safety trial of hAADC gene therapy for Parkinson's disease. *Neurology*, **70**, 1980–1983.

Eriksson, P.S., Perfilieva, E., Bjork-Eriksson, T. *et al.* (1998) Neurogenesis in the adult human hippocampus. *Nature Medicine*, **4**, 1313–1317.

Fan, D.S., Ogawa, M., Fujimoto, K.I. *et al.* (1998) Behavioral recovery in 6-hydroxydopamine-lesioned rats by cotransduction of striatum with tyrosine hydroxylase and aromatic L-amino acid decarboxylase genes using two separate adeno-associated virus vectors. *Human Gene Therapy*, **9**, 2527–2535.

Freed, C.R., Breeze, R.E., Fahn, S. and Eidelberg, D. (2004) Preoperative response to levodopa is the best predictor of transplant outcome. *Annals of Neurology*, **55**, 896–897.

Freed, C.R., Greene, P.E., Breeze, R.E. *et al.* (2001) Transplantation of embryonic dopamine neurons for severe Parkinson's disease. *The New England Journal of Medicine*, **344**, 710–719.

Gage, F.H. (2000) Mammalian neural stem cells. *Science (New York, NY)*, **287**, 1433–1438.

Gage, F.H., Ray, J. and Fisher, L.J. (1995) Isolation, characterization, and use of stem cells from the CNS. *Annual Review of Neuroscience*, **18**, 159–192.

Gill, S.S., Patel, N.K., Hotton, G.R. *et al.* (2003) Direct brain infusion of glial cell line-derived neurotrophic factor in Parkinson's disease. *Nature Medicine*, **9**, 589–595.

Goetz, C.G., Stebbins, G.T., 3rd Klawans, H.L. *et al.* (1991) United Parkinson Foundation Neurotransplantation Registry on adrenal medullary transplants: presurgical, and 1- and 2-year follow-up. *Neurology*, **41**, 1719–1722.

Hagell, P. and Cenci, M.A. (2005) Dyskinesias and dopamine cell replacement in Parkinson's disease: a clinical perspective. *Brain Research Bulletin*, **68**, 4–15.

Hagell, P., Piccini, P., Bjorklund, A. *et al.* (2002) Dyskinesias following neural transplantation in Parkinson's disease. *Nature Neuroscience*, **5**, 627–628.

Ichinose, H., Ohye, T., Takahashi, E. *et al.* (1994) Hereditary progressive dystonia with marked diurnal fluctuation caused by mutations in the GTP cyclohydrolase I gene. *Nature Genetics*, **8**, 236–242.

Kanda, S., Tamada, Y., Yoshidome, A. *et al.* (2004) Over-expression of bHLH genes facilitate neural formation of mouse embryonic stem (ES) cells *in vitro*. *International Journal of Developmental Neuroscience*, **22**, 149–156.

Kaplitt, M.G., Feigin, A., Tang, C. *et al.* (2007) Safety and tolerability of gene therapy with an adeno-associated virus (AAV) borne GAD gene for Parkinson's disease: an open label, phase I trial. *Lancet*, **369**, 2097–2105.

Kawasaki, H., Mizuseki, K., Nishikawa, S. *et al.* (2000) Induction of midbrain dopaminergic neurons from ES cells by stromal cell-derived inducing activity. *Neuron*, **28**, 31–40.

Kim, D.W., Chung, S., Hwang, M. *et al.* (2006) Stromal cell-derived inducing activity, Nurr1, and signaling molecules synergistically induce dopaminergic neurons from mouse embryonic stem cells. *Stem Cells (Dayton, Ohio)*, **24**, 557–567.

Kim, H.J., Sugimori, M., Nakafuku, M. and Svendsen, C.N. (2007) Control of neurogenesis and tyrosine hydroxylase expression in neural progenitor cells through bHLH proteins and Nurr1. *Experimental Neurology*, **203**, 394–405.

Kim, J.H., Auerbach, J.M., Rodriguez-Gomez, J.A. *et al.* (2002) Dopamine neurons derived from embryonic stem cells function in an animal model of Parkinson's disease. *Nature*, **418**, 50–56.

Kirik, D., Georgievska, B., Burger, C. *et al.* (2002) Reversal of motor impairments in parkinsonian rats by continuous intrastriatal delivery of L-dopa using rAAV-mediated gene transfer. *Proceedings of the National Academy of Sciences of the United States of America*, **99**, 4708–4713.

Kishima, H., Poyot, T., Bloch, J. *et al.* (2004) Encapsulated GDNF-producing C2C12 cells for Parkinson's disease: a pre-clinical study in chronic MPTP-treated baboons. *Neurobiology of Disease*, 16, 428–439.

Kordower, J.H., Freeman, T.B., Chen, E.Y. *et al.* (1998) Fetal nigral grafts survive and mediate clinical benefit in a patient with Parkinson's disease. *Movement Disorders*, 13, 383–393.

Kordower, J.H., Palfi, S., Chen, E.Y. *et al.* (1999) Clinicopathological findings following intraventricular glial-derived neurotrophic factor treatment in a patient with Parkinson's disease. *Annals of Neurology*, 46, 419–424.

Lane, E.L., Winkler, C., Brundin, P. and Cenci, M.A. (2006) The impact of graft size on the development of dyskinesia following intrastriatal grafting of embryonic dopamine neurons in the rat. *Neurobiology of Disease*, 22, 334–345.

Lang, A.E., Gill, S., Patel, N.K. *et al.* (2006) Randomized controlled trial of intraputamenal glial cell line-derived neurotrophic factor infusion in Parkinson's disease. *Annals of Neurology*, 59, 459–466.

LEAPS (2005) Michael J Fox foundation: Encapsulated GDNF-Producing Cells for Neuroprotection in Parkinson's Disease, http://www.michaeljfox.org/research_MJFFfunding-Portfolio_searchableAwardedGrants_3.cfm?ID=134.

Lee, S.H., Lumelsky, N., Studer, L. *et al.* (2000) Efficient generation of midbrain and hindbrain neurons from mouse embryonic stem cells. *Nature Biotechnology*, 18, 675–679.

Leff, S.E., Rendahl, K.G., Spratt, S.K. *et al.* (1998) *In vivo* L-DOPA production by genetically modified primary rat fibroblast or 9L gliosarcoma cell grafts via coexpression of GTPcyclohydrolase I with tyrosine hydroxylase. *Experimental Neurology*, 151, 249–264.

Levitt, P., Moore, R.Y. and Garber, B.B. (1976) Selective cell association of catecholamine neurons in brain aggregates *in vitro*. *Brain Research*, 111, 311–320.

Lindvall, O. and Hagell, P. (2000) Clinical observations after neural transplantation in Parkinson's disease. *Prog Brain Res*, 127, 299–320.

Lindvall, O., Backlund, E.O., Farde, L. *et al.* (1987) Transplantation in Parkinson's disease: two cases of adrenal medullary grafts to the putamen. *Annals of Neurology*, 22, 457–468.

Love, S., Plaha, P., Patel, N.K. *et al.* (2005) Glial cell line-derived neurotrophic factor induces neuronal sprouting in human brain. *Nature Medicine*, 11, 703–704.

Madrazo, I., Drucker-Colin, R., Diaz, V. *et al.* (1987) Open microsurgical autograft of adrenal medulla to the right caudate nucleus in two patients with intractable Parkinson's disease. *The New England Journal of Medicine*, 316, 831–834.

Maherali, N., Sridharan, R., Xie, W. *et al.* (2007) Directly reprogrammed fibroblasts show global epigenetic remodeling and widespread tissue contribution. *Cell Stem Cell*, 1, 55–70.

Marks, W.J., Jr., Ostrem, J.L., Verhagen, L. *et al.* (2008) Safety and tolerability of intraputaminal delivery of CERE-120 (adeno-associated virus serotype 2-neurturin) to patients with idiopathic Parkinson's disease: an open-label, Phase I trial. *Lancet Neurology*, 7, 400–408.

McPhee, S.W., Janson, C.G., Li, C. *et al.* (2006) Immune responses to AAV in a phase I study for Canavan disease. *The Journal of Gene Medicine*, 8, 577–588.

Mendez, I., Sanchez-Pernaute, R., Cooper, O. *et al.* (2005) Cell type analysis of functional fetal dopamine cell suspension transplants in the striatum and substantia nigra of patients with Parkinson's disease. *Brain: A Journal of Neurology*, 128, 1498–1510.

Moffat, M., Harmon, S., Haycock, J. and O'Malley, K.L. (1997) L-Dopa and dopamine-producing gene cassettes for gene therapy approaches to Parkinson's disease. *Experimental Neurology*, 144, 69–73.

Mouradian, M.M., Heuser, I.J., Baronti, F. and Chase, T.N. (1990) Modification of central dopaminergic mechanisms by continuous levodopa therapy for advanced Parkinson's disease. *Annals of Neurology*, 27, 18–23.

Muramatsu, S., Fujimoto, K., Ikeguchi, K. *et al.* (2002) Behavioral recovery in a primate model of Parkinson's disease by triple transduction of striatal cells with adeno-associated viral vectors expressing dopamine-synthesizing enzymes. *Human Gene Therapy*, 13, 345–354.

Nutt, J.G., Obeso, J.A. and Stocchi, F. (2000) Continuous dopamine-receptor stimulation in advanced Parkinson's disease. *Trends in Neurosciences*, 23, S109–115.

Nutt, J.G., Burchiel, K.J., Comella, C.L. *et al.* (2003) Randomized, double-blind trial of glial cell line-derived neurotrophic factor (GDNF) in PD. *Neurology*, 60, 69–73.

Okita, K., Ichisaka, T. and Yamanaka, S. (2007) Generation of germline-competent induced pluripotent stem cells. *Nature*, 448, 313–317.

Olanow, C.W., Obeso, J.A. and Stocchi, F. (2006) Continuous dopamine-receptor treatment of Parkinson's disease: scientific rationale and clinical implications. *Lancet Neurol*, 5, 677–687.

Olanow, C.W., Goetz, C.G., Kordower, J.H. *et al.* (2003) A double-blind controlled trial of bilateral fetal nigral transplantation in Parkinson's disease. *Annals of Neurology*, 54, 403–414.

Olson, L. and Malmfors, T. (1970) Growth characteristics of adrenergic nerves in the adult rat. Fluorescence histochemical and 3H-noradrenaline uptake studies using tissue transplantations to the anterior chamber of the eye. *Acta Physiologica Scandinavica Supplement*, 348, 1–112.

Olson, L. and Seiger, A. (1972) Brain tissue transplanted to the anterior chamber of the eye. 1. Fluorescence histochemistry of immature catecholamine and 5-hydroxytryptamine neurons reinnervating the rat iris. *Zeitschrift fur Zellforschung und Mikroskopische Anatomie*, 135, 175–194.

Ostenfeld, T., Caldwell, M.A., Prowse, K.R. *et al.* (2000) Human neural precursor cells express low levels of telomerase *in vitro* and show diminishing cell proliferation with extensive axonal outgrowth following transplantation. *Experimental Neurology*, 164, 215–226.

Park, C.H., Kang, J.S., Shin, Y.H. *et al.* (2006) Acquisition of *in vitro* and *in vivo* functionality of Nurr1-induced dopamine neurons. *The FASEB Journal*, 20, 2553–2555.

Peden, C.S., Burger, C., Muzyczka, N. and Mandel, R.J. (2004) Circulating anti-wild-type adeno-associated virus type 2 (AAV2) antibodies inhibit recombinant AAV2 (rAAV2)-mediated, but not rAAV5-mediated, gene transfer in the brain. *Journal of Virology*, 78, 6344–6359.

Perrier, A.L., Tabar, V., Barberi, T. *et al.* (2004) Derivation of midbrain dopamine neurons from human embryonic stem cells. *Proceedings of the National Academy of Sciences of the United States of America*, 101, 12543–12548.

Piccini, P., Brooks, D.J., Bjorklund, A. *et al.* (1999) Dopamine release from nigral transplants visualized *in vivo* in a Parkinson's patient. *Nature Neuroscience*, 2, 1137–1140.

Piccini, P., Lindvall, O., Bjorklund, A. *et al.* (2000) Delayed recovery of movement-related cortical function in Parkinson's disease after striatal dopaminergic grafts. *Annals of Neurology*, 48, 689–695.

Priller, J., Persons, D.A., Klett, F.F. *et al.* (2001) Neogenesis of cerebellar Purkinje neurons from gene-marked bone marrow cells *in vivo*. *The Journal of Cell Biology*, 155, 733–738.

ProSavin (2007) Oxford BioMedica: Oxford Biomedica Presents Encouraging Preclinical Efficacy Data With Prosavin In Parkinson's Disease, http://www.oxfordbiomedica.co.uk/news/2006-ob-24.htm.

Rice, C.M. and Scolding, N.J. (2004) Adult stem cells–reprogramming neurological repair? *Lancet*, **364**, 193–199.

Roy, N.S., Cleren, C., Singh, S.K. *et al.* (2006) Functional engraftment of human ES cell-derived dopaminergic neurons enriched by coculture with telomerase-immortalized midbrain astrocytes. *Nature Medicine*, **12**, 1259–1268.

Roybon, L., Brundin, P. and Li, J.Y. (2005) Stromal cell-derived inducing activity does not promote dopaminergic differentiation, but enhances differentiation and proliferation of neural stem cell-derived astrocytes. *Experimental Neurology*, **196**, 373–380.

Roybon, L., Hjalt, T., Christophersen, N.S. *et al.* (2008) Effects on differentiation of embryonic ventral midbrain progenitors by Lmx1a, Msx1, Ngn2, and Pitx3. *J Neurosci*, **28**, 3644–3656.

Sanftner, L.M., Suzuki, B.M., Doroudchi, M.M. *et al.* (2004) Striatal delivery of rAAV-hAADC to rats with preexisting immunity to AAV. *Molecular Therapy: The Journal of the American Society of Gene Therapy*, **9**, 403–409.

Schnepp, B.C., Jensen, R.L., Chen, C.L. *et al.* (2005) Characterization of adeno-associated virus genomes isolated from human tissues. *Journal of Virology*, **79**, 14793–14803.

Shen, Y., Muramatsu, S.I., Ikeguchi, K. *et al.* (2000) Triple transduction with adeno-associated virus vectors expressing tyrosine hydroxylase, aromatic-L-amino-acid decarboxylase, and GTP cyclohydrolase I for gene therapy of Parkinson's disease. *Human Gene Therapy*, **11**, 1509–1519.

Sherer, T.B., Fiske, B.K., Svendsen, C.N. *et al.* (2006) Crossroads in GDNF therapy for Parkinson's disease. *Movement Disorders*, **21**, 136–141.

Slevin, J.T., Gerhardt, G.A., Smith, C.D. *et al.* (2005) Improvement of bilateral motor functions in patients with Parkinson's disease through the unilateral intraputaminal infusion of glial cell line-derived neurotrophic factor. *Journal of Neurosurgery*, **102**, 216–222.

Slevin, J.T., Gash, D.M., Smith, C.D. *et al.* (2007) Unilateral intraputamenal glial cell line-derived neurotrophic factor in patients with Parkinson's disease: response to 1 year of treatment and 1 year of withdrawal. *Journal of Neurosurgery*, **106**, 614–620.

Spheramine (2008) Titan Pharmaceuticals Announces Spheramine(R) Initial Phase IIb Results. http://phx.corporate-ir.net/phoenix.zhtml?c =95579&p=irol-newsArticle&ID=1171417. Titan Pharmaceuticals, Inc.

Stoessl, A.J. (2007) Gene therapy for Parkinson's disease: early data. *Lancet*, **369**, 2056–2058.

Takahashi, K. and Yamanaka, S. (2006) Induction of pluripotent stem cells from mouse embryonic and adult fibroblast cultures by defined factors. *Cell*, **126**, 663–676.

Takahashi, K., Tanabe, K., Ohnuki, M., *et al.* (2007) Induction of pluripotent stem cells from adult human fibroblasts by defined factors. *Cell*, **131**, 861–872.

Weimann, J.M., Johansson, C.B., Trejo, A. and Blau, H.M. (2003) Stable reprogrammed heterokaryons form spontaneously in Purkinje neurons after bone marrow transplant. *Nature Cell Biology*, **5**, 959–966.

Wernig, M., Meissner, A., Foreman, R. *et al.* (2007) *In vitro* reprogramming of fibroblasts into a pluripotent ES-cell-like state. *Nature*, **448**, 553–560.

Widner, H. and Brundin, P. (1988) Immunological aspects of grafting in the mammalian central nervous system. A review and speculative synthesis. *Brain Research*, **472**, 287–324.

Yang, M., Donaldson, A.E., Marshall, C.E. *et al.* (2004) Studies on the differentiation of dopaminergic traits in human neural progenitor cells *in vitro* and *in vivo*. *Cell Transplantation*, **13**, 535–547.

9

Parkinson-Plus Disorders

Martin Köllensperger and Gregor K. Wenning

Movement Disorders Unit, Clinical Department of Neurology, Innsbruck Medical University, Austria

The term "parkinson-plus disorders" or the synonymously used "atypical parkinsonian disorders" embraces a heterogeneous group of movement disorders all characterized by prominent parkinsonism, accompanied by specific additional ("plus") features such as cerebellar ataxia, pyramidal tract signs, myoclonus, supranuclear gaze palsy and apraxia, which are atypical for idiopathic Parkinson's disease (PD). Other features, like dysautonomia or dementia, are more pronounced than in PD and occur much earlier in the disease. Beside these additional features, rapid disease progression and poor or absent response to L-Dopa therapy is a commonality which raises the suspicion of an atypical parkinsonian disorder (APD). Currently, multiple system atrophy (MSA), progressive supranuclear palsy (PSP), corticobasal degeneration (CBD) and dementia with Lewy Bodies (DLB) are referred to as APDs. In this chapter we will focus on available therapeutic evidence and management of these disorders.

MULTIPLE SYSTEM ATROPHY

Definition and Clinical features

Multiple system atrophy (MSA) is a degenerative disorder of the central and autonomic nervous systems characterized by abnormal α-synuclein aggregation in oligodendroglia and neurons.

Clinically, cardinal features include autonomic failure, parkinsonism, cerebellar ataxia, and pyramidal signs, in any combination. Two major motor presentations can be distinguished. In the Western hemisphere, parkinsonian features predominate in 66% of patients (MSA-P subtype), cerebellar ataxia is the major motor feature in 34% of patients (MSA-C sub-type) (Geser et al., 2005). The reverse distribution is observed in the Eastern Hemisphere (Watanabe et al., 2002). MSA-associated parkinsonism is dominated by progressive akinesia and rigidity, whereas tremor is less common than in PD. Postural stability is compromised early on; however, recurrent falls at disease onset are unusual, in contrast to PSP. The cerebellar disorder of MSA is composed of gait ataxia, limb kinetic ataxia, and scanning dysarthria, as well as cerebellar oculomotor disturbances. Dysautonomia develops in virtually all patients with MSA. Clinically most important is urogenital dysfunction. Early impotence (erectile dysfunction) is virtually universal in men, and urinary incontinence (77%) or incomplete bladder emptying (60%), often early in the course or as presenting symptoms, are frequent. Orthostatic hypotension is present in 71% (Geser et al., 2005).

The clinical diagnosis of MSA rests largely on history and physical examination. The consensus criteria (Gilman et al., 2008) specify three diagnostic categories of increasing certainty: possible, probable and definite. Whereas a definite diagnosis requires histopathological examination, the diagnosis of possible and probable MSA is based on the presence of clinical criteria (Table 9.1) and supportive features (Table 9.2).

Prevalence

MSA affects both men and women; it usually starts in the sixth decade and relentlessly progresses, with death occurring after an average of nine years (Wenning et al., 1994). There are only few epidemiological surveys suggesting that MSA is an orphan disease with a prevalence rate of 4.4/100 000 and an incidence rate of 3/100 000/year (Bower et al., 1997; Schrag, Ben Shlomo and Quinn, 1999).

Pathophysiology and Clinicopathological Correlations

The cardinal features of MSA correlate with the distribution of oligodendroglial and neuronal pathology (Wenning et al., 1997). Severity of parkinsonism reflects neuronal loss in substantia nigra pars compacta resulting in profound

Table 9.1 MSA Consensus Criteria.

Criteria for the Diagnosis of Definite MSA
   Neuropathological findings of widespread and abundant
   CNS α-synuclein positive glial cytoplasmic inclusions
   (Papp–Lantos inclusions) in association with
   neurodegenerative changes in striatonigral or
   olivopontocerebellar structures.

Criteria for the Diagnosis of Probable MSA
   A sporadic, progressive, adult (>30 yr)-onset disease
   characterized by:
      -Autonomic failure involving urinary incontinence
       (inability to control the release of urine from the
       bladder, with ED in males) or an orthostatic fall of
       blood pressure within three min of standing by at
       least 30 mm Hg systolic or 15 mm Hg diastolic *and*
      -Poorly levodopa-responsive parkinsonism
       (bradykinesia with rigidity, tremor or postural
       instability) *or*
      -A cerebellar syndrome (gait ataxia with cerebellar
       dysarthria, limb ataxia or cerebellar oculomotor
       dysfunction)

Criteria for Autonomic Failure
      -Orthostatic fall in BP (30 systolic or 15 diastolic
       mmHg) *or*
      -Urinary incontinence (accompanied by erectile
       dysfunction in men)

Criteria for Possible MSA
   A sporadic, progressive adult (>30 yr)-onset disease
   characterized by:
      -Parkinsonism (bradykinesia with rigidity, tremor or
       postural instability) *or*
      -A cerebellar syndrome (gait ataxia with cerebellar
       dysarthria, limb ataxia, or cerebellar oculomotor
       dysfunction *and*
      -At least one feature suggesting autonomic
       dysfunction (otherwise unexplained urinary
       urgency, frequency or incomplete bladder emptying,
       erectile dysfunction in males, or significant
       orthostatic blood pressure decline that does not meet
       the level required in probable MSA) *and*
      -At least one of the additional features shown in
       Table 9.2B

(Adapted from Gilman, S. *et al.* (2008) Second consensus statement on the diagnosis of multiple system atrophy. *Neurology*,
71 (9): 670–676). Copyright © 2008, Lippincott Williams &
Wilkins.

striatal dopamine depletion, lack of L-Dopa response relates
to striatal and brainstem pathology, severity of cerebellar
ataxia correlates with OPCA, cardiovascular autonomic
failure is associated with neuronal cell loss in the intermediolateral cell column, and pyramidal signs appear to be

Table 9.2 Additional Features of Possible MSA.

A. Possible MSA-P or MSA-C:
      -Babinski sign with hyperreflexia
      -Stridor

B. Possible MSA-P
      -Rapidly progressive parkinsonism
      -Poor response to levodopa
      -Postural instability within 3 yr of motor onset
      -Gait ataxia, cerebellar dysarthria, limb ataxia, or
       cerebellar oculomotor dysfunction
      -Dysphagia within 5 yr of motor onset
      -Atrophy on MRI of putamen, middle cerebellar
       peduncle, pons or cerebellum
      -Hypometabolism on FDG-PET in putamen,
       brainstem or cerebellum

C. Possible MSA-C
      -Parkinsonism (bradykinesia and rigidity)
      -Atrophy on MRI of putamen, middle cerebellar
       peduncle or pons
      -Hypometabolism on FDG-PET in putamen
      -Presynaptic nigrostriatal dopaminergic denervation
       on SPECT or PET

(Adapted from Gilman, S. *et al.* (2008) Second consensus statement on the diagnosis of multiple system atrophy. *Neurology*,
71 (9): 670–676). Copyright © 2008, Lippincott Williams &
Wilkins.

associated with corticospinal tract degeneration. The role of
oligodendroglial α-synuclein inclusions in MSA-associated neurodegeneration is unclear at present, however, recent
clinicopathological (Ozawa *et al.*, 2004) as well as experimental (Shults *et al.*, 2005; Stefanova *et al.*, 2005; Yazawa
et al., 2005) data suggest that neuronal loss in MSA may
result from primary glial inclusion pathology.

Principles of Management

Currently, there is no effective neuroprotective therapy in
MSA. Symptomatic treatment is largely restricted to parkinsonism and dysautonomia. Other features, such as cerebellar ataxia, appear to be unresponsive to drug treatment.

Neuroprotective Therapy

A placebo-controlled double-blind pilot trial of recombinant human growth hormone (r-HGH) conducted by the
European MSA Study Group (EMSA-SG) has shown a
trend towards reduction of motor progression (measured
both with UPDRS and UMSARS) which, however, failed to
reach significance (Holmberg *et al.*, 2007).

   More recently, minocycline, an antibiotic with neuroprotective effects in a transgenic MSA mouse model
(Stefanova *et al.*, 2007), as well as models of related

neurodegenerative disorders (Zhu *et al.*, 2002; Casarejos *et al.*, 2006) proved ineffective in a phase II neuroprotection trial by EMSA-SG and the German Parkinson Network (KNP) (Dodel *et al.*, personal communication).

The recent NNIPPS (Neuroprotection and Natural History in Parkinson Plus Syndromes) trial investigating the effects of riluzole, an antiglutamatergic agent, on mortality and disease progression in atypical parkinsonian disorders, including MSA, was negative (Leigh *et al.*, 2007) A small randomized, controlled trial excluded symptomatic benefit of riluzole in MSA-P patients (Seppi *et al.*, 2006).

The success of further neuroprotection trials in MSA crucially depends on defining appropriate pathogenetic targets that are likely to mediate the progression of the disease.

Symptomatic Therapy

Parkinsonism

Only a small number of randomized controlled trials have been conducted in MSA, the practical management is largely based on empirical evidence or single randomized studies.

Dopaminergic Agents

L-Dopa is widely regarded the anti-parkinsonian therapy of choice in MSA, although a randomized controlled trial of L-Dopa has never been performed. Despite MSA patients being commonly believed to be non- or poorly responsive to dopaminergic therapy, efficacy has been documented in up to 40%, often lasting up to a few years (Wenning *et al.*, 2004). However, the benefit is transient in most of these subjects, leaving 90% of the MSA-P patients L-Dopa-unresponsive in the long term (Geser and Wenning, 2006). L-Dopa responsiveness should be tested by administering escalating doses over a three-month period up to a least 1000 mg per day (if necessary and if tolerated) (Gilman 1998). L-Dopa-induced dyskinesias affecting orofacial and neck muscles occur in 50% of MSA-P patients, sometimes in the absence of motor benefit (Boesch *et al.*, 2002).

No controlled trials with dopamine agonists are available, these compounds seem no more effective than L-Dopa and often poorly tolerated. Lisuride was effective in only one of seven MSA patients (Lees and Bannister, 1981). Heinz *et al.* reported the benefit of continuous subcutaneous lisuride infusion in four patients with sporadic olivopontocerebellar atrophy (OPCA) and severe signs of parkinsonism (Heinz *et al.*, 1992). Goetz and colleagues, using doses of 10–80 mg daily of bromocriptine, reported a benefit in five patients who had previously responded to L-Dopa and one patient who had failed to respond to L-Dopa (Goetz, Tanner and Klawans, 1984). There are no reports on

other ergolene or non-ergolene dopamine agonists, such as pergolide, cabergoline, ropinirole or pramipexole.

Pathological hypersexuality predominantly linked to adjuvant dopamine agonist therapy has been reported in two patients with MSA (Klos *et al.*, 2005).

MSA patients frequently report the appearance or worsening of postural hypotension after initiation of dopaminergic therapy, which may limit further increase in dosage.

Anti-cholinergic Agents

Anti-cholinergics usually do not improve motor symptoms, but they may be helpful when sialorrhea is severe and disturbing.

NMDA Receptor Antagonists

Despite anecdotal benefit in single cases (Wenning *et al.*, 1994), a short-term open trial with amantadine at high doses (400–600 mg/day) in five patients with MSA unresponsive to L-Dopa was negative (Colosimo, Merello and Pontieri, 1996). These disappointing results were confirmed more recently in a randomized placebo-controlled trial (Wenning, 2005).

SSRIs

In a recent randomized controlled trial of 19 MSA patients, paroxetine (PXT) 30 mg tid resulted in a significant improvement of the motor abilities of the upper limbs and speech when compared to placebo. The treatment with PXT was generally well tolerated. The degree of depressive symptoms was not significantly influenced by PXT or placebo during the observation period (Friess *et al.*, 2006).

Surgical Therapy

Whereas ablative neurosurgical procedures such as medial pallidotomy fail to improve parkinsonism in MSA (Lang *et al.*, 1997), bilateral subthalamic stimulation has been reported beneficial in four patients with MSA-P (Visser-Vandewalle *et al.*, 2003), whereas a poor response was seen in other cases (Lezcano *et al.*, 2004; Santens *et al.*, 2006). At present there is no role for DBS procedures in the routine management of MSA patients.

Non-Pharmacological Treatments

Because of the poor efficacy of anti-parkinsonian therapies in MSA, non-pharmacological interventions, such as physiotherapy, speech and occupational therapy are all the more important. Indeed, a recent study showed substantial benefit of occupational therapy in a series of 17 MSA patients (Jain *et al.*, 2004). Treated patients showed a reduction of 20% in UPDRS-ADL scores, as well as the PDQ-39 index score, whereas the control group deteriorated significantly over the two months study period.

Dystonia

Local injections of botulinum toxin are effective in orofacial as well as limb dystonia associated with MSA (Muller et al., 2002). Severe dysphagia with the necessity of nasogastric feeding has been reported after treatment of disproportionate antecollis with botulinum toxin and this type of treatment is not currently recommended (Thobois et al., 2001).

In addition, local botulinum toxin injections into parotid and submandibular glands have been effective in PD-associated sialorrhea in two double-blind placebo-controlled trials (Mancini et al., 2003; Lagalla et al., 2006). In contrast to anti-cholinergics, central side effects can be avoided.

Autonomic Symptoms

Treatment of autonomic dysfunction is crucial to avoid complications like ascending urinary tract infections or orthostatic hypotension (OH), which could lead to falls. In addition, autonomic dysfunction is associated with reduced quality of life (Schrag et al., 2006; Kollensperger et al., 2007). Unfortunately, most of the available therapies have not been evaluated in randomized-controlled trials.

Orthostatic Hypotension

Non-pharmacological options to treat OH include sufficient fluid intake, high-salt diet, more frequent, but smaller, meals per day to reduce post-prandial hypotension by spreading the total carbohydrate intake, compression stockings or custom-made elastic body garments. Ingestion of approx. 0.5 L of water in less then 5 min has been shown to substantially raise blood pressure in patients with autonomic failure, including MSA (Shannon et al., 2002; Young and Mathias, 2004). During the night, head-up tilt, not only reduces hypertensive cerebral perfusion pressure, but also increases intravasal volume up to 1 L within a week, which is particularly helpful to improve hypotension early in the morning. Constipation can affect the overall well-being and is relieved by an increase in intraluminal fluid, which may be achieved by macrogol-water solution (Eichhorn and Oertel, 2001).

Midodrine showed significant benefit in randomized placebo-controlled trials (Jankovic et al., 1993; Low et al., 1997) in patients with OH, but may exacerbate urinary retention. Comparable effects to midodrine can also be obtained with phenylpropanolamine in low doses or yohimbine or indomethacin in moderate doses (Jordan et al., 1998). Another promising drug seems to be the norepinephrine precursor L-threodihydroxy-phenylserine

(L-threo-DOPS), which has been used for this indication in Japan for years, and whose efficacy has now been shown by two double-blind placebo-controlled trials including patients with MSA (Mathias et al., 2001; Kaufmann et al., 2003).

The somatostatin analog, octreotide, has been shown to be beneficial in post-prandial hypotension in patients with pure autonomic failure (Alam et al., 1995), presumably because it inhibits release of vasodilatory gastrointestinal peptides (Raimbach et al., 1989); importantly, it does not enhance nocturnal hypertension (Alam et al., 1995).

Urinary Dysfunction

Whereas pro-cholinergic substances are usually not successful to adequately reduce post-void residual volume in MSA, anti-cholinergics like oxybutynin can improve symptoms of detrusor hyperreflexia or sphincter-detrusor dyssynergy in the early course of the disease (Beck, Betts and Fowler, 1994). However, central side effects may be limiting. In a large multi-centre randomized, controlled study in patients with detrusor hyperreflexia, trospium chloride, a peripherally acting quaternary anti-cholinergic, has been shown to be equally effective with better tolerability (Halaska et al., 2003). However, trospium has not been investigated in MSA and, further, it appears that central and peripheral anti-cholinergics are equally effective and tolerated in non-demented PD patients (2002). At present, there is no evidence for ranking the efficacy and safety of anti-cholinergics in the management of detrusor hyperreflexia associated with MSA. α-Adrenergic receptor antagonists like prazosin and moxisylyte have been shown to improve voiding, with reduction of residual volumes in MSA patients (Sakakibara et al., 2000).

The vasopressin analog, desmopressin, which acts on renal tubular vasopressin-2 receptors, reduces nocturnal polyuria and improves morning postural hypotension (Mathias et al., 1986).

The peptide erythropoietin may be beneficial in some patients by raising red cell mass, secondarily improving cerebral oxygenation (Perera, Isola and Kaufmann, 1995; Winkler et al., 2001).

Surgical therapies for neurogenic bladder problems should be avoided in MSA, because post-operative worsening of bladder control is very likely (Beck, Betts and Fowler, 1994), but, for example, severe prostate hypertrophy with urinary retention and secondary hydronephrosis can not be left untreated.

With post-micturition volumes >150 ml, clean intermittent catheterization three to four times per day may be necessary to prevent secondary consequences. A permanent transcutaneous suprapubic catheter may become necessary if mechanical obstruction in the urethra or motor symptoms of MSA prevent uncomplicated catheterization.

Erectile Dysfunction

After an initial report on the efficacy in the treatment of erectile dysfunction in PD (Zesiewicz, Helal and Hauser, 2000), sildenafil citrate has been shown to be effective in a double-blind placebo-controlled randomized trial in patients with PD and MSA (Hussain *et al.*, 2001). Since it may unmask or exacerbate orthostatic hypotension, measurement of lying and standing blood pressure before prescribing sildenafil to men with parkinsonism is recommended. Erectile failure in MSA may also be improved by oral yohimbine or by intracavernosal injection of papaverine or a penis implant (Beck, Betts and Fowler, 1994).

Inspiratory Stridor

Inspiratory stridor develops in about 30% of patients. Continuous positive airway pressure (CPAP) may be helpful in some of these patients, suitable as long-term therapy (Iranzo *et al.*, 2004; Ghorayeb *et al.*, 2005; Nonaka *et al.*, 2006). A tracheostomy is rarely needed and performed.

Non-Medical Therapy

Because the results of drug treatment for MSA are generally poor, other therapies are all the more important. Physiotherapy helps maintain mobility and prevent contractures, and speech therapy can improve speech and swallowing and provide communication aids (Jain *et al.*, 2004). Dysphagia may require feeding by means of a nasogastric tube or even percutaneous endoscopic gastrostomy. Occupational therapy helps to limit the handicap resulting from the patient's disabilities and should include a home visit. Provision of a wheelchair is usually dictated by the liability to falls because of postural instability and gait ataxia, but not by akinesia and rigidity per se. Psychological support for patients and partners needs to be stressed (Table 9.3).

PROGRESSIVE SUPRANUCLEAR PALSY

Definition and Clinical Features

Progressive supranuclear palsy (PSP) is a chronic progressive neurodegenerative disorder characterized by supranuclear vertical gaze palsy, postural instability and frontolimbic dementia (Steele, Richardson and Oslzewski, 1964).

Patients with PSP classically present with symmetric parkinsonism unresponsive to L-Dopa with prominent extensor rigidity and dystonia of neck muscles resulting in an erect posture with neck hyperextension. Postural stability is severely impaired resulting in recurrent falls, typically backwards, early in the course of the disease (Litvan *et al.*, 1996; Nath *et al.*, 2003).

Table 9.3 Pragmatic Management of MSA.

The management of MSA is largely empirical in the absence of evidence from randomized placebo-controlled drug trials and it is targeted at the following clinical features:

Parkinsonism
First choice: L-Dopa (up to 1000 mg/day, if tolerated and necessary)
Second choice: Dopamine agonists (PD titration schemes)
Third choice: Amantadine: (100 mg tid)
Physiotherapy
Occupational therapy
Speech therapy

Dytonia (orofacial and limb, antecollis excluded)
First choice: Botulinum toxin

Cerebellar Ataxia
No drug therapy available
Physiotherapy
Occupational therapy
Speech therapy

Autonomic Symptoms
Orthostatic Hypotension
First choice: Non-pharmacological strategies: elastic support stockings or tights, high-salt diet, frequent small meals, head-up tilt of the bed at night
If needed: add fludrocortisone (0.1–0.3 mg) at night.
If needed: add midodrine (2.5–10 mg tid) (combined with fludrocortisone)
If needed: replace midodrine by ephedrine (15–45 mg tid) or L-threo-DOPS (100 mg tid)

Urinary failure—urge incontinence
Trospium chloride (20 mg bid or 15 mg tid)
Oxybutynin (2.5–5 mg bid to tid) NB: central side effects
Tolterodine (2 mg bid)

Urinary failure—incomplete bladder emptying
Post-micturition residue of >100 ml is an indication for intermittent self-catheterization
In the advanced stages of MSA a urethral or suprapubic catheter may become necessary.

Erectile failure
First choice: Sildenafil (50–100 mg)
Second choice: Oral yohimbine (2.5–5 mg)
Third choice: Intracavernosal injection of papaverine

Palliative Therapy
Botulinum toxin for sialorrhea
CPAP (for prominent stridor)
PEG
Tracheostomy (rarely needed)

Supranuclear vertical gaze palsy with complete loss of vertical eye movements, slowing of vertical and horizontal saccades and hypometric saccades are considered pathognomonic features. This leads, in combination with facial immobility and elevated eyebrows, to a characteristic staring facial expression. Pseudobulbar syndromes lead to a characteristic growling and groaning speech.

PSP is also characterized by a "subcortical" or "frontal lobe-type" dementia with cognitive slowing, dysexecutive syndrome and other frontal lobe deficits including utilization behavior.

The NINDS diagnostic criteria for PSP, primarily developed as clinical research criteria, have been established as gold standard over the last 10 years (Litvan *et al.*, 1996) (Table 9.4), although highly specific sensitivity is rather low (Osaki *et al.*, 2004) possibly reflecting phenotypic variation. Recent findings (Williams *et al.*, 2005) suggest that there may be two sub-types of the disease, with two-thirds of patients showing classical features (Richardson's syndrome) and one-third a more benign PD-like phenotype with asymmetric onset, rest tremor and a moderate therapeutic response to levodopa (PSP-P sub-type).

Prevalence

The mean age at disease onset is around 60 years and mean survival is six years (Litvan *et al.*, 1996). The disease is rapidly progressive and leads to wheelchair- and bed-bound later stages.

Prevalence rates lie between 5.0 and 6.4/100 000 (Schrag, Ben Shlomo and Quinn, 1999; Nath *et al.*, 2001), but might be higher due under-recognition and misdiagnosis (Nath *et al.*, 2001; Williams *et al.*, 2005). The cause is unknown; genetic studies have indicated that a specific haplotype of the tau gene is over-represented in PSP and CBD, indicating a common genetic background of these tauopathies (Di Maria *et al.*, 2000).

Pathophysiology and Clinicopathological Correlations

The progressive axial motor disorder and frontal dementia syndrome associated with PSP reflects multi-focal neuronal pathology including neurofibrillary tangles containing abnormally phosphorylated tau protein in the basal ganglia, brainstem and frontal cortex (Steele, Richardson and Oslzewski, 1964; Morris *et al.*, 2002). Neuropil threads, tufted astrocytes and glial tau inclusions are also found in these brain areas. In addition to these changes, there are multiple neurotransmitter abnormalities, including dopamine, acetylcholine, γ-aminobutyric acid and noradrenaline systems (Rajput and Rajput, 2001).

Principles of Management

Neuroprotective Therapy

Currently disease-modifying agents are not available for PSP. The results of the NNIPPS trial indicate no neuroprotective effects of Riluzole (Leigh *et al.*, 2007). Other targets for neuroprotective in PSP currently investigated include abnormal tau phosphorylation by glycogen synthase kinase 3 (GSK-3), which can be suppressed by lithium, suppression of microglial activation and more experimental strategies like reduction of four-repeat tau by RNA interference or delivery of trophic factors (Burn and Warren, 2005). In a recent short-term randomized placebo-controlled trial co-enzyme Q10 not only provided mild clinical benefit but also improved cerebral energy metabolism which may lead to long-term benefit. (Stamelou *et al.*, 2008).

Symptomatic Therapy

Since only few controlled trials have been performed in PSP, symptomatic therapy is largely based on empirical evidence (van Balken and Litvan, 2006).

Dopaminergic Agents

Treatment with L-Dopa is indicated, since up to 35% of patients show at least a partial response, even though transient in most cases (Litvan *et al.*, 1996; Kompoliti *et al.*, 1998; Nath *et al.*, 2003). More recent clinicopathological studies suggest that PSP-P with an L-Dopa-responsive PD-like syndrome may also show a distinct tau phenotype (Williams *et al.*, 2005; Williams *et al.*, 2007) Dopamine receptor agonists proved partially effective in the overall PSP population with an response of 24% (van Balken and Litvan, 2006). Modest transient anti-parkinsonian efficacy has been observed for bromocriptine (Kompoliti *et al.*, 1998) and pergolide (Jankovic, 1983). In contrast, lack of anti-parkinsonian efficacy was reported for lisuride (Neophytides *et al.*, 1982) and pramipexole (Weiner, Minagar and Shulman, 1999) in two small open-label studies.

The monoamine oxidase B inhibitor selegeline has been described retrospectively as similarly effective.

Serotonergic Agents

Amitryptiline has been shown to improve, not only quality of life, but also parkinsonian features in a double-blind placebo-controlled trial; however, only four patients were studied. (Newman, 1985). Tandospirone citrate, a 5HT-1A agonist currently available only in Japan and China, also has been described as effective on motor symptoms in PSP (Fujino *et al.*, 2002).

Table 9.4 NINDS-SPSP clinical criteria for the diagnosis of PSP.

PSP	Mandatory inclusion criteria	Mandatory exclusion criteria	Supportive criteria
Possible	Gradually progressive disorder	Recent history of encephalitis	Symmetric akinesia or rigidity, proximal more than distal
	Onset at age 40 or later	Alien limb syndrome, cortical deficits, focal frontal or temporoparietal atrophy	Abnormal neck posture, especially retrocollis
	Either vertical (upward or downward gaze) supranuclear palsy or both slowing of vertical saccades and prominent postural instability with falls in the first year of disease onset	Hallucinations or delusions unrelated to dopaminergic therapy	Poor or absent response of parkinsonism to levodopa therapy
		Cortical dementia of Alzheimer's (severe amnesia and aphasia or agnosia, according to NINCDS-ADRA criteria)	Early dysphagia and dysarthria
	No evidence of other diseases that could explain the fore-going features, as indicated by mandatory exclusion criteria	Prominent, early cerebellar symptoms or prominent, early unexplained dysautonomia (marked hypotension and urinary disturbances)	Early onset of cognitive impairment including at least two of the following: apathy, impairment in abstract thought, decreased verbal fluency, utilization or imitation behavior, or frontal release signs
Probable	Gradually progressive disorder	Severe, asymmetric parkinsonian signs (i.e., bradykinesia)	
	Onset at age 40 or later	Neuroradiologic evidence of relevant structural abnormality (i.e., basal gangliam or brainstem infarcts, lobar atrophy)	
	Vertical (upward or downward gaze) supranuclear palsy *and* prominent postural instability with falls in the first year of disease onset	Whipple's disease, confirmed by polymerase chain reaction, if indicated	
	No evidence of other diseases that could explain the fore-going features, as indicated by mandatory exclusion criteria		
Definite[a]	Clinically probable or possible PSP *and* histopathologic evidence of typical PSP		

Modified from Litvan, I. *et al.* (1996) Clinical research criteria for the diagnosis of progressive supranuclear palsy (Steele-Richardson-Olszewski syndrome): report of the NINDS-SPSP international workshop. *Neurology*, **47** (1), 1–9. Copyright © 1996, Lippincott Williams & Wilkins.
[a]Definite PSP is a clinicopathologic diagnosis.

Serotonin Antagonists

Methysergide has been reported to improve swallowing, speech, parkinsonian features and oculomotor disturbances in an open-label study of 12 patients (Rafal and Grimm, 1981), but this observation could not be confirmed by others (Paulson, Lowery and Taylor, 1981; Duncombe and Lees, 1985) and there is concern about the risk of fibrosis.

Noradrenergic Agents

Double-blind placebo-controlled trials reported benefits on mobility, balance, gait, and finger dexterity for the α-adrenergic antagonist idazoxan (Ghika et al., 1991), but not for the more potent and selective efaroxan (Rascol et al., 1998). Desipramin showed an improvement preferentially on apraxia of eyelid opening in two out of four patients in a double-blind placebo-controlled trial (Newman, 1985).

Glutamatergic Agents

Zolpidem was shown to improve saccadic eye movements and parkinsonism in a double-blind cross-over study of 10 patients with probable PSP; however, the benefit was limited by drowsiness, particularly at dosages higher than 5 mg/d (Daniele, Moro and Bentivoglio, 1999).

Cholinergic Agents

Administration of cholinergic agents is not beneficial; they may actually worsen both motor and cognitive function, as reported for donepezil, a centrally acting cholinesterase inhibitor, in a double-blind placebo-controlled trial with 21 PSP patients (Litvan et al., 2001). Fabbrini and colleagues also reported lack of efficacy for donepezil in an open-label trial of six PSP patients (Fabbrini et al., 2001). Physostigmine showed efficacy on oculomotor (Blin et al., 1995) and cognitive function (Kertzman, Robinson and Litvan, 1990) in two double-blind placebo-controlled trials; however, it was ineffective in another trial (Litvan et al., 1994). RS-86, an M1–M2 muscarinic agonist, also showed no effect on motor and cognitive function in 10 PSP patients during a nine-week double-blind randomized, controlled trial (Foster et al., 1989).

Anti-cholinergics

Whereas case reports on benztropine describe minor positive anti-parkinsonian effects for benztropine (Haldeman et al., 1981), there was motor and cognitive worsening on scopolamine (Litvan et al., 1994)

Botulinum Toxin A

Botulinum toxin A has been reported effective for cervical and limb dystonia, as well as orofacial dystonia, especially involuntary eye closure (Piccione et al., 1997; Muller et al., 2002).

Surgical Therapies

Anecdotal experiences with patients misclassified as PD have produced negative results for deep brain stimulation (Okun et al., 2005).

Implantation of adrenal medullary tissue into the caudate nucleus has been performed in a few PSP patients; however, the procedure proved to be ineffective, as well as hazardous, with substantial peri-operative morbidity and mortality (Koller et al., 1989; Waxman et al., 1991).

Non-Medical Therapy

Since gait instability shows only minimal or no response to drug therapy, weighted walkers should be considered. Swallowing disturbances should be regularly evaluated by speech therapists to avoid aspiration pneumonia. Dysphagia can be managed by the use of straws, food thickeners, or soft processed food. The question of whether a nasogastric tube or percutaneous endoscopic gastrostomy could reduce the chances of aspiration pneumonia needs further assessment. Patients can also be helped by a variety of communication aids. Visual prisms are rarely of help; patients may instead resort to books on tape. Artificial tears are useful to avoid exposure keratitis secondary to decreased eye blink rate (Table 9.5).

DEMENTIA WITH LEWY BODIES

Definition and Clinical Features

Dementia with Lewy bodies (DLB) is characterized by co-existent parkinsonism and progressive cognitive decline, with particular deficits of visuospatial ability and frontal executive function, accompanied by spontaneous recurrent visual hallucinations and marked fluctuations in alertness and cognitive performance (McKeith et al., 2005).

Psychotic symptoms, in particular hallucinations and visual delusions have been found in between 25 and 80% of patients in various series (Ballard et al., 1998; Morris, Olichney and Corey-Bloom, 1998). Despite the differences between studies, it is probably correct to estimate that two-thirds of DLB patients will have prominent psychotic behavior in the course of their illness. Hallucinatory psychosis often goes along with confusion, agitation, and sleep disorders and constitutes a major therapeutic challenge (Lauterbach, 2004).

The two main differential diagnoses for DLB include Alzheimer's disease (AD) and PD. AD is accompanied by extrapyramidal motor features in up to 30% of cases, and most patients diagnosed with DLB also show some Alzheimer change on post-mortem brain examination. On

Table 9.5 Pragmatic Management of PSP.

Due to the small number of randomized controlled trials the practical management of PSP is largely based on empirical evidence. Treatment is largely targeted at the motor presentation.

Parkinsonism
  L-dopa (up to 1000 mg/day, if tolerated – benefit in up to 35% of patients with higher rates in the PSP-P subtype)
  Amitriptyline (orally up to 25 mg tid – benefit in 35% of patients ($n = 20$))
  Zolpidem (5–10 mg od – benefit in 100% of patients ($n = 10$))
  Physiotherapy
  Occupational therapy
  Speech therapy

Dysphagia
  Consider nasogastric tube or PEG

Dystonia
  Botulinum toxin (tarsal and pretarsal blepharospasm, limb dystonia).

Urinary Failure
  As for MSA (see Table 9.3)

---

the other hand, between 20 and 40% of patients with PD will become demented in the course of their illness (Emre, 2003). To improve the differential diagnosis of DLB, consensus criteria have been developed that establish possible and probable levels of diagnostic accuracy, restricting a diagnosis of DLB only to patients with parkinsonism who have dementia develop within 12 months of the onset of motor symptoms (McKeith *et al.*, 2005) (Table 9.6).

Prevalence

Brain bank data suggested that DLB may represent the second most frequent cause of dementia in the elderly, after Alzheimer's disease, accounting for up to 30.5% of cases (Zaccai, McCracken and Brayne, 2005). Prevalence rates from prospective door-to-door surveys range from 0.1% in the general population to 5% in the population aged $75 +$. (Yamada *et al.*, 2001; Stevens *et al.*, 2002; Rahkonen *et al.*, 2003).

Pathophysiology and Clinicopathological Correlations

The pathological hallmark is diffuse Lewy-body deposition in limbic and neocortical areas, commonly associated with Alzheimer-type pathology in addition to nigral deposition,

as found in PD. Although the correlation between Lewy-body pathology and severity of dementia is inconsistent and variable, Lewy bodies prominently expressing α-synuclein plays a key role in the pathophysiology of DLB-related cognitive and motor features (Cummings, 1995). In addition, several studies have found cholinergic denervation similar to that in AD (Perry *et al.*, 1999). Nigrostriatal dopaminergic denervation accounts for parkinsonian features in DLB and appears to progress more rapidly compared to PD (Ransmayr *et al.*, 2001). The lack of sustained L-Dopa benefit in DLB may reflect aggressive nigral Lewy-body pathology, a limited therapeutic window due to autonomic and/or psychiatric side effects as well as dopamine receptor dysfunction due to putaminal Lewy neuritic pathology (Walker *et al.*, 2002).

Principles of Management

Neuroprotective Therapy

Up to now studies aimed at disease modification have not been conducted in DLB. Since DLB shares its underlying α-synuclein pathology with PD, candidate neuroprotective agents for PD are also highly relevant for DLB. A detailed discussion of neuroprotective strategies in PD and related disorders is given elsewhere (Chapter 8).

Symptomatic Therapy

Progressive parkinsonism, dementia and associated psychiatric features, as well as autonomic symptoms, are at the centre of therapeutic needs in this disorder. Although there is no satisfying treatment yet available, a number of important advances have been made in recent years.

Dementia and Psychiatric Features

Cholinesterase Inhibitors

Rivastigmine is the only cholinesterase inhibitor (ChEI) tested in a prospective placebo-controlled double-blind trial in 92 patients with probable DLB and mild to moderately severe dementia. Significantly more patients in the treatment arm (63% vs 32%) showed a >30% improvement in cognitive function. Adverse effects (nausea, vomiting, anorexia, and somnolence) were slightly more frequent (92% vs 75%) than with placebo. Parkinsonian symptoms, as assessed by the UPDRS, did not change (McKeith *et al.*, 2000). A three-month open-label extension study in 11 of these patients showed a significant reduction of NPI scores over baseline. In 5 of these 11 patients, clinical improvement was judged very relevant. In addition, parkinsonism, as assessed by the UPDRS, also showed some improvement (McKeith *et al.*, 2000). A recent study showed that

Table 9.6 Revised criteria for the clinical diagnosis of dementia with Lewy bodies (DLB).

1. *Central feature* (essential for a diagnosis of possible or probable DLB)

   Dementia defined as progressive cognitive decline of sufficient magnitude to interfere with normal social or occupational function.

   Prominent or persistent memory impairment may not necessarily occur in the early stages but is usually evident with progression.

   Deficits on tests of attention, executive function, and visuospatial ability may be especially prominent.

2. *Core features* (two core features are sufficient for a diagnosis of probable DLB, one for possible DLB)

   Fluctuating cognition with pronounced variations in attention and alertness

   Recurrent visual hallucinations that are typically well formed and detailed

   Spontaneous features of parkinsonism

3. *Suggestive features* (If one or more of these is present in the presence of one or more core features, a diagnosis of probable DLB can be made. In the absence of any core features, one or more suggestive features is sufficient for possible DLB. Probable DLB should not be diagnosed on the basis of suggestive features alone.)

   REM sleep behavior disorder

   Severe neuroleptic sensitivity

   Low dopamine transporter uptake in basal ganglia demonstrated by SPECT or PET imaging

4. *Supportive features* (commonly present but not proven to have diagnostic specificity)

   Repeated falls and syncope

   Transient, unexplained loss of consciousness

   Severe autonomic dysfunction, for example, orthostatic hypotension, urinary incontinence

   Hallucinations in other modalities

   Systematized delusions

   Depression

   Relative preservation of medial temporal lobe structures on CT/MRI scan

   Generalized low uptake on SPECT/PET perfusion scan with reduced occipital activity

   Abnormal (low uptake) MIBG myocardial scintigraphy

   Prominent slow wave activity on EEG with temporal lobe transient sharp waves

5. A diagnosis of DLB is *less likely*

   In the presence of cerebrovascular disease evident as focal neurologic signs or on brain imaging

   In the presence of any other physical illness or brain disorder sufficient to account in part or in total for the clinical picture

   If parkinsonism only appears for the first time at a stage of severe dementia

6. *Temporal sequence* of symptoms

   DLB should be diagnosed when dementia occurs before or concurrently with parkinsonism (if it is present). The term Parkinson's disease dementia (PDD) should be used to describe dementia that occurs in the context of well-established Parkinson's disease. In a practice setting the term that is most appropriate to the clinical situation should be used and generic terms such as LB disease are often helpful. In research studies in which distinction needs to be made between DLB and PDD, *the existing one-year rule between the onset of dementia and parkinsonism DLB continues to be recommended.* Adoption of other time periods will simply confound data pooling or comparison between studies. In other research settings that may include clinicopathological studies and clinical trials, both clinical phenotypes may be considered collectively under categories such as LB disease or alpha-synucleinopathy.

Adapted from McKeith, I.G., Dickson, D.W., Lowe, J., Emre, M., O'Brien, J.T., Feldman, H. *et al.* (2005). Diagnosis and management of dementia with Lewy bodies: third report of the DLB Consortium. *Neurology*, **65** (12): 1863–1872. Copyright © 2005, Lippincott Williams & Wilkins

rivastigmine produces comparable cognitive benefits in patients with DLB and AD, and, in addition, a significant improvement of behavioral disorders (Rozzini *et al.*, 2007).

Donepezil is another ChEI with proven efficacy in AD. Contrary to rivastigmine, it has not been tested in a controlled fashion in DLB. However, several open-label observational studies and case reports describe improvements in cognitive function, as well as behavioral benefits with reduced agitation and aggressive behavior (Lanctot and Herrmann, 2000; Skjerve and Nygaard, 2000; Rojas-Fernandez, 2001; Thomas *et al.*, 2005; Mori *et al.*, 2006; Rowan *et al.*, 2007). Several reports emphasize improvements in pre-existing hallucinations and delusions (Aarsland *et al.*, 1999; Fergusson and Howard, 2000; Samuel *et al.*, 2000), but there are also observations on worsening of parkinsonism (Shea, MacKnight and Rockwood, 1998).

A few small-scale open-label uncontrolled studies have been conducted on the use of tacrine in DLB (Levy *et al.*, 1994; Lebert *et al.*, 1998; Querfurth *et al.*, 2000). Doses were between 80 and 120 mg/day and results varied considerably.

One multi-centre open-label study of the ChEI galantamine has shown significant improvement in NPI scores, as well as Clinician's Global Impression of Change in 25 patients with DLB. In addition, there was significant improvement in cognitive function, activities of daily living, sleep and confusion assessments without adverse effects on parkinsonism (Edwards *et al.*, 2004; Edwards *et al.*, 2007).

ChEIs are effective symptomatic treatments in DLB. In addition there may also be additional disease-modifying effects by reducing cortical β-amyloid deposition, which may be relevant to the disease course of dementia patients (Ballard *et al.*, 2007).

Neuroleptics

Neuroleptic drugs can induce severe complications, including marked increases in parkinsonism with rigidity, postural imbalance and falls, sometimes accompanied by mental status changes and other features of the neuroleptic malignant syndrome associated with increased mortality (McKeith *et al.*, 1992). Risperidone is a benzisoxazole derivative with both 5HT-2 and D2 receptor affinity. Open-label retrospective observations in small series suggest that it can induce marked worsening of parkinsonism even aggravate confusion and agitation (McKeith, Ballard and Harrison, 1995), even at low doses (Rich *et al.*, 1995; Ballard *et al.*, 1998). Its general use in DLB is not recommended despite favorable case reports (Kato *et al.*, 2002).

Clozapine is a dibenzodiazepine derivative with potent anti-psychotic properties and is virtually free of extrapyramidal side effects when used in schizophrenic patients (Kane *et al.*, 1988). There are no controlled trials of clozapine in the treatment of psychosis in DLB. Whereas two patients, who had worsening of parkinsonism and confusion after treatment with risperidone, were reported to improve with clozapine (Rich *et al.*, 1995); increase in confusion and psychotic behavior, but no worsening of parkinsonism, could be observed in two patients of another series (Burke, Pfeiffer and McComb, 1998).

Olanzapine is a thienobenzodiazepine similar to clozapine with preferential affinity to 5HT-2 over D2 receptors and selective affinity to mesolimbic over striatal dopamine receptors. Contrary to clozapine, its use does not require blood count monitoring. In a small open-label study in eight DLB patients with psychosis and behavioral disturbances, low doses of 2.5–7.5 mg of olanzapine led to unacceptable worsening of parkinsonism or postural instability, whereas there was no or only marginal improvement of psychosis in the others (Walker *et al.*, 1999). This is in line with the results from a double-blind prospective clozapine-controlled study in PD patients with drug-induced psychosis (Goetz *et al.*, 2000), and argues against the use of this drug in DLB. A post hoc analysis of 29 patients with DLB in a larger placebo-controlled double-blind nursing home study, however, showed the benefit of olanzapine on psychosis without evidence of worsening of parkinsonism (Cummings *et al.*, 2002).

Quetiapine is another dibenzodiazepine with close pharmacological resemblance to clozapine. One small, uncontrolled study in 10 patients with DLB-associated psychosis reported improvement on the brief psychiatric rating scale in all patients after six months of follow-up without negative impact on motor function (Parsa and Bastani, 1998). A randomized, controlled multi-centre trial in 23 patients with DLB failed to show any significant effects of quetiapine over placebo (Kurlan *et al.*, 2007).

NMDA Receptor Antagonists

Since amantadine can also induce or increase psychosis and has only limited anti-parkinsonian effects, its use should be avoided in DLB.

Anti-depressants

Treatment of depression in patients with DLB is entirely empirically based, without any controlled trial data. Selective serotonin reuptake inhibitors (SSRIs) are frequently used with sufficient success. Anti-muscarinic agents should be avoided because of their anti-cholinergic properties and potential to aggravate cognitive dysfunction. There are no data on the use of newer anti-depressants like mirtazepine or roboxetine in patients with DLB.

Parkinsonism

Although parkinsonism is a main feature of the disease, no therapeutic intervention has been specifically assessed in a controlled trial specifically in DLB patients. Treatment decisions are therefore generally based on experience in other diseases like PD or MSA with L-Dopa as the "gold standard." Doses are usually in the low to middle range between 300 and 500 mg per day; visual hallucinations and psychotic behavior can be dose-limiting. Up to 75% of DLB patients can show a long-term response to L-Dopa (Bonelli *et al.*, 2004). Dopamine agonists do not offer significant advantages over L-Dopa in DLB, but have a greater risk of inducing psychotic side effects.

Autonomic Symptoms

Both urogenital features, including urge incontinence, incomplete bladder emptying and erectile failure, as well as orthostatic hypotension with or without postural syncope are common sequelae in DLB. Recent studies have shown that orthostatic hypotension significantly exacerbates both cognitive and motor function (Allcock, Kenny and Burn, 2006; Peralta *et al.*, 2007). Therefore, identification of significant postural blood pressure drop and rigorous treatment can have a profound impact on the overall functioning of DLB patients. Considering the wide range of effective therapeutic interventions to control neurogenic bladder disturbances, it is also vital to address these disabling and stigmatizing aspects of the disease. The management principals both for orthostatic hypotension and urogenital failure have already been summarized in the section on MSA.

Non-Medical Therapy

Patients with significant dysarthria and dysphagia should receive speech therapy. Postural imbalance and falls are also symptoms generally not responsive to drug therapy and require physiotherapy. Home placement will be required for patients with persistent psychiatric complications unresponsive to drug therapy (Table 9.7).

CORTICOBASAL DEGENERATION

Definition and Clinical Features

First described by Rebeiz and colleagues in 1967 (Rebeiz, Kolodny and Richardson, 1967) as "corticodentatonigral degeneration with neuronal achromasia," almost 20 years elapsed before corticobasal degeneration (CBD), a rare multi-system tauopathy, received renewed attention (Mahapatra *et al.*, 2004).

Classically patients present in the sixth or seventh decade with a strikingly asymmetrical akinetic-rigid parkinsonian syndrome associated with other movement disorders—most often dystonia and myoclonus—in combination with cortical signs. These include apraxia and "alien limb" phenomena, cortical sensory loss, and variable degrees of dysphasia. Depression and frontal lobe-type behavioral changes, including apathy or disinhibition, impulsiveness, and irritability, develop in 30–50% of patients (Rinne *et al.*, 1994; Wenning *et al.*, 1998; Cummings and Litvan, 2000) and up to 25% may become demented (Kompoliti *et al.*, 1998). Symptoms usually remain clearly asymmetrical,

Table 9.7 Pragmatic Management of DLB.

Therapy in DLB is guided by its major presentations including parkinsonism, early onset dementia with or without psychosis, and autonomic failure.

Parkinsonism
  First choice: L-Dopa (up to 1000 mg, if tolerated—NB: hallucinations)
  DA as well as amantadine should be avoided (hallucinations)
  Physiotherapy
  Speech therapy
  Occupational therapy

Dementia
  First choice: Rivastigmine: 3–12 mg/day
  Second choice: Donezepil: 5–10 mg/day
  Third choice: Galantamine: 8–16 mg/day
Cognitive training

Depression
  SSRIs may be tried on an empirical basis

Psychosis
  Clozapine: 6.25–50 mg/day (may be more effective than quetiapine, needs blood monitoring)
  Quetiapine: 25–150 mg/day (may be less effective than clozapine, no need for blood monitoring)

Autonomic failure
  as for MSA (see Table 9.3)

eventually spreading from the affected arm to the ipsilateral leg and progress steadily until death, which usually occurs 4 to 8 years after disease onset.

Several schemes for diagnostic criteria for CBD have been proposed and mostly focus on the presence of a markedly asymmetrical parkinsonian syndrome with relentless progression and various combinations of movement disorders and cortical dysfunction. Table 9.8 summarizes clinical diagnostic criteria proposed by (Kumar, Bergeron and Lang, 2002). Overall, diagnostic sensitivity to CBD is sub-optimal even among expert neurologists, who only detected 30% of post-mortem-confirmed CBD cases on the basis of clinical presentation at first visit (Litvan, 1997).

Prevalence

The incidence and prevalence of CBD are largely unknown, accounting for only some 3% of patients with degenerative parkinsonism (Hughes *et al.*, 2002); prevalence in the

Table 9.8 Clinical Diagnostic Criteria For CBD.

1. *Marked asymmetry at onset* (includes motor and cortical sensory signs, apraxia and dysphasia)
2. *Progressive course*
3. *Presence of:*
   (a) Movement disorder
      Akinetic-rigid parkinsonism
      Limb dystonia
      Focal myoclonus
      Cortical sensory loss
   (b) Cortical dysfunction
      Alien-limb phenomena (levitation only excluded)
      Apraxia
4. *Exclusion of:*
   Early dementia
   Levodopa responsiveness
   Down gaze palsy
   Typical rest tremor
   Severe dysautonomia
   Alternative pathology accounting for clinical features on appropriate imaging studies

general population might be well below 1 per 100 000 (Schrag, Ben Shlomo and Quinn, 2000).

Pathophysiology and Clinicopathological Correlations

The tauopathy CBD is a multi-system disorder affecting the nigrostriatal motor system plus a variety of other subcortical structures, including variable cell loss in the thalamus, subthalamic nucleus, the pallidum, red nucleus, dentate nucleus and scattered changes in other brainstem nuclei. In addition there is prominent and usually asymmetrical cortical degeneration involving frontoparietal areas. These neuropathological features account for the cardinal clinical signs including L-dopa refractory parkinsonism, dystonia, myoclonus and apraxia (Murray *et al.*, 2007). CBD might present with cognitive impairment and there is some controversy that frontotemporal dementia and CBD may represent different ends of a single disease spectrum (Kertesz *et al.*, 2000). The etiology and pathogenesis of CBD remain to be resolved. There is abnormal tau aggregation affecting both basal ganglia and motor cortex. Recent evidence suggests that there may be a genetic predisposition towards tau accumulation that is shared by PSP patients (Di Maria *et al.*, 2000). Whether CBD and PSP are distinct clinicopathological entities or phenotypic variants of one tauopathy remains debatable (Sha *et al.*, 2006).

Principles of Management

Neuroprotective Therapy

Currently disease-modifying agents are not available for CBD.

Symptomatic Therapy

Because of the rarity of CBD, to date there has been no single controlled or even uncontrolled prospective clinical trial of any intervention. Medical treatment is based on retrospective uncontrolled case series, mainly on the series of Kompoliti and colleagues analyzing 147 patients from eight movement disorder centres (Kompoliti *et al.*, 1998).

Dopaminergic Agents

Eighty-seven percent of all 147 cases in the series by Kompoliti and colleagues had been exposed to therapeutic trials of L-Dopa, with a mean daily dose of 300 mg (range, 100–2000 mg) (Kompoliti *et al.*, 1998). Some clinical improvement, especially of rigidity and bradykinesia was noted in 26% of patients, but there are no data on the magnitude or duration of this response. However, 5% had some degree of worsening, either of parkinsonism or gait dysfunction or dystonia and myoclonus. L-Dopa-induced dyskinesias were not observed in this series, even with high-dose treatment, and there are also no other reports in the literature noting the occurrence of dyskinesias in response to L-Dopa in CBD (Kompoliti and Goetz, 2000).

Dopamine agonists are less commonly used than L-Dopa to treat parkinsonian features of CBD. Twenty-five percent of the 147 patients collected by Kompoliti and colleagues had been treated with low doses of either pergolide or bromocriptine. Only 6% of patients showed some improvement. Agonist-induced confusion was relatively common, affecting 14% of patients, whereas gastrointestinal side effects or dizziness was noted in 11% each. Selegeline improved parkinsonism in 3 out of 30 patients (Kompoliti *et al.*, 1998).

Anti-cholinergics

Thirty-eight patients (27%) of the series had been exposed to anti-cholinergics—either trihexiphenidyl or benztropine—and four of these (10%) had improvements in rigidity or tremor (Kompoliti *et al.*, 1998). There is no report on side effects, specifically cognitive dysfunction, in the literature.

Anti-cholinergics and baclofen were reported to have improved dystonia in individual cases (Kompoliti *et al.*, 1998; Vanek and Jankovic, 2000).

NMDA Receptor Antagonists

Amantadine produced some benefit in 3 out of 24 patients treated. Other than tremor and rigidity, gait was

Table 9.9 Pragmatic Management of CBD.

Due to the small number of randomized controlled trials the practical management of CBD is largely based on empirical evidence. Treatment is largely targeted at the motor presentation.

Parkinsonism
  L-Dopa (up to 1000 mg, if tolerated and necessary)
  Physiotherapy
  Speech therapy
  Occupational therapy

Postural limb deformities
  Baclofen (up to 40 mg/d)
  Botulinum toxin

Myoclonus
  Clonazepam (0.5–6 mg/day).

Cognitive impairment including apraxia
  Cognitive training
  Occupational therapy

---

reported to improve following amantadine (Kompoliti *et al.*, 1998).

Benzodiazepines

The use of benzodiazepines to treat myoclonic jerks has been reported in a number of studies (Litvan, 1997; Kompoliti *et al.*, 1998; Vanek and Jankovic, 2000). Results are inconsistent, and the drug most often reported as beneficial is clonazepam, ameliorating myoclonic jerking in 23% of patients, with sedation as most common side effect, affecting 26% of patients (Kompoliti *et al.*, 1998).

Botulinum Toxin A

Of nine patients in the large series reported by Kompoliti *et al.* who received local botulinum toxin injections to treat focal limb dystonia, six (67%) reported some improvement (Kompoliti *et al.*, 1998). All six patients in the series of 66 cases reported by Vanek and Jankovic had some response of their focal dystonic symptoms to botulinum toxin injections—two of these experienced marked degrees of improvement of both dystonia and pain with this form of therapy (Vanek and Jankovic, 2000). Müller and colleagues reported on two patients with CBD who received successful treatment with botulinum toxin injections for focal limb dystonia (Muller *et al.*, 2002). Dosages used were 40–120 units Dysport for finger flexor muscles, 80–120 units Dysport for wrist flexor and extensor muscles, and 160–240 units Dysport for elbow flexor muscles.

Non-Medical Therapy

There is no evidence available that various methods of physiotherapy, occupational therapy, or speech therapy significantly reduce disability. Limb apraxia may show a limited response for a limited period of time to physiotherapy, and occupational therapy may increase functional hand use, particularly when combined with anti-parkinsonian and anti-dystonic pharmacotherapy.

Speech and swallowing problems are common as CBD progresses and should be treated with speech therapy; nasogastric or gastrostomy tube feeding for severe dysphagia are rarely necessary, but should be considered in case of silent aspirations (Table 9.9).

References

Movement Disorder Society task force (2002) Drugs to treat autonomic dysfunction in Parkinson's disease. *Movement Disorders*, **17** (Suppl. 4), S103–S111.

Aarsland, D., Larsen, J.P., Lim, N.G. and Tandberg, E. (1999) Olanzapine for psychosis in patients with Parkinson's disease with and without dementia. *Journal of Neuropsychiatry and Clinical Neurosciences*, **11** (3), 392–394.

Alam, M., Smith, G., Bleasdale-Barr, K., Pavitt, D.V. and Mathias, C.J. (1995) Effects of the peptide release inhibitor, octreotide, on daytime hypotension and on nocturnal hypertension in primary autonomic failure. *Journal of Hypertension*, **13** (12 Pt 2), 1664–1669.

Allcock, L.M., Kenny, R.A. and Burn, D.J. (2006) Clinical phenotype of subjects with Parkinson's disease and orthostatic hypotension: autonomic symptom and demographic comparison. *Movement Disorders*, **21** (11), 1851–1855.

Ballard, C., Grace, J., McKeith, I. and Holmes, C. (1998) Neuroleptic sensitivity in dementia with Lewy bodies and Alzheimer's disease. *Lancet*, **351** (9108), 1032–1033.

Ballard, C.G., Chalmers, K.A., Todd, C., McKeith, I.G., O'Brien, J.T., Wilcock, G. *et al.* (2007) Cholinesterase inhibitors reduce cortical Abeta in dementia with Lewy bodies. *Neurology*, **68** (20), 1726–1729.

Beck, R.O., Betts, C.D. and Fowler, C.J. (1994) Genitourinary dysfunction in multiple system atrophy: clinical features and treatment in 62 cases. *The Journal of Urology*, **151** (5), 1336–1341.

Blin, J., Mazetti, P., Mazoyer, B., Rivaud, S., Ben Ayed, S., Malapani, C. *et al.* (1995) Does the enhancement of cholinergic neurotransmission influence brain glucose kinetics and clinical symptomatology in progressive supranuclear palsy? *Brain: A Journal of Neurology*, **118** (Pt 6), 1485–1495.

Boesch, S.M., Wenning, G.K., Ransmayr, G. and Poewe, W. (2002) Dystonia in multiple system atrophy. *Journal of Neurology, Neurosurgery, and Psychiatry*, **72** (3), 300–303.

Bonelli, S.B., Ransmayr, G., Steffelbauer, M., Lukas, T., Lampl, C. and Deibl, M. (2004) L-dopa responsiveness in dementia with Lewy bodies, Parkinson's disease with and without dementia. *Neurology*, **63** (2), 376–378.

Bower, J.H., Maraganore, D.M., McDonnell, S.K. and Rocca, W.A. (1997) Incidence of progressive supranuclear palsy and multiple system atrophy in Olmsted County, Minnesota, 1976 to 1990. *Neurology*, **49** (5), 1284–1288.

Burke, W.J., Pfeiffer, R.F. and McComb, R.D. (1998) Neuroleptic sensitivity to clozapine in dementia with Lewy bodies. *Journal* of Neuropsychiatry and Clinical Neurosciences, **10** (2), 227–229.

Burn, D.J. and Warren, N.M. (2005) Toward future therapies in progressive supranuclear palsy. *Movement Disorders*, **20** (Suppl 12), S92–S98.

Casarejos, M.J., Menendez, J., Solano, R.M., Rodriguez-Navarro, J.A., Garcia de Yebenes, J. and Mena, M.A. (2006) Susceptibility to rotenone is increased in neurons from parkin null mice and is reduced by minocycline. *Journal of Neurochemistry*, **97** (4), 934–946.

Colosimo, C., Merello, M. and Pontieri, F.E. (1996) Amantadine in parkinsonian patients unresponsive to levodopa: a pilot study. *Journal of Neurology*, **243** (5), 422–425.

Cummings, J.L. (1995) Lewy body diseases with dementia: pathophysiology and treatment. *Brain Cognition*, **28** (3), 266–280.

Cummings, J.L. and Litvan, I. (2000) Neuropsychiatric aspects of corticobasal degeneration. *Advances in Neurology*, **82**, 147–152.

Cummings, J.L., Street, J., Masterman, D. and Clark, W.S. (2002) Efficacy of olanzapine in the treatment of psychosis in dementia with lewy bodies. *Dementia and Geriatric Cognitive Disorders*, **13** (2), 67–73.

Daniele, A., Moro, E. and Bentivoglio, A.R. (1999) Zolpidem in progressive supranuclear palsy. *The New England Journal of Medicine*, **341** (7), 543–544.

Di Maria, E., Tabaton, M., Vigo, T., Abbruzzese, G., Bellone, E., Donati, C. *et al.* (2000) Corticobasal degeneration shares a common genetic background with progressive supranuclear palsy. *Annals of Neurology*, **47** (3), 374–377.

Duncombe, A.S. and Lees, A.J. (1985) Methysergide in progressive supranuclear palsy. *Neurology*, **35** (6), 936–937.

Edwards, K., Royall, D., Hershey, L., Lichter, D., Hake, A., Farlow, M. *et al.* (2007) Efficacy and safety of galantamine in patients with dementia with Lewy bodies: a 24-week open-label study. *Dementia and Geriatric Cognitive Disorders*, **23** (6), 401–405.

Edwards, K.R., Hershey, L., Wray, L., Bednarczyk, E.M., Lichter, D., Farlow, M. *et al.* (2004) Efficacy and safety of galantamine in patients with dementia with Lewy bodies: a 12-week interim analysis. *Dementia and Geriatric Cognitive Disorders*, **17** (Suppl 1), 40–48.

Eichhorn, T.E. and Oertel, W.H. (2001) Macrogol 3350/electrolyte improves constipation in Parkinson's disease and multiple system atrophy. *Movement Disorders*, **16** (6), 1176–1177.

Emre, M. (2003) Dementia associated with Parkinson's disease. *Lancet Neurol*, **2** (4), 229–237.

Fabbrini, G., Barbanti, P., Bonifati, V., Colosimo, C., Gasparini, M., Vanacore, N. *et al.* (2001) Donepezil in the treatment of progressive supranuclear palsy. *Acta Neurologica Scandinavica*, **103** (2), 123–125.

Fergusson, E. and Howard, R. (2000) Donepezil for the treatment of psychosis in dementia with Lewy bodies. *International Journal of Geriatric Psychiatry*, **15** (3), 280–281.

Foster, N.L., Aldrich, M.S., Bluemlein, L., White, R.F. and Berent, S. (1989) Failure of cholinergic agonist RS-86 to improve cognition and movement in PSP despite effects on sleep. *Neurology*, **39** (2 Pt 1), 257–261.

Friess, E., Kuempfel, T., Modell, S., Winkelmann, J., Holsboer, F., Ising, M. *et al.* (2006) Paroxetine treatment improves motor symptoms in patients with multiple system atrophy. *Parkinsonism & Related Disorders*, **12** (7), 432–437.

Fujino, Y., Nakajima, M., Tsuboi, Y., Baba, Y. and Yamada, T. (2002) [Clinical effectiveness of tandospirone citrate (5-HT1A agonist) on patients with progressive supranuclear palsy]. *Rinsho Shinkeigaku*, **42** (1), 42–44.

Geser, F., Seppi, K., Stampfer-Kountchev, M., Kollensperger, M., Diem, A., Ndayisaba, J.P. *et al.* (2005) The European Multiple System Atrophy-Study Group (EMSA-SG). *Journal of Neural Transmission*, **112** (12), 1677–1686.

Geser, F. and Wenning, G.K. (2006) The diagnosis of multiple system atrophy. *Journal of Neurology*, **253** (Suppl 3), iii2–iii15.

Ghika, J., Tennis, M., Hoffman, E., Schoenfeld, D. and Growdon, J. (1991) Idazoxan treatment in progressive supranuclear palsy. *Neurology*, **41** (7), 986–991.

Ghorayeb, I., Yekhlef, F., Bioulac, B. and Tison, F. (2005) Continuous positive airway pressure for sleep-related breathing disorders in multiple system atrophy: long-term acceptance. *Sleep Medicine*, **6** (4), 359–362.

Gilman, S., Wenning, G.K., Low, P.A., *et al.* (2008) Second consensus statement on the diagnosis of multiple system atrophy. *Neurology*, **71** (9), 670–676.

Gilman, S. http://www.ncbi.nlm.nih.gov/pubmed/9869555?ordinalpos=2&itool=EntrezSystem2. PEntrez.Pubmed.Pubmed_ResultsPanel.Pubmed_RVDocSum.

Goetz, C.G., Blasucci, L.M., Leurgans, S. and Pappert, E.J. (2000) Olanzapine and clozapine: comparative effects on motor function in hallucinating PD patients. *Neurology*, **55** (6), 789–794.

Goetz, C.G., Tanner, C.M. and Klawans, H.L. (1984) The pharmacology of olivopontocerebellar atrophy. *Advances in Neurology*, **41**, 143–148.

Halaska, M., Ralph, G., Wiedemann, A., Primus, G., Ballering-Bruhl, B., Hofner, K. *et al.* (2003) Controlled, double-blind, multicentre clinical trial to investigate long-term tolerability and efficacy of trospium chloride in patients with detrusor instability. *World Journal of Urology*, **20** (6), 392–399.

Haldeman, S., Goldman, J.W., Hyde, J. and Pribram, H.F. (1981) Progressive supranuclear palsy, computed tomography, and response to antiparkinsonian drugs. *Neurology*, **31** (4), 442–445.

Heinz, A., Wohrle, J., Schols, L., Klotz, P., Kuhn, W. and Przuntek, H. (1992) Continuous subcutaneous lisuride infusion in OPCA. *Journal of Neural Transmission. General Section*, **90** (2), 145–150.

Holmberg, B., Johansson, J.O., Poewe, W., Wenning, G., Quinn, N. P., Mathias, C. *et al.* (2007) Safety and tolerability of growth hormone therapy in multiple system atrophy: A double-blind, placebo-controlled study. *Movement Disorders*, **22** (8), 1138–1144.

Hughes, A.J., Daniel, S.E., Ben Shlomo, Y. and Lees, A.J. (2002) The accuracy of diagnosis of parkinsonian syndromes in a specialist movement disorder service. *Brain: A Journal of Neurology*, **125** (Pt 4), 861–870.

Hussain, I.F., Brady, C.M., Swinn, M.J., Mathias, C.J. and Fowler, C.J. (2001) Treatment of erectile dysfunction with sildenafil citrate (Viagra) in parkinsonism due to Parkinson's disease or multiple system atrophy with observations on orthostatic hypotension. *Journal of Neurology, Neurosurgery, and Psychiatry*, **71** (3), 371–374.

Iranzo, A., Santamaria, J., Tolosa, E., Vilaseca, I., Valldeoriola, F., Marti, M.J. *et al.* (2004) Long-term effect of CPAP in the treatment of nocturnal stridor in multiple system atrophy. *Neurology*, **63** (5), 930–932.

Jain, S., Dawson, J., Quinn, N.P. and Playford, E.D. (2004) Occupational therapy in multiple system atrophy: a pilot randomized controlled trial. *Movement Disorders*, **19** (11), 1360–1364.

Jankovic, J. (1983) Controlled trial of pergolide mesylate in Parkinson's disease and progressive supranuclear palsy. *Neurology*, **33** (4), 505–507.

Jankovic, J., Gilden, J.L., Hiner, B.C., Kaufmann, H., Brown, D.C., Coghlan, C.H. *et al.* (1993) Neurogenic orthostatic hypotension:

a double-blind, placebo-controlled study with midodrine. *The American Journal of Medicine*, **95** (1), 38–48.

Jordan, J., Shannon, J.R., Biaggioni, I., Norman, R., Black, B.K. and Robertson, D. (1998) Contrasting actions of pressor agents in severe autonomic failure. *The American Journal of Medicine*, **105** (2), 116–124.

Kane, J., Honigfeld, G., Singer, J. and Meltzer, H. (1988) Clozapine for the treatment-resistant schizophrenic. A double-blind comparison with chlorpromazine. *Archives of General Psychiatry*, **45** (9), 789–796.

Kato, K., Wada, T., Kawakatsu, S. and Otani, K. (2002) Improvement of both psychotic symptoms and Parkinsonism in a case of dementia with Lewy bodies by the combination therapy of risperidone and L-DOPA. *Progress in Neuro-Psychopharmacology & Biological Psychiatry*, **26** (1), 201–203.

Kaufmann, H., Saadia, D., Voustianiouk, A., Goldstein, D.S., Holmes, C., Yahr, M.D. *et al.* (2003) Norepinephrine precursor therapy in neurogenic orthostatic hypotension. *Circulation*, **108** (6), 724–728.

Kertesz, A., Martinez-Lage, P., Davidson, W. and Munoz, D.G. (2000) The corticobasal degeneration syndrome overlaps progressive aphasia and frontotemporal dementia. *Neurology*, **55** (9), 1368–1375.

Kertzman, C., Robinson, D.L. and Litvan, I. (1990) Effects of physostigmine on spatial attention in patients with progressive supranuclear palsy. *Archives of Neurology*, **47** (12), 1346–1350.

Klos, K.J., Bower, J.H., Josephs, K.A., Matsumoto, J.Y. and Ahlskog, J.E. (2005) Pathological hypersexuality predominantly linked to adjuvant dopamine agonist therapy in Parkinson's disease and multiple system atrophy. *Parkinsonism & Related Disorders*, **11** (6), 381–386.

Kollensperger, M., Stampfer-Kountchev, M., Seppi, K., Geser, F., Frick, C., Del Sorbo, F. *et al.* (2007) Progression of dysautonomia in multiple system atrophy: a prospective study of self-perceived impairment. *European Journal of Neurology*, **14** (1), 66–72.

Koller, W.C., Morantz, R., Vetere-Overfield, B. and Waxman, M. (1989) Autologous adrenal medullary transplant in progressive supranuclear palsy. *Neurology*, **39** (8), 1066–1068.

Kompoliti, K. and Goetz, C.G. (2000) Therapeutic approaches. *Advances in Neurology*, **82**, 217–221.

Kompoliti, K., Goetz, C.G., Boeve, B.F., Maraganore, D.M., Ahlskog, J.E., Marsden, C.D. *et al.* (1998) Clinical presentation and pharmacological therapy in corticobasal degeneration. *Archives of Neurology*, **55** (7), 957–961.

Kompoliti, K., Goetz, C.G., Litvan, I., Jellinger, K. and Verny, M. (1998) Pharmacological therapy in progressive supranuclear palsy. *Archives of Neurology*, **55** (8), 1099–1102.

Kumar, R., Bergeron, C. and Lang, A.E. (2002) Corticobasal degeneration, in Parkinson's disease and movement disorders, (eds J.C. Janssen and E. Tolosa), Lippincott, Williams & Wilkins, Philadelphia, pp. 185–198.

Kurlan, R., Cummings, J., Raman, R. and Thal, L. (2007) Quetiapine for agitation or psychosis in patients with dementia and parkinsonism. *Neurology*, **68** (17), 1356–1363.

Lagalla, G., Millevolte, M., Capecci, M., Provinciali, L. and Ceravolo, M.G. (2006) Botulinum toxin type A for drooling in Parkinson's disease: a double-blind, randomized, placebo-controlled study. *Movement Disorders*, **21** (5), 704–707.

Lanctot, K.L. and Herrmann, N. (2000) Donepezil for behavioural disorders associated with Lewy bodies: a case series. *International Journal of Geriatric Psychiatry*, **15** (4), 338–345.

Lang, A.E., Lozano, A., Duff, J., Tasker, R., Miyasaki, J., Galvez-Jimenez, N. *et al.* (1997) Medial pallidotomy in late-stage

Parkinson's disease and striatonigral degeneration. *Advances in Neurology*, **74**, 199–211.

Lauterbach, E.C. (2004) The neuropsychiatry of Parkinson's disease and related disorders. *Psychiatr Clin North Am*, **27** (4), 801–825.

Lebert, F., Pasquier, F., Souliez, L. and Petit, H. (1998) Tacrine efficacy in Lewy body dementia. *International Journal of Geriatric Psychiatry*, **13** (8), 516–519.

Lees, A.J. and Bannister, R. (1981) The use of lisuride in the treatment of multiple system atrophy with autonomic failure (Shy-Drager syndrome). *Journal of Neurology, Neurosurgery, and Psychiatry*, **44** (4), 347–351.

Leigh, P.N., Ludolph, A., Agid, Y. and Bensimon, G. (2007) Neuroprotection and Natural History in parkinson Plus Syndromes (NNIPPS): Results of a randomized placebo-controlled trial of riluzole in PSP and MSA. *Movement Disorders*, **22** (16), 2.

Levy, R., Eagger, S., Griffiths, M., Perry, E., Honavar, M., Dean, A. *et al.* (1994) Lewy bodies and response to tacrine in Alzheimer's disease. *Lancet*, **343** (8890), 176.

Lezcano, E., Gomez-Esteban, J.C., Zarranz, J.J., Alcaraz, R., Atares, B., Bilbao, G. *et al.* (2004) Parkinson's disease-like presentation of multiple system atrophy with poor response to STN stimulation: a clinicopathological case report. *Movement Disorders*, **19** (8), 973–977.

Litvan, I. (1997) Progressive supranuclear palsy and corticobasal degeneration. *Baillieres Clinical Neurology*, **6** (1), 167–185.

Litvan, I., Agid, Y., Calne, D., Campbell, G., Dubois, B., Duvoisin, R.C. *et al.* (1996) Clinical research criteria for the diagnosis of progressive supranuclear palsy (Steele-Richardson-Olszewski syndrome): report of the NINDS-SPSP international workshop. *Neurology*, **47** (1), 1–9.

Litvan, I., Blesa, R., Clark, K., Nichelli, P., Atack, J.R., Mouradian, M.M. *et al.* (1994) Pharmacological evaluation of the cholinergic system in progressive supranuclear palsy. *Annals of Neurology*, **36** (1), 55–61.

Litvan, I., Mangone, C.A., McKee, A., Verny, M., Parsa, A., Jellinger, K. *et al.* (1996) Natural history of progressive supranuclear palsy (Steele-Richardson-Olszewski syndrome) and clinical predictors of survival: a clinicopathological study. *Journal of Neurology, Neurosurgery, and Psychiatry*, **60** (6), 615–620.

Litvan, I., Phipps, M., Pharr, V.L., Hallett, M., Grafman, J. and Salazar, A. (2001) Randomized placebo-controlled trial of donepezil in patients with progressive supranuclear palsy. *Neurology*, **57** (3), 467–473.

Low, P.A., Gilden, J.L., Freeman, R., Sheng, K.N. and McElligott, M.A. (1997) Efficacy of midodrine vs placebo in neurogenic orthostatic hypotension. A randomized, double-blind multicenter study. Midodrine Study Group. *The Journal of the American Medical Association*, **277** (13), 1046–1051.

Mahapatra, R.K., Edwards, M.J., Schott, J.M. and Bhatia, K.P. (2004) Corticobasal degeneration. *Lancet Neurology*, **3** (12), 736–743.

Mancini, F., Zangaglia, R., Cristina, S., Sommaruga, M.G., Martignoni, E., Nappi, G. *et al.* (2003) Double-blind, placebo-controlled study to evaluate the efficacy and safety of botulinum toxin type A in the treatment of drooling in parkinsonism. *Movement Disorders*, **18** (6), 685–688.

Mathias, C.J., Fosbraey, P., da Costa, D.F., Thornley, A. and Bannister, R. (1986) The effect of desmopressin on nocturnal polyuria, overnight weight loss, and morning postural hypotension in patients with autonomic failure. *British Medical Journal (Clinical Research Ed.)*, **293** (6543), 353–354.

Mathias, C.J., Senard, J.M., Braune, S., Watson, L., Aragishi, A., Keeling, J.E. *et al.* (2001) L-threo-dihydroxyphenylserine

(L-threo-DOPS; droxidopa) in the management of neurogenic orthostatic hypotension: a multi-national, multi-center, dose-ranging study in multiple system atrophy and pure autonomic failure. *Clinical Autonomic Research*, **11** (4), 235–242.

McKeith, I., Del Ser, T., Spano, P., Emre, M., Wesnes, K., Anand, R. *et al.* (2000) Efficacy of rivastigmine in dementia with Lewy bodies: a randomised, double-blind, placebo-controlled international study. *Lancet*, **356** (9247), 2031–2036.

McKeith, I., Fairbairn, A., Perry, R., Thompson, P. and Perry, E. (1992) Neuroleptic sensitivity in patients with senile dementia of Lewy body type. *BMJ (Clinical Research Ed)*, **305** (6855), 673–678.

McKeith, I.G., Ballard, C.G. and Harrison, R.W. (1995) Neuroleptic sensitivity to risperidone in Lewy body dementia. *Lancet*, **346** (8976), 699.

McKeith, I.G., Dickson, D.W., Lowe, J., Emre, M., O'Brien, J.T., Feldman, H. *et al.* (2005) Diagnosis and management of dementia with Lewy bodies: third report of the DLB Consortium. *Neurology*, **65** (12), 1863–1872.

McKeith, I.G., Grace, J.B., Walker, Z., Byrne, E.J., Wilkinson, D., Stevens, T. *et al.* (2000) Rivastigmine in the treatment of dementia with Lewy bodies: preliminary findings from an open trial. *International Journal of Geriatric Psychiatry*, **15** (5), 387–392.

Mori, S., Mori, E., Iseki, E. and Kosaka, K. (2006) Efficacy and safety of donepezil in patients with dementia with Lewy bodies: preliminary findings from an open-label study. *Psychiatry and Clinical Neurosciences*, **60** (2), 190–195.

Morris, H.R., Gibb, G., Katzenschlager, R., Wood, N.W., Hanger, D.P., Strand, C. *et al.* (2002) Pathological, clinical and genetic heterogeneity in progressive supranuclear palsy. *Brain: A Journal of Neurology*, **125** (Pt 5), 969–975.

Morris, S.K., Olichney, J.M. and Corey-Bloom, J. (1998) Psychosis in Dementia With Lewy Bodies. *Seminars in Clinical Neuropsychiatry*, **3** (1), 51–60.

Muller, J., Wenning, G.K., Wissel, J., Seppi, K. and Poewe, W. (2002) Botulinum toxin treatment in atypical parkinsonian disorders associated with disabling focal dystonia. *Journal of Neurology*, **249** (3), 300–304.

Murray, R., Neumann, M., Forman, M.S., Farmer, J., Massimo, L., Rice, A. *et al.* (2007) Cognitive and motor assessment in autopsy-proven corticobasal degeneration. *Neurology*, **68** (16), 1274–1283.

Nath, U., Ben Shlomo, Y., Thomson, R.G., Lees, A.J. and Burn, D. J. (2003) Clinical features and natural history of progressive supranuclear palsy: a clinical cohort study. *Neurology*, **60** (6), 910–916.

Nath, U., Ben Shlomo, Y., Thomson, R.G., Morris, H.R., Wood, N. W., Lees, A.J. *et al.* (2001) The prevalence of progressive supranuclear palsy (Steele-Richardson-Olszewski syndrome) in the UK. *Brain: A Journal of Neurology*, **124** (Pt 7), 1438–1449.

Neophytides, A., Lieberman, A.N., Goldstein, M., Gopinathan, G., Leibowitz, M., Bock, J. *et al.* (1982) The use of lisuride, a potent dopamine and serotonin agonist, in the treatment of progressive supranuclear palsy. *Journal of Neurology, Neurosurgery, and Psychiatry*, **45** (3), 261–263.

Newman, G.C. (1985) Treatment of progressive supranuclear palsy with tricyclic antidepressants. *Neurology*, **35** (8), 1189–1193.

Nonaka, M., Imai, T., Shintani, T., Kawamata, M., Chiba, S. and Matsumoto, H. (2006) Non-invasive positive pressure ventilation for laryngeal contraction disorder during sleep in multiple system atrophy. *Journal of the Neurological Sciences*, **247** (1), 53–58.

Okun, M.S., Tagliati, M., Pourfar, M., Fernandez, H.H., Rodriguez, R.L., Alterman, R.L. *et al.* (2005) Management of referred deep brain stimulation failures: a retrospective analysis from 2 movement disorders centers. *Archives of Neurology*, **62** (8), 1250–1255.

Osaki, Y., Ben Shlomo, Y., Lees, A.J., Daniel, S.E., Colosimo, C., Wenning, G. *et al.* (2004) Accuracy of clinical diagnosis of progressive supranuclear palsy. *Movement Disorders*, **19** (2), 181–189.

Ozawa, T., Paviour, D., Quinn, N.P., Josephs, K.A., Sangha, H., Kilford, L. *et al.* (2004) The spectrum of pathological involvement of the striatonigral and olivopontocerebellar systems in multiple system atrophy: clinicopathological correlations. *Brain: A Journal of Neurology*, **127** (Pt 2), 2657–2671.

Parsa, M.A. and Bastani, B. (1998) Quetiapine (Seroquel) in the treatment of psychosis in patients with Parkinson's disease. *Journal of Neuropsychiatry and Clinical Neurosciences*, **10** (2), 216–219.

Paulson, G.W., Lowery, H.W. and Taylor, G.C. (1981) Progressive supranuclear palsy: pneumoencephalography, electronystagmography and treatment with methysergide. *European Neurology*, **20** (1), 13–16.

Peralta, C., Stampfer-Kountchev, M., Karner, E., Kollensperger, M., Geser, F., Wolf, E. *et al.* (2007) Orthostatic hypotension and attention in Parkinson's disease with and without dementia. *Journal of Neural Transmission*, **114**, 585–588.

Perera, R., Isola, L. and Kaufmann, H. (1995) Effect of recombinant erythropoietin on anemia and orthostatic hypotension in primary autonomic failure. *Clinical Autonomic Research*, **5** (4), 211–213.

Perry, E., Walker, M., Grace, J. and Perry, R. (1999) Acetylcholine in mind: a neurotransmitter correlate of consciousness? *Trends in Neurosciences*, **22** (6), 273–280.

Piccione, F., Mancini, E., Tonin, P. and Bizzarini, M. (1997) Botulinum toxin treatment of apraxia of eyelid opening in progressive supranuclear palsy: report of two cases. *Archives of Physical Medicine and Rehabilitation*, **78** (5), 525–529.

Querfurth, H.W., Allam, G.J., Geffroy, M.A., Schiff, H.B. and Kaplan, R.F. (2000) Acetylcholinesterase inhibition in dementia with Lewy bodies: results of a prospective pilot trial. *Dementia and Geriatric Cognitive Disorders*, **11** (6), 314–321.

Rafal, R.D. and Grimm, R.J. (1981) Progressive supranuclear palsy: functional analysis of the response to methysergide and antiparkinsonian agents. *Neurology*, **31** (12), 1507–1518.

Rahkonen, T., Eloniemi-Sulkava, U., Rissanen, S., Vatanen, A., Viramo, P. and Sulkava, R. (2003) Dementia with Lewy bodies according to the consensus criteria in a general population aged 75 years or older. *Journal of Neurology, Neurosurgery, and Psychiatry*, **74** (6), 720–724.

Raimbach, S.J., Cortelli, P., Kooner, J.S., Bannister, R., Bloom, S. R. and Mathias, C.J. (1989) Prevention of glucose-induced hypotension by the somatostatin analogue octreotide (SMS 201-995) in chronic autonomic failure: haemodynamic and hormonal changes. *Clinical Science (London, England: 1979)*, **77** (6), 623–628.

Rajput, A. and Rajput, A.H. (2001) Progressive supranuclear palsy: clinical features, pathophysiology and management. *Drugs Aging*, **18** (12), 913–925.

Ransmayr, G., Seppi, K., Donnemiller, E., Luginger, E., Marksteiner, J., Riccabona, G. *et al.* (2001) Striatal dopamine transporter function in dementia with Lewy bodies and Parkinson's disease. *European Journal of Nuclear Medicine*, **28** (10), 1523–1528.

Rascol, O., Sieradzan, K., Peyro-Saint-Paul, H., Thalamas, C., Brefel-Courbon, C., Senard, J.M. *et al.* (1998) Efaroxan, an alpha-2 antagonist, in the treatment of progressive supranuclear palsy. *Movement Disorders*, **13** (4), 673–676.

Rebeiz, J.J., Kolodny, E.H. and Richardson, E.P., Jr (1967) Corticodentatonigral degeneration with neuronal achromasia: a progressive disorder of late adult life. *Transactions of the American Neurological Association*, **92**, 23–26.

Rich, S.S., Friedman, J.H. and Ott, B.R. (1995) Risperidone versus clozapine in the treatment of psychosis in six patients with Parkinson's disease and other akinetic-rigid syndromes. *Journal of Clinical Psychiatry*, **56** (12), 556–559.

Rinne, J.O., Lee, M.S., Thompson, P.D. and Marsden, C.D. (1994) Corticobasal degeneration. A clinical study of 36 cases. *Brain: A Journal of Neurology*, **117** (Pt 5), 1183–1196.

Rojas-Fernandez, C.H. (2001) Successful use of donepezil for the treatment of dementia with Lewy bodies. *Annals of Pharmacotherapy*, **35** (2), 202–205.

Rowan, E., McKeith, I.G., Saxby, B.K., O'Brien, J.T., Burn, D., Mosimann, U. *et al.* (2007) Effects of donepezil on central processing speed and attentional measures in Parkinson's disease with dementia and dementia with Lewy bodies. *Dementia and Geriatric Cognitive Disorders*, **23** (3), 161–167.

Rozzini, L., Chilovi, B.V., Bertoletti, E., Conti, M., Delrio, I., Trabucchi, M. *et al.* (2007) Cognitive and psychopathologic response to rivastigmine in dementia with Lewy bodies compared to Alzheimer's disease: a case control study. *American Journal of Alzheimer's Disease and Other Dementias*, **22** (1), 42–47.

Sakakibara, R., Hattori, T., Uchiyama, T., Kita, K., Asahina, M., Suzuki, A. *et al.* (2000) Urinary dysfunction and orthostatic hypotension in multiple system atrophy: which is the more common and earlier manifestation? *Journal of Neurology, Neurosurgery, and Psychiatry*, **68** (1), 65–69.

Samuel, W., Caligiuri, M., Galasko, D., Lacro, J., Marini, M., McClure, F.S. *et al.* (2000) Better cognitive and psychopathologic response to donepezil in patients prospectively diagnosed as dementia with Lewy bodies: a preliminary study. *International Journal of Geriatric Psychiatry*, **15** (9), 794–802.

Santens, P., Vonck, K., De Letter, M., Van Driessche, K., Sieben, A., De Reuck, J. *et al.* (2006) Deep brain stimulation of the internal pallidum in multiple system atrophy. *Parkinsonism & Related Disorders*, **12** (3), 181–183.

Schrag, A., Ben Shlomo, Y. and Quinn, N.P. (1999) Prevalence of progressive supranuclear palsy and multiple system atrophy: a cross-sectional study. *Lancet*, **354** (9192), 1771–1775.

Schrag, A., Ben Shlomo, Y. and Quinn, N.P. (2000) Cross sectional prevalence survey of idiopathic Parkinson's disease and Parkinsonism in London. *BMJ (Clinical Research Ed)*, **321** (7252), 21–22.

Schrag, A., Geser, F., Stampfer-Kountchev, M., Seppi, K., Sawires, M., Kollensperger, M. *et al.* (2006) Health-related quality of life in multiple system atrophy. *Movement Disorders*, **21**, 809–815.

Seppi, K., Peralta, C., Diem-Zangerl, A., Puschban, Z., Mueller, J., Poewe, W. *et al.* (2006) Placebo-controlled trial of riluzole in multiple system atrophy. *European Journal of Neurology*, **13** (10), 1146–1148.

Sha, S., Hou, C., Viskontas, I.V. and Miller, B.L. (2006) Are frontotemporal lobar degeneration, progressive supranuclear palsy and corticobasal degeneration distinct diseases? *Nature Clinical Pracicet Neurology*, **2** (12), 658–665.

Shannon, J.R., Diedrich, A., Biaggioni, I., Tank, J., Robertson, R.M., Robertson, D. *et al.* (2002) Water drinking as a treatment for orthostatic syndromes. *The American Journal of Medicine*, **112** (5), 355–360.

Shea, C., MacKnight, C. and Rockwood, K. (1998) Donepezil for treatment of dementia with Lewy bodies: a case series of nine patients. *International Psychogeriatrics*, **10** (3), 229–238.

Shults, C.W., Rockenstein, E., Crews, L., Adame, A., Mante, M., Larrea, G. *et al.* (2005) Neurological and neurodegenerative alterations in a transgenic mouse model expressing human alpha-synuclein under oligodendrocyte promoter: implications for multiple system atrophy. *The Journal of Neuroscience*, **25** (46), 10689–10699.

Skjerve, A. and Nygaard, H.A. (2000) Improvement in sundowning in dementia with Lewy bodies after treatment with donepezil. *International Journal of Geriatric Psychiatry*, **15** (12), 1147–1151.

Stamelou, M., Reuss, A., Pilatus, U., Magerkurth, J., Niklowitz, P., Eggert, K.M., Krisp, A., Menke, T., Schade-Brittinger, C., Oertel, W.H. and Höglinger, G.U. (2008) Short-term effects of coenzyme Q10 in progressive supranuclear palsy: a randomized, placebo-controlled trial. *Movement Disorders*, **23** (7), 942–949.

Steele, J.C., Richardson, J. and Oslzewski, J. (1964) Progressive supranuclear palsy. A heterogeneous degeneration involving the brain stem, basal ganglia and cerebellum with vertical gaze and pseudobulbar palsy, nuchal dystonia and dementia. *Archives of Neurology*, **10**, 333–359.

Stefanova, N., Reindl, M., Neumann, M., Haass, C., Poewe, W., Kahle, P.J. *et al.* (2005) Oxidative stress in transgenic mice with oligodendroglial alpha-synuclein overexpression replicates the characteristic neuropathology of multiple system atrophy. *The American Journal of Pathology*, **166** (3), 869–876.

Stefanova, N., Reindl, M., Neumann, M., Kahle, P.J., Poewe, W. and Wenning, G.K. (2007) Microglial activation mediates neurodegeneration related to oligodendroglial alpha-synucleinopathy: implications for multiple system atrophy. *Movement Disorders*, **22** (15), 2196–2203.

Stevens, T., Livingston, G., Kitchen, G., Manela, M., Walker, Z. and Katona, C. (2002) Islington study of dementia subtypes in the community. *British Journal of Psychiatry*, **180**, 270–276.

Thobois, S., Broussolle, E., Toureille, L. and Vial, C. (2001) Severe dysphagia after botulinum toxin injection for cervical dystonia in multiple system atrophy. *Movement Disorders*, **16** (4), 764–765.

Thomas, A.J., Burn, D.J., Rowan, E.N., Littlewood, E., Newby, J., Cousins, D. *et al.* (2005) A comparison of the efficacy of donepezil in Parkinson's disease with dementia and dementia with Lewy bodies. *International Journal of Geriatric Psychiatry*, **20** (10), 938–944.

van Balken, I. and Litvan, I. (2006) Current and future treatments in progressive supranuclear palsy. *Current Treatment Options in Neurology*, **8** (3), 211–223.

Vanek, Z.F. and Jankovic, J. (2000) Dystonia in corticobasal degeneration. *Advances in Neurology*, **82**, 61–67.

Visser-Vandewalle, V., Temel, Y., Colle, H. and van der, L.C. (2003) Bilateral high-frequency stimulation of the subthalamic nucleus in patients with multiple system atrophy–parkinsonism. Report of four cases. *Journal of Neurosurgery*, **98** (4), 882–887.

Walker, Z., Costa, D.C., Walker, R.W., Shaw, K., Gacinovic, S., Stevens, T. *et al.* (2002) Differentiation of dementia with Lewy bodies from Alzheimer's disease using a dopaminergic presynaptic ligand. *Journal of Neurology, Neurosurgery, and Psychiatry*, **73** (2), 134–140.

Walker, Z., Grace, J., Overshot, R., Satarasinghe, S., Swan, A., Katona, C.L. *et al.* (1999) Olanzapine in dementia with Lewy bodies: a clinical study. *International Journal of Geriatric Psychiatry*, **14** (6), 459–466.

Watanabe, H., Saito, Y., Terao, S., Ando, T., Kachi, T., Mukai, E. *et al.* (2002) Progression and prognosis in multiple system atrophy: an analysis of 230 Japanese patients. *Brain: A Journal of Neurology*, **125** (Pt 5), 1070–1083.

Waxman, M.J., Morantz, R.A., Koller, W.C., Paone, D.B. and Nelson, P.W. (1991) High incidence of cardiopulmonary complications associated with implantation of adrenal medullary tissue into the caudate nucleus in patients with advanced neurologic disease. *Critical Care Medicine*, **19** (2), 181–186.

Weiner, W.J., Minagar, A. and Shulman, L.M. (1999) Pramipexole in progressive supranuclear palsy. *Neurology*, **52** (4), 873–874.

Wenning, G.K. (2005) Placebo-controlled trial of amantadine in multiple-system atrophy. *Clinical Neuropharmacology*, **28** (5), 225–227.

Wenning, G.K., Ben Shlomo, Y., Magalhaes, M., Daniel, S.E. and Quinn, N.P. (1994) Clinical features and natural history of multiple system atrophy. An analysis of 100 cases. *Brain: A Journal of Neurology*, **117** (Pt 4), 835–845.

Wenning, G.K., Colosimo, C., Geser, F. and Poewe, W. (2004) Multiple system atrophy. *Lancet Neurology*, **3** (2), 93–103.

Wenning, G.K., Litvan, I., Jankovic, J., Granata, R., Mangone, C. A., McKee, A. *et al.* (1998) Natural history and survival of 14 patients with corticobasal degeneration confirmed at postmortem examination. *Journal of Neurology, Neurosurgery, and Psychiatry*, **64** (2), 184–189.

Wenning, G.K., Tison, F., Ben Shlomo, Y., Daniel, S.E. and Quinn, N.P. (1997) Multiple system atrophy: a review of 203 pathologically proven cases. *Movement Disorders*, **12** (2), 133–147.

Williams, D.R., de Silva, R., Paviour, D.C., Pittman, A., Watt, H.C., Kilford, L. *et al.* (2005) Characteristics of two distinct clinical phenotypes in pathologically proven progressive supranuclear palsy: Richardson's syndrome and PSP-parkinsonism. *Brain: A Journal of Neurology*, **128** (Pt 6), 1247–1258.

Williams, D.R., Holton, J.L., Strand, C., Pittman, A., de Silva, R., Lees, A.J. *et al.* (2007) Pathological tau burden and distribution distinguishes progressive supranuclear palsy-parkinsonism from Richardson's syndrome. *Brain: A Journal of Neurology*, **130** (Pt 6), 1566–1576.

Winkler, A.S., Marsden, J., Parton, M., Watkins, P.J. and Chaudhuri, K.R. (2001) Erythropoietin deficiency and anaemia in multiple system atrophy. *Movement Disorders*, **16** (2), 233–239.

Yamada, T., Hattori, H., Miura, A., Tanabe, M. and Yamori, Y. (2001) Prevalence of Alzheimer's disease, vascular dementia and dementia with Lewy bodies in a Japanese population. *Psychiatry and Clinical Neurosciences*, **55** (1), 21–25.

Yazawa, I., Giasson, B.I., Sasaki, R., Zhang, B., Joyce, S., Uryu, K. *et al.* (2005) Mouse model of multiple system atrophy alpha-synuclein expression in oligodendrocytes causes glial and neuronal degeneration. *Neuron*, **45** (6), 847–859.

Young, T.M. and Mathias, C.J. (2004) The effects of water ingestion on orthostatic hypotension in two groups of chronic autonomic failure: multiple system atrophy and pure autonomic failure. *Journal of Neurology, Neurosurgery, and Psychiatry*, **75** (12), 1737–1741.

Zaccai, J., McCracken, C. and Brayne, C. (2005) A systematic review of prevalence and incidence studies of dementia with Lewy bodies. *Age and Ageing*, **34** (6), 561–566.

Zesiewicz, T.A., Helal, M. and Hauser, R.A. (2000) Sildenafil citrate (Viagra) for the treatment of erectile dysfunction in men with Parkinson's disease. *Movement Disorders*, **15** (2), 305–308.

Zhu, S., Stavrovskaya, I.G., Drozda, M., Kim, B.Y., Ona, V., Li, M. *et al.* (2002) Minocycline inhibits cytochrome c release and delays progression of amyotrophic lateral sclerosis in mice. *Nature*, **417** (6884), 74–78.

Part II

TREMOR DISORDERS

10

Essential Tremor

Rodger J. Elble

Department of Neurology, Southern Illinois University School of Medicine, Springfield, IL, USA

BACKGROUND

Clinical Characteristics of Essential Tremor

Essential tremor (ET) is a common movement disorder that affects the upper limbs (at least 95% of patients) and less commonly the head (at least 30%), voice (at least 20%), face/jaw (approximately 10%), tongue (approximately 20%), trunk (approximately 5%), and lower limbs (approximately 10%) (Elble, 2000; Hardesty et al., 2004; Hsu et al., 1990; Whaley et al., 2007). Tremor in the upper limbs is commonly asymmetric, but it is rarely, if ever, strictly unilateral (Louis et al., 1998a; Whaley et al., 2007). Tremors in the tongue, trunk and lower limbs may be found by examination, but are usually not the primary reason for seeking medical attention.

ET is an action tremor that occurs when patients voluntarily attempt to maintain a steady posture (postural tremor) or move (kinetic tremor). Patients with advanced ET frequently exhibit crescendo accentuation as the hand approaches its target (intention tremor) (Deuschl et al., 2000). Advanced patients also occasionally exhibit rest tremor in the hands (Cohen et al., 2003; Rajput, Robinson and Rajput, 2004; Whaley et al., 2007), but other signs of parkinsonism (bradykinesia and rigidity) are not seen. Furthermore, rest tremor without prominent action in the upper limbs is never seen, nor is rest tremor seen in the lower limbs. The rest tremor in ET is produced by rotation of the forearm and extension-flexion of the wrist. The classic pill rolling hand tremor of Parkinson's disease is not seen in ET, and frequently the "rest tremor" of ET is actually a postural tremor that is caused by incomplete muscle relaxation. This common diagnostic error can be avoided by examining patients in recumbent and seated positions with complete body support. Monosymptomatic rest tremor is nearly always a sign of Parkinson's disease or some other form of parkinsonism (Brooks et al., 1992; Ghaemi et al., 2002; Tolosa, Wenning and Poewe, 2006).

Approximately 5–15% of new essential tremor cases arise during childhood (Louis, Dure and Pullman, 2001; Paulson, 1976; Tan, Lum and Prakash, 2006), but its prevalence and incidence increase with age. At least 5% of people 65 years of age and older have essential tremor (Benito-Leon et al., 2003; Bergareche et al., 2001; Dogu et al., 2003; Elble, 1998; Louis et al., 1995). The annual incidence in this age group is approximately 616 per 100 000 person-years (Benito-Leon, Bermejo-Pareja and Louis, 2005). Essential tremor has been found in all ethnic groups studied, and men and women are affected equally. Cases beginning before age 20 are usually familial (Louis and Ottman, 2006). Most patients with essential tremor have not been diagnosed by a physician, but the majority of these patients report functional disability (Benito-Leon, Bermejo-Pareja and Louis, 2005; Dogu et al., 2005).

Pathophysiology of ET

Many cases are inherited in a Mendelian dominant fashion with a high genetic penetrance by age 65 years (Bain et al., 1994; Lorenz et al., 2004). Nevertheless, a specific gene for ET has not been found. Studies of autosomal dominant pedigrees have identified candidate loci on chromosome 3q13 (hereditary essential tremor, type 1) (Gulcher et al., 1997), chromosome 2p22–p25 (Higgins, Pho and Nee, 1997), and elsewhere (Ma et al., 2006; Shatunov et al., 2006). Higgins and co-workers reported an association between essential tremor and an Ala265Gly variant of the HS1-BP3 gene located in the 2p24 chromosomal region (Higgins et al., 2005; Higgins et al., 2006), and Jeanneteau and co-workers (Jeanneteau et al., 2006) found that the Ser9Gly variant of the dopamine D3 receptor (DRD3) gene on chromosome 3q13.3 co-segregates with essential tremor in 23 of 30 French families studied. However, both gene variants are common in the general population, so the role of these genes is unclear (Deng, Le and Jankovic, 2007;

Deng *et al.*, 2005; Jeanneteau *et al.*, 2006; Shatunov *et al.*, 2005).

The elusiveness of the ET gene is a subject of considerable discussion and speculation (Elble, 2006). Genetic heterogeneity in essential tremor is virtually certain, and given the high prevalence and non-specificity of the essential tremor phenotype, large families with dominantly inherited ET could contain a second gene or phenocopy that would confound genetic linkage studies. Polygenic inheritance is a possible source of difficulty (Ma *et al.*, 2006), and misdiagnosis and environmental factors could introduce confounding ET phenocopies into large families being studied.

Sporadic cases of ET are common, and it is becoming increasingly apparent that essential tremor is a clinically defined syndrome, not a specific disease. Most patients exhibit monosymptomatic tremor for a lifetime. However, it is widely recognized that the clinical and electrophysiologic characteristics of the action tremor in ET are not unique, and patients with other diseases may exhibit similar tremor for years before they exhibit diagnostic signs and symptoms of their neurologic disease. Diseases that occasionally present with ET-like tremor include Parkinson's (Lee *et al.*, 1999; Pellecchia *et al.*, 2006), dystonia (Jedynak, Bonnet and Agid, 1991; Münchau *et al.*, 2001; Schrag *et al.*, 2000; Yanagisawa, Goto and Narabayashi, 1972), spinocerebellar ataxia (Schöls *et al.*, 2004), and fragile X pre-mutation (Berry-Kravis *et al.*, 2003; Leehey *et al.*, 2003). Furthermore, it is clear that ET is a common disorder and will therefore occur commonly with other conditions. The relationship between essential tremor and other neurologic disorders can only be established through genetic testing or some other specific biological marker or neurophysiologic test for ET, which unfortunately does not exist.

Routine post-mortem studies have revealed no consistent abnormalities in patients with ET (Rajput, Robinson and Rajput, 2004). This could be the result of genetic and pathophysiologic heterogeneity, a failure of neuropathologists to find the abnormalities, or possibly the absence of visible structural abnormalities. Isolated Lewy bodies in the locus ceruleus, torpedoes in Purkinje cell axons, segmental Purkinje cell loss and cell loss in the dentate have been found in isolated patients or small groups of patients (Louis *et al.*, 2005; Louis *et al.*, 2006b; Louis *et al.*, 2006c). The interpretation of autopsy data from very elderly patients is difficult, and studies of younger patients and multiple affected people in the same family are needed to distinguish spurious or coincidental pathology from the pathology of ET.

Many clinical observations suggest that essential tremor emerges from abnormal oscillation within thalamocortical and olivocerebellar loops. Lesions in the cerebellum and thalamus greatly reduce essential tremor (Deuschl and Elble, 2000). Tremor-correlated neuronal discharge occurs in the ventrolateral thalamus, especially in the nucleus ventralis intermedius, and electrophysiologic studies have demonstrated enhanced cortical rhythmicity (Hellwig *et al.*, 2003; Hellwig *et al.*, 2001; Hua and Lenz, 2005). Contralateral limb tremor is suppressed by ablation, high-frequency stimulation and muscimol microinjection of the ventralis intermedius (Pahapill *et al.*, 1999; Schuurman *et al.*, 2000). PET studies have revealed bilaterally increased olivary glucose utilization and bilaterally increased blood flow in the cerebellum, red nucleus and thalamus, and functional MRI studies have disclosed increased blood flow bilaterally in the cerebellar hemispheres, dentate nucleus, and red nucleus and contralaterally in the globus pallidus, thalamus, and primary sensorimotor cortex (Boecker and Brooks, 1998). The cerebellar signs of intention tremor (Deuschl *et al.*, 2000) and unsteady tandem gait (Stolze *et al.*, 2001) in some essential tremor patients could be interpreted as evidence for cerebellar neurodegeneration, but Klebe and co-workers found that orally administered ethanol improved intention tremor and tandem gait in patients with essential tremor (Klebe *et al.*, 2005), which suggests that the cerebellar signs are reversible and not the result of neurodegeneration. The harmaline model of ET supports the notion of increased thalamocortical and olivocerebellar rhythmicity in ET, but this model and the more recent GABA-A receptor α-1 sub-unit knockout mouse model (Kralic *et al.*, 2005) illustrate that ET could be caused by a fairly widespread electrophysiologic disturbance with no discernible microscopic pathology.

Diagnosis and Differential Diagnosis of ET

The similarities between ET and the action tremors in other conditions have led virtually all students of ET to propose fairly restrictive diagnostic criteria, which are summarized in Table 10.1. Disagreement exists as to whether patients with isolated head tremor without evidence of dystonia should be classified as classic (i.e., "definite") ET. Tremulous cervical dystonia is frequently mistaken for ET, and nearly all patients with ET have hand tremor. Thus, the exclusion of patients with isolated head tremor does not affect many patients. Ultimately, this controversy will be resolved with the discovery of one or more genes or biologic markers for ET.

The Washington Heights-Inwood Genetic Study of ET (WHIGET) (Louis *et al.*, 1998b) and National Institute of Neurological Diseases and Stroke (NINDS) (Brin and Koller, 1998) criteria (Table 10.1) include minimum tremor amplitude requirements that will exclude cases of enhanced physiologic tremor, but will also exclude some cases of very mild ET. Unfortunately, there is no established method for distinguishing very mild ET from physiologic tremor (Elble, 2003; Elble and Deuschl, 2002; Elble, Higgins and

Table 10.1 Diagnostic criteria for classic (definite) ET.

	Inclusion criteria	Exclusion criteria
TRIG[a]	**Definite ET** 1. Bilateral postural hand tremor with or without kinetic tremor that is visible and persistent 2. May be asymmetric and may involve other body parts 3. Duration of at least 5 yr Isolated head tremor was classified as probable ET.	1. Other abnormal neurologic signs except Froment's sign (cogwheeling without rigidity during passive manipulation of the limb) 2. Presence of known causes of enhanced physiologic tremor (e.g., drugs, anxiety, hyperthyroidism) 3. Concurrent or recent exposure to tremorogenic drugs or presence of a drug withdrawal state 4. Trauma to the nervous system within three months of tremor onset 5. History or presence of psychogenic tremor 6. Sudden onset or stepwise progression 7. Primary orthostatic tremor 8. Isolated position-specific or task-specific tremors, including occupational tremors and primary writing tremor 9. Isolated tremor in the voice, tongue, chin or legs
Kiel Consensus Criteria[b]	1. Bilateral, largely symmetrical postural or kinetic tremor involving the hands and forearms that is visible and persistent. Intention tremor may be present in advanced cases, and rest tremor is rarely seen. 2. Additional or isolated tremor of the head may occur but in the absence of abnormal posturing	1. Other abnormal neurologic signs, especially dystonia 2. Presence of known causes of enhanced physiologic tremor 3. Historic or clinical evidence of psychogenic tremor 4. Sudden onset or stepwise progression 5. Primary orthostatic tremor 6. Isolated voice tremor 7. Isolated position-specific or task-specific tremors, including occupational tremors and primary writing tremor 8. Isolated tongue or chin tremor 9. Isolated leg tremor
WHIGET[c]	1. A 2+ (0–3 point scale) postural tremor of at least one arm (head tremor may be present but is not sufficient for the diagnosis) 2. A 2+ kinetic tremor in at least four tasks or a 3+ tremor on a second task. Tasks include pouring water, using a spoon to drink water, drinking water from a cup, finger-to-nose, and drawing a spiral 3. If tremor is present in the dominant hand, then by report, it must interfere with at least one activity of daily living (e.g., eating, drinking, writing). This criterion is irrelevant if tremor is not present in the dominant hand.	1. Medications, hyperthyroidism, alcohol and dystonia are not potential etiologic factors. 2. Not psychogenic

(continued)

Table 10.1 (*Continued*)

	Inclusion criteria	Exclusion criteria
NINDS[d]	1. 2 + action tremor in both arms (0–4 point scale), or 2 + in one arm and 1 + in the other, or 1 + in one arm and predominant cranial-cervical tremor. Predominant cranial-cervical means rhythmic tremor with no directional preponderance or asymmetric cervical muscles (i.e., no evidence of dystonia)	1. No evidence of enhanced physiologic tremor, parkinsonism, endocrine abnormalities, tremorogenic drugs, and so on.

[a] Findley and Koller (1995).
[b] Deuschl *et al.* (1998a).
[c] Louis *et al.* (1998b).
[d] Brin and Koller (1998).

Elble, 2005). The frequently dramatic suppression of tremor by ethanol ingestion is not sufficiently sensitive or specific to be used diagnostically (Rajput, 1996; Rajput *et al.*, 1975).

Generally accepted exclusion criteria for classic ET are: (i) other abnormal neurologic signs; (ii) recent neurologic trauma preceding the onset of tremor; (iii) presence of known causes of enhanced physiologic tremor (e.g., drugs, anxiety, depression, hyperthyroidism); (iv) history or presence of psychogenic tremor; (v) sudden onset or stepwise progression; (vi) primary orthostatic tremor; (vii) isolated position-specific or task-specific tremors (e.g., occupational tremors, primary writing tremor); and (viii) isolated tremor in the voice, tongue, face, jaw, or legs. Isolated head tremor should raise the suspicion of focal cervical dystonia.

Thus, classic ET is essentially a monosymptomatic tremor disorder with no other neurologic signs. Some patients with advanced essential tremor have mild impairment of balance and tandem walking (Stolze *et al.*, 2001). Other reported neurologic deficits are not detectable by routine neurologic examination. These deficits include decreased initial ocular smooth pursuit acceleration and impaired reduction of the time constant of post-rotatory vestibular nystagmus (Helmchen *et al.*, 2003), sub-clinical deficits in cognitive function (Benito-Leon, Louis and Bermejo-Pareja, 2006; Gasparini *et al.*, 2001; Lombardi *et al.*, 2001; Sahin *et al.*, 2006), and conflicting evidence of mild olfactory impairment (Applegate and Louis, 2005; Shah *et al.*, 2005). These sub-clinical deficits are important from a scientific standpoint, but they are not severe enough to affect the clinical presentation of patients with ET. Consequently, neurologic abnormalities other than tremor should be regarded as "red flags" that some other disorder is present, either in isolation or in combination with essential tremor (Elble, 2002).

The inclusion and exclusion criteria for classic ET are incorporated into the diagnostic flow diagram in Figure 10.1. Tremulous cervical dystonia is often suppressed by sensory tricks (*geste antagoniste*), whereas ET is not (Deuschl *et al.*, 1992; Masuhr *et al.*, 2000). The relationship of ET to other task-specific and focal tremors such as isolated chin tremor, writing tremor, and vocal tremor is doubtful (Soland *et al.*, 1996). ET in the jaw tends to occur in patients with head tremor, voice tremor and more severe upper extremity tremor (Louis *et al.*, 2006a), so isolated jaw tremor or the combination of jaw tremor and rest tremor in the hands should raise the suspicion of Parkinson's. Drug- and toxin-induced tremor, cortical tremor (rhythmic cortical myoclonus), cerebellar outflow tremor (intention tremor with terminal dysmetria and other signs of ataxia), tardive tremor, focal dystonia, neuropathic tremor, post-traumatic tremor, mild Parkinson's and psychogenic tremor are frequently misdiagnosed as ET (Jain, Lo and Louis, 2006; Schrag *et al.*, 2000).

Psychogenic tremors exhibit erratic frequency and amplitude fluctuations, and they frequently resolve and recur spontaneously. Tremor is usually reduced or abolished when the patient is distracted with motor or cognitive tasks. In many patients, the frequency of psychogenic tremor changes to the frequency of voluntary repetitive movements, performed with the ipsilateral or contralateral limb, or the patient exhibits a peculiar inability to perform the voluntary repetitive movements at the requested frequency (Kim, Pakiam and Lang, 1999; O'Suilleabhain and Matsumoto, 1998). Some patients produce psychogenic tremor simply by consciously or sub-consciously co-activating the flexor and extensor muscles of the wrist, without voluntary wrist oscillation, and this form of psychogenic tremor fluctuates with the degree of co-activation (Deuschl *et al.*, 1998b; Raethjen *et al.*, 2004).

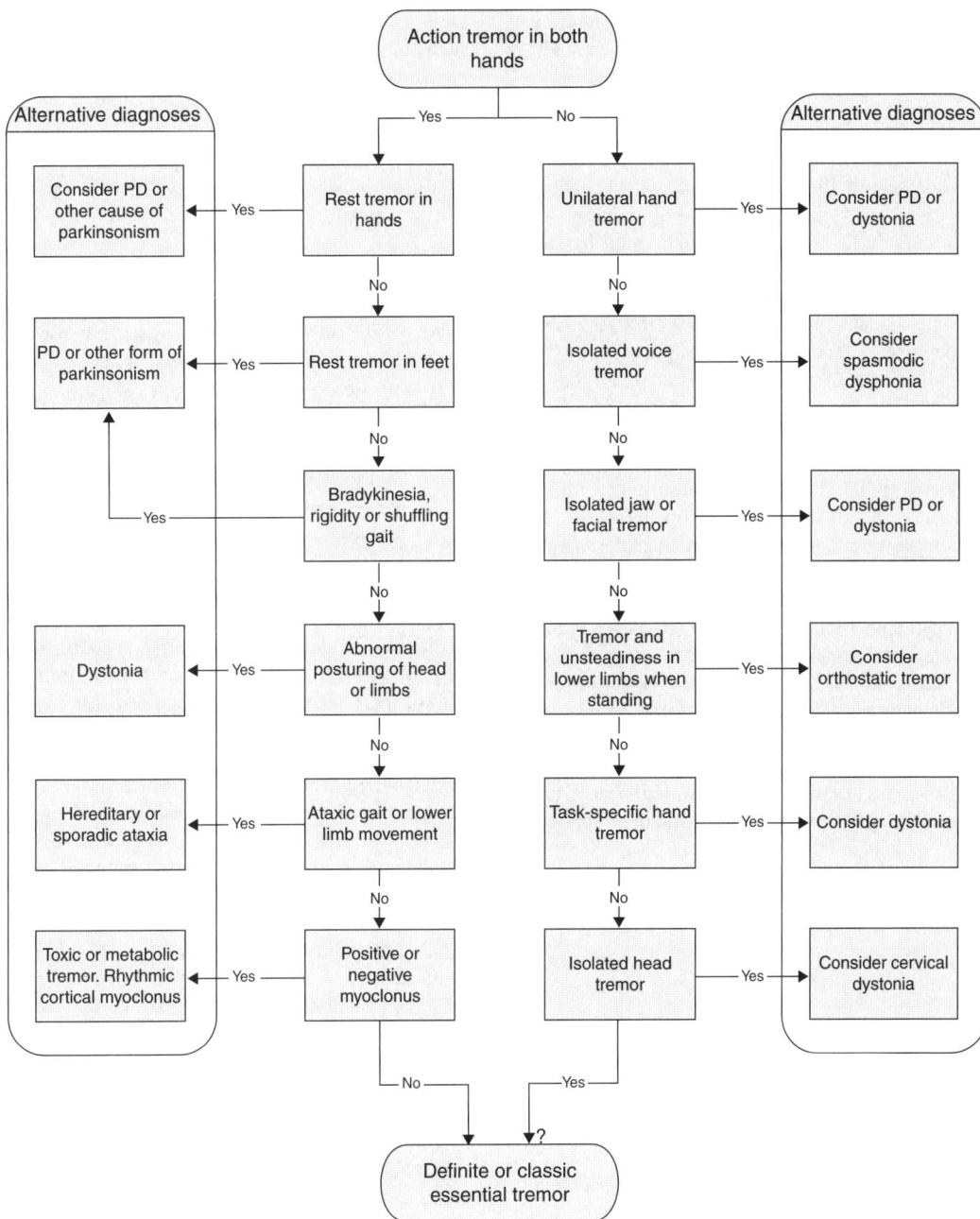

Figure 10.1 Differential diagnosis of essential tremor.

TREATMENT

Pharmacologic Treatment

Many patients with ET require or desire nothing more than an accurate diagnosis and assurance that a more sinister disease is not present. Social embarrassment, depression and anxiety may contribute significantly to a patient's disability, and these factors should be carefully considered, particularly in patients that complain vehemently of relatively mild tremor. The avoidance of stimulants such as caffeine and the judicious consumption of ethanol at meal-times or at social events are helpful to some patients. The prevalence of alcoholism in ET is probably not greater than in the general population (Koller, 1983; Rautakorpi, Marttila and Rinne, 1983), but no-one has studied the long-term risk of alcoholism and alcohol-related adverse events in patients who are prescribed ethanol for ET. The benefit of ethanol is less than two hours, and the well-known social limitations and side effects limit its use during much of the day. At least a third of all patients notice no benefit from ethanol, even when their blood levels approach legal intoxication, and many responders experience comparable benefit from much safer medications (Rajput et al., 1975). Consequently, we do not recommend ethanol for ET, but do not discourage its use in patients who derive benefit at mealtimes.

Many drugs have been used to treat essential tremor. The pathophysiology of ET is poorly understood, but the role of abnormal neuronal oscillation and entrainment is clear. The serendipitous discovery of efficacy from ethanol, propranolol and primidone has led many investigators to try other beta blockers, anti-convulsants, GABA agonists, and any other medication that might disrupt the abnormal oscillation in motor circuits. Consequently, numerous controlled and uncontrolled studies have been done, and many promising anecdotal observations and uncontrolled studies have led to disappointingly negative results in controlled studies. The average number of patients per study has been less than 25, and the methods of assessment have varied so much that comparison of results across studies is difficult or impossible (Zesiewicz et al., 2005).

Relevant studies published in English were recently reviewed and published by a sub-committee of the American Academy of Neurology (Zesiewicz et al., 2005). This report and the results of a few more recent studies are summarized in Table 10.2. Studies were classified as follows:

Class I: A prospective, randomized, controlled clinical trial with masked outcome assessment, in a representative population, and all of the following:

(a) primary outcome(s) clearly defined
(b) exclusion and inclusion criteria clearly defined
(c) adequate accounting for drop-outs and cross-overs with numbers sufficiently low to have minimal potential for bias
(d) relevant baseline characteristics are presented and substantially equivalent among treatment groups or there is appropriate statistical adjustment for differences.

Class II: A prospective matched group cohort study in a representative population with masked outcome assessment that meets requirements (a)–(d) of a class I study, or a randomized, controlled trial in a representative population that lacks one of the criteria (a)–(d)

Class III: All other controlled trials including well-defined natural history controls or patients serving as own controls in a representative population, where outcome is independently assessed or independently derived by objective outcome measurement.

The levels of evidence in Table 10.2 are as follows:

A: Established as effective, ineffective or harmful, based on at least two consistent class I studies
B: Probably effective, ineffective or harmful, based on at least one class I study or at least two consistent class II studies
C: Possibly effective, ineffective or harmful, based on at least one class II study or two consistent class III studies.

Propranolol (regular and long-acting forms) and primidone are the only two medications with level A evidence of efficacy (Zesiewicz et al., 2005). Approximately 50% of patients with essential tremor benefit from one or both of these medications, and the response to one does not predict the response to the other. The average reduction in tremor is about 50%, and complete suppression of tremor is rare. The beneficial effect is largely limited to hand tremor. Fatigue, lightheadedness, and bradycardia are the most common side effects. Erectile dysfunction and depression are often emphasized, but their occurrence is probably overstated (Silvestri et al., 2003; Van Melle et al., 2006).

Other beta blockers have been studied (Table 10.2), but none has been shown to be more effective than propranolol. Some mildly affected patients take the short-acting formulation on an as-needed basis (e.g., 10–40 mg, 30 minutes before an anticipated need), but most patients prefer the long-acting formulation, taken once daily. Patients may respond to as little as 60 mg per day and rarely benefit from more that 240 mg per day. Therefore, we recommend the long-acting formulation unless patients prefer as-needed administration because of side effects or limited disability. The total daily dosage is increased each week in 60 mg increments as tolerated and as needed, not exceeding 240 mg. Propranolol and other beta blockers should be avoided in patients with asthma, heart block, unstable heart failure and bradycardia, and these drugs should be discontinued by gradual taper over 1–2 weeks in cardiac patients.

Many patients experience mild sedation and dizziness when they start primidone. These side effects usually resolve in a week or so, but an occasional patient will experience a

Table 10.2 Non-surgical treatment of essential tremor.

Level of evidence	Drug	Daily dose range (mg)	Common side effects[a]	Severe uncommon side effects
A	Primidone	25–750	Sedation, dizziness	Severe acute dizziness and sedation with nausea and vomiting
	Propranolol	60–800	Fatigue, lightheadedness, bradycardia, erectile dysfunction, depression	Bradycardia, exacerbation of asthma or congestive heart failure. Abrupt cessation may exacerbate angina or ventricular arrhythmias
B	Alprazolam	0.125–3	Sedation	Dependency, abuse
	Atenolol	50–150	Fatigue, lightheadedness, bradycardia, erectile dysfunction, depression	Bradycardia, exacerbation of asthma or congestive heart failure. Abrupt cessation may exacerbate angina or ventricular arrhythmias
	Gabapentin monotherapy	1200–1800	Sedation, dizziness, nausea	
	Sotalol	75–200	Fatigue, lightheadedness, bradycardia	Bradycardia, exacerbation of asthma or congestive heart failure. Abrupt cessation may exacerbate angina or ventricular arrhythmias
	Topiramate	100–400	Anorexia, weight loss, cognitive impairment, paresthesias, distorted taste, somnolence	Kidney stones, acute narrow angle glaucoma
C	Clonazepam	0.5–6	Sedation	
	Clozapine	6–75	Sedation	Agranulocytosis, cardiorespiratory collapse
	Nadolol	120–240	Fatigue, lightheadedness, bradycardia, erectile dysfunction, depression	Bradycardia, exacerbation of asthma or congestive heart failure. Abrupt cessation may exacerbate angina or ventricular arrhythmias
	Nimodipine	120	Hypotension, headache, gastrointestinal distress	Cardiac arrhythmias, exacerbation of congestive heart failure
	Botulinum toxin A (hand tremor)	50–100 U	Muscle weakness, injection site pain	
	Botulinum toxin A (head tremor)	40–400 U	Muscle weakness, injection site pain, dysphagia	Severe dysphagia
	Botulinum toxin A (voice tremor)	0.6–15	Weak voice, dysphagia	Severe dysphagia

[a] Consult the package insert, online.ePocrates.com or medlineplus.gov for a more comprehensive list of side effects.

more severe and frequently intolerable first-dose reaction consisting of drowsiness, dizziness, dysequilibrium and nausea. Consequently, most physicians prescribe an initial dosage of one-quarter or one-half of a 50 mg tablet at bedtime, even though a randomized, controlled trial of 40 patients revealed no benefit of initiating much smaller dosages (O'Suilleabhain and Dewey, 2002). We routinely start with a dosage of 25 mg at bedtime and titrate the dosage each week in 25 mg increments, as tolerated and as needed. The usual dosage is 50–350 mg per day in 1–3 divided doses, but total daily dosages greater than 250 mg frequently produce little or no additional benefit (Serrano-Duenas, 2003).

Of the drugs with level B evidence, only topiramate has been studied in a large number of patients and was found to be moderately effective (Ondo *et al.*, 2006). Adverse events limited treatment in 32% of patients, and nearly 20% of patients taking topiramate dropped out due to side effects. Although gabapentin monotherapy produced largely positive results, gabapentin was largely ineffective in patients taking other anti-tremor medications (Zesiewicz *et al.*, 2005). Therefore, the response to this drug is usually disappointing.

The drugs in Table 10.2 with level C evidence require additional study to determine efficacy. Despite encouraging initial anecdotal reports, clonazepam, methazolamide, flunarizine, nimodipine, clonidine, low-dose theophylline, amantadine, verapamil, nifedipine, acetazolamide, isoniazid, pindolol, L-tryptophan/pyridoxine, metoprolol, nicardipine, olanzapine, Phenobarbital, quetiapine, clozapine, glutethimide and mirtazapine have been tried with inconclusive or negative results (Zesiewicz *et al.*, 2005). In addition, levetiracetam (Handforth and Martin, 2004), amantadine (Gironell *et al.*, 2006), 3,4-diaminopyridine (Lorenz *et al.*, 2006) and zonisamide (Zesiewicz *et al.*, 2006b) were found ineffective in randomized, controlled trials performed since the 2005 review by Zesiewicz and co-workers (Zesiewicz *et al.*, 2005).

Given the frequently dramatic response of essential tremor to ethanol, other forms of alcohol and GABA agonists have been sought for therapeutic trials. Pilot studies of 1-octanol revealed that this eight-carbon alcohol suppresses essential hand tremor, but additional controlled studies are needed to examine the safety, tolerability and efficacy of long-term treatment (Bushara *et al.*, 2004; Shill *et al.*, 2004). In two pilot studies, Frucht and co-workers found an impressive response of essential tremor to oxybate, which is approved in the United States for the treatment of narcolepsy (Frucht *et al.*, 2005a; Frucht *et al.*, 2005b). Oxybate is a central nervous system depressant with abuse potential (schedule III drug) and is available only through a central pharmacy (see www.xyrem.com). Two patients recently experienced benefit from pregabalin

in an open-label trial (Zesiewicz *et al.*, 2006a). Benefit from 1,3-dimethoxymethyl-5,5-diphenyl-barbituric acid was found in two small controlled trials (Melmed, Moros and Rutman, 2007).

Botulinum toxin injections into the forearm muscles produce little if any improvement in most patients, and finger or wrist weakness is a common side effect (Zesiewicz *et al.*, 2005). Greater efficacy has been reported occasionally in patients with disabling head tremor (Wissel *et al.*, 1997) and voice tremor (Adler *et al.*, 2004), but this experience is largely anecdotal (Lyons *et al.*, 2003; Zesiewicz *et al.*, 2005). Nevertheless, a cautious trial of botulinum toxin is appropriate in disabled patients who do not respond to oral medications and who understand the risks (Table 10.2), particularly in those patients with possible underlying dystonia (e.g., subtle head tilt, abnormal hand postures, and response to sensory tricks—*geste antagoniste*).

Surgical Treatment

Stereotactic surgery in the ventrolateral thalamus is an effective treatment for disabling drug-resistant essential tremor (Zesiewicz *et al.*, 2005). There have been no placebo-controlled (sham surgery) randomized trials of thalamotomy or thalamic deep brain stimulation (DBS), which explains the level C evidence in Table 10.2. Nevertheless, thalamic DBS is widely recognized as the most effective treatment for ET.

The optimum thalamic target is nucleus ventralis intermedius (Papavassiliou *et al.*, 2004). Destructive thalamotomy and high-frequency DBS produce comparable improvement, but DBS can be programmed to provide optimum functional improvement with fewer side effects (Schuurman *et al.*, 2000). The reversibility of DBS has made this the surgical procedure preferred by most surgeons (Benabid *et al.*, 1996; Zesiewicz *et al.*, 2005).

The efficacy of thalamic DBS is unquestioned, but the absence of long-term randomized, controlled trials casts some uncertainty on magnitude and duration of efficacy and the incidence of side effects, in particular. Problems related to lead placement (skin erosion, lead breakage) and stimulator malfunction are not uncommon (Pahwa *et al.*, 2006; Slowinski *et al.*, 2007; Sydow *et al.*, 2003), and thalamic DBS, like thalamotomy, may cause dysarthria, dysphagia, somatosensory loss, paresthesias, cognitive impairment, dysequilibrium, ataxia, infection, intracranial hemorrhage and, rarely, death. One or more side effects occur in at least 20% of patients undergoing unilateral DBS (Zesiewicz *et al.*, 2005). Most side effects caused by thalamic DBS are reduced or abolished by adjusting the stimulus parameters, but these adjustments may result in reduced tremor suppression.

Bilateral thalamotomy is contraindicated due to the high incidence of complications, but bilateral thalamic DBS is possible with an overall complication rate of about 30%, dysarthria and impaired balance being most common (Zesiewicz *et al.*, 2005). Marked suppression of limb tremor is achieved in approximately 70–90% of patients. Good control of limb tremor with thalamic deep brain stimulation is maintained for more than five years in most patients, but efficacy is gradually lost in some (Kumar *et al.*, 2003; Sydow *et al.*, 2003). The reason for lost efficacy is believed to be sub-optimal lead placement in many patients, but other patients seem to develop a true physiological tolerance to deep brain stimulation (Papavassiliou *et al.*, 2004).

The role of thalamic DBS in the treatment of midline tremor (head and voice) is less certain (Zesiewicz *et al.*, 2005). Many patients undergo bilateral surgery for their hand tremor, and many of these patients have experienced a substantial reduction in head and voice tremor (Putzke *et al.*, 2005; Slowinski *et al.*, 2007). However, some reports have not been encouraging (Limousin *et al.*, 1999), and it is unclear whether disabling midline tremor is ever a primary indication for DBS (Zesiewicz *et al.*, 2005).

Ventralis intermedius has been such an effective target for ET that there has been little incentive to look for alternative targets. Nevertheless, some patients with severe proximal tremor respond poorly to thalamic DBS, and patients with both ET and Parkinson's (PD) are not uncommon. Two groups found that ET responds to deep brain stimulation in the posteromedial subthalamic area, and the magnitude of improvement was comparable to that derived from thalamic DBS (Murata *et al.*, 2003; Plaha, Patel and Gill, 2004). Midline tremors also improved (bilateral DBS). The critical target in this anatomically compact area is unclear but is possibly the zona incerta and prelemniscal radiation, which carry cerebellar and somatosensory afferents to the ventrolateral thalamus (Murata *et al.*, 2003; Plaha, Patel and Gill, 2004). Parkinson tremor and ET may both respond to subthalamic DBS when these diseases occur in the same patient (Stover *et al.*, 2005). Targeting the subthalamus in patients with PD and ET makes sense because the bradykinesia, rigidity and gait impairment of PD respond poorly to thalamic DBS. However, the role of subthalamic DBS in pure ET is unestablished.

The mechanism of thalamic DBS is uncertain (Mcintyre *et al.*, 2004; Perlmutter and Mink, 2006). Most investigators believe that DBS drives motor circuits at high frequencies, so as to preclude low-frequency tremorogenic neuronal firing, but other mechanisms are probably also at play. Thalamic and subthalamic stimulation frequencies greater than 60 Hz are needed to suppress tremor, and stimulation frequencies below 60 Hz can be tremorogenic (Constantoyannis *et al.*, 2004; Plaha, Patel and Gill, 2004; Ushe *et al.*, 2006; Ushe *et al.*, 2004).

Therapeutic stimulation parameters in current use have been derived by trial-and-error clinical programming of the neurostimulators. Thousands of combinations of pulse width, stimulation frequency and pulse voltage are available, and the quadripolar electrodes can be selected to deliver monopolar cathodic or bipolar stimulation. The optimum stimulation parameters appear to be frequencies of 90–130 Hz, pulse widths of 60–120 μs, and voltages of 1–3.5 V (Kuncel *et al.*, 2006; O'Suilleabhain *et al.*, 2003; Ushe *et al.*, 2004). The optimum electrode contact should be the negative pole in a monopolar or bipolar configuration, depending upon the clinical response and side effects.

Some reports suggest that stereotactic gamma-knife thalamotomy is a relatively safe and effective alternative to radiofrequency thalamotomy and thalamic stimulation (Ohye, Shibazaki and Sato, 2005; Ohye *et al.*, 2002; Young *et al.*, 2000). However, the response to treatment is delayed, taking months to a year or more, depending on the dose of radiation (Ohye, Shibazaki and Sato, 2005; Ohye *et al.*, 2002). Disturbing long-term complications have been reported (Okun *et al.*, 2001; Siderowf *et al.*, 2001), and controlled multi-center trials are lacking (Zesiewicz *et al.*, 2005). Consequently, there is insufficient evidence to recommend this procedure.

Practical Management

An algorithm for the treatment of ET is proposed in Figure 10.2. Failure to respond to medications is not uncommon. Accurate diagnosis is necessary to maximize success. Unrecognized PD, dystonia and drug-induced tremor are the most common errors in diagnosis (Jain, Lo and Louis, 2006; Schrag *et al.*, 2000).

Level C drugs with dangerous side effects (e.g., clozapine) should be used very cautiously or not at all. Thalamic DBS is a viable option for patients who have disabling drug-refractory tremor. Patients should understand the risks and the need for long-term monitoring and re-programming of the stimulator. Most, but not all, patients are pleased that they underwent thalamic DBS.

The mechanisms of action of beneficial and possibly beneficial medications are unknown because the pathophysiology of ET is poorly understood. The harmaline model and GABA-A receptor α-1 subunit knockout mouse have provided some insight, but more animal models are needed, and the identification of one or more ET genes is crucial to solving this disorder (Elble, 2006).

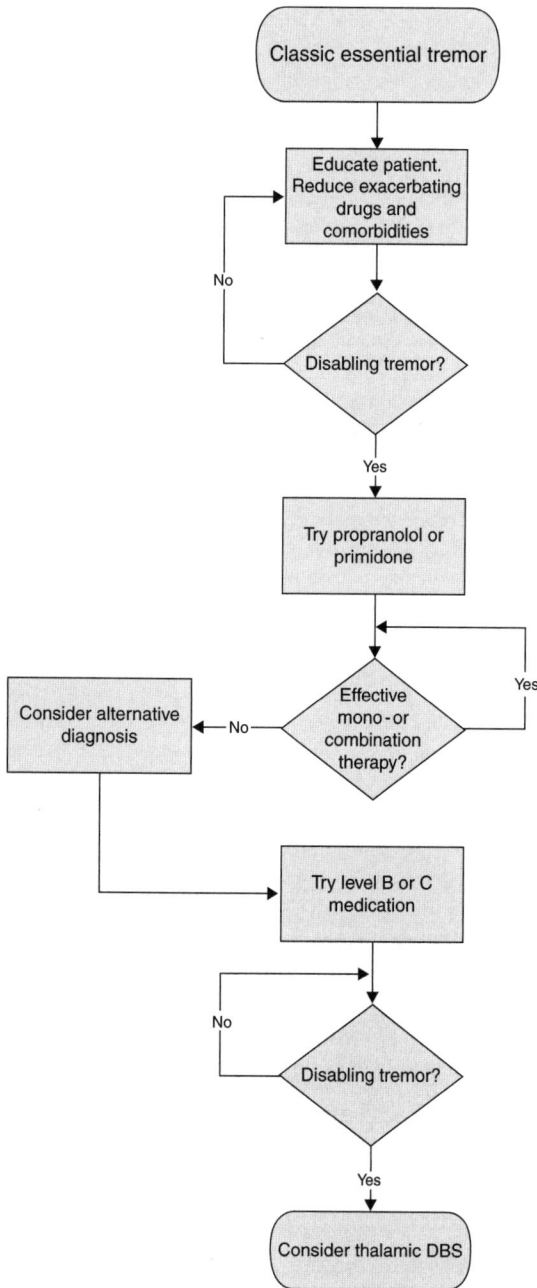

Figure 10.2 Treatment algorithm for essential tremor.

References

Adler, C.H., Bansberg, S.F., Hentz, J.G. et al. (2004) Botulinum toxin type A for treating voice tremor. *Archives of Neurology*, **61**, 1416–1420.

Applegate, L.M. and Louis, E.D. (2005) Essential tremor: mild olfactory dysfunction in a cerebellar disorder. *Parkinsonism & Related Disorders*, **11**, 399–402.

Bain, P.G., Findley, L.J., Thompson, P.D. et al. (1994) A study of hereditary essential tremor. *Brain*, **117**, 805–824.

Benabid, A.L., Pollak, P., Gao, D. et al. (1996) Chronic electrical stimulation of the ventralis intermedius nucleus of the thalamus as a treatment of movement disorders. *Journal of Neurosurgery*, **84**, 203–214.

Benito-Leon, J., Bermejo-Pareja, F. and Louis, E.D. (2005) Incidence of essential tremor in three elderly populations of central Spain. *Neurology*, **64**, 1721–1725.

Benito-Leon, J., Louis, E.D. and Bermejo-Pareja, F. (2006) Population-based case-control study of cognitive function in essential tremor. *Neurology*, **66**, 69–74.

Benito-Leon, J., Bermejo-Pareja, F., Morales, J.M. et al. (2003) Prevalence of essential tremor in three elderly populations of central Spain. *Movement Disorders*, **18**, 389–394.

Bergareche, A., De La Puente, E., Lopez De Munain, A. et al. (2001) Prevalence of essential tremor: a door-to-door survey in Bidasoa, Spain. *Neuroepidemiology*, **20**, 125–128.

Berry-Kravis, E., Lewin, F., Wuu, J. et al. (2003) Tremor and ataxia in fragile X premutation carriers: blinded videotape study. *Annals of Neurology*, **53**, 616–623.

Boecker, H. and Brooks, D.J. (1998) Functional imaging of tremor. *Movement Disorders*, **13**, 64–72.

Brin, M.F. and Koller, W. (1998) Epidemiology and genetics of essential tremor. *Movement Disorders*, **13**, 55–63.

Brooks, D.J., Playford, E.D., Ibanez, V. et al. (1992) Isolated tremor and disruption of the nigrostriatal dopaminergic system: an 18F-dopa PET study. *Neurology*, **42**, 1554–1560.

Bushara, K.O., Goldstein, S.R., Grimes, G.J., Jr et al. (2004) Pilot trial of 1-octanol in essential tremor. *Neurology*, **62**, 122–124.

Cohen, O., Pullman, S., Jurewicz, E. et al. (2003) Rest tremor in patients with essential tremor: prevalence, clinical correlates, and electrophysiologic characteristics. *Archives of Neurology*, **60**, 405–410.

Constantoyannis, C., Kumar, A., Stoessl, A.J. and Honey, C.R. (2004) Tremor induced by thalamic deep brain stimulation in patients with complex regional facial pain. *Movement Disorders*, **19**, 933–936.

Deng, H., Le, W. and Jankovic, J. (2007) Genetics of essential tremor. *Brain*, **130**, 1456–1464.

Deng, H., Le, W.D., Guo, Y. et al. (2005) Extended study of A265G variant of HS1BP3 in essential tremor and Parkinson's disease. *Neurology*, **65**, 651–652.

Deuschl, G. and Elble, R.J. (2000) The pathophysiology of essential tremor. *Neurology*, **54**, S14–S20.

Deuschl, G., Bain, P. and Brin, M. (1998a) Consensus statement of the movement disorder society on tremor. Ad Hoc Scientific Committee. *Movement Disorders*, **13**, 2–23.

Deuschl, G., Köster, B., Lücking, C.H. and Scheidt, C. (1998b) Diagnostic and pathophysiological aspects of psychogenic tremors. *Movement Disorders*, **13**, 294–302.

Deuschl, G., Wenzelburger, R., Loffler, K. et al. (2000) Essential tremor and cerebellar dysfunction clinical and kinematic analysis of intention tremor. *Brain*, **123**, 1568–1580.

Deuschl, G., Heinen, F., Kleedorfer, B. et al. (1992) Clinical and polymyographic investigation of spasmodic torticollis. *Journal of Neurology*, **239**, 9–15.

Dogu, O., Louis, E.D., Sevim, S. et al. (2005) Clinical characteristics of essential tremor in Mersin, Turkey--a population-based door-to-door study. *Journal of Neurology*, **252**, 570–574.

Dogu, O., Sevim, S., Camdeviren, H. et al. (2003) Prevalence of essential tremor: door-to-door neurologic exams in Mersin Province, Turkey. *Neurology*, **61**, 1804–1806.

Elble, R.J. (1998) Tremor in ostensibly normal elderly people. *Movement Disorders*, **13**, 457–464.

Elble, R.J. (2000) Diagnostic criteria for essential tremor and differential diagnosis. *Neurology*, **54**, S2–S6.

Elble, R.J. (2002) Essential tremor is a monosymptomatic disorder. *Movement Disorders*, **17**, 633–637.

Elble, R.J. (2003) Characteristics of physiologic tremor in young and elderly adults. *Clinical Neurophysiology*, **114**, 624–635.

Elble, R.J. (2006) Report from a U.S. conference on essential tremor. *Movement Disorders*, **21**, 2052–2061.

Elble, R.J. and Deuschl, G. (2002) Tremor, in *Neuromuscular Function and Disease: Basic, Clinical and Electrodiagnostic Aspects* (eds W.F. Brown, C.F. Bolton and M. Aminoff), W.B. Saunders Co., Philadelphia.

Elble, R.J., Higgins, C. and Elble, S. (2005) Electrophysiologic transition from physiologic tremor to essential tremor. *Movement Disorders*, **20**, 1038–1042.

Findley, L.J. and Koller, W.C. (1995) Definitions and behavioral classifications, in *Handbook of Tremor Disorders* (eds L.J. Findley and W.C. Koller) Marcel Dekker, Inc., New York.

Frucht, S.J., Bordelon, Y., Houghton, W.H. and Reardan, D. (2005a) A pilot tolerability and efficacy trial of sodium oxybate in ethanol-responsive movement disorders. *Movement Disorders*, **20**, 1330–1337.

Frucht, S.J., Houghton, W.C., Bordelon, Y. *et al.* (2005b) A single-blind, open-label trial of sodium oxybate for myoclonus and essential tremor. *Neurology*, **65**, 1967–1969.

Gasparini, M., Bonifati, V., Fabrizio, E. *et al.* (2001) Frontal lobe dysfunction in essential tremor: a preliminary study. *Journal of Neurology*, **248**, 399–402.

Ghaemi, M., Raethjen, J., Hilker, R. *et al.* (2002) Monosymptomatic resting tremor and Parkinson's disease: a multitracer positron emission tomographic study. *Movement Disorders*, **17**, 782–788.

Gironell, A., Kulisevsky, J., Pascual-Sedano, B. and Flamarich, D. (2006) Effect of amantadine in essential tremor: a randomized, placebo-controlled trial. *Movement Disorders*, **21**, 441–445.

Gulcher, J.R., Jonsson, P., Kong, A. *et al.* (1997) Mapping of a familial essential tremor gene, FET1, to chromosome 3q13. *Nature Genetics*, **17**, 84–87.

Handforth, A. and Martin, F.C. (2004) Pilot efficacy and tolerability: a randomized, placebo-controlled trial of levetiracetam for essential tremor. *Movement Disorders*, **19**, 1215–1221.

Hardesty, D.E., Maraganore, D.M., Matsumoto, J.Y. and Louis, E.D. (2004) Increased risk of head tremor in women with essential tremor: longitudinal data from the Rochester Epidemiology Project. *Movement Disorders*, **19**, 529–533.

Hellwig, B., Schelter, B., Guschlbauer, B. *et al.* (2003) Dynamic synchronisation of central oscillators in essential tremor. *Clinical Neurophysiology*, **114**, 1462–1467.

Hellwig, B., Häussler, S., Schelter, B. *et al.* (2001) Tremor-correlated cortical activity in essential tremor. *Lancet*, **357**, 519–523.

Helmchen, C., Hagenow, A., Miesner, J. *et al.* (2003) Eye movement abnormalities in essential tremor may indicate cerebellar dysfunction. *Brain*, **126**, 1319–1332.

Higgins, J.J., Pho, L.T. and Nee, L.E. (1997) A gene (ETM) for essential tremor maps to chromosome 2p22–p25. *Movement Disorders*, **12**, 859–864.

Higgins, J.J., Lombardi, R.Q., Pucilowska, J. *et al.* (2005) A variant in the HS1-BP3 gene is associated with familial essential tremor. *Neurology*, **64**, 417–421.

Higgins, J.J., Lombardi, R.Q., Pucilowska, J. *et al.* (2006) HS1-BP3 gene variant is common in familial essential tremor. *Movement Disorders*, **21**, 306–309.

Hsu, Y.D., Chang, M.K., Sung, S.C. *et al.* (1990) Essential tremor: clinical, electromyographical and pharmacological studies in 146 Chinese patients. *Chung Hua I Hsueh Tsa Chih (Taipei)*, **45**, 93–99.

Hua, S.E. and Lenz, F.A. (2005) Posture-related oscillations in human cerebellar thalamus in essential tremor are enabled by voluntary motor circuits. *Journal of Neurophysiology*, **93**, 117–127.

Jain, S., Lo, S.E. and Louis, E.D. (2006) Common misdiagnosis of a common neurological disorder: how are we misdiagnosing essential tremor? *Archives of Neurology*, **63**, 1100–1104.

Jeanneteau, F., Funalot, B., Jankovic, J. *et al.* (2006) A functional variant of the dopamine D3 receptor is associated with risk and age-at-onset of essential tremor. *Proceedings of the National Academy of Sciences of the United States of America*, **103**, 10753–10758.

Jedynak, C.P., Bonnet, A.M. and Agid, Y. (1991) Tremor and idiopathic dystonia. *Movement Disorders*, **6**, 230–236.

Kim, Y.J., Pakiam, A.S.-I. and Lang, A.E. (1999) Historical and clinical features of psychogenic tremor: a review of 70 cases. *Canadian Journal Neurological Sciences*, **26**, 190–195.

Klebe, S., Stolze, H., Grensing, K. *et al.* (2005) Influence of alcohol on gait in patients with essential tremor. *Neurology*, **65**, 96–101.

Koller, W.C. (1983) Alcoholism in essential tremor. *Neurology*, **33**, 1074–1076.

Kralic, J.E., Criswell, H.E., Osterman, J.L. *et al.* (2005) Genetic essential tremor in gamma-aminobutyric acid A receptor alpha1 subunit knockout mice. *The Journal of Clinical Investigation*, **115**, 774–779.

Kumar, R., Lozano, A.M., Sime, E. and Lang, A.E. (2003) Long-term follow-up of thalamic deep brain stimulation for essential and parkinsonian tremor. *Neurology*, **61**, 1601–1604.

Kuncel, A.M., Cooper, S.E., Wolgamuth, B.R. *et al.* (2006) Clinical response to varying the stimulus parameters in deep brain stimulation for essential tremor. *Movement Disorders*, **21**, 1920–1928.

Lee, M.S., Kim, Y.D., Im, J.H. *et al.* (1999) 123I-IPT brain SPECT study in essential tremor and Parkinson's disease. *Neurology*, **52**, 1422–1426.

Leehey, M.A., Munhoz, R.P., Lang, A.E. *et al.* (2003) The fragile X premutation presenting as essential tremor. *Archives of Neurology*, **60**, 117–121.

Limousin, P., Speelman, J.D., Gielen, F. and Janssens, M. (1999) Multicentre European study of thalamic stimulation in parkinsonian and essential tremor. *Journal of Neurology, Neurosurgery, and Psychiatry*, **66**, 289–296.

Lombardi, W.J., Woolston, D.J., Roberts, J.W. and Gross, R.E. (2001) Cognitive deficits in patients with essential tremor. *Neurology*, **57**, 785–790.

Lorenz, D., Frederiksen, H., Moises, H. *et al.* (2004) High concordance for essential tremor in monozygotic twins of old age. *Neurology*, **62**, 208–211.

Lorenz, D., Hagen, K., Ufer, M. *et al.* (2006) No benefit of 3,4-diaminopyridine in essential tremor: a placebo-controlled crossover study. *Neurology*, **66**, 1753–1755.

Louis, E.D. and Ottman, R. (2006) Study of possible factors associated with age of onset in essential tremor. *Movement Disorders*, **21**, 1980–1986.

Louis, E.D., Dure, L.S. and Pullman, S. (2001) Essential tremor in childhood: a series of nineteen cases. *Movement Disorders*, **16**, 921–923.

Louis, E.D., Wendt, K.J., Pullman, S.L. and Ford, B. (1998a) Is essential tremor symmetric? Observational data from a community-based study of essential tremor. *Archives of Neurology*, **55**, 1553–1559.

Louis, E.D., Ford, B., Lee, H. *et al.* (1998b) Diagnostic criteria for essential tremor: a population perspective. *Archives of Neurology*, **55**, 823–828.

Louis, E.D., Rios, E., Applegate, L.M. *et al.* (2006a) Jaw tremor: prevalence and clinical correlates in three essential tremor case samples. *Movement Disorders*, **21**, 1872–1878.

Louis, E.D., Honig, L.S., Vonsattel, J.P. *et al.* (2005) Essential tremor associated with focal nonnigral Lewy bodies: a clinicopathologic study. *Archives of Neurology*, **62**, 1004–1007.

Louis, E.D., Vonsattel, J.P., Honig, L.S. *et al.* (2006b) Neuropathologic findings in essential tremor. *Neurology*, **66**, 1756–1759.

Louis, E.D., Vonsattel, J.P., Honig, L.S. *et al.* (2006c) Essential tremor associated with pathologic changes in the cerebellum. *Archives of Neurology*, **63**, 1189–1193.

Louis, E.D., Marder, K., Cote, L. *et al.* (1995) Differences in the prevalence of essential tremor among elderly African Americans, whites, and Hispanics in northern Manhattan, NY. *Archives of Neurology*, **52**, 1201–1205.

Lyons, K.E., Pahwa, R., Comella, C.L. *et al.* (2003) Benefits and risks of pharmacological treatments for essential tremor. *Drug Safety*, **26**, 461–481.

Ma, S., Davis, T.L., Blair, M.A. *et al.* (2006) Familial essential tremor with apparent autosomal dominant inheritance: should we also consider other inheritance modes? *Movement Disorders*, **21**, 1368–1374.

Masuhr, F., Wissel, J., Muller, J. *et al.* (2000) Quantification of sensory trick impact on tremor amplitude and frequency in 60 patients with head tremor. *Movement Disorders*, **15**, 960–964.

Mcintyre, C.C., Savasta, M., Walter, B.L. and Vitek, J.L. (2004) How does deep brain stimulation work? Present understanding and future questions. *Journal of Clinical Neurophysiology*, **21**, 40–50.

Melmed, C., Moros, D. and Rutman, H. (2007) Treatment of essential tremor with the barbiturate t2000 (1,3-dimethoxymethyl-5,5-diphenyl-barbituric acid). *Movement Disorders*, **22**, 723–727.

Münchau, A., Schrag, A., Chuang, C. *et al.* (2001) Arm tremor in cervical dystonia differs from essential tremor and can be classified by onset age and spread of symptoms. *Brain*, **124**, 1765–1776.

Murata, J., Kitagawa, M., Uesugi, H. *et al.* (2003) Electrical stimulation of the posterior subthalamic area for the treatment of intractable proximal tremor. *Journal of Neurosurgery*, **99**, 708–715.

Ohye, C., Shibazaki, T. and Sato, S. (2005) Gamma knife thalamotomy for movement disorders: evaluation of the thalamic lesion and clinical results. *Journal of Neurosurgery*, **102** (Suppl), 234–240.

Ohye, C., Shibazaki, T., Zhang, J. and Andou, Y. (2002) Thalamic lesions produced by gamma thalamotomy for movement disorders. *Journal of Neurosurgery*, **97**, 600–606.

Okun, M.S., Stover, N.P., Subramanian, T. *et al.* (2001) Complications of gamma knife surgery for Parkinson's disease. *Archives of Neurology*, **58**, 1995–2002.

Ondo, W.G., Jankovic, J., Connor, G.S. *et al.* (2006) Topiramate in essential tremor: a double-blind, placebo-controlled trial. *Neurology*, **66**, 672–677.

O'Suilleabhain, P. and Dewey, R.B., Jr (2002) Randomized trial comparing primidone initiation schedules for treating essential tremor. *Movement Disorders*, **17**, 382–386.

O'Suilleabhain, P.E. and Matsumoto, J.Y. (1998) Time-frequency analysis of tremors. *Brain*, **121**, 2127–2134.

O'Suilleabhain, P.E., Frawley, W., Giller, C. and Dewey, R.B., Jr (2003) Tremor response to polarity, voltage, pulsewidth and frequency of thalamic stimulation. *Neurology*, **60**, 786–790.

Pahapill, P.A., Levy, R., Dostrovsky, J.O. *et al.* (1999) Tremor arrest with thalamic microinjections of muscimol in patients with essential tremor. *Annals of Neurology*, **46**, 249–252.

Pahwa, R., Lyons, K.E., Wilkinson, S.B. *et al.* (2006) Long-term evaluation of deep brain stimulation of the thalamus. *Journal of Neurosurgery*, **104**, 506–512.

Papavassiliou, E., Rau, G., Heath, S. *et al.* (2004) Thalamic deep brain stimulation for essential tremor: relation of lead location to outcome. *Neurosurgery*, **54**, 1120–1129 discussion 1129–30.

Paulson, G.W. (1976) Benign essential tremor in childhood: Symptoms, pathogenesis, treatment. *Clinical Pediatrics*, **15**, 67–70.

Pellecchia, M.T., Varrone, A., Annesi, G. *et al.* (2006) Parkinsonism and essential tremor in a family with pseudo-dominant inheritance of PARK2: An FP-CIT SPECT study. *Movement Disorders*, **22**, 559–563.

Perlmutter, J.S. and Mink, J.W. (2006) Deep brain stimulation. *Annual Review of Neuroscience*, **29**, 229–257.

Plaha, P., Patel, N.K. and Gill, S.S. (2004) Stimulation of the subthalamic region for essential tremor. *Journal of Neurosurgery*, **101**, 48–54.

Putzke, J.D., Uitti, R.J., Obwegeser, A.A. *et al.* (2005) Bilateral thalamic deep brain stimulation: midline tremor control. *Journal of Neurology, Neurosurgery, and Psychiatry*, **76**, 684–690.

Raethjen, J., Kopper, F., Govindan, R.B. *et al.* (2004) Two different pathogenetic mechanisms in psychogenic tremor. *Neurology*, **63**, 812–815.

Rajput, A., Robinson, C.A. and Rajput, A.H. (2004) Essential tremor course and disability: a clinicopathologic study of 20 cases. *Neurology*, **62**, 932–936.

Rajput, A.H. (1996) Specificity of ethanol in essential tremor [letter; comment]. *Annals of Neurology*, **40**, 950–951.

Rajput, A.H., Jamieson, H., Hirsh, S. and Quraishi, A. (1975) Relative efficacy of alcohol and propranolol in action tremor. *The Canadian Journal of Neurological Sciences*, **2**, 31–35.

Rautakorpi, I., Marttila, R.J. and Rinne, U.K. (1983) Alcohol consumption of patients with essential tremor. *Acta Neurologica Scandinavica*, **68**, 177–179.

Sahin, H.A., Terzi, M., Ucak, S. *et al.* (2006) Frontal functions in young patients with essential tremor: a case comparison study. *The Journal of Neuropsychiatry and Clinical Neurosciences*, **18**, 64–72.

Schöls, L., Bauer, P., Schmidt, T. *et al.* (2004) Autosomal dominant cerebellar ataxias: clinical features, genetics, and pathogenesis. *The Lancet Neurology*, **3**, 291–304.

Schrag, A., Münchau, A., Bhatia, K.P. *et al.* (2000) Essential tremor: an overdiagnosed condition? *Journal of Neurology*, **247**, 955–959.

Schuurman, P.R., Bosch, D.A., Bossuyt, P.M. *et al.* (2000) A comparison of continuous thalamic stimulation and thalamotomy for suppression of severe tremor [see comments]. *The New England Journal of Medicine*, **342**, 461–468.

Serrano-Duenas, M. (2003) Use of primidone in low doses (250 mg/day) versus high doses (750 mg/day) in the management of essential tremor. Double-blind comparative study with one-year follow-up. *Parkinsonism & Related Disorders*, **10**, 29–33.

Shah, M., Findley, L., Muhammed, N. and Hawkes, C. (2005) Olfaction is normal in essential tremor and can be used to distinguish it from Parkinson's disease. *Movement Disorders*, **20**, S166.

Shatunov, A., Jankovic, J., Elble, R. *et al.* (2005) A variant in the HS1-BP3 gene is associated with familial essential tremor. *Neurology*, **65**, 1995; author reply 1995.

Shatunov, A., Sambuughin, N., Jankovic, J. *et al.* (2006) Genome-wide scans in North American families reveal genetic linkage of essential tremor to a region on chromosome 6p23. *Brain*, **129**, 2318–2331.

Shill, H.A., Bushara, K.O., Mari, Z. *et al.* (2004) Open-label dose-escalation study of oral 1-octanol in patients with essential tremor. *Neurology*, **62**, 2320–2322.

Siderowf, A., Gollump, S.M., Stern, M.B. *et al.* (2001) Emergence of complex, involuntary movements after gamma knife radio-surgery for essential tremor. *Movement Disorders*, **16**, 965–967.

Silvestri, A., Galetta, P., Cerquetani, E. *et al.* (2003) Report of erectile dysfunction after therapy with beta-blockers is related to patient knowledge of side effects and is reversed by placebo. *European Heart Journal*, **24**, 1928–1932.

Slowinski, J., Uitti, R.J., Putzke, J.D. and Wharen, R.E., Jr (2007) Deep brain stimulation. *Journal of Neurosurgery*, **106**, 192–193 author reply 193–4.

Soland, V.L., Bhatia, K.P., Volonte, M.A. and Marsden, C.D. (1996) Focal task-specific tremors. *Movement Disorders*, **11**, 665–670.

Stolze, H., Petersen, G., Raethjen, J. *et al.* (2001) The gait disorder of advanced essential tremor. *Brain*, **124**, 2278–2286.

Stover, N.P., Okun, M.S., Evatt, M.L. *et al.* (2005) Stimulation of the subthalamic nucleus in a patient with Parkinson's disease and essential tremor. *Archives of Neurology*, **62**, 141–143.

Sydow, O., Thobois, S., Alesch, F. and Speelman, J.D. (2003) Multicentre European study of thalamic stimulation in essential tremor: a six year follow up. *Journal of Neurology, Neurosurgery, and Psychiatry*, **74**, 1387–1391.

Tan, E.K., Lum, S.Y. and Prakash, K.M. (2006) Clinical features of childhood onset essential tremor. *European Journal of Neurology*, **13**, 1302–1305.

Tolosa, E., Wenning, G. and Poewe, W. (2006) The diagnosis of Parkinson's disease. *The Lancet Neurology*, **5**, 75–86.

Ushe, M., Mink, J.W., Tabbal, S.D. *et al.* (2006) Postural tremor suppression is dependent on thalamic stimulation frequency. *Movement Disorders*, **21**, 1290–1292.

Ushe, M., Mink, J.W., Revilla, F.J. *et al.* (2004) Effect of stimulation frequency on tremor suppression in essential tremor. *Movement Disorders*, **19**, 1163–1168.

Van Melle, J.P., Verbeek, D.E., Van Den Berg, M.P. *et al.* (2006) Beta-blockers and depression after myocardial infarction: a multicenter prospective study. *Journal of the American College of Cardiology*, **48**, 2209–2214.

Whaley, N.R., Putzke, J.D. Baba, Y. *et al.* (2007) Essential tremor: Phenotypic expression in a clinical cohort. *Parkinsonism & Related Disorders*, **13**, 33–339.

Wissel, J., Masuhr, F., Schelosky, L. *et al.* (1997) Quantitative assessment of botulinum toxin treatment in 43 patients with head tremor. *Movement Disorders*, **12**, 722–726.

Yanagisawa, N., Goto, A. and Narabayashi, H. (1972) Familial dystonia musculorum deformans and tremor. *Journal of the Neurological Sciences*, **16**, 125–136.

Young, R.F., Jacques, S., Mark, R. *et al.* (2000) Gamma knife thalamotomy for treatment of tremor: long-term results. *Journal of Neurosurgery*, **93** (Suppl. 3), 128–135.

Zesiewicz, T.A., Ward, C.L., Hauser, R.A. *et al.* (2006a) Pregabalin (Lyrica) in the treatment of essential tremor. *Movement Disorders*, **22**, 139–141.

Zesiewicz, T.A., Ward, C.L., Hauser, R.A. *et al.* (2006b) A double-blind placebo-controlled trial of zonisamide (zonegran) in the treatment of essential tremor. *Movement Disorders*, **22**, 279–282.

Zesiewicz, T.A., Elble, R., Louis, E.D. *et al.* (2005) Practice parameter: therapies for essential tremor: report of the Quality Standards Subcommittee of the American Academy of Neurology. *Neurology*, **64**, 2008–2020.

11

Other Tremor Disorders

Günther Deuschl

Christian-Albrechts-University Kiel, Germany

INTRODUCTION

Tremor denotes a rhythmic involuntary movement of one or more regions of the body. Normal tremor is present in every subject and related to physiologic mechanisms of movement (Vallbo and Wessberg, 1993). Pathologic tremor is clinically defined on the basis of visibility to the naked eye, but activation conditions and frequencies are also often different. The three most common pathologic tremors are enhanced physiologic tremor, essential tremor and tremor of Parkinson's disease. Other important tremors are cerebellar tremor, dystonic tremor and orthostatic tremor. The disabilities caused by these tremors differ as much as their clinical appearance, pathophysiology and etiology. Some tremors can be successfully medically treated, but others not, and therefore, for severely incapacitating tremors, refined stereotactic surgical approaches have become increasingly important. This chapter will cover tremors except essential and parkinsonian tremor.

ENHANCED PHYSIOLOGICAL TREMOR

This term was originally used by neurophysiologists to label a form of tremor characterized by frequency and activation features of normal physiologic tremor but with larger amplitude. It is a visible postural and action tremor that can be cumbersome, particularly on action. In most cases a cause can be identified. This form of tremor is considered to be reversible if the cause of the tremor is corrected for. There may be many causes for this enhancement of normal physiologic tremor (Table 11.1). The exclusion of other neurological symptoms or diseases that could cause tremor is mandatory for the diagnosis (Deuschl et al., 1998a).

A recent cross-sectional population-based study in Tyrolia has found the prevalence of enhanced physiological tremor (EPT) to be 9.5% in subjects over 50 years of age. EPT was much more common than essential tremor

(3.06%), parkinsonian tremor (2.05%) or Parkinson's disease (4.49%) (Wenning et al., 2005). There are no studies available on the natural cause of the condition. As most of the causes (a side effect of drugs, endogenous intoxications, etc.) of EPT are treatable and/or reversible, it is believed that it can be corrected for many causes.

The pathophysiologic mechanisms underlying the enhancement of these physiologic reflex conditions may either be activation of the reflex loops, which has been shown for thyrotoxic tremor (Elble, 1996) or the activation of a central oscillator which has been shown for amitriptyline (Raethjen et al., 2001).

The causes of an enhancement of one or both of the physiological tremor components are diverse. Trembling with excitement, fear or anxiety is common which may be cumbersome for performing artists or persons who need a high accuracy of dexterity, such as surgeons. It is thought to be mediated through an increased sympathetic tone, which results in a β-adrenergically driven sensitization of the muscle spindles increasing the gain in the reflex loops (Marsden and Meadows, 1968). A similar origin via the sympathetic nervous system has been proposed for the tremor in reflex sympathetic dystrophy. Metabolic abnormalities or drugs and toxin or withdrawal from such substances are common causes of EPT. The pathophysiology can be peripheral or central depending on the cause.

As both EPT and early essential tremor (ET), are not accompanied by any other neurological symptoms they can sometimes be difficult to distinguish. The positive family history in ET, its chronic course and the lack of an overt cause for the tremor are important hints. Sometimes the diagnosis can only be made after having observed the patient for an extended time period. EPT is usually bilateral and thus, any tremor presenting unilaterally, even with a high frequency and a pure postural component, must be suspected to be a symptomatic tremor. Spectral analysis of accelerometric and EMG signals can be helpful to demonstrate a centrally driven component in ET (Raethjen et al.,

Therapeutics of Parkinson's Disease and Other Movement Disorders Edited by Mark Hallett and Werner Poewe
© 2008 John Wiley & Sons, Ltd.

Table 11.1 Causes of enhanced physiologic tremor.

Metabolic disturbances (Hyperthyroidism, Hyperparathyroidism, Hypoglycaemia, Hepatic encephalopathy, Magnesium deficiency, Hypocalcaemia, Hyponatraemia)

Toxins (Mercury, Lead, Manganese, Alcohol, DDT, Lindan)

Drugs (Neuroleptics, Metoclopramide, Antidepressants (tricyclics), Lithium, Cocaine, Alcohol, Sympathomimetics, Steroids, Valproate, Antiarrhythmics (Amiodarone), Thyroid-hormones, Cytostatics, Immunodepressants)

Others (anxiety, fatigue, sympathetic reflex dystrophy, withdrawal of alcohol or drugs)

2004). A frequency below 8 Hz, which can be seen in the very early stages of ET, seems to be in favour of ET rather than EPT (Elble, Higgins and Elble, 2005).

Treatment

Depending on the etiology of EPT in a particular patient, causative treatment is always the first step. There are only a few studies on symptomatic treatment of EPT and only for a minority of etiologies. Treatment of thyrotoxic tremor with propranolol (<160 mg daily) is recommended, but other β-blockers (atenolol (<200 mg daily), metoprolol (<200 mg daily), acebutolol (<400 mg daily), oxprenolol (<160 mg daily), nadolol (<80 mg daily) and timolol (<20 mg daily) have a similar effect (Feely and Peden, 1984). Propranolol improves the tremor of ophthalmic surgeons when given prior to surgery (Elman *et al.*, 1998). Although a study of acetazolamide for the treatment of valproate tremors was positive, many tremor specialists use propranolol for this condition. Interestingly, it has been shown that introduction of slow-release compared to conventional valproate elicits no significant tremor (Rinnerthaler *et al.*, 2005). Other treatment recommendations are based on expert opinions only. A single dose of a β-blocking agent (e.g., propranolol 10–60 mg) 30 minutes before a stressful situation is recommended to suppress transient tremor that is known in a pre-disposed subject to interfere with important (e.g., professional) activities.

PRIMARY ORTHOSTATIC TREMOR

Primary orthostatic tremor is a unique tremor syndrome (Heilman, 1984) characterized by a subjective feeling of unsteadiness during stance, but only in severe cases during gait. Some patients show sudden falls. None of the patients has problems when sitting and lying. The only clinical finding is sometimes visible, but mostly only palpable, fine-amplitude rippling of leg muscles. Listening to the muscles with the bell of the stethoscope can also reveal the tremor. Thus, this tremor is suspected, mainly based on the complaints of the patients rather than clinical findings. The diagnosis can only be confirmed with electromyography as the surface electromyography (e.g., from the quadriceps femoris muscle) while standing shows a pathognomic 13–18 Hz burst pattern. All the leg, trunk and even arm muscles show this pattern, which is, in many cases, absent during tonic innervation when sitting and lying (McManis and Sharbrough, 1993).

Orthostatic tremor (OT) is a relatively rare condition (only small case series have been published adding up to less than 200 cases), and epidemiological data are lacking. The condition occurs only in patients above 40 years and in one series (Gerschlager *et al.*, 2004) the mean age at onset was lower for women (50 years) compared with men (60 years). So far it is not considered a hereditary disease, but one familial case has been reported (Contarino *et al.*, 2006).

OT is considered an idiopathic condition. Other movement disorders often occur together with it for unknown reasons. Parkinson's disease, vascular parkinsonism, and restless legs syndrome have all been described in OT, but none of these conditions are apparently pathophysiologically related. It is of special interest that dopaminergic terminals are significantly reduced in this condition, but clinical trials with L-dopa and dopamine agonists are mostly unsuccessful (Katzenschlager *et al.*, 2003).

Arm tremor may occur in roughly half of the patients and is usually more evident during stance (Boroojerdi *et al.*, 1999; McAuley *et al.*, 2000). The high-frequency EMG pattern is coherent in all the muscles of the body (Britton and Thompson, 1995), leading to the hypothesis that a bilaterally descending system must underlie OT. Such projections originate only from the brainstem and not from the hemispheres. Therefore, the generator for this tremor is assumed to be located within the brainstem or cerebellum (Wu *et al.*, 2001). The differential diagnosis is broad, as other idiopathic tremors, like essential tremor and cerebellar tremor, can present with similar complaints. The most important test to separate them is electromyography.

Treatment

Orthostatic tremor has been documented to be responsive to clonazepam and primidone. Valproate and propranolol were applied in single cases with variable success. Abnormalities of dopaminergic innervation of the striatum have been described although L-Dopa has not consistently shown efficiency (Katzenschlager *et al.*, 2003; Wills *et al.*, 1999). Pramipexol has been useful in one case (Finkel, 2000). According to small, double-blind studies (Evidente *et al.*, 1998; Onofrj *et al.*, 1998) gabapentin seems to have an excellent and most consistent beneficial effect, confirmed by objective measurements (Rodrigues *et al.*, 2006; Rodrigues *et al.*, 2005). Meanwhile I recommend it as the drug of first choice for orthostatic tremor (1800–2400 mg daily). The drug of second choice is clonazepam in our hands. Deep brain stimulation was never reported, but one case responded to spinal cord stimulation at the thoracic level (Krauss *et al.*, 2006).

DYSTONIC TREMOR SYNDROMES

Dystonic tremor is still an entity that is under debate and different definitions have been proposed by clinicians (Jedynak *et al.*, 1991; Vidailhet *et al.*, 1998). Its pathophysiology is largely unknown, but is likely related to the CNS (basal ganglia) abnormality postulated for dystonia itself (Deuschl, 2003). Tremor associated with dystonia may be a "forme fruste" of essential tremor (Marsden, 1976).

Typical dystonic tremor occurs in the body region affected by dystonia. It is defined (Deuschl, 2003) as a postural/kinetic tremor usually not seen during complete rest. At onset and sometimes during the course of the disease, dystonic tremor is focal and limited to one or two extremities with irregular amplitudes and variable frequencies (mostly below 7 Hz). Some patients exhibit focal tremors even without overt signs of dystonia. They have been included among dystonic tremors (Rivest and Marsden, 1990) because some of them later develop dystonia. Special forms of dystonic tremor are task-specific tremors like dystonic voice tremor (Koda and Ludlow, 1992) or dystonic writing tremor (Elble, Moody and Higgins, 1990; Bain *et al.*, 1995). Dystonic jaw tremor has been proposed to be a specific entity (Schneider and Bhatia, 2007).

Tremor associated with dystonia is a more generalized form of tremor in extremities that are not affected by the dystonia. This is a relatively symmetric, postural and kinetic tremor usually showing higher frequencies than actual dystonic tremor, often seen in the upper limbs in patients with spasmodic torticollis (Munchau *et al.*, 2001).

The prevalence of dystonic tremor is unknown. In one Brasilian cross-sectional study it was estimated to be around 20% of patients with primary or secondary dystonia (Ferraz *et al.*, 1994), but seems to be more common in cervical dystonia (Bartolome *et al.*, 2003). In a large survey among patients from a large Indian movement-disorder center, dystonic tremor was diagnosed in 20% of all patients, excluding Parkinson's disease and ET (Shukla and Behari, 2004).

In patients with dystonic tremors, antagonistic gestures can lead to a reduction of the tremor amplitude. This is well known for dystonic head tremor in the setting of spasmodic torticollis. A reduction in tremor is seen when the patient touches the head or only lifts the arm (Masuhr *et al.*, 2000). As this sign is absent in essential head tremor it can be an important differential diagnostic hint in unclear head tremors in which the dystonic posture is not obvious. The effect of these maneuvers can sometimes be difficult to observe clinically and it can be helpful to record surface EMG from the affected muscles and look for EMG suppression (Masuhr *et al.*, 2000). Although almost exclusively seen in dystonic tremor the sensitivity of the sign is unknown. Other important, but less specific differential diagnostic clues are the focal nature and relatively low frequency of dystonic tremor. The tremor associated with dystonia is more difficult to separate from ET, especially when the accompanying dystonia has not evolved completely.

Treatment

No controlled study of oral medication is available. A positive effect of propranolol has been described earlier in studies of dystonic head tremor. The efficacy of botulinum toxin for dystonic head (Jankovic *et al.*, 1991) tremor and for tremulous spasmodic dysphonia is well documented. A double blind study has also documented the efficacy of botulinum toxin for hand tremor (Brin *et al.*, 2001), but the use of this drug for this indication is limited because of the associated paresis. Dystonic tremor in the setting of segmental or generalized dystonia has been successfully treated with deep-brain-stimulation of the pallidum in a controlled study (Kupsch *et al.*, 2006). Stimulation of the ventrolateral thalamus can also alleviate the tremor but can occasionally lead to worsening of the dystonia itself. Tremor associated with dystonia often responds to the medication for classical essential tremor.

Experts sometimes recommend the use of anticholinergics or propranolol/primidone. For drug dosages see Table 11.2.

CEREBELLAR TREMOR SYNDROMES

The classical cerebellar tremor is an intention tremor occurring uni- or bilaterally depending on the underlying cerebellar disease. The tremor frequency is almost always below 5 Hz. Simple kinetic and postural tremor may be present. Some patients with a mild cerebellar ataxia present with an isolated postural and simple kinetic tremor above 5 Hz, resembling essential tremor (Deuschl *et al.*, 1998b). Titubation is another tremor manifestation of cerebellar disease and is a low-frequency oscillation (around 3 Hz) of the head and trunk depending on postural innervation. If the low frequency action tremor is severe it may sometimes be seen in a seemingly resting position because the patient is unable to completely relax.

Table 11.2 Dosages of various substances applied for the treatment of tremor.

	Initial dose	Increase in steps of	High dose
L-Dopa and dopamine agonists			
L-Dopa + dopadecarboxylase inhibitor	50 mg	50 mg/d	600 mg
Bromocriptine	5 mg	5 mg/w	20 mg
Lisuride	0.1 mg	0.1 mg/w	1.2 mg
α-Dihydroergocryptin	10 mg	10 mg/w	90 mg
Pergolide	0.15 mg	0.10 mg/d	3.0 mg
Pramipexole	1.5 mg	0.5 mg/w	4.5 mg
Ropinirole	3 mg	1.5 mg/d	15 mg
Cabergoline	2 mg	1 mg/w	6 mg
Rotigotine (patch)	2 mg	2 mg	8 mg
Anti-cholinergics			
Bornaprine	3 mg	3 mg/w	12 mg
Metixen	7.5 mg	7.5 mg/w	60 mg
Trihexyphenidyl	1 mg	2 mg/w	10 mg
β-Blockers			
Propranolol	30 mg	30 mg/w	240 mg
Nadolol	10 mg	30 mg/w	120 mg
Miscellaneous			
Primidone	62.5 mg	125 mg/d	500 mg
Clonazepam	0.5 mg	0.5 mg/d	6 mg
Gabapentine	300	600 mg/w	2400 mg daily
Topiramate	20	20 mg/d	300 mg/d
Botulinum toxin	Depending on muscle and product		
Clozapine	12.5 mg	12.5 mg/d	75 mg
Amantadine	100 mg	100 mg/d	300 mg
Alprazolam	0.75 mg	0.75 mg/d	4 mg

For some substances (e.g., anti-cholinergics) a slow titration is strongly recommended.

Intention tremor is a characteristic form of tremor that can usually be separated from other tremors clinically. But intention tremor can also occur in advanced ET. In this case the most important clinical clue is the degree to which ataxia is present and the absence of clinically detectable oculomotor abnormalities in ET. While in ET only a mild dysmetria and tandem gait disturbance (Stolze et al., 2001) have been described, this dominates the cerebellar syndrome, in which lesions or atrophy can often be seen in brain imaging studies.

As this type of tremor can be caused by various etiologies, no epidemiologic data is available. One of the most common causes of cerebellar tremor certainly is demyelinating lesions in multiple sclerosis (Alusi et al., 2001a). Cerebellar strokes can also present with tremor especially when the brainstem is involved (Louis et al., 1996). Degenerations of cerebellar neurones of various etiologies often produce tremor. Hereditary ataxias, particularly SCA 12, 16, and 21, can produce tremor. Toxic cerebellar degeneration due to alcohol abuse predominantly of the anterior lobe is common and often presents with low frequency (2–3 Hz) stance tremor in the anterior-posterior direction (Neiman et al., 1990).

The pathophysiology of the classical cerebellar intention tremor seems to be distinct from the other central tremors, as it is not believed to be due to a central oscillator, but to alterations of feedback loops. One of the striking abnormalities in cerebellar dysfunction is a delay of the second and third phase of the triphasic EMG pattern in ballistic movements (Hallett et al., 1975) or a delay of the reflexes regulating stance control (Mauritz et al., 1981). During goal-directed movements, this will cause the breaking movement to occur too late and thereby produce an overshoot with a subsequent abnormal correction movement, thus producing a quasi-rhythmic movement which is compatible with intention tremor. However, the higher frequency postural and action tremors in some patients with cerebellar disease more likely reflect the existence of a separate central oscillator.

Treatment

Cerebellar tremors are difficult to treat and good results are rare. Double-blind studies are lacking. Studies with cholinergic substances (physostigmine, lecithine) have shown improvement in some patients, but failed in the majority. Isoniazid failed to show significant results (Hallett et al., 1991). 5-HTP has been found to be effective in some patients (Rascol et al., 1981; Trouillas et al., 1995). Open studies or single case observations have shown favorable results with amantadine, propranolol, clonazepam, carbamazepine, tetrahydrocannabiol and trihexyphenidyl. Levetiracetam (50 mg/kg/day) was positively tested in a pilot trial (Striano et al., 2006). Cannabis is not effective (Fox et al., 2004). Probably the best symptomatic improvement can be obtained with deep-brain stimulation of the thalamus or thalamotomy in selected patients (Alusi et al., 2001b; Lozano, 2000; Schuurman et al., 2000). Thalamic stimulation was found to be superior to thalamotomy. Functional outcome after surgery, however, greatly varies and depends on the presence of other motor symptoms of the disease. Patients with MS-tremor with a frequency above 3 Hz and significant tremor-related disabilities were found to respond favorably (Alusi et al., 2001b). Thus accelerometric tremor recordings and frequency analysis may help to distinguish patients with predominant MS tremor from those with tremor and ataxia. Long-term follow-up studies of larger cohorts are lacking.

Limited improvements have been observed after loading of the shaking extremity, but most clinicians do not use it because the patients adapt rapidly to the new weight. Recommendations also often include physiotherapy.

HOLMES' TREMOR

This is a rare symptomatic tremor due to a lesion. It has been labelled under different names in the past (rubral tremor, midbrain tremor, myorhythmia, tremor of Benedikt's syndrome). It is the only tremor with resting, postural and intentional components. It typically shows low frequencies (<4.5 Hz) and is often irregular and not as rhythmic as other tremors. If the date of the lesion is known (e.g., in case of a cerebrovascular accident) a variable delay between the lesion and the first occurrence of the tremor is typical (mostly two weeks to two years). This is among the most disabling forms of tremor because it disturbs rest and all kinds of voluntary

and involuntary movements. It mainly affects the hand and proximal arm and is mostly unilateral.

This unique tremor form is caused by a combined lesion of the cerebellothalamic and nigrostriatal systems as suggested by autopsy data (Masucci, Kurtzke and Saini, 1984), PET data (Remy et al., 1995) and clinical observations (Deuschl et al., 1999; Krack et al., 1994). Any lesion involving fiber tracts from both systems can produce this tremor. Thus, the exact location of the lesions seen in these patients may vary.

Thalamic tremor (Miwa et al., 1996) can be difficult to differentiate from Holmes' tremor. This tremor is part of a spectrum of symptoms including variable combinations of dystonia, chorea and action tremor following lateral-posterior thalamic insults, mostly strokes (Kim, 2001; Lehericy et al., 2001). The "thalamic" tremor itself is a mixture of action tremor with an intentional component and dystonia in the setting of a well-recovered severe hemiparesis. Proximal segments are often involved. This tremor syndrome also develops with a certain delay after the initial insult. The combination of tremor, dystonia and a severe sensory loss is an important clue for the diagnosis, but imaging is usually necessary.

Cerebellar tremor that continues under seemingly resting conditions due to a lack of relaxation can be mistaken for Holmes' tremor. The irregularity, the lower frequency and an accompanying parkinsonian syndrome can help to recognize Holmes' tremor in this situation.

Treatment

No generally accepted therapy is available. Nevertheless, treatment is successful in a higher percentage than for patients with cerebellar tremor. Some patients respond to levodopa, anti-cholinergics or clonazepam. For drug dosages see Table 10.2. The effect of functional neurosurgery for this tremor syndrome is poorly documented. Such patients have been operated on, but they were diagnosed as post-traumatic tremors or post-stroke tremors and the clinical features are not described in detail. Several patients received thalamic surgery either with lesion or DBS (Kim et al., 2002; Kudo et al., 2001; Nikkhah et al., 2004) with some improvement.

PALATAL TREMOR SYNDROMES

Palatal tremors are rare tremor syndromes and can be separated into two forms (Deuschl et al., 1990; Deuschl, Toro and Hallett, 1994). Symptomatic palatal tremor (SPT) is characterized by rhythmic movements of the soft palate (levator veli palatini). This is clinically visible as a rhythmic movement of the edge of the palate. Other brainstem-innervated (leading to oscillopsia in case of eye muscle involvement) or extremity muscles can also be involved

(Masucci, Kurtzke and Saini, 1984). It typically follows a brainstem/cerebellar lesion with a variable delay (Deuschl and Wilms, 2002; Samuel *et al.*, 2004) and is often associated with a cerebellar syndrome (Deuschl, Jost and Schumacher, 1996). Essential palatal tremor (EPaT) occurs without any overt central nervous pathology and is characterized by rhythmic movements of the soft palate (tensor veli palatini), usually with an ear click. The tensor contraction is visible as a movement of the roof of the palate. Extremity or eye muscles are not involved.

While the pathophysiologic basis of EPaT is unknown, the emergence of SPT has been studied in detail and carries important implications for central mechanisms of tremors in general. After the cerebellar/brainstem lesion, an inferior olivary pseudohypertrophy (which can be demonstrated by MRI) develops most likely as a consequence of an interruption of inhibitory GABAergic fibres terminating in the inferior olive. Inferior olivary neurones are prone to oscillate spontaneously and can be easily synchronized through gap junctions (Llinas and Welsh, 1993). Thus, the disinhibition and hypertrophy will lead to enhanced synchronized oscillations and builds the basis for the rhythmic movement disorder. Interestingly this rhythm is also reflected in rhythmic EMG inhibition in extremity muscles, sometimes leading to a mild postural tremor (Deuschl *et al.*, 1994). Therefore it has been postulated that the inferior olive (and the olivocerebellar system) may be a key structure in producing postural tremors (Deuschl *et al.*, 2001) and that these tremors are characterized by a rhythmic inhibition of ongoing contractions rather than rhythmic activation which may be the basis of the etiologically different resting tremors (Deuschl *et al.*, 1994).

Treatment

The disability of patients with SPT is mostly due to other clinical symptoms of the underlying cerebellar lesion. The rhythmic palatal movement in SPT does not cause discomfort or disability for the patient except when the eyes are involved or when there is an extremity tremor.

Oscillopsia is difficult to treat. Single cases have been described with a favorable response to clonazepam. Other oral drugs that have been proposed are trihexyphenidyl and valproate. Botulinum toxin has been used for the treatment of oscillopsia. The toxin can either be injected into the retrobulbar fat tissue or individual eye muscles can be targeted selectively (Leigh *et al.*, 1994; Repka, Savino and Reinecke, 1994). So far no controlled studies are available. In our hands this treatment is helpful for some patients, but is not always accepted for long-term use.

For the treatment of extremity tremors, single cases have been reported to respond to clonazepam (Bakheit and Behan, 1990) or trihexiphenidyl (Jabbari *et al.*, 1989).

The only complaint of patients with EPaT is the ear click. A number of medications have been reported to be successful: valproate (Borggreve and Hageman, 1991), trihexyphenidyl (Jabbari *et al.*, 1989) and flunarizine (Cakmur *et al.*, 1997). Recently sumatriptane has been found to be effective in a few patients (Gambardella and Quattrone, 1998; Scott, Evans and Jankovic, 1996), but was unsuccessful in others (Pakiam and Lang, 1999). The antagonism of 5-HT receptors may thus play a role, at least for some of the patients. As a long-term therapy this drug is not applicable for various reasons. Presently the most established therapy is the treatment of the click by injection of botulinum toxin into the tensor veli palatini (Deuschl *et al.*, 1991). Low dosages of botulinum toxin (e.g., 4–10 units Botox) are injected under electromyographic guidance. The critical point is to ascertain with endoscopy and electromyography, through an EMG-injection needle isolated until the tip, that the needle is definitely placed within the tensor muscle. Spread of botulinum toxin in the soft palate or too large dosages can otherwise cause severe side effects of dysphagia. Although we have never seen any such complications in our patients, it must be mentioned that injection of botulinum toxin into the palatal muscles in rabbits has been introduced as an animal model for middle ear infections.

TREMOR SYNDROMES IN PERIPHERAL NEUROPATHY

Several peripheral neuropathies regularly present with tremors. The tremors are mostly postural and action tremors. The frequency in hand muscles can be lower than in proximal arm muscles. Abnormal position sense need not be present.

Dysgammaglobulinaemia and chronic Guillain–Barré syndrome are the acquired neuropathies presenting most frequently with tremor. In a series of 62 patients with dysgammaglobulinaemic polyneuropathy, postural and action tremor of the hands was present in 70–80% of the cases (Yeung *et al.*, 1991). However, it only rarely represents the dominant source of disability in these patients (Busby *et al.*, 2003). A similar type of tremor can be observed in around 40% of patients with hereditary polyneuropathy (HMSN). Many of these patients have a family history of tremor (Cardoso and Jankovic, 1993).

The tremor in dysimmune neuropathies seems to be somewhat related to the severity of the peripheral neuronal damage and it has been postulated that an abnormal peripheral feedback to central tremor-generating structures could be the basis for the tremor enhancement in this situation (Bain *et al.*, 1996).

The tremor in HMSN seems to be largely unrelated to the severity of neuropathic syndromes and it may also occur in family members without a neuropathy. Thus it has been suggested that it is genetically related to ET (Cardoso and Jankovic, 1993). There is an ongoing debate as to whether the combination of a hereditary neuropathy with postural tremor (Roussy–Levy syndrome) actually constitutes a distinct disease entity (Plante-Bordeneuve *et al.*, 1999).

Treatment

No convincing therapies are reported for this type of tremor. Successful treatment of the underlying neuropathy can improve the tremor in some of the patients (Dalakas, Teravainen and Engel, 1984). In our hands, propranolol and primidone have been helpful for some patients at similar dosages as for essential tremor. One patient was successfully implanted with DBS electrodes (Ruzicka *et al.*, 2003).

PSYCHOGENIC TREMOR

Psychogenic tremors have very diverse clinical presentations and are a specific variant of psychogenic movement disorders (see Chapter 31 on psychogenic movement disorders). Most of these tremors are action tremors, but many also remain during rest and often show very unusual combinations of rest/postural and intention tremors (Kim, Pakiam and Lang, 1999). Typical clinical features are a sudden onset and sometimes spontaneous remissions, decrease of tremor amplitude or variable frequency during distraction, selective disability and a positive "co-activation sign." This is tested as with rigidity testing at the wrist. Variable, voluntary-like force exertion can be felt in both movement directions (Deuschl *et al.*, 1998c). Some of the patients have a history of somatizations in the past, or additional, unrelated (psychogenic) neurologic symptoms and signs (Deuschl *et al.*, 1998c).

In a large series of 842 patients presenting with a movement disorder, only 3.3% were diagnosed with psychogenic movement disorders. Among those psychogenic tremor was the most common diagnosis (50%) (Factor, Podskalny and Molho, 1995).

Pathophysiology and Etiology

Two pathogenetic mechanisms seem to play a role in psychogenic tremor. Voluntary-like rhythmic movements can be detected by coupled (coherent) tremor oscillations in different limbs. This resembles the situation in voluntarily sustained rhythmic movements in normal subjects, as it is extremely difficult to keep up two completely independent rhythms in different limbs (Brown and Thompson, 2001; McAuley *et al.*, 1998). In pathologic, organic tremor (clearly involuntary rhythmic movements) the oscillations are typically independent between different limbs (Lauk *et al.*, 1999; Raethjen *et al.*, 2000) but generally not in psychogenic tremor. Such independent rhythms can rarely be found in psychogenic tremor patients (Raethjen *et al.*, 2004b). They most likely represent physiological oscillations based on a clonus-like mechanism, which is enhanced by the ongoing co-contraction of antagonistic muscles detected as the co-activation sign. These findings may easily explain the motor control mechanisms underlying these tremors. They do not allow conclusions on the underlying psychological mechanisms.

Psychogenic tremor has a very variable presentation and can mimic virtually all organic tremors. Thus, the tremor phenomenology does not help to differentiate them. The typical conditions of tremor appearance or disappearance, enhancement or attenuation described above are important clinical clues. The coupling between the oscillations in both arms, which is only present in psychogenic tremor and is absent in organic tremors (other than OT), can be used as an electrophysiological diagnostic tool. The surface EMG from both arm muscles can be analyzed using "coherence" which is a reliable mathematical measure of the oscillatory coupling. If the patients only show unilateral tremor, a voluntarily sustained rhythmic hand movement on the unaffected side is related with the tremor on the affected side ("coherence entrainment test") (McAuley and Rothwell, 2004). This test is very specific and the "entrainment" of psychogenic tremor by a contralateral rhythmic movement can sometimes be visible even clinically. However, it is not very sensitive, as some psychogenic tremor patients show unrelated rhythms in different limbs, resembling organic tremors (Raethjen *et al.*, 2004b). An accelerometric quantification of the distractibility can also be helpful (Zeuner *et al.*, 2003).

Treatment

Studies on the treatment effects in psychogenic tremor are rare (Koller *et al.*, 1989). Anti-depressants may be helpful (Voon and Lang, 2005). Psychotherapy is helpful only in the minority of patients. We recommend physiotherapy aiming to avoid co-contraction of the muscles during voluntary movements. Additionally we administer propranolol at medium or high dosages to desensitize the muscle spindles, which are necessary to maintain the clonus mechanism in these patients. Conclusive data on the prognosis and long-term outcome in these patients are lacking (see also Chapter 13), but the prognosis is generally believed to be poor (Feinstein *et al.*, 2001).

References

Alusi, S.H., Worthington, J., Glickman, S., Bain, P.G. (2001a) A study of tremor in multiple sclerosis. *Brain*, **124** (Pt 4), 720–730.

Alusi, S.H., Aziz, T.Z., Glickman, S., Jahanshahi, M., Stein, J.F., Bain, P.G. (2001b) Stereotactic lesional surgery for the treatment of tremor in multiple sclerosis: a prospective case-controlled study. *Brain*, **124** (Pt 8), 1576–1589.

Bain, P.G., Findley, L.J., Britton, T.C. *et al.* (1995) Primary writing tremor. *Brain*, **116**, 203–209.

Bain, P.G., Britton, T.C., Jenkins, I.H. *et al.* (1996) Tremor associated with benign IgM paraproteinaemic neuropathy. *Brain*, **119** (Pt 3), 789–799.

Bakheit, A.M. and Behan, P.O. (1990) Palatal myoclonus successfully treated with clonazepam [letter] [see comments]. *Journal of Neurology, Neurosurgery, and Psychiatry*, **53** (9), 806.

Bartolome, F.M., Fanjul, S., Cantarero, S., Hernandez, J. and Garcia Ruiz, P.J. (2003) [Primary focal dystonia: descriptive study of 205 patients]. *Neurologia*, **18** (2), 59–65.

Borggreve, F. and Hageman, G. (1991) A case of idiopathic palatal myoclonus: treatment with sodium valproate. *European Neurology*, **31** (6), 403–404.

Boroojerdi, B., Ferbert, A., Foltys, H., Kosinski, C.M., Noth, J. and Schwarz, M. (1999) Evidence for a non-orthostatic origin of orthostatic tremor. *Journal of Neurology, Neurosurgery, and Psychiatry*, **66** (3), 284–288.

Brin, M.F., Lyons, K.E., Doucette, J. *et al.* (2001) A randomized, double masked, controlled trial of botulinum toxin type A in essential hand tremor. *Neurology*, **56** (11), 1523–1528.

Britton, T.C. and Thompson, P.D. (1995) Primary orthostatic tremor. *Bmj*, **310** (6973), 143–144.

Brown, P. and Thompson, P.D. (2001) Electrophysiological aids to the diagnosis of psychogenic jerks, spasms, and tremor. *Movement Disorders*, **16** (4), 595–599.

Busby, M., Nithi, K., Mills, K. and Donaghy, M. (2003) The tremor associated with non-paraproteinaemic acquired demyelinating polyneuropathy – a case study. *Journal of Neurology*, **250** (4), 486–487.

Cakmur, R., Idiman, E., Idiman, F., Baklan, B. and Ozkiziltan, S. (1997) Essential palatal tremor successfully treated with lunarizine. *European Neurology*, **38** (2), 133–134.

Cardoso, F.E. and Jankovic, J. (1993) Hereditary motor-sensory neuropathy and movement disorders. *Muscle & Nerve*, **16** (9), 904–910.

Contarino, M.F., Welter, M.L., Agid, Y. and Hartmann, A. (2006) Orthostatic tremor in monozygotic twins. *Neurology*, **66** (10), 1600–1601.

Dalakas, M.C., Teravainen, H. and Engel, W.K. (1984) Tremor as a feature of chronic relapsing and dysgammaglobulinemic polyneuropathies. Incidence and management. *Archives of Neurology*, **41** (7), 711–714.

Deuschl, G. (2003) Dystonic tremor. *Revue Neurologique*, **159** (10 Pt 1), 900–905.

Deuschl, G. and Wilms, H. (2002) Clinical spectrum and physiology of palatal tremor. *Movement Disorders*, **17** (Suppl 2), S63–S66.

Deuschl, G., Mischke, G., Schenck, E., Schulte-Mönting, J. and Lücking, C.H. (1990) Symptomatic and essential rhythmic palatal myoclonus. *Brain*, **113**, 1645–1672.

Deuschl, G., Lohle, E., Heinen, F. and Lücking, C. (1991) Ear click in palatal tremor: its origin and treatment with botulinum toxin. *Neurology*, **41** (10), 1677–1679.

Deuschl, G., Toro, C. and Hallett, M. (1994) Symptomatic and essential palatal tremor. 2. Differences of palatal movements. *Movement Disorders*, **9** (6), 676–678.

Deuschl, G., Toro, C., Valls, S.J., Zeffiro, T., Zee, D.S. and Hallett, M. (1994) Symptomatic and essential palatal tremor. 1. Clinical, physiological and MRI analysis. *Brain*, **117**, 775–788.

Deuschl, G., Jost, S. and Schumacher, M. (1996) Symptomatic palatal tremor is associated with signs of cerebellar dysfunction. *Journal of Neurology*, **243** (7), 553–556.

Deuschl, G., Bain, P. and Brin, M. (1998) Adhoc-Scientific-Committee Consensus statement of the Movement Disorder Society on Tremor. *Movement Disorders*, **13** (Suppl 3), 2–23.

Deuschl, G., Bain, P., Brin, M. and Committee AHS (1998b) Consensus statement of the Movement Disorder Society on Tremor. *Movement Disorders*, **13** (Suppl 3), 2–23.

Deuschl, G., Koster, B., Lucking, C.H. and Scheidt, C. (1998c) Diagnostic and pathophysiological aspects of psychogenic tremors. *Movement Disorders*, **13** (2), 294–302.

Deuschl, G., Wilms, H., Krack, P., Wurker, M. and Heiss, W.D. (1999) Function of the cerebellum in Parkinsonian rest tremor and Holmes' tremor. *Annals of Neurology*, **46** (1), 126–128.

Deuschl, G., Raethjen, J., Lindemann, M. and Krack, P. (2001) The pathophysiology of tremor. *Muscle & Nerve*, **24** (6), 716–735.

Elble, R.J. (1996) Central mechanisms of tremor. *Journal of Clinical Neurophysiology*, **13**, 133–144.

Elble, R.J., Moody, C. and Higgins, C. (1990) Primary writing tremor. A form of focal dystonia? *Movement Disorders*, **5** (2), 118–126.

Elble, R.J., Higgins, C. and Elble, S. (2005) Electrophysiologic transition from physiologic tremor to essential tremor. *Movement Disorders*, **20** (8), 1038–1042.

Elman, M.J., Sugar, J., Fiscella, R. *et al.* (1998) The effect of propranolol versus placebo on resident surgical performance. *Transactions of the American Ophthalmological Society*, **96**, 283–291.

Evidente, V.G., Adler, C.H., Caviness, J.N. and Gwinn, K.A. (1998) Effective treatment of orthostatic tremor with gabapentin. *Movement Disorders*, **13** (5), 829–831.

Factor, S.A., Podskalny, G.D. and Molho, E.S. (1995) Psychogenic movement disorders: Frequency, clinical profile, and characteristics. *Journal of Neurology, Neurosurgery and Psychiatry*, **59** (4), 406–412.

Feely, J. and Peden, N. (1984) Use of β-adrenoceptor blocking drugs in hyperthyroidism. *Drugs*, **27** (5), 425–446.

Feinstein, A., Stergiopoulos, V., Fine, J. and Lang, A.E. (2001) Psychiatric outcome in patients with a psychogenic movement disorder: a prospective study. *Neuropsychiatry Neuropsychology and Behavioral Neurology*, **14** (3), 169–176.

Ferraz, H.B., De Andrade, L.A., Silva, S.M., Borges, V. and Rocha, M.S. (1994) [Postural tremor and dystonia. Clinical aspects and physiopathological considerations]. *Arquivos de Neuro-Psiquiatria*, **52** (4), 466–470.

Finkel, M.F. (2000) Pramipexole is a possible effective treatment for primary orthostatic tremor (shaky leg syndrome). *Archives of Neurology*, **57** (10), 1519–1520.

Fox, P., Bain, P.G., Glickman, S., Carroll, C. and Zajicek, J. (2004) The effect of cannabis on tremor in patients with multiple sclerosis. *Neurology*, **62** (7), 1105–1109.

Gambardella, A. and Quattrone, A. (1998) Treatment of palatal myoclonus with sumatriptan [letter]. *Movement Disorders*, **13** (1), 195.

Gerschlager, W., Munchau, A., Katzenschlager, R. *et al.* (2004) Natural history and syndromic associations of orthostatic tremor: a review of 41 patients. *Movement Disorders*, **19** (7), 788–795.

Hallett, M., Shahani, B.T. and Young, R.R. (1975) EMG analysis of patients with cerebellar deficits. *Journal of Neurology, Neurosurgery, and Psychiatry*, **38** (12), 1163–1169.

Hallett, M., Ravits, J., Dubinsky, R.M., Gillespie, M.M. and Moinfar, A. (1991) A double-blind trial of isoniazid for essential tremor and other action tremors. *Movement Disorders*, **6** (3), 253–256.

Heilman, K.M. (1984) Orthostatic tremor. *Archives of Neurology*, **41** (8), 880–881.

Jabbari, B., Scherokman, B., Gunderson, C.H., Rosenberg, M.L. and Miller, J. (1989) Treatment of movement disorders with trihexyphenidyl. *Movement Disorders*, **4** (3), 202–212.

Jankovic, J., Leder, S., Warner, D. and Schwartz, K. (1991) Cervical dystonia: clinical findings and associated movement disorders. *Neurology*, **41** (7), 1088–1091.

Jedynak, C.P., Bonnet, A.M. and Agid, Y. (1991) Tremor and idiopathic dystonia. *Movement Disorders*, **6** (3), 230–236.

Katzenschlager, R., Costa, D., Gerschlager, W. *et al.* (2003) [123I]-FP-CIT-SPECT demonstrates dopaminergic deficit in orthostatic tremor. *Annals of Neurology*, **53** (4), 489–496.

Kim, J.S. (2001) Delayed onset mixed involuntary movements after thalamic stroke: clinical, radiological and pathophysiological findings. *Brain*, **124** (Pt 2), 299–309.

Kim, Y.J., Pakiam, A.S. and Lang, A.E. (1999) Historical and clinical features of psychogenic tremor: a review of 70 cases. *The Canadian Journal of Neurological Sciences*, **26** (3), 190–195.

Kim, M.C., Son, B.C., Miyagi, Y. and Kang, J.K. (2002) Vim thalamotomy for Holmes' tremor secondary to midbrain tumour. *Journal of Neurology, Neurosurgery, and Psychiatry*, **73** (4), 453–455.

Koda, J. and Ludlow, C.L. (1992) An evaluation of laryngeal muscle activation in patients with voice tremor. *Otolaryngology Head & Neck Surgery*, **107** (5), 684–696.

Koller, W., Lang, A., Vetere, O.B. *et al.* (1989) Psychogenic tremors. *Neurology*, **39** (8), 1094–1099.

Krack, P., Deuschl, G., Kaps, M., Warnke, P., Schneider, S. and Traupe, H. (1994) Delayed onset of "rubral tremor" 23 years after brainstem trauma. *Movement Disorders*, **9** (2), 240–242.

Krauss, J.K., Weigel, R., Blahak, C. *et al.* (2006) Chronic spinal cord stimulation in medically intractable orthostatic tremor. *Journal of Neurology, Neurosurgery, and Psychiatry*, **77** (9), 1013–1016.

Kudo, M., Goto, S., Nishikawa, S. *et al.* (2001) Bilateral thalamic stimulation for Holmes' tremor caused by unilateral brainstem lesion. *Movement Disorders*, **16** (1), 170–174.

Kupsch, A., Benecke, R., Muller, J. *et al.* (2006) Pallidal deep-brain stimulation in primary generalized or segmental dystonia. *The New England Journal of Medicine*, **355** (19), 1978–1990.

Lauk, M., Koster, B., Timmer, J., Guschlbauer, B., Deuschl, G. and Lucking, C.H. (1999) Side-to-side correlation of muscle activity in physiological and pathological human tremors. *Clinical Neurophysiology*, **110** (10), 1774–1783.

Lehericy, S., Grand, S., Pollak, P. *et al.* (2001) Clinical characteristics and topography of lesions in movement disorders due to thalamic lesions. *Neurology*, **57** (6), 1055–1066.

Leigh, R.J., Averbuch, H.L., Tomsak, R.L., Remler, B.F., Yaniglos, S.S. and Dell'Osso, L.F. (1994) Treatment of abnormal eye movements that impair vision: strategies based on current concepts of physiology and pharmacology. *Annals of Neurology*, **36** (2), 129–141.

Llinas, R. and Welsh, J.P. (1993) On the cerebellum and motor learning. *Current Opinion in Neurobiology*, **3** (6), 958–965.

Louis, E.D., Lynch, T., Ford, B., Greene, P., Bressman, S.B. and Fahn, S. (1996) Delayed-onset cerebellar syndrome. *Archives of Neurology*, **53** (5), 450–454.

Lozano, A.M. (2000) Vim thalamic stimulation for tremor. *Archives of Medical Research*, **31** (3), 266–269.

Marsden, C.D. (1976) Dystonia: the spectrum of the disease. *Res Publ Assoc Res Nerv Ment Dis*, **55**, 351–367.

Marsden, C.D. and Meadows, J.C. (1968) The effect of adrenaline on the contraction of human muscle – one mechanism whereby adrenaline increases the amplitude of physiological tremor. *The Journal of Physiology*, **194** (2), 70–71.

Masucci, E.F., Kurtzke, J.F. and Saini, N. (1984) Myorhythmia: a widespread movement disorder. Clinicopathological correlations. *Brain*, **107**, 53–79.

Masuhr, F., Wissel, J., Muller, J., Scholz, U. and Poewe, W. (2000) Quantification of sensory trick impact on tremor amplitude and frequency in 60 patients with head tremor. *Movement Disorders*, **15** (5), 960–964.

Mauritz, K.H., Schmitt, C. and Dichgans, J. (1981) Delayed and enhanced long latency reflexes as the possible cause of postural tremor in late cerebellar atrophy. *Brain*, **104** (Pt 1), 97–116.

McAuley, J. and Rothwell, J. (2004) Identification of psychogenic, dystonic, and other organic tremors by a coherence entrainment test. *Movement Disorders*, **19** (3), 253–267.

McAuley, J.H., Rothwell, J.C., Marsden, C.D. and Findley, L.J. (1998) Electrophysiological aids in distinguishing organic from psychogenic tremor. *Neurology*, **50** (6), 1882–1884.

McAuley, J.H., Britton, T.C., Rothwell, J.C., Findley, L.J. and Marsden, C.D. (2000) The timing of primary orthostatic tremor bursts has a task-specific plasticity. *Brain*, **123** (Pt 2), 254–266.

McManis, P.G. and Sharbrough, F.W. (1993) Orthostatic tremor: clinical and electrophysiologic characteristics. *Muscle & Nerve*, **16** (11), 1254–1260.

Miwa, H., Hatori, K., Kondo, T., Imai, H. and Mizuno, Y. (1996) Thalamic tremor: case reports and implications of the tremor-generating mechanism. *Neurology*, **46** (1), 75–79.

Munchau, A., Schrag, A., Chuang, C. *et al.* (2001) Arm tremor in cervical dystonia differs from essential tremor and can be classified by onset age and spread of symptoms. *Brain*, **124** (Pt 9), 1765–1776.

Neiman, J., Lang, A.E., Fornazzari, L. and Carlen, P.L. (1990) Movement disorders in alcoholism: a review. *Neurology*, **40** (5), 741–746.

Nikkhah, G., Prokop, T., Hellwig, B., Lucking, C.H. and Ostertag, C.B. (2004) Deep brain stimulation of the nucleus ventralis intermedius for Holmes (rubral) tremor and associated dystonia caused by upper brainstem lesions. Report of two cases. *Journal of Neurosurgery*, **100** (6), 1079–1083.

Onofrj, M., Thomas, A., Paci, C. and D'Andreamatteo, G. (1998) Gabapentin in orthostatic tremor: results of a double-blind crossover with placebo in four patients. *Neurology*, **51** (3), 880–882.

Pakiam, A.S. and Lang, A.E. (1999) Essential palatal tremor: evidence of heterogeneity based on clinical features and response to Sumatriptan. *Movement Disorders*, **14** (1), 179–180.

Plante-Bordeneuve, V., Guiochon-Mantel, A., Lacroix, C., Lapresle, J. and Said, G. (1999) The Roussy-Levy family: from the original description to the gene. *Annals of Neurology*, **46** (5), 770–773.

Raethjen, J., Pawlas, F., Lindemann, M., Wenzelburger, R. and Deuschl, G. (2000) Determinants of physiologic tremor in a large normal population. *Clinical Neurophysiology*, **111** (10), 1825–1837.

Raethjen, J., Lemke, M.R., Lindemann, M., Wenzelburger, R., Krack, P. and Deuschl, G. (2001) Amitriptyline enhances the central component of physiological tremor. *Journal of Neurology, Neurosurgery, and Psychiatry*, **70** (1), 78–82.

Raethjen, J., Lauk, M., Koster, B. *et al.* (2004a) Tremor analysis in two normal cohorts. *Clinical Neurophysiology*, **115** (9), 2151–2156.

Raethjen, J., Kopper, F., Govindan, R.B., Volkmann, J. and Deuschl, G. (2004b) Two different pathogenetic mechanisms in psychogenic tremor. *Neurology*, **63** (5), 812–815.

Rascol, A., Clanet, M., Montastruc, J.L., Delage, W. and Guiraud-Chaumeil, B. (1981) L5H tryptophan in the cerebellar syndrome treatment. *Biomedicine*, **35** (4), 112–113.

Remy, P., de Recondo, A., Defer, G. *et al.* (1995) Peduncular 'rubral' tremor and dopaminergic denervation: a PET study [see comments]. *Neurology*, **45** (3 Pt 1), 472–477.

Repka, M.X., Savino, P.J. and Reinecke, R.D. (1994) Treatment of acquired nystagmus with botulinum neurotoxin A. *Archives of Ophthalmology*, **112** (10), 1320–1324.

Rinnerthaler, M., Luef, G., Mueller, J. *et al.* (2005) Computerized tremor analysis of valproate-induced tremor: a comparative study of controlled-release versus conventional valproate. *Epilepsia*, **46** (2), 320–323.

Rivest, J. and Marsden, C.D. (1990) Trunk and head tremor as isolated manifestations of dystonia. *Movement Disorders*, **5** (1), 60–65.

Rodrigues, J.P., Edwards, D.J., Walters, S.E. *et al.* (2005) Gabapentin can improve postural stability and quality of life in primary orthostatic tremor. *Movement Disorders*, **20** (7), 865–870.

Rodrigues, J.P., Edwards, D.J., Walters, S.E. *et al.* (2006) Blinded placebo crossover study of gabapentin in primary orthostatic tremor. *Movement Disorders*, **21** (7), 900–905.

Ruzicka, E., Jech, R., Zarubova, K., Roth, J. and Urgosik, D. (2003) VIM thalamic stimulation for tremor in a patient with IgM paraproteinaemic demyelinating neuropathy. *Movement Disorders*, **18** (10), 1192–1195.

Samuel, M., Torun, N., Tuite, P.J., Sharpe, J.A. and Lang, A.E. (2004) Progressive ataxia and palatal tremor (PAPT): clinical and MRI assessment with review of palatal tremors. *Brain*, **127** (Pt 6), 1252–1268.

Schneider, S.A. and Bhatia, K.P. (2007) The entity of jaw tremor and dystonia. *Movement Disorders*, **22**, 1491–1495.

Schuurman, P.R., Bosch, D.A., Bossuyt, P.M. *et al.* (2000) A comparison of continuous thalamic stimulation and thalamotomy for suppression of severe tremor. *The New England Journal of Medicine*, **342** (7), 461–468.

Scott, B.L., Evans, R.W. and Jankovic, J. (1996) Treatment of palatal myoclonus with sumatriptan. *Movement Disorders*, **11** (6), 748–751.

Shukla, G. and Behari, M. (2004) A clinical study of non-parkinsonian and non-cerebellar tremor at a specialty movement disorders clinic. *Neurology India*, **52** (2), 200–202.

Stolze, H., Petersen, G., Raethjen, J., Wenzelburger, R. and Deuschl, G. (2001) The gait disorder of advanced essential tremor. *Brain*, **124** (Pt 11), 2278–2286.

Striano, P., Coppola, A., Vacca, G. *et al.* (2006) Levetiracetam for cerebellar tremor in multiple sclerosis: An open-label pilot tolerability and efficacy study. *Journal of Neurology*, **253** (6), 762–766.

Trouillas, P., Serratrice, G., Laplane, D. *et al.* (1995) Levorotatory form of 5-hydroxytryptophan in Friedreich's ataxia. Results of a double-blind drug-placebo cooperative study. *Archives of Neurology*, **52** (5), 456–460.

Vallbo, A.B. and Wessberg, J. (1993) Organization of motor output in slow finger movements in man. *Journal of Physiology London*, **469** (673), 673–691.

Vidailhet, M., Jedynak, C.P., Pollak, P. and Agid, Y. (1998) Pathology of symptomatic tremors. *Movement Disorders*, **13** (Suppl 3), 49–54.

Voon, V. and Lang, A.E. (2005) Antidepressant treatment outcomes of psychogenic movement disorder. *Journal of Clinical Psychiatry*, **66** (12), 1529–1534.

Wenning, G.K., Kiechl, S., Seppi, K. *et al.* (2005) Prevalence of movement disorders in men and women aged 50–89 years (Bruneck Study cohort): a population-based study. *Lancet Neurology*, **4** (12), 815–820.

Wills, A.J., Brusa, L., Wang, H.C., Brown, P. and Marsden, C.D. (1999) Levodopa may improve orthostatic tremor: case report and trial of treatment. *Journal of Neurology, Neurosurgery, and Psychiatry*, **66** (5), 681–684.

Wu, Y.R., Ashby, P. and Lang, A.E. (2001) Orthostatic tremor arises from an oscillator in the posterior fossa. *Movement Disorders*, **16** (2), 272–279.

Yeung, K.B., Thomas, P.K., King, R.H. *et al.* (1991) The clinical spectrum of peripheral neuropathies associated with benign monoclonal IgM, IgG and IgA paraproteinaemia. Comparative clinical, immunological and nerve biopsy findings. *Journal of Neurology*, **238** (7), 383–391.

Zeuner, K.E., Shoge, R.O., Goldstein, S.R., Dambrosia, J.M. and Hallett, M. (2003) Accelerometry to distinguish psychogenic from essential or parkinsonian tremor. *Neurology*, **61** (4), 548–550.

Part III

DYSTONIA, CRAMPS, AND SPASMS

12

Pathophysiology of Dystonia

Mark Hallett

Human Motor Control Section, NINDS, NIH, Bethesda, MD, USA

DEFINITION AND CLINICAL CLASSIFICATION

Dystonia is a disorder characterized by involuntary movements of sustained muscle contractions, causing prolonged movements or abnormal postures. Movements are often twisting in nature, meaning rotatory about the long axis of a body part. Some patients may also have quick movements, called myoclonic dystonia, or tremor, but ordinarily there will have to be some sustained movements for dystonia to be recognized as such. Dystonia can be present during rest, but in general is more likely to appear when the patient is engaged in voluntary activity, called action dystonia. Voluntary movements are slow, clumsy and characterized by overflow (excessive activity in muscles not needed for the task). Sometimes sensory input can ameliorate the dystonia, at least briefly; this phenomenon is referred to as a sensory trick or geste antagoniste. The most common sensory trick is seen in cervical dystonia where a finger placed on the side of the face will alleviate the dystonia.

Dystonia can be present in any part of the body, and can be classified as focal, segmental, multi-focal, generalized, or hemidystonia. Focal means that one body part is affected and includes conditions such as blepharospasm, cranial dystonia, spasmodic dysphonia, cervical dystonia, and writer's cramp. Cranial dystonia encompasses blepharospasm, oromandibular dystonia and lingual dystonia. Spasmodic dysphonia comes in two varieties, adductor, the more common, causing a strained, strangled voice, and abductor, causing a breathy voice. Cervical dystonia involves different movements of the neck; torticollis or twisting is most common. Segmental implies two or more contiguous regions, such as involvement of a whole limb with the associated part of the trunk. Multi-focal is multiple non-contiguous regions. Hemidystonia denotes one side of the body. Generalized implies a whole body affection.

There is no laboratory test to prove that a patient has dystonia, it is a clinical diagnosis. At least in the primary forms, there are no routine imaging abnormalities, and no blood or CSF findings (Albanese *et al.*, 2006).

ETIOLOGIC CLASSIFICATION

Genetic Etiologies

Dystonia can be primary, meaning largely genetic in origin, or secondary. Genes for the dystonias are being identified on a regular basis, and the genetic classification and genes or linkages are listed in Table 12.1 (de Carvalho Aguiar and Ozelius, 2002; Bressman, 2003; Tarsy and Simon, 2006).

Hereditary childhood onset dystonia (idiopathic torsion dystonia, DYT1) most commonly starts between 6 and 12 years of age with dystonia of the foot while walking. The illness is then slowly progressive and becomes generalized. The onset is before age 28 in the majority of cases. The disorder is usually autosomal dominant with reduced penetrance both in Jews and non-Jews (Bressman *et al.*, 1994a). The abnormal gene, located on chromosome 9q, produces a protein called torsin A, whose function is not yet known (Ozelius *et al.*, 1997). Most mutations are a GAG deletion, but a second mutation has been identified (Leung *et al.*, 2001), and there will likely be others. Genetic testing is possible (Albanese *et al.*, 2006).

There is a good deal of work trying to identify what torsin A does and how a mutation in it causes disease. Torsin A is closely associated with the nuclear envelope. There is some evidence that the mutation causes a loss of function (Goodchild, Kim and Dauer, 2005), and other evidence that it causes a gain of function (Hewett *et al.*, 2006; Kock *et al.*, 2006). Animal models can be made with mutant torsin A, and physiological studies of these animals should be helpful (Pisani *et al.*, 2006).

There is now demonstrated pathology in DYT1 dystonia, although, surprisingly, not in the basal ganglia. Perinuclear inclusion bodies in the midbrain reticular formation and periaqueductal gray were seen in four clinically documented

Table 12.1 The genetic dystonias.

Locus	Designation	Mode of Inheritance	Chromosome location	Protein
DYT1/TOR1A	Early-onset primary torsion dystonia, Oppenheim's dystonia	AD	9q34	TorsinA
DYT2	Autosomal recessive primary torsion dystonia (uncertain)	AR	Unknown	Unknown
DYT3	X-linked dystonia-parkinsonism, Lubag	X-linked	Xq13.1	Multiple transcript system called DYT3
DYT4	Non-DYT1 primary torsion dystonia, predominant whispering dysphonia	AD	Unknown	Unknown
DYT5/GCH1	Dopa-responsive dystonia, Segawa syndrome	AD	14q22.1–q22.2	GCH1
DYT5	Dopa-responsive dystonia	AR		Tyrosine hydroxylase
DYT6	Adolescent onset primary torsion dystonia of mixed type, German-Mennonite origin	AD	8p21–8q22	Unknown
DYT7	Adult-onset focal primary torsion dystonia (uncertain)	AD	18p11.3	Unknown
DYT8/PNKD	Paroxysmal dystonic choreoathetosis/non-kinesiogenic dyskinesia	AD	2q25–q33	Myofibrillogenesis regulator 1
DYT9/CSE	Paroxysmal choreoathetosis with episodic ataxia and spasticity	AD	1p13.3–p21	Unknown
DYT10/PKD	Paroxysmal kinesiogenic dystonia/choreoathetosis	AD	16p11.2–q12.1	Unknown
DYT10	Paroxysmal kinesiogenic dystonia/choreoathetosis		16q13–q22.1	Unknown
DYT11	Myoclonus dystonia	AD	7q21–q31	ε-sarcoglycan
DYT11	Myoclonus dystonia (uncertain)	AD	11q23	Dopamine D2 receptor
DYT12	Rapid-onset dystonia-parkinsonism	AD	19q13	ATP 1A3
DYT13	Early and late-onset focal or segmental dystonia	AD	1p36.13	Unknown
DYT15	Myoclonus dystonia	AD	18p11	Unknown

and genetically confirmed DYT1 patients, but not in controls (McNaught *et al.*, 2004). The inclusions were located within cholinergic and other neurons in the pedunculopontine nucleus, cuneiform nucleus and griseum centrale mesencephali and stained positively for ubiquitin, torsinA, and the nuclear envelope protein lamin A/C. There were also tau/ubiquitin-immunoreactive aggregates in pigmented neurons of the substantia nigra pars compacta and locus coeruleus in all four DYT1 dystonia cases, but not in controls. How this pathology relates to disease genesis is not yet clear.

There are also other genes for autosomal dominant dystonia, even with clinically similar presentations (Bressman *et al.*, 1994b). These include DYT4, DYT6, DYT7 and DYT13 (de Carvalho Aguiar and Ozelius, 2002). Of course,

there are many clinically similar patients for whom the gene is not yet identified (Elia *et al.*, 2006; Fasano *et al.*, 2006).

Dopa-responsive dystonia (DYT5), also known as Segawa's disease or hereditary progressive dystonia with marked diurnal fluctuation, is another childhood-onset, autosomal-dominant disorder with a number of clinical characteristics that are helpful in diagnosis. The disorder is much better in the morning and after a rest. Signs and symptoms are generalized and there is often an appearance of spasticity as well as dystonia. These patients respond well to small doses of levodopa. The etiology for the disorder is most commonly a mutation in the GTP cyclohydrolase I gene which leads to a deficiency in the production of dopamine (Ichinose, Ohye and Takahashi, 1994; Segawa, Nomura and Nishiyama, 2003; Furukawa, 2004).

Synthesis of Dopamine

Tyrosine

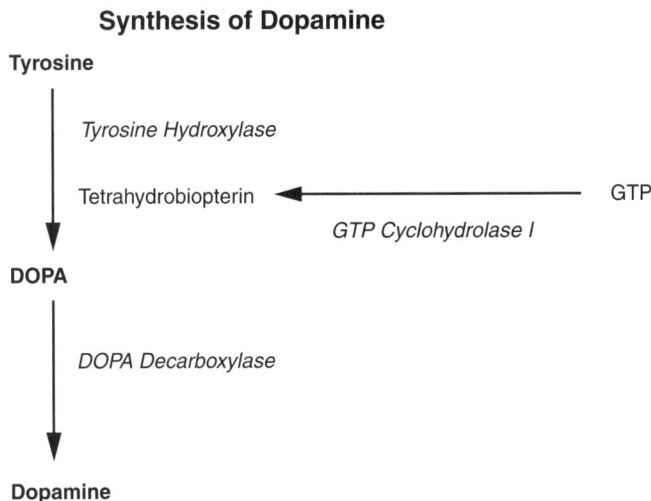

Figure 12.1 Biochemical pathway for the synthesis of dopamine, illustrating the role of GTP cyclohydrolase I.

GTP cyclohydrolase I is the rate-limiting enzyme in the synthesis of tetrahydrobiopterin from GTP (Figure 12.1). Tetrahydrobiopterin, in turn, is a co-factor for tyrosine hydroxylase in the synthesis of levodopa from tyrosine. Since the gene has been identified, the clinical spectrum of the disorder has been expanded to include adult-onset parkinsonism, oromandibular dystonia, spontaneously remitting dystonia, spasticity with developmental delay mimicking cerebral palsy and generalized hypotonia with proximal weakness (de Carvalho Aguiar and Ozelius, 2002). There have been so many individual mutations found that it is not possible to do genetic testing easily.

Mutations in the tyrosine hydroxylase gene can also be responsible for an autosomal recessive form of the disorder, which is still included under the designation of DYT5 (Ludecke, Dworniczak and Bartholome, 1995; de Carvalho Aguiar and Ozelius, 2002; Furukawa, Kish and Fahn, 2004). There is also a severe form of tyrosine hydroxylase deficiency with non-responsive dystonia and encephalopathy (Hoffmann et al., 2003).

DYT14 was another described genetic defect that could lead to dopa-responsive dystonia, but the gene was not known (Grotzsch et al., 2002). In a more recent report, it has now been identified that this was a mistake, and the genetic defect was really DYT5 (Wider et al., 2008).

Myoclonus dystonia (DYT11) is an autosomal dominant syndrome where symptoms include dystonic myoclonus as well as more prolonged spasms (Gasser et al., 1996). Tremor, similar to essential tremor, may also be present. There is often a marked response to ethanol. In many families, the genetic abnormality has been identified to be in the protein ε-sarcoglycan (Zimprich et al., 2001; Asmus et al., 2002). Interestingly, this gene is maternally

imprinted, that is, the maternal gene is more likely to be expressed in the brain (Grabowski et al., 2003). This finding is an example of how genetic disorders can be modified by other factors that are not environmental. There is only little information on how the mutation might cause disease (Esapa et al., 2007). The spectrum of DYT11 includes obsessive-compulsive disorder (Hess et al., 2007), and possibly even depression (Misbahuddin et al., 2007).

There is certainly genetic heterogeneity (Grimes et al., 2001; Han et al., 2003; Schule et al., 2004), and at least one family is linked to another site and has been designated DYT15 (Grimes et al., 2002; Han et al., 2007). There has been some consideration of the D2 receptor also, but this is likely just a polymorphism.

Lubag is an X-linked, recessive dystonia-parkinsonism syndrome (Waters et al., 1993) primarily found in the Philippine Islands. The disorder appears to originate from mutations in a multiple transcript system called DYT3 (Nolte, Niemann and Muller, 2003). There are at least 16 exons and 4 transcripts. The pathology of this disorder is particularly interesting. The striosome compartment of the striatum is severely depleted of neurons, but the matrix is relatively spared (Goto et al., 2005). This could give rise to an imbalance of output from the basal ganglia.

Rapid-onset dystonia-parkinsonism (DYT12) is a striking autosomal-dominant disorder characterized by abrupt onset of dystonia, usually accompanied by signs of parkinsonism. In families, there is variable expressivity and reduced penetrance. The sudden onset of symptoms over hours to a few weeks, often associated with physical or emotional stress, suggests a trigger initiating a nervous system insult that results in permanent neurologic disability. In seven unrelated families, there were six missense mutations in the gene for the Na+/K+ -ATPase α3 subunit

(ATP1A3) (de Carvalho Aguiar *et al.*, 2004). These muta-tions likely impair enzyme activity or stability.

The focal dystonias are usually sporadic and occur in later life. Patients may have more than one focal dystonia (Weiss *et al.*, 2006), although progression to generalized disease is uncommon. There is likely a genetic basis, with reduced penetrance (Defazio *et al.*, 2003a, 2003b; Defazio, Berardelli and Hallett, 2007). One family with spasmodic torticollis (DYT7) has a genetic linkage to chromosome 18p (Leube *et al.*, 1996), but this linkage has not been confirmed. A polymorphism in the dopamine D5 receptor has been associated with focal dystonia, but this also has not been confirmed (Brancati *et al.*, 2003). Torsin A haplotypes may predispose to primary dystonia also (Clarimon *et al.*, 2005; Kamm *et al.*, 2006; Clarimon *et al.*, 2007), but this has not been seen in studies of all groups (Hague *et al.*, 2006).

The hope, of course, is that a solid understanding of the genetic abnormalities and resultant cell biological derange-ments can be reversed by specific therapies. Etiological treatment is to be preferred. Pre-natal testing, at least for DYT1 dystonia, can be used to prevent dystonia.

Secondary Etiologies

Secondary dystonia can be caused by a variety of neurologic disorders including Parkinson's disease, Wilson's disease, gangliosidoses, leukodystrophies, Leigh's disease, Pantothe-nate Kinase Deficiency, the juvenile form of Huntington's disease, corticobasal ganglionic degeneration and structural brain lesions (Table 12.2). Patients with cerebral palsy commonly have dystonia. The overwhelming preponderance of lesions that cause dystonia is in the basal ganglia or its pathways. Lesions in the putamen, caudate and thalamus can give rise to dystonia (Marsden *et al.*, 1985; Pettigrew and Jankovic, 1985; Bathia and Marsden, 1994). It is this ana-tomical fact that has led to the widespread view that dystonias arise from abnormalities of the basal ganglia, even when no pathology is evident. One form of secondary dystonia is post-hemiplegic dystonia. In this situation, a stroke or other brain lesion, which manifests with early hemiplegia, also produces dystonia months or years later (Scott and Jankovic, 1996). The etiology is not clear, but this must be a manifestation of some aberrant plasticity.

There is also some evidence that dystonia might arise from cerebellar abnormalities (Jinnah and Hess, 2006). Patients have been described with ataxia and dystonia who have cerebellar, but not obvious basal ganglia abnormali-ties (Le Ber *et al.*, 2006). Additionally, there are some animal models of dystonia where the pathological process appears to involve primarily the cerebellum.

Dystonia apparently can also result from peripheral trauma. This is somewhat controversial, but it does seem more frequent than chance that dystonia develops in a

Table 12.2 Heredodegenerative and metabolic disorders sometimes causing dystonia.

Wilson's disease
Parkinsonian syndromes
  Parkinson's disease
  Juvenile parkinsonism (PARKIN mutations)
  Multi-system atrophy
  Corticobasal degeneration
  Progressive supranuclear palsy
Globus pallidus degenerations
Pantothenate kinase deficiency due to PANK2 mutations
Familial basal ganglia calcifications
Huntington's disease
Spinocerebellar degenerations
Lysosomal storage disorders
  Dystonic lipidosis
  Ceroid lipofuscinosis
  Metachromatic leukodystrophy
  GM1 and GM2 gangliosidosis
  Neimann–Pick disease type C
  Krabbe's disease
  Pelizaeus–Merzbacher disease
Organic aminoacidurias
  Glutaric acidemia
  Homocysteinuria
  Hartnup's disease
  Methylmalonic aciduria
Mitochondrial disorders
  Leigh's disease
  Leber's plus dystonia
  X-linked dystonia-deafness
  Neuroacanthocytosis
Lesch–Nyhan syndrome
Ataxia–telangiectasia

(From Tarsy and Simon (2006) with permission.)

traumatized body part (Jankovic, 2001). Nerve injury does not seem necessary. This type of post-traumatic dystonia can be associated with complex regional pain syndrome (CRPS), which itself is a controversial outcome of periph-eral trauma (Bhatia, Bhatt and Marsden, 1993; Verdugo and Ochoa, 2000). CRPS is divided into CRPS I, where there is no nerve injury, also called reflex sympathetic dystrophy, and CRPS II, where there is nerve injury, also called causalgia.

Dystonia can also be psychogenic (Lang, 1995). Of the psychogenic movement disorders, dystonia is one of the frequent sub-types. Psychogenic movement disorders are dealt with in Chapter 26, but, briefly, clinical charac-teristics include sudden onset and remission, paroxysmal nature, fixed postures, improvement with distraction, and lack of a sensory trick (Hallett, 2006c). Despite the fact that there are physiological abnormalities seen in dystonia that will be described below, surprisingly, many of these are shared in psychogenic dystonia (Espay *et al.*, 2006). Perhaps this indicates that if there is a certain type of physiological abnormality, this can, in the right circumstances, lead to either organic or psychogenic dystonia. In any event, physiological testing, at present, cannot separate the two etiologies.

PHYSIOLOGY OF DYSTONIA

There has been a considerable amount of work trying to understand the pathophysiology of focal dystonia on an integrative level. The abnormalities identified can be of two types: (i) a reflection of the genetic abnormality indicating the substrate on which the dystonia develops, and (ii) a reflection of the developed dystonia on the background substrate. As most of the abnormalities found characterize not only the affected body part, but also non-affected body parts, it is thought that these likely represent the background substrate. There are three general lines of work at the present time that may indicate the physiological substrate for dystonia, loss of inhibition, increased plasticity and abnormal sensory function. All three are persuasive and it is not clear whether they are related to each other or whether one is more fundamental than the others.

Loss of Inhibition

A principal finding in focal dystonia is that of loss of inhibition (Hallett, 2004). Loss of inhibition is likely responsible for the excessive movement seen in dystonia patients. Excessive movement includes abnormally long bursts of EMG activity, co-contraction of antagonist muscles, and overflow of activity into muscles not intended for the task (Cohen and Hallett, 1988). Loss of inhibition can be demonstrated in spinal and brainstem reflexes. Examples are the loss of reciprocal inhibition in the arm in patients with focal hand dystonia (Nakashima *et al.*, 1989; Panizza *et al.*, 1990) and abnormalities of blink reflex recovery in blepharospasm (Berardelli *et al.*, 1985). Loss of reciprocal inhibition can be partly responsible for the presence of co-contraction of antagonist muscles that characterizes voluntary movement in dystonia.

Loss of inhibition can also be demonstrated for motor cortical function, including short intracortical inhibition, long intracortical inhibition and the silent period. Short intracortical inhibition (SICI) is obtained with paired pulse methods and reflects interneuron influences in the cortex. (Ziemann, Rothwell and Ridding, 1996) In such studies, an initial conditioning stimulus is given, enough to activate cortical neurons, but small enough that no descending influence on the spinal cord can be detected. A second test stimulus, at suprathreshold level, follows at a short interval. Intracortical influences initiated by the conditioning stimulus modulate the amplitude of the motor evoked potential (MEP) produced by the test stimulus. At short intervals, less than 5 ms, there is inhibition that is likely largely a GABAergic effect, specifically GABA-A (Di Lazzaro *et al.*, 2000). (At intervals between 8 and 30 ms, there is facilitation, called intracortical facilitation, ICF). There is a loss of intracortical inhibition in patients with focal hand dystonia (Ridding *et al.*, 1995). Inhibition was less in both hemispheres of patients with focal hand dystonia, and this indicates that this abnormality is more consistent as a substrate for dystonia.

The silent period (SP) is a pause in ongoing voluntary EMG activity produced by TMS. While the first part of the SP is due in part to spinal cord refractoriness, the latter part is entirely due to cortical inhibition (Fuhr, Agostino and Hallett, 1991). This type of inhibition is likely mediated by GABA-B receptors (Werhahn *et al.*, 1999). SICI and the SP show different modulation in different circumstances and clearly reflect different aspects of cortical inhibition. The SP is shortened in focal dystonia.

Intracortical inhibition can also be assessed with paired suprathreshold TMS pulses at intervals from 50 to 200 ms (Valls-Solé *et al.*, 1992). This is called long intracortical inhibition, or LICI, to differentiate it from SICI as noted above. LICI and SICI differ as demonstrated by the facts that, with increasing test pulse strength, LICI decreases, but SICI tends to increase, and that there is no correlation between the degree of SICI and LICI in different individuals (Sanger, Garg and Chen, 2001). The mechanisms of LICI and the SP may be similar in that both seem to depend on GABA-B receptors. Chen *et al.*, (1997) investigated long intracortical inhibition in patients with writer's cramp and found a deficiency only in the symptomatic hand and only with background contraction. This abnormality is particularly interesting since it is restricted to the symptomatic setting, and therefore might be a correlate of the development of the dystonia.

There is also neuroimaging evidence consistent with a loss of inhibition. Using positron emission tomography (PET), dopamine D2 receptors have been found deficient in focal dystonias (Perlmutter *et al.*, 1997). There is also direct evidence using magnetic resonance spectroscopy (MRS) for reduced GABA concentration both in basal ganglia and motor cortex (Levy and Hallett, 2002). Another possible technique for looking at inhibition in the sensory system is the investigation of the high-frequency oscillations after sensory stimulation. These are thought to reflect inhibitory neuron function. These oscillations may be decreased in patients with focal hand dystonia (Cimatti *et al.*, 2007).

Loss of cortical inhibition in the motor cortex can give rise to dystonic-like movements in primates. Matsumura *et al.* showed that local application of bicuculline, a GABA antagonist, onto the motor cortex led to disordered movement and changed the movement pattern from reciprocal inhibition of antagonist muscles to co-contraction (Matsumura *et al.*, 1991). In a second study, they showed that bicuculline caused cells to lose their crisp directionality, converted unidirectional cells to bidirectional cells, and increased firing rates of most cells, including making silent cells into active ones (Matsumura, Sawaguchi and Kubota, 1992).

There is a valuable animal model for blepharospasm that supports the idea of a combination of genetics and environment, and, specifically, that the background for the development of dystonia could be a loss of inhibition (Schicatano, Basso and Evinger, 1997). In this model, rats were lesioned to cause a depletion of dopamine; this reduces inhibition. Then the orbicularis oculi muscle was weakened. This causes an increase in the blink reflex drive in order to produce an adequate blink. Together, but not separately, these two interventions produced spasms of eyelid closure, similar to blepharospasm. Shortly after the animal model was presented, several patients with blepharospasm after a Bell's palsy were reported (Chuke, Baker and Porter, 1996; Baker *et al.*, 1997). This could be a human analog of the animal experiments. The idea is that those patients who developed blepharospasm were in some way predisposed. A gold weight implanted into the weak lid of one patient, aiding lid closure, improved the condition, suggesting that when the abnormal increase in reflex drive was removed, the dystonia could be ameliorated (Chuke, Baker and Porter, 1996).

A principle for function of the motor system may be "surround inhibition." Surround inhibition is a concept well accepted in sensory physiology (Angelucci, Levitt and Lund, 2002). Surround inhibition is not so well known in the motor system, but it is a logical concept. When making a movement, the brain must activate the motor system. It is possible that the brain just activates the specific movement. On the other hand, it is more likely that the one specific movement is generated, and, simultaneously, other possible movements are suppressed. The suppression of unwanted movements would be surround inhibition, and this should produce a more precise movement, just as surround inhibition in sensory systems produces more precise perceptions. For dystonia, a failure of "surround inhibition" may be particularly important, since overflow movement is often seen and is a principal abnormality.

There is now good evidence for surround inhibition in human movement. Sohn *et al.*, (2003) have shown that with movement of one finger there is widespread inhibition of muscles in the contralateral limb. Significant suppression

of MEP amplitudes was observed when TMS was applied between 35 and 70 ms after EMG onset. Sohn and Hallett, (2004b) have also shown that there is some inhibition of muscles in the ipsilateral limb when those muscles are not involved in any way in the movement. TMS was delivered to the left motor cortex from 3 ms to 1000 ms after EMG onset in the flexor digitorum superficialis muscle. MEPs from abductor digiti minimi were slightly suppressed during the movement of the index finger in the face of increased F-wave amplitude and persistence, indicating that cortical excitability is reduced.

Surround inhibition was studied similarly in patients with focal hand dystonia (Sohn and Hallett, 2004a). The MEPs were enhanced similarly in the flexor digitorum superficialis and abductor digiti minimi indicating a failure of surround inhibition (Figure 12.2). Using another experimental paradigm, Stinear and Byblow have also found a loss of surround inhibition in the hand (Stinear and Byblow, 2004) .

Increased Plasticity

There is an abnormal plasticity of the motor cortex in patients with focal hand dystonia (Quartarone *et al.*, 2003). This has been demonstrated using the technique of paired associative stimulation (PAS) (Stefan *et al.*, 2000). In PAS a median nerve shock is paired with a TMS pulse to the sensorimotor cortex timed to be immediately after the arrival of the sensory volley. This intervention increases the amplitude of the MEP produced by TMS to the motor cortex. It has been demonstrated that the process of PAS produces motor learning similar to long-term potentiation (LTP). In patients with dystonia, PAS produces a larger increase in the MEP than that seen in normal subjects. In PAS, if the timing of the peripheral stimulus is such that the volley reaches the sensorimotor cortex about 10 ms prior to the TMS pulse, then the amplitude of the MEP will be suppressed, and this process is likely similar to long-term depression (LTD). Patients who have dystonia also have a more marked inhibition compared to normal subjects (Weise *et al.*, 2006).

Another technique that shows increased plasticity is the pairing of high-frequency stimulation of the supraorbital nerve during the R2 of the blink reflex (Mao and Evinger, 2001). This leads to an increase in the R2, and this increase is exaggerated in patients with blepharospasm (Quartarone *et al.*, 2006).

Plasticity of the motor system can also be assessed using a method called theta-burst stimulation. This is a form of rapid repetitive TMS where brief bursts at 50 Hz are delivered every 200 ms. If given continuously for 300 pulses, this will cause inhibition of the MEP. This inhibition is abnormally prolonged in patients with DYT1 dystonia or with cervical dystonia (Edwards *et al.*, 2006). However, there was no abnormality seen in asymptomatic carriers of

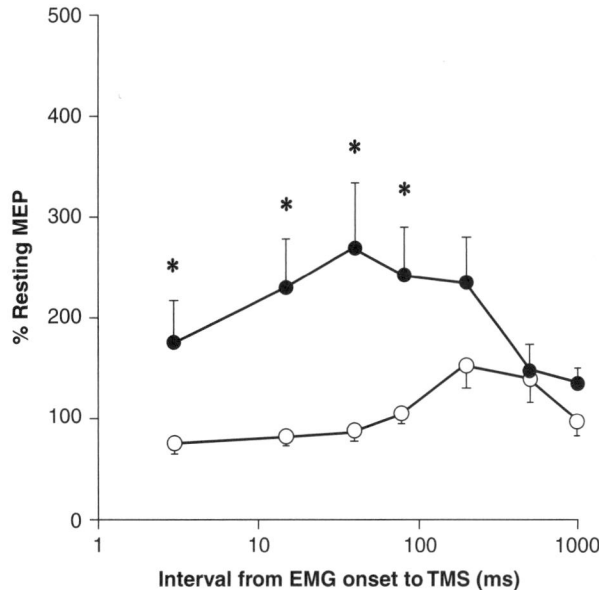

Figure 12.2 Changes in motor-evoked potential (MEP) amplitude in the abductor digiti minimi (ADM) muscle in self-triggered transcranial magnetic stimulation (TMS) at each interval (3, 15, 40, 80, 200, 500, and 1000 ms) from electromyography (EMG) onset of flexor digitorum superficialis (FDS) to TMS, compared with the resting state. (*asterisk*) Significant difference between patients (filled circles) and healthy subjects (open circles) ($p < 0.05$). Note that the MEP amplitudes of ADM are significantly suppressed in healthy subjects, but are enhanced in patients during voluntary flexion of the index finger. From Sohn and Hallett, 2004a.

the DYT1 mutation. This suggests that the development of abnormal plasticity is highly relevant in the genesis of symptoms.

Another aspect of the abnormal plasticity is that not only is the plasticity increased, but there is a failure of its homeostatic property (Quartarone *et al.*, 2005). The homeostatic property is that plasticity ordinarily increases and decreases within bounds. If, for example, the excitability of the motor cortex is high, then it cannot be driven higher, only lower. The recent finding, using several types of brain stimulation, is that plasticity in dystonia may not be properly bounded and may increase abnormally.

Increased plasticity may arise from decreased inhibition so the inhibitory problem may well be more fundamental. This abnormality may be an important link in demonstrating how environmental influences can trigger dystonia.

The possibility of increased plasticity in dystonia had been suspected for some time given that repetitive activity over long periods seems to be a trigger for its development. An animal model supported this idea (Byl, Merzenich and Jenkins, 1996). Monkeys were trained to hold a vibrating manipulandum for long periods. After some time, they became unable to do so, and this motor control abnormality was interpreted as a possible dystonia. The sensory cortex of these animals was studied, and sensory receptive fields were found to be large. The interpretation of these results

was that the synchronous sensory input caused the receptive field enlargement, and that the abnormal sensory function led to abnormal motor function. The results suggested that the same thing might be happening in human focal dystonia; repetitive activity causes sensory receptive field changes and leads to the motor disorder.

Sensory Abnormality

Stimulated by the findings of sensory dysfunction in the primate model, investigators began examining sensory function in patients with focal hand dystonia and found it to be abnormal. Although there is no apparent sensory loss on a clinical level, detailed testing of spatial and temporal discrimination revealed subtle impairments (Molloy *et al.*, 2003). The abnormality is present on both hands of patients with unilateral hand dystonia and also on hands of patients with cervical dystonia and blepharospasm. Kinesthesia is also abnormal (Putzki *et al.*, 2006). The identification of abnormality of sensation beyond the symptomatic body parts indicated that the sensory abnormality could not be a consequence of abnormal learning, but is more likely a preexisting physiological state. Further evidence for this point comes from studies of patients who are asymptomatic carriers of the DYT1 mutation and show abnormal temporal discrimination (Fiorio *et al.*, 2007).

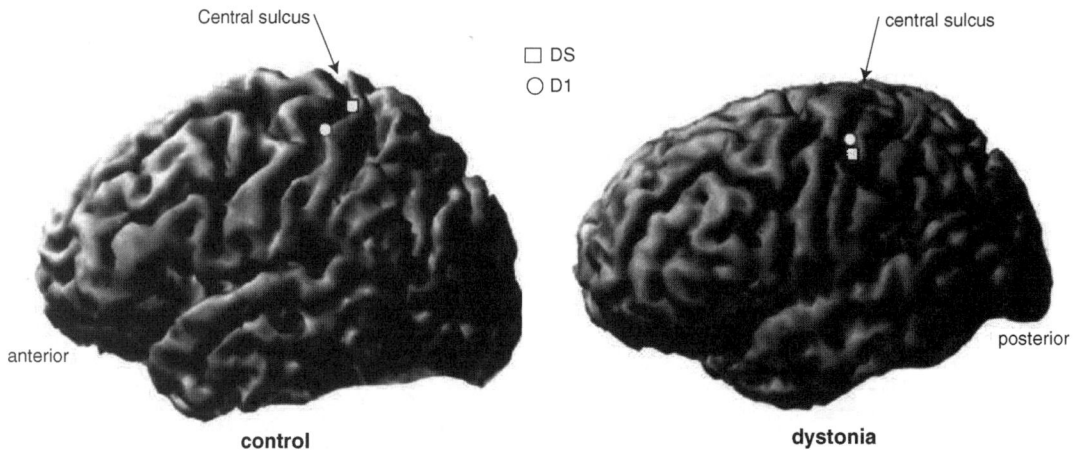

Figure 12.3 Somatosensory evoked potential (SEP) dipoles indicating position in the primary sensory cortex for stimulation of the thumb (D1) and little finger (D5) in a single control subject, and a patient with focal hand dystonia. As in the control subject, the D1 dipole should be about 1.5 cm lateral to the D5 dipole. In the patient, the dipoles are closer together and in the wrong orientation with respect to each other. From Bara-Jimenez *et al.* 1998.

Sensory dysfunction can also be demonstrated with somatosensory-evoked potential (SEP) testing. The dipoles of the N20 from stimulation of individual fingers show disordered representation in the primary sensory cortex, (Bara-Jimenez *et al.*, 1998) (Figure 12.3) and these abnormalities are present on both hands of patients with focal hand dystonia (Meunier *et al.*, 2001). The bilateral SEP abnormality was the first indication in the literature that the sensory abnormality was more likely endophenotypic than a consequence of repetitive activity. PET studies show that the sensory cortex is more activated than normal with writing and is more activated when patients are experiencing more dystonia (Lerner *et al.*, 2004). fMRI studies show an increase in basal ganglia activation in patients when doing spatial discrimination assessment, and this has been interpreted as a loss of surround inhibition in sensory processing (Peller *et al.*, 2006). Voxel-based morphometry studies in patients with focal hand dystonia show an increase in gray matter in the primary sensory cortex (Garraux *et al.*, 2004). Such observations indicate that dystonia is a sensory disorder as well as a motor disorder.

There have been other implications that sensorimotor integration is abnormal. One piece of evidence comes from evoked potential studies during a reaction-time task (Murase *et al.*, 2000). In this experiment, the imperative stimulus was a median nerve stimulus used to trigger the movement. In normal subjects the N30 peak is gated in the reaction time, but this does not happen in patients with focal hand dystonia. Other evidence comes from studies of the influence of a sensory stimulus on the MEP induced by TMS (Abbruzzese *et al.*, 2001). At intervals of about 200 ms between a median nerve stimulus and the

TMS, there is a normal inhibition of the MEP (called long afferent inhibition, LAI). In patients with focal hand dystonia, the inhibition is converted to facilitation. It is conceivable that a loss of inhibition in sensory systems could give rise to this abnormality so that, once again, loss of inhibition could possibly be the most fundamental disorder.

There are data from sensory function that are compatible with loss of surround inhibition. Tinazzi *et al.* (Tinazzi *et al.*, 2000) studied median and ulnar nerve SEPs in patients who had dystonia involving at least one upper limb. They compared the amplitude of SEP components obtained by stimulating the median and ulnar nerves simultaneously (MU), the amplitude value being obtained from the arithmetic sum of the SEPs elicited by stimulating the same nerves separately (M + U). The ratio of MU:(M + U) indicates the interaction between afferent inputs from the two peripheral nerves. No significant difference was found between SEP amplitudes and latencies for individually stimulated median and ulnar nerves in dystonic patients and normal subjects, but recordings in patients yielded a significantly higher percentage ratio for spinal N13, brainstem P14 and cortical N20, P27 and N30 components. The authors state that "these findings suggest that the inhibitory integration of afferent inputs, mainly proprioceptive inputs, coming from adjacent body parts is abnormal in dystonia. This inefficient integration, which is probably due to altered surrounding inhibition, could give rise to an abnormal motor output and might therefore contribute to the motor impairment present in dystonia."

An indication of loss of surround inhibition in sensorimotor integration is a finding from PAS studies. In normal subjects, LTP-like PAS with median nerve stimulation increases the MEP only in median nerve innervated muscles, but in patients with dystonia the abnormal increase is also seen in ulnar nerve innervated muscles (Quartarone *et al.*, 2003). Similar abnormal spread of LTD-like PAS is also seen in patients with dystonia (Weise *et al.*, 2006).

All of the results of these physiological investigations have been used to guide therapy. In general terms, there have been attempts to increase inhibition, improve sensory deficits, and to reverse the abnormal plastic changes with new motor learning. The therapeutic approaches will be described in subsequent chapters.

ACKNOWLEDGEMENT

Portions of the text are similar to other reviews I have written, (Hallett, 2006a, 2006b) and are modified and updated as appropriate. Work of the US Government, there is no copyright.

References

Abbruzzese, G., Marchese, R., Buccolieri, A. *et al.* (2001) Abnormalities of sensorimotor integration in focal dystonia: a transcranial magnetic stimulation study. *Brain*, **124**, 537–545.

Albanese, A., Barnes, M.P., Bhatia, K.P. *et al.* (2006) A systematic review on the diagnosis and treatment of primary (idiopathic) dystonia and dystonia plus syndromes: report of an EFNS/MDS-ES Task Force. *European Journal of Neurology*, **13**, 433–444.

Angelucci, A., Levitt, J.B. and Lund, J.S. (2002) Anatomical origins of the classical receptive field and modulatory surround field of single neurons in macaque visual cortical area V1. *Progress in Brain Research*, **136**, 373–388.

Asmus, F., Zimprich, A., Tezenas Du Montcel, S. *et al.* (2002) Myoclonus-dystonia syndrome: epsilon-sarcoglycan mutations and phenotype. *Annals of Neurology*, **52**, 489–492.

Baker, R.S., Sun, W.S., Hasan, S.A. *et al.* (1997) Maladaptive neural compensatory mechanisms in Bell's palsy-induced blepharospasm. *Neurology*, **49**, 223–229.

Bara-Jimenez, W., Catalan, M.J., Hallett, M. and Gerloff, C. (1998) Abnormal somatosensory homunculus in dystonia of the hand. *Annals of Neurology*, **44**, 828–831.

Bathia, K.P. and Marsden, C.D. (1994) The behavioural and motor consequences of focal lesions of the basal ganglia in man. *Brain*, **117**, 859–876.

Berardelli, A., Rothwell, J.C., Day, B.L. and Marsden, C.D. (1985) Pathophysiology of blepharospasm and oromandibular dystonia. *Brain*, **108**, 593–608.

Bhatia, K.P., Bhatt, M.H. and Marsden, C.D. (1993) The causalgia-dystonia syndrome. *Brain*, **116**, 843–851.

Brancati, F., Valente, E.M., Castori, M. *et al.* (2003) Role of the dopamine D5 receptor (DRD5) as a susceptibility gene for cervical dystonia. *Journal of Neurology, Neurosurgery, and Psychiatry*, **74**, 665–666.

Bressman, S.B. (2003) Dystonia: phenotypes and genotypes. *Revue Neurologique*, **159**, 849–856.

Bressman, S.B. (2004) Dystonia genotypes, phenotypes, and classification. *Advances in Neurology*, **94**, 101–107.

Bressman, S.B., de Leon, D., Kramer, P.L. *et al.* (1994a) Dystonia in Ashkenazi Jews: clinical characterization of a founder mutation. *Annals of Neurology*, **36**, 771–777.

Bressman, S.B., Hunt, A.L., Heiman, G.A. *et al.* (1994b) Exclusion of the DYT1 locus in a non-Jewish family with early-onset dystonia. *Movement Disorders*, **9**, 626–632.

Byl, N., Merzenich, M.M. and Jenkins, W.M. (1996) A primate genesis model of focal dystonia and repetitive strain injury: I. Learning-induced dedifferentiation of the representation of the hand in the primary somatosensory cortex in adult monkeys. *Neurology*, **47**, 508–520.

Chen, R., Wassermann, E., Caños, M. and Hallett, M. (1997) Impaired inhibition in writer's cramp during voluntary muscle activation. *Neurology*, **49**, 1054–1059.

Chuke, J.C., Baker, R.S. and Porter, J.D. (1996) Bell's Palsy-associated blepharospasm relieved by aiding eyelid closure. *Annals of Neurology*, **39**, 263–268.

Cimatti, Z., Schwartz, D.P., Bourdain, F. *et al.* (2007) Time-frequency analysis reveals decreased high-frequency oscillations in writer's cramp. *Brain*, **130**, 198–205.

Clarimon, J., Asgeirsson, H., Singleton, A. *et al.* (2005) Torsin A haplotype predisposes to idiopathic dystonia. *Annals of Neurology*, **57**, 765–767.

Clarimon, J., Brancati, F., Peckham, E. *et al.* (2007) Assessing the role of DRD5 and DYT1 in two different case-control series with primary blepharospasm. *Movement Disorders*, **22**, 162–166.

Cohen, L.G. and Hallett, M. (1988) Hand cramps: clinical features and electromyographic patterns in a focal dystonia. *Neurology*, **38**, 1005–1012.

de Carvalho Aguiar, P., Sweadner, K.J., Penniston, J.T. *et al.* (2004) Mutations in the Na+/K+ -ATPase alpha3 gene ATP1A3 are associated with rapid-onset dystonia parkinsonism. *Neuron*, **43**, 169–175.

de Carvalho Aguiar, P.M. and Ozelius, L.J. (2002) Classification and genetics of dystonia. *Lancet Neurology*, **1**, 316–325.

Defazio, G., Aniello, M.S., Masi, G. *et al.* (2003a) Frequency of familial aggregation in primary adult-onset cranial cervical dystonia. *Neurological Sciences*, **24**, 168–169.

Defazio, G., Brancati, F., Valente, E.M. *et al.* (2003b) Familial blepharospasm is inherited as an autosomal dominant trait and relates to a novel unassigned gene. *Movement Disorders*, **18**, 207–212.

Defazio, G., Berardelli, A. and Hallett, M. (2007) Do primary adult-onset focal dystonias share aetiological factors? *Brain*, **130**, 1183–1193.

Di Lazzaro, V., Oliviero, A., Meglio, M. *et al.* (2000) Direct demonstration of the effect of lorazepam on the excitability of the human motor cortex. *Clinical Neurophysiology*, **111**, 794–799.

Edwards, M.J., Huang, Y.Z., Mir, P. *et al.* (2006) Abnormalities in motor cortical plasticity differentiate manifesting and nonmanifesting DYT1 carriers. *Movement Disorders*, **21**, 2181–2186.

Elia, A.E., Filippini, G., Bentivoglio, A.R. *et al.* (2006) Onset and progression of primary torsion dystonia in sporadic and familial cases. *European Journal of Neurology*, **13**, 1083–1088.

Esapa, C.T., Waite, A., Locke, M. *et al.* (2007) SGCE missense mutations that cause myoclonus-dystonia syndrome impair epsilon-sarcoglycan trafficking to the plasma membrane: modulation by ubiquitination and torsinA. *Human Molecular Genetics*, **16**, 327–342.

Espay, A.J., Morgante, F., Purzner, J. *et al.* (2006) Cortical and spinal abnormalities in psychogenic dystonia. *Annals of Neurology*, **59**, 825–834.

Fasano, A., Nardocci, N., Elia, A.E. *et al.* (2006) Non-DYT1 early-onset primary torsion dystonia: comparison with DYT1 phenotype and review of the literature. *Movement Disorders*, **21**, 1411–1418.

Fiorio, M., Gambarin, M., Valente, E.M. *et al.* (2007) Defective temporal processing of sensory stimuli in DYT1 mutation carriers: a new endophenotype of dystonia? *Brain*, **130**, 134–142.

Fuhr, P., Agostino, R. and Hallett, M. (1991) Spinal motor neuron excitability during the silent period after cortical stimulation. *Electroencephalography and Clinical Neurophysiology*, **81**, 257–262.

Furukawa, Y. (2004) Update on dopa-responsive dystonia: locus heterogeneity and biochemical features. *Advances in Neurology*, **94**, 127–138.

Furukawa, Y., Kish, S.J. and Fahn, S. (2004) Dopa-responsive dystonia due to mild tyrosine hydroxylase deficiency. *Annals of Neurology*, **55**, 147–148.

Garraux, G., Bauer, A., Hanakawa, T. *et al.* (2004) Changes in brain anatomy in focal hand dystonia. *Annals of Neurology*, **55**, 736–739.

Gasser, T., Bereznai, B., Muller, B. *et al.* (1996) Linkage studies in alcohol-responsive myoclonic dystonia. *Movement Disorders*, **11**, 363–370.

Goodchild, R.E., Kim, C.E. and Dauer, W.T. (2005) Loss of the dystonia-associated protein torsinA selectively disrupts the neuronal nuclear envelope. *Neuron*, **48**, 923–932.

Goto, S., Lee, L.V., Munoz, E.L. *et al.* (2005) Functional anatomy of the basal ganglia in X-linked recessive dystonia-parkinsonism. *Annals of Neurology*, **58**, 7–17.

Grabowski, M., Zimprich, A., Lorenz-Depiereux, B. *et al.* (2003) The epsilon-sarcoglycan gene (SGCE), mutated in myoclonus-dystonia syndrome, is maternally imprinted. *European Journal of Human Genetics*, **11**, 138–144.

Grimes, D.A., Bulman, D., George-Hyslop, P.S. and Lang, A.E. (2001) Inherited myoclonus-dystonia: evidence supporting genetic heterogeneity. *Movement Disorders*, **16**, 106–110.

Grimes, D.A., Han, F., Lang, A.E. *et al.* (2002) A novel locus for inherited myoclonus-dystonia on 18p11. *Neurology*, **59**, 1183–1186.

Grotzsch, H., Pizzolato, G.P., Ghika, J. *et al.* (2002) Neuropathology of a case of dopa-responsive dystonia associated with a new genetic locus, DYT14. *Neurology*, **58**, 1839–1842.

Hague, S., Klaffke, S., Clarimon, J. *et al.* (2006) Lack of association with TorsinA haplotype in German patients with sporadic dystonia. *Neurology*, **66**, 951–952.

Hallett, M. (2004) Dystonia: abnormal movements result from loss of inhibition. *Advances in Neurology*, **94**, 1–9.

Hallett, M. (2006a) Pathophysiology of dystonia. *Journal of Neural Transmission. Supplementum*, 485–488.

Hallett, M. (2006b) Pathophysiology of writer's cramp. *Human Movement Science*, **25**, 454–463.

Hallett, M. (2006c) Psychogenic movement disorders: a crisis for neurology. *Current Neurology and Neuroscience Reports*, **6**, 269–271.

Han, F., Lang, A.E., Racacho, L. *et al.* (2003) Mutations in the epsilon-sarcoglycan gene found to be uncommon in seven myoclonus-dystonia families. *Neurology*, **61**, 244–246.

Han, F., Racacho, L., Lang, A.E. *et al.* (2007) Refinement of the DYT15 locus in myoclonus dystonia. *Movement Disorders*, **22**, 888–892.

Hess, C.W., Raymond, D., Aguiar Pde, C. *et al.* (2007) Myoclonus-dystonia, obsessive-compulsive disorder, and alcohol dependence in SGCE mutation carriers. *Neurology*, **68**, 522–524.

Hewett, J.W., Zeng, J., Niland, B.P. *et al.* (2006) Dystonia-causing mutant torsinA inhibits cell adhesion and neurite extension through interference with cytoskeletal dynamics. *Neurobiology of Disease*, **22**, 98–111.

Hoffmann, G.F., Assmann, B., Brautigam, C. *et al.* (2003) Tyrosine hydroxylase deficiency causes progressive encephalopathy and dopa-nonresponsive dystonia. *Annals of Neurology*, **54** (Suppl 6), S56–S65.

Ichinose, H., Ohye, T. and Takahashi, E. (1994) Hereditary progressive dystonia with marked diurnal fluctuation caused by mutations in the GTP cyclohydrolase I gene. *Nature Genetics*, **8**, 236–242.

Jankovic, J. (2001) Can peripheral trauma induce dystonia and other movement disorders? Yes! *Movement Disorders*, **16**, 7–12.

Jinnah, H.A. and Hess, E.J. (2006) A new twist on the anatomy of dystonia: the basal ganglia and the cerebellum? *Neurology*, **67**, 1740–1741.

Kamm, C., Asmus, F., Mueller, J. *et al.* (2006) Strong genetic evidence for association of TOR1A/TOR1B with idiopathic dystonia. *Neurology*, **67**, 1857–1859.

Kock, N., Allchorne, A.J., Sena-Esteves, M. *et al.* (2006) RNAi blocks DYT1 mutant torsinA inclusions in neurons. *Neuroscience Letters*, **395**, 201–205.

Lang, A.E. (1995) Psychogenic dystonia: a review of 18 cases. *The Canadian Journal of Neurological Sciences*, **22**, 136–143.

Le Ber, I., Clot, F., Vercueil, L. *et al.* (2006) Predominant dystonia with marked cerebellar atrophy: a rare phenotype in familial dystonia. *Neurology*, **67**, 1769–1773.

Lerner, A., Shill, H., Hanakawa, T. *et al.* (2004) Regional cerebral blood flow correlates of the severity of writer's cramp symptoms. *NeuroImage*, **21**, 904–913.

Leube, B., Rudnicki, D., Ratzlaff, T. *et al.* (1996) Idiopathic torsion dystonia: assignment of a gene to chromosome 18p in a German family with adult onset, autosomal dominant inheritance and purely focal distribution. *Human Molecular Genetics*, **5**, 1673–1677.

Leung, J.C., Klein, C., Friedman, J. *et al.* (2001) Novel mutation in the TOR1A (DYT1) gene in atypical early onset dystonia and polymorphisms in dystonia and early onset parkinsonism. *Neurogenetics*, **3**, 133–143.

Levy, L.M. and Hallett, M. (2002) Impaired brain GABA in focal dystonia. *Annals of Neurology*, **51**, 93–101.

Ludecke, B., Dworniczak, B. and Bartholome, K. (1995) A point mutation in the tyrosine hydroxylase gene associated with Segawa's syndrome. *Human Genetics*, **95**, 123–125.

Mao, J.B. and Evinger, C. (2001) Long-term potentiation of the human blink reflex. *The Journal of Neuroscience*, **21**, RC151.

Marsden, C.D., Obeso, J.A., Zarranz, J.J. and Lang, A.E. (1985) The anatomical basis of symptomatic hemidystonia. *Brain*, **108**, 463–483.

Matsumura, M., Sawaguchi, T. and Kubota, K. (1992) GABAergic inhibition of neuronal activity in the primate motor and premotor cortex during voluntary movement. *Journal of Neurophysiology*, **68**, 692–702.

Matsumura, M., Sawaguchi, T., Oishi, T. *et al.* (1991) Behavioral deficits induced by local injection of bicuculline and muscimol into the primate motor and premotor cortex. *Journal of Neurophysiology*, **65**, 1542–1553.

McNaught, K.S., Kapustin, A., Jackson, T. *et al.* (2004) Brainstem pathology in DYT1 primary torsion dystonia. *Annals of Neurology*, **56**, 540–547.

Meunier, S., Garnero, L., Ducorps, A. *et al.* (2001) Human brain mapping in dystonia reveals both endophenotypic traits and adaptive reorganization. *Annals of Neurology*, **50**, 521–527.

Misbahuddin, A., Placzek, M., Lennox, G. *et al.* (2007) Myoclonus-dystonia syndrome with severe depression is caused by an exon-skipping mutation in the epsilon-sarcoglycan gene. *Movement Disorders*, **22**, 1173–1175.

Molloy, F.M., Carr, T.D., Zeuner, K.E. *et al.* (2003) Abnormalities of spatial discrimination in focal and generalized dystonia. *Brain*, **126**, 2175–2182.

Murase, N., Kaji, R., Shimazu, H. *et al.* (2000) Abnormal pre-movement gating of somatosensory input in writer's cramp. *Brain*, **123** Pt (9), 1813–1829.

Nakashima, K., Rothwell, J.C., Day, B.L. *et al.* (1989) Reciprocal inhibition in writer's and other occupational cramps and hemiparesis due to stroke. *Brain*, **112**, 681–697.

Nolte, D., Niemann, S. and Muller, U. (2003) Specific sequence changes in multiple transcript system DYT3 are associated with X-linked dystonia parkinsonism. *Proceedings of the National Academy of Sciences of the United States of America*, **100**, 10347–10352.

Ozelius, L.J., Hewett, J.W., Page, C.E. *et al.* (1997) The early onset torsion dystonia gene (DYT1) encodes an ATP-binding protein. *Nature Genetics*, **17**, 40–48.

Panizza, M., Lelli, S., Nilsson, J. and Hallett, M. (1990) H-reflex recovery curve and reciprocal inhibition of H-reflex in different kinds of dystonia. *Neurology*, **40**, 824–828.

Peller, M., Zeuner, K.E., Munchau, A. *et al.* (2006) The basal ganglia are hyperactive during the discrimination of tactile stimuli in writer's cramp. *Brain*, **129**, 2697–2708.

Perlmutter, J.S., Stambuk, M.K., Markham, J. *et al.* (1997) Decreased [18F]spiperone binding in putamen in idiopathic focal dystonia. *The Journal of Neuroscience*, **17**, 843–850.

Pettigrew, L.C. and Jankovic, J. (1985) Hemidystonia: a report of 22 patients and review of the literature. *Journal of Neurology, Neurosurgery, and Psychiatry*, **48**, 650–657.

Pisani, A., Martella, G., Tscherter, A. *et al.* (2006) Altered responses to dopaminergic D2 receptor activation and N-type calcium currents in striatal cholinergic interneurons in a mouse model of DYT1 dystonia. *Neurobiology of Disease*, **24**, 318–325.

Putzki, N., Stude, P., Konczak, J. *et al.* (2006) Kinesthesia is impaired in focal dystonia. *Movement Disorders*, **21**, 754–760.

Quartarone, A., Bagnato, S., Rizzo, V. *et al.* (2003) Abnormal associative plasticity of the human motor cortex in writer's cramp. *Brain*, **126**, 2586–2596.

Quartarone, A., Rizzo, V., Bagnato, S. *et al.* (2005) Homeostatic-like plasticity of the primary motor hand area is impaired in focal hand dystonia. *Brain*, **128**, 1943–1950.

Quartarone, A., Sant'Angelo, A., Battaglia, F. *et al.* (2006) Enhanced long-term potentiation-like plasticity of the trigeminal blink reflex circuit in blepharospasm. *The Journal of Neuroscience*, **26**, 716–721.

Ridding, M.C., Sheean, G., Rothwell, J.C. *et al.* (1995) Changes in the balance between motor cortical excitation and inhibition in focal, task specific dystonia. *Journal of Neurology, Neurosurgery, and Psychiatry*, **59**, 493–498.

Sanger, T.D., Garg, R.R. and Chen, R. (2001) Interactions between two different inhibitory systems in the human motor cortex. *The Journal of Physiology*, **530**, 307–317.

Schicatano, E.J., Basso, M.A. and Evinger, C. (1997) Animal model explains the origins of the cranial dystonia benign essential blepharospasm. *Journal of Neurophysiology*, **77**, 2842–2846.

Schule, B., Kock, N., Svetel, M. *et al.* (2004) Genetic heterogeneity in ten families with myoclonus-dystonia. *Journal of Neurology, Neurosurgery, and Psychiatry*, **75**, 1181–1185.

Scott, B.L. and Jankovic, J. (1996) Delayed-onset progressive movement disorders after static brain lesions. *Neurology*, **46**, 68–74.

Segawa, M., Nomura, Y. and Nishiyama, N. (2003) Autosomal dominant guanosine triphosphate cyclohydrolase I deficiency (Segawa disease). *Annals of Neurology*, **54** (Suppl 6), S32–S45.

Sohn, Y.H. and Hallett, M. (2004a) Disturbed surround inhibition in focal hand dystonia. *Annals of Neurology*, **56**, 595–599.

Sohn, Y.H. and Hallett, M. (2004b) Surround inhibition in human motor system. *Experimental Brain Research*, **158**, 397–404.

Sohn, Y.H., Jung, H.Y., Kaelin-Lang, A. and Hallett, M. (2003) Excitability of the ipsilateral motor cortex during phasic voluntary hand movement. *Experimental Brain Research*, **148**, 176–185.

Stefan, K., Kunesch, E., Cohen, L.G. *et al.* (2000) Induction of plasticity in the human motor cortex by paired associative stimulation. *Brain*, **123** (Pt 3), 572–584.

Stinear, C.M. and Byblow, W.D. (2004) Impaired modulation of intracortical inhibition in focal hand dystonia. *Cerebral Cortex*, **14**, 555–561.

Tarsy, D. and Simon, D.K. (2006) Dystonia. *The New England Journal of Medicine*, **355**, 818–829.

Tinazzi, M., Priori, A., Bertolasi, L. *et al.* (2000) Abnormal central integration of a dual somatosensory input in dystonia. Evidence for sensory overflow. *Brain*, **123**, 42–50.

Valls-Solé, J., Pascual-Leone, A., Wassermann, E.M. and Hallett, M. (1992) Human motor evoked responses to paired transcranial magnetic stimuli. *Electroencephalography and Clinical Neurophysiology*, **85**, 355–364.

Verdugo, R.J. and Ochoa, J.L. (2000) Abnormal movements in complex regional pain syndrome: assessment of their nature. *Muscle & Nerve*, **23**, 198–205.

Waters, C.H., Faust, P.L., Powers, J. *et al.* (1993) Neuropathology of lubag (x-linked dystonia parkinsonism). *Movement Disorders*, **8**, 387–390.

Weise, D., Schramm, A., Stefan, K. *et al.* (2006) The two sides of associative plasticity in writer's cramp. *Brain*, **129**, 2709–2721.

Weiss, E.M., Hershey, T., Karimi, M. *et al.* (2006) Relative risk of spread of symptoms among the focal onset primary dystonias. *Movement Disorders*, **21**, 1175–1181.

Werhahn, K.J., Kunesch, E., Noachtar, S. *et al.* (1999) Differential effects on motorcortical inhibition induced by blockade of GABA uptake in humans. *Journal of Physiology-London*, **517**, 591–597.

Wider, C., Melquist, S., Hauf, M. *et al.* (2008) Study of a Swiss dopa-responsive dystonia family with a deletion in GCH1: redefining DYT14 as DYT5. *Neurology*, **70**, 1377–1383.

Ziemann, U., Rothwell, J.C. and Ridding, M.C. (1996) Interaction between intracortical inhibition and facilitation in human motor cortex. *Journal of Physiology-London*, **496**, 873–881.

Zimprich, A., Grabowski, M., Asmus, F. *et al.* (2001) Mutations in the gene encoding epsilon-sarcoglycan cause myoclonus-dystonia syndrome. *Nature Genetics*, **29**, 66–69.

13

General Management Approach to Dystonia

Cynthia L. Comella

Rush University Medical Center, Chicago, IL, USA

INTRODUCTION

In the absence of curative therapies, the treatment of dystonia is primarily aimed towards improvement of abnormal postures, reduction in pain and enhancement in functional capacity and quality of life. The treatment options available for dystonia have recently been reviewed (Balash and Giladi, 2004; Jankovic, 2006) and have changed substantially with the introduction of botulinum toxin for focal dystonia and deep brain stimulation for intractable generalized dystonia. These areas will be addressed in subsequent chapters. In contrast, progress has been slower in the development of clinically practical non-pharmacologic and pharmacologic treatments for dystonia. The evidence supporting the use of any of these therapeutic interventions is largely based on open clinical trials, retrospective studies, case reports, clinical experience or small controlled trials. There are many factors that have hampered progress in these areas. One of the most important impediments to development of new drugs for dystonia is the absence of a clear understanding of the basic pharmacology of dystonia and the failure to identify specific neurotransmitter abnormalities that could provide targets for pharmacologic interventions. Other factors contributing to the slow progress in this area include the heterogeneity of dystonia, a disorder that has numerous different causes, variable clinical features, and inconsistent responsiveness to medications; the relatively low prevalence of dystonia; and the availability of other effective interventions (botulinum toxin and DBS). This chapter will review the non-pharmacologic and medical therapeutics of dystonia. Subsequent chapters will address chemodenervation and surgical interventions.

NON-PHARMACOLOGIC INTERVENTIONS

The non-pharmacologic interventions for dystonia are based on clinical observations and current understandings of the neurological mechanisms of dystonia. From observations of sensory tricks, and elucidation of the electrophysiological abnormalities detailed in the previous chapter, innovative interventions have been suggested to increase central inhibition, reduce sensory abnormalities and normalize changes in central plasticity. Experimental non-pharmacologic therapies, while currently under investigation, have not been established as practical, widely applicable interventions, but will be summarized. Most studies are open-label, providing class IV evidence. Despite the lack of evidence, the utility of these ancillary methods of improving dystonia should be evaluated in individual patients.

Maximizing Sensory Tricks

The effect of sensory tricks (geste antagoniste) in alleviating dystonia is a feature of dystonia (Jahanshahi, 2000). Several anecdotal reports indicate that tricks may be useful as a therapeutic intervention. Examples of these include an appropriately fitted ankle-foot orthotic (Hurvitz et al., 1988), dental devices for oromandibular dystonia (Frucht et al., 1999) and a variety of writing devices for writer's cramp (Ranawaya and Lang, 1991; Tas et al., 2001; Baur et al., 2006). Occupational therapists with knowledge of dystonia may be able to optimize sensory tricks and avoid the need for more invasive therapies.

Limb Cooling

Cooling of the involved limb has been reported to be of benefit in some patients with hand dystonia (Pohl *et al.*, 2002). Limb cooling requires immersion in 15 °C cold water for five minutes. In 10 patients with writer's cramp, limb cooling improved the writing performance for up to 25 minutes following cold-water immersion. This improvement was postulated to arise from a reduction in muscle spindle afferent activity due to lowered temperatures.

Repetitive Transcranial Magnetic Stimulation

Repetitive transcranial magnetic stimulation (rTMS) provides a method for producing cortical effects that are either excitatory (at high rates of stimulation: >5 Hz) or inhibitory (at low stimulation frequencies: <1 Hz) (Chen, 2000). These excitatory or inhibitory effects can be directed towards particular cortical regions through appropriate placement of the TMS coil. Application of inhibitory stimulation using rTMS at 1 Hz to the hand area of the contralateral motor cortex in 16 patients with simple or dystonic writer's cramp showed improvement in handwriting in 8 out of 16 patients, with marked improvement in 6. The benefit in these patients was sustained for more than three hours, with two patients having persistent improvement after several days. Sham stimulation with the coil placed anterior to the motor cortex did not result in any improvement (Siebner *et al.*, 1999). A subsequent study in nine right-handed patients with dystonic writer's cramp using rTMS at 0.2 Hz delivered in random order to the motor cortex (MC), premotor cortex (PMC) and supplementary motor cortex (SMC) showed significant improvement following PMC stimulation but not after SMC, MC or sham stimulation (Murase *et al.*, 2005).

Repetitive transcutaneous electrical nerve stimulation (TENS) of the forearm flexor muscles has been shown to improve handwriting in patients with writer's cramp. This was associated with a reduction in the motor-evoked potentials in the flexor carpi radialis muscle after TMS, suggesting alterations in cortical excitability through manipulation of peripheral sensory inputs (Tinazzi *et al.*, 2005; Tinazzi *et al.*, 2006). Whether practical therapeutic approaches can be derived from these observations remains to be shown.

Sensory Motor Retuning and Constraint Therapies

Sensory motor retuning (SMR), also called constraint induced movement therapy (CI), has shown promise as an effective intervention for rehabilitation following stroke (Taub *et al.*, 2003) and is considered a potential therapy for other motor disorders, including hand dystonia (Taub *et al.*, 2006). In stroke, the technique of SMR involves constraining movements of the unaffected limb while intensively training use of the affected limb for prolonged periods of weeks to months (Taub *et al.*, 1999). In hand dystonia, the non-dystonic finger(s) are immobilized by splinting, forcing the dystonic finger to work in concert with the other fingers in carrying out the desired activity. In one study, musicians were splinted to immobilize the non-dystonic fingers and instructed to play their instruments for $1\frac{1}{2}$ to $2\frac{1}{2}$ hours per day for eight consecutive days and then to use the splint for one hour per day for up to one year. In this study, SMR improved dystonia in six pianists and two guitarists, and showed modest benefit in wind instrument players other than flutists (Candia *et al.*, 2002). Associated with improvement in skills was a modification of the abnormal representation of the dystonic fingers in the somatosensory cortex (Candia *et al.*, 2005). However, application of this technique to writer's cramp in which there is involvement of more than one finger, showed only modest effects in 50% of subjects, and no changes in cortical excitability (Zeuner *et al.*, 2005). A more complex, intensive program of sensorimotor retuning with and without biofeedback demonstrated improvement in occupational hand dystonia in an open-label, prospective study (Byl and McKenzie, 2000; Byl *et al.*, 2003), but controlled studies of this technique have not yet been completed.

Conversely, other investigators have applied the opposite technique, in which the dystonic arm is immobilized by splinting for periods of 4–5 weeks, followed by a period of retraining of the dystonic arm. This technique was used in an open-label study of eight patients with occupational hand dystonia. Following the splinting period, all patients had initial clumsiness and weakness that recovered in approximately four weeks with improvement in dystonia that was sustained for up to 24 weeks in seven patients (Priori *et al.*, 2001). This was followed by a larger study that included 19 patients with either writer's cramp or musician's dystonia. This study found variable outcome, with 20% reporting no benefit and approximately 45% reporting moderate to marked benefit. The factors associated with a good outcome included more severe dystonia at the beginning of the trial, a transient improvement after fatiguing contraction, a younger age, an onset related to overuse and no prior treatment with botulinum toxin (Pesenti *et al.*, 2004). A controlled study has not yet confirmed these findings. As a cautionary note, dystonia has also been elicited by prolonged immobilization with casting (Okun *et al.*, 2002).

Some patients with dystonia have sensory abnormalities with deficits in spatial discrimination (Bara-Jimenez *et al.*, 2000a, 2000b). Based on this observation and others, sensory training (e.g., reading braille) has been proposed as a treatment for hand dystonia. In one study, 10 patients with hand dystonia were trained to read braille and demonstrated improvements in both sensory perception and hand posturing (Zeuner *et al.*, 2002). With ongoing training, improvements were sustained over one year. However, benefit was reduced or lost if practice was discontinued (Zeuner and Hallett, 2003). Controlled trials have not been done.

PHARMACOLOGIC TREATMENTS: ORAL MEDICATIONS (TABLE 13.1)

Anti-cholinergic Drugs

Anti-cholinergic drugs, in particular trihexyphenidyl, may be useful for treatment of dystonia, particularly in younger patients with generalized dystonia (Level B). The anti-cholinergic agents that have been used include trihexyphenidyl, benztropine, biperiden, atropine, procyclidine, orphenadrine, scopolamine and ethopropazine. Most studies were not placebo controlled and many were retrospective without validated outcome measures (Class III and IV). One placebo-controlled double blind, crossover study in 31 patients with predominantly generalized dystonia showed that 71% of patients improved after the 18-week treatment period (Class II). In the 68% of patients who continued trihexyphenidyl over 2.4 years of follow-up, 42% reported sustained substantial improvement using trihexyphenidyl doses from 5 to 120 mg per day. Trihexyphenidyl was well tolerated in the young patients (age range 9–32 years) included in the study, with the two most frequent side effects being blurred vision and dry mouth (Burke, 1986).

A second placebo-controlled trial assessed outcome following intravenous injections of atropine, benztropine, chlorpheniramine and normal saline in random order. This study did not show significant improvement with any active drug in focal dystonia, although individual patients may have shown improvement (Class II) (Lang *et al.*, 1982). In a trial comparing botulinum toxin to trihexyphenidyl using a randomized, double-blinded, parallel-arm design in 66 CD patients, there was no improvement in the trihexyphenidyl group at a mean dose of 16.25 mg (range 4–24 mg), with 13 of the 32 patients having worsened symptoms, and frequent adverse effects (Brans *et al.*, 1996) (Class II).

In one prospective, open-label study, patients were treated with trihexyphenidyl or ethopropazine. This study reported benefit in 61% of 23 children and 38% of 52 adults with dystonia. Over half of the adults discontinued the anti-cholinergic drugs as a result of adverse effects. The children tolerated the drugs without significant side effects and were able to be treated at higher doses than the adults (Fahn, 1983) (Class III). Similar open-label and retrospective reports using a variety of anti-cholinergic agents have confirmed these results (Marsden, 1984; Greene, 1988) (Class IV).

The lack of a consistent response to anti-cholinergic agents suggests that cholinergic mechanisms are not primary in dystonia (Lang *et al.*, 1982; Lang *et al.*, 1983; Lang, 1982). However, in some patients there may be clear improvement of dystonic symptoms with anti-cholinergic therapy (Greene *et al.*, 1988). High doses of anti-cholinergic agents are usually necessary for benefit. It is important, however, to initiate treatment at the lowest possible dose of a given agent and to escalate the dose slowly over a period of weeks to months. Anti-cholinergic dosing should be divided into three or four daily doses. Improvement is often delayed, thus dose adjustments should be made slowly, allowing a week or two at a dose level. Adults are usually unable to tolerate high doses because of side effects. Children, although tolerant of high doses, should be monitored for side effects as they mature.

One of the greatest limitations to the use of this class of agents is the frequent occurrence of adverse effects. Adverse effects from anti-cholinergic agents are not correlated with serum levels, but rather increase with increasing age (Fahn, 1983; Burke and Fahn, 1985). Peripheral side effects, such as dry mouth, blurred vision and urinary retention may be reversed using a peripheral cholinesterase inhibitor (glycopyrrolate). The central side effects are dose limiting, and include memory loss, confusion and sedation, psychiatric disorders, chorea and insomnia. If side effects occur with one anti-cholinergic agent, it may be possible to change to another agent. Ethopropazine has fewer peripheral side effects than most other anti-cholinergic agents, but it is not available in the United States. If side effects occur in the absence of benefit, anti-cholinergic treatment should be discontinued. Discontinuation of anti-cholinergic agents should be done gradually, as withdrawal effects may occur (Fahn, 1983).

Dopaminergic Drugs

The use of levodopa in dopa-responsive dystonia is essentially an etiologic treatment and, in low dose, rapidly leads to a complete normalization of symptoms. In other forms of primary dystonia, carbidopa/levodopa and other dopamine agonist drugs can be useful, but have not been sufficiently evaluated. Most evidence is Class III–IV. Early observations were inconsistent, with some open-label studies suggesting benefit (Coleman, 1970; Fletcher *et al.*, 1993) and others reporting no improvement or worsening (Barrett *et al.*, 1970; Mandell, 1970). In a retrospective study, approximately 12% of 41 dystonic patients treated with dopamine agonists were found to have a good response (Greene *et al.*, 1988). Direct dopamine agonists, including bromocriptine, lisuride and apomorphine have not been promising (Lang, 1988). Although there is insufficient evidence to support the use of levodopa for primary dystonia, the tolerability of the drug, the rapidity of a test trial and the expanding phenotype of dopa-responsive dystonia (Nygaard *et al.*, 1990; Bandmann *et al.*, 1998b; Schneider *et al.*, 2006), support an empiric trial in patients with primary generalized and focal dystonia (Albanese *et al.*, 2006). Levodopa in combination with carbidopa is started at low doses (50–100 mg per day) and increased gradually to a maximum dose of 600–1000 mg. The most frequent adverse effect of levodopa is nausea, particularly at initiation of therapy, that can be treated with supplemental carbidopa. If there is no improvement with levodopa

Table 13.1 Oral medications useful for the treatment of dystonia.

Pharmacological agent	Efficacy and comment (level of evidence)	Side effects
Anti-cholinergic/ Anti-histaminic Trihexyphenidyl (Artane) Benztropine (Cogentin) Procyclidine (Kemadrin) Diphenhydramine (Benedryl) Ethopropazine (Parsidol)	Effective in approximately 40% of young onset, generalized dystonia (Class I) May be effective in focal and segmental dystonia (Class II, III, IV) Benefit limited by side effects Requires slow upward titration	Dry mouth May lead to dental caries Blurred vision Exacerbation of acute angle glaucoma Urinary retention Memory problems Sedation Confusion Hallucinations Heat intolerance
Baclofen (Lioresal)	Effective in approximately 20% (Class III and IV) High doses tolerated in children (Class III) Benefits limited by side effects; intrathecal baclofen minimally successful	Nausea Sedation Dysphoria Muscle weakness (in those with spasticity associated) Withdrawal effects on sudden discontinuation
Clonazepam (Klonipin)	Effective in approximately 15% (Class IV) Possibility for addiction Withdrawal effects on sudden discontinuation	Sedation Depression Confusion Dependence
Dopamine agonists Carbidopa/Levodopa (Sinemet)	Dramatic response in the dopa-responsive form of dystonia Effective in 12% of primary dystonia (Class IV) Test for levodopa response in young-onset generalized and focal dystonia to rule out DRD	Nausea (especially at initiation of therapy) May worsen dystonia Rapid discontinuation possible
Muscle relaxants Tizanidine (Zanaflex) Cyclobenzaprine (Flexoril)	Limited benefit in some patients Side effects frequent (Class IV)	Sedation Dysphoria
Anti-epileptic medications Carbamazepine (Tegretol) Gabapentin (Neurontin)	Benefit in <10% (Class IV)	Ataxia Sedation
Dopamine Depleting agents Tetrabenazine	Benefit for dystonia (Class IV) Requires a very slow upward titration	Depression Dysphoria Parkinsonism

Table 13.1 (*Continued*)

Pharmacological agent	Efficacy and comment (level of evidence)	Side effects
Dopamine antagonists (anti-psychotics)	Effective in up to 25% (Class IV)	Atypical anti-psychotics:
Atypical	Clozapine requires weekly blood counts and may cause life threatening agranulocytosis	Sedation, orthostatic hypotension, metabolic syndrome, sudden death, seizures
Clozapine (Clozaril)		Clozapine: agranulocytosis (requires monitoring). Typical anti-psychotics possibility of tardive dyskinesia and the other adverse effects from this class of medications severely limits usefulness. Not recommended for dystonia
Quetiapine (Seroquel) Typical Pimozide Haloperidol		

dose at 600 mg for four weeks, the drug can be stopped (Bandmann *et al.*, 1998a).

Dopamine Receptor Antagonists and Dopamine Depletion

Dopamine receptor antagonists (anti-psychotic agents), have not been adequately studied as a treatment for dystonia. Open-label studies have shown good response in 35% of 26 patients treated chronically (Greene *et al.*, 1988). Combination therapy with pimozide, an anti-cholinergic agent and tetrabenazine was suggested to be useful in severe disabling axial or generalized dystonia in open-label observational studies (Marsden *et al.*, 1984). Other typical DA antagonists, including haloperidol and phenothiazines, have anecdotally been observed to improve dystonia (Lang, 1988), but controlled trials are lacking. Side effects of the typical antipsychotics include reversible drug-induced parkinsonism and potentially permanent tardive dyskinesia. Atypical antipsychotics, including clozapine and quetiapine may be useful in generalized dystonia, craniofacial dystonias and oromandibular dystonia, although results have not been consistent in the small number of open-label studies conducted. (Thiel *et al.*, 1994; Trugman *et al.*, 1994; Burbaud *et al.*, 1998; Karp *et al.*, 1999; Hanagasi *et al.*, 2004). The side effects of clozapine include sedation and agranulocytosis requiring frequent blood monitoring. Quetiapine is another atypical anti-psychotic that does not require hematological monitoring. There are only case reports of its effect in primary dystonia (Reeves and Liberto, 2003). Side effects of the atypical anti-psychotics include sedation, orthostatic hypotension, lowered seizure threshold and metabolic

syndrome (diabetes, dyslipidemia and hypertension, with associated obesity) (Shirzadi and Ghaemi, 2006).

Tetrabenazine depletes monoamines, including dopamine, through its action as an inhibitor of vesicular monoamine transporter 2 (VMAT2) and has additional dopamine receptor antagonist properties (Kenney *et al.*, 2006). Tetrabenazine is reported to be beneficial in a variety of hyperkinetic movement disorders, including tardive dyskinesia, Tourette's syndrome and Huntington's disease (HSG, 2006). Early case series and retrospective chart reviews found benefit with tetrabenazine, alone or in combination with other agents, in 25% of dystonia patients (Marsden *et al.*, 1984; Greene *et al.*, 1988; Jankovic and Beach, 1997; Paleacu *et al.*, 2004). One randomized, placebo-controlled study showed improvement in dystonia in four out of six with cranial dystonia (Meige syndrome), and five out of six patients with other forms of dystonia (Jankovic, 1982). A retrospective chart study showed improvement in 64% of 108 idiopathic dystonia patients (Jankovic and Orman, 1988; Jankovic and Beach, 1997). A more recent retrospective chart review in 132 dystonia patients reported that 67% had a marked or moderate reduction in movements with 50–75 mg of tetrabenazine. The improvement was sustained over approximately three years of follow-up in the 44% of patients who continued the drug (Kenney and Jankovic, 2006). Side effects are common and include sedation, depression, parkinsonism, akathisia, nervousness and insomnia (Kenney *et al.*, 2006; Kenney and Jankovic, 2006). Tetrabenazine is now approved in the United States (for Huntington's disease), and has been available in other countries. A trial of tetrabenazine is time consuming. Typically, the drug is initiated at very low doses and increased quite slowly. Tetrabenazine can cause a drug-induced depression at any dose, but particularly at doses of 75 mg or greater.

Benzodiazepine Drugs: Clonazepam

Clonazepam is a benzodiazepine that is used frequently for dystonia but has not been evaluated in controlled studies. Clonazepam was observed to be beneficial in retrospective studies for 21% of CD patients at doses ranging from 1.5 to 12 mg per day (Greene *et al.*, 1988). This drug may be particularly useful to treat CD with predominant dystonic head tremor (Hughes *et al.*, 1991; Davis *et al.*, 1995). Small case series have observed benefit for blepharospasm (Jankovic and Ford, 1983). Modest benefit for dystonia has been reported with intravenous clonazepam (Povlsen and Pakkenberg, 1990). Benzodiazepines may be particularly useful in patients with myoclonic dystonia (Asmus and Gasser, 2004). The usual starting dose is 0.5 mg in the evening. Clonazepam is gradually escalated to benefit or side effects. Doses up to 8 mg can be used. The adverse effects include sedation, depression, confusion and dependence.

Baclofen

Baclofen, a pre-synaptic GABA-B receptor agonist, has been administered by both oral and intrathecal routes for the treatment of dystonia and spasticity. For dystonia, there are no controlled studies, and most reports are from retrospective chart studies or case series. In retrospective studies, approximately 20% of dystonia patients reported a good response (Greene *et al.*, 1988). In a case series of children with primary generalized dystonia, 7 out of 16 patients had substantial or moderate improvement with baclofen, when added to other agents at doses up to 120 mg, (Greene and Fahn, 1992). A subsequent review showed that 14 out of 31 children with dystonia improved using a dose range from 40 to 180 mg per day (Greene, 1992). Adults did not fare as well. For cranial dystonia and blepharospasm, initial benefit was seen in 28 of 60 patients, however only 11 continued on baclofen with the primary reason for discontinuation being side effects (Greene, 1992). Patients with cervical dystonia were the least likely to benefit, with only 11% obtaining a good response at a dose range of 25–200 mg per day (Greene, 1992). Baclofen is initiated with small doses of 5 mg three times a day. Dose escalation is done slowly, allowing a week between dose increases. The most common side effects from baclofen are dizziness, sedation, nausea and urinary symptoms. Confusion, hallucinations and paranoia have been reported, but are rare. Sudden withdrawal of baclofen may precipitate psychosis or seizures or dramatic increase in dystonia.

In contrast to oral administration, intrathecal administration of baclofen (ITB), using an infusion pump, allows high spinal fluid levels with the highest concentration of baclofen in the lower thecal sac (Kroin, 1993). Theoretically, this method of treatment could reduce the occurrence of central side effects of baclofen. ITB has been shown to be effective for the treatment of spasticity and spasticity associated with dystonia (Meythaler *et al.*, 1999). Its usefulness as a treatment for primary generalized or focal dystonia has yet to be established, and there are conflicting results from case reports (Narayan *et al.*, 1991; Ford *et al.*, 1996; Diederich *et al.*, 1997; Walker *et al.*, 2000; Jaffe and Nienstedt, 2001). When administered in the high cervical spine or into the cerebral ventricles, there may be benefit (Dykstra *et al.*, 2005). Intrathecal baclofen has numerous potentially serious complications, including surgical complications and malfunction of the pump causing sudden withdrawal (Santiago-Palma *et al.*, 2004; Vender *et al.*, 2006). ITB is not currently viewed as a treatment option for primary dystonia.

Other Treatments

Local injections of lidocaine, an anesthetic drug, improves symptoms of focal dystonia transiently (Jacome, 1988; Mubaidin, 2000; Yoshida *et al.*, 2002). Mexiletine is a lidocaine derivative that is used to treat cardiac ventricular arrhythmias. Mexiletine has been assessed in open-label trials for the treatment of cervical and generalized dystonia using oral doses of 450–1200 mg per day (Ohara *et al.*, 1997; Ohara *et al.*, 1998; Lucetti *et al.*, 2000). Although the results have been promising, with sustained improvement in dystonic symptoms, controlled trials have not yet been published. Mexiletine is well tolerated, with the most frequent side effects being upper gastrointestinal symptoms, dizziness, ataxia and dysarthria.

Other treatments have been reported anecdotally. Muscle relaxants such as tizanidine, cyclobenzaprine, orphenadrine and methocarbamol have been used for dystonia, but evidence for improvement is lacking (Lang and Riley, 1992). Anti-convulsants, although beneficial for paroxysmal dyskinesia, have not been adequately studied in primary dystonia. These agents include carbamazepine (Geller *et al.*, 1976; Garg, 1982), topiramate (Papapetropoulos and Singer, 2006) and gabapentin. A small open trial of riluzole demonstrated benefit in cervical dystonia. (Muller *et al.*, 2002).

TREATMENT GUIDELINES FOR DYSTONIA

With the paucity of controlled trials for treatments of dystonia, the initial choice of therapy is largely dependent on the body regions involved, the age of the patient, the

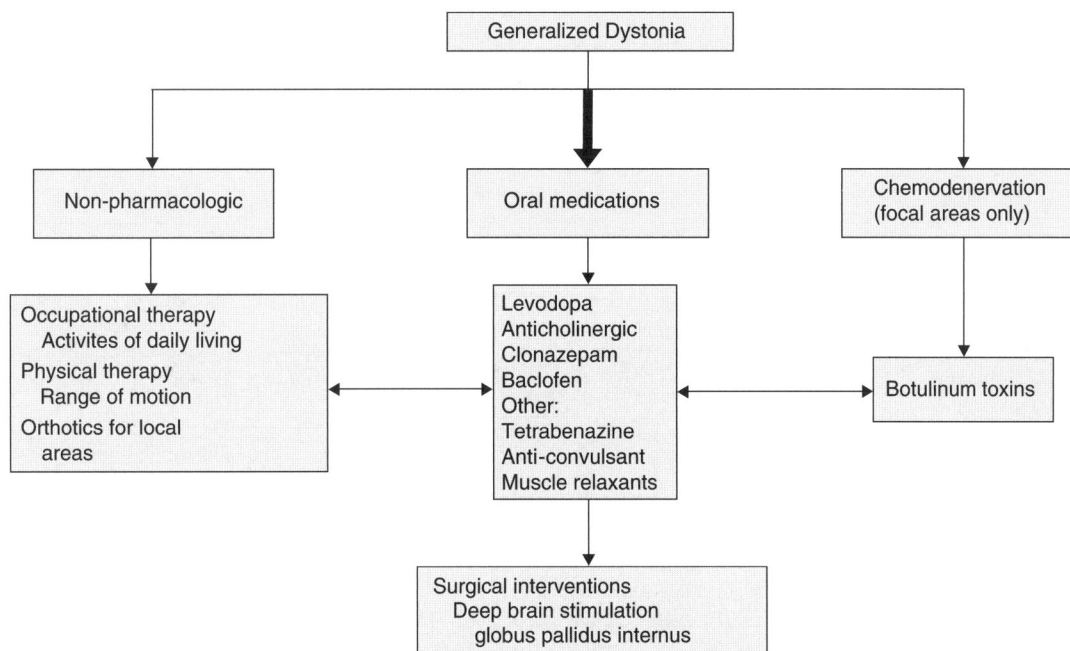

Figure 13.1 Guidelines for treatment of generalized dystonia. The thick arrow indicates the primary treatment option. The therapies indicated should be modified to the specific patient.

tolerability of the medications, the availability of medications and the experience of the physician.

Generalized Dystonia (Figure 13.1)

In children with generalized dystonia, oral medications are the first line of treatment. Levodopa in combination with carbidopa administered in doses up to 1000 mg is recommended as the first drug. Marked response to levodopa suggests a diagnosis of dopa-responsive dystonia, and other treatments will not be necessary. Failing levodopa, anti-cholinergic agents are often used as the oral agent. Anti-cholinergic agents can be very effective at high doses and are well tolerated in children. If there is inadequate benefit from anti-cholinergic agents alone, then combination therapy with the addition of tetrabenazine (if available), baclofen or clonazepam may be useful.

The role of rehabilitation therapy, although not established in studies, is a valuable adjunct to pharmacologic treatments. By preventing and treating muscle contractures, optimizing function and testing the effectiveness of prosthetic devices, such as shoe inserts, and specialized keyboards, the physical and occupational therapists can play an important role in management.

Botulinum toxins and deep brain stimulation surgery will be discussed in the following chapters. These treatment modalities are considered second line, but may provide benefit if oral medications fail.

Focal Dystonia (Figure 13.2)

Focal and segmental dystonia typically affects adults. The treatment of choice for most focal dystonia is botulinum toxin. However, oral medications are useful in those patients who are not candidates for botulinum toxin, those who fail to benefit from botulinum toxin or in combination with botulinum toxin to enhance outcomes and perhaps prolong the interval between injections. The limitation of most oral medications is the lack of tolerability to these agents in adults.

Physical rehabilitation may be useful in maintaining range of motion and flexibility and in providing useful adjunctive treatments. In patients with foot dystonia, specially designed shoes or an ankle-foot orthotic may take advantage of the sensory "trick." In writer's cramp, a thick pen or one with a special grip may improve function. Other techniques described previously, including constraint therapy, sensorimotor retraining and sensory training, may be considered if carefully administered by a trained therapist and monitored by the physician.

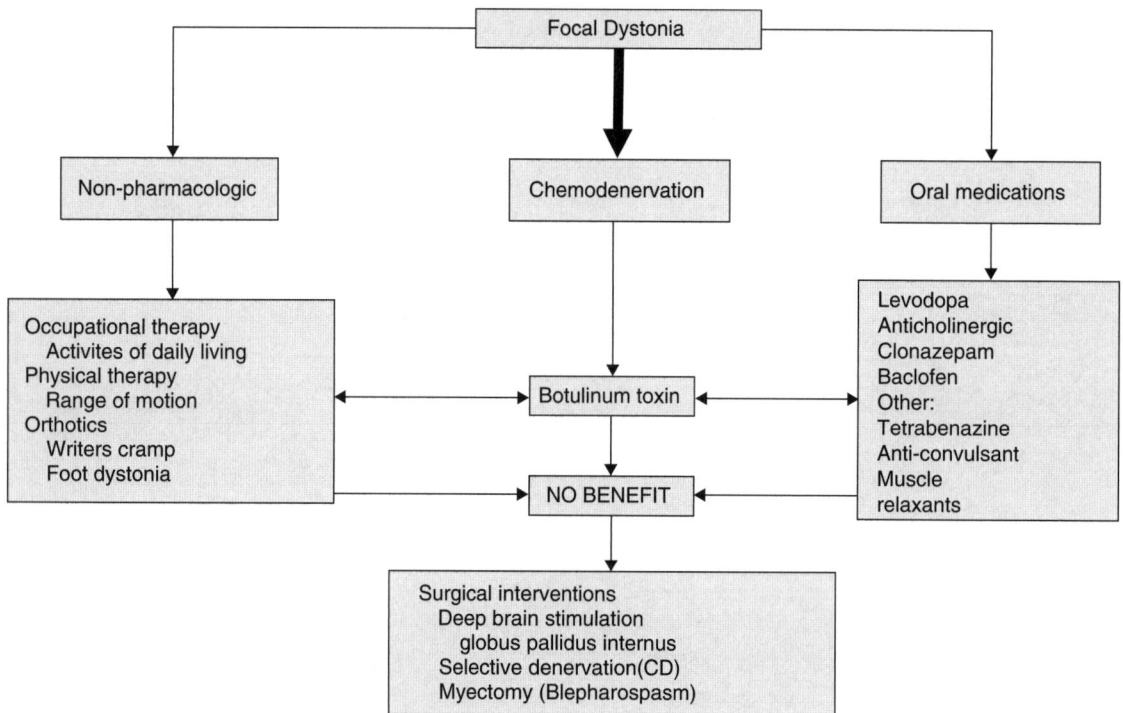

Figure 13.2 Guidelines for treatment of focal and segmental dystonia. The thick arrow indicates the primary treatment option. The therapies indicated should be modified to the specific patient.

References

Albanese, A., Barnes, M.P. *et al.* (2006) A systematic review on the diagnosis and treatment of primary (idiopathic) dystonia and dystonia plus syndromes: report of an EFNS/MDS-ES Task Force. *European Journal of Neurology*, **13** (5), 433–444.

Asmus, F. and Gasser, T. (2004) Inherited myoclonus-dystonia. *Advances in Neurology*, **94**, 113–119.

Balash, Y. and Giladi, N. (2004) Efficacy of pharmacological treatment of dystonia: evidence-based review including meta-analysis of the effect of botulinum toxin and other cure options. *European Journal of Neurology*, **11** (6), 361–370.

Bandmann, O., Marsden, C.D. *et al.* (1998a) Atypical presentations of dopa-responsive dystonia. *Advances in Neurology*, **78**, 283–290.

Bandmann, O., Valente, E.M. *et al.* (1998b) Dopa-responsive dystonia: a clinical and molecular genetic study. *Annals of Neurology*, **44** (4), 649–656.

Bara-Jimenez, W., Shelton, P. *et al.* (2000a) Spatial discrimination is abnormal in focal hand dystonia. *Neurology*, **55** (12), 1869–1873.

Bara-Jimenez, W., Shelton, P. *et al.* (2000b) Sensory discrimination capabilities in patients with focal hand dystonia. *Annals of Neurology*, **47** (3), 377–380.

Barrett, R.E., Yahr, M.D. *et al.* (1970) Torsion dystonia and spasmodic torticollis – results of treatment with L-dopa. *Neurology*, **20** (11), 107–113.

Baur, B., Schenk, T. *et al.* (2006) Modified pen grip in the treatment of Writer's Cramp. *Human Movement Science*, **25** (4–5), 464–473.

Brans, J.W., Lindeboom, R. *et al.* (1996) Botulinum toxin versus trihexyphenidyl in cervical dystonia: a prospective, randomized, double-blind controlled trial. *Neurology*, **46** (4), 1066–1072.

Burbaud, P., Guehl, D. *et al.* (1998) A pilot trial of clozapine in the treatment of cervical dystonia. *Journal of Neurology*, **245** (6–7), 329–331.

Burke, R.E. and Fahn, S. (1985) Serum trihexyphenidyl levels in the treatment of torsion dystonia. *Neurology*, **35** (7), 1066–1069.

Burke, R.E., Fahn, S. and Marsden, C.D. (1986) Torsion dystonia: a double-blind, prospective trial of high-dosage trihexyphenidyl. *Neurology*, **33** (2), 160–164.

Byl, N.N. and McKenzie, A. (2000) Treatment effectiveness for patients with a history of repetitive hand use and focal hand dystonia: a planned, prospective follow-up study. *Journal of Hand Therapy*, **13** (4), 289–301.

Byl, N.N., Nagajaran, S. *et al.* (2003) Effect of sensory discrimination training on structure and function in patients with focal hand dystonia: a case series. *Archives of Physical Medicine and Rehabilitation*, **84** (10), 1505–1514.

Candia, V., Rosset-Llobet, J. *et al.* (2005) Changing the brain through therapy for musicians' hand dystonia. *Annals of the New York Academy of Sciences*, **1060**, 335–342.

Candia, V., Schafer, T. *et al.* (2002) Sensory motor retuning: a behavioral treatment for focal hand dystonia of pianists and guitarists. *Archives of Physical Medicine and Rehabilitation*, **83** (10), 1342–1348.

Chen, R. (2000) Studies of human motor physiology with transcranial magnetic stimulation. *Muscle Nerve Suppl*, **9**, S26–S32.

Coleman, M. (1970) Preliminary remarks on the L-dopa therapy of dystonia. *Neurology*, **20** (11), 114–121.

Davis, T.L., Charles, P.D. *et al.* (1995) Clonazepam-sensitive intermittent dystonic tremor. *Southern Medical Journal*, **88** (10), 1069–1071.

Diederich, N.J., Comella, C.L. *et al.* (1997) Sustained effect of high-dose intrathecal baclofen in primary generalized dystonia: a 2-year follow-up study. *Movement Disorders*, **12** (6), 1100–1102.

Dykstra, D.D., Mendez, A. *et al.* (2005) Treatment of cervical dystonia and focal hand dystonia by high cervical continuously infused intrathecal baclofen: a report of 2 cases. *Archives of Physical Medicine and Rehabilitation*, **86** (4), 830–833.

Fahn, S. (1983) High dosage anticholinergic therapy in dystonia. *Neurology*, **33** (10), 1255–1261.

Fletcher, N.A., Thompson, P.D. *et al.* (1993) Successful treatment of childhood onset symptomatic dystonia with levodopa. *Journal of Neurology, Neurosurgery, and Psychiatry*, **56** (8), 865–867.

Ford, B., Greene, P. *et al.* (1996) Use of intrathecal baclofen in the treatment of patients with dystonia. *Archives of Neurology*, **53** (12), 1241–1246.

Frucht, S., Fahn, S. *et al.* (1999) A geste antagoniste device to treat jaw-closing dystonia. *Movement Disorders*, **14** (5), 883–886.

Garg, B.P. (1982) Dystonia musculorum deformans: implications of therapeutic response to levodopa and carbamazepine. *Archives of Neurology*, **39** (6), 376–377.

Geller, M., Kaplan, B. *et al.* (1976) Treatment of dystonic symptoms with carbamazepine. *Advances in Neurology*, **14**, 403–410.

Greene, P. (1992) Baclofen in the treatment of dystonia. *Clinical Neuropharmacology*, **15** (4), 276–288.

Greene, P., Shale, H. *et al.* (1988) Experience with high dosages of anticholinergic and other drugs in the treatment of torsion dystonia. *Advances in Neurology*, **50**, 547–556.

Greene, P.E. and Fahn, S. (1992) Baclofen in the treatment of idiopathic dystonia in children. *Movement Disorders*, **7** (1), 48–52.

Hanagasi, H.A., Bilgic, B. *et al.* (2004) Clozapine treatment in oromandibular dystonia. *Clinical Neuropharmacology*, **27** (2), 84–86.

HSG (2006) Tetrabenazine as antichorea therapy in Huntington disease: a randomized controlled trial. *Neurology*, **66** (3), 366–372.

Hughes, A.J., Lees, A.J. *et al.* (1991) Paroxysmal dystonic head tremor. *Movement Disorders*, **6** (1), 85–86.

Hurvitz, E.A., Ellenberg, M.R. *et al.* (1988) Orthotic technique for dystonia musculorum deformans. *Archives of Physical Medicine and Rehabilitation*, **69** (10), 892–894.

Jacome, D.E. (1988) Writing tremor myoclonus. *European Neurology*, **28** (3), 126–130.

Jaffe, M.S. and Nienstedt, L.J. (2001) Intrathecal baclofen for generalized dystonia: a case report. *Archives of Physical Medicine and Rehabilitation*, **82** (6), 853–855.

Jahanshahi, M. (2000) Factors that ameliorate or aggravate spasmodic torticollis. *Journal of Neurology, Neurosurgery, and Psychiatry*, **68** (2), 227–229.

Jankovic, J. (1982) Treatment of hyperkinetic movement disorders with tetrabenazine: a double-blind crossover study. *Annals of Neurology*, **11** (1), 41–47.

Jankovic, J. (2006) Treatment of dystonia. *The Lancet Neurology*, **5** (10), 864–872.

Jankovic, J. and Beach, J. (1997) Long-term effects of tetrabenazine in hyperkinetic movement disorders. *Neurology*, **48** (2), 358–362.

Jankovic, J. and Ford, J. (1983) Blepharospasm and orofacial-cervical dystonia: clinical and pharmacological findings in 100 patients. *Annals of Neurology*, **13** (4), 402–411.

Jankovic, J. and Orman, J. (1988) Tetrabenazine therapy of dystonia, chorea, tics, and other dyskinesias. *Neurology*, **38** (3), 391–394.

Karp, B.I., Goldstein, S.R. *et al.* (1999) An open trial of clozapine for dystonia. *Movement Disorders*, **14** (4), 652–657.

Kenney, C., Hunter, C. *et al.* (2006) Long-term tolerability of tetrabenazine in the treatment of hyperkinetic movement disorders. *Movement Disorders*, **22** (2), 193–197.

Kenney, C. and Jankovic, J. (2006) Tetrabenazine in the treatment of hyperkinetic movement disorders. *Expert Review of Neurotherapeutics*, **6** (1), 7–17.

Kroin J.S., Ali, A., York, M. and Penn, R.D. (1993) The distribution of medication along the spinal canal after chronic intrathecal administration. *Neurosurgery*, **33** (2), 226–230.

Lang, A.E. (1988) Dopamine agonists and antagonists in the treatment of idiopathic dystonia. *Advances in Neurology*, **50**, 561–570.

Lang, A.E. and Riley, D.E. (1992) Tizanidine in cranial dystonia. *Clinical Neuropharmacology*, **15** (2), 142–147.

Lang, A.E., Sheehy, M.P. *et al.* (1982) Anticholinergics in adult-onset focal dystonia. *The Canadian Journal of Neurological Sciences*, **9** (3), 313–319.

Lang, A.E., Sheehy, M.P. *et al.* (1983) Acute anticholinergic action in focal dystonia. *Advances in Neurology*, **37**, 193–200.

Lucetti, C., Nuti, A. *et al.* (2000) Mexiletine in the treatment of torticollis and generalized dystonia. *Clinical Neuropharmacology*, **23** (4), 186–189.

Mandell, S. (1970) The treatment of dystonia with L-dopa and haloperidol. *Neurology*, **20** (11), 103–106.

Marsden, C.D., Marion, M.H. *et al.* (1984) The treatment of severe dystonia in children and adults. *Journal of Neurology, Neurosurgery, and Psychiatry*, **47** (11), 1166–1173.

Meythaler, J.M., Guin-Renfroe, S. *et al.* (1999) Long-term continuously infused intrathecal baclofen for spastic-dystonic hypertonia in traumatic brain injury: 1-year experience. *Archives of Physical Medicine and Rehabilitation*, **80** (1), 13–19.

Mubaidin, A.F. (2000) Alcohol with xylocaine for treatment of eyelid dystonia. *European Journal of Neurology*, **7** (2), 213–215.

Muller, J., Wenning, G.K. *et al.* (2002) Riluzole therapy in cervical dystonia. *Movement Disorders*, **17** (1), 198–200.

Murase, N., Rothwell, J.C. *et al.* (2005) Subthreshold low-frequency repetitive transcranial magnetic stimulation over the premotor cortex modulates writer's cramp. *Brain*, **128** (Pt 1), 104–115.

Narayan, R.K., Loubser, P.G. *et al.* (1991) Intrathecal baclofen for intractable axial dystonia. *Neurology*, **41** (7), 1141–1142.

Nygaard, T.G., Trugman, J.M. *et al.* (1990) Dopa-responsive dystonia: the spectrum of clinical manifestations in a large North American family. *Neurology*, **40** (1), 66–69.

Ohara, S., Hayashi, R. *et al.* (1998) Mexiletine in the treatment of spasmodic torticollis. *Movement Disorders*, **13** (6), 934–940.

Ohara, S., Miki, J. *et al.* (1997) Treatment of spasmodic torticollis with mexiletine: a case report. *Movement Disorders*, **12** (3), 466–469.

Okun, M.S., Nadeau, S.E. *et al.* (2002) Immobilization dystonia. *Journal of the Neurological Sciences*, **201** (1–2), 79–83.

Paleacu, D., Giladi, N. *et al.* (2004) Tetrabenazine treatment in movement disorders. *Clinical Neuropharmacology*, **27** (5), 230–233.

Papapetropoulos, S. and Singer, C. (2006) Improvement of cervico-trunco-brachial segmental dystonia with topiramate. *Journal of Neurology*, **253** (4), 535–536.

Pesenti, A., Barbieri, S. *et al.* (2004) Limb immobilization for occupational dystonia: a possible alternative treatment for selected patients. *Advances in Neurology*, **94**, 247–254.

Pohl, C., Happe, J. *et al.* (2002) Cooling improves the writing performance of patients with writer's cramp. *Movement Disorders*, **17** (6), 1341–1344.

Povlsen, U.J. and Pakkenberg, H. (1990) Effect of intravenous injection of biperiden and clonazepam in dystonia. *Movement Disorders*, **5** (1), 27–31.

Priori, A., Pesenti, A. *et al.* (2001) Limb immobilization for the treatment of focal occupational dystonia. *Neurology*, **57** (3), 405–409.

Ranawaya, R. and Lang, A. (1991) Usefulness of a writing device in writer's cramp. *Neurology*, **41** (7), 1136–1138.

Reeves, R.R. and Liberto, V. (2003) Treatment of essential blepharospasm with quetiapine. *Movement Disorders*, **18** (9), 1072–1073.

Santiago-Palma, J., Hord, E.D. *et al.* (2004) Respiratory distress after intrathecal baclofen withdrawal. *Anesthesia and Analgesia*, **99** (1), 227–229.

Schneider, S.A., Mohire, M.D. *et al.* (2006) Familial dopa-responsive cervical dystonia. *Neurology*, **66** (4), 599–601.

Shirzadi, A.A. and Ghaemi, S.N. (2006) Side effects of atypical antipsychotics: extrapyramidal symptoms and the metabolic syndrome. *Harvard Review of Psychiatry*, **14** (3), 152–164.

Siebner, H.R., Tormos, J.M. *et al.* (1999) Low-frequency repetitive transcranial magnetic stimulation of the motor cortex in writer's cramp. *Neurology*, **52** (3), 529–537.

Tas, N., Karatas, G.K. *et al.* (2001) Hand orthosis as a writing aid in writer's cramp. *Movement Disorders*, **16** (6), 1185–1189.

Taub, E., Uswatte, G. *et al.* (2006) The learned nonuse phenomenon: implications for rehabilitation. *Eura Medicophys*, **42** (3), 241–256.

Taub, E., Uswatte, G. *et al.* (2003) Improved motor recovery after stroke and massive cortical reorganization following Constraint-Induced Movement therapy. *Physical Medicine and Rehabilitation Clinics of North America*, **14** (1 Suppl), S77–S91 ix.

Taub, E., Uswatte, G. *et al.* (1999) Constraint-Induced Movement Therapy: a new family of techniques with broad application to physical rehabilitation – a clinical review. *Journal of Rehabilitation Research & Development*, **36** (3), 237–251.

Thiel, A., Dressler, D. *et al.* (1994) Clozapine treatment of spasmodic torticollis. *Neurology*, **44** (5), 957–958.

Tinazzi, M., Zarattini, S. *et al.* (2005) Long-lasting modulation of human motor cortex following prolonged transcutaneous electrical nerve stimulation (TENS) of forearm muscles: evidence of reciprocal inhibition and facilitation. *Experimental Brain Research*, **161** (4), 457–464.

Tinazzi, M., Zarattini, S. *et al.* (2006) Effects of transcutaneous electrical nerve stimulation on motor cortex excitability in writer's cramp: neurophysiological and clinical correlations. *Movement Disorders*, **21** (11), 1908–1913.

Trugman, J.M., Leadbetter, R. *et al.* (1994) Treatment of severe axial tardive dystonia with clozapine: case report and hypothesis. *Movement Disorders*, **9** (4), 441–446.

Vender, J.R., Hester, S. *et al.* (2006) Identification and management of intrathecal baclofen pump complications: a comparison of pediatric and adult patients. *Journal of Neurosurgery*, **104** (1 Suppl), 9–15.

Walker, R.H., Danisi, F.O. *et al.* (2000) Intrathecal baclofen for dystonia: benefits and complications during six years of experience. *Movement Disorders*, **15** (6), 1242–1247.

Yoshida, K., Kaji, R. *et al.* (2002) Factors influencing the therapeutic effect of muscle afferent block for oromandibular dystonia and dyskinesia: implications for their distinct pathophysiology. *International Journal of Oral and Maxillofacial Surgery*, **31** (5), 499–505.

Zeuner, K.E., Bara-Jimenez, W. *et al.* (2002) Sensory training for patients with focal hand dystonia. *Annals of Neurology*, **51** (5), 593–598.

Zeuner, K.E. and Hallett, M. (2003) Sensory training as treatment for focal hand dystonia: a 1-year follow-up. *Movement Disorders*, **18** (9), 1044–1047.

Zeuner, K.E., Shill, H.A. *et al.* (2005) Motor training as treatment in focal hand dystonia. *Movement Disorders*, **20** (3), 335–341.

14

Botulinum Toxin for Treatment of Dystonia

Dirk Dressler

Department of Neurology, Hannover Medical School, Hannover, Germany

HISTORY

Botulinum toxin (BT) is infamous for being the compound with the highest toxic potential of any natural or man-made substance, causing the clinical picture of botulism in man and animals. More than 20 years ago this perception changed completely, when BT was first used by Alan B Scott to treat strabismus in children (Scott, Rosenbaum and Collins, 1973; Scott, 1980). After these first courageous trials it became clear that this had established a novel therapeutic principle that could be used in various other pathological conditions caused by muscle hyperactivity. Subsequently BT was used in blepharospasm, hemifacial spasm and cervical dystonia, thus reaching neurology (Frueh *et al.*, 1984; Tsui *et al.*, 1985). Here its use exploded and reached numerous other medical specialties. With its use in crocodile tears, pioneered by M. Mayer in Zurich, exocrine glands became a second principal target tissue. BT's use for treatment of pain syndromes is currently being explored, with some promising perspectives. For most of its indications, BT therapy is the therapy of choice (Dressler, 2000c; Moore and Naumann, 2003). For some it has revolutionized therapy altogether. This, together with its exploding use in cosmetics, has generated an industry with annual sales in excess of 1 billion US dollars. BT's use in dystonia, however, is still one of the most important indications for BT, both with respect to the amount of BT used, as well as with respect to the therapeutic impact generated.

PHARMACOLOGY OF BOTULINUM TOXIN DRUGS

Structure

As shown in Figure 14.1, BT drugs consist of the BT component and of excipients. The BT component, with a molecular weight of 450 kD is formed by botulinum neurotoxin (BNT) and by non-toxic proteins, also known as complexing proteins or complex proteins. BNT consists of a heavy amino acid chain with a molecular weight of 100 kD and a light amino acid chain with a molecular weight of 50 kD interconnected by a single disulfide bridge. Two BT molecules associate to a dimer with a molecular weight of 900 kD (Dressler and Benecke, 2007). In Xeomin®, a BT type A drug, the complexing proteins are removed during the manufacturing process so that Xeomin contains isolated monomenric BNT only. Drugs based on other BT types, including B, contain different complexing protein aggregates, resulting in different molecular weights.

Mode of Action

When a BT drug is injected into a target tissue, it is bound with astounding selectivity to glycoprotein structures located on the cholinergic nerve terminal. Subsequently BNT's light chain is internalized by using synaptic vesicle proteins and syntagmins of the neuron's acetylcholine vesicle recycling mechanism (Dong *et al.*, 2003; Rummel *et al.*, 2004; Mahrhold *et al.*, 2006; Dong *et al.*, 2006). Intracellularly, BT cleaves different proteins of the acetylcholine transport protein cascade (soluble *N*-ethylmaleimide-sensitive fusion attachment protein receptor, SNARE proteins) which transports the acetylcholine vesicle from the intracellular space into the synaptic cleft (Pellizzari *et al.*, 1999). Different BT types target different SNARE proteins. BT interrupts synaptic transmission only temporarily. Structural neuronal changes or functional neuronal impairment other than the synaptic blockade itself cannot be detected. Recently, we therefore suggested classifying BT not as a neurotoxin, but as a temporary

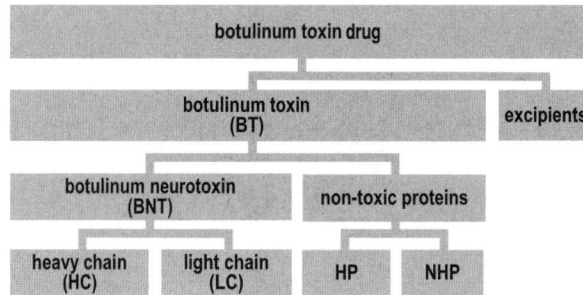

HP: hemagglutinating protein
NHP: non-hemagglutinating protein

Figure 14.1 Contents of botulinum toxin drugs.

neuromodulator (Brin, Dressler and Aoki, 2004). BT can block cholinergic neuromuscular transmission, but also the cholinergic autonomic innervation of the sweat glands, the tear glands, the salivary glands and the smooth muscles, depending on the target tissue selected.

Apart from a direct action upon striated muscles, BT can act upon the muscle spindle organ reducing its centripetal information traffic (Filippi *et al.*, 1993; Dressler *et al.*, 1993; Rosales *et al.*, 1996). Whether this is relevant to BT's therapeutic action remains unclear (Kaji *et al.*, 1995a, 1995b). Although BT can produce numerous indirect central nervous system effects, direct central nervous system effects beyond the α motoneuron have not been described after intramuscular injection (Wiegand, Erdmann and Wellhoner, 1976). Although BT is transported centripetally by mechanisms of retrograde axonal transport, BT is inactivated by the time it reaches the central nervous system. Affection of the central nervous system via transport through the blood–brain barrier is excluded due to BTs molecular size.

Time Course of Action

After intramuscular injection, initial BT effects can be detected within two to three days, depending on the detection method used. BT reaches its maximal effect after about two weeks, maintains this effect and then gradually starts to decline after two to two and a half months. BT injections into glandular tissue can exert prolonged effects of up to six or nine months. BTs action follows a dose–effect correlation (Dressler and Rothwell, 2000). An additional dose–duration correlation can also be assumed. Both correlations are valid only within certain limits. Although there may be considerable interindividual variability of the duration of action there is remarkable intraindividual reproducibility of the duration of action throughout years of continued treatment.

In addition to the blockade of the acetylcholine secretion, animal experiments indicate BT-induced blockades of transmitters involved in pain perception, pain transmission and pain processing (Shone and Melling, 1992; McMahon, Foran and Dolly, 1992; Ishikawa *et al.*, 2000; Purkiss *et al.*, 2000; Welch, Purkiss and Foster, 2000; Morris, Jobling and Gibbins, 2001; Cui *et al.*, 2002). Whether these data can be translated into genuine clinical nociceptive effects in humans remains open at this point in time.

Botulinum Toxin Drugs

BT drugs are either based upon BT-A, such as Botox® (Allergan Inc., Irvine, CA, USA), Dysport® (Ipsen Ltd, Slough, Berks, UK) and Xeomin (Merz Pharmaceuticals, Frankfurt/M, Germany), or upon BT-B, such as Neurobloc/MyoBloc® (Solstice Neurosciences Inc., Malvern, PA, USA). Additional BT drugs are being distributed in fringe markets. As shown in Table 14.1 the properties of the different BT drugs are similar. Differences include antigenicity, adverse effect profiles, adverse effect frequency, injection site pain, storage conditions, mode of preparation, pharmacological stability and potency labelling. Although all these drugs are based upon BT they are not generics. They can be compared in principle and they can be interchanged in an ongoing therapy, but certain differences have to be taken into account. By no means can this comparison be unimodal. Current understanding suggests that Botox and Xeomin have similar therapeutic effects and adverse effect profiles (Benecke *et al.*, 2005; Dressler and Adib Saberi, 2006). Their potency labelling is identical, making exchanges between the two products particularly easy. Based upon previous observations (Jankovic etc) Xeomin should have a reduced antigenicity as compared to conventional BT drugs. Dysport also has a similar therapeutic profile to Botox. Its potency labelling is still a matter of debate. Compared conversion ratio

Table 14.1 Properties of different botulinum toxin drugs.

	Botox	Dysport	Xeomin	NeuroBloc Myobloc
Manufacturer	Allergan Inc.	Ipsen Ltd	Merz Pharmaceuticals	Solstice Neurosciences Inc.
Pharmaceutical preparation	Powder	Powder	Powder	Ready-to-use solution 5000 MU-E/ml
Storage conditions	Below 8 °C	Below 8 °C	Below 25 °C	Below 8 °C
Shelf life	36 months	24 months	36 months	24 months
Botulinum toxin type	A	A	A	B
SNARE target	SNAP25	SNAP25	SNAP25	VAMP
pH-value of the reconstituted preparation	7.4	7.4	7.4	5.6
Stabilization	Vacuum drying	Freeze-drying (lyophilisate)	Vacuum drying	pH-reduction
Excipients	Human serum albumin 500 ug/vial NaCl 900 ug/vial Buffer system	Human serum albumin 125 ug/vial Lactose 2500 ug/vial Buffer system	Human serum albumin 1000 µg/vial Sucrose 4.7 mg/vial Buffer system	Human serum albumin 500 µg/ml Disodium succinate 0.01 M Sodium chloride 0.1 M H_2O Hydrochloric acid
Biological activity	100 MU-A/vial	500 MU-I/vial	100 MU-M/vial	1.0/2.5/10.0 kMU-E/vial
Biological activity in relation to Botox	1	1/3	1	1/40
Specific biological activity	60 MU-EV/ngBNT	100 MU-EV/ngBNT	167 MU-EV/ngBNT	5 MU-EV/ngBNT

BNT: botulinum neurotoxin; MU-A: mouse unit in the Allergan mouse lethality assay; MU-E: mouse unit in the Solstice mouse lethality assay; MU-I: mouse unit in the Ipsen mouse lethality assay; MU-M: mouse unit in the Merz mouse lethality assay; MU-EV: approximate equivalence mouse unit, 1 MU-EV = 1 MU-A = 1 MU-M = 3 MU-I = 40 MU-E.

between the mouse units measured by Allergan for Botox and the mouse units measured by Ipsen for Dysport of 1:3 is currently assumed. Adverse effect differences between Botox and Dysport will be discussed below. Neurobloc/ MyoBloc's potency labelling can be compared to that of Botox by using an approximate conversion ratio of 1:40. It has a high antigenicity (Dressler, Benecke and Bigalke, 2003; Dressler and Bigalke, 2004). Its disadvantageous adverse effect profile will also be discussed below. Therefore, Neurobloc/MyoBloc can only be recommended for those dystonia patients with complete secondary therapy failure due to formation of antibodies against BT-A.

Antigenicity

Since BT consists of foreign proteins, antibodies can be formed against both BNT and the non-toxic proteins. Antibodies formed against BNT (BNT-AB) block the biological activity and, thus, produce antibody-induced

therapy failure (ABTF). BNT-AB are therefore called blocking or neutralizing antibodies. BNT-AB and BT are in a functional balance (Dressler et al., 2002). The therapeutic relevance of BNT-AB titres therefore depend on their titres. Antibodies formed against the non-toxic proteins do not interfere with BTs biological activity and are called non-neutralizing antibodies.

Risk factors for ABTF include the amount of BT applied at each injection series (single dose), the interinjection interval (Dressler and Dirnberger, 2000) and the immunological quality of the BT drug, as described by their specific biological activity. The specific biological activity varies substantially between different therapeutic preparations, as shown in Table 14.1 (Jankovic, Vuong and Ahsan, 2003; Pickett, Panjwani and O'Keeffe, Nov. 2003; Setler, 2000; Dressler and Benecke, 2006). A probable risk factor for ABTF is the reaginability of the immune system of the individual patient (Dressler, 2000; Dressler, 2004). Potential risk factors include the target tissue, that is, intradermal, intramuscular or intraglandular injections, and female sex. Cumulative dose, treatment time and patient age have been explicitly excluded as risk factors. Recent analysis revealed that ABTF usually develops within the first two to three years of BT therapy (Dressler, 2002a). After a treatment time of more than five years ABTF becomes extremely rare.

Safety Aspects and Adverse Effects

Based upon a broad therapeutic window and strictly local effects, avoiding contact with excretion organs, BT excels with a remarkably advantageous adverse effects profile. Adverse effects can be classified as obligate, local or systemic. Obligate adverse effects are inborn effects caused by the therapeutic principle itself. Local adverse effects are caused by diffusion of BT from the target tissue into adjacent tissues. Systemic adverse effects are adverse effects in tissues distant from the injection site requiring a BT transport within the blood circulation. BT adverse effects occur in a typical time window, starting one week after BT application and usually lasting for one to two weeks. Severity and duration of adverse effects depend on the BT dose applied, the target tissue and the adjacent tissues. Central nervous system adverse effects have not been reported so far.

After intramuscular application BT is transported centripetally (Wiegand, Erdmann and Wellhoner, 1976). However, this transport is so slow that BT is inactivated by the time it reaches the spinal cord. A transsynaptic transport beyond the α motoneuron has not been demonstrated. Systemic spread of BT becomes clinically relevant only when the doses applied are very high. The use of BT during pregnancy is contraindicated as a precautionary measure until further experience is gained. A few accidental BT applications during pregnancies, however, did not induce any developmental abnormalities. Extremely rarely, BT applications appear to trigger acute autoimmune reactions with brachial plexopathies or with dermatomyositis (Probst et al., 2002). If plexopathies occur, continuation of BT therapy seems to be safe, since re-occurrence is rare.

Caution is required when using BT in patients with pre-existing pareses, as in amyotrophic lateral sclerosis, myopathies and motor polyneuropathies, or in patients with impaired neuromuscular transmission, such as myasthenia gravis and Lambert–Eaton syndrome (Erbguth et al., 1993). Warnings not to use BT in patients receiving aminoglycoside antibiotics seem theoretical.

With large numbers of patients being treated over prolonged periods of time, long-term experience is ample, and does not indicate additional adverse effects (Naumann et al., 2006).

All therapeutic BT-A preparations have similar adverse effect profiles. However, observations suggest an increased frequency of local adverse effects after Dysport as compared to Botox (Dressler, 2002b). In doses of more than 1500 MU, Dysport can produce systemic motor adverse effects not seen with other BT-A drugs. Reasons for these observations are unclear, but may include increased diffusion, as demonstrated in animal experiments (Brin, Dressler and Aoki, 2004), or conversion factors incorrectly underestimating Dysport's biological activity. Based upon a conversion factor of 1:1, the adverse effect profiles of Xeomin and of Botox are identical (Benecke et al., 2005; Dressler and Adib Saberi, 2006). The adverse effect profiles of therapeutic BT-B drugs are substantially different from the adverse effect profiles of therapeutic BT-A drugs. Whereas even low and intermediate BT-B doses frequently produce autonomic adverse effects, including dryness of mouth, corneal irritation, accommodation difficulties and irritation of the nasal or genital mucosa, the frequencies of motor adverse effects are similar after BT-B and BT-A (Dressler and Benecke, 2003). Comparison of injection sites and localization of autonomic adverse effects suggests a systemic spread of BT-B. Whereas BT-A has a relatively strong effect on the motor system and a relatively weak effect on the autonomic nervous system, this correlation is reversed in BT-B (Dressler and Benecke, 2006). Because of its systemic autonomic adverse effects BT-B should be used with caution in patients with pre-existing autonomic dysfunction or in connection with anticholinergics.

Therapeutic Profile

With the features described above the therapeutic profile of BT can be summarized as shown in Table 14.2. BT can be used in muscles, exocrine glands and, potentially, structures associated with pain. BT's therapeutic effect follows a time course that is remarkably reproducible in the individual patient, but shows considerable interindividual variability. When BT is injected into muscle tissue it produces a peripheral paresis. This paresis manifests clinically after a few days, reaches its maximum after one to two weeks, is usually stable for six to twelve weeks and then gradually resolves over several weeks. The extent of the therapeutic effect is well controlled by the amount of BT applied and its duration can be controlled within limits. Adverse effects are benign and fully reversible. With BT-B, systemic anticholinergic adverse effects and ABTF are frequent.

BASIC PRINCIPLES OF BOTULINUM TOXIN THERAPY

The Multi-Layer Concept of Dystonia Treatment

BT therapy is an entirely symptomatic treatment. Nevertheless, its use may change the long-term perspective of

Table 14.2 Therapeutic profile of botulinum toxin drugs.

Target tissues	Striate and smooth muscles ("neuromuscular junction")
	Exocrine glands
	Structures involved in generation, perception or transmission of pain
Therapeutic effect	Localized
	Predictable time course
	Fully reversible
	Extent well controllable
	Duration controllable within limits
Adverse effects	Fully reversible
	Obligate adverse effects manageable
	Local adverse effects few
	Systemic adverse effects:
	BT-A: extremely rare
	BT-B: frequent anti-cholinergic adverse effects

Table 14.3 The multi-layer concept of comprehensive dystonia therapy.

Layer	Description	Modalities
1	Anti-dystonic treatment	Botulinum toxin therapy
		Oral drugs
		Intrathecal baclofen
		Surgical interventions
2	Adjuvant drugs	Analgesics
		Anxiolytics
3	Adjuvant treatment	Physiotherapy psychotherapy
4	Adjuvant measures	Social support
		Providing information
		Patient support groups

patient affected. In children, symptomatic suppression of dystonic muscle activity may allow certain motor developments otherwise prevented. In adults it can avoid development of complications that my otherwise dominate the clinical picture. Use of BT therapy early in the course of the condition being treated therefore seems advisable. With its benign adverse effect profile and predominantly peripheral mode of action, it can easily be combined with other anti-dystonic treatment modalities, including oral drug therapy, intrathecal baclofen, and peripheral or central surgical interventions including deep brain stimulation. Adjuvant drugs including analgesics and anxiolytics can become necessary, when the effects of the anti-dystonic drugs are unsatisfactory. Amongst the adjuvant treatments, physiotherapy plays a major role: stretching exercises can increase and maintain joint mobility and training of antagonistic muscles can improve functional capabilities. Re-training the impaired patient's self-perception in space is often essential when BT therapy for cervical dystonia is initiated (Barth and Dressler, 1993). Relaxation exercises can break the vicious circle of motor induction in dystonia. Adjuvant measures include adequate information for the patient and his family about the BT therapy as well as about the treated condition. Sharing a solid information base is a prerequisite for a stable patient–physician relationship, which seems particularly important since dystonia is a chronic condition. Patient support groups have a role to play here. Social support gives advice to the patient about available social

benefits. All this together adds up to the multi-layer treatment concept shown in Table 14.3.

Dosing

BT is a local therapy. Dosing, therefore, depends on two elements, that is, the number of dystonic muscles requiring treatment (target muscles) and the degree of their dystonic involvement. Given the enormous variability of dystonia with respect to localization and intensity, communication of the total dose per patient is mostly irrelevant. Unfortunately, most regulatory authorities and reimbursement authorities have not acknowledged this basic principle, either due to lack of insight or for obvious economic reasons. Only with respect to systemic adverse effects total doses may become relevant. Recently, it has been demonstrated that the use of Xeomin, in total doses of up to 840 MU, is free of any clinically detectable motor or autonomic systemic adverse effects (Dressler and Adib Saberi, 2006). Indirect evidence suggests the same safety margins for Botox (Dressler and Adib Saberi, 2006). With Dysport, occasionally total doses of 1500 MU may produce systemic motor adverse effects. Contrary to these extremely wide safety margins of BT-A drugs, BT-B produces systemic autonomic adverse effects even when low or intermediate doses are applied (Dressler and Benecke, 2003). Although total doses vary substantially between studies treating the same condition, as well as amongst individual patients within the same study, a relatively broad consensus has been reached with respect to the dose range in individual target muscles.

Within these dose ranges the individual dose has to be selected according to the degree of dystonic involvement. Additionally, the individual strength of the patient's target

Table 14.4 Dose modyfyers for botulinum toxin therapy.

Sex	Male	Dose increase
	Female	Dose reduction
Age	Young age	Dose increase
	Old age	Dose reduction
Body weight	High	Dose increase
	Low	Dose reduction
Proportional	High	Dose increase
muscle mass	Low	Dose reduction

These factors, when present, modify the botulinum toxin dose within the recommended dose ranges.

muscles has to be taken into account. It can be predicted by the body weight, sex, age and the proportional muscle mass. These factors can be used as general dose modifiers, as shown in Table 14.4. When neuromuscular transmission is impaired or when underlying paresis is present, dosages need to be reduced further. The individual sensitivity of the target muscles has been corrected for in the tables showing the recommended BT doses.

Planning of Botulinum Toxin Therapy

Planning of BT therapy is based upon identification of target muscles and upon their degree of dystonic involvement. This information can be obtained clinically by describing the dystonic movements or postures. Based upon physiological activation patterns dystonic muscles can be deduced. However, with unphysiological co-activation of agonistic and antagonistic muscles as a key feature of dystonia, this clinical approach obviously has its limitations. An additional problem arises from compensatory muscle activity, which is difficult to identify if the patient is unable to suppress it. Occasionally patients maintain preventive postures to avoid certain postures triggering dystonic muscle activity. The clinical approach does not allow determination of the degree of dystonic involvement. Electromyography may help to plan botulinum toxin therapy (Dressler 2000a). Needle electromyography allows precise target muscle identification and comparison between maximal muscle activation and spontaneous, that is, dystonic, muscle activity, allows calculation of the dystonic involvement. Still, identification of compensatory muscle activation can sometimes be a problem. However, recording of prolonged periods of electromyographic activity often separates between initial dystonic activity and secondary compensatory muscle activity. Target muscle selection by estimation of muscle hypertrophy using tomographic imaging techniques seems inadequate, since muscle hypertrophy is not a necessary feature of dystonic muscle involvement and precise measurement of hypertro-

phy would require muscle relaxation, which dystonic patients usually cannot perform. The planning yields the injection scheme outlining the target muscles with their respective BT doses. This injection scheme is a prediction of the patient's therapeutic response. Based on the individual experience of the injector it may or may not be optimal. Subsequent treatment sessions with a careful evaluation of the previous therapeutic response may improve the original injection scheme. The patient should be aware of this process in order to avoid frustration. If the injector has doubts about the injection scheme, often the decision arises either to use lower doses with reduced efficacy, but reduced adverse effects, or to use higher doses with improved efficacy, but increased adverse effects. If patients are informed about potential adverse effects and their transient and generally benign character, they usually prefer the second option, especially when they have experienced prolonged and frustrating previous treatments. Recommendations occasionally formulated by regulatory authorities not to exceed certain initial total doses and to very gradually build them up, are counterproductive and endanger the patient's compliance.

Once the injection scheme is optimized it should be adhered to unless there is evidence of major changes in the treated symptomatology.

Intramuscular Placement of Botulinum Toxin Drugs

Once the injection scheme has been developed, the BT drugs have to be placed within the target muscles. This can be done by palpation, ideally under voluntary activation of the target muscle, by using surface landmarks or by backtracing the muscle tendons. To identify individual finger muscles repetitive active or passive finger movements may palpation of the target muscles facilitate. In target muscles, in which this is difficult, such as the iliopsoas or the piriformis muscles, or when selective injection of individual finger muscles is required, electromyography using a special injection needle may be required. Simultaneous electric stimulation may be of additional benefit. General use of electromyography to place BT drugs does not seem to be necessary. Whether electromyography-guided BT placement allows a dose reduction needs to be demonstrated. Tomographic imaging has also been suggested for target muscles which are difficult to identify otherwise. Since magnetic resonance imaging may be disturbed by the injection needle, X-ray tomography has been applied. Application of substantial radiation doses, however, limits the use of X-ray techniques, esp. in chronic therapies. Ultrasound techniques seem to be more helpful, especially in children, who may be uncooperative and particularly pain sensitive (Berweck et al., 2002).

The effects of dilution and number of injection sites within a given target muscle have not been well studied so far. It is believed that increased dilution increases diffusion. The injection volumes at each injection site should be manageable. In our experience, injection volumes of 0.5–1.0 ml and 0.1–0.3 ml in facial muscles seem reasonable.

Monitoring of the Therapeutic Effect

Usually the therapeutic effect of BT therapy is evaluated two to four weeks after application by a pre-treatment/post-treatment comparison. Apart from subjective scores reflecting overall outcome or dystonic pain, various objective dystonia rating scales, such as the Tsui Scale (Tsui *et al.*, 1986), the Toronto Western Spasmodic Torticollis Rating Scale (TWSTRS) (Consky *et al.*, 1990) or the Burke–Fahn–Marsden Scale (Burke *et al.*, 1985), have been introduced. The disadvantage of these measurements, taken at discrete time points, is that they do not describe the dynamics of BT therapy, that is, the time it takes for the therapeutic effect to build up and the time when it is waning. In order to construct the integral of the therapeutic effect, we introduced the treatment calendar shown in Figure 14.2.

SPECIFIC INDICATIONS FOR BOTULINUM TOXIN THERAPY IN DYSTONIA

Cranial Dystonias

Cranial dystonias can affect periocular muscles, mandibular muscles and perioral muscles. Rarely, scalp muscles or periauricular muscles are affected (Alonso-Navarro *et al.*, 2007). BT therapy can be used in all of these conditions successfully, either when they occur in isolation or when they occur in various combinations. Cranial target muscles with their recommended doses are shown in Tables 14.5 and 14.6. For anatomical information referral to anatomic atlases or special electromyographer's handbooks is advisable.

In periocular dystonia, producing the classical clinical picture of blepharospasm, BT is injected into the orbicularis oculi muscle responsible for eyelid closure (Frueh *et al.*, 1984; Costa *et al.*, 2005). Additional target muscles include the procerus and the corrugator supercilii muscles which form the horizontal and vertical nasal root folds and narrow the eyebrows. They may produce tension, but don't have much influence on eyelid function. The nasalis muscle forms the longitudinal nasal dorsum fold and can be injected when the patient complains of irritation, especially when wearing glasses. The frontalis muscle is an accessory eyelid opening muscle and, therefore, should not be injected in blepharospasm against occasional contrary belief. Doses, dilutions and injection points for the treatment of blepharopsasm vary considerably, whereas results and adverse effects are surprisingly similar. Adverse effects include ptosis, double vision, lagophthalmus and hema-

toma. They are rare and transient. Ptosis can almost certainly be avoided by sparing the midline part of the upper eyelid. Some patients with blepharospasm, especially those with progressive supranuclear palsy, have a varying degree of additional apraxia of eyelid opening (Aramideh *et al.*, 1994), that is, a supranuclear impairment of the eyelid opening mechanism. In those patients, additional BT injections close to the rim of the eyelid are helpful (Jankovic, 1996). If this strategy does not produce satisfactory results, a bilateral suspension operation connecting the upper eyelid to the frontalis muscle by a subcutaneous non-resorbable thread is helpful (Roggenkämper and Nüssgens, 1993). In mild cases, a wire spring attached to a glass's frame can have a similar effect.

In perioral dystonia, muscles above the oral orifice should generally be injected with special care, in order to avoid drooping of the mouth. BT injections into the upper lip may produce paresthesias for unknown reasons. The risorius muscle can be injected safely 2 cm lateral to the corner of the mouth, whereas injections into the depressor labii inferioris bear the risk of instability of the lower lip.

In mandibular dystonia, a jaw-opening form can be distinguished from a jaw-closing form (Marsden, 1976). Combined activation of opening and closing muscles, however, are not infrequent. Additional jaw movements include jaw protrusion and lateral shifts of the jaw. Jaw closing is caused by activation of the masseter, the temporalis and—to a minor extent—the medial pterygoid muscles. Jaw opening is the result of activation of the lateral pterygoid muscle and the the suprahyoid muscles forming the muscular floor of the cavity of the mouth. Protrusion and lateral shifts are caused by the pterygoid muscles, mainly the lateral ones. Whereas treatment of the jaw-closing type produces excellent results with only rare adverse effects, treatment of the jaw-opening type is less rewarding. Our experience indicates that BT injections into the pterygoid muscles through the incisura mandibulae together with injections of the suprahyoid muscles seem to work best in this situation. Attempts to inject the lateral and the medial pterygoid muscles separately cause major technical problems and discomfort for the patient. Local spread and frequent co-activation of both muscles question the logic of this approach.

Pharyngolaryngeal Dystonia

Tonic or clonic dystonia of the pharynx can produce dysphagia and dyspnea (Zwirner and Dressler, 1995). They can occur spontaneously or in an action-induced fashion. BT injections into the posterior pharynx can easily be placed transorally and are effective. Doses range between 20–40 MU of Botox. Laryngeal dystonia produces the clinical picture of spasmodic dysphonia, either in the adductor form with a strained-strangled voice or in the much less

DAY	DYSTONIA-SYMPTOMS (in percent of maximal untreated dystonia symptoms)	REMARKS
1	0 5 10 15 20 25 30 35 40 45 50 55 60 65 70 75 80 85 90 95 100	
2	0 5 10 15 20 25 30 35 40 45 50 55 60 65 70 75 80 85 90 95 100	
3	0 5 10 15 20 25 30 35 40 45 50 55 60 65 70 75 80 85 90 95 100	
4	0 5 10 15 20 25 30 35 40 45 50 55 60 65 70 75 80 85 90 95 100	
5	0 5 10 15 20 25 30 35 40 45 50 55 60 65 70 75 80 85 90 95 100	
6	0 5 10 15 20 25 30 35 40 45 50 55 60 65 70 75 80 85 90 95 100	
7	0 5 10 15 20 25 30 35 40 45 50 55 60 65 70 75 80 85 90 95 100	
8	0 5 10 15 20 25 30 35 40 45 50 55 60 65 70 75 80 85 90 95 100	
9	0 5 10 15 20 25 30 35 40 45 50 55 60 65 70 75 80 85 90 95 100	
10	0 5 10 15 20 25 30 35 40 45 50 55 60 65 70 75 80 85 90 95 100	
11	0 5 10 15 20 25 30 35 40 45 50 55 60 65 70 75 80 85 90 95 100	
12	0 5 10 15 20 25 30 35 40 45 50 55 60 65 70 75 80 85 90 95 100	
13	0 5 10 15 20 25 30 35 40 45 50 55 60 65 70 75 80 85 90 95 100	
14	0 5 10 15 20 25 30 35 40 45 50 55 60 65 70 75 80 85 90 95 100	
15	0 5 10 15 20 25 30 35 40 45 50 55 60 65 70 75 80 85 90 95 100	
16	0 5 10 15 20 25 30 35 40 45 50 55 60 65 70 75 80 85 90 95 100	
17	0 5 10 15 20 25 30 35 40 45 50 55 60 65 70 75 80 85 90 95 100	
18	0 5 10 15 20 25 30 35 40 45 50 55 60 65 70 75 80 85 90 95 100	
19	0 5 10 15 20 25 30 35 40 45 50 55 60 65 70 75 80 85 90 95 100	
20	0 5 10 15 20 25 30 35 40 45 50 55 60 65 70 75 80 85 90 95 100	
21	0 5 10 15 20 25 30 35 40 45 50 55 60 65 70 75 80 85 90 95 100	
22	0 5 10 15 20 25 30 35 40 45 50 55 60 65 70 75 80 85 90 95 100	
23	0 5 10 15 20 25 30 35 40 45 50 55 60 65 70 75 80 85 90 95 100	
24	0 5 10 15 20 25 30 35 40 45 50 55 60 65 70 75 80 85 90 95 100	
25	0 5 10 15 20 25 30 35 40 45 50 55 60 65 70 75 80 85 90 95 100	
26	0 5 10 15 20 25 30 35 40 45 50 55 60 65 70 75 80 85 90 95 100	
27	0 5 10 15 20 25 30 35 40 45 50 55 60 65 70 75 80 85 90 95 100	
28	0 5 10 15 20 25 30 35 40 45 50 55 60 65 70 75 80 85 90 95 100	
29	0 5 10 15 20 25 30 35 40 45 50 55 60 65 70 75 80 85 90 95 100	
30	0 5 10 15 20 25 30 35 40 45 50 55 60 65 70 75 80 85 90 95 100	
31	0 5 10 15 20 25 30 35 40 45 50 55 60 65 70 75 80 85 90 95 100	

Figure 14.2 Patient diary to monitor the effects of botulinum toxin therapy over time.

frequent abductor form with hypophonia (Marsden and Sheehy, 1982). In adductor forms, 2.5–10 MU of Botox are administered into the thyroarytenoid (vocalis) muscle. Unilateral application appears to produce fewer adverse effects than when the same amount is distributed over both sides. In abductor forms, 2.5–10 MU of Botox are administered into the posterior cricoarytenoid muscle unilaterally in order to avoid dyspnea. BT application can be performed perorally or transcutaneously using electromyographic guidance. The transoral approach allows detection of additional dystonic muscle activities in the pharynx or the larynx and, therefore, seems to be the superior method.

For the patient and for the physician, BT therapy of spasmodic dysphonia represents a very satisfying indication (Whurr, Nye and Lorch, 1998). Practically all patients benefit, and the degree of improvement is astonishing. In many cases almost normal speech patterns can be regained. In patients with abductor forms, the treatment results are less favorable. Adverse effects include difficulties with swallowing liquids or solid food and dyspnea.

Injections also can induce weakness of coughing and some pain at the injection side. In treatment of adductor forms, hoarseness, breathiness of voice and hypophonia can occur. For this reason BT therapies for abductor forms should only be carried out by qualified personnel in selected institutions.

Spasmodic laryngeal dyspnea describes spontaneously occurring or respiration-induced muscle hyperactivity of laryngeal muscles (Zwirner, Dressler and Kruse, 1997). This condition is very rare and may affect both glottic and supraglottic muscles, but can also be treated with BT therapy.

Cervical Dystonia

Cervical dystonia consists of torticollis, that is, rotation of the head on a transversal plane, antecollis or retrocollis, that is, flexion or extension of the head in a sagittal plane, and laterocollis, that is, flexion of the head in a frontal plane. Protrusion describes an anterior shift of the head on a

Table 14.5 Recommended botulinum toxin doses in cranial muscles.

Muscle	Function	Recommended dose [MU-A Botox]
Orbicularis oculi	Eyelid closure	12–64
Procerus	Formation of horizontal nasal root fold	4–12
Corrugator supercilii	Eyebrow adduction	8–16
Nasalis (transversal part)	Formation of longitudinal nasal dorsum fold	8–12
Risorius	Corner of mouth abduction	4–8
Depressor anguli oris	Corner of mouth depression	4–12
Depressor labii inferioris	Stabilisation of lower lip	4–8
Mentalis	Formation of chin dimples	8–12
Platysma	Formation of neck skin profile	20–60

MU-A: mouse unit of the mouse bioassay of Allergan Inc.
Dilution: 100 MU-A in 2.5 ml 0.9% NaCl/H$_2$O.

Table 14.6 Recommended botulinum toxin doses in mandibular muscles.

Muscle	Function	Recommended dose [MU-A Botox]
Masseter	Jaw closing	20–60
Temporalis	Jaw closing	40–80
Pterygoidei (per side)	Jaw protrusion Jaw lateralization Jaw opening Jaw closing	20–40
Supra- and infrahyoid muscles (per side)	Jaw opening	20–60

MU-A: mouse unit of the mouse bioassay of Allergan Inc.
Dilution: 100 MU-A in 2.5 ml 0.9% NaCl/H$_2$O.

transversal plane. Isolated occurrence of these elements is rare. Most patients suffer from a combination of two or more of these elements.

Torticollis is caused by activation of the ipsilateral splenius capitis and the contralateral sternocleidomastoid muscles and the ipsilateral trapezius/semispinalis capitis muscle complex. Deep posterior neck muscles arising from the atlas and the axis, including the obliquus capitis inferior, the rectus capitis posterior major and the rectus capitis posterior minor muscles, are strong ipsilateral head rotators. The levator scapulae muscle is an additional, but weaker, ipsilateral head rotator. In torticollis the role of the sternocleidomastoid is often overestimated, whereas the role of the splenius capitis muscle and the deep posterior neck muscles is often underestimated. Antecollis is caused by activation of the supra- and infrahyoid muscles, the scalenii and deep anterior neck muscles, including the longus colli, the longus capitis and the rectus capitis anterior muscles. Retrocollis originates from bilateral activation of the trapezius/semispinalis capitis muscle complex, the splenius capitis muscle and

the deep posterior neck muscles. Laterocollis originates from ipsilateral activation of the sternocleidomastoid, scalenii, levator scapulae, splenius capitis muscles and the trapezius/semispinalis capitis muscle complex. Protrusion is the consequence of bilateral sternocleidomastoid muscle activation.

Planning of BT therapy for cervical dystonia includes careful examination of the spontaneous head position, the head position under motor and stress activation, the slow active head movement and the passive head mobility. When dystonia occurs in waves, or when it can be suppressed by gestes antagonistes, the time course of a dystonic build up helps to identify compensatory muscle activity. Slow active movements can identify trigger postures and therefore potential preventive postures. Testing for pre-existent dysphagia identifies patients in which BT application into anterior neck muscles should be performed with caution.

Target muscles and recommended BT doses for cervical muscles are shown in Table 14.7.

Dystonic pain as the leading complaint in most patients with cervical dystonia can almost always be reduced markedly by BT therapy. Residual pain may be caused by secondary degenerative processes or by radicular irritation. Head posture can also be improved substantially. Often, patients report the effects of the first BT applications enthusiastically, most likely due to the contrast to the sometimes prolonged period of insufficient treatment. When they realize that BT therapy is a symptomatic treatment requiring perpetual re-injections, with all their logistic and financial burdens, this honeymoon effect wanes and patients may complain. In those situations demonstrating the untreated symptomatology on video

Table 14.7 Recommended botulinum toxin doses for cervical muscles.

Muscle	Function	Recommended dose [MU-A Botox]
Sternocleidomastoid	Contralateral horizontal head rotation Sagittal head flexion Frontal head flexion	20–80
Splenius capitis	Ipsilateral horizontal Head rotation	20–100
Scalenii	Frontal head flexion Sagittal head flexion	20–60
Levator scapulae	Shoulder elevation Ipsilateral head rotation Frontal head extension	20–80
Trapezius/semispinalis capitis complex	Sagittal head extension Ipsilateral head rotation	20–80
Trapezius, horizontal part	Shoulder elevation Frontal head flexion	40–100

MU-A: mouse unit of the mouse bioassay of Allergan Inc.
Dilution: 100 MU-A in 2.5 ml 0.9% NaCl/H$_2$O.

recordings is helpful. Especially in the treatment of cervical dystonia, additional physiotherapy following the above discussed guidelines is necessary (Barth and Dressler, 1993). Certain forms of cervical dystonia respond less favorably to BT therapy. Antecollis is especially difficult to treat when deep anterior neck muscles are involved, but also alternating types of cervical dystonia may present a therapeutic challenge. In tremor types, sometimes reduced BT doses can be helpful.

The most common adverse effect of BT therapy of cervical dystonia is dysphagia. Depending on the definition of dysphagia and the effort to search for it, its incidence varies greatly. Applying current treatment standards, certainly less than 5% of patients experience dysphagia constantly after each injection series. Occasional dysphagia may be more frequent. Another adverse effect is head instability, especially due to impaired head extension. When these adverse effects occur, their duration is usually limited to one or two weeks. Injection of the scalenii muscles can produce needle contacts with brachial plexus nerve fibers eliciting short-lasting electric sensations.

Arm Dystonia

Arm dystonia can be divided into action-induced and non-action-induced forms. Action-induced forms occur only during certain activities, which can sometimes be highly specific. Non-action-induced forms are not associated with specific activities, although they may be increased by unspecific

physical activity. Writer's cramp is the most common action-induced dystonia (Sheehy, Rothwell and Marsden, 1988). Other highly specific and sometimes peculiar activities can also trigger dystonia, such as playing musical instruments or performing sports. Especially when these activities are performed under professional conditions, dystonia can result and the term occupational cramp can be applied.

In writer's cramp a wrist-flexor and a wrist-extensor type can be distinguished. Additionally, elbow and shoulder muscles may be involved. However, abnormal elbow and shoulder postures may be compensatory, in order to change the writing position and to reduce dystonia. Planning of BT therapy for writer's cramp is based on careful examination of the clinical symptoms. Electromyography can be confusing, since normal writing already generates widespread muscle activation. In experienced hands, however, it can be helpful. Sometimes, asking the patient to write with the contralateral hand produces the dystonic pattern in the dystonic hand without contamination of normal or compensatory muscle activity.

Target muscles and recommended BT doses for arm dystonia are shown in Table 14.8.

Results of BT therapy of writer's cramp are limited, because of narrow therapeutic windows for the potential target muscles (Das, Dressler and Hallett, 2006). This is a problem especially in the finger extensors. Apart from this, writer's cramp frequently affects a large number of forearm muscles. BT therapy targeting all of these muscles would induce major paretic adverse effects. Additionally, distinc-

Table 14.8 Recommended botulinum toxin doses for arm muscles.

Muscle	Function	Recommended dose [MU-A Botox]
Deltoideus	Shoulder abduction	40–120
Pectoralis major et minor	Shoulder adduction	40–120
Teres major	Shoulder inward rotation	40–100
Triceps brachii	Elbow extension	40–100
Biceps brachii	Elbow flexion	40–120
Bachialis	Elbow flexion	40–100
Brachioradialis	Elbow flexion	40–100
Extensor carpi radialis	Wrist extension	20–40
Flexor carpi radialis	Wrist flexion	40–80
Flexor carpi ulnaris	Wrist flexion	40–100
Extensor digitorum profundus et superficialis	Finger extension	20–60
Flexor digitorum profundus et superficialis	Finger flexion	40–200
Interosseus	Metacarpophalangeal adduction Metacarpophalangeal abduction	20
Abductor digiti quinti	Little finger Metacarpophal- angeal abduction	20–40
Flexor pollicis longus	Thumb flexion	20–60

MU-A: mouse unit of the mouse bioassay of Allergan Inc.
Dilution: 100 MU-A in 2.5 ml 0.9% NaCl/H$_2$O.

tion between physiological and dystonic muscle activity and identification of compensatory muscle activity may be difficult. Our experience indicates that even after several modifications of the injection scheme only about one-third of the patients benefit from BT therapy and continue treatment. Results are better when the finger muscles are not involved, that is, when the symptoms are restricted to the wrist or elbow muscles. When finger muscles are involved, the outcome is better when individual finger muscles and when finger flexors rather than finger exten-

sors are dystonic. If the symptoms are restricted to individual finger muscles, electromyography, possibly with additional electric stimulation, may facilitate BT placement. If BT therapy is not successful in treatment of writer's cramp, the patient can shift writing to the contralateral hand. Many patients can permanently use the contralateral hand for writing, whereas some develop writer's cramp in this hand as well within one or two years. Increased use of keyboards is also one option to circumvent writer's cramp. Re-training exercises may also become a therapeutic option in the future (Zeuner *et al.*, 2002).

Treatment of other action-induced arm dystonias, especially when they are occupational, is even more problematic, since the motor performance expected by the patient is usually so high that it cannot be met, either due to dystonic residues or due to therapy-induced paresis (Jabusch *et al.*, 2005).

Non-action-induced arm dystonia usually occurs as part of a spasticity-dystonia syndrome or as idiopathic dystonia. Typical postures include finger flexion, thumb flexion, wrist flexion, elbow flexion and shoulder adduction or abduction. In spasticity-dystonia syndrome, treatment is focused on pain and prevention of contractures. Functional improvement may result, but is often restricted by the underlying paresis.

Leg Dystonia

Leg dystonia can occur in idiopathic, and in symptomatic dystonia, mostly as part of a spasticity-dystonia syndrome due to stroke or cerebral palsy. Action-induced forms are less common. Typical postures include hip adduction, knee flexion, equinovarus posture, that is, the combination of ankle plantar flexion, foot supination and toe flexion, ankle plantar flexion and isolated toe flexion. Hip extension occurs less frequently. Hip adduction is caused by activation of the adductor muscle group (adductor magnus, minimus, longus, brevis and gracilis muscles), knee flexion by activation of the hamstrings (semimembranosus, semitendinosus, biceps femoris muscles) and the equinovarus posture by activation of the tibialis posterior, triceps surae, flexor hallucis and digitorum longus muscles. Ankle plantar flexion is the result of activation of triceps surae, peroneus longus and brevis and flexor digitorum longus muscles, toe flexion of the activation of the flexor digitorum longus and brevis muscles.

Target muscles and recommended BT doses for leg dystonia are shown in Table 14.9.

Hip adduction, ankle plantar flexion and equinovarus postures respond well to BT therapy. Doses, however, may be high, especially when bilateral injections are necessary. BT therapy for knee extension bears the risk of knee weakness, especially in patients with additional paresis as in spasticity-dystonia syndrome after stroke. Toe and great

Table 14.9 Recommended botulinum toxin doses for leg muscles.

Muscle	Function	Recommended dose [MU-A Botox]
Iliopsoas	Hip flexion	100–200
Adductor muscle group	Hip adduction	100–300
Quadriceps femoris	Knee extension	100–300
Hamstring muscles	Knee flexion	100–400
Triceps surae	Ankle plantar flexion	100–200
Tibialis anterior	Ankle dorsiflexion	40–200
Tibialis posterior	Foot supination	60–200
Extensor digitorum longus	Toe extension Ankle dorsiflexion	40–100
Flexor digitorum longus	Toe flexion	40–100
Extensor hallucis longus	Great toe extension Ankle dorsiflexion	40–60
Flexor hallucis longus	Great toe flexion Ankle plantar flexion	60–100

MU-A: mouse unit of the mouse bioassay of Allergan Inc.
Dilution: 100 MU-A in 2.5 ml 0.9% NaCl/H$_2$O.

toe flexion often requires combined treatment of short and long toe and great toe flexors.

Segmental Dystonia, Generalized Dystonia

BT therapy of extended dystonic symptoms usually requires selection of those target muscles that play a major role in functional impairment, pain and prevention of complications. Less relevant target muscles may need to be left untreated in order not to exceed total BT doses that are safe with respect to toxicological and immunological adverse effects. Paravertebral muscles require 40–60 MU Botox per segment per side, the rectus abdominis 40–80 MU Botox per segment per side and the abdominal wall muscle complex (obliqus internus abdominis, obliqus externus abdominis and transversus abdominis muscles) 80–200 MU Botox per side.

Toxicological and immunological safety margins have been discussed above. When safety margins are exploited to their full extent, BT therapy can improve even extended symptoms substantially. In patients requiring excess BT doses, deep brain stimulation may offer a treatment alternative. Combinations of BT therapy and deep brain therapy or intrathecal baclofen are possible.

OUTLOOK

BT therapy presents a novel therapeutic concept. It has revolutionized many medical fields. In dystonia, for the first time, it offers help to large numbers of patients with focal dystonia. In segmental and generalized dystonia, high BT doses are necessary, but emerging experience suggests these can be immunologically and toxicologically safe. The recent introduction of low antigenicity BT drugs may allow booster injections for rapid dose adaptation, reduced inter-injection intervals for improved dynamic adjustment and increased dose for treatment of extended symptoms. High affinity BT drugs may improve antigenicity even further. They may reduce the threshold for systemic toxicology so that higher total BT doses may be applied.

References

Alonso-Navarro, H., Puertas, I., Cabrera-Valdivia, F., de Toledo-Heras, M., García-Albea, E. and Jiménez-Jiménez, F.J. (2007) Posterior auricular muscle 'dystonia'. *European Journal of Neurology*, **14**, e14–e15.

Aramideh, M., Ongerboer de Visser, B.W., Koelman, J.H., Bour, L.J., Devriese, P.P. and Speelman, J.D. (1994) Clinical and electromyographic features of levator palpebrae superioris muscle dysfunction in involuntary eyelid closure. *Movement Disorders*, **9**, 395–402.

Barth, K. and Dressler, D. (1993) Die krankengymnastische Zusammenarbeit mit Schiefhalspatienten nach der Behandlung mit Botulinum Toxin. *Krankengymnastik*, **45**, 134–142.

Benecke, R., Jost, W.H., Kanovsky, P., Ruzicka, E., Comes, G. and Grafe, S. (2005) A new botulinum toxin type A free of complexing proteins for treatment of cervical dystonia. *Neurology*, **64**, 1949–1951.

Berweck, S., Feldkamp, A., Francke, A., Nehles, J., Schwerin, A. and Heinen, F. (2002) Sonography-guided injection of botulinum toxin A in children with cerebral palsy. *Neuropediatrics*, **2002**, **33**, 221–223.

Brin, M.F., Dressler, D. and Aoki, R. (2004) Pharmacology of botulinum toxin therapy, in *Dystonia: Etiology, Clinical Features, and Treatment* (eds J. Jankovic, C. Comella and M.F. Brin), Lippincott Williams & Wilkins, Philadelphia, pp. 93–112.

Burke, R.E., Fahn, S., Marsden, C.D., Bressman, S.B., Moskowitz, C. and Friedman, J. (1985) Validity and reliability of a rating scale for the primary torsion dystonias. *Neurology*, **35**, 73–77.

Consky, E.S., Basinki, A., Belle, L., Ranawaya, R. and Lang, A.E. (1990) The Toronto Westrn Spasmodic Torticollis Rating Scale (TWSTRS): assessment of validity and inter-rater reliability. *Neurology*, **40** (Suppl 1), 445.

Costa, J., Espírito-Santo, C., Borges, A., Ferreira, J.J., Coelho, M., Moore, P. and Sampaio, C. (2005) Botulinum toxin type A therapy for blepharospasm. *Cochrane Database of Systematic Reviews*, **1**, CD004900.

Cui, M., Li, Z., You, S., Khanijou, S. and Aoki, R. (2002) Mechanisms of the antinociceptive effect of subcutaneous Botox: inhibition of peripheral and central nociceptive processing. *Archives of Pharmacology*, **365**, R17.

Das, C.P., Dressler, D. and Hallett, M. (2006) Botulinum toxin therapy of writer's cramp. *European Journal of Neurology*, **13** (Suppl 1), 55–59.

Dong, M., Yeh, F., Tepp, W.H., Dean, C., Johnson, E.A., Janz, R. and Chapman, E.R. (2006) SV2 is the protein receptor for botulinum neurotoxin A. *Science*, **312**, 592–596.

Dong, M., Richards, D.A., Goodnough, M.C., Tepp, W.H., Johnson, E.A. and Chapman, E.R. (2003) Synaptotagmins I and II mediate entry of botulinum neurotoxin B into cells. *The Journal of Cell Biology*, **162**, 1293–1303.

Dressler, D. (2000a) Electromyographic evaluation of cervical dystonia for planning of botulinum toxin therapy. *European Journal of Neurology*, **7**, 713–718.

Dressler, D. (2000b) Complete secondary botulinum toxin therapy failure in blepharospasm. *Journal of Neurology*, **247**, 809–810.

Dressler, D. (2000c) *Botulinum Toxin Therapy*, Thieme Verlag, Stuttgart, New York.

Dressler, D. (2002a) Clinical features of secondary failure of botulinum toxin therapy. *European Neurology*, **48**, 26–29.

Dressler, D. (2002b) Dysport produces intrinsically more swallowing problems than Botox: Unexpected results from a conversion factor study in cervical dystonia. *Journal of Neurology, Neurosurgery, and Psychiatry*, **73**, 604.

Dressler, D. (2004) New formulation of BOTOX: Complete antibody-induced therapy failure in hemifacial spasm. *Journal of Neurology*, **251**, 360.

Dressler, D. and Adib Saberi, F. (2006) Safety aspects of high dose Xeomin therapy. *Journal of Neurology*, **253** (Suppl 2), II/141.

Dressler, D. and Benecke, R. (2003) Autonomic side effects of botulinum toxin type B treatment of cervical dystonia and hyperhidrosis. *European Neurology*, **49**, 34–38.

Dressler, D. and Benecke, R. (2006) Xeomin eine neue therapeutische Botulinum Toxin Typ A-Präparation. *Aktuelle Neurologie*, **33**, 138–141.

Dressler, D. and Benecke, R. (2007) Pharmacology of therapeutic botulinum toxin preparations. *Disability and Rehabilitation*, **29**, 1761–1768.

Dressler, D. and Bigalke, H. (2004) Antibody-induced failure of botulinum toxin type B therapy in de novo patients. *European Neurology*, **52**, 132–135.

Dressler, D. and Dirnberger, G. (2000) Botulinum toxin therapy: Risk factors for therapy failure. *Movement Disorders*, **15** (Suppl 2), 51.

Dressler, D. and Eleopra, R. (2006) Clinical use of non-A botulinum toxins: Botulinum toxin type B. *Neurotoxicity Research*, **9**, 121–125.

Dressler, D. and Rothwell, J.C. (2000) Electromyographic quantification of the paralysing effect of botulinum toxin. *European Neurology*, **43**, 13–16.

Dressler, D., Benecke, R. and Bigalke, H. (2003) Botulinum toxin type B (NeuroBloc) in patients with botulinum toxin type A antibody-induced therapy failure. *Journal of Neurology*, **250**, 967–969.

Dressler, D., Eckert, J., Kukowski, B. and Meyer, B.U. (1993) Somatosensorisch Evozierte Potentiale bei Schreibkrampf: Normalisierung pathologischer Befunde unter Botulinum Toxin Therapie. *Zeitschrift für Elektroenzephalographie und Elektromyographie*, **24**, 191.

Dressler, D., Muenchau, A., Bhatia, K.P., Quinn, N.P. and Bigalke, H. (2002) Antibody induced botulinum toxin therapy failure: Can it be overcome by increased botulinum toxin doses? *European Neurology*, **47**, 118–121.

Erbguth, F., Claus, D., Engelhardt, A. and Dressler, D. (1993) Systemic effect of local botulinum toxin injections unmasks subclinical Lambert-Eaton myasthenic syndrome. *Journal of Neurology, Neurosurgery, and Psychiatry*, **56**, 1235–1236.

Filippi, G.M., Errico, P., Santarelli, R., Bagolini, B. and Manni, E. (1993) Botulinum A toxin effects on rat jaw muscle spindles. *Acta Oto-Laryngologica*, **113**, 400–404.

Frueh, B.R., Felt, D.P., Wojno, T.H. and Musch, D.C. (1984) Treatment of blepharospasm with botulinum toxin. A preliminary report. *Archives of Ophthalmology*, **102**, 1464–1468.

Ishikawa, H., Mitsui, Y., Yoshitomi, T., Mashimo, K., Aoki, S., Mukuno, K. and Shimizu, K. (2000) Presynaptic effects of botulinum toxin type A on the neuronally evoked response of albino and pigmented rabbit iris sphincter and dilator muscles. *Japanese Journal of Ophthalmology*, **44**, 106–109.

Jabusch, H.C., Zschucke, D., Schmidt, A., Schuele, S. and Altenmüller, E. (2005) Focal dystonia in musicians: treatment strategies and long-term outcome in 144 patients. *Movement Disorders*, **20**, 1623–1626.

Jankovic, J. (1996) Pretarsal injection of botulinum toxin for blepharospasm and apraxia of eyelid opening. *Journal of Neurology, Neurosurgery, and Psychiatry*, **60**, 704.

Jankovic, J., Vuong, K.D. and Ahsan, J. (2003) Comparison of efficacy and immunogenicity of original versus current botulinum toxin in cervical dystonia. *Neurology*, **60**, 1186–1188.

Kaji, R., Kohara, N., Katayama, M., Kubori, T., Mezaki, T., Shibasaki, H. and Kimura, J. (1995a) Muscle afferent block by intramuscular injection of lidocaine for the treatment of writer's cramp. *Muscle & Nerve*, **18**, 234–235.

Kaji, R., Rothwell, J.C., Katayama, M., Ikeda, T., Kubori, T., Kohara, N., Mezaki, T., Shibasaki, H. and Kimura, J. (1995b) Tonic vibration reflex and muscle afferent block in writer's cramp. *Annals of Neurology*, **138**, 155–162.

Mahrhold, S., Rummel, A., Bigalke, H., Davletov, B. and Binz, T. (2006) The synaptic vesicle protein 2C mediates the uptake of botulinum neurotoxin A into phrenic nerves. *FEBS Letters*, **580**, 2011–2014.

Marsden, C.D. (1976) The problem of adult-onset idiopathic torsion dystonia and other isolated dyskinesias in adult life (including blepharospasm, oromandibular dystonia, dystonic writer's cramp, and torticollis, or axial dystonia). *Advances in Neurology*, **14**, 259–276.

Marsden, C.D. and Sheehy, M.P. (1982) Spastic dysphonia, Meige disease, and torsion dystonia. *Neurology*, **32**, 1202–1203.

McMahon, H., Foran, P. and Dolly, J. (1992) Tetanus toxin and botulinum toxins type A and B inhibit glutamate, gamma-aminobutyric acid, aspartate, and met-enkephalin release from synaptosomes: clues to the locus of action. *The Journal of Biological Chemistry*, **267**, 21338–21343.

Moore, A.P. and Naumann, M. (2003) *Handbook of Botulinum Toxin Treatment*, 2nd edn, Blackwell Science, Malden, MA, USA.

Morris, J., Jobling, P. and Gibbins, I. (2001) Differential inhibition by botulinum neurotoxin A of cotransmitters released from autonomic vasodilator neurons. *American Journal of Physiology. Heart and Circulatory Physiology*, **281**, 2124–2132.

Naumann, M., Albanese, A., Heinen, F., Molenaers, G. and Relja, M. (2006) Safety and efficacy of botulinum toxin type A following long-term use. *European Journal of Neurology*, **13** (Suppl 4), 35–40.

Pellizzari, R., Rossetto, O., Schiavo, G. and Montecucco, C. (1999) Tetanus and botulinum neurotoxins: mechanism of action and therapeutic uses. *Philosophical Transactions of the Royal Society of London. Series B, Biological Sciences*, **354**, 259–268.

Pickett, A., Panjwani, N. and O'Keeffe, R.S. (Nov. 2003) Potency of Type A Botulinum Toxin Preparations in Clinical Use. 40th Annual Meeting of the Interagency Botulism Research Coordinating Committee (IBRCC), Atlanta, USA.

Probst, T.E., Heise, H., Heise, P., Benecke, R. and Dressler, D. (2002) Rare immunologic side effects of botulinum toxin therapy: brachial plexus neuropathy and dermatomyositis. *Movement Disorders*, **17** (Suppl 5), S49.

Purkiss, J., Welch, M., Doward, S. and Foster, K. (2000) Capsaicin-stimulated release of substance P from cultured dorsal root ganglion neurons: involvement of two distinct mechanisms. *Biochemical Pharmacology*, **59**, 1403–1406.

Roggenkämper, P. and Nüssgens, Z. (1993) Frontalis suspension for essential blepharospasm unresponsive to botulinum toxin therapy. First results. *German Journal of Ophthalmology*, **2**, 426–428.

Rosales, R.L., Arimura, K., Takenaga, S. and Osame, M. (1996) Extrafusal and intrafusal muscle effects in experimental botulinum toxin-A injection. *Muscle & Nerve*, **19**, 488–496.

Rummel, A., Karnath, T., Henke, T., Bigalke, H. and Binz, T. (2004) Synaptotagmins I and II act as nerve cell receptors for botulinum neurotoxin G. *The Journal of Biological Chemistry*, **279**, 30865–30870.

Scott, A.B., Rosenbaum, A. and Collins, C.C. (1973) Pharmacologic weakening of extraocular muscles. *Investigative Ophthalmology and Visual Science*, **12**, 924–927.

Scott, A.B. (1980) Botulinum toxin injection into extraocular muscles as an alternative to strabismus surgery. *Journal of Pediatric Ophthalmology & Strabismus*, **17**, 21–25.

Setler, P. (2000) The biochemistry of botulinum toxin type B. *Neurology*, **55** (Suppl 5), S22–S28.

Sheehy, M.P., Rothwell, J.C. and Marsden, C.D. (1988) Writer's cramp. *Advances in Neurology*, **50**, 457–472.

Shone, C.C. and Melling, J. (1992) Inhibition of calcium-dependent release of noradrenaline from PC12 cells by botulinum type-A neurotoxin. Long-term effects of the neurotoxin on intact cells. *European Journal of Biochemistry*, **207**, 1009–1016.

Tsui, J.K., Eisen, A., Mak, E., Carruthers, J., Scott, A. and Calne, D.B. (1985) A pilot study on the use of botulinum toxin in spasmodic torticollis. *The Canadian Journal of Neurological Sciences*, **12**, 314–316.

Tsui, J.K., Eisen, A., Stoessl, A.J., Calne, S. and Calne, D.B. (1986) Double-blind study of botulinum toxin in spasmodic torticollis. *Lancet*, **2** (8501), 245–247.

Welch, M.J., Purkiss, J.R. and Foster, K.A. (2000) Sensitivity of embryonic rat dorsal root ganglia neurons to Clostridium botulinum neurotoxins. *Toxicon*, **38**, 245–258.

Whurr, R., Nye, C. and Lorch, M. (1998) Meta-analysis of botulinum toxin treatment of spasmodic dysphonia: a review of 22 studies. *International Journal of Language and Communication Disorders*, **33** (Suppl), 327–329.

Wiegand, H., Erdmann, G. and Wellhoner, H.H. (1976) 125I-labelled botulinum A neurotoxin: pharmacokinetics in cats after intramuscular injection. *Naunyn-Schmiedeberg's Archives of Pharmacology*, **292**, 161–165.

Zeuner, K.E., Bara-Jimenez, W., Noguchi, P.S., Goldstein, S.R., Dambrosia, J.M. and Hallett, M. (2002) Sensory training for patients with focal hand dystonia. *Annals of Neurology*, **51**, 593–598.

Zwirner, P. and Dressler, D. (1995) Dystonie als Ursache pharyngo-laryngealer Motilitätsstörungen. *HNO*, **43**, 498–501.

Zwirner, P., Dressler, D. and Kruse, E. (1997) Spasmodic laryngeal dyspnea: a rare manifestation of laryngeal dystonia. *European Archives of Oto-Rhino-Laryngology*, **254**, 242–245.

15

Surgical Treatments of Dystonia

Christopher Kenney and Joseph Jankovic

Parkinson's Disease Center and Movement Disorders Clinic,
Department of Neurology, Baylor College of Medicine, Houston, USA

BACKGROUND AND RATIONALE

Numerous surgical interventions have been attempted to control the excessive muscle contractions and significant disability associated with dystonia, especially in medically refractory cases. The history of surgery for dystonia is complex and probably dates back to Minnius in 1641, who sectioned the sternocleidomastoid muscle in an attempt to treat cervical dystonia (Putnam, Herz and Glaser, 1949; Lang, 1998). In the 1950s, Cooper first used an anterior dorsomedial pallidotomy to treat primary generalized dystonia, but eventually determined that lesions involving the medial ventrolateral thalamus were more effective (Cooper, 1976). Over the past decade, there has been a resurgence of interest in surgical options to treat medically refractory dystonia, partly as a result of better understanding of the pathophysiology of dystonia and improved safety and efficacy of deep brain stimulation (DBS) (Kenney et al., 2007).

INTRATHECAL BACLOFEN

Baclofen is a γ-aminobutyric acid (GABA) analog administered orally for a variety of reasons, including dystonia. For dystonic patients that fail to respond to oral medications, intrathecal baclofen (ITB) has been used as an alternative since the first report in 1991, treating a patient with axial dystonia (Narayan et al., 1991). Subsequent studies confirmed the benefits of ITB to treat segmental dystonia, generalized dystonia and secondary dystonia from cerebral palsy, stroke, head trauma and medications (tardive dystonia) (Albright, 1996; Albright et al., 1996; Dressler, Oeljeschlager and Ruther, 1997; Albright et al., 1998; Walker et al., 2000). ITB may be particularly useful when patients display dystonia accompanied by spasticity, such as occurs with cerebral palsy, head trauma and stroke, especially when attempting to improve function of the lower extremities (Meythaler, Guin-Renfroe and Hadley, 1999; Butler and Campbell, 2000). Interestingly, a negative or positive response to oral baclofen does not predict its utility when administered into the intrathecal space (Walker et al., 2000). The medical literature on the use of ITB for dystonia, mostly a decade or more old, discusses small case series, and is not very compelling with regard to efficacy (Narayan et al., 1991; Albright et al., 1996; Ford et al., 1996; Paret et al., 1996; Dressler, Oeljeschlager and Ruther, 1997; Albright et al., 1998; Dalvi, Fahn and Ford, 1998; Siebner et al., 1998; Awaad, Munoz and Nigro, 1999). A relatively small proportion (20–30%) of patients improved objectively using validated clinical scales for dystonia, and predictors of response are not well established. ITB appears to be equally effective for several types of dystonia, regardless of cause (primary generalized, secondary, generalized, and segmental), though patients with tardive dystonia may respond the best (Walker et al., 2000). The use of ITB for dystonia has declined as the popularity of DBS has increased, largely as a function of better efficacy (Vidailhet et al., 2005; Kupsch et al., 2006) and tolerability (Kenney et al., 2007).

Standard procedures at centers implanting ITB dictate proof of unresponsiveness to maximal doses of medications that may improve dystonia: dopaminergic (levodopa), anticholinergic (trihexyphenidyl), GABAergic (benzodiazepine) or dopamine-depleting drug (tetrabenazine) (Jankovic, 2006; Kenney, Hunter and Jankovic 2007). Patients evaluated for ITB should then undergo a trial bolus of baclofen administered directly into the intrathecal space (25–200 µg) which may be repeated on as many as three occasions, if initial trials reveal a lack of response (Walker et al., 2000). A subjective and/or objective improvement is usually necessary to proceed with implantation, but patients have been reported to improve after implantation despite lack of response during the trial infusion (Hou, Ondo and Jankovic, 2001). ITB is then titrated in increments of about

Therapeutics of Parkinson's Disease and Other Movement Disorders   Edited by Mark Hallett and Werner Poewe
© 2008 John Wiley & Sons, Ltd.

10% until the patient experiences a sufficient clinical response or dose-limiting side effects. A maximal ITB dose is approximately 1000 µg/day. Recommendations for optimizing surgical technique are published as the result of a multi-disciplinary conference entitled "ITB Therapy Best Practice Forum" (Albright, Turner and Pattisapu, 2006). The authors suggest subfascial pump placement, insertion of Tuohy needle in an oblique, paramedian trajectory and catheter placement at the spinal cord consistent with the therapeutic indication (C1–4 for generalized dystonia). Other aspects are also addressed including techniques to minimize cerebrospinal fluid leak and prevent infection.

Albright reviewed their six-year, open-label experience with 77 patients treated with ITB for severe generalized dystonia (Albright et al., 2001). Dystonia was graded by the Barry–Albright Scale (Barry, VanSwearingen and Albright, 1999), which revealed improvement that was maintained for two years of follow-up. Quality of life (85%), ease of care (86%) and speech (33%) also improved after ITB. Dystonia improved more in patients with intrathecal catheters positioned at T4 or higher when compared to catheters at T6 or lower. Side effects occurred in 26% of participants: constipation (19%), weakness (8%) and drowsiness (6%). Surgical complications, on the other hand, developed in 38%: catheter malfunction (21%), infection (14%) and cerebrospinal fluid (CSF) leak (8%).

In a more recent publication, Walker and colleagues presented their experience with 14 dystonia patients treated with ITB (primary generalized, $n = 8$; idiopathic cranial segmental dystonia, $n = 1$; and secondary dystonia, $n = 5$) (Walker et al., 2000) They reported a mean dose of patients remaining on ITB of 590 ug/day (range: 50–1000 ug/day). A previous response to oral baclofen did not predict the response to ITB. Some patients responded to oral baclofen, but not ITB and vice versa. The patient that benefited the most had tardive dystonia, but primary and secondary dystonia of various causes responded similarly. Specifically, of the 14 patients, 5 showed objective improvement using blinded video-raters, two unequivocally and the reminder to a lesser degree. Interestingly, four patients with subjective improvement showed either no change or worsening as judged by the Burke–Fahn–Marsden Dystonia Scale (BFMDS). In five patients the BFMDS scores worsened on ITB. It was not clear whether this reflected disease progression or a direct effect of ITB. Six patients experienced complications, two of which required revisions. By the end of the follow-up period (mean: 29 months; range: 6–64 months), only four patients remained on ITB therapy.

In one of the few randomized, double-blind, placebo-controlled studies, Van Hilten studied the efficacy of ITB to treat dystonia in sic patients with reflex sympathetic dystrophy using a crossover trial design (van Hilten et al.,

2000). Each patient received five intrathecal injections: two with placebo and one each with three different doses of ITB (25 ug, 50 ug, and 75 ug). Using a visual analog scale to assess dystonia severity, patients improved more when receiving ITB when compared to placebo. Overall benefit was better with 50 ug compared to 25 ug, but no difference was noted between 50 ug and 75 ug. In the open-label phase, dystonia of the arms improved markedly in six out of seven patients receiving bolus ITB, leg dystonia to a lesser degree. Three patients regained normal hand function, and two regained the ability to walk.

PERIPHERAL SURGERY

Before botulinum toxin revolutionized the treatment of blepharospasm, surgical treatments directed to either nerve or muscle were often employed. Peripheral facial neurectomy involved damaging the nerve with various techniques including alcohol injections, thermolysis, sectioning and avulsion (Lang, 1998). High recurrence and/or complication rates (inability to close eye, excessive tearing and weakness) were fairly high (Bates et al., 1991). As a result of these difficulties, myectomy then became the surgical procedure of choice with partial or complete removal of procerus, corrugator and upper orbicularis oris (Gillum and Anderson, 1981; Grivet et al., 2005). A second procedure (lower myectomy) was performed with resection of tarsal, septal and orbital portions of orbicularis oculi in those not responding to the first (22–35%) (McCord et al., 1984; Jones, Waller and Samples, 1985; Frueh, Musch and Bersani, 1992). In a large series of 400 patients treated with myectomy, approximately 90% experienced improvement of visual disability (Patel and Anderson, 1993). These procedures have been mostly abandoned in light of the robust response that most experience with botulinum toxin injections, although some patients who fail to obtain satisfactory relief with the injections may require myectomy to enable them to keep their eyes open (Figure 15.1) (Kenney and Jankovic, 2007). Patients with co-existing apraxia of eye-lid opening may benefit from blepharoplasty with or without frontalis suspension (De Groot et al., 2000; Kerty and Eidal, 2006).

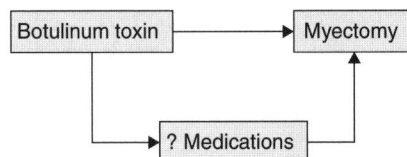

Figure 15.1 Algorithm for the treatment of blepharospasm.

A wide variety of surgical techniques have been attempted to improve cervical dystonia, including myotomy, myectomy, spinal accessory nerve section, anterior cervical rhizotomy, epidural cervical cord stimulation and microvascular decompression of spinal accessory nerve roots (Lang, 1998; Kraus, Grossman and Jankovic, 2001; Meyer, 2001; Taira and Hori, 2001; Braun and Richter, 2002). Surgical sectioning of the sternocleidomastoid was one of the earliest attempts to improve torticollis, but was abandoned because of morbidity and recurrence of symptoms. In 46 patients with cervical dystonia undergoing 70 procedures with intradural denervation approaches in 33 instances, extradural denervation approaches in 21 and myectomy sections (singly or combined) in 22 instances, the global outcome was rated as excellent in nine (21%), marked in 12 (27%), moderate in nine (21%), mild in nine (21%) and no improvement in five (11%) (Krauss et al., 1997). There was a statistically significant improvement for almost all sub-scores of the Toronto Western Spasmodic Torticollis Scale (TWSTRS); also functional disability and pain improved. During the mean duration of long-term follow up of 6.5 years, post-operative complications occurred in 10% of the procedures, and usually resolved shortly after surgery. One patient had a persistent side effect consisting of mild difficulty with balance. In another study involving 15 patients with cervical dystonia, excellent benefit was reported in 13 of the patients after partial resection of upper trapezius, splenius and semispinalis bilaterally while preserving normal posture and mobility during 3–10 years of follow-up (Chen et al., 1991). Neurectomy, and specifically bilateral anterior cervical rhizotomy combined with partial section of the spinal accessory nerve has been employed in most of the peripheral surgeries to treat cervical dystonia with studies ranging from 8 to 58 patients revealing improvement in 0–90% (average 65%) (Meares, 1971; Fabinyi and Dutton, 1980; Hernesniemi and Keranen, 1990; Friedman et al., 1993). Complications of anterior rhizotomies can be fairly disabling, with neck weakness, neck instability (sometimes requiring cervical fusion) shoulder weakness, pain and dysphagia. Barium swallow examinations before anterior rhizotomy revealed mild abnormalities in 68.3% of patients ($n = 41$) increasing to 95.1% showing radiologic abnormalities, which were moderate to severe in one-third (Horner et al., 1992). Because of this morbidity, other investigators have favored a more selective denervation procedure, ramisectomy, which entails lesioning the posterior rami (C1–C6) along with sectioning of the spinal accessory nerve (Bertrand, Molina-Negro and Martinez, 1978; Bertrand et al., 1987). Good to excellent responses have been reported in 87–88% of patients (Bouvier, 1989; Bertrand and Lenz, 1995). In a prospective study of 31 cervical dystonia patients undergoing selective peripheral denervation, a 30% decrease was noted in the TWSTRS at 12 months in patients with a history of responding to botulinum toxin (Munchau et al., 2001). Non-responders to botulinum toxin showed no improvement. This procedure has been better tolerated, but does cause sensory loss in the distribution of the occipital nerve along with less frequent trapezius weakness and dysphagia. Retrospective studies indicated that patients with rotational torticollis responded better than those with laterocollis or retrocollis (Bouvier, 1989). Many problems exist with the literature that discusses peripheral surgical treatment options to treat dystonia: (i) most of the literature is 10–30 years old, before botulinum toxin became first-line treatment; (ii) none of the studies have a control population and long-term follow-up is lacking; (iii) evaluations are not blinded; (iv) many clinical assessments did not include a reliable scale that has been validated in a systematic fashion. At Baylor College of Medicine, we no longer utilize peripheral surgical treatments or ITB for cervical dystonia, but rather rely on mostly botulinum toxin, medications in some and DBS for patients refractory to these treatments (Figure 15.2).

CENTRAL SURGERY/ABLATION

Generalized Dystonia

Primary

Stereotactic surgical techniques have been used to target various regions in the brain to improve dystonia, including the internal capsule, dentate nucleus, cerebral peduncle, putamen, subthalamic nucleus, globus pallidus and thalamus. Cooper focused on thalamic lesioning for dystonia, claiming that 69.7% of 208 patients with generalized dystonia improved with a mean follow-up of 7.9 years (Cooper, 1976). Initially, he lesioned the posterior ventrolateralis (VL) nucleus and observed the patient for several months. If the dystonia worsened, or did not improve to a satisfactory degree, the lesion was extended to VL anterior or even the pulvinar nucleus leading to multiple operations in many cases. Of the 208 patients, 69 had two operations, 41 had three, 24 had four, 5 had five, 1 had six and 2 had seven (Bronte-Stewart, 2003). Jewish patients with a family

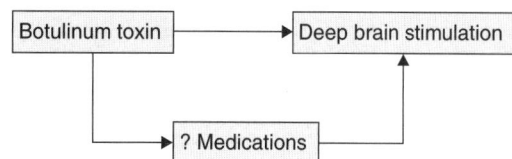

Figure 15.2 Algorithm for the treatment of cervical dystonia.

history of dystonia responded most favorably, but even Jewish patients without a family history had a good response in 75% of the cases, probably reflecting primary dystonia with a genetic basis and low penetrance (DYT1). In contrast to other reports, Cardoso and colleagues found that only 43% of patients with primary dystonia improved after VL thalamotomy, less than those with secondary dystonia (50%) (Cardoso et al., 1995). Subsequent studies over the next two decades revealed moderate to marked improvement in 33–80% of patients with generalized dystonia using thalamotomy (Gros et al., 1976; Andrew, Fowler and Harrison, 1983; Tasker, Doorly and Yamashiro, 1988; Cardoso et al., 1995). In one of these series, 3 out of 16 patients with generalized dystonia died within one year of surgical intervention, but these patients were also severely disabled prior to ablation (Andrew, Fowler and Harrison, 1983). Cooper quoted a mortality rate of 2% in his series of 208 patients (Cooper, 1976). Morbidity has been one of the major limiting factors for bilateral thalamotomy associated with frequent speech difficulty in 20–80% (Cooper, 1976; Andrew, Fowler and Harrison, 1983; Tasker, Doorly and Yamashiro, 1988). Other side effects have included hemiparesis, dysphonia, numbness and ataxia.

Historically, Cooper and other investigators favored thalamic ablation over pallidotomy, which offered less side effects, but more inconsistent benefits. Pallidotomy made a slight re-emergence in use for dystonia, with the findings that pallidotomy improved dystonia in Parkinson's disease (PD), if properly targeted to the posterolateral portion of the GPi rather than the anteromedial (non-motor) portion (Vitek, Bakay and DeLong, 1997; Eskandar et al., 1998; Gross et al., 1999; Bronte-Stewart, 2003). Recordings from the pallidum in patients with dystonia identified regular, irregular, bursting and clustering patterns of discharge (Sanghera et al., 2003). It has been postulated that either ablation or stimulation of the pallidum at least partially abolishes the abnormal patterns of discharge.

In small series pallidotomy improved primary generalized dystonia by 60–80% over several months of observation, unlike the immediate improvement occurring in PD (Iacono et al., 1996; Lozano et al., 1997; Lin et al., 1998; Ondo et al., 1998; Vitek et al., 1998). Unilateral pallidotomy appears to be both safe and efficacious. Some investigators caution about increased adverse events such as dysphagia and dysarthria after a bilateral pallidotomy (Kishore et al., 1997). Unfortunately no prospective, randomized study has been performed comparing pallidotomy to thalamotomy. However, in a retrospective comparison of 32 patients undergoing ablative surgery for dystonia, thalamotomy ($n = 18$) and pallidotomy ($n = 14$), the authors concluded that patients with primary dystonia who underwent pallidotomy demonstrated significantly better long-term outcomes than patients who underwent thalamotomy ($p = 0.05$) (Yoshor et al., 2001).

Secondary

Thalamotomy has been reported to improve secondary generalized dystonia from a moderate to a marked degree in 30 out of 54 patients, with most undergoing unilateral ablation (Tasker, Doorly and Yamashiro, 1988). Appendicular dystonia improved more than axial dystonia. Four of the five patients who underwent bilateral thalamotomy developed persistent dysarthria and dysphagia, and functional improvements waned over time. Three separate series have indicated that thalamotomy is not very effective for secondary dystonia caused by cerebral palsy (Van Manan, 1965; Narabayashi, 1977; Kandel, 1989). No prospective, randomized studies have been completed to date, but in a retrospective analysis, patients with secondary dystonia tended to do better with thalamotomy when compared to pallidotomy, though these differences were not statistically significant (Yoshor et al., 2001).

Focal Dystonia

Cervical

Cooper reported on a series of 160 cervical dystonia patients treated with bilateral thalamotomy; an improvement of 60% occurred with 20% experiencing speech difficulty (Cooper, 1977). Andrew noted improvement in 10 out of 16 cervical dystonia patients after bilateral thalamotomy, but persistent dysarthria was high (Andrew, Fowler and Harrison, 1983). Unilateral thalamotomy was not found to be beneficial.

Writer's Cramp

There are only few reports of ablative procedures to treat task-specific focal hand dystonia (writer's cramp), but this literature does date back to 1969 (Siegfried, Crowell and Perret, 1969; Mempel, Kucinski and Witkiewicz, 1986; Goto et al., 1997; Taira, Harashima and Hori, 2003; Taira and Hori, 2003). The largest series reported to date included 12 patients with medically intractable task-specific focal dystonia of the hand who underwent thalamotomy (nucleus ventrooralis) (Taira and Hori, 2003). Seven patients were professionals who stopped their careers because of excessive dystonic symptoms. The mean sub-score on the writer's cramp rating scale improved from 13.1 to 0.8 ($p < 0.001$). Two patients developed transient hemiparesis and dysarthria, which resolved within three weeks, while another patient developed a possible pulmonary air embolism without clinical sequelae.

CENTRAL SURGERY/DEEP BRAIN STIMULATION

Mudinger reported the use of thalamic stimulation in 1977 for cervical dystonia (Mundinger, 1977), but the major shift from ablative surgery to DBS occurred after Benabid reported the use of thalamic DBS to control tremor in 1987 (Benabid *et al.*, 1987). In comparison to ablative procedures, DBS has several advantages (Tagliati *et al.*, 2004). First, implantation is reversible, allowing patients to be eligible for future therapies that may require intact basal ganglia structures. Second, programming parameters are adjustable. Third, the overall side effect profile is more benign, especially for bilateral procedures commonly used in dystonic patients (Kenney *et al.*, 2007). Serious adverse events reported include intracerebral hemorrhage in 1%, infection in 4% and seizure in 1% (Kenney *et al.*, 2007). Ideal candidates have primary generalized dystonia that has not responded to medications or botulinum toxin along with significant disability from motor dysfunction (Table 15.1). Segmental dystonia, hemidystonia and some forms of focal dystonia (cervical) also respond, but to a lesser degree; primary dystonia, in particular DYT1 positive dystonia, responds more favorably than secondary dystonia (Volkmann and Benecke, 2002; Eltahawy *et al.*, 2004; Krause *et al.*, 2004; Vidailhet *et al.*, 2007). The Food and Drug Administration (FDA) granted Medtronic a Humanitarian Device Exemption for the treatment of primary generalized dystonia in 2003.

Generalized Dystonia

Primary

Benabid reported that thalamic DBS improved flexion of the limbs in two patients with primary dystonia (Benabid *et al.*, 1996). Thalamic DBS did not improve dystonic symptoms appreciably in a patient with inherited myoclonus dystonia (Trottenberg *et al.*, 2001). While thalamic DBS appeared to provide some benefit, early reports favored GPi-DBS because of superior efficacy (Vercueil *et al.*, 2001). In a retrospective study of nine primary dystonia patients, the authors noted improvement of global functional improvement, but not dystonia movement or disability scores with thalamic DBS targeted to the VL nucleus (Vercueil *et al.*, 2001). Because of modest improvements with thalamic DBS to treat primary dystonia, the authors began treating this patient population solely with GPi-DBS.

Several small, open-label studies conclude that bilateral GPi-DBS improves primary dystonia 60–100% using the Unified Dystonia Rating Scale (UDRS) BFMDRS (Kumar *et al.*, 1999; Coubes *et al.*, 2000; Tronnier and Fogel, 2000; Yianni *et al.*, 2003; Zorzi *et al.*, 2005; Diamond *et al.*, 2006). Amelioration of dystonia tends to be delayed, gradual and cumulative, as seen after pallidotomy (Vidailhet *et al.*, 2005). DBS settings are usually adjusted regularly during the first year after implantation with minimal adjustments required during follow-up (Kumar, 2002). Batteries may deplete as quickly as two years in patients with dystonia, as energy consumption is much higher given the need for larger pulse width and voltage to optimize symptomatic improvement (Bhidayasiri and Tarsy, 2006). In contrast to PD and essential tremor, in which DBS frequency is around 150, in patients with dystonia with the electrode placed posteroventrally within the internal globus pallidus, nearer the internal capsule, much lower frequency, perhaps as low as 60 Hz, may enhance the efficacy and tolerability of chronic stimulation (Alterman *et al.*, 2007). In contrast to thalamotomy, no signs of regression usually occur after GPi-DBS, although patients with progressive dystonia, such as DYT1 dystonia, may continue to deteriorate after a period of stabilization as part of the natural history of the disease. Medications can be reduced in patients with generalized dystonia after GPi-DBS resulting in improved alertness and cognitive function. No deterioration in cognition has been detected after GPi-DBS (Halbig *et al.*, 2005). GPi-DBS is gaining acceptance as the surgical treatment of choice, not only in adult patients with dystonia, but also in children (Figure 15.3) (Alterman and Tagliati, 2007).

The largest published experience with GPi-DBS for dystonia reported on 53 patients, including 15 with DYT1 positive generalized dystonia, 17 with DYT1 negative dystonia and the remainder with secondary dystonia (Cif *et al.*, 2003). One year after implantation, dystonia improved 71% in the DYT1 positive group and 74% in the DYT1 negative group using BFMDS scores. Secondary dystonia improved, on average, to a lesser degree, 31%. Adverse events were limited to delayed infection in three cases and a single lead fracture. The best controlled study to date enrolled 40 patients (primary dystonia, $n = 26$; segmental dystonia, $n = 14$) in a prospective, multi-center study; patients were randomized 1:1 to neurostimulation or sham stimulation (Kupsch *et al.*, 2006). At three months the BFMDS scores improved 39.3% in the treatment group and only 4.9% in the sham group ($p < 0.001$). Interestingly, patients with generalized dystonia and segmental dystonia experienced similar symptomatic benefit after six months of stimulation. Infection at the simulator site occurred in three patients, requiring removal in two cases. In a prospective study of 22 patients with primary generalized dystonia, seven of whom were DYT1 positive, bilateral GPi-DBS improved dystonia by 54.6% ($p < 0.001$) at 12 months, according to a blinded rater using the BFMDS (Vidailhet *et al.*, 2005); the disability score improved by 42%. Maximum benefit was not achieved in some patients until 3–6 months after implantation. Five adverse events occurred in three patients, all of which resolved without permanent sequelae, including one case of sub-clinical

Table 15.1 Selected studies using deep brain stimulation for dystonia.

Investigator	Year	N	Type of Dystonia	Study Design	Procedure	Efficacy
Krauss et al. (1999)	1999	3	Cervical	Open label	Bilateral GPi-DBS	Improved TWSTRS 60.3%
Bereznai et al. (2002)	2002	6	Segmental, $n=3$ Primary generalized, $n=1$ Cervical, $n=1$	Open label	Bilateral GPi-DBS	Improved BFMDRS 72.5% Improved Tsui scale 45%
Yianni et al. (2003)	2003	25	Generalized, $n=12$ Cervical, $n=7$ Secondary, $n=6$	Open label	Bilateral GPi-DBS	Improved BFMDRS 46% Improved TWSTRS 59% Improved AIMS 37%
Cif et al. (2003)	2003	53	Primary generalized, $n=32$ Secondary generalized, $n=21$	Open label	Bilateral GPi-DBS	Improved BFMDRS 71–74% Improved BFMDRS 31%
Krauss et al. (2003)	2003	6	Primary generalized, $n=2$ Secondary generalized, $n=4$	Open label	Bilateral GPi-DBS	Improved BFMDRS 71% Improved BFMDRS 21%
Coubes et al. (2004)	2004	31	Primary generalized	Open label	Bilateral GPi-DBS	Improved BFMDRS 78.2%
Trottenberg et al. (2005)	2005	5	Secondary generalized (tardive)	Open label	Bilateral GPi-DBS	Improved BFMDRS 87%
Vidailhet et al. (2005)	2005	22	Primary generalized	Prospective study with "blinded" rater	Bilateral GPi-DBS	Improved BFMDS 54.6%
Diamond et al. (2006)	2006	11	Primary generalized, $n=10$ Hemidystonia, $n=1$	Open-label with "blinded" rater	Bilateral GPi-DBS ($n=9$) Unilateral GPi-DBS ($n=2$)	Improved UDRS 38.3%
Kupsch et al. (2006)	2006	40	Primary generalized, $n=24$ Segmental, $n=16$	Prospective, randomized to stimulation off/on	Bilateral GPi-DBS	Improved BFMDRS 39.3–4.9% without stimulation
Hung et al. (2007)	2007	10	Cervical	Open label	Bilateral GPi-DBS	Improved TWSTRS 56.8%
Ostrem et al. (2007)	2007	6	Segmental (Meige)	Open label	Bilateral GPi-DBS	Improved BFMDRS 72%
Vidailhet et al. (2007)	2007	22	Primary generalized	Prospective study with "blinded" rater	Bilateral GPi-DBS	Improved BFMDRS 58%

GPi – globus pallidus interna; DBS – deep brain stimulation; TWSTRS – Toronto Western Spasmodic Torticollis Rating Scale; BFMDS – Burke–Fahn–Marsden Dystonia Scale; AIMS – Abnormal Involuntary Movement Scale; UDRS – Unified Dystonia Rating Scale.

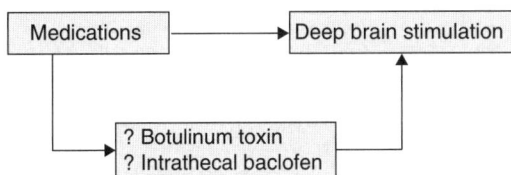

Figure 15.3 Algorithm for the treatment of generalized dystonia.

frontal lobe edema, a fractured lead, two skin infections and one hematoma near the neurostimulator. In one series of 16 patients treated for dystonia with GPi-DBS, two patients committed suicide, an occurrence noted with other indications as well (Burkhard *et al.*, 2004; Foncke, Schuurman and Speelman, 2006). Overall current data supports the conclusion that GPi is the preferred target for patients with primary generalized dystonia. The best improvement has been achieved in DYT1 positive dystonia, but remarkable improvement has also been attained in non-DYT1 patients (Vidailhet *et al.*, 2005).

Secondary

Thalamic DBS may be more effective for secondary dystonia, as reported in a case of hemidystonia caused by an extradural hematoma (Sellal *et al.*, 1993). The unilateral electrode was targeted to the ventroposterolateral nucleus. Another report of four patients with post-anoxic dystonia noted little improvement after GPi-DBS; one patient eventually underwent bilateral thalamic DBS with substantial functional improvement (Ghika *et al.*, 2002).

Although some reports indicate that thalamotomy may be more effective for secondary than primary dystonia, GPi-DBS has produced less dramatic results. In three patients with secondary dystonia the BFMDRS improved 23.7% after 6–12 months of follow-up (Bronte-Stewart, 2003). In one patient with secondary generalized dystonia, bilateral GPi-DBS improved dystonia only 14% after six months (Tronnier and Fogel, 2000). In another case of post-traumatic hemidystonia, bilateral GPi-DBS led to a remarkable improvement in pain, dystonia and function, which maintained after four years of follow-up (Loher *et al.*, 2000). In a case report of tardive dystonia, the patient was implanted with GPi-DBS on one side and Vim-DBS on the other (Trottenberg *et al.*, 2001). The authors found only the GPi-DBS to be effective.

Focal Dystonia

Cervical

Patients who have failed first-line treatment with botulinum toxin and with medications may be candidates for DBS (Goto, Mita and Ushio, 2002). Mundinger pioneered the use of thalamic DBS for cervical dystonia in a report of seven patients who underwent 30–40 minutes of stimulation resulting in relief of dystonia for 3–4 hours (Mundinger, 1977). Krauss reported excellent clinical outcomes in five patients with cervical dystonia 20 months after bilateral GPi-DBS (Krauss *et al.*, 2002). Using the TWSTRS, a statistical improvement was observed starting three months after implantation, which persisted throughout the period of observation. At the 20-month time point, the severity score improved 63%, while the disability and pain scores improved 69% and 50%, respectively. Hung reported experience with bilateral GPi-DBS to treat severe cervical dystonia in 10 patients (Hung *et al.*, 2007). Long-term follow-up (1–5 years) revealed improvement of 56.8% using the TWSTRS. The severity score, disability score and pain score all improved to a similar degree. As with generalized dystonia, phasic movements improved more rapidly than tonic movements. The results from this largest series to date of patients with medication-refractory cervical dystonia treated with GPi-DBS confirms findings from previous case series by demonstrating improvements in dystonic movements and disability, however, must be interpreted cautiously as this was an open-label study and the TWSTRS assessments were not performed by a blinded rater. Further, it is unclear whether all patients received the maximum tolerated dosage of medications, including optimal treatment with botulinum toxin. Improvement of cervical dystonia with GPi-DBS is consistent with the finding of others that axial regions (e.g., trunk and neck) improve more than distal areas (Diamond *et al.*, 2006).

CONCLUSION

Most patients with focal or segmental dystonia respond sufficiently to botulinum toxin injections such that surgical options are not needed. For those patients with medically refractory segmental dystonia, hemidystonia and generalized dystonia, DBS offers a relatively safe treatment option. Primary dystonia patients, particularly DYT1 positive, respond most favorably. Less consistent results have been obtained with secondary dystonia, but few alternative treatments exist for these patients. With the advent of DBS, peripheral surgeries, ITB and ablative surgeries are being performed much less frequently. However, a large body of evidence supports their utilization in the appropriate patient population.

References

Albright, A.L. (1996) Baclofen in the treatment of cerebral palsy. *Journal of Child Neurology*, **11**, 77–83.

Albright, A.L., Barry, M.J., Fasick, P. *et al.* (1996) Continuous intrathecal baclofen infusion for symptomatic generalized dystonia. *Neurosurgery*, **38**, 934–938; discussion 938–39.

Albright, A.L., Barry, M.J., Painter, M.J. and Shultz, B. (1998) Infusion of intrathecal baclofen for generalized dystonia in cerebral palsy. *Journal of Neurosurgery*, **88**, 73–76.

Albright, A.L., Barry, M.J., Shafton, D.H. and Ferson, S.S. (2001) Intrathecal baclofen for generalized dystonia. *Developmental Medicine and Child Neurology*, **43**, 652–657.

Albright, A.L., Turner, M. and Pattisapu, J.V. (2006) Best-practice surgical techniques for intrathecal baclofen therapy. *Journal of Neurosurgery*, **104**, 233–239.

Alterman, R.L., Shils, J.L., Miravite, J. and Tagliati, M. (2007) Lower stimulation frequency can enhance tolerability and efficacy of pallidal deep brain stimulation for dystonia. *Movement Disorders*, **22**, 366–368.

Alterman, R.L. and Tagliati, M. Deep brain stimulation for torsion dystonia in children. (2007) Child's Nervous System, (Epub ahead of print).

Andrew, J., Fowler, C.J. and Harrison, M.J. (1983) Stereotaxic thalamotomy in 55 cases of dystonia. *Brain: A Journal of Neurology*, **106** (Pt 4), 981–1000.

Awaad, Y., Munoz, S. and Nigro, M. (1999) Progressive dystonia in a child with chromosome 18p deletion, treated with intrathecal baclofen. *Journal of Child Neurology*, **14**, 75–77.

Barry, M.J., VanSwearingen, J.M. and Albright, A.L. (1999) Reliability and responsiveness of the Barry–Albright Dystonia Scale. *Developmental Medicine and Child Neurology*, **41**, 404–411.

Bates, A.K., Halliday, B.L., Bailey, C.S. *et al.* (1991) Surgical management of essential blepharospasm. *The British Journal of Ophthalmology*, **75**, 487–490.

Benabid, A.L., Pollak, P., Gao, D. *et al.* (1996) Chronic electrical stimulation of the ventralis intermedius nucleus of the thalamus as a treatment of movement disorders. *Journal of Neurosurgery*, **84**, 203–214.

Benabid, A.L., Pollak, P., Louveau, A. *et al.* (1987) Combined (thalamotomy and stimulation) stereotactic surgery of the VIM thalamic nucleus for bilateral Parkinson's disease. *Applied Neurophysiology*, **50**, 344–346.

Bereznai, B., Steude, U., Seelos, K. and Botzel, K. (2002) Chronic high-frequency globus pallidus internus stimulation in different types of dystonia: a clinical, video, and MRI report of six patients presenting with segmental, cervical, and generalized dystonia. *Movement Disorders*, **17**, 138–144.

Bertrand, C. and Lenz, F. (1995) in *Handbook of dystonia*, (eds J. Tsui and D. Calne), Marcel Dekker, New York, pp. 329–345.

Bertrand, C., Molina-Negro, P., Bouvier, G. and Gorczyca, W. (1987) Observations and analysis of results in 131 cases of spasmodic torticollis after selective denervation. *Applied Neurophysiology*, **50**, 319–323.

Bertrand, C., Molina-Negro, P. and Martinez, S.N. (1978) Combined stereotactic and peripheral surgical approach for spasmodic torticollis. *Applied Neurophysiology*, **41**, 122–133.

Bhidayasiri, R. and Tarsy, D. (2006) Treatment of dystonia. *Expert Review of Neurotherapeutics*, **6**, 863–886.

Bouvier, G. (1989) The use of selective denervation for spasmodic torticollis in cervical dystonias. *The Canadian Journal of Neurological Sciences*, **16**, 242.

Braun, V. and Richter, H.P. (2002) Selective peripheral denervation for spasmodic torticollis: 13-year experience with 155 patients. *Journal of Neurosurgery*, **97**, 207–212.

Bronte-Stewart, H. (2003) Surgical therapy for dystonia. *Current Neurology and Neuroscience Reports*, **3**, 296–305.

Burkhard, P.R., Vingerhoets, F.J., Berney, A. *et al.* (2004) Suicide after successful deep brain stimulation for movement disorders. *Neurology*, **63**, 2170–2172.

Butler, C. and Campbell, S. (2000) Evidence of the effects of intrathecal baclofen for spastic and dystonic cerebral palsy. AACPDM Treatment Outcomes Committee Review Panel. *Developmental Medicine and Child Neurology*, **42**, 634–645.

Cardoso, F., Jankovic, J., Grossman, R.G. and Hamilton, W.J. (1995) Outcome after stereotactic thalamotomy for dystonia and hemiballismus. *Neurosurgery*, **36**, 501–507; discussion 507–08.

Chen, X.K., Ji, S.X., Zhu, G.H. and Ma, A.B. (1991) Operative treatment of bilateral retrocollis. *Acta Neurochirurgica*, **113**, 180–183.

Cif, L., El Fertit, H., Vayssiere, N. *et al.* (2003) Treatment of dystonic syndromes by chronic electrical stimulation of the internal globus pallidus. *Journal of Neurosurgical Sciences*, **47**, 52–55.

Cooper, I.S. (1976) 20-year followup study of the neurosurgical treatment of dystonia musculorum deformans. *Advances in Neurology*, **14**, 423–452.

Cooper, I.S. (1976) *Dystonia: Surgical approaches to treatment and physiologic implications*, Raven Press, New York.

Cooper, I.S. (1977) Neurosurgical treatment of the dyskinesias. *Clinical Neurosurgery*, **24**, 367–390.

Coubes, P., Cif, L., El Fertit, H. *et al.* (2004) Electrical stimulation of the globus pallidus internus in patients with primary generalized dystonia: long-term results. *Journal of Neurosurgery*, **101**, 189–194.

Coubes, P., Roubertie, A., Vayssiere, N. *et al.* (2000) Treatment of DYT1-generalised dystonia by stimulation of the internal globus pallidus. *Lancet*, **355**, 2220–2221.

Dalvi, A., Fahn, S. and Ford, B. (1998) Intrathecal baclofen in the treatment of dystonic storm. *Movement Disorders*, **13**, 611–612.

De Groot, V., De Wilde, F., Smet, L. and Tassignon, M.J. (2000) Frontalis suspension combined with blepharoplasty as an effective treatment for blepharospasm associated with apraxia of eyelid opening. *Ophthalmic Plastic and Reconstructive Surgery*, **16**, 34–38.

Diamond, A., Shahed, J., Azher, S. *et al.* (2006) Globus pallidus deep brain stimulation in dystonia. *Movement Disorders*, **21**, 692–695.

Dressler, D., Oeljeschlager, R.O. and Ruther, E. (1997) Severe tardive dystonia: treatment with continuous intrathecal baclofen administration. *Movement Disorders*, **12**, 585–587.

Eltahawy, H.A., Saint-Cyr, J., Giladi, N. *et al.* (2004) Primary dystonia is more responsive than secondary dystonia to pallidal interventions: outcome after pallidotomy or pallidal deep brain stimulation. *Neurosurgery*, **54**, 613–619; discussion 619–21.

Eskandar, E.N., Cosgrove, G.R., Shinobu, L.A. and Penney, J.B. Jr (1998) The importance of accurate lesion placement in posteroventral pallidotomy. Report of two cases. *Journal of Neurosurgery*, **89**, 630–634.

Fabinyi, G. and Dutton, J. (1980) The surgical treatment of spasmodic torticollis. *Australian and New Zealand Journal of Surgery*, **50**, 155–157.

Foncke, E.M., Schuurman, P.R. and Speelman, J.D. (2006) Suicide after deep brain stimulation of the internal globus pallidus for dystonia. *Neurology*, **66**, 142–143.

Ford, B., Greene, P., Louis, E.D. *et al.* (1996) Use of intrathecal baclofen in the treatment of patients with dystonia. *Archives of Neurology*, **53**, 1241–1246.

Friedman, A.H., Nashold, B.S. Jr Sharp, R. *et al.* (1993) Treatment of spasmodic torticollis with intradural selective rhizotomies. *Journal of Neurosurgery*, **78**, 46–53.

Frueh, B.R., Musch, D.C. and Bersani, T.A. (1992) Effects of eyelid protractor excision for the treatment of benign essential blepharospasm. *American Journal of Ophthalmology*, **113**, 681–686.

Ghika, J., Villemure, J.G., Miklossy, J. *et al.* (2002) Postanoxic generalized dystonia improved by bilateral Voa thalamic deep brain stimulation. *Neurology*, **58**, 311–313.

Gillum, W.N. and Anderson, R.L. (1981) Blepharospasm surgery. An anatomical approach. *Archives of Ophthalmology*, **99**, 1056–1062.

Goto, S., Mita, S. and Ushio, Y. (2002) Bilateral pallidal stimulation for cervical dystonia. An optimal paradigm from our experiences. *Stereotactic and Functional Neurosurgery*, **79**, 221–227.

Goto, S., Tsuiki, H., Soyama, N. *et al.* (1997) Stereotactic selective Vo-complex thalamotomy in a patient with dystonic writer's cramp. *Neurology*, **49**, 1173–1174.

Grivet, D., Robert, P.Y., Thuret, G. *et al.* (2005) Assessment of blepharospasm surgery using an improved disability scale: study of 138 patients. *Ophthalmic Plastic and Reconstructive Surgery*, **21**, 230–234.

Gros, C., Frerebeau, P., Perez-Dominguez, E. *et al.* (1976) Long term results of stereotaxic surgery for infantile dystonia and dyskinesia. *Neurochirurgia (Stuttg)*, **19**, 171–178.

Gross, R.E., Lombardi, W.J., Lang, A.E. *et al.* (1999) Relationship of lesion location to clinical outcome following microelectrode-guided pallidotomy for Parkinson's disease. *Brain: A Journal of Neurology*, **122** (Pt 3), 405–416.

Halbig, T.D., Gruber, D., Kopp, U.A. *et al.* (2005) Pallidal stimulation in dystonia: effects on cognition, mood, and quality of life. *Journal of Neurology, Neurosurgery, and Psychiatry*, **76**, 1713–1716.

Hernesniemi, J. and Keranen, T. (1990) Long-term outcome after surgery for spasmodic torticollis. *Acta Neurochirurgica*, **103**, 128–130.

Horner, J., Riski, J.E., Ovelmen-Levitt, J. and Nashold, B.S. Jr (1992) Swallowing in torticollis before and after rhizotomy. *Dysphagia*, **7**, 117–125.

Hou, J.G., Ondo, W. and Jankovic, J. (2001) Intrathecal baclofen for dystonia. *Movement Disorders*, **16**, 1201–1202.

Hung, S.W., Hamani, C., Lozano, A.M. *et al.* (2007) Long-term outcome of bilateral pallidal deep brain stimulation for primary cervical dystonia. *Neurology*, **68**, 457–459.

Iacono, R.P., Kuniyoshi, S.M., Lonser, R.R. *et al.* (1996) Simultaneous bilateral pallidoansotomy for idiopathic dystonia musculorum deformans. *Pediatric Neurology*, **14**, 145–148.

Jankovic, J. (2006) Treatment of dystonia. *Lancet Neurology*, **5**, 864–872.

Jones, T.W., Jr Waller, R.R. and Samples, J.R. (1985) Myectomy for essential blepharospasm. *Mayo Clinic Proceedings*, **60**, 663–666.

Kandel, E. (1989) *Functional and Stereotactic Neurosurgery*, Plenum Press, New York.

Kenney, C., Hunter, C. and Jankovic, J. (2007) Long-term tolerability of tetrabenazine in the treatment of hyperkinetic movement disorders. *Movement Disorders*, **22**, 193–197.

Kenney, C. and Jankovic, J. (2007) Botulinum toxin in the treatment of blepharospasm and hemifacial spasm. *Journal of Neural Transmission*, **115**, 585–591.

Kenney, C., Simpson, R. and Hunter, C. *et al.* (2007) Short-term and long-term safety of deep brain stimulation for the treatment of movement disorders. *Journal of Neurosurgery*, **106**, 621–625.

Kerty, E. and Eidal, K. (2006) Apraxia of eyelid opening: clinical features and therapy. *European Journal of Ophthalmology*, **16**, 204–208.

Kishore, A., Turnbull, I.M. and Snow, B.J. *et al.* (1997) Efficacy, stability and predictors of outcome of pallidotomy for Parkinson's disease. Six-month follow-up with additional 1-year observations. *Brain: A Journal of Neurology*, **120** (Pt 5), 729–737.

Kraus, J., Grossman, R. and Jankovic, J. (2001) Treatment options for surgery of cervical dystonia, in *Surgery for Parkinson's Disease and Movement Disorders* (eds J. Kraus, J. Jankovic and

R. Grossman), Lippincott Williams & Wilkins, Philadelphia, pp. 323–334.

Krause, M., Fogel, W., Kloss, M. *et al.* (2004) Pallidal stimulation for dystonia. *Neurosurgery*, **55**, 1361–1368; discussion 1368–70.

Krauss, J.K., Loher, T.J., Pohle, T. *et al.* (2002) Pallidal deep brain stimulation in patients with cervical dystonia and severe cervical dyskinesias with cervical myelopathy. *Journal of Neurology, Neurosurgery, and Psychiatry*, **72**, 249–256.

Krauss, J.K., Loher, T.J., Weigel, R. *et al.* (2003) Chronic stimulation of the globus pallidus internus for treatment of non-dYT1 generalized dystonia and choreoathetosis: 2-year follow up. *Journal of Neurosurgery*, **98**, 785–792.

Krauss, J.K., Pohle, T., Weber, S. *et al.* (1999) Bilateral stimulation of globus pallidus internus for treatment of cervical dystonia. *Lancet*, **354**, 837–838.

Krauss, J.K., Toups, E.G., Jankovic, J. and Grossman, R.G. (1997) Symptomatic and functional outcome of surgical treatment of cervical dystonia. *Journal of Neurology, Neurosurgery, and Psychiatry*, **63**, 642–648.

Kumar, R. (2002) Methods for programming and patient management with deep brain stimulation of the globus pallidus for the treatment of advanced Parkinson's disease and dystonia. *Movement Disorders*, **17** (Suppl 3), S198–S207.

Kumar, R., Dagher, A., Hutchison, W.D. *et al.* (1999) Globus pallidus deep brain stimulation for generalized dystonia: clinical and PET investigation. *Neurology*, **53**, 871–874.

Kupsch, A., Benecke, R., Muller, J. *et al.* (2006) Pallidal deep-brain stimulation in primary generalized or segmental dystonia. *The New England Journal of Medicine*, **355**, 1978–1990.

Lang, A.E. (1998) Surgical treatment of dystonia. *Advances in Neurology*, **78**, 185–198.

Lin, J.J., Lin, S.Z., Lin, G.Y. *et al.* (1998) Application of bilateral sequential pallidotomy to treat a patient with generalized dystonia. *European Neurology*, **40**, 108–110.

Loher, T.J., Hasdemir, M.G., Burgunder, J.M. and Krauss, J.K. (2000) Long-term follow-up study of chronic globus pallidus internus stimulation for posttraumatic hemidystonia. *Journal of Neurosurgery*, **92**, 457–460.

Lozano, A.M., Kumar, R., Gross, R.E. *et al.* (1997) Globus pallidus internus pallidotomy for generalized dystonia. *Movement Disorders*, **12**, 865–870.

McCord, C.D., Jr Coles, W.H., Shore, J.W. *et al.* (1984) Treatment of essential blepharospasm. I. Comparison of facial nerve avulsion and eyebrow-eyelid muscle stripping procedure. *Archives of Ophthalmology*, **102**, 266–268.

Meares, R. (1971) Natural history of spasmodic torticollis, and effect of surgery. *Lancet*, **2**, 149–150.

Mempel, E., Kucinski, L. and Witkiewicz, B. (1986) Writer's cramp syndrome treated successfully by thalamotomy. *Neurologia i Neurochirurgia Polska*, **20**, 475–480.

Meyer, C.H. (2001) Outcome of selective peripheral denervation for cervical dystonia. *Stereotactic and Functional Neurosurgery*, **77**, 44–47.

Meythaler, J.M., Guin-Renfroe, S., Grabb, P. and Hadley, M.N. (1999) Long-term continuously infused intrathecal baclofen for spastic-dystonic hypertonia in traumatic brain injury: 1-year experience. *Archives of Physical Medicine and Rehabilitation*, **80**, 13–19.

Meythaler, J.M., Guin-Renfroe, S. and Hadley, M.N. (1999) Continuously infused intrathecal baclofen for spastic/dystonic hemiplegia: a preliminary report. *American Journal of Physical Medicine & Rehabilitation*, **78**, 247–254.

Munchau, A., Palmer, J.D., Dressler, D. *et al.* (2001) Prospective study of selective peripheral denervation for botulinum-toxin resistant patients with cervical dystonia. *Brain: A Journal of Neurology*, **124**, 769–783.

Mundinger, F. (1977) New stereotactic treatment of spasmodic torticollis with a brain stimulation system (author's transl). *Medizinische Klinik (Munich, Germany: 1983)*, **72**, 1982–1986.

Narabayashi, H. (1977) Experiences of stereotaxic surgery on cerebral palsy patients. *Acta Neurochirurgica*, (Suppl 24), 3–10.

Narayan, R.K., Loubser, P.G., Jankovic, J. *et al.* (1991) Intrathecal baclofen for intractable axial dystonia. *Neurology*, **41**, 1141–1142.

Ondo, W.G., Desaloms, J.M., Jankovic, J. and Grossman, R.G. (1998) Pallidotomy for generalized dystonia. *Movement Disorders*, **13**, 693–698.

Ostrem, J.L., Marks, W.J., Jr Volz, M.M. *et al.* (2007) Pallidal deep brain stimulation in patients with cranial-cervical dystonia (Meige syndrome). *Movement Disorders*, **22**, 1885–1891.

Paret, G., Tirosh, R., Ben Zeev, B. *et al.* (1996) Intrathecal baclofen for severe torsion dystonia in a child. *Acta Paediatrica (Oslo, Norway: 1992)*, **85**, 635–637.

Patel, B. and Anderson, R. (1993) Diagnosis and management of essential blepharospasm. *Ophthalmic Practice*, **11**, 293–302.

Putnam, T., Herz, E. and Glaser, G. (1949) Spasmodic torticollis. *Archives of Neurology and Psychiatry*, **61**, 240–247.

Sanghera, M.K., Grossman, R.G., Kalhorn, C.G. *et al.* (2003) Basal ganglia neuronal discharge in primary and secondary dystonia in patients undergoing pallidotomy. *Neurosurgery*, **52**, 1358–1370; discussion 1370–73.

Sellal, F., Hirsch, E., Barth, P. *et al.* (1993) A case of symptomatic hemidystonia improved by ventroposterolateral thalamic electrostimulation. *Movement Disorders*, **8**, 515–518.

Siebner, H.R., Dressnandt, J., Auer, C. and Conrad, B. (1998) Continuous intrathecal baclofen infusions induced a marked increase of the transcranially evoked silent period in a patient with generalized dystonia. *Muscle & Nerve*, **21**, 1209–1212.

Siegfried, J., Crowell, R. and Perret, E. (1969) Cure of tremulous writer's cramp by stereotaxic thalamotomy. Case report. *Journal of Neurosurgery*, **30**, 182–185.

Tagliati, M., Shils, J., Sun, C. and Alterman, R. (2004) Deep brain stimulation for dystonia. *Expert Review of Medical Devices*, **1**, 33–41.

Taira, T., Harashima, S. and Hori, T. (2003) Neurosurgical treatment for writer's cramp. *Acta Neurochirurgica. Supplement*, **87**, 129–131.

Taira, T. and Hori, T. (2001) Peripheral neurotomy for torticollis: a new approach. *Stereotactic and Functional Neurosurgery*, **77**, 40–43.

Taira, T. and Hori, T. (2003) Stereotactic ventrooralis thalamotomy for task-specific focal hand dystonia (writer's cramp). *Stereotactic and Functional Neurosurgery*, **80**, 88–91.

Tasker, R.R., Doorly, T. and Yamashiro, K. (1988) Thalamotomy in generalized dystonia. *Advances in Neurology*, **50**, 615–631.

Tronnier, V.M. and Fogel, W. (2000) Pallidal stimulation for generalized dystonia. Report of three cases. *Journal of Neurosurgery*, **92**, 453–456.

Trottenberg, T., Meissner, W., Kabus, C. *et al.* (2001) Neurostimulation of the ventral intermediate thalamic nucleus in inherited myoclonus-dystonia syndrome. *Movement Disorders*, **16**, 769–771.

Trottenberg, T., Paul, G., Meissner, W. *et al.* (2001) Pallidal and thalamic neurostimulation in severe tardive dystonia. *Journal of Neurology, Neurosurgery, and Psychiatry*, **70**, 557–559.

Trottenberg, T., Volkmann, J., Deuschl, G. *et al.* (2005) Treatment of severe tardive dystonia with pallidal deep brain stimulation. *Neurology*, **64**, 344–346.

van Hilten, B.J., van de Beek, W.J., Hoff, J.I. *et al.* (2000) Intrathecal baclofen for the treatment of dystonia in patients with reflex sympathetic dystrophy. *The New England Journal of Medicine*, **343**, 625–630.

Van Manan, J. (1965) Indications for stereotaxic operations in cerebral palsy. *Confinia Neurologica*, **26**, 254–257.

Vercueil, L., Pollak, P., Fraix, V. *et al.* (2001) Deep brain stimulation in the treatment of severe dystonia. *Journal of Neurology*, **248**, 695–700.

Vidailhet, M., Vercueil, L., Houeto, J.L. *et al.* (2005) Bilateral deep-brain stimulation of the globus pallidus in primary generalized dystonia. *The New England Journal of Medicine*, **352**, 459–467.

Vidailhet, M., Vercueil, L., Houeto, J.L. *et al.* (2007) Bilateral, pallidal, deep-brain stimulation in primary generalised dystonia: a prospective 3 year follow-up study. *Lancet Neurology*, **6**, 223–229.

Vitek, J.L., Bakay, R.A. and DeLong, M.R. (1997) Microelectrode-guided pallidotomy for medically intractable Parkinson's disease. *Advances in Neurology*, **74**, 183–198.

Vitek, J.L., Zhang, J., Evatt, M. *et al.* (1998) GPi pallidotomy for dystonia: clinical outcome and neuronal activity. *Advances in Neurology*, **78**, 211–219.

Volkmann, J. and Benecke, R. (2002) Deep brain stimulation for dystonia: patient selection and evaluation. *Movement Disorders*, **17** (Suppl 3), S112–S115.

Walker, R.H., Danisi, F.O., Swope, D.M. *et al.* (2000) Intrathecal baclofen for dystonia: benefits and complications during six years of experience. *Movement Disorders*, **15**, 1242–1247.

Yianni, J., Bain, P., Giladi, N. *et al.* (2003) Globus pallidus internus deep brain stimulation for dystonic conditions: a prospective audit. *Movement Disorders*, **18**, 436–442.

Yianni, J., Bain, P.G., Gregory, R.P. *et al.* (2003) Post-operative progress of dystonia patients following globus pallidus internus deep brain stimulation. *European Journal of Neurology*, **10**, 239–247.

Yoshor, D., Hamilton, W.J., Ondo, W. *et al.* (2001) Comparison of thalamotomy and pallidotomy for the treatment of dystonia. *Neurosurgery*, **48**, 818–824; discussion 824–26.

Zorzi, G., Marras, C., Nardocci, N. *et al.* (2005) Stimulation of the globus pallidus internus for childhood-onset dystonia. *Movement Disorders*, **20**, 1194–1200.

16

Wilson's Disease

George J. Brewer

Department of Human Genetics, Department of Internal Medicine, University of Michigan Medical School, Michigan, USA

INTRODUCTION TO THE DISEASE

Wilson's disease (WD) is a rare disease of copper accumulation and copper toxicity (Brewer and Yuzbasiyan-Gurkan, 1992; Brewer, 2000, 2001, 2004; Hoogenraad, 1996; Scheinberg and Sternlieb, 1984). It is inherited as an autosomal recessive disease. In most populations the disease frequency is about 1 in 30 000 to 40 000 births. The disease is due to mutations in both copies of the ATP7B gene (Bull et al., 1993; Tanzi et al., 1993; Yamaguchi, Heiny and Gitlin, 1993), which is involved in excreting excessive copper into the bile for loss in the stool. Copper is an essential trace element, but the average diet contains about 1 mg of copper, which is in excess of needs by about 0.25 mg. This excess copper, if not excreted in the bile, gradually accumulates. It is primarily stored in the liver, but as the liver's storage capacity is exceeded, the liver is damaged. This probably begins as early as three years of age. Excess copper begins to accumulate in other parts of the body, and the next most sensitive areas are those parts of the brain that coordinate movement.

Patients present in roughly equal numbers with liver disease or neurologic disease. In Western countries the age of presentation of both types is generally from age 10–40 years, with a peak at about 20 years. In countries such as India and the Far East, the age of presentation tends to be much younger.

The liver disease presentation can take several forms (Brewer and Yuzbasiyan-Gurkan, 1992; Brewer, 2000, 2001, 2004; Hoogenraad, 1996; Scheinberg and Sternlieb, 1984). It may present with an episode of hepatitis, with jaundice. Usually such patients are viral negative, although viral positivity can coincide with WD. If a diagnosis is not made, the hepatitis may subside, but then recur, perhaps several times. In between episodes, the serum transaminase enzymes tend to remain elevated. The liver damage may remain sub-clinical, and the patient develops cirrhosis. The cirrhosis may be discovered on a routine scan, or when portal hypertension causes thrombocytopenia and/or leukopenia, or when the patient bleeds from esophageal or gastric varices. Some patients will present with liver failure, with elevated serum bilirubin, low serum albumin, ascites and/or peripheral edema, abnormal serum clotting factors and even hepatic encephalopathy.

The neurologic presentation includes one or more symptoms of a movement disorder (Starosta-Rubinstein et al., 1987). Symptoms that can occur include dysarthria, tremor, incoordination, muscle cramps or stiffness from dystonia, postural or gait abnormalities from dystonia, dysphagia and drooling. One symptom may occur in isolation for a long period of time (such as tremor), or many symptoms may occur at about the same time. About half of patients who present with neurologic disease have had sufficient psychiatric/behavioral disturbances to have seen a health care worker for these problems (Brewer, 2005). Such behavioral disturbances may antedate neurologic symptoms by 2–3 years. The behavioral problems are quite wide-ranging and include loss of emotional control, depression, impulsiveness, delusions, disinhibition and other bizarre behaviors.

Because the disease is inherited, once a case is diagnosed, it is important to work up full siblings, because each has a 25% chance of being affected, but at a pre-symptomatic state. The disease is close to 100% penetrant, so it is important to treat these pre-symptomatic patients prophylactically. Pre-symptomatic patients may also be occasionally diagnosed by workup after a routine screening reveals elevation of transaminase enzymes, or by chance ophthalmological detection of copper deposits in the cornea, called Kayser–Fleischer (KF) rings.

It is important that WD be diagnosed as early as possible because it is very treatable, and severe irreversible changes can largely be prevented if treatment starts early enough. The key to diagnosis is for physicians to screen patients who present with hepatitis, cirrhosis, liver failure, tremor, early age Parkinson's syndrome or other symptoms of a movement disorder, for WD (Brewer, 2001, 2004). The

Therapeutics of Parkinson's Disease and Other Movement Disorders Edited by Mark Hallett and Werner Poewe
© 2008 John Wiley & Sons, Ltd.

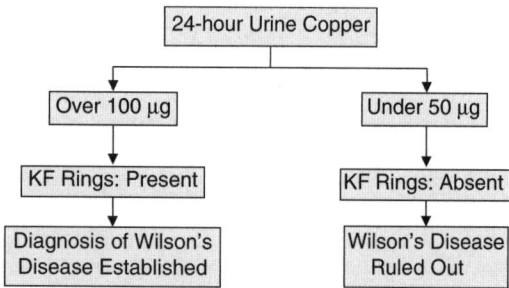

If tests are discordant, i.e. urine copper over 100µg and KF rings negative, or KF rings positive and urine copper under 50 µg, do liver biopsy and measure hepatic copper

Figure 16.1 Screening and diagnosis in patients with the neurologic/psychiatric presentation.

negative, WD (in a patient with neurologic symptoms) is excluded. In the rare instance where these two tests are discordant, a liver biopsy with quantitative assay for copper will settle the matter (Figure 16.1).

Occasionally, magnetic resonance imaging (MRI) or computed tomography (CT) brain scans may be helpful in diagnosing patients with neurologic Wilson's disease. These scans are usually abnormal in patients with neurologic symptoms from Wilson's disease. While they are not specific enough to be diagnostic, they can support the diagnosis, and occasionally may suggest it in the first place, for example, in patients with primarily psychiatric symptoms.

Screening for, and definitive diagnosis of, WD with a hepatic presentation is illustrated in Figure 16.2. Screening and diagnosis is not as straightforward as with the neurologic presentation, because KF rings are only present about half the time, and because other hepatic diseases can also elevate urine copper (Brewer, 2001, 2004). Chronic obstructive liver disease (marked by very high alkaline phosphatase levels) is a particularly difficult differential because it can elevate liver copper and urine copper into the Wilson's range, and even result in KF rings. However, in the absence of chronic obstructive liver disease, the presence of KF rings and a urine copper over 100 µg are pretty strong indications of WD. However, a liver biopsy with

problem is that there are many more patients with viral hepatitis, alcoholic cirrhosis, steatohepatitis, essential tremor, real Parkinson's disease and so on, than there are who have WD. Thus, it is critical for physicians and specialists who see these kinds of patients to be ever vigilant for, and rigorously screen for, WD.

Screening for, and definitive diagnosis of, WD with a neurologic presentation, is shown in Figure 16.1. The patient, with one or more symptoms of a movement disorder, should have an ophthalmologic examination by slit lamp for KF rings, and a 24-hour urine copper study. KF rings were present in 178 of 179 of our patients who had neurologic disease, so they are an excellent indicator of WD in this type of patient. Only very rarely have KF-like rings been seen in the absence of WD (one exception is chronic obstructive liver disease). In our experience, 24-hour urine copper is always over 100 µg (normal 20–50) in symptomatic, untreated WD patients. Thus, the presence of both KF rings and a 24-hour urine copper over 100 µg in a neurologic patient establishes the diagnosis, and further workup is unnecessary (Brewer, 2001, 2004). We like to have positive results in both tests because occasionally an inexperienced ophthalmologist will make an error in diagnosing KF rings (in either direction) and a 24-hour urine copper can be faulty because of contamination or inexperience with the assay. If both these tests are

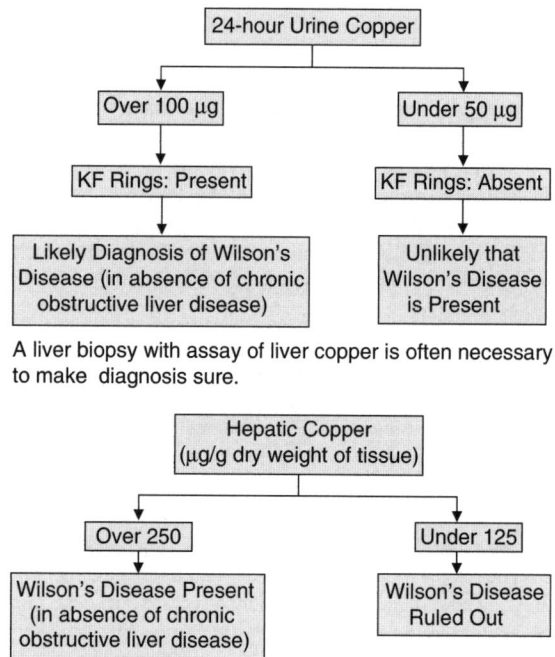

A liver biopsy with assay of liver copper is often necessary to make diagnosis sure.

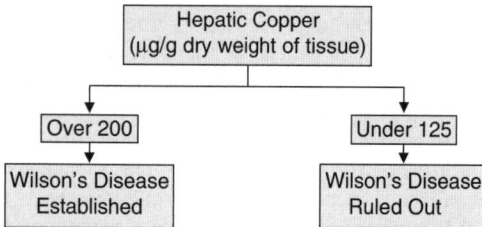

Figure 16.2 Screening and diagnosis in patients with the hepatic presentation.

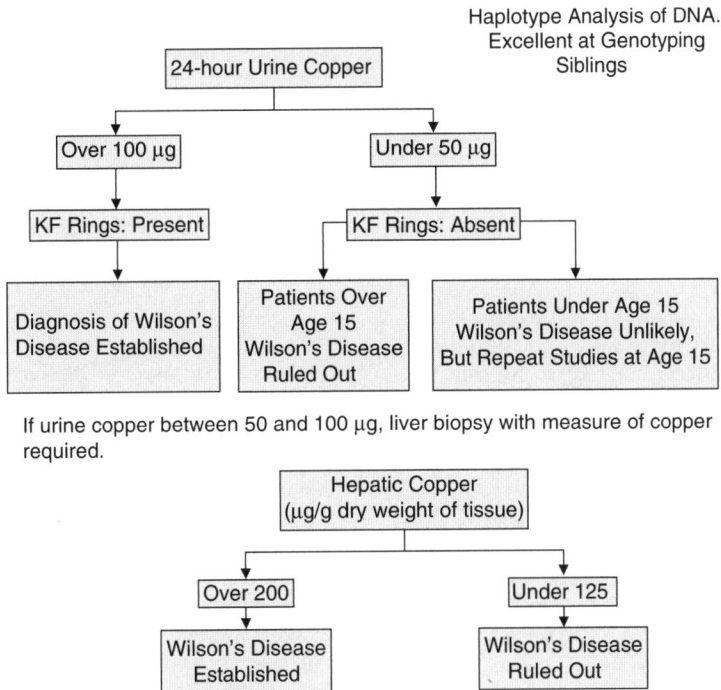

Figure 16.3 Screening and diagnosis of pre-symptomatic siblings.

quantitative assay for copper usually needs to be carried out, to confirm the diagnosis. The same specimen can be used to assess liver histology.

Screening for, and definitive diagnosis of, WD in the pre-symptomatic patient (siblings of an affected) is shown in Figure 16.3. About one-third of such patients have KF rings, and about two-thirds have 24-hour urine copper values over 100 µg (Brewer and Yuzbasiyan-Gurkan, 1992). Such patients have WD. If KF rings are absent, and 24-hour urine copper is normal (20–50 µg), in our experience the diagnosis is excluded. If the patient is younger than 15 years, we repeat the study at age 15 just in case copper hasn't had time to accumulate in a young patient. If KF rings are absent and urine copper between 50 and 100 µg/24 hour, a liver biopsy with quantitative assay for copper is required to settle the matter. This is because the 50–100 µg region of 24-hour urine copper values is an overlap region between gene carriers and pre-symptomatic affected siblings (Yuzbasiyan-Gurkan, Johnson and Brewer, 1991).

Another approach to diagnosing siblings of an affected is a DNA-based approach called haplotyping. In this approach, genetic markers on each side of the ATP7B gene are compared between the affected and siblings. In this way, it can be determined if the sibling shares both of the chromosomes carrying ATP7B with the affected, in which case the sibling is affected, only one chromosome shared, in which case the sibling is a carrier, or none, in which case the sibling is completely normal. This is a very reliable approach for diagnosing siblings of an affected patient, and commercial services are available.

The above discussion of screening and diagnosis leaves out measuring serum ceruloplasmin (Cp) because we have never found it to be definitive in any situation. It is low in 80–90% of WD patients, but also low in 20% of gene carriers (Brewer and Yuzbasiyan-Gurkan, 1992). Thus, if low, it can be used to affect index of suspicion, but shouldn't be used as a definitive diagnostic aid. Similarly, serum copper is not very useful in diagnosis. Because Cp-bound copper accounts for the majority of serum copper, the serum copper can be low, normal or high, dependent upon the Cp level.

Analysis of DNA for mutations in the ATP7B gene in order to diagnose Wilson's disease is still in its infancy. There are so many causative mutations that it is very difficult to detect all of them, and thus a negative test may be negative because the testing simply didn't reveal the mutation. While efforts are being made to use this approach, it isn't yet ready for practical use. This should not be confused with the haplotype approach of DNA analysis, which is very accurate for diagnosing siblings of an affected, as already discussed.

THERAPEUTICS OF WILSON'S DISEASE

Introduction

Since WD is a disease of copper accumulation and copper toxicity, therapy of this disease centers on treatment with anti-copper drugs. Most physicians have been educated in a period when penicillamine was the only anti-copper drug available, or was at least the only first line anti-copper therapy available. However, gone are the days when a diagnosis of WD simply means pushing the penicillamine treatment button. We now have different therapies available which are generally better than penicillamine and very much less toxic. In fact, we rarely use penicillamine any more. It is important to use the right drug, or combination of drugs, in specific situations, and it behooves the physician who is going to treat a patient with WD to know which drugs to use, and when. We will begin with a discussion of each of the anti-copper drugs and include a discussion of their mechanism of action, their toxicities, and how to monitor for efficacy and toxicity. We will then turn to the treatment of each of the various phases and presentations of WD.

It is not within the scope of this review to consider ancillary therapies for the various symptoms and complications of WD, such as for neurologic or psychiatric symptoms or for the various problems of liver failure or portal hypertension in these patients. In general, these problems should be treated as in other diseases causing these complications.

The Anti-Copper Drugs

Zinc

Zinc is becoming the mainstay of the treatment of WD, either as sole therapy, or as joint therapy in specific situations. Zinc was first used in two patients in the Netherlands, by Schouwink (Schouwink, 1961), whose work has largely gone unnoticed because it was published only in a thesis, and not in the literature. His work was later followed up in the Netherlands by Hoogenraad and colleagues (Hoogenraad et al., 1978, Hoogenraad, Koevoet and de Ruyter Korver, 1979, Hoogenraad, Van Hattum and Van den Hamer, 1987). We initiated studies of zinc independently (Brewer et al., 1983) after observing copper deficiency in zinc-treated patients with sickle cell anemia (Brewer et al., 1977; Prasad et al., 1978). In our sickle cell studies, we had established that zinc had to be given separate from food, in order to get significant absorption. There are many substances in food that bind zinc and prevent it from entering the intestinal cell.

Subsequently it was shown in rats by two groups that the anti-copper mechanism of zinc action is through induction of intestinal cell metallothionein (Hall, Young and

Bremner, 1979; Menard, McCormick and Cousins, 1981; Oestreicher and Cousins, 1985), which binds food and endogenously secreted copper with high affinity, and prevents its transfer into blood. Mucosal cells are sloughed with about a six-day turnover time, and the complexed copper is excreted in the stool. We subsequently showed that the metallothionein mechanism was true for humans as well (Yuzbasiyan-Gurkan et al., 1992). In the WD patient, it takes about two weeks of oral zinc therapy to fully induce metallothionein, and block copper absorption.

We carried out extensive copper balance studies, supplemented with measuring uptake of orally administered ^{64}Cu to establish dose response (Brewer, Yuzbasiyan-Gurkanand Dick, 1990, Brewer et al., 1993a; Hill et al., 1986, 1987). We found that the minimally effective dose was 75 mg/day, but it had to be given in two or three divided doses. We ended up recommending 50 mg three times/day to provide a safety factor, each dose separated from food and beverages other than water by at least one hour.

Various possible zinc toxicities have been evaluated. It has been suggested that zinc has an adverse effect on cholesterol levels, and on lymphocyte function (Chandra, 1984), but this has been shown not to be the case in Wilson's disease (Brewer, Yuzbasiyan-Gurkanand and Johnson, 1991, Brewer, Johnson and Kaplan, 1997). Zinc therapy results in mildly elevated levels of blood amylase and lipase, raising the possibility of zinc-induced pancreatitis. However, studies have not shown pancreatitis (Yuzbasiyan-Gurkan et al., 1989). It appears zinc induces higher levels of these enzymes in the pancreas, increasing their benign release into the blood. The sole remaining toxicity of zinc is gastric irritation, which occurs in about 10% of patients (Brewer et al., 1998). The zinc acetate we have used is better tolerated than the zinc sulfate used elsewhere. In most patients, the gastric irritation subsides after a few days of zinc administration. In some patients, it occurs only with the first morning dose. Often, simply having the patient take the first dose of the day at midmorning, a couple of hours after breakfast, solves this problem. In recalcitrant cases, offending doses can be taken with a little protein (no bread), such as hamburger, lunchmeat, cheese or jello. Protein interferes with zinc absorption the least of various foods.

Monitoring for zinc efficacy and compliance is the simplest of all the anti-copper drugs (Brewer et al., 1998). Since zinc doesn't act by causing urine copper excretion, the urinary excretion of copper is a good measure of body loading of mobilizable copper. During maintenance therapy with zinc, 24-hour urine copper will generally decrease after the first year to 50–125 μg (normal 20–50). This value will tend to be maintained for years, as stored hepatic copper is gradually mobilized, maintaining a somewhat elevated value. It should be monitored every 6–12 months, and an increasing value, say by more than

25%, is a warning of poor compliance. The value of urine monitoring is strongly enhanced by also measuring zinc in the same 24-hour sample (Brewer *et al.*, 1998). In an adequately treated, well complying, patient, 24-hour urine zinc should be at least 2.0 mg (normal 0.2–0.5 mg). Fall off in this value gives an early warning of poor compliance, because it happens sooner than an increase in urine copper.

The interaction of zinc with the other anti-copper drugs, penicillamine and trientine, has been looked at in maintenance-phase patients (Brewer *et al.*, 1993b). It was determined that the combination of zinc with either of these drugs does not increase negative copper balance over zinc alone, probably because in the absence of excessive available copper, these chelators bind some zinc, and thus the zinc and chelator partially inactivate each other. Therefore, during the maintenance phase, only one anti-copper drug should be given.

After the multiple studies described above, the FDA approved zinc therapy for the maintenance treatment of WD in 1997.

Trientine

Trientine was introduced into WD therapy by Walshe in 1982 (Walshe, 1982). It is a copper chelator that acts primarily by increasing copper excretion in the urine. There is also some evidence that it increases the fecal excretion of copper. Its original use was as a substitute for penicillamine in the face of penicillamine intolerance.

The dose of trientine is 1.0 g/day in two to four divided doses. During maintenance treatment it is often possible to decrease the dose to 750 to 500 mg/day. Each dose should be given at least one half hour before, or two hours after, meals.

Trientine has a fairly large number of toxicities that include bone marrow suppression, proteinuria and, later in therapy, autoimmune-like diseases, such as systemic lupus erythematosis and Goodpasture's syndrome.

Early in therapy with trientine, blood counts, basic blood biochemistries and urinalysis should be carried out regularly to monitor for toxicity. Weekly monitoring can be decreased to biweekly, monthly, every three months, every six months and, ultimately, annually, as evidence accumulates that the drug is tolerated.

Monitoring efficacy is complicated by the fact that trientine acts by increasing urinary excretion of copper. Thus the 24-hour urine excretion of copper is a composite of both the body loading of copper and the therapeutic effect of the drug. Nonetheless, 24-hour urine copper is usually monitored, and starts out at 1 mg or more during early treatment and decreases to 500 µg or so during maintenance therapy. However, a better way to monitor efficacy is to follow blood "free"-copper levels. Free copper refers to easily mobilizable copper, and in the blood, is the non-ceruloplasmin copper. Ceruloplasmin (Cp) is the major copper-containing protein in the blood. The copper in Cp is covalently bound, and not toxic. The rest of the copper in the blood is more loosely bound to albumin and other molecules, and is the potentially toxic copper pool in WD. This "free" copper is determined by simultaneously measuring serum copper and ceruloplasmin on the same sample. Each mg/dl of Cp contains 3 µg/ml of copper. This value is subtracted from total serum copper. The normal value of "free" copper is 10–15 µg/dl, and this is the desired value in well-treated WD patients during maintenance therapy. If it trends upward, problems with compliance should be suspected.

Tetrathiomolybdate

Tetrathiomolybdate (TM) came to attention as a result of observations in Australia and New Zealand, in which ruminants, but not non-ruminants, grazing in certain pastures, developed a disease later shown to be severe copper deficiency (Dick and Bull, 1945; Ferguson, Lewis and Waterson, 1943; Miller and Engel, 1960). The soil of the pastures was found to have a high molybdenum content. Feeding molybdenum to ruminants, but not to non-ruminants, reproduced the disease syndrome (Marcilese Ammerman *et al.*, 1969; Mason, 1990). Later it was found that the rumen converted the molybdenum to thiomolybdate compounds. These compounds, given to rats, produced strong anti-copper effects with the tetra-substituted compound, tetrathiomolybdate, being the most potent (Bremner, Mills and Young, 1982; McQuaid and Mason, 1991; Mills, El-Gallad and Bremner, 1981, Mills *et al.*, 1981). Tetrathiomolybdate has seen use in veterinary medicine, where it has been used to save copper-poisoned sheep, who often die of acute liver failure (Gooneratne, Howell and Gawthorne, 1981).

Tetrathiomolybdate has a unique mechanism of action. It forms a stable tripartite complex with copper and protein (Bremner, Mills and Young, 1982; Gooneratne, Howell and Gawthorne, 1981; Mills, El-Gallad and Bremner, 1981, Mills *et al.*, 1981). Used clinically, it can have two mechanisms of action (Brewer *et al.*, 1991, 1994a, 1996, 2003, 2006). Given with food, it forms the complex with food copper and endogenously secreted copper from saliva and gastric juice, plus food protein. This complex does not allow the absorption of the copper, and it passes out in the stool. Thus, given this way, TM causes an immediate negative copper balance. Given away from food, TM is well absorbed, and forms the complex with "free" copper and albumin in the blood. This complexed copper is not available for cellular uptake, it accumulates to a certain extent, and is metabolized primarily by the liver. In this way the "free", or potentially toxic, copper of the blood is rapidly titrated. TM, used for initial treatment in WD, can titrate copper toxicity in two weeks or less (Brewer *et al.*, 1994a).

The dose of TM used in most of the initial work for initial treatment of WD is 120 mg given for eight weeks (Brewer *et al.*, 1991, 1994a, 1996, 2003, 2006). This daily dose is broken down as 20 mg three times/day with meals, and either 20 mg three times/day between meals, or 60 mg away from food, usually at bedtime given as a single dose.

TM has two toxicities in WD (Brewer *et al.*, 2006). One is anemia and/or leukopenia, which appear to be due to bone marrow depletion of copper, copper being required to make cells. It occurs in about 10–15% of patients, and is quickly responsive to a 2–5 day drug holiday followed by halving the dose. The other toxicity is a further elevation of serum transaminase enzymes. This also occurs in 10–15% of patients and may be due to TMs ability to remove copper from metallothionein stores, further exacerbating hepatitis. This too is quickly responsive to a 2–5 day drug holiday followed by halving the dose.

There is no efficacy monitoring for TM, but because of the two above toxicities, blood counts and serum biochemistries should be done weekly.

Penicillamine

Penicillamine was the first effective oral anti-copper drug and was introduced in 1956 by Walshe (Walshe, 1956). It is effective and for 40 years was essentially the main treatment for WD, and a couple of generations of WD patients owe their lives to this drug.

Penicillamine's mechanism of action is that of a reductive chelator. It reduces copper, decreasing its binding affinity to proteins, and then chelating the copper and causing its excretion in the urine. Penicillamine is a very aggressive mobilizer of "free" copper. It is not uncommon for initial urinary excretion of copper to reach 10 mg/day.

The dose of penicillamine is similar to trientine, 1.0 g/day in two or four divided doses. As with trientine, it should be given at least one half hour before, or at least two hours after, meals.

Penicillamine is an extremely toxic drug (Brewer and Yuzbasiyan-Gurkan, 1992; Physicians Desk Reference, 2007). Upon initial administration, 20–25% of patients exhibit a hypersensitivity syndrome with hives or rash and fever. This can be overcome often by stopping the drug and restarting at very low doses and working up, or by using concomitant corticosteroid therapy.

Sub-acute and chronic toxicities include bone marrow suppression, proteinuria, initiation of autoimmune diseases, susceptibility to infection, arthralgias and numerous skin manifestations such as skin wrinkling, abnormal scar formation and elastosis perforans serpiginosa. Animal studies have shown defective collagen formation in blood vessels leading to risk of aneurysms (Nimni and Bavetta, 1965; Ronchetti *et al.*, 1986).

Penicillamine is such a toxic drug we no longer recommend its use in WD, now that we have effective and safer alternatives. If penicillamine is used, there should be frequent blood draws during early use, much as with trientine, to monitor for toxicity. Its efficacy, and compliance, can be monitored by following non-ceruloplasmin serum copper, as with trientine.

Other Anti-copper Drugs

A drug called British antilewisite (BAL) saw some early use in Wilson's disease and occasionally some practitioners still use it. We don't recommend its use because it has to be injected, the injections are often painful and it has never been shown that it is more effective than the orally administered anti-copper drugs.

Treatment of the Various Phases of Wilson's Disease

Initial Treatment of the Hepatic Presentation (see Figure 16.4)

Hepatic Failure

For our purposes, hepatic failure is defined as the liver not keeping up with its normal functions such as to result in hyperbilirubinemia, and reduced synthetic functions. The latter leads to a low blood albumin and lower levels of clotting factors, and a prolonged prothrombin time. It is often accompanied by fluid accumulation in the form of ascites or peripheral edema, and if severe, hepatic encephalopathy.

If Wilson's disease is diagnosed in such a patient, the first step is to triage the patient in terms of whether a liver transplant will almost certainly be required to save the patient's life (Figure 16.4). We have used the Nazer prognostic index (Nazer *et al.*, 1986) for this purpose and find it very useful (Table 16.1). The scoring systems in use by hepatologists for other liver diseases, such as the MELD score, are not appropriate for triaging Wilson's disease patients, because they often dictate transplantation in patients who can be better treated medically. A patient with

---

Hepatic Failure
    Triage Using Nazer Score
        10–12: Refer for liver transplant
          7–9: Use clinical judgment re-transplantation
          1–6: Treat medically
    Medical Treatment
        Trientine, 1.0 g/day for 4–6 months (in 2–4 divided dose)
        Zinc, 50 mg 3x/day

Hepatitis or Cirrhosis Without Liver Failure
    Zinc 50 mg 3x/day

Figure 16.4 Initial treatment of the hepatic presentation.

Table 16.1 Prognostic index of Nazer *et al.*, 1986 (modified with permission).

Laboratory Measurement	Normal Value	Score (in Points)				
		0	1	2	3	4
Serum bilirubin	0.2–1.2 mg/dl	<5.8	5.8–8.8	8.8–11.7	11.7–17.5	>17.5
Serum aspartate transferase (AST)	10–35 IU/L	<100	100–150	151–200	201–300	>300
Prolongation of prothrombin time (seconds)	—	<4	4–8	9–12	13–20	>20

Modified from Brewer, G.J. (2001) *Wilson's Disease: A Clinician's Guide to Recognition, Diagnosis, and Management*, Chapter 6, page 91, Table 6.2, with kind permission of Springer Science and Business Media.

a Nazer score of 10–12 will almost certainly require transplantation, while a score of 1–6 means the patient should do well on medical therapy. A score of 7–9 indicates judgment should be used as to whether to treat the patient medically or not. If such a patient is treated medically, they should be watched carefully for deterioration, which might mandate transplantation. A new scoring system (Dhawan *et al.*, 2005), said to have improved specificity and sensitivity, has recently been published. It should be emphasized again that it is important to use one of these WD-specific scoring systems.

Our recommended therapy for liver failure patients to be treated medically is a combination of 1.0 g of trientine/day, in two to four divided doses, with 150 mg of zinc in three divided doses (Figure 16.4) (Askari *et al.*, 2003). These medications should be separated from food and from each other by at least one hour. This combination is given for 4–6 months, then the trientine stopped, and zinc continued as maintenance therapy. The length of time of giving trientine can be varied depending on the recovery of liver function tests (LFTs). If they are well on their road to recovery at four months, trientine can be stopped then. Otherwise it can be continued until the six-month point.

Hepatitis or Cirrhosis

If the presentation is that of hepatitis, with elevated serum transaminase enzymes and perhaps a mildly elevated serum bilirubin, but a normal serum albumin, the patient can be treated from the beginning with 150 mg zinc, in three divided doses/day, and kept on this dose as maintenance therapy (Brewer *et al.*, 1998).

The same is true for the patient diagnosed with chronic cirrhosis, whose LFTs are normal, aside from elevated transaminase enzymes. Again, maintenance zinc therapy can be initiated from the beginning.

Initial Treatment of the Neurologic/Psychiatric Presentation (see Figure 16.5)

The Problems with Chelators

After developing zinc for maintenance therapy, we began to get numerous patient referrals to switch to zinc from current therapy, usually penicillamine. Many of these patients had severe irreversible neurologic damage. As we delved into the history of these patients, we began to realize that many of them had been diagnosed having mild neurologic disease, but upon treatment with penicillamine, had worsened neurologically, and never recovered. We did a retrospective survey, and of 26 patients presenting neurologically and treated with penicillamine, 13 had worsened neurologically, and 6 never recovered to their penicillamine baseline (Brewer *et al.*, 1987). These data indicate there is a 50% risk of worsening, and about a 25% risk of permanent loss of function from penicillamine therapy. While such survey numbers are somewhat soft, it is clear that there is a substantial risk of permanent neurological worsening with penicillamine treatment of neurologically presenting patients.

Subsequently, we carried out a double-blind trial of trientine, the other chelator on the market, in neurologically presenting patients. We found a rate of neurological worsening with trientine of 26% (Brewer *et al.*, 2006).

The mechanism of this chelator-induced neurologic worsening may involve mobilization of copper from the liver to the bloodstream, in order to accomplish urinary excretion. This flush of extra copper in the blood may further elevate brain copper, causing the neurologic worsening.

The Development of Tetrathiomolybdate (TM)

The problems with chelators in treating the neurologic presentation left us with the problem of how to treat these

```
┌─────────────────────────────────────────────────────────────┐
│   Initial Treatment of the Neurologic/Psychiatric Presentation│
│  Depending upon the Availability of Tetrathiomolybdate (TM)   │
└─────────────────────────────────────────────────────────────┘
```

TM Available	TM Not Available

```
                                          ┌──────────────────────────┐
                                          │ Zinc, 150 mg/day in 3 doses│
                                          └──────────────────────────┘
```

Standard Regimen	Alternate Regimen
120 mg TM Daily	120 mg TM Daily
20 mg 3 X/day with meals	20 mg 3 X/day with meals
60 mg away from food	60 mg away from food
+	For 2 weeks; then
150 mg Zinc/day in 3 doses	60 mg TM Daily
For 8 weeks, then continue	10 mg 3 X/day with meals
on zinc	30 mg away from food
	For 14 weeks,
	+
	150 mg Zinc/day in 3 doses
	After 16 weeks, continue on
	zinc

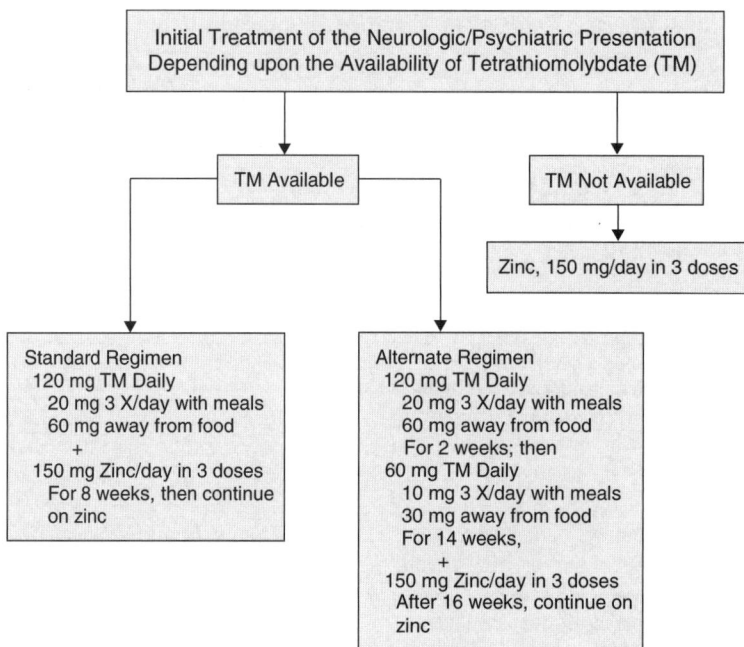

Figure 16.5 Initial treatment of the neurologic/psychiatric presentation. depending upon the availability of tetrathiomolybdate (TM).

patients, because we felt that zinc was too slow acting for these acutely ill patients. We estimate that it takes up to six months for zinc as sole therapy to gain control over copper toxicity, and during that period, the disease can progress. Indeed, in one of three neurologically presenting patients we treated with zinc alone, tremor progressed to a near disabling level.

This caused us to look for another drug. The properties of TM, reviewed earlier, seemed ideal for this purpose. Fortunately, there had been enough animal and veterinary work with TM so that the FDA allowed us to use it for the initial treatment of neurologically presenting WD. We developed semiquantitative neurologic and speech scoring systems, so that these patients' neurologic function could be evaluated weekly.

In a 55 patient open-label study, only 2 (3.6%) of neurologically presenting patients treated with TM for eight weeks reached criteria for neurologic deterioration (Brewer *et al.*, 2003). We believe that an occasional patient will deteriorate because of the natural course of the disease, while the penicillamine and trientine deteriorations are due to a drug-catalyzed effect. In this study, we settled on a standard dose of 120 mg of TM/day, given as 20 mg 3×/day with meals, and 60 mg away from food, given for eight weeks, usually together with 50 mg zinc twice daily.

Subsequently, we did a double-blind trial of TM vs trientine in the treatment of neurologically presenting patients (this is the study referred to earlier, in connection with trientine). We confirmed the low rate of neurologic worsening with TM (less than 4%) and observed the 26% rate of worsening with trientine (Brewer *et al.*, 2006). These differences were statistically significant ($p = 0.05$). These patients also received 50 mg of zinc twice daily while on TM or trientine.

Side effects of TM include a 10–15% rate of anemia/leukopenia and a 10–15% rate of further increase in transaminase enzymes (Brewer *et al.*, 2006). These do not occur prior to about four weeks of treatment, and both are responsive to halving the dose. Given this data, we are currently evaluating an alternate regimen of TM, where a loading dose of 120 mg/day is given for two weeks, then a half dose of 60 mg/day for an additional 14 weeks. The objective is to retain the efficacy of the standard dose regimen and reduce the side effects. It is too early in this trial to know if these objectives will be accomplished.

It is anticipated that TM will become commercially available in late 2009. Figure 16.5 lays out the options. Until TM becomes available, we recommend zinc therapy alone, thus avoiding the drug-catalyzed neurologic worsening with the chelators. After TM becomes available, we recommend using either the standard regimen for eight weeks, or the alternate regimen for 16 weeks, followed by maintenance zinc therapy.

In general, with TM therapy followed by maintenance zinc, improvement in symptoms begins at about 5–6 months after therapy initiation and continues for another

Maintenance Treatment

	1st Choice	2nd Choice
After treatment of clinical presentation	Zinc	Trientine
Presymptomatic patients	Zinc	Trientine
Pediatric patients	Zinc	Trientine
Pregnant patients	Zinc	Trientine

Figure 16.6 Maintenance Treatment.

18 months. Defects present after two years will probably be permanent. Overall, improvement is very substantial. Those patients with the most severe defects to begin with will have the most residual deficit.

Maintenance Therapy (see Figure 16.6)

The long-term therapy of WD is aimed at countering the positive copper balance these patients have by enhancing the excretion of copper. Since the pathologic tendency to a positive copper balance is a lifelong constant, the anti-copper therapy aimed at enhancing excretion must also be a lifelong constant. Thus, these patients must take anti-copper medication daily for the rest of their lives. This is called maintenance therapy.

All three of the anti-copper medications currently on the market, zinc, trientine and penicillamine, are effective, if taken faithfully and taken properly. Thus, the choice comes down to the safety profile. Because of this, zinc, which has only gastric intolerance in a small percentage of patients, is the first choice, and trientine, which has many fewer side effects than penicillamine, is second choice.

Zinc has been very well studied as a maintenance therapy. A central paper (Brewer *et al.*, 1998) involved 141 patients, many of them followed for 10 years, and most of them for five years. This is the largest and longest study of an anti-copper maintenance therapy and provides guidance in the dosing, monitoring, and results of zinc maintenance therapy. Studies of zinc maintenance therapy have also come from Hoogenraad's group (Hoogenraad, Van Hattum and Van den Hamer, 1987) in the Netherlands, Czlonkowska's group (Czlonkowska, Gajda and Rodo, 1996) in Poland and Nobili's (Marcellini *et al.*, 2005) group in Italy.

Trientine has not been as well studied, but observations by a number of investigators, and our own observations (Askari *et al.*, 2003), indicate that it is better tolerated than penicillamine.

There are several different settings for maintenance therapy and each of these will be briefly discussed.

Maintenance Therapy after Initial Therapy

After initial medical therapy for hepatic failure, or for the neurologic/psychiatric presentation, the patient then goes on maintenance therapy for the rest of their lives (Figure 16.6). Zinc is our first choice (Brewer *et al.*, 1998), with trientine second.

Treatment of Pre-Symptomatic Patients From the Beginning

Most of these patients are siblings of an affected patient in which family workup resulted in a diagnosis of an affected patient in the pre-symptomatic state. Occasionally pre-symptomatic patients will be diagnosed after chance observation of KF rings during an eye examination, or from workup of a patient in which elevated serum transaminase levels were observed from routine blood screening.

It is believed that WD is close to 100% penetrant, which means that if you have the genotype, you will become ill from copper toxicity at some point. This mandates prophylactic anti-copper therapy.

Because these patients are pre-symptomatic they are relatively comparable to patients who have presented clinically, received initial therapy and are now in the maintenance phase of therapy. Thus, these pre-symptomatic patients can be treated from the beginning with maintenance therapy. We recommend zinc (Brewer *et al.*, 1998), with trientine as second choice. A paper on the treatment of 13 pre-symptomatic patients with zinc from the time of diagnosis has been published (Brewer *et al.*, 1994b).

Treatment of the Pediatric Patient

If a pediatric patient presents clinically with liver failure or neurologic/psychiatric disease, they should be treated initially as discussed previously in those sections. After that, they require maintenance therapy. However, many of these patients will be diagnosed in the pre-symptomatic state as a result of family workup.

We have worked out a reduced dose of zinc for pediatric patients which is 25 mg ×2/day from age 1 until age 6, 25 mg ×3/day until age 15 or a body weight of 125 pounds, then the adult dose of 50 mg ×3/day. In addition to our published work (Brewer *et al.*, 2001), these doses were used in a study of maintenance therapy in 22 pediatric patients, and worked very well (Marcellini *et al.*, 2005). These pediatric patients were followed for 10 years during which time there was very good efficacy and lack of toxicity. Interestingly, they found improvement in liver histology, including less fibrosis, in these zinc-treated patients (Marcellini *et al.*, 2005).

Treatment of the Pregnant Patient

A woman with WD who becomes pregnant will almost invariably be in maintenance therapy, because acute copper toxicity usually prevents menstrual periods and fertility. Once copper toxicity is controlled, menstrual periods will usually begin again and the woman becomes fertile. There is no contraindication to pregnancy in such women, assuming their liver function is relatively normal.

It is important for pregnant WD patients to continue their anti-copper therapy to protect their own health. In the days when penicillamine was the only therapy available, a number of pregnant patients stopped their treatment because of the teratogenicity of penicillamine, usually leading to relapse of their WD and often death (Brewer and Yuzbasiyan-Gurkan, 1992).

We have reported on 26 pregnancies treated with zinc in which the health of the mother was fully protected (Brewer *et al.*, 2000). Two of the babies had birth defects. This could be chance, but it was interesting that copper control was among the best in these two women. This suggests that the fetus may have suffered from inadequate copper, which is known to be teratogenic. At this time we recommend that the zinc dose be adjusted to maintain urine copper between 75 and 150 μg/day, compared to the usual recommendation of 50–125 μg/day.

Trientine has also been used successfully during pregnancy, and from scattered reports, appears to be a reasonable choice.

References

Askari, F.K., Greenson, J., Dick, R.D. *et al.* (2003) Treatment of Wilson's disease with zinc. XVIII. Initial treatment of the hepatic decompensation presentation with trientine and zinc. *The Journal of Laboratory and Clinical Medicine*, **142**, 385–390.

Bremner, I., Mills, C.F. and Young, B.W. (1982) Copper metabolism in rats given di- or trithiomolybdates. *Journal of Inorganic Biochemistry*, **16**, 109–119.

Brewer, G.J., Schoomaker, E.B., Leichtman, D.A. *et al.* (1977) The uses of pharmacologic doses of zinc in the treatment of sickle cell anemia, in *Zinc Metabolism: Current Aspects in Health and Disease* (eds G.J. Brewer and A.S. Prasad), Allan R. Liss, Inc., New York.

Brewer, G.J., Hill, G.M., Prasad, A.S. *et al.* (1983) Oral zinc therapy for Wilson's disease. *Annals of Internal Medicine*, **99**, 314–319.

Brewer, G.J., Terry, C.A., Aisen, A.M. and Hill, G.M. (1987) Worsening of neurologic syndrome in patients with Wilson's disease with initial penicillamine therapy. *Archives of Neurology*, **44**, 490–493.

Brewer, G.J., Yuzbasiyan-Gurkan, V. and Dick, R. (1990) Zinc therapy of Wilson's disease: VIII. Dose response studies. *The*

Journal of Trace Elements in Experimental Medicine, **3**, 227–234.

Brewer, G.J., Dick, R.D., Yuzbasiyan-Gurkan, V. *et al.* (1991) Initial therapy of patients with Wilson's disease with tetrathiomolybdate. *Archives of Neurology*, **48**, 42–47.

Brewer, G.J., Yuzbasiyan-Gurkan, V. and Johnson, V. (1991) Treatment of Wilson's disease with zinc. IX: Response of serum lipids. *The Journal of Laboratory and Clinical Medicine*, **118**, 466–470.

Brewer, G.J. and Yuzbasiyan-Gurkan, V. (1992) Wilson's disease. *Medicine*, **71**, 139–164.

Brewer, G.J., Yuzbasiyan-Gurkan, V., Johnson, V. *et al.* (1993a) Treatment of Wilson's disease with zinc XII: dose regimen requirements. *The American Journal of the Medical Sciences*, **305**, 199–202.

Brewer, G.J., Yuzbasiyan-Gurkan, V., Johnson, V. *et al.* (1993b) Treatment of Wilson's disease with zinc: XI. Interaction with other anticopper agents. *Journal of the American College of Nutrition*, **12**, 26–30.

Brewer, G.J., Dick, R.D., Johnson, V. *et al.* (1994a) Treatment of Wilson's disease with ammonium tetrathiomolybdate. I. Initial therapy in 17 neurologically affected patients. *Archives of Neurology*, **51**, 545–554.

Brewer, G.J., Dick, R.D., Yuzbasiyan-Gurkan, V. *et al.* (1994b) Treatment of Wilson's disease with zinc. XIII: Therapy with zinc in presymptomatic patients from the time of diagnosis. *The Journal of Laboratory and Clinical Medicine*, **123**, 849–858.

Brewer, G.J., Johnson, V., Dick, R.D. *et al.* (1996) Treatment of Wilson's disease with ammonium tetrathiomolybdate. II. Initial therapy in 33 neurologically affected patients and follow-up with zinc therapy. *Archives of Neurology*, **53**, 1017–1025.

Brewer, G.J., Johnson, V. and Kaplan, J. (1997) Treatment of Wilson's disease with zinc: XIV. Studies of the effect of zinc on lymphocyte function. *The Journal of Laboratory and Clinical Medicine*, **129**, 649–652.

Brewer, G.J., Dick, R.D., Johnson, V.D. *et al.* (1998) Treatment of Wilson's disease with zinc: XV long-term follow-up studies. *The Journal of Laboratory and Clinical Medicine*, **132**, 264–278.

Brewer, G.J. (2000) Recognition, diagnosis, and management of Wilson's disease. *Experimental Biology and Medicine*, **223**, 39–46.

Brewer, G.J., Johnson, V.D., Dick, R.D. *et al.* (2000) Treatment of Wilson's disease with zinc XVII: Treatment during pregnancy. *Hepatology*, **31**, 364–370.

Brewer, G.J. (2001) *Wilson's Disease: A Clinician's Guide to Recognition, Diagnosis, and Management*, Kluwer Academic Publishers, Boston, MA.

Brewer, G.J., Dick, R.D., Johnson, V.D. *et al.* (2001) Treatment of Wilson's disease with zinc XVI: treatment during the pediatric years. *The Journal of Laboratory and Clinical Medicine*, **137**, 191–198.

Brewer, G.J., Hedera, P., Kluin, K.J. *et al.* (2003) Treatment of Wilson's disease with ammonium tetrathiomolybdate: III. Initial therapy in a total of 55 neurologically affected patients and follow-up with zinc therapy. *Archives of Neurology*, **60**, 379–385.

Brewer, G.J. (2004) Wilson's disease, in *Harrison's Principles of Internal Medicine*, 16th edn, (eds D.L. Kasper E. Braunward A.S. Fauci S.L. Hauser D.L. Longo and J.L. Jameson), McGraw-Hill Companies, Inc., New York, NY.

Brewer, G.J. (2005) Behavioral abnormalities in Wilson's disease, in *Behavioral Neurology of Movement Disorders* 2nd edn, (eds W.J. Weiner A.E. Lang and K.E. Anderson), Lippincott, Williams & Wilkins, Philadelphia.

Brewer, G.J., Askari, F., Lorincz, M.T. *et al.* (2006) Treatment of Wilson's disease with ammonium tetrathiomolybdate: IV. Comparison of tetrathiomolybdate and trientine in a double-blind study of treatment of the neurologic presentation of Wilson's disease. *Archives of Neurology*, **63**, 521–527.

Bull, P.C., Thomas, G.R., Rommens, J.M. *et al.* (1993) The Wilson's disease gene is a putative copper transporting P-type ATPase similar to the Menkes gene. *Nature Genetics*, **5**, 327–337.

Chandra, R.K. (1984) Excessive intake of zinc impairs immune responses. *Journal of the American Medical Association*, **252**, 1443–1446.

Czlonkowska, A., Gajda, J. and Rodo, M. (1996) Effects of long-term treatment in Wilson's disease with D-penicillamine and zinc sulphate. *Journal of Neurology*, **243**, 269–273.

Dhawan, A., Taylor, R.M., Cheeseman, P. *et al.* (2005) Wilson's disease in children: 37-year experience and revised King's score for liver transplantation. *Liver Transplantation*, **11**, 441–448.

Dick, A.T. and Bull, L.B. (1945) Some preliminary observations of the effect of molybdenum on copper metabolism in herbivorous animals. *Australian Veterinary Journal*, **21**, 70–72.

Ferguson, W.S., Lewis, A.L. and Waterson, S.J. (1943) The teart pastures of Somerset, I:the cause and cure of teartness. *Journal of Agriculture Science*, **33**, 44.

Gooneratne, S.R., Howell, J.M. and Gawthorne, J.M. (1981) An investigation of the effects of intravenous administration of thiomolybdate on copper metabolism in chronic Cu-poisoned sheep. *The British Journal of Nutrition*, **46**, 469–480.

Hall, A.C., Young, B.W. and Bremner, I. (1979) Intestinal metallothionein and the mutual antagonism between copper and zinc in the rat. *Journal of Inorganic Biochemistry*, **11**, 57–66.

Hill, G.M., Brewer, G.J., Juni, J.E. *et al.* (1986) Treatment of Wilson's disease with zinc. II. Validation of oral 64copper with copper balance. *The American Journal of the Medical Sciences*, **292**, 344–349.

Hill, G.M., Brewer, G.J., Prasad, A.S. *et al.* (1987) Treatment of Wilson's disease with zinc. I. Oral zinc therapy regimens. *Hepatology*, **7**, 522–528.

Hoogenraad, T.U., Van den Hammer, C.J.A., Koevoet, R. and De Ruyter Korver, E.G.W.M. (1978) Oral zinc in Wilson's disease. *Lancet*, **2**, 1262–1263.

Hoogenraad, T.U., Koevoet, R. and de Ruyter Korver, E.G. (1979) Oral zinc sulphate as long-term treatment in Wilson's disease (hepatolenticular degeneration). *European Neurology*, **18**, 205–211.

Hoogenraad, T.U., Van Hattum, J. and Van den Hamer, C.J.A. (1987) Management of Wilson's disease with zinc sulfate. Experience in a series of 27 patients. *Journal of the Neurological Sciences*, **77**, 137–146.

Hoogenraad, T.U. (1996) *Wilson's Disease*, Saunders, London.

Marcellini, M., Di Ciommo, V., Callea, F. *et al.* (2005) Treatment of Wilson's disease with zinc from the time of diagnosis in pediatric patients: a single-hospital, 10-year follow-up study. *The Journal of Laboratory and Clinical Medicine*, **145**, 139–143.

Marcilese Ammerman, C.B., Valsecchi, R.M., Dunavant, B.G. and Davis, G.K. (1969) Effect of dietary molybdenum and sulfate upon copper metabolism in sheep. *Journal of Nutrition*, **99**, 177–183.

Mason, J. (1990) The biochemical pathogenesis of molybdenum-induced copper deficiency syndromes in ruminants: towards the final chapter. *Irish Veterinary Journal*, **43**, 18–21.

McQuaid, A. and Mason, J. (1991) A comparison of the effects of penicillamine, trientine, and trithiomolybdate on [35S]-labeled metallothionein in vitro; implications for Wilson's disease therapy. *Journal of Inorganic Biochemistry*, **41**, 87–92.

Menard, M.P., McCormick, C.C. and Cousins, R.J. (1981) Regulation of intestinal metallothionein biosynthesis in rats by dietary zinc. *The Journal of Nutrition*, **111**, 1353–1361.

Miller, R.F. and Engel, R.W. (1960) Interrelations of copper, molybdenum and sulfate sulfur in nutrition. *Federation Proceedings*, **19**, 666–677.

Mills, C.F., El-Gallad, T.T. and Bremner, I. (1981) Effects of molybdate, sulfide, and tetrathiomolybdate on copper metabolism in rats. *Journal of Inorganic Biochemistry*, **14**, 189–207.

Mills, C.F., El-Gallad, T.T., Bremner, I. and Weham, G. (1981) Copper and molybdenum absorption by rats given ammonium tetrathiomolybdate. *Journal of Inorganic Biochemistry*, **14**, 163–175.

Nazer, H., Ede, R.J., Mowat, A.P. and Williams, R. (1986) Wilson's disease: clinical presentation and use of prognostic index. *Gut*, **27**, 1377–1381.

Nimni, M.E. and Bavetta, L.A. (1965) Collagen defect induced by penicillamine. *Science*, **150**, 905–907.

Oestreicher, P. and Cousins, R.J. (1985) Copper and zinc absorption in the rat: mechanism of mutual antagonism. *The Journal of Nutrition*, **115**, 159–166.

Physicians Desk Reference (2007) Montvale, NJ, Thomson PDR.

Prasad, A.S., Brewer, G.J., Schoomaker, E.B. and Rabbini, P. (1978) Hypocupremia induced by zinc therapy in adults. *The Journal of the American Medical Association*, **240**, 2166–2168.

Ronchetti, I.P., Fornieri, C., Contri, M.B. *et al.* (1986) Effect of DL-penicillamine on the aorta of growing chickens. *American Journal of Pathology*, **124**, 436–447.

Scheinberg, I.H. and Sternlieb, I. (1984) Wilson's disease, in *Major Problems in Internal Medicine* (ed. L.H.J. Smith), W.B. Saunders Company, Philadelphia.

Schouwink, G. (1961) De hepatocecerebrale degeneratie, met een onderzoek naar de zonkstrofwisseling. MD thesis (with a summary in English, French, and German). University of Amsterdam.

Starosta-Rubinstein, S., Young, A.B., Kluin, K. *et al.* (1987) Clinical assessment of 31 patients with Wilson's disease. Correlations with structural changes on magnetic resonance imaging. *Archives of Neurology*, **44**, 365–370.

Tanzi, R.E., Petrukhin, K., Chernov, I. *et al.* (1993) The Wilson's disease gene is a copper transporting ATPase with homology to the Menkes disease gene. *Nature Genetics*, **5**, 344–350.

Walshe, J.M. (1956) Penicillamine, a new oral therapy for Wilson's disease. *American Journal of Medicine*, **21**, 487–495.

Walshe, J.M. (1982) Treatment of Wilson's disease with trientine (triethylene tetramine) dihydrochloride. *Lancet*, **1**, 643–647.

Yamaguchi, Y., Heiny, M.E. and Gitlin, J.D. (1993) Isolation and characterization of a human liver cDNA as a candidate gene for Wilson's disease. *Biochemical and Biophysical Research Communications*, **197**, 271–277.

Yuzbasiyan-Gurkan, V., Brewer, G.J., Abrams, G.D. *et al.* (1989) Treatment of Wilson's disease with zinc. V. Changes in serum levels of lipase, amylase, and alkaline phosphatase in patients with Wilson's disease. *The Journal of Laboratory and Clinical Medicine*, **114**, 520–526.

Yuzbasiyan-Gurkan, V., Johnson, V. and Brewer, G.J. (1991) Diagnosis and characterization of presymptomatic patients with Wilson's disease and the use of molecular genetics to aid in the diagnosis. *Journal of Laboratory & Clinical Medicine*, **118**, 458–465.

Yuzbasiyan-Gurkan, V., Grider, A., Nostrant, T. *et al.* (1992) Treatment of Wilson's disease with zinc: X. Intestinal metallothionein induction. *The Journal of Laboratory and Clinical Medicine*, **120**, 380–386.

17

Cramps and Spasms

Christine D. Esper, Pratibha G. Aia, Leslie J. Cloud and Stewart A. Factor

Emory University School of Medicine, Department of Neurology, Atlanta, GA, USA

Cramps and spasms are common medical ailments that may be seen in a movement disorders clinic. Some of these conditions are benign and self-limited, and fall into the realm of typical movement disorders. In contrast, we also review some less common neuromuscular disorders that have some overlap with such movement disorders. This chapter discusses these disorders in detail, in addition to prevalence, clinical characteristics, diagnostic testing and treatment modalities. When evaluating patients in a movement disorders clinic, applying information provided in this chapter will be useful in recognizing specific disorders underlying the symptoms of spasms, in addition to muscle cramps.

HEMIFACIAL SPASM

Hemifacial spasm (HFS) is a syndrome of unilateral, involuntary, intermittent, tonic or clonic contractions of one or more muscles innervated by cranial nerve VII. Rare cases of bilateral HFS have been reported (Tan and Jankovic, 1999). The two sides behave independently in such cases. HFS most often initially affects the periorbital muscles (orbicularis oculi) unilaterally. Over time, other ipsilateral facial muscles (corrugator, frontalis, zygomaticus, risorius and platysma) become affected, and brief clonic twitching can progress to more sustained tonic contractions (see Figure 17.1). The facial nerve also innervates the stapedius muscle in the middle ear, and clonic contractions of that muscle can lead to a pulsating sound in the ear. Although the occurrence of spasms is unpredictable, triggers including fatigue, anxiety, stress, reading, exposure to bright light or fluorescent lights and driving have been reported. Spasms may persist in sleep (Montagna *et al.*, 1986). HFS is sometimes associated with pain, and ipsilateral facial weakness can occur in chronic cases. There is no sensory loss. HFS occurs almost exclusively in adults. Although rare cases of familial HFS have been reported (Friedman, Jamrozik and Bojakowski, 1989;

Micheli *et al.*, 1994; Miwa, Mizuno and Kondo, 2002), it is ordinarily not considered to be a hereditary disorder. A non-spontaneous form of HFS, known as "post-paralytic HFS" occurs as a sequela of Bell's palsy or trauma to the seventh nerve (Martinelli, Giuliani and Ippoliti, 1992; Valls-Sole and Montero, 2003). This is more appropriately referred to as synkinesis.

Because HFS is an episodic disorder, there may be no signs on physical exam; however, the spasms can often be provoked by having the patient voluntarily close and then open his or her eyes, puff out their cheeks or smile. The classic findings are irregular periorbital spasms that cause eyelid squinting or closure and lower facial spasms that pull the cheek or chin or lift the corner of the mouth along with platysma spasms.

Electromyography and blink reflex studies may help to differentiate HFS from other involuntary facial movements. The presence of characteristic high-frequency discharges on EMG, in association with the lateral spread response and variable synkinesis on blink reflex, constitutes the electrophysiologic hallmark of HFS (Nielsen, 1984; Nielsen, 1985).

While HFS is far more common than the other disorders discussed in this chapter, there is a paucity of epidemiologic data. One epidemiologic study in Olmstead County, Minnesota found an average age-adjusted annual incidence of HFS for all ages of 0.78/100 000. The prevalence was 14.5/100 000 in women and 7.4/100 000 in men (Auger and Whisnant, 1990). HFS is particularly common in Asians.

HFS probably results from a peripheral injury to the facial nerve. In a notable fraction of cases, HFS can be attributed to vascular compression of the facial nerve at the root exit zone (REZ), although the exact prevalence is not well documented in the literature. Modern neuroimaging techniques and surgical visualization often demonstrate neurovascular compression (Figure 17.2). The offending vessel is usually an atherosclerotic, aberrant or ectatic intracranial artery, most commonly the anterior or posterior

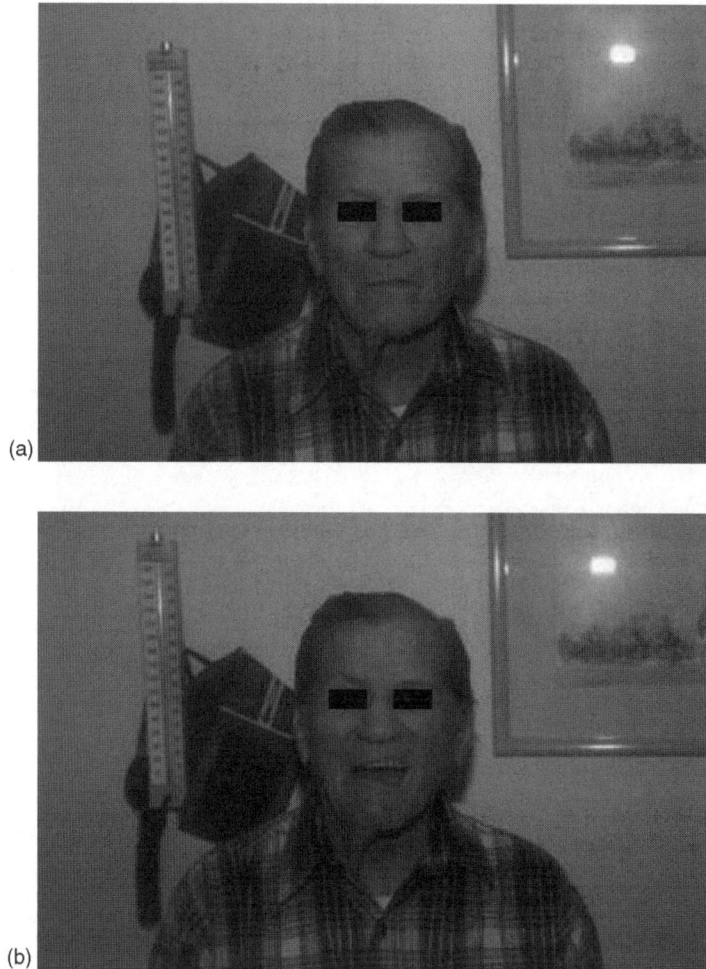

Figure 17.1 (a) Patient shown with right hemifacial spasm demonstrating elevation of the eyebrow, squinting of the eye, pulling of the corner of the mouth and tightness of the platysma; (b) The spasm is further activated by smiling.

cerebellar artery or the vertebral artery. Various space-occupying lesions in the cerebellopontine angle(epidermoid tumors, lipomas and meningiomas) have also rarely been associated with HFS (Auger *et al.*, 1981; Digre and Corbett, 1988; Galvez-Jimenez, Hanson and Desai, 2001).

Electrophysiologic evidence also implicates compression of the nerve at the REZ as the cause for HFS. The theory of "ectopic" excitation and "ephaptic" transmission, proposed by Gardner (1966) and later by Nielson (Nielsen, 1984, 1985), asserts that nerve compression and the resulting demyelination cause a "false" synapse at which ectopic activity may be triggered. Mechanical irritation or flow of extracellular current during passage of nerve impulses in adjacent nerves leads to aberrant activity. Nielson demonstrated that stimulation of the zygomatic branch of the compressed facial nerve results in the expected response in the orbicularis oculi and also a simultaneous response in the mentalis muscle, which is supplied by the mandibular branch. This phenomenon, which was absent in controls, disappeared after surgical decompression of the facial nerve. Moller and Jannetta (1984) examined intraoperative intracranial recordings of the facial muscles and the facial nerve near its entrance into the brainstem in HFS patients. They proposed an alternate hypothesis that the REZ becomes a trigger where impulses are generated orthodromically as well as antidromically. They further postulated that antidromic impulses activate facial nuclei motoneurons, which in turn send impulses down the seventh cranial nerve. Subsequently, spontaneous activity of the motoneurons developed and was considered similar to "kindling."

MRI and MRA are warranted in all HFS patients, but especially those with atypical features, such as facial

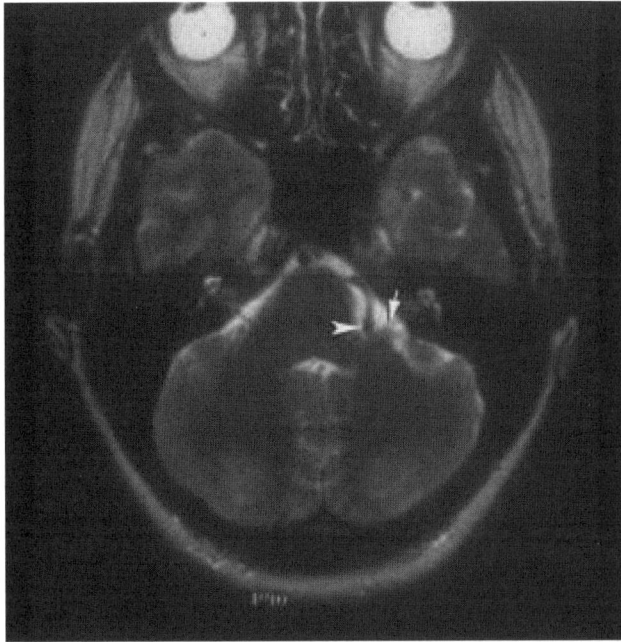

Figure 17.2 MRI scan demonstrating vascular compression of the facial nerve (arrow) in the cerebellopontine angle by an ectatic vessel (arrowhead).

numbness and weakness. In patients with an underlying structural mass lesion, treatment should be directed against the identified lesion. However, most patients with HFS do not fall into this category and must be treated medically.

Oral medical treatment is by "trial and error". The efficacy of oral medications is often modest and transient, and, for this reason, this approach is not the first choice. Carbamazepine, baclofen, clonazepam, haloperidol and orphenadrine have all been studied in HFS (Alexander and Moses, 1982; Hughes, Brackman and Weinstein, 1980; Iacono *et al.*, 1987). A cautious interpretation of the results is needed due to very small numbers of patients in these open-label, non-randomized treatment trials. More recently, gabapentin has been added to the list of potentially useful agents (Daniele *et al.*, 2001; Bandini and Mazzella, 1999). Sedation is a common side effect of all of these medications, especially at higher doses.

For most patients with HFS, injections of botulinum toxin (BoNT) into the involved facial muscles is the treatment of choice. There is most experience with botulinum toxin type A (BoNT/A). BoNT acts by inhibiting the release of acetylcholine pre-synaptically at the neuromuscular junction, which results in muscle weakening and reduction in muscle spasms. Long-term open trials have demonstrated that 92–97% of patients respond to the injections and that, with repeated injections approximately every three months, the response was maintained for years (Mauriello *et al.*, 1996; Kraft and Lang, 1988). The doses

utilized for BoNT/A (Botox) are 7.5–40 units on one side of the face and injections can be placed in ocular and lower facial muscles depending on the needs of the patient. The dose does not change very much over time. In many patients with upper and lower face spasms, injections in the periocular area may be enough to control spasms on the entire face. If not, injections can be given in whatever muscles require it. The onset of action is 3–7 days and the mean duration of benefit is 3–6 months. Transient side effects are local and include ptosis, weakness of eyebrow elevation or eyelid closure, lacrimation abnormalities, blurry vision, diplopia and facial weakness with an asymmetric smile. (An asymmetrical smile might be avoided by not injecting the zygomaticus muscle.) These side effects usually resolve in a few days or weeks but the therapeutic benefit lasts a few months (Van den Bergh *et al.*, 1995; Brin *et al.*, 1988; Defazio *et al.*, 2002). Botulinum toxin type B has also been found to be useful in HFS (Trosch, Adler and Pappert, 2007) particularly in those patients who develop antibodies to type A. However, its use is limited due to burning pain with injections and the rarity of immune resistance to BoNT/A in part because of the use of low doses.

Surgical treatment of HFS is an option for some patients who fail medical and BoNT/A management. Microvascular decompression of the facial nerve at the cerebellopontine angle has emerged as a potentially useful surgical procedure for HFS. The procedure involves placing a sponge between the REZ of cranial nerve VII and any adjacent tortuous or dilated blood vessels that may be found to compress the region. In a retrospective review of 1200 patients that underwent microvascular decompression for HFS, follow-up for 2–10 years showed that 88.7% of the patients were cured and 5.6% were relieved with an effective rate of 94.3%. Recurrence rate was 3.2%, and the procedure was ineffective in 2.6% (Yuan *et al.*, 2005). Common complications include temporary or permanent dysfunction of the facial or auditory nerves (Barker *et al.*, 1995; Auger *et al.*, 1981; Yuan *et al.*, 2005). Intraoperative monitoring of the facial and auditory nerves may reduce the frequency of these complications. EMG recording of spontaneous activity from several facial muscles is used to monitor facial nerve function intraoperatively. Brainstem auditory evoked potentials, electrocochleography or direct recording of nerve action potentials are used to intraoperatively monitor the function of cranial nerve VIII.

EPISODIC FOCAL LINGUAL SPASMS

An unusual form of muscle spasm was reported by Edwards *et al.* in a 33 year old woman who presented with episodic tightening of the left side of her tongue (Edwards, Schott and Bhatia, 2003). The episodes had no clear precipitants and occurred over 100 times per day, lasting 20 to 120 seconds. These spasms resulted in difficulty articulating and swallowing. During such spasms, the tongue would pucker, become ridged and bulge. She also had a mild postural tremor of the hands and investigations were unremarkable. Two other very similar cases were reported by Lees *et al.* in 1986 and referred to as hemiglossal twisting (Lees, Blau and Schon, 1986). Edwards *et al.* suggested that these movements were the result of dystonia, although the puckering movements were not characteristic and the nature of the spasms remained unclear. Some have suggested that the pathophysiology may be similar to hemifacial spasm, and the prevalence of this disorder is unknown. Additionally, while botulinum toxin therapy is a reasonable option, there is no clinical experience to support this.

RIPPLING MUSCLE DISEASE

Rippling muscle disease (RMD) is not a movement disorder, but actually a rare benign myopathy characterized by muscle hyperexcitability that is distinct from myotonia. It is included in this chapter because its presentation is frequently associated with muscle cramping. It was first reported in 1975 in a family with five affected members in three generations (Torbergsen, 1975). Since then, several other cases and families have been described and the etiology has been discerned.

Hereditary cases of RMD generally have an age of onset in the first and second decade (Torbergsen, 2002), while sporadic autoimmune cases occur in the fourth decade and

beyond (Schulte-Mattler *et al.*, 2005). The syndrome is generally benign and non-progressive (Torbergsen, 2002). Clinically, the earliest features are muscle stiffness and slowness of movement after prolonged rest or sleep (Torbergsen, 2002; Dotti *et al.*, 2006). This stiffness often leads to toe walking in the early morning (Madrid, Kubisch and Hays, 2005; So *et al.*, 2001), which disappears with activity. In one family with 11 affected members, muscle stiffness and myalgias were the most prominent symptoms (So *et al.*, 2001). Patients also complain of exercise-induced muscle pain and muscle cramping (Torbergsen, 2002; Dotti *et al.*, 2006), which is most pronounced in the proximal leg muscles. There is also calf hypertrophy (Dotti *et al.*, 2006; So *et al.*, 2001). The most characteristic feature is mounding of muscle (also referred to as myoedema) in response to mechanical stimulation such as percussion with a reflex hammer, called percussion induced rapid muscle contraction (PIRC). There is also a rolling or rippling contraction of muscle (Dotti *et al.*, 2006; Kubisch *et al.*, 2003; Kubisch *et al.*, 2005; Lamb, 2005; Lorenzoni *et al.*, 2007; Torbergsen, 2002). The velocity of movement in these rippling muscles is 10 times slower than the propagation velocity of muscle fiber action potentials. Muscle strength is generally normal (Torbergsen, 2002), although there have been reports of muscle weakness in more severe cases (Kubisch *et al.*, 2003; Kubisch *et al.*, 2005; Roberts *et al.*, 2006; Lorenzoni *et al.*, 2007; Madrid, Kubisch and Hays, 2005). Other features include muscle fatigue and sensitivity to cold. In one report, extraocular muscle paresis was present (Ueyama *et al.*, 2007). There have also been reports of hypertrophic cardiomyopathy (Dotti *et al.*, 2006). There is some phenotypic variability from case to case, even within families (Vorgerd *et al.*, 1999; So *et al.*, 2001).

Laboratory findings include a moderate elevation of creatine kinase (CK) in the hundreds to thousands. Electromyography shows normal recruitment and motor unit potentials in most cases (Torbergsen, 2002), but some reports of myopathic potentials have also been published (Dotti *et al.*, 2006; Roberts *et al.*, 2006). The rippling contractions are electrically silent. One hypothesis is that the abnormal muscle contractions are evoked by "silent" action potentials traveling in the muscle's tubular system (Lamb, 2005). Recommended diagnostic criteria include PIRCs, mounding and rippling contractions and elevated CK (Torbergsen, 2002).

RMD is genetically heterogeneous and has been seen in dominant, recessive and sporadic forms. Autosomal dominant inheritance is most common. A single autosomal dominant family was linked to chromosome 1q41 in 1994 (Stephan *et al.*, 1994). There have been no other RMD families linked to this locus. The most common linkage has been to the gene CAV3 on chromosome 3q25, which codes for a sarcolemmal protein caveolin 3 (Betz *et al.*, 2001). Caveolin 3 is a muscle specific protein product expressed in skeletal, cardiac and smooth muscle, and is located in the sarcolemma and T-tubules. It is involved in sarcolemmal trafficking, sorting, transport and signal transduction (Lorenzoni *et al.*, 2007). A mutation in CAV3 results in T-tubule system derangement, sarcolemmal membrane alterations and subsarcolemmal vesicle formation (Woodman *et al.*, 2004). Thus far, more than 10 mutations (missense and deletions) have been described (Torbergsen, 2002; Dotti *et al.*, 2006; Lorenzoni *et al.*, 2007; Ueyama *et al.*, 2007; Roberts *et al.*, 2006). Recessive mutations in CAV3 have also been reported, and these homozygous cases are the ones who experience muscle weakness and extraocular muscle paresis as previously described (Kubisch *et al.*, 2003; Kubisch *et al.*, 2005; Ueyama *et al.*, 2007). The CAV3 gene is also linked to three other disorders: limb-girdle muscular dystrophy type 1C, distal myopathy and hyperCKemia without neuromuscular symptoms, indicating phenotypic variability for the CAV3 mutations.

There is an autoimmune form of RMD that has an onset in middle age. It has been associated with myasthenia gravis (MG). In some cases, the rippling comes first, as does the antibody to high molecular weight sarcolemmal proteins that are functionally related to ion channels (Torbergsen, 2002; Schulte-Mattler *et al.*, 2005). The MG subsequently develops, and as with other cases of MG, these patients develop thymomas and respond to their removal.

While several muscle biopsy reports were considered negative for myopathic changes (Kubisch *et al.*, 2003; Kubisch *et al.*, 2005), others have found proliferation of the endomesial connective tissue, variation in fiber size with centralization of nuclei and foci of necrosis (Roberts *et al.*, 2006; Dotti *et al.*, 2006; Lorenzoni *et al.*, 2007; Madrid, Kubisch and Hays, 2005). Immunostaining has demonstrated the absence of CAV3 in the sarcolemma (Madrid, Kubisch and Hays, 2005; Lorenzoni *et al.*, 2007; Roberts *et al.*, 2006; Dotti *et al.*, 2006). Electron microscopy demonstrates absence of caveolae in the sarcolemma, subsarcolemmal vacuoles, plasmalemmal discontinuities, abnormal papillary projections and dilated T-tubules (Kubisch *et al.*, 2003; Dotti *et al.*, 2006). In autoimmune cases, immunoglobulin deposition is seen in the sarcolemma along with inflammatory change, and the CAV3 loss is irregular and appears in a mosaic pattern (Schulte-Mattler *et al.*, 2005). The mechanism of the hyperexcitability in RMD is presumed to be the result of abnormalities of the sarcoplasmic reticulum and calcium channels (Torbergsen, 2002).

RMD is a rare disorder with a generally benign outcome and for that reason there is little written on the treatment of this disorder. Some investigators have suggested treatment with dantrolene and calcium-channel blockers (Ricker, Moxley and Rohkamm, 1989; Torbergsen, 2002). The use of such agents requires confirmation.

For the autoimmune type, thymectomy and immunosuppressive therapy such as azathioprine are recommended (Torbergsen, 2002; Muller-Felber *et al.*, 1999).

SCHWARTZ–JAMPEL SYNDROME

The Schwartz–Jampel syndrome (SJS) is a rare, inherited disorder characterized by generalized myotonia, short stature, skeletal abnormalities and a characteristic facies. SJS has several synonyms including chondrodystrophic myotonia, osteochondromuscular dystrophy and Aberfield's syndrome. Although the exact prevalence of SJS is unknown, more than 80 cases have been reported in the medical literature. Inheritance is usually autosomal recessive, although dominant inheritance has been suggested in some family reports (Pascuzzi *et al.*, 1990). Symptoms become apparent in the first three years of life, but could be seen even at birth. There are case reports of pre-natal diagnosis of SJS using ultrasonography (Hunziker *et al.*, 1989).

Height is typically below the 10th percentile in all age groups. Several characteristic skeletal anomalies contribute to the short stature. These include: bony dysplasia with metaphyseal enlargement and cortical thickening, bowing and shortening of the long bones of the extremities, arachnodactyly, hip dysplasia with acetabular abnormalities, kyphoscoliosis, platyspondyly with coronally cleft vertebrae, lumbar lordosis and pectus carinatum (Mereu and Porter,1969; Pavone *et al.*, 1978; Schwartz and Jampel, 1962; Spranger *et al.*, 2000; Viljoen and Beighton, 1992). Patients have a waddling gait and a crouched stance. Contractures of major joints are common and progressive until mid-adolescence when they peak and thereafter remain static.

Myotonia results in a fixed facial expression with pursed lips and narrowed palpebral fissures. Additional facial anomalies include blepharophimosis, micronathia, upward slanting eyes, exotropia, microcornea, low set ears with folded helices and medial displacement of the outer canthi. Other dysmorphic features include prominent eyebrows, short neck, hypoplastic larynx and hypertrichosis. Patients with SJS may have prominent proximal muscle hypertrophy and distal-predominant generalized weakness and atrophy (Pascuzzi *et al.*, 1990; Lehmann-Horn *et al.*, 1990). Myotonia is evident on thenar percussion. Tendon reflexes are generally depressed although muscle tone is increased. Intelligence is normal in most cases, although several cases with mental retardation have been described (Giedion *et al.*, 1997).

Due to the clinical and radiologic heterogeneity in SJS, Giedion *et al.* proposed a classification scheme (Giedion *et al.*, 1997). Type 1A exhibits moderate myotonia, bone dysplasia, muscle hypertrophy and dysmorphic facies in childhood. Type 1B is similar to type 1A but is apparent at birth and is associated with more severe skeletal anomalies, particularly short-limbed dysplasia with dumbbell shaped femora (Kniest dysplasia-like). Type 2 is the most severe. It manifests at birth with contractures, prominent myotonia, camptomelia (severe long bone bowing), and severe facial and pharyngeal anomalies that preclude normal feeding and result in infantile death. Due to the similarities between type 2 SJS and Stuve–Wiedemann syndrome, some authors have suggested that they may represent the same disease (Cormier-Daire *et al.*, 1998). Life expectancy appears to be normal in patients with type 1A SJS, whereas life expectancy for patients with type 1B is probably reduced.

When SJS is suspected based on clinical and radiographic appearance, electromyography can be a useful confirmatory procedure. Motor and sensory nerve conduction studies are normal (Lehmann-Horn *et al.*, 1990). Concentric needle electromyography (CNEMG) shows persistent spontaneous activity that is uninfluenced by curare or ischemia (Lehmann-Horn *et al.*, 1990; Taylor *et al.*, 1972). The spontaneous activity is in the form of high-frequency, low-voltage discharges that wax and wane in frequency and amplitude (myotonic discharges) as well as high-frequency discharges that do not vary in frequency or amplitude (complex repetitive discharges) (Pascuzzi *et al.*, 1990; Schwartz and Jampel, 1962; Lehmann-Horn *et al.*, 1990; Taylor *et al.*, 1972; Squires and Prangley, 1996; Jablecki and Schultz, 1982). Single fiber electromyography (SFEMG) shows rather stable, sometimes intermittent, discharge series with occasional amplitude and/or frequency fluctuations (Jablecki and Schultz, 1982; Lehmann-Horn *et al.*, 1990).

No pathognomonic histopathologic tests are available. Light microscopy usually reveals normal skeletal muscle (Lehmann-Horn *et al.*, 1990; Pascuzzi *et al.*, 1990; Squires and Prangley, 1996). Mild myopathic features, including excessive variability in fiber size, may occasionally be observed (Scribanu and Ionasescu, 1981). Electron microscopy reveals subsarcolemmal membrane abnormalities and mild changes in intracellular organelles (Lehmann-Horn *et al.*, 1990; Squires and Prangley, 1996). Although the myofibrils have a normal configuration, the distribution of isoforms of myosin, myosin light chains, and other contractile or structural proteins are altered in SJS (Soussi-Yanicostas *et al.*, 1991). Serum CK may be modestly elevated.

Inheritance of SJS is usually autosomal recessive. Localization of the SJS locus to chromosome 1p34-p36.1 by homozygosity mapping has been reported (Nicole *et al.*, 1995). However, there are also reports of families with neonatal SJS who do not map to human chromosome 1p34-p36.1, suggesting genetic heterogeneity (Brown *et al.*, 1997). The proteins that are altered are not known.

The pathophysiology of the myotonia in SJS is poorly understood. *In vitro* studies of skeletal muscle fibers from a patient with SJS (using the cell-attached patch clamp mode) implicated a defect in sodium-channel gating as a potential cause (Lehmann-Horn *et al.*, 1990). Depolarizing pulses elicited delayed synchronous sodium-channel openings that persisted after the surface membrane repolarized. The delayed openings suggest that the transition from the closed to the open state of the sodium channel is altered. Repeated openings during depolarization suggest a destabilization of the fast-inactivated state so that channels can repeatedly jump between the inactivated and open-channel states. This destabilization of the fast-inactivated state increases membrane excitability, thus contributing to the genesis of myotonia (Lehmann-Horn *et al.*, 1990).

Treatment is appropriate if SJS is symptomatic. Orthopedic surgery may be needed for skeletal deformities. Cosmetic repair of narrowed palpebral fissures may be necessary to facilitate normal vision. Ophthalmologic treatment of myopia and juvenile cataract is sometimes warranted. Numerous drugs have been used in attempts to abolish the continuous muscle activity associated with SJS. Diazepam, barbiturates, phenytoin and quinine have all been used without success (Seay and Ziter, 1978; Topaloglu *et al.*, 1993; Fariello *et al.*, 1978). Procainamide (Lehmann-Horn *et al.*, 1990) and carbamazepine (Squires and Prangley, 1996) have been shown to reduce myotonia and muscle stiffness in SJS. Early and aggressive treatment of myotonia may reduce the development of some skeletal anomalies, such as bowing of the long bones (Squires and Prangley, 1996). Because patients with SJS are susceptible to malignant hyperthermia, depolarizing muscle relaxants are best avoided during anesthesia (Seay and Ziter, 1978).

HEREDITARY DISTAL MUSCLE CRAMPS WITHOUT NEUROPATHY

Hereditary distal muscle cramps without neuropathy is a rare disease characterized by persistent cramping involving distal muscle groups. The trait is autosomal dominant. Within affected families, anticipation is observed (an earlier age of onset and increased severity of symptoms are described with each successive generation). Patients present in childhood or early adolescence with painful muscle cramps predominantly affecting distal muscles, with only rare cramps reported in more proximal ones. In affected individuals, symptoms occur during activity, at rest and even in sleep. Cramps are made worse by cold or a sudden change in temperature, but can also be present at normal temperature and in hot weather. After a period of strong cramps, subjective weakness or tiredness occurs, but no paralysis. The symptoms may progress slightly with advancing age. Physical examination is unremarkable except for the observation of dramatic muscle cramps.

The first and best description of the clinical phenotype came from Jusic, Dogan and Stojanovic (1972) who described the disease occurring in 12 members of the same family. Their propositus held her hands "in a more or less flexed position with fingers moving in accordance with more tonic or jerky painful contractions of the intrinsic hand or forearm muscles. Tonic thumb opposition was especially frequent and painful." In her legs, visible contractions were seen in the gastrocnemius and anterior tibial compartment. Her feet were flexed in the equinovarus position or moved repetitively in the opposite direction with irregular jerky or tonic movements. Her cramps were exaggerated by repeated voluntary contractions and relieved by pressing and twisting the hands and feet.

The prevalence is unknown. After the Jusic *et al.* description, Lazaro, Rollinson and Fenichel (1981) published a description of a very similar clinical entity occurring in 16 members of another family. To date, these are the only two affected families reported in the English medical literature. Both families were of Yugoslavian origin.

The pathophysiology of this disease is unknown. Muscle biopsies were essentially normal (Lazaro, Rollinson and Fenichel, 1981; Jusic, Dogan and Stojanovic, 1972). The forearm ischemic exercise test produced a normal generation of lactate and ammonia, without elevation of creatine kinase levels and no cramping. Urine was negative for hemoglobin and myoglobin during and immediately after the ischemic exercise test (Lazaro, Rollinson and Fenichel, 1981).

Electrophysiologic data differed significantly between the two reported families. Jusic, Dogan and Stojanovic (1972) found no evidence for an underlying neuropathy or neuronopathy. They found no myotonic response on insertion. Motor unit potentials were normal. Continual waxing and waning electrical discharges corresponding to clinically visible cramps were present. Motor and afferent nerve conduction velocities were normal. Repetitive nerve stimulation demonstrated no effect on the amplitude of evoked muscle potentials. With spinal anesthesia or nerve block, the muscle contractions continued, but became painless. The muscle cramps were only stopped by local infiltration of anesthetic into the muscle.

The lack of neurogenic EMG findings by Jusic, Dogan and Stojanovic (1972) should be contrasted with the EMG findings by Lazaro, Rollinson and Fenichel (1981). They found borderline slow nerve conduction velocities, prolonged motor distal latencies, prolonged F wave latencies, occasional large amplitude prolonged polyphasic motor unit potentials and occasional fasciculations. These findings would localize the disorder to the motor neuron. Despite the differences in the electrophysiologic data between the two families, Lazaro *et al.* felt their family did indeed suffer from the same disease because the clinical presentations were so strikingly similar. The discrepancies

between the electrophysiologic data of the two groups have not yet been reconciled.

The only available treatment data comes from Jusic, Dogan and Stojanovic (1972), who reported the results of drug studies in their propositus. Carbamazepine at 200 mg three times daily and diazepam at 5 mg three times daily had no effect on symptoms. Meprobamate 400 mg three times daily improved the nocturnal cramps, but only transiently. Ten days later, the cramps returned at a lesser degree than before administration of the drug and increased dosage provided no further effect. Corticotropin (ACTH) 100 i.u. daily for two weeks did not influence the symptoms. Hydrochlorthiazide, prescribed in addition to the ACTH at a dose of 25 mg twice daily, made the symptoms worse. Neostigmine 1.5 mg IM and biperidol 5 mg IM three times daily had no effect. Potassium chloride 2 mg daily resulted in two days with substantial reduction and finally total disappearance of cramps. After 10 days, the therapy was discontinued, but the condition continued to be controlled until three months later when the cramps reappeared. Resumption of the potassium had no substantial influence on the symptoms (Jusic, Dogan and Stojanovic, 1972).

NEUROMYOTONIA

Neuromyotonia, or Isaacs' syndrome, is a rare condition of generalized peripheral nerve hyperexcitability. It manifests as spontaneous, continuous, muscle activity of peripheral nerve origin. Although it has been described in infants (Black *et al.*, 1972) it more commonly occurs in adults. Clinically, it is characterized by the gradual onset of muscle stiffness at rest, with continuous twitching (fasciculations) or quivering (myokymia) of muscles, and cramps following voluntary contractions due to delay in muscle relaxation (pseudomyotonia) (Isaacs, 1961). The distribution of muscle involvement is usually distal; however, it can also involve the proximal extremities, trunk and facial muscles. Involvement can be focal, as one case report described a patient with finger flexion resembling focal hand dystonia (Jamora, Umapathi and Tan, 2006). There may be associated hyperhidrosis and reddening of the skin. Pain is rare, but muscle aching is common. Persistent contraction often occurs after exercise; and, a rippling of continuously contracting muscles can be seen (Gutmann, 2002).

The electrophysiologic characteristics of peripheral nerve hyperexcitability, first described by Denny-Brown in 1948, are characterized by spontaneous high-frequency (neuromyotonic) motor unit discharges and myokymic discharges (doublet or multiplet motor unit discharges) (Denny-Brown and Folley, 1948). It wasn't until 1961 that Isaacs made the first full description of "continuous muscle-fiber activity" and established the peripheral nerve origin of the spontaneously occurring discharges (Isaacs, 1961). He demonstrated that: (i) there was persistence of abnormal EMG activity after proximal nerve brachial block; (ii) there was no change in spontaneous muscle activity during general anesthesia with thiopentone; (iii) the depolarizing muscle relaxant succinylcholine and neuromuscular blocking agent curare produced electrical silence after a few minutes (Maddison, 2006).

Neuromyotonia can be sporadic (Gardner-Medwin and Walton, 1969; Isaacs, 1961) or inherited (Ashizawa et al., 1983; Falace et al., 2007). Many of these sporadic cases appear to have an autoimmune or paraneoplastic etiology. It has also been found in association with myasthenia gravis (Martinelli et al., 1996), thymoma (Garcia-Merino et al., 1991), Addison's disease (Vilchez et al., 1980), vitiligo (Vilchez et al., 1980), Hashimoto's thyroiditis, vitamin B12 deficiency (Vasilescu, Alexianu and Dan, 1984), celiac disease (Hadjivassiliou et al., 1997), rheumatoid arthritis (Le Gars et al., 1997), systemic sclerosis (Benito-Leon et al., 1999) and following bone marrow transplantation (Liguori et al., 2000). Neuromyotonia has also been reported in patients with small-cell lung cancer (Partanen et al., 1980), suggesting a possible paraneoplastic cause. A number of hematological malignancies have also been found in association with neuromyotonia (Caress et al., 1997; Gutmann, Gutmann and Schochet, 1996; Zifko et al., 1994), and these tend to be tumors known for their propensity to develop paraneoplastic disorders (Maddison, 2006). Neuromyotonic discharges have also been reported in association with inherited (Hahn et al., 1991; Vasilescu, Alexianu and Dan, 1984), inflammatory (Valenstein, Watson and Parker, 1978; Vasilescu, Alexianu and Dan, 1984), or metabolic (Vasilescu and Florescu, 1982; Wallis, Van Poznak and Plum, 1970) peripheral neuropathies.

There is considerable evidence that an abnormality of axonal voltage-gated potassium channels (VGKCs) is the basis of the abnormal discharges occurring in most of the neuromyotonic syndromes. Antibodies to VGKCs have been described in cases of generalized neuromyotonia (Shillito et al., 1995; Vernino et al., 1999; Vincent, 2000). Up to 50% of patients with acquired neuromyotonia have antibodies to VGKCs (Barber, Anderson and Vincent, 2000; Lee et al., 1998).

The symptoms of peripheral nerve excitability often respond well to anti-convulsants such as phenytoin, carbamazepine, sodium valproate, lamotrigine, gabapentin, and acetazolamide (Celebisoy et al., 1998; Dhand, 2006; Auger, 1994; Jamieson and Katirji, 1994; Isaacs, 1961; Mertens and Zschocke, 1965; Vasilescu, Alexianu and Dan, 1987), many of which work by altering channel properties in peripheral nerves and reducing spontaneous discharges. When the disorder is autoimmune, plasmaphe-

resis may be effective (Hayat et al., 2000; Nakatsuji et al., 2000), as well as IVIg (Alessi et al., 2000). The role of prednisone and other immunosuppressive agents has not been fully evaluated. The association with thymoma, small-cell lung cancer and lymphoma (Caress et al., 1997; Hart et al., 2002) should prompt the search for an underlying malignancy when neuromyotonia is diagnosed, along with the appropriate treatment plan.

In Isaacs' original patients, as well as others, response to medication and alleviation in symptoms was reported (Isaacs, 1961; Welch, Appenzeller and Bicknell, 1972). Resolution or reduction of electrophysiologic abnormalities has also been documented (Gutmann, 2002). A 14-year follow-up of Isaacs' original patients showed continued response to phenytoin, with eventual remission (Isaacs and Heffron, 1974). However, the long period of follow-up of Isaacs' patients has not been duplicated in the literature.

JUMPY STUMPS

As early as 1872, S. Weir Mitchell described causalgia after gunshot wounds injuring peripheral nerves and, in addition, reported tremor, jerks and spasms of the remaining stump following amputation (Hallett, 2007). However, Colles and Hancock (Hancock, 1852) are actually credited with the first descriptions of "convulsive movements of stumps;" and later in the early twentieth century, spasms of stumps was the subject of a thesis entitled "Les convulsions des moignons" (Amyot, 1929). The "jumpy stump" has been further described by others more recently (Kulisevsky, Marti-Fabregas and Grau, 1992; Marion, Gledhill and Thompson, 1989; Steiner, Dejesus and Mancall, 1974).

These movements are varied in nature, consisting of jerking, tremulousness or spasms of the stump, and they are often associated with severe stump pain (Steiner, Dejesus and Mancall, 1974). It has been reported that only 1% of post-amputation patients will experience these spontaneous, involuntary, autonomous movements of the stump (Carlen et al., 1978; Iacono et al., 1987). In the majority of cases with limb amputation, the motor disability relates directly to the loss of the limb, and the associated difficulty with acquiring voluntary control over the stump (Marion, Gledhill and Thompson, 1989). Jerking of the stump, when it occurs, is often preceded by severe pain, and upper or lower limb stumps could be affected. The stump jerks are usually induced by voluntary movement, but can also be triggered by cutaneous stimuli (Zadikoff, Mailis-Gagnon and Lang, 2006).

Jerking of the amputation stump with associated neuralgic pain can sometimes occur in the immediate postoperative period and settle over weeks to months, but may also develop gradually after a variable latent period and persist indefinitely (Zadikoff, Mailis-Gagnon and Lang, 2006). The movement phenomenon has been referred to as "jactitation" (Henderson and Smyth, 1948; Russell, 1970). In one case, a patient was described to experience symptoms for up to 40 years (Marion, Gledhill and Thompson, 1989). Phantom limb pain alone is a common sequela of amputation, occurring in up to 80% of people who undergo the procedure (Flor, 2002). In contrast, spasm of amputation stumps appears to be a rare phenomenon, judging by the sparse literature in standard neurology and orthopedics texts. This may be due to the improvement in surgical technique with less tissue damage during amputation, suggesting that traumatic amputation and extensive soft tissue injury may contribute to the development of these spasms (Marion, Gledhill and Thompson, 1989).

The pathophysiology of jumpy stumps is unknown. Some consider involuntary stump movements to be a form of segmental myoclonus, caused by afferent impulses arising from severed nerves (Steiner, Dejesus and Mancall, 1974). Marion and colleagues proposed an alteration in the processing of afferent sensory input as a contributing factor. This may occur as a result of functional changes in the spinal cord (or cortical) circuitry, leading to structural reorganization of local neuronal circuitry by axonal sprouting following nerve injury (Marion, Gledhill and Thompson, 1989). Another hypothesis suggests that following nerve injury, there is a loss of tonic inhibition, hence promoting autonomous, self-sustaining neural activity (Lang, Sittl and Erbguth, 1997). Most recently, some have suggested that spasms of the stump represent another variant within the spectrum of movement disorders associated with peripheral nerve injury (Jankovic, 2001).

There are no large-scale studies addressing the management of post-amputation stump movements, and treatment, if necessary, is difficult and often unsuccessful, although some isolated case reports have been promising. Iacono and colleagues reported that Baclofen at 20–40 mg per day successfully treated two post-amputation patients who developed continuous complex involuntary movements of the proximal extremity (Iacono et al., 1987); similar results have been reported by others (Carlen et al., 1978). Another case report found that doxepin provided dramatic relief in both post-amputation pain and involuntary autonomous movements in a 40-year-old man (Iacono et al., 1987). Most recently, it has been reported that gabapentin at 300 mg three times daily provided dramatic relief of both phantom limb pain and stump movements in a patient, with complete resolution in 24 hours (Mera et al., 2004). Injections of botulinum neurotoxin might be used in this circumstance, although there are no reports of this.

BELLY DANCER'S DYSKINESIA

The term "belly dancer's dyskinesia (BDD)," (also known as the moving umbilicus syndrome), was first used in 1990 in an article describing five patients with focal dyskinesias affecting the abdominal wall (Iliceto et al., 1990). The clinical characteristics of this syndrome include writhing movements and contractions of the abdominal muscles (Caviness et al., 1994; Iliceto et al., 1990). The onset is usually gradual, and the movements cannot be voluntarily suppressed (Linazasoro et al., 2005). In the original report, electrophysiologic studies revealed bilaterally synchronous 800–1000 ms bursts in the upper and lower abdominal recti that alternated with bursts in the external oblique muscles with a frequency of 30–40 per minute (Iliceto et al., 1990). This pattern of activation accounted for the circular movement of the umbilicus. The clinical course is long-lasting or permanent.

There are other focal dyskinesias that may resemble BDD. The physiology might be similar to that of spinal myoclonus (Jankovic and Pardo, 1986). Inghilleri and colleagues reported a case of spinal myoclonus resembling BDD in an 85 year-old woman with a T10 disk herniation (Inghilleri et al., 2006). Another case reported spinal myoclonus resembling BDD involving abdominal, thoracic and lumbar paraspinal muscles, and the involuntary movements became stimulus-sensitive in the later phase of the clinical course (Kono et al., 1994). The EMG discharges lasted 50–200 ms, and the interval of the successive discharges was at least 500 ms. Diaphragmatic flutter is a different, also rare, movement disorder that is associated with dyspnea, thoracic or abdominal wall pain, and epigastric pulsations resulting from involuntary contractions of the diaphragm with a frequency of 0.5–8.0 Hz (Vantrappen, Decramer and Harlet, 1992).

The cause of BDD is unknown. Investigations, such as spinal and abdominal imaging often fail to reveal any abnormality that could explain the movement disorder (Linazasoro et al., 2005). One report describes a woman who developed abdominal movements following childbirth, which fluctuated with her menstrual cycle (Linazasoro et al., 2005). A prior history of local trauma or surgical procedures of the abdomen may be present in up to half the cases (Linazasoro et al., 2005). One hypothesis is that peripheral trauma may alter the afferent signals from the periphery to the spinal cord and more rostral structures. This may lead to alterations in the central processing of sensory information and result in an abdominal motor output (Marsden et al., 1984; Nathan, 1978; Schott, 1985). Other reports have suggested that dopamine receptor blockers caused the involuntary muscle movements, including clebopride (Linazasoro et al., 2005) haloperidol and sulpiride (Shan, Liao and Fuh, 1998). A recent case report described a woman with central pontine myelinolysis who presented with BDD five months after severe hyponatremia (Roggendorf *et al.*, 2007).

There are no large-scale studies addressing the management of BDD, in part because of its rarity, and, as no definitive effective treatment exists, the prognosis is generally not favorable. However, one case report presented a woman with BDD who had a dramatic response to transcutaneous electrical nerve stimulation (TENS) (Linazasoro *et al.*, 2005). Specifically, the effect of TENS (at a rate of 80–100 Hz) was immediate and dramatic, with a subjective improvement of more than 90% in the number and intensity of the episodes. In another case, benzhexol provided some relief in the involuntary pelvic and abdominal movements in a woman (Caviness *et al.*, 1994). And, in two patients who developed involuntary abdominal movements after chronic use of haloperidol and sulpiride, there was dramatic improvement with reserpine (Shan, Liao and Fuh, 1998). Injections of botulinum neurotoxin might be used in this circumstance, although there are no reports of this.

PAINFUL LEGS AND MOVING TOES

In 1971, Spillane *et al.* first described this "syndrome of pain in the feet or lower limbs with spontaneous movements of the toes" (Spillane *et al.*, 1971). With the description of additional cases it has been found that the age of onset is usually middle or late life (Hallett, 2007). The syndrome consists of pain in the affected limb associated with spontaneous, involuntary, slow, wriggling movements of the toes (Mark, 2004). The movements may be unilateral or bilateral, intermittent or continuous, occasionally stopping completely for minutes (Barrett, Singh and Fahn, 1981; Nathan, 1978; Schoenen, Gonce and Delwaide, 1984; Schott, 1981; Spillane *et al.*, 1971; Wulff, 1982). Specifically, the toe movements consist of complex sequences of flexion, extension, abduction and adduction, in various combinations, at frequencies of 1–2 Hz (Dressler *et al.*, 1994). In a case series of 20 new patients diagnosed with this syndrome, electromyographic recordings performed in nine of them revealed the movements to be produced by long-duration (500 ms to 2 s) bursts of activity comprised of normal motor units and normal recruitment patterns; none exhibited EMG findings characteristic of neuromyotonia (Dressler *et al.*, 1994). In rare cases, the upper limbs may be involved instead of, or in addition to, the lower limbs, and in this situation the disorder is referred to as "painful arms and moving fingers" (Ebersbach *et al.*, 1998; Funakawa, Mano and Takayanagi, 1987; Verhagen, Horstink and Notermans, 1985).

The disability of the disorder is largely related to pain rather than the involuntary movements. The pain is diffuse, intractable, aching and deep (Yoon, Crabtree and Botek, 2001), and is usually the first symptom, preceding the onset of movement by days to years (Dressler *et al.*, 1994). The distribution of the pain is typically non-dermatomal (Dressler *et al.*, 1994). In many patients, the pain and movement appear to be closely linked, with an increase in the severity of the movement associated by exacerbations of pain (Dressler *et al.*, 1994). However, on rare occasions, identical movements are seen without pain, referred to as "painless legs and moving toes".

Many more reports have been published since the original literature by Spillane, but no single etiology or specific pathophysiological mechanism has been found. The syndrome has been reported to occur after spinal cord or cauda equina trauma, lumbar radiculopathy, peripheral neuropathy (including HIV-related axonal neuropathy), traumatic lesions of the soft tissue and bone in the foot, during treatment with neuroleptics or without any antecedents (Barrett, Singh and Fahn, 1981; Dressler *et al.*, 1994; Montagna *et al.*, 1983; Nathan, 1978; Pitagoras de Mattos, Oliveira and Andre, 1999; Ansevin and Agamanolis, 1996; Sandyk, 1990; Schott, 1981; Spillane *et al.*, 1971; Wulff, 1982; Yoon, Crabtree and Botek, 2001). Nathan has suggested that the posterior nerve root or dorsal root ganglion could be implicated in the generation of frequent and spontaneous impulses contributing to painful legs and moving toes (Nathan, 1978). These inputs from posterior root fibers would then excite local spinal interneurons and lead to simultaneous abnormal movements and pain (Pitagoras de Mattos, Oliveira and Andre, 1999). Afferent stimulation would trigger this phenomenon in lesions of the peripheral nerves, root nerve fibers or even limb soft tissue and bone. Other authors (Dressler *et al.*, 1994; Ansevin and Agamanolis, 1996; Schott, 1981; Verhagen, Horstink and Notermans, 1985) implicate the involvement of other structures above the spinal segmental level in the genesis of painful legs and moving toes. The pain and toe movements often subside briefly after a lumbar sympathetic blockade (Dressler *et al.*, 1994; Guieu *et al.*, 1990; Spillane *et al.*, 1971), but can return within a few days despite the absence of sympathetic function (Nathan, 1978), implying that abnormal sympathetic function may be incidental rather than causal (Drummond and Finch, 2004). It has been suggested that the complex nature of the toe movements cannot be adequately explained by a spinal cord mechanisms and suggests some participation of cerebral neurons in its genesis (Dressler *et al.*, 1994; Verhagen, Horstink and Notermans, 1985). This model suggests that the abnormal sensory inputs from the periphery to the spinal cord could lead to a reorganization of subsequent processing and generate pain and involuntary movements (Pitagoras de Mattos, Oliveira and Andre, 1999).

Treatment of this syndrome is difficult. Drugs such as carbamazepine (Dressler *et al.*, 1994; Schott, 1981), tricyclic anti-depressants (Dressler *et al.*, 1994; Mosek *et al.*, 1996; Schott, 1981), diazepam (Dressler *et al.*, 1994;

Funakawa, Mano and Takayanagi, 1987; Schott, 1981), baclofen (Dressler *et al.*, 1994; Funakawa, Mano and Takayanagi, 1987; Schott, 1981), beta-blockers (Funakawa, Mano and Takayanagi, 1987), corticosteroids (Schott, 1981) and analgesics (Schott, 1981) have been tried in different combinations with variable results. There is one report that adenosine may be useful (Guieu *et al.*, 1994). One patient responded to gabapentin 600 mg three times daily (Villarejo *et al.*, 2004). Dual combination of TENS and vibratory stimulation provided significant relief of pain in one patient (Guieu *et al.*, 1990). Lumbar sympathetic blockade with guanethidine or aqueous phenol resulted only transient remission of the symptoms in a few cases (Dressler *et al.*, 1994; Nathan, 1978; Schott, 1981; Spillane *et al.*, 1971). Reports have demonstrated that even sympathectomy may only lead to transient remission (Dressler *et al.*, 1994; Spillane *et al.*, 1971). Epidural block may be helpful (Okuda *et al.*, 1998), as well as epidural spinal cord stimulation (Takahashi *et al.*, 2002). Injections of botulinum neurotoxin have not been useful.

PERIPHERAL DYSTONIA, REFLEX SYMPATHETIC DYSTROPHY (RSD) DYSTONIA, CAUSALGIA DYSTONIA, CRPS DYSTONIA

The terms peripheral dystonia, RSD dystonia, causalgia dystonia and CRPS dystonia have been used interchangeably and for what appears to be one and the same syndrome. The clinical definition and scientific understanding of this condition is still evolving and controversial. The International Association for the Study of Pain (IASP) (1979) defines causalgia as "a syndrome of sustained burning pain after a traumatic nerve injury combined with vasomotor and pseudomotor dysfunction and later trophic changes".

"Reflex sympathetic dystrophy" (RSD) and "causalgia" are classified by the IASP as Complex Regional Pain Syndromes (CRPS) I and II respectively (Walker and Cousins, 1997). Implicit in the definition of reflex sympathetic dystrophy is the notion that there is dysfunction of the sympathetic nervous system (Bonica, 1979). This is based on reports that in some cases sympathetic block may provide temporary relief. Bonica had advanced nerve blocks to a standard therapy in these patients (Bonica, 1990). But the link between nociceptive neurons and postganglionic sympathetic activity is tenuous, with sympathetic blocks sometimes altering the syndrome at least temporarily and sometimes not. Surgical sympathetomy hardly ever provides relief (Eccles, Kosak and Westerman, 1962).

There is confusion with regard to what is meant by RSD (Wilson, 1992; Janig, 1990) and it has lost usefulness as a clinical designation due to its indiscriminate use. Hence

IASP (1994) revised the criteria under the umbrella term Complex Regional Pain Syndrome (CPRS) (Stanton-Hicks *et al.*, 1995).

CRPS Type I (RSD) criteria:

1. Type I is a syndrome that develops after an initiating noxious event.
2. Spontaneous pain or allodynia/hyperalgesia occurs, is not limited to the territory of a single peripheral nerve, and is disproportionate to the inciting event.
3. There is or has been evidence of edema, skin blood-flow abnormality, or abnormal sudomotor activity in the region of the pain since the inciting event.
4. This diagnosis is excluded by the existence of conditions that would otherwise account for the degree of pain and dysfunction.

CRPS Type II (causalgia) criteria:

1. Type II is a syndrome that develops after a nerve injury.
2. Spontaneous pain or allodynia/hyperalgesia occurs and is not necessarily limited to the territory of the injured nerve.
3. There is or has been evidence of edema, skin blood flow abnormality, or abnormal sudomotor activity in the region of the pain since the inciting event.
4. This diagnosis is excluded by the existence of conditions that would otherwise account for the degree of pain and dysfunction.

The clinical features of the two types of CRPS are identical. The distinguishing feature is the presence of a peripheral nerve injury in patients with type II (Rho *et al.*, 2002).

Various movement disorders that accompany CRPS I and II have been described which include, but are not limited to tremor, dystonia and spasm (Bhatia, Bhatt and Marsden, 1993; Jankovic and Van der Linden, 1988; Koller, Wong and Lang, 1989; Marsden *et al.*, 1984; Schwartzman and Kerrigan, 1990). Clinical features of dystonia accompanying the above condition are based on a few well-described, but heterogeneous cases. There is some question as to whether the spasms seen in these cases represent actual dystonia, but because of the similarities, that term is utilized.

When occurring with causalgia/RSD, dystonia usually begins in the upper or lower limbs in adulthood. The upper limb is affected distally and typically produces flexion of the fingers and wrist, but there may be relative sparing of the thumb and index finger. The hand may be swollen with mottling of the skin, especially in those cases associated with RSD (Figure 17.3). In the lower limbs, fixed inversion and plantar flexion of the foot commonly occurs, sometimes with clawing of the toes. There have also been cases

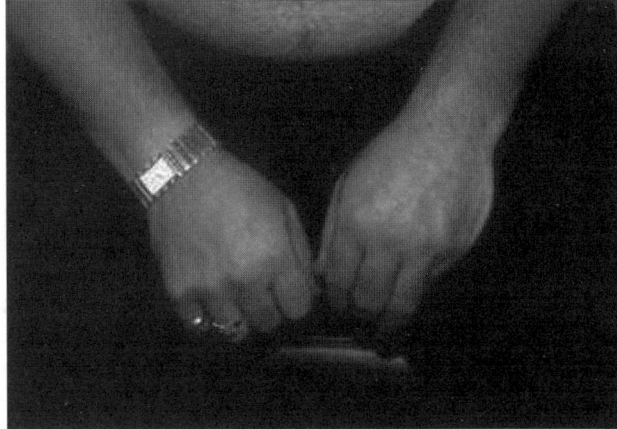

Figure 17.3 Peripheral dystonia of the left hand. Note the flexion of the last finger, hand swelling and mottling of the skin.

of post-traumatic torticollis which is the result of a minor neck injury such as whiplash. In these cases patients have an abrupt onset painful laterocollis with shoulder elevation (Figure 17.4). Other features are decreased range of motion, hypertrophy of lateral muscles, absence of spasmodic movements and unresponsiveness to botulinum toxin injections (Goldman and Ahlskog, 1993; Tarsy, 1998; Truong *et al.*, 1991). Tarsy demonstrated that this syndrome often occurs within weeks of the injury. The dystonia in the neck and limbs is usually characterized by abrupt-onset, rapidly progressive to peak, early fixed posture present at rest often with underlying contracture, limitation of passive range of movement and absence of sensory tricks (geste antagonistique), particularly in post-traumatic torticollis. However, the fixed posture is not a consistent finding and the dystonia may occasionally be clinically indistinguishable from primary torsion dystonia. The dystonia may spread proximally, become multi-focal or more generalized (Betz *et al.*, 2001; Bhatia, Bhatt and Marsden, 1993; Jankovic, 1994; Krauss and Jankovic, 2002; Schott, 2007). Pain and tenderness is a key factor.

It has also been noted that these patients tend to be younger than adult-onset dystonia patients. The onset of dystonia is most often abrupt, but may be gradual, may precede the pain and may be present in a mirror distribution on the contralateral side of the body (Schwartzman and Kerrigan, 1990).

Diagnostic criteria have been suggested for peripherally induced movement disorder/post-traumatic peripheral dystonia: (Jankovic, 1994)

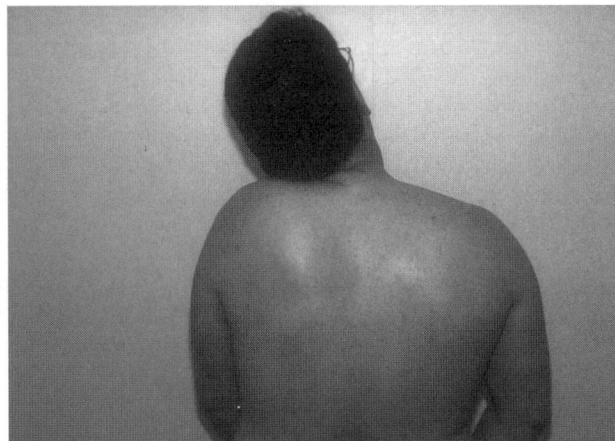

Figure 17.4 Post-traumatic torticollis viewed from behind demonstrating neck lateroflexion and elevation of the shoulder.

1. Injury must be severe enough to cause local symptoms persistent for at least two weeks or requiring medical evaluation within two weeks after the peripheral injury.
2. The onset of the movement disorder must have occurred within a few days or months (up to one year) after the injury.
3. The onset of the movement disorder must have been anatomically related to the site of the injury.

But these criteria are arbitrary, not specific or based on known pathophysiology (Weiner, 2001). The onset latency in cases varied from five weeks to five years in reported cases (van Rijn et al., 2007) although Tarsy suggested that only those with onset within a month were post-traumatic, while those with onset later had typical idiopathic dystonia (Tarsy, 1998). Occasionally causalgia may tend to get better while the dystonia gets worse. All of these findings indicate that likely separate mechanisms underlie the pain and dystonia in this condition and these mechanisms need not be purely peripheral or central, rather may be a combination of the two.

Up until 1984, when the paper describing causalgia dystonia by Marsden et al. (1984) was published, very few reports had mentioned this condition. At this point it is difficult to estimate the true prevalence of this condition, as case reports are heterogeneous and authors tend to lump together a variety of movement disorders that are associated with peripheral injury. In addition, the criteria used to define causalgia/RSD itself is variable.

van Rijn et al. (2007) retrospectively analyzed 185 patients who met IASP criteria for CRPS I (RSD) in one or more extremities. Patients were predominantly female 160 (86.5%), and 121 (65.4%) had a movement disorder. Of the patients with a movement disorder, 110 (90.9%) had dystonia. The dystonia of this disorder was predominantly characterized by tonic flexion postures. In the majority of patients, dystonia was limited to the distal extremity and mostly involved flexion of digits and wrist in the upper extremity, and inversion and flexion postures of the feet in the lower. In a minority of patients, dystonia extended proximally to either elbows or shoulders, and knees or hips. The time interval between the onset of CRPS and dystonia varied, with 56% developing the dystonia more than a month after the onset of CRPS, for 27% the dystonia appeared more than a year later and three patients developed it after a five-year interval (van Rijn et al., 2007).

Briklein et al. have described neurological findings in 145 patients with CRPS of which 122 (84.1%) had CRPS I, and 23 (15.9%) had CRPS II. They reported that 44 (30.3%) patients had dystonia/myoclonic jerks. The dystonia and myoclonic jerks were lumped together with no clear distinction. Of these 48% had CRPS II and 27% CRPS I (Birklein et al., 2000).

Jankovic (Jankovic and Van der Linden, 1988) studied 23 patients, 18 of which had focal dystonia after peripheral nerve injury and half had RSD with a movement disorder that was similar to idiopathic dystonia. One difference was that their dystonia persisted at rest and was not action induced.

Schwartzman and Kerrigan (1990) studied 200 patients with causalgia and RSD and collected 43 patients with various forms of movement disorders, which included dystonia, spasms and tremors. No further description of the dystonia was provided. Bhatia, Bhatt and Marsden (1993) studied 18 patients with fixed focal dystonia at the original site of causalgia. In 15 of these patients injury was the precipitating event. In eight patients the dystonia remained focal, and in the remaining 10 patients it spread.

The pathophysiology of causalgia and RSD is not well understood and has been subject to much speculation. Their relevance to the pathophysiology of dystonia and other movement disorders that accompany these conditions is unclear. What these conditions seem to have in common is that both can be triggered peripherally and result in a phenomenon mediated by the central nervous system.

The prevailing discussions encompass a broad range of issues, from peripheral vs. central mechanisms, to organic vs. psychogenic origin of the movement disorder.

Primary sympathetic dysfunction seems to be an unlikely explanation for the development of dystonia. A majority of cases of causalgia dystonia/RSD dystonia have a preceding event, which is usually a minor trauma. Whether this is causative is controversial. Proponents of this theory draw support from experimental models that reveal that peripheral injury including pain can lead to plastic changes in the cortex representing the body part affected which, in turn, lead to dystonia. It is also stated that central reorganization may explain why peripherally induced movement disorders have a tendency to spread beyond the original site of injury. It has been shown that de-afferentation of the spinal cord in cats and humans results in neuronal and reflex hyperexcitability that spreads beyond the involved segment and a similar mechanism may be involved in spread of peripheral dystonia (Eccles, Kosak and Westerman, 1962; Loeser, Ward and White, 1968). However, the relevance of this data has been questioned (Weiner, 2001).

A particular recurring issue is that soft tissue trauma is a frequent occurrence, whereas causalgia/RSD dystonia is a rare entity (Weiner, 2001). To explain this fact the popular hypothesis is that individuals who develop the condition have an underlying susceptibility to develop the dystonia after trauma. Suggested predisposing factors include family history of dystonia, family history of essential tremor or tics, consanguinity, previous exposure to dopamine-receptor blocking agents, pre-existing movement disorders (essential tremor, focal dystonia elsewhere), delayed developmental milestones and previous surgery at the site of onset of dystonia (Jankovic and van der Linden, 1988; Schott, 1985). None of these predisposing factors have been validated (Weiner, 2001). Bressman *et al.* (1998) have investigated the role of DYT1 in secondary dystonia including those related to trauma and failed to find an association. van Hilten *et al.* (2000) have reported increased prevalence of tissue type HLA-DR13 in patients with causalgia dystonia, an observation that needs to be confirmed.

Some reports have suggested that causalgia/RSD dystonia is a functional neurological disorder or the consequence of a psychological disorder (Ecker, 1990; Lang and Fahn, 1990). The clinical features that support this being a psychogenic dystonia is the abrupt onset, fixed posture, onset of limb dystonia, particularly foot, in an adult, non-physiological sensory findings in these cases and the frequent association with litigation (Factor, Podskalny and Molho, 1995; Lang, 1995). This is seen with limb as well as cervical forms of peripheral dystonia. Schwartzmann and Kerrigan's report has been re-interpreted as psychogenic dystonia by some authors (Cagliani *et al.*, 2003; Lang and Fahn, 1990; Schrag *et al.*, 2004). Many of the patients with post-traumatic RSD dystonia have pending law suits that make it difficult to ascertain whether the dystonia is precipitated by secondary gain. Furthermore, cases of video-proven malingering support the notion that these cases are psychogenic (Kurlan, Brin and Fahn, 1997; Schrag *et al.*, 2004; Verdugo and Ochoa, 2000).

Schrag *et al.* (2004) studied 103 patients with fixed dystonia, 62 retrospectively and 41 prospectively. Peripheral injury preceded dystonia in 63% of cases and spread to other body parts occurred in 56%. Most of the cases were limbs with a minority affecting the neck and shoulder. Pain was present in most patients and the major issue in 41%. Of those followed prospectively, nearly 40% met criteria for established psychogenic movement disorder, and 30% met criteria for a diagnosis of somatization disorder. In the rest no definitive features of psychogenic disorder was seen. Fifteen of the 18 patients with CRPS in the prospectively studied group had probable or definite psychogenic disorder. Affective and dissociative disorders were much more common in the fixed dystonia cases compared to typical idiopathic dystonia (Schrag *et al.*, 2004).

Sa *et al.* (Cagliani *et al.*, 2003) examined 16 patients with post-traumatic torticollis due to work-related injuries or motor vehicle accidents. They all had the typical fixed painful posture. All 16 had litigation pending. Sodium amytal improved 13 of 13 cases, and general anesthesia in five patients allowed for normal range of motion. These authors demonstrated significant psychological factors in this group of patients.

The treatment of co-existing CRPS and dystonia remains extremely unsatisfactory. There have been no controlled trials. Bhatia *et al.* tried several different therapies on their 18 patients. Despite the use of splints and casts the dystonia returned once the use of these devices was discontinued. Athrodesis of joints splints or tendon transfers were not helpful. Eight patients were given sympathetic blocks, had sympathectomies and guanethidine infusions, which on occasion provided temporary relief, but no long-term benefit was noted. Epidural anesthesia was tried in three patients with no benefit. Various medications including benzhexol, baclofen, levodopa, carabamazepine, diazepam, cloanazepam and amitryptline provided no sustained benefit (Bhatia, Bhatt and Marsden, 1993). Two patients had spontaneous recovery after four and nine years of illness (Bhatia, Bhatt and Marsden, 1993).

Verdugo and Ochoa (2000) studied 686 patients with CRPS I and II, 58 of these patients had abnormal movements. In three patients with sustained dystonic posture of the affected extremity, the movement disorders completely reversed after placebo injection.

van Hilten *et al.* (2000) conducted a double-blind, randomized crossover trial comparing intrathecal baclofen, a GABA-receptor agonist (type B), with placebo for the treatment of multi-focal or generalized dystonia in patients with reflex sympathetic dystrophy. In six out of seven patients, bolus injections of 50 and 75 µg of baclofen resulted in complete or partial resolution of dystonia of the hands, but little improvement was noted in dystonia of the legs. The patients whose hands were affected regained normal function with prolonged therapy. Pain and violent spasms were also relieved in some patients. The results of this study strongly support the role of GABAergic inhibitory neurons in the pathophysiology of reflex sympathetic dystrophy. Baclofen was tried in two patients with generalized dystonia at a dose of 90–120 mg and was noted to be effective by Schwartzman and colleagues (Schwartzman and Kerrigan, 1990). These patients did continue to have plantar flexion and inversion of the feet and dystonic posturing of the hands though they were able to carry out activities of daily living. Other studies have not reported success with intrathecal baclofen (Schrag *et al.*, 2004). Sympathectomies have not been reported to provide sustained relief in these patients (Schrag *et al.*, 2004; Verdugo and Ochoa, 1994).

Conservative multi-disciplinary approaches, including a combination of rehabilitation, physical and occupational therapy incorporated with psychotherapy and, when appropriate, psychiatric treatment, have proven successful in some cases, and are probably particularly effective in those with psychogenic forms (Bhatia, Bhatt and Marsden, 1993; Schrag *et al.*, 2004).

References

Alessi, G., de Reuck, J., de Bleecker, J. and Vancayzeele, S. (2000) Successful immunoglobulin treatment in a patient with neuromyotonia. *Clinical Neurology and Neurosurgery*, **102**, 173–175.

Alexander, G.E. and Moses, H. III (1982) Carbamazepine for hemifacial spasm. *Neurology*, **32**, 286–287.

Amyot, R. (1929) *Les convulsions des moignons d'amputees*, Librairie Louis Arnette, Paris.

Ansevin, C.F. and Agamanolis, D.P. (1996) Rippling muscles and myasthenia gravis with rippling muscles. *Archives of Neurology*, **53**, 197–199.

Ashizawa, T., Butler, I.J., Harati, Y. and Roongta, S.M. (1983) A dominantly inherited syndrome with continuous motor neuron discharges. *Annals of Neurology*, **13**, 285–290.

Auger, R.G. (1994) AAEM minimonograph #44: diseases associated with excess motor unit activity. *Muscle & Nerve*, **17**, 1250–1263.

Auger, R.G. and Whisnant, J. (1990) Hemifacial spasm in Rochester and Olmstead county, Minnesota, 1960 to 1984. *Archives of Neurology*, **47**, 1233–1234.

Auger, R.G., Piepgras, D.G., Laws, E.R. and Miller, R.H. (1981) Microvascular decompression of the facial nerve for hemifacial spasm: clinical and electrophysiologic observations. *Neurology*, **31**, 346–350.

Bandini, F. and Mazzella, L. (1999) Gabapentin as treatment for hemifacial spasm. *European Neurology*, **42**, 49–51.

Barber, P.A., Anderson, N.E. and Vincent, A. (2000) Morvan's syndrome associated with voltage-gated K+ channel antibodies. *Neurology*, **54**, 771–772.

Barker, F.G., Jannetta, P.J., Bissonette, D.J., Shields, P.T., Larkins, M.V. and Jho, H.D. (1995) Microvascular decompression for hemifacial spasm. *Journal of Neurosurgery*, **82**, 201–210.

Barrett, R., Singh, N. and Fahn, S. (1981) The syndrome of painful legs and moving toes. *Neurology*, **31** (Suppl 1), 4179–4180.

Benito-Leon, J., Miguelez, R., Vincent, A., Masjuan, J. and de Blas, G. (1999) Neuromyotonia in association with systemic sclerosis. *Journal of Neurology*, **246**, 976–977.

Betz, R.C., Schoser, B.G., Kasper, D., Ricker, K., Ramirez, A., Stein, V., Torbergsen, T., Lee, Y.A., Nothen, M.M., Wienker, T. F., Malin, J.P., Propping, P., Reis, A., Mortier, W., Jentsch, T.J., Vorgerd, M. and Kubisch, C. (2001) Mutations in CAV3 cause mechanical hyperirritability of skeletal muscle in rippling muscle disease. *Nature Genetics*, **28**, 218–219.

Bhatia, K.P., Bhatt, M.H. and Marsden, C.D. (1993) The causalgia-dystonia syndrome. *Brain: A Journal of Neurology*, **116** (Pt 4), 843–851.

Birklein, F., Riedl, B., Sieweke, N., Weber, M. and Neundorfer, B. (2000) Neurological findings in complex regional pain syndromes – analysis of 145 cases. *Acta Neurologica Scandinavica*, **101**, 262–269.

Black, J.T., Garcia-Mullin, R., Good, E. and Brown, S. (1972) Muscle rigidity in a newborn due to continuous peripheral nerve hyperactivity. *Archives of Neurology*, **27**, 413–425.

Bonica, J.J. (1979) The relation of injury to pain. *Pain*, **7**, 203–207.

Bonica, J.J. (1990) Causalgia and other reflex sympathetic dystrophies, *The Management of Pain*, 2nd edn Lea & Febiger, Philadelphia, PA.

Bressman, S.B., de Leon, D., Raymond, D., Greene, P.E., Brin, M. F., Fahn, S., Ozelius, L.J., Breakefield, X.O., Kramer, P.L. and Risch, N.J. (1998) The role of the DYT1 gene in secondary dystonia. *Advances in Neurology*, **78**, 107–115.

Brin, M.F., Fhan, S., Moskowitz, C., Friedman, A., Shale, H., Greene, P., Blitzer, A., List, T., Lange, D., Lovelace, R. and Mcmahon, D. (1988) Localized injections of botulinum toxin for the treatment of focal dystonia and hemifacial spasm. *Advances in Neurology*, **50**, 599–608.

Brown, K.A., Al-Gazali, L.I., Moynihan, L.M., Lench, N.J., Markham, A.F. and Mueller, R.F. (1997) Genetic heterogeneity in Schwartz-Jampel syndrome: two families with neonatal Schwartz-Jampel syndrome do not map to human chromosome 1p34-p36.1. *Journal of Medical Genetics*, **34**, 685–687.

Cagliani, R., Bresolin, N., Prelle, A., Gallanti, A., Fortunato, F., Sironi, M., Ciscato, P., Fagiolari, G., Bonato, S., Galbiati, S., Corti, S., Lamperti, C., Moggio, M. and Comi, G.P. (2003) A CAV3 microdeletion differentially affects skeletal muscle and myocardium. *Neurology*, **61**, 1513–1519.

Caress, J.B., Abend, W.K., Preston, D.C. and Logigian, E.L. (1997) A case of Hodgkin's lymphoma producing neuromyotonia. *Neurology*, **49**, 258–259.

Carlen, P.L., Wall, P.D., Nadvorna, H. and Steinbach, T. (1978) Phantom limbs and related phenomena in recent traumatic amputations. *Neurology*, **28**, 211–217.

Caviness, J.N., Gabellini, A., Kneebone, C.S., Thompson, P.D., Lees, A.J. and Marsden, C.D. (1994) Unusual focal dyskinesias: the ears, the shoulders, the back, and the abdomen. *Movement Disorders*, **9**, 531–538.

Celebisoy, N., Colakoglu, Z., Akbaba, Y. and Yuceyar, N. (1998) Continuous muscle fibre activity: a case treated with acetazolamide. *Journal of Neurology, Neurosurgery, and Psychiatry*, **64**, 256–258.

Cormier-Daire, V., Superti-Furga, A., Munnich, A., Lyonnet, S., Rustin, P., Delezoide, A.L., de Lonlay, P., Giedion, A., Maroteaux, P. and Le Merrer, M. (1998) Clinical homogeneity of the Stuve-Wiedemann syndrome and overlap with the Schwartz-Jampel syndrome type 2. *American Journal of Medical Genetics*, **78**, 146–149.

Daniele, O., Caravaglios, G., Marchini, C., Mucchiut, L., Capus, P. and Natale, E. (2001) Gabapentin in the treatment of hemifacial spasm. *Acta Neurologica Scandinavica*, **104**, 110–112.

Defazio, G., Abbruzzese, G., Girlanda, P., Vacca, L., Curra, A., de Salvia, R., Marchese, R., Raineri, R., Roselli, F., Livrea, P. and Berardelli, A. (2002) Botulinum toxin A treatment for primary hemifacial spasm. A 10-year multicenter study. *Archives of Neurology*, **59**, 418–420.

Denny-Brown, D. and Folley, J.M. (1948) Myokymia and the benign fasciculations of muscular cramps. *Transactions of the Association of American Physicians*, **61**, 88–96.

Dhand, U.K. (2006) Isaacs' syndrome: clinical and electrophysiological response to gabapentin. *Muscle & Nerve*, **34**, 646–650.

Digre, K. and Corbett, J. (1988) Hemifacial spasm: differential diagnosis, mechanism, and treatment. *Advances in Neurology*, **49**, 151–176.

Dotti, M.T., Malandrini, A., Gambelli, S., Salvadori, C., de Stefano, N. and Federico, A. (2006) A new missense mutation in caveolin-3 gene causes rippling muscle disease. *Journal of the Neurological Sciences*, **243**, 61–64.

Dressler, D., Thompson, P.D., Gledhill, R.F. and Marsden, C.D. (1994) The syndrome of painful legs and moving toes. *Movement Disorders*, **9**, 13–21.

Drummond, P.D. and Finch, P.M. (2004) Sympathetic nervous system involvement in the syndrome of painful legs and moving toes. *Clinical Journal of Pain*, **20**, 370–374.

Ebersbach, G., Schelosky, L., Schenkel, A., Scholz, U. and Poewe, W. (1998) Unilateral painful legs and moving toes syndrome with moving fingers – evidence for distinct oscillators. *Movement Disorders*, **13**, 965–968.

Eccles, R.M., Kosak, W. and Westerman, R.A. (1962) Enhancement of spinal monosynaptic reflex responses after denervation of synergic hindlimb muscles. *Experimental Neurology*, **6**, 451–464.

Ecker, A. (1990) The movement disorder of reflex sympathetic dystrophy. *Neurology*, **40**, 1477.

Edwards, M., Schott, G. and Bhatia, K. (2003) Episodic focal lingual dystonic spasms. *Movement Disorders*, **18**, 836–837.

Factor, S.A., Podskalny, G.D. and Molho, E.S. (1995) Psychogenic movement disorders: frequency, clinical profile, and characteristics. *Journal of Neurology, Neurosurgery, and Psychiatry*, **59**, 406–412.

Falace, A., Striano, P., Manganelli, F., Coppola, A., Striano, S., Minetti, C. and Zara, F. (2007) Inherited neuromyotonia: a clinical and genetic study of a family. *Neuromuscular Disorders*, **17**, 23–27.

Fariello, R., Meloff, K., Murphy, E., Reilly, B. and Armstrong, D. (1978) A case of Schwartz-Jampel syndrome with unusual muscle biopsy findings. *Annals of Neurology*, **3**, 93–96.

Flor, H. (2002) Phantom-limb pain: characteristics, causes treatment. *Lancet Neurology*, **1**, 182–189.

Friedman, A., Jamrozik, Z. and Bojakowski, J. (1989) Familial hemifacial spasm. *Movement Disorders*, **4**, 213–218.

Funakawa, I., Mano, Y. and Takayanagi, T. (1987) Painful hand and moving fingers. A case report. *Journal of Neurology*, **234**, 342–343.

Galvez-Jimenez, N., Hanson, M. and Desai, M. (2001) Unusual causes of hemifacial spasm. *Seminars in Neurology*, **21**, 75–83.

Garcia-Merino, A., Cabello, A., Mora, J.S. and Liano, H. (1991) Continuous muscle fiber activity, peripheral neuropathy, and thymoma. *Annals of Neurology*, **29**, 215–218.

Gardner, W. (1966) Cross talk – the paradoxical transmission of a nerve impulse. *Archives of Neurology*, **14**, 149–156.

Gardner-Medwin, D. and Walton, J.N. (1969) Myokymia with impaired muscular relaxation. *Lancet*, **1**, 943–944.

Giedion, A., Boltshauser, E., Briner, J., Eich, G., Exner, G., Fendel, H., Kaufmann, L., Steinmann, B., Spranger, J. and Superti-Furga, A. (1997) Heterogeneity in Schwartz-Jampel chondrodystrophic myotonia. *European Journal of Pediatrics*, **156**, 214–223.

Goldman, S. and Ahlskog, J.E. (1993) Posttraumatic cervical dystonia. *Mayo Clinic Proceedings*, **68**, 443–448.

Guieu, R., Tardy-Gervet, M.F., Blin, O. and Pouget, J. (1990) Pain relief achieved by transcutaneous electrical nerve stimulation and/or vibratory stimulation in a case of painful legs and moving toes. *Pain*, **42**, 43–48.

Guieu, R., Sampieri, F., Pouget, J., Guy, B. and Rochat, H. (1994) Adenosine in painful legs and moving toes syndrome. *Clinical Neuropharmacology*, **17**, 460–469.

Gutmann, L. (2002) *Nerve Hyperexcitability Syndromes*, Butterworth-Heinemann, Woburn.

Gutmann, L., Gutmann, L. and Schochet, S.S. (1996) Neuromyotonia and type I myofiber predominance in amyloidosis. *Muscle & Nerve*, **19**, 1338–1341.

Hadjivassiliou, M., Chattopadhyay, A.K., Davies-Jones, G.A., Gibson, A., Grunewald, R.A. and Lobo, A.J. (1997) Neuromuscular disorder as a presenting feature of coeliac disease. *Journal of Neurology, Neurosurgery, and Psychiatry*, **63**, 770–775.

Hahn, A.F., Parkes, A.W., Bolton, C.F. and Stewart, S.A. (1991) Neuromyotonia in hereditary motor neuropathy. *Journal of Neurology, Neurosurgery, and Psychiatry*, **54**, 230–235.

Hallett, M. (2007) Restless Legs Syndrome and Peripheral Movement Disorders, Churchill Livingstone.

Hancock, H. (1852) Convulsive movements of the stump. *Lancet*, **i**, 281–283.

Hart, I.K., Maddison, P., Newsom-Davis, J., Vincent, A. and Mills, K.R. (2002) Phenotypic variants of autoimmune peripheral nerve hyperexcitability. *Brain: A Journal of Neurology*, **125**, 1887–1895.

Hayat, G.R., Kulkantrakorn, K., Campbell, W.W. and Giuliani, M.J. (2000) Neuromyotonia: autoimmune pathogenesis and response to immune modulating therapy. *Journal of the Neurological Sciences*, **181**, 38–43.

Henderson, W. and Smyth, G.E. (1948) Phantom limbs. *Journal of Neurology Neurosurgery and Psychiatry*, **11**, 88–112.

Hughes, E., Brackman, D. and Weinstein, R. (1980) Seventh nerve spasm: effect of modification of cholinergic balance. *Otolaryngology and Head and Neck Surgery*, **88**, 491–499.

Hunziker, U.A., Savoldelli, G., Boltshauser, E., Giedion, A. and Schinzel, A. (1989) Prenatal diagnosis of Schwartz-Jampel syndrome with early manifestation. *Prenatal Diagnosis*, **9**, 127–131.

Iacono, R.P., Linford, J., Tourian, A. and Sandyk, R. (1987) Baclofen in the treatment of post-amputation autonomous stump movements. *European Neurology*, **26**, 141–144.

Iliceto, G., Thompson, P.D., Day, B.L., Rothwell, J.C., Lees, A.J. and Marsden, C.D. (1990) Diaphragmatic flutter, the moving umbilicus syndrome, and "belly dancer's" dyskinesia. *Movement Disorders*, **5**, 15–22.

Inghilleri, M., Conte, A., Frasca, V., Vaudano, A.E. and Meco, G. (2006) Belly dance syndrome due to spinal myoclonus. *Movement Disorders*, **21**, 394–396.

Isaacs, H. (1961) A syndrome of continuous muscle-fibre activity. *Journal of Neurology Neurosurgery and Psychiatry*, **24**, 319–325.

Isaacs, H. and Heffron, J.J. (1974) The syndrome of 'continuous muscle-fibre activity' cured: further studies. *Journal of Neurology, Neurosurgery, and Psychiatry*, **37**, 1231–1235.

Jablecki, C. and Schultz, P. (1982) Single muscle fiber recordings in the Schwartz-Jampel syndrome. *Muscle & Nerve*, **5**, S64–S69.

Jamieson, P.W. and Katirji, M.B. (1994) Idiopathic generalized myokymia. *Muscle & Nerve*, **17**, 42–51.

Jamora, R.D., Umapathi, T. and Tan, L.C. (2006) Finger flexion resembling focal dystonia in Isaacs' syndrome. *Parkinsonism & Related Disorders*, **12**, 61–63.

Janig, W. (1990) The sympathetic nervous system in pain: physiology and pathophysiology, in *Pain and the Sympathetic Nervous System* (ed. M. Stanton-Hicks), Kluwer Academic, Boston.

Jankovic, J. (1994) Post-traumatic movement disorders: central and peripheral mechanisms. *Neurology*, **44**, 2006–2014.

Jankovic, J. (2001) Can peripheral trauma induce dystonia and other movement disorders? Yes! *Movement Disorders*, **16**, 7–12.

Jankovic, J. and Pardo, R. (1986) Segmental myoclonus. Clinical and pharmacologic study. *Archives of Neurology*, **43**, 1025–1031.

Jankovic, J. and Van der Linden, C. (1988) Dystonia and tremor induced by peripheral trauma: predisposing factors. *Journal of Neurology, Neurosurgery, and Psychiatry*, **51**, 1512–1519.

Jusic, A., Dogan, S. and Stojanovic, V. (1972) Hereditary persistant distal cramps. *Journal of Neurology, Neurosurgery, and Psychiatry*, **35**, 379–384.

Koller, W.C., Wong, G.F. and Lang, A. (1989) Posttraumatic movement disorders: a review. *Movement Disorders*, **4**, 20–36.

Kono, I., Ueda, Y., Araki, K., Nakajima, K. and Shibasaki, H. (1994) Spinal myoclonus resembling belly dance. *Movement Disorders*, **9**, 325–329.

Kraft, S. and Lang, A. (1988) Botulinum toxin injections in the treatment of blepharospasm, hemifacial spasm, and eyelid fasciculations. *The Canadian Journal of Neurological Sciences*, **15**, 276–280.

Krauss, J.K. and Jankovic, J. (2002) Head injury and posttraumatic movement disorders. *Neurosurgery*, **50**, 927–939 discussion 939-40.

Kubisch, C., Schoser, B.G., von During, M., Betz, R.C., Goebel, H. H., Zahn, S., Ehrbrecht, A., Aasly, J., Schroers, A., Popovic, N., Lochmuller, H., Schroder, J.M., Bruning, T., Malin, J.P., Fricke, B., Meinck, H.M., Torbergsen, T., Engels, H., Voss, B. and Vorgerd, M. (2003) Homozygous mutations in caveolin-3 cause a severe form of rippling muscle disease. *Annals of Neurology*, **53**, 512–520.

Kubisch, C., Ketelsen, U.P., Goebel, I. and Omran, H. (2005) Autosomal recessive rippling muscle disease with homozygous CAV3 mutations. *Annals of Neurology*, **57**, 303–304.

Kulisevsky, J., Marti-Fabregas, J. and Grau, J.M. (1992) Spasms of amputation stumps. *Journal of Neurology, Neurosurgery, and Psychiatry*, **55**, 626–627.

Kurlan, R., Brin, M.F. and Fahn, S. (1997) Movement disorder in reflex sympathetic dystrophy: a case proven to be psychogenic by surveillance video monitoring. *Movement Disorders*, **12**, 243–245.

Lamb, G.D. (2005) Rippling muscle disease may be caused by "silent" action potentials in the tubular system of skeletal muscle fibers. *Muscle & Nerve*, **31**, 652–658.

Lang, A.E. (1995) Psychogenic dystonia: a review of 18 cases. *The Canadian Journal of Neurological Sciences*, **22**, 136–143.

Lang, A. and Fahn, S. (1990) The movement disorder of reflex sympathetic dystrophy. *Neurology*, **40**, 1476–1477.

Lang, C.J., Sittl, H. and Erbguth, F. (1997) Autonomous stump movements in brain death. *European Neurology*, **37**, 249.

Lazaro, R.P., Rollinson, R.D. and Fenichel, G.M. (1981) Familial cramps and muscle pain. *Archives of Neurology*, **38**, 22–24.

Le Gars, L., Clerc, D., Cariou, D., Lavabre, C., Metral, S. and Bisson, M. (1997) Systemic juvenile rheumatoid arthritis and associated Isaacs' syndrome. *The Journal of Rheumatology*, **24**, 178–180.

Lee, E.K., Maselli, R.A., Ellis, W.G. and Agius, M.A. (1998) Morvan's fibrillary chorea: a paraneoplastic manifestation of thymoma. *Journal of Neurology, Neurosurgery, and Psychiatry*, **65**, 857–862.

Lees, A.J., Blau, J.N. and Schon, F. (1986) Paroxysmal hemiglossal twisting. *Lancet*, **2**, 812–813.

Lehmann-Horn, F., Iaizzo, P.A., Franke, C., Hatt, H. and Spaans, F. (1990) Schwartz-Jampel syndrome: II. Na+ channel defect causes myotonia. *Muscle & Nerve*, **13**, 528–535.

Liguori, R., Vincent, A., Avoni, P., Valentino, M.L., D'alessandro, R., Zaccaria, A., Bandini, G. and Montagna, P. (2000) Acquired neuromyotonia after bone marrow transplantation. *Neurology*, **54**, 1390–1391.

Linazasoro, G., van Blercom, N., Lasa, A., Fernandez, J.M. and Aranzabal, I. (2005) Etiological and therapeutic observations in a case of belly dancer's dyskinesia. *Movement Disorders*, **20**, 251–253.

Loeser, J.D., Ward, A.A. Jr and White, L.E. Jr (1968) Chronic deafferentation of human spinal cord neurons. *Journal of Neurosurgery*, **29**, 48–50.

Lorenzoni, P.J., Scola, R.H., Vieira, N., Vainzof, M., Carsten, A.L. and Werneck, L.C. (2007) A novel missense mutation in the caveolin-3 gene in rippling muscle disease. *Muscle & Nerve*, **36**, 258–260.

Maddison, P. (2006) Neuromyotonia. *Clinical Neurophysiology*, **117**, 2118–2127.

Madrid, R.E., Kubisch, C. and Hays, A.P. (2005) Early-onset toe walking in rippling muscle disease due to a new caveolin-3 gene mutation. *Neurology*, **65**, 1301–1303.

Marion, M.H., Gledhill, R.F. and Thompson, P.D. (1989) Spasms of amputation stumps: a report of 2 cases. *Movement Disorders*, **4**, 354–358.

Mark, M.H. (2004) Other choreatic disorders, in *Movement Disorders: Neurologic Principles & Practice*, 2nd edn (eds R.L. Watts and W.C. Koller), McGraw-Hill Companies, New York.

Marsden, C.D., Obeso, J.A., Traub, M.M., Rothwell, J.C., Kranz, H. and La Cruz, F. (1984) Muscle spasms associated with Sudeck's atrophy after injury. *British Medical Journal (Clinical Research Ed.)*, **288**, 173–176.

Martinelli, P., Giuliani, S. and Ippoliti, M. (1992) Hemifacial spasm due to peripheral injury of facial nerve: a nuclear syndrome? *Movement Disorders*, **7**, 181–184.

Martinelli, P., Patuelli, A., Minardi, C., Cau, A., Riviera, A.M. and Dal Pozzo, F. (1996) Neuromyotonia, peripheral neuropathy and myasthenia gravis. *Muscle & Nerve*, **19**, 505–510.

Mauriello, J.A., Leone, T., Dhillon, S., Pakeman, B., Mostafavi, R. and Yepez, M.C. (1996) Treatment choices of 119 patients with hemifacial spasm over 11 years. *Clinical Neurology and Neurosurgery*, **98**, 213–216.

Mera, J., Martinez-Castrillo, J.C., Mariscal, A., Herrero, A. and Alvarez-Cermeno, J.C. (2004) Autonomous stump movements responsive to gabapentin. *Journal of Neurology*, **251**, 346–347.

Mereu, T.R. and Porter, I.H. (1969) Mytonotia, shortness of stature and hip dysplasia. *American Journal of Diseases of Children*, **117**, 470–478.

Mertens, H.-G. and Zschocke, S. (1965) Neuromyotonie. *Klinische Wochenschrift*, 43, 917–925.

Micheli, F., Scorticati, M.C., Gatto, E., Cersosimo, G. and Adi, J. (1994) Familial hemifacial spasm. *Movement Disorders*, **9**, 330–332.

Miwa, H., Mizuno, Y. and Kondo, T. (2002) Familial hemifacial spasm: report of cases and review of the literature. *Jornal of the Neurological Sciences*, **193**, 97–102.

Moller, A. and Jannetta, P.J. (1984) On the origin of synkinesis in hemifacial spasm: result of intracranial recording. *Journal of Neurosurgery*, **61**, 569–576.

Montagna, P., Cirignotta, F., Sacquegna, T., Martinelli, P., Ambrosetto, G. and Lugaresi, E. (1983) "Painful legs and moving toes" associated with polyneuropathy. *Journal of Neurology, Neurosurgery, and Psychiatry*, **46**, 399–403.

Montagna, P., Imbriaco, A., Zucconi, R., Liguori, R., Cirignotta, F. and Lugaresi, E. (1986) Hemifacial spasm in sleep. *Neurology*, **36**, 270–273.

Mosek, A., Rabey, J.M., Kushnir, M. and Korczyn, A.D. (1996) Painful calf, moving foot. *Movement Disorders*, **11**, 339–340.

Muller-Felber, W., Ansevin, C.F., Ricker, K., Muller-Jenssen, A., Topfer, M., Goebel, H.H. and Pongratz, D.E. (1999) Immuno-suppressive treatment of rippling muscles in patients with myasthenia gravis. *Neuromuscular Disorders*, **9**, 604–607.

Nakatsuji, Y., Kaido, M., Sugai, F., Nakamori, M., Abe, K., Watanabe, O., Arimura, K. and Sakoda, S. (2000) Isaacs' syndrome successfully treated by immunoadsorption plasmapheresis. *Acta Neurologica Scandinavica*, **102**, 271–273.

Nathan, P.W. (1978) Painful legs and moving toes: evidence on the site of the lesion. *Journal of Neurology, Neurosurgery, and Psychiatry*, **41**, 934–939.

Nicole, S., Ben Hamida, C., Beighton, P., Bakouri, S., Belal, S., Romero, N., Viljoen, D., Ponsot, G., Sammoud, A., Weissenbach, J., Fardeau, M., Ben Hamida, M., Fontaine, B. and Hentati, F. (1995) Localization of the Schwartz-Jampel syndrome locus to chromosome 1p34-p36.1 by homozygosity mapping. *Human Molecular Genetics*, **4**, 1633–1636.

Nielsen, V.K. (1984) Pathophysiology of Hemifacial Spasm: II. Lateral Spread of the Supraorbital Nerve Reflex. *Neurology*, **34**, 427–431.

Nielsen, V.K. (1985) Electrophysiology of the facial nerve in hemifacial spasm: ectopic/ephaptic excitation. *Muscle & Nerve*, **8**, 545–555.

Okuda, Y., Suzuki, K., Kitajima, T., Masuda, R. and Asai, T. (1998) Lumbar epidural block for 'painful legs and moving toes' syndrome: a report of three cases. *Pain*, **78**, 145–147.

Partanen, V.S., Soininen, H., Saksa, M. and Riekkinen, P. (1980) Electromyographic and nerve conduction findings in a patient with neuromyotonia, normocalcemic tetany and small-cell lung cancer. *Acta Neurologica Scandinavica*, **61**, 216–226.

Pascuzzi, R.M., Gratianne, R., Azzarelli, B. and Kincaid, J.C. (1990) Schwartz-Jampel syndrome with dominant inheritance. *Muscle & Nerve*, **13**, 1152–1163.

Pavone, L., Mollica, F, Grasso, A., Cao, A. and Gullotta, F. (1978) Schwartz-Jampel syndrome in two daughters of first cousins. *Journal of Neurology, Neurosurgery and Psychiatry*, **41**, 161–169.

Pitagoras de Mattos, J., Oliveira, M. and Andre, C. (1999) Painful legs and moving toes associated with neuropathy in HIV-infected patients. *Movement Disorders*, **14**, 1053–1054.

Rho, R.H., Brewer, R.P., Lamer, T.J. and Wilson, P.R. (2002) Complex regional pain syndrome. *Mayo Clinic Proceedings*, **77**, 174–180.

Ricker, K., Moxley, R.T. and Rohkamm, R. (1989) Rippling muscle disease. *Archives of Neurology*, **46**, 405–408.

Roberts, H.L., Day, B., Lo, H., Mclean, C. and North, K. (2006) Rippling muscle disease. *Journal of Clinical Neuroscience*, **13**, 576–578.

Roggendorf, J., Burghaus, L., Liu, W.C., Weisenbach, S., Eggers, C., Fink, G.R. and Hilker, R. (2007) Belly dancer's syndrome following central pontine and extrapontine myelinolysis. *Movement Disorders*, **22**, 892–894.

Russell, W. (1970) Neurological sequelae of amputation. *British Journal of Hospital Medicine*, **6**, 607–609.

Sandyk, R. (1990) Neuroleptic-induced "painful legs and moving toes" syndrome: successful treatment with clonazepam and baclofen. *Italian Journal of Neurological Sciences*, **11**, 573–576.

Schoenen, J., Gonce, M. and Delwaide, P.J. (1984) Painful legs and moving toes: a syndrome with different physiopathologic mechanisms. *Neurology*, **34**, 1108–1112.

Schott, G.D. (1981) "Painful legs and moving toes": the role of trauma. *Journal of Neurology, Neurosurgery, and Psychiatry*, **44**, 344–346.

Schott, G.D. (1985) The relationship of peripheral trauma and pain to dystonia. *Journal of Neurology, Neurosurgery, and Psychiatry*, **48**, 698–701.

Schott, G.D. (2007) Peripherally-triggered CRPS and dystonia. *Pain*, **130**, 203–207.

Schrag, A., Trimble, M., Quinn, N. and Bhatia, K. (2004) The syndrome of fixed dystonia: an evaluation of 103 patients. *Brain: A Journal of Neurology*, **127**, 2360–2372.

Schulte-Mattler, W.J., Kley, R.A., Rothenfusser-Korber, E., Bohm, S., Bruning, T., Hackemann, J., Steinbrecher, A., During, M.V., Voss, B. and Vorgerd, M. (2005) Immune-mediated rippling muscle disease. *Neurology*, **64**, 364–367.

Schwartz, O. and Jampel, R. (1962) Congenital blepharophimosis associated with a unique generalized myopathy. *Archives of Opthalmology*, **68**, 82–87.

Schwartzman, R.J. and Kerrigan, J. (1990) The movement disorder of reflex sympathetic dystrophy. *Neurology*, **40**, 57–61.

Scribanu, N. and Ionasescu, V. (1981) Schwartz-Jampel syndrome: a case report stimulatory effect of calcium and A23187 calcioum ionophore for protein synthesis in muscle cell cultures. *European Neurology*, **20**, 46–51.

Seay, A. and Ziter, F. (1978) Malignant hyperpyrexia in a patient with Schwartz-Jampel syndrome. *The Journal of Pediatrics*, **93**, 83–84.

Shan, D.E., Liao, K.K. and Fuh, J.L. (1998) Clinical manifestations of tardive truncal dystonia – abdominal movements: report of two cases. *Zhonghua Yi Xue Za Zhi (Taipei)*, **61**, 545–550.

Shillito, P., Molenaar, P.C., Vincent, A., Leys, K., Zheng, W., Van Den Berg, R.J., Plomp, J.J., Van Kempen, G.T., Chauplannaz, G., Wintzen, A.R. *et al.* (1995) Acquired neuromyotonia: evidence for autoantibodies directed against K+ channels of peripheral nerves. *Annals of Neurology*, **38**, 714–722.

So, Y.T., Zu, L., Barraza, C., Figueroa, K.P. and Pulst, S.M. (2001) Rippling muscle disease: evidence for phenotypic and genetic heterogeneity. *Muscle & Nerve*, **24**, 340–344.

Soussi-Yanicostas, N., Ben Hamida, C., Butler-Browne, G.S., Hentati, F., Bejaoui, K. and Ben Hamida, M. (1991) Modification in the expression and localization of contractile and cyto-skeletal proteins in Schwartz-Jampel syndrome. *Journal of the Neurological Sciences*, **104**, 64–73.

Spillane, J.D., Nathan, P.W., Kelly, R.E. and Marsden, C.D. (1971) Painful legs and moving toes. *Brain: A Journal of Neurology*, **94**, 541–556.

Spranger, J., Hall, B.D., Hane, B., Srivastava, A. and Stevenson, R.E. (2000) Spectrum of Schwartz–Jampel syndrome includes micromelic chondrodysplasia, kyphomelic dysplasia, and Burton disease. *American Journal of Medical Genetics*, **94**, 287–295.

Squires, L.A. and Prangley, J. (1996) Neonatal Diagnosis of Schwartz-Jampel Syndrome With Dramatic Response to Carbamazepine. *Pediatric Neurology*, **15**, 172–174.

Stanton-Hicks, M., Janig, W., Hassenbusch, S., Haddox, J.D., Boas, R. and Wilson, P. (1995) Reflex sympathetic dystrophy: changing concepts and taxonomy. *Pain*, **63**, 127–133.

Steiner, J.C., Dejesus, P.V. and Mancall, E.L. (1974) Painful jumping amputation stumps: pathophysiology of a "sore circuit". *Transactions of the American Neurological Association*, **99**, 253–255.

Stephan, D.A., Buist, N.R., Chittenden, A.B., Ricker, K., Zhou, J. and Hoffman, E.P. (1994) A rippling muscle disease gene is localized to 1q41: evidence for multiple genes. *Neurology*, **44**, 1915–1920.

Takahashi, H., Saitoh, C., Iwata, O., Nanbu, T., Takada, S. and Morita, S. (2002) Epidural spinal cord stimulation for the treatment of painful legs and moving toes syndrome. *Pain*, **96**, 343–345.

Tan, E.K. and Jankovic, J. (1999) Bilateral hemifacial spasm: a report of five cases and a literature review. *Movement Disorders*, **14**, 345–349.

Tarsy, D. (1998) Comparison of acute- and delayed-onset posttraumatic cervical dystonia. *Movement Disorders*, **13**, 481–485.

Taylor, R., Layzer, R., Davis, H. and Fowler, W. (1972) Continuous muscle fiber activity in the Schwartz-Jampel syndrome. *Electroencephalography and Clinical Neurophysiology*, **33**, 497–509.

Topaloglu, H., Serdaroglu, A., Okan, M., Gucuyener, K. and Topcu, M. (1993) Improvement of myotonia withcarbamazepine in three cases with the Schwartz-Jampel syndrome. *Neuropediatrics*, **24**, 232–234.

Torbergsen, T. (1975) A family with dominant hereditary myotonia, muscular hypertrophy, and increased muscular irritability, distinct from myotonia congenita thomsen. *Acta Neurologica Scandinavica*, **51**, 225–232.

Torbergsen, T. (2002) Rippling muscle disease: a review. *Muscle & Nerve* (Suppl 11), S103–S107.

Trosch, R.M., Adler, C.H. and Pappert, E.J. (2007) Botulinum toxin type B (Myobloc) in subjects with hemifacial spasm: results from an open-label, dose-escalation safety study. *Movement Disorders*, **22**, 1258–1264.

Truong, D.D., Dubinsky, R., Hermanowicz, N., Olson, W.L., Silverman, B. and Koller, W.C. (1991) Posttraumatic torticollis. *Archives of Neurology*, **48**, 221–223.

Ueyama, H., Horinouchi, H., Obayashi, K., Hashinaga, M., Okazaki, T. and Kumamoto, T. (2007) Novel homozygous mutation of the caveolin-3 gene in rippling muscle disease with extraocular muscle paresis. *Neuromuscular Disorders*, **17**, 558–561.

Valenstein, E., Watson, R.T. and Parker, J.L. (1978) Myokymia, muscle hypertrophy and percussion "myotonia" in chronic recurrent polyneuropathy. *Neurology*, **28**, 1130–1134.

Valls-Sole, J. and Montero, J. (2003) Movement Disorders in Patients with Peripheral Facial Palsy. *Movement Disorders*, **18**, 1424–1435.

Van den Bergh, P., Francart, J., Mourin, S., Kollman, P. and Laterre, E.C. (1995) Five-year experience in the treatment of focal movement disorders with low-dose dysport botulinum toxin. *Muscle & Nerve*, **18**, 720–729.

van Hilten, B.J., van de Beek, W.J., Hoff, J.I., Voormolen, J.H. and Delhaas, E.M. (2000) Intrathecal baclofen for the treatment of dystonia in patients with reflex sympathetic dystrophy. *The New England Journal of Medicine*, **343**, 625–630.

van Rijn, M.A., Marinus, J., Putter, H. and Van Hilten, J.J. (2007) Onset and progression of dystonia in complex regional pain syndrome. *Pain*, **130**, 287–293.

Vantrappen, G., Decramer, M. and Harlet, R. (1992) High-frequency diaphragmatic flutter: symptoms and treatment by carbamazepine. *Lancet*, **339**, 265–267.

Vasilescu, C. and Florescu, A. (1982) Peripheral neuropathy with a syndrome of continuous motor unit activity. *Journal of Neurology*, **226**, 275–282.

Vasilescu, C., Alexianu, M. and Dan, A. (1984) Muscle hypertrophy and a syndrome of continuous motor unit activity in prednisone-responsive Guillain-Barre polyneuropathy. *Journal of Neurology*, **231**, 276–279.

Vasilescu, C., Alexianu, M. and Dan, A. (1987) Valproic acid in Isaacs-Mertens syndrome. *Clinical Neuropharmacology*, **10**, 215–224.

Verdugo, R.J. and Ochoa, J.L. (1994) 'Sympathetically maintained pain.' I. Phentolamine block questions the concept. *Neurology*, **44**, 1003–1010.

Verdugo, R.J. and Ochoa, J.L. (2000) Abnormal movements in complex regional pain syndrome: assessment of their nature. *Muscle & Nerve*, **23**, 198–205.

Verhagen, W.I., Horstink, M.W. and Notermans, S.L. (1985) Painful arm and moving fingers. *Journal of Neurology, Neurosurgery, and Psychiatry*, **48**, 384–385.

Vernino, S., Auger, R.G., Emslie-Smith, A.M., Harper, C.M. and Lennon, V.A. (1999) Myasthenia, thymoma, presynaptic antibodies, and a continuum of neuromuscular hyperexcitability. *Neurology*, **53**, 1233–1239.

Vilchez, J.J., Cabello, A., Benedito, J. and Villarroya, T. (1980) Hyperkalaemic paralysis, neuropathy and persistent motor neuron discharges at rest in Addison's disease. *Journal of Neurology, Neurosurgery, and Psychiatry*, **43**, 818–822.

Viljoen, D. and Beighton, P. (1992) Schwartz–Jampel syndrome (chondrodystophic myotonia). *Journal of Medical Genetics*, **29**, 58–62.

Villarejo, A., Porta-Etessam, J., Camacho, A., Gonzalez de La Aleja, J., Martinez-Salio, A. and Penas, M. (2004) Gabapentin for painful legs and moving toes syndrome. *European Neurology*, **51**, 180–181.

Vincent, A. (2000) Understanding neuromyotonia. *Muscle & Nerve*, **23**, 655–657.

Vorgerd, M., Bolz, H., Patzold, T., Kubisch, C., Malin, J.P. and Mortier, W. (1999) Phenotypic variability in rippling muscle disease. *Neurology*, **52**, 1453–1459.

Walker, S.M. and Cousins, M.J. (1997) Complex regional pain syndromes: including "reflex sympathetic dystrophy" and "causalgia". *Anaesth Intensive Care*, **25**, 113–125.

Wallis, W.E., Van Poznak, A. and Plum, F. (1970) Generalized muscular stiffness, fasciculations, and myokymia of peripheral nerve origin. *Archives of Neurology*, **22**, 430–439.

Weiner, W.J. (2001) Can peripheral trauma induce dystonia? No! *Movement Disorders*, **16**, 13–22.

Welch, L.K., Appenzeller, O. and Bicknell, J.M. (1972) Peripheral neuropathy with myokymia, sustained muscular contraction, and continuous motor unit activity. *Neurology*, **22**, 161–169.

Wilson, P.R. (1992) Reflex'? Sympathetic'? Dystrophy'? Paradigm shift'? (editorial). *Clinical Journal of Pain*, **8**, 281–284.

Woodman, S.E., Sotgia, F., Galbiati, F., Minetti, C. and Lisanti, M.P. (2004) Caveolinopathies: mutations in caveolin-3 cause four distinct autosomal dominant muscle diseases. *Neurology*, **62**, 538–543.

Wulff, C.H. (1982) Painful legs and moving toes. A report of 3 cases with neurophysiological studies. *Acta Neurologica Scandinavica*, **66**, 283–287.

Yoon, J., Crabtree, C. and Botek, G. (2001) Syndrome of painful legs and moving toes: a case study. *Journal of the American Podiatric Medical Association*, **91**, 361–364.

Yuan, Y., Wang, Y., Zhang, S.-X., Zhang, L., Li, R. and Guo, J. (2005) Microvascular decompression in patients with hemifacial spasm: report of 1200 cases. *Chinese Medical Journal*, **118**, 833–836.

Zadikoff, C., Mailis-Gagnon, A. and Lang, A.E. (2006) A case of a psychogenic "jumpy stump". *Journal of Neurology, Neurosurgery, and Psychiatry*, **77**, 1101.

Zifko, U., Drlicek, M., Machacek, E., Jellinger, K. and Grisold, W. (1994) Syndrome of continuous muscle fiber activity and plasmacytoma with IgM paraproteinemia. *Neurology*, **44**, 560–561.

18

Stiff Person Syndrome

Philip D. Thompson and Hans-Michael Meinck

University Department of Medicine, University of Adelaide and Department of Neurology, Royal Adelaide Hospital, Adelaide, Australia
Department of Neurology, University of Heidelberg, Heidelberg, Germany

Moersch and Woltman introduced the term "stiff man syndrome" to describe a condition in which the principal clinical features were "progressive fluctuating muscular rigidity and spasm" with marked sensitivity to external stimuli (Moersch and Woltman, 1956). Since females are more commonly affected than males, the name of the condition was subtly changed to "stiff person syndrome" (SPS) to reflect this (Blum and Jankovic, 1991). The condition is generally regarded as rare, but with greater awareness of the clinical features is increasingly recognized, though the prevalence remains unknown.

CLINICAL PRESENTATION

The presenting features of SPS are muscle stiffness, rigidity and spasms affecting the trunk, particularly the thoracolumbar region and one or both legs with associated difficulties in walking. The onset is insidious, usually in the fifth decade, and symptoms are progressive. The stiffness is produced by continuous motor unit activity and persistent muscle contraction despite attempted relaxation. Antagonist muscle groups are equally affected further contributing to the rigidity. The muscle activity and rigidity lessen or even disappear during sleep and narcosis. Paraspinal muscle contraction produces an exaggerated lumbar lordosis (Figure 18.1) and trunkal rigidity. Contraction of anterior abdominal muscles results in "board-like" rigidity of the abdominal wall. Rigidity of the trunkal and proximal leg muscles limits the range of voluntary movement of the trunk and legs. Movements, particularly walking, become slow and labored with loss of the normal fluid flowing motion of the leg and trunk with each step. The muscular rigidity fluctuates from a mild increase in tone to painful prolonged muscle contractions.

Stimulus-induced or apparently spontaneous spasms result in sudden and dramatic increases in stiffness superimposed on the background rigidity. Spasms are one of the most characteristic features of SPS. Any sudden and unexpected stimulus, particularly noise and touch, but also voluntary movement, fear, anger and other strong emotions may trigger a spasm. Spasms begin with a short myoclonic jerk that is often difficult to see because the amplitude of limb and trunk movement is limited by the background rigidity, followed by a prolonged contraction with tonic activity that persists for several seconds before gradually settling. Reflex spasms may spread from one leg to the other with motor patterns that resemble either extensor thrusts, including opisthotonus, or flexor spasms with crossed leg extension. Surface electromyography (EMG) recordings are very useful in identifying this pattern of enhanced exteroceptive reflex response (see below) which is virtually diagnostic of SPS (Meinck, Ricker and Conrad, 1984). Prolonged spasms may be accompanied by pain and autonomic disturbances, particularly profuse sweating. Brisk tendon reflexes may be the only other abnormal neurological sign.

VARIATION IN CLINICAL PRESENTATION

Patients may present with brief stimulus-induced spasms or progressive rigidity and stiffness confined to one leg. Asymmetry of leg involvement and greater limb than trunkal rigidity is not uncommon in the earlier stages (Barker et al., 1998; Saiz et al., 1998; Dalakas et al., 2000; Meinck and Thompson, 2002). An exaggerated startle response and myoclonus of brainstem origin is present in many cases, in addition to the stimulus-induced spasms and rigidity. This has been referred to as the "jerking stiff man syndrome" (Leigh et al., 1980; Alberca, Remero and Chaparro, 1982). Stimulus-induced jerks, spasms and enhanced startle responses are frequently associated with sudden incapacitating increases in muscle

Therapeutics of Parkinson's Disease and Other Movement Disorders Edited by Mark Hallett and Werner Poewe
© 2008 John Wiley & Sons, Ltd.

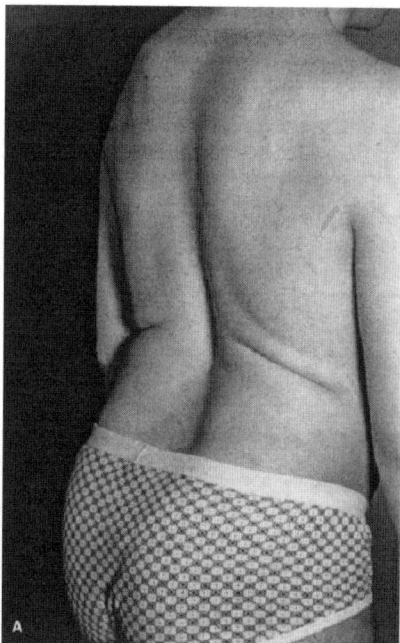

Figure 18.1 Exaggerated lumbar lordosis in SPS. Note the accentuated contour of the paraspinal musculature and the transverse skin crease reflecting contraction of the oblique truncal muscles. (Reproduced from Meinck, H.M. and Thompson, P.D. (2002), with permission from John Wiley & Sons Inc).

stiffness and prolonged rigidity leading to falls and a loss of confidence in walking, particularly in open environments without support, or in crowded busy areas with unpredictable ambient noise and traffic. These factors may contribute to a fear of open spaces and phobic avoidance behavior that is misinterpreted as agoraphobia or considered psychogenic or hysterical in origin (Henningsen and Meinck, 2003).

PATHOPHYSIOLOGY

Neurophysiology

Neurophysiological studies reveal continuous motor unit activity in axial and proximal muscles, comprising normal motor unit potentials. Several lines of evidence indicate this activity is driven by changes in excitability of spinal interneurones and their descending control from the brainstem, though the precise mechanism remains obscure (Meinck and Thompson, 2002). One of the hallmarks of the SPS is the presence of enhanced non-habituating exteroceptive or cutaneomuscular reflexes (Figure 18.2) (Meinck, Ricker and Conrad, 1984). These reflexes are assumed to be responsible for the spasms of SPS that spread from one limb to another and to the trunk. Enhancement of

the blink reflex (Meinck, Ricker and Conrad, 1984; Molloy, Dalakas and Floeter, 2002) and startle responses (Figure 18.3) (Meinck, Ricker and Conrad, 1984; Berger and Meinck, 2003; Khasani, Becker and Meinck, 2004) indicate increased excitability of the descending control of polysynaptic brainstem and spinal interneuronal pathways. Spinal inhibitory reflex responses such as vibration-induced inhibition are impaired, though pre-synaptic inhibition, recurrent inhibition and reciprocal inhibition are normal or variable (Floeter et al., 1998). Motor cortex hyperexcitability has also been demonstrated (Sandbrink et al., 2000; Koerner et al., 2004). These physiological changes indicating enhanced neuronal excitability at different levels of the central nervous system may be a consequence of impaired inhibitory function of γ-aminobutyric acid (GABA) pathways.

IMMUNOPATHOLOGY

Anti-GAD Antibodies

There is now strong evidence that SPS has an autoimmune basis. Oligoclonal bands are found in the cerebrospinal fluid in 60%, but a cellular response in cerebrospinal fluid is rare (Dalakas et al., 2001; Meinck and Thompson, 2002). Antibodies directed against glutamic acid decarboxylase (antiGADab) are found in 60–80% of cases (Solimena et al., 1990; Walikonis and Lennon, 1998). Radioimmunoassay is the most specific and sensitive method for detection (Dinkel et al., 1998; Murinson et al., 2004). AntiGADab in SPS are similar to those in type 1 diabetes mellitus, but differ in epitope recognition, the antibody titer is much higher in SPS and antibodies are detected in both serum and cerebrospinal fluid in SPS (Daw et al., 1996; Raju et al., 2005). The role of GAD autoimmunity in SPS has been the subject of debate since some other disorders such as cerebellar ataxia, palatal myoclonus and epilepsy may also have detectable antiGADab (Honnorat, Saiz and Giometto, 2001). Evidence of intrathecal synthesis of antiGADab that block GABA synthesis (Raju et al., 2005), inflammatory pathological changes in SPS (discussed below) and the induction of continuous motor unit activity and enhanced exteroceptive reflexes in rats (mimicking SPS) following intrathecal injection of IgG from patients with antiGADab all suggest that the antibodies are pathogenic in an immune-mediated encephalomyelitis (Manto et al., 2007). Antibodies against gephyrin, a post-synaptic protein important in receptor clustering in inhibitory GABAergic and glycinergic synapses (Yu et al., 2007), have also been reported (Butler et al., 2000). Anti-amphiphysin antibodies have been found in association with paraneoplastic SPS, particularly breast cancer (Rosin et al., 1998).

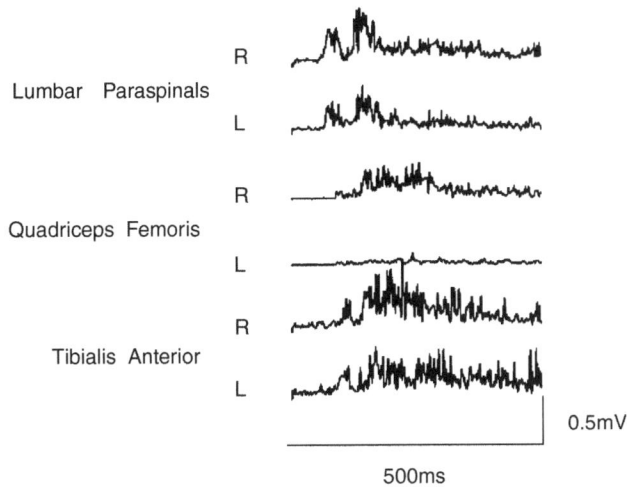

Figure 18.2 Rectified surface electromyographic recordings from axial and leg muscles after stimulation of the digital nerve of the index finger (delivered at the start of the sweep) in a man with the SPS. After stimulation there is an initial burst of myoclonic activity followed by a prolonged tonic increase in muscle activity. The initial burst in the lumbar paraspinal muscles occurred approximately 60 ms after the stimulus. (Reproduced from Meinck, H.M. and Thompson, P.D. (2002), with permission from John Wiley & Sons Inc).

ANTIBODY-MEDIATED ENDOCRINOPATHIES

Pancreatic islet cell (60%), gastric parietal cell (50%) and thyroid microsomal (40%) antibodies are commonly detected and autoimmune endocrine disease is present in about 50% (Meinck and Thompson, 2002). An association with diabetes mellitus was noted in the original description,

and 30–60% of patients have diabetes mellitus (for references see Meinck and Thompson, 2002).

NEUROPATHOLOGY

The published neuropathological studies of SPS were recently reviewed (Meinck and Thompson 2002). Perivascular lymphocytic cuffing and variable neuronal loss were

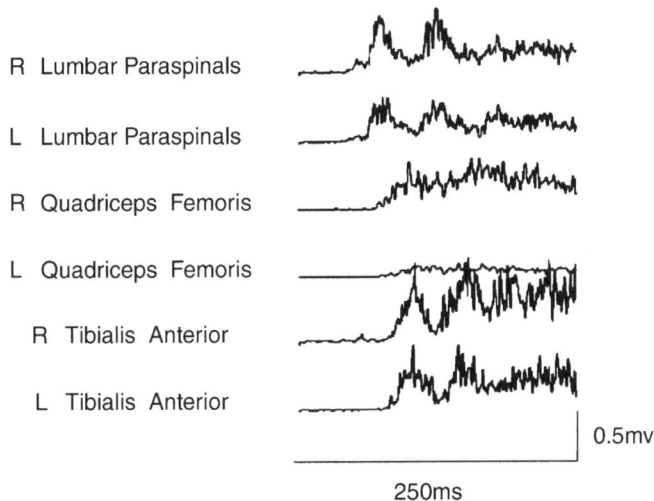

Figure 18.3 Rectified surface electromyographic recordings from axial and leg muscles after auditory stimulation delivered at the start of the sweep (same patient as in Figure 18.2). Brief myoclonic bursts of activity (beginning in lumbar paraspinal muscles approximately 50 ms after the tone) are followed by prolonged tonic discharge similar to that seen after cutaneous stimulation. (Reproduced from Meinck, H.M. and Thompson, P.D. (2002), with permission from John Wiley & Sons Inc).

evident in the brainstem and spinal cord in cases with and without known antibody status. The significance of these changes and the relationship to progressive encephalomyelitis with rigidity (PER) (Whiteley, Swash and Urich, 1976; Armon *et al.*, 1996; Warren *et al.*, 2002) remains the subject of debate.

PHARMACOLOGY

As discussed above, a number of physiological studies point towards impairment of inhibitory function in the central nervous system. Pharmacological manipulation of adrenergic and GABA transmission adds weight to the suggestion that these systems are involved in the physiological mechanisms responsible for rigidity and spasms. Central α-adrenergic agonists (clonidine, tizanidine) and GABA agonists (diazepam, baclofen) reduce spasms and exteroceptive reflex activity (Meinck, Ricker and Conrad, 1984). The effect of diazepam is particularly striking and this is discussed further below.

SPS VARIANTS

Progressive Encephalomyelitis with Rigidity (PER)

This condition presents with the sub-acute onset of rigidity and spasm (that may be violent and myoclonic) associated with vertigo, ataxia, diplopia, dysarthria or sensory symptoms. Signs of brainstem (ophthalmoplegia, nystagmus, deafness and bulbar palsy) and spinal (muscle wasting weakness, areflexia, extensor plantar responses) involvement distinguish PER from the SPS (Kasperek and Zebrowski 1971; Whiteley, Swash and Urich, 1976; Howell, Lees and Toghill, 1979). Severe rigidity of all limbs, prominent myoclonus (Campbell and Garland 1956; Rothwell, Obeso and Marsden, 1986; Brown *et al.*, 1991), autonomic crises, cerebrospinal fluid lymphocytic pleocytosis, abnormal brainstem and spinal cord imaging (McCombe *et al.*, 1989) and a rapidly progressive course are further distinctive features. Spinal inflammation, interneuronal cell loss and ascending tract degeneration have lead to the designation spinal "neuronitis" or "interneuronitis".

The distinction between SPS and PER is straightforward where there is rapid progression and the accumulation of bulbar, cerebellar and spinal signs. However, it is increasingly recognized that some cases of otherwise typical SPS have bulbar involvement (Dalakas *et al.*, 2000; personal observation) or develop additional signs with the passage of time (Mitsumoto *et al.*, 1991; Warren *et al.*, 2002) while others are found to have an encephalomyelitis on pathological examination (Meinck *et al.*, 1994; Armon *et al.*, 1996; Warren *et al.*, 2002). Moreover, many cases of PER have antiGADab (Brown *et al.*, 1991;

Meinck and Thompson 2002). One conclusion from these observations is that SPS and PER are closely related.

PARANEOPLASTIC ENCEPHALOMYELITIS

Segmental rigidity, spasm and myoclonus have been described as paraneoplastic manifestations of breast (Rosin *et al.*, 1998) and small-cell lung cancer (Roobol, Kazzaz and Vecht, 1987; Bateman, Weller and Kennedy, 1990). Clinical features suggesting a paraneoplastic etiology include rigidity confined to one upper limb, rapid progression and the early appearance of joint deformity (Rosin *et al.*, 1998). Other paraneoplastic syndromes, such as sensory ganglionopathy may co-exist (Stingele *et al.*, 1998). Neurological signs may appear well before presentation of the neoplasm. Anti-amphiphysin antibodies have been identified in cases with paraneoplastic rigidity associated with breast cancer (Folli *et al.*, 1993; Dropcho 1996) and may co-exist with antiGADab (Rosin *et al.*, 1998). Personal observations suggest that paraneoplastic SPS may be associated with antiGADab and screening for cancer is always indicated in SPS in the first years after presentation.

DIFFERENTIAL DIAGNOSIS

From a practical point of view the commonest differential diagnosis is fibromyalgic chronic low back pain with associated restriction of mobility. Continuous motor unit activity, rigidity and enhanced exteroceptive reflexes are not present in chronic low back pain. Back pain may be a feature of SPS, but this is usually paroxysmal in association with spasm. Abnormal lumbar posturing is present in axial dystonia and certain myopathies. Dystonia occurs on standing and walking, but the abnormal posturing settles on lying down. The exaggerated lumbar lordosis of SPS is present when standing and usually persists on lying down. Myopathies, such as the rigid spine syndrome, inflammatory myopathies and myositis ossificans, may produce an abnormal lumbar posture due to fibrotic contracture of paraspinal muscles that persists when standing, lying down and during sleep. Muscle weakness and wasting is usually evident and needle electromyography will reveal myopathic units and a low-amplitude dense interference pattern in contrast to the continuous motor unit activity of SPS. Cramps may be confused with the spasms of SPS. Benign physiological cramps affect one muscle and can be "broken" by stretching the affected muscle, in contrast to the more widespread recruitment of muscles in a spasm that typically involves both legs and the trunk. Peripheral nerve hyperexcitability syndromes produce distal and proximal muscle stiffness, delayed muscle relaxation, depressed tendon reflexes and characteristic spontaneous high-frequency discharges, myokymia and after-discharges on needle electromyography. Brief paroxysms of muscle stiffness and rigidity in early SPS pose a difficult diagnostic problem since the precipitating stimuli (anxiety, emotion, noise) may escape notice. Accordingly, SPS should be considered in the differential diagnosis of tonic spasms in demyelinating disease, tonic seizures and paroxysmal dyskinesias. Segmental rigidity with spasms affecting one limb may complicate a variety of spinal cord pathologies (Penry et al., 1960; Tarlov 1967; Davis et al., 1981). The presence of other signs points toward a structural spinal lesion and imaging of the spinal cord should be undertaken if there is any doubt. A small number of patients with rigidity confined to one limb have no identifiable cause. The term "stiff leg syndrome" was originally used to describe such cases and it was suggested these represent a form of chronic spinal interneuronitis (Brown, Rothwell and Marsden, 1997).

DIAGNOSIS OF SPS

The clinical features of trunkal rigidity due to continuous motor unit activity with superimposed spasm form a distinctive pattern. The absence of other neurological signs is an important additional criterion. Earlier descriptions of SPS listed a number of diagnostic criteria encompassing these essential features. Today, these clinical features, coupled with neurophysiological demonstration of characteristic reflex enhancement and the presence of antiGADab are invaluable in forming the basis for diagnosis, though the latter are not essential for diagnosis, since antiGADab are detected in only 60–80% of cases. Conversely, interpretation of serum antiGADab also requires caution since they are present in 1% of the normal population and about 5% of unselected neurologic diseases (Meinck et al., 2001).

TREATMENT

A number of symptomatic drug therapies have been reported, mostly as therapeutic observations in the form of case reports or limited series without controlled trials. More recently immunomodulatory strategies to modify the immune response and disease progression have been studied. Physiotherapy also provides a valuable adjunct to pharmacological treatments.

Diazepam was one of the first drugs reported to be of benefit (Cohen, 1966) and remains the most widely used. The acute response to intravenous diazepam is so dramatic that it is a useful diagnostic test, though this is not specific. An infusion of 5 mg diazepam (prepared as 20 mg of diazepam diluted in 100 ml normal saline) administered over five minutes reduces muscle tone with relief of

stiffness and restriction of movement (Meinck and Conrad, 1986).

Oral diazepam is particularly effective in relieving the muscle spasms, but background muscle rigidity due to continuous muscle activity frequently persists. Therapeutic benefit from maintenance oral diazepam usually requires increasing doses because of habituation and carries the risk of addiction. The same considerations apply to clonazepam. Sedative and cognitive side effects also limit the use of long-term high-dose benzodiazepines. Because of this, diazepam is usually given in combination with baclofen or other GABAergic drugs. The use of oral baclofen is also limited by side effects at higher doses and intrathecal administration of baclofen has been proposed as one method of providing higher central nervous system concentrations of the drug than is possible with oral administration (Penn and Mangieri, 1993). Significant improvements have been reported with this technique (Seitz et al., 1995; Stayer et al., 1997). In the case reported by Seitz et al. (1995) intrathecal baclofen was combined with azathioprine for 24 months, during which time a decrease in continuous muscle activity, muscle tone and rigidity was accompanied by a return to independent walking. Withdrawal of intrathecal baclofen was followed within 18 hours by reappearance of continuous muscle activity and deteriorating gait, which again improved after resumption of the infusion. In a double-blind placebo-controlled trial of intrathecal baclofen in three patients, a reduction in reflex excitability was accompanied by clinical improvement in only one patient (Silbert et al., 1995). The use of intrathecal baclofen must be approached with caution, since the sudden withdrawal of baclofen due to catheter breakage or pump failure can lead to an acute baclofen-withdrawal syndrome with autonomic crises that can be fatal (Stayer et al., 1997).

The benefits of drugs that enhance GABAergic transmission, such as valproate (Spehlmann et al., 1981), levetiracetam (Ruegg, Steck and Fuhr, 2004), tiagibine (Murinson and Rizzo 2001) and vigabatrin (Ligouri et al., 1993; Vermeij et al., 1996; Prevett, Brown and Duncan, 1997), have been dramatic in individual case reports. This usually reflects the improvement in functional capacity that follows a reduction in stimulus-induced jerks, spasms and enhanced startle responses. Patients who were previously unable to walk outside or go shopping because of fear of falling during a prolonged spasm may be able to do so if spasms are dampened by treatment. The effect on continuous muscle contraction and axial rigidity seems more variable and is difficult to quantify, though a reduction in axial rigidity may also contribute to improved mobility. In many cases, the reduction in spasms from the additional medication allows a significant reduction in concurrent benzodiazepine use with a corresponding improvement in sedative and cognitive side effects of high-dose benzodiazepine use.

Drugs that modify central adrenergic transmission such as clonidine and tizanidine are also useful adjuncts in reducing spasms, though the beneficial effects are limited by sedation and hypotension (Meinck and Conrad, 1986).

Botulinum toxin injections have relieved painful paraspinal and proximal leg muscle stiffness and continuous motor unit activity, with effects lasting four to seven months at a time (Davis and Jabbari, 1993; Ligouri et al., 1997). Spasms, rigidity and mobility were improved. Whether the toxin can improve function by diminishing the spread of a regional spasm remains to be determined.

Because of the immune-mediated inflammatory basis for SPS a number of immunomodulatory therapies have been tried. Anecdotal reports of varying degrees of benefit with plasma exchange in association with other immune therapies have not been followed by systematic study. All these cases had experienced sub-optimal responses to pharmacological therapies usually in multiple combinations. Improvement in mobility, a reduction in continuous motor unit activity, exteroceptive reflexes and serum GAD-like immunoreactivity (Brashear and Phillips, 1991), improvement in clinical symptoms and continuous motor unit activity with (Hau et al., 1999) and without change in antiGADab (Vicari et al., 1989) and marginal (Shariatmadar and Noto 2001) or no discernible effect (Harding et al., 1989) have been described. In many of these cases, varying forms of immunosuppression were coincident with plasma exchange. There have been no reports on the efficacy on individual immunosuppressive drugs beyond anecdotal mention of their use in these reports.

High-dose methylprednisolone (500 mg intravenous for five days) can be useful, but maintenance steroid therapy is often required for long-term suppression of symptoms (Meinck, 2000). Steroids are generally used in concert with other forms of immunomodulation. The value of long-term high-dose steroids is limited by the potential to exacerbate or unmask co-existing or latent diabetes mellitus.

Case reports of improvement in spasms and continuous motor unit activity after intravenous immunoglobulin (IVIg) allowing a reduction in the doses of diazepam and related drugs (Amato, Cornman and Kissel, 1994; Barker and Marsden 1997; Souza-Lima et al., 2000) were followed by the only controlled trial involving any form of treatment in SPS. Sixteen antiGADab positive patients randomly received high-dose intravenous immunoglobulin (2 gm per kilogram body weight) or placebo in a double blind cross-over design monthly for three months before one-month washout and then three months with the other treatment (Dalakas et al., 2001). Monthly assessments showed that IVIg reduced stiffness and spasms, the number of falls and improved walking. These functional gains were lost during the one-month washout period and scores declined back to baseline on placebo (Figure 18.4). This study used a higher dose of IVIg than is normally employed for other neurological immunomodulatory therapies.

A single case report of a patient refractory to treatment with various immunomodulatory therapies including IVIg, cyclophosphamide and mycophenolate documented the efficacy of rituximab, a monoclonal anti B cell antibody in reducing continuous motor unit activity and stiffness with an improvement in functional capacity and reduction in antiGADab (Baker et al., 2005). Diazepam, baclofen and dantrolene were continued, but at reduced doses.

CONCLUDING REMARKS

The therapeutic approach for the initial treatment of SPS can be summarized in two categories (Table 18.1). First, symptomatic treatment to reduce spasms and stiffness. Second, disease modification by immunomodulatory therapies. In practice, the approach taken will depend on the severity of symptoms. Symptomatic treatment with a combination of diazepam and baclofen is recommended to reduce spasms. It is desirable, though not always possible, to keep the dose of diazepam as low as possible. If spasms remain troublesome, other drugs can be added. It is evident that most patients with SPS are eventually treated with a range of drugs with similar actions, often in combination, in an effort to provide symptomatic relief from the stiffness and spasm. Lack of efficacy and side effects are common. Excessive sedation from combinations of benzodiazepines and anti-convulsants is often exacerbated by the injudicious addition of opiates for painful spasm further interfering with cognitive function and the ability to conduct daily activities. Such adverse effects may be as disabling as the spasms and stiffness.

In contrast, immunomodulatory therapies, particularly IVIg appear promising in terms of efficacy and, although expensive, seems to have relatively few side effects. When starting immunomodulation we recommend minimizing the doses of other drugs so the efficacy of immunomodulation can be assessed, and to establish whether maintenance immunomodulation is necessary. The beneficial effects of immunomodulation on the disease course in the longer term are not known. It does appear that disease modification can reduce muscle contraction and stiffness. In severe cases, combinations of therapy will inevitably be used.

If there is significant evidence of inflammatory disease of the central nervous system (and if the question of PER is raised) then pulse intravenous methylprednisolone followed by maintenance corticosteroids should be considered. Whether other forms of immunosuppression will prove helpful remains to be determined.

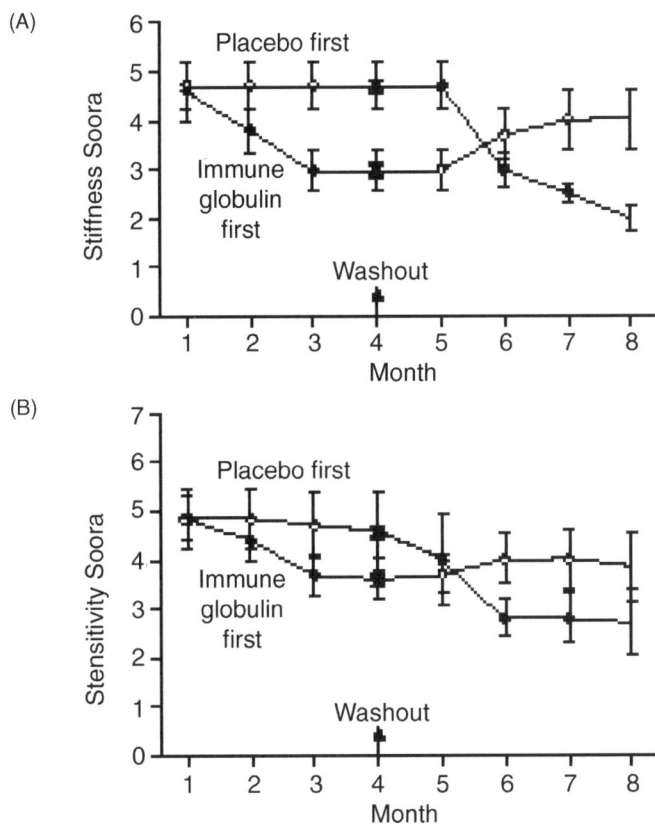

Figure 18.4 The effect of immunoglobulin on scores representing the extent of stiffness on clinical examination (A) and stimulus sensitive spasms (B) in a randomized double-blind placebo-controlled crossover trial in 16 patients with SPS. Patients received immunoglobulin (solid symbols) or placebo (open symbols) and were examined monthly. Higher scores indicate greater impairment for both scales, i.e., more widespread stiffness and more frequent spasms. Values are mean score ±SE. Stiffness scores were significantly improved at three, four and five months after immunoglobulin, then deteriorated significantly during placebo at seven and eight months (A). Stimulus-sensitive spasms were significantly worse at six and seven months during treatment with placebo (B). Reproduced from Dalakas, *et al.* (2001) with permission. Copyright © 2001, Massachusetts Medical Society. All rights reserved.

Table 18.1 Therapeutic options in SPS.

A: Symptomatic treatment (for spasms)
  Benzodiazepines, e.g. (diazepam)
  Baclofen
  Tizanindine, Clonidine

Also reported to be effective (see text for references)
  Valproate
  Vigabatrin
  Tiagibine
  Levetiracetam

B: Disease modifying—Immunomodulatory treatment
  (reduces muscle contraction and stiffness)
  Immune globulin
  Intravenous methyl prednisolone
  Plasma exchange
  Rituximab

References

Alberca, R., Remero, M. and Chaparro, J. (1982) Jerking stiff-man syndrome. *Journal of Neurology, Neurosurgery, and Psychiatry*, **45**, 1159–1160.

Amato, A.A., Cornman, E.W. and Kissel, J.T. (1994) Treatment of stiff-man syndrome with intravenous immunoglobulin. *Neurology*, **44**, 1652–1654.

Armon, C., Swanson, J.W., McLean, J.M. *et al.* (1996) Subacute encephalomyelitis presenting as stiff-person syndrome: clinical, polygraphic and pathologic correlations. *Movement Disorders*, **11**, 701–709.

Baker, M.R., Das, M., Isaacs, J., Fawcett, P.R.W. and Bates, D. (2005) Treatment of stiff person syndrome with rituximab. *Journal of Neurology Neurosurgery and Psychiatry*, **76**, 999–1001.

Barker, R.A. and Marsden, C.D. (1997) Successful treatment of stiff man syndrome with intravenous immunoglobulin. *Journal of Neurology Neurosurgery and Psychiatry*, **62**, 426–427.

Barker, R.A., Revesz, T., Thom, M., Marsden, C.D. and Brown, P. (1998) Review of 23 patients affected by the stiff man syndrome: clinical subdivision into stiff trunk (man) syndrome, stiff limb syndrome, and progressive encephalomyelitis with rigidity. *Journal of Neurology Neurosurgery and Psychiatry*, **65**, 633–640.

Bateman, D.E., Weller, R.O. and Kennedy, P. (1990) Stiffman syndrome: a rare paraneoplastic disorder? *Journal of Neurology, Neurosurgery and Psychiatry*, **53**, 695–696.

Berger, C. and Meinck, H.M. (2003) Head retraction reflex in stiff man syndrome and related disorders. *Movement Disorders*, **8**, 906–911.

Blum, P. and Jankovic, J. (1991) Stiff Person Syndrome: An autoimmune disease. *Movement Disorders*, **6**, 12–20.

Brashear, H.R. and Phillips, L.H. (1991) Autoantibodies to GABAergic neurons and response to plasmapheresis in stiff-man syndrome. *Neurology*, **41**, 1588–1592.

Brown, P., Rothwell, J.C., Thompson, P.D., Britton, T.C., Day, B.L. and Marsden, C.D. (1991) The hyperekplexias and their relationship to the normal startle reflex. *Brain*, **114**, 1903–1928.

Brown, P., Rothwell, J.C. and Marsden, C.D. (1997) The stiff leg syndrome. *Journal of Neurology Neurosurgery and Psychiatry*, **62**, 31–37.

Burn, D.J., Ball, J., Lees, A.J., Behan, P.O. and Morgan-Hughes, J.A. (1991) A case of progressive encephalomyelitis with rigidity and positive antiglutamic acid dehydrogenase antibodies. *Journal of Neurology Neurosurgery and Psychiatry*, **54**, 449–451.

Butler, H.M., Hatashi, A., Ohkoshi, N. *et al.* (2000) Autoimmunity to gephyrin in stiff-man syndrome. *Neuron*, **26**, 307–312.

Campbell, A.M.G. and Garland, H. (1956) Subacute myoclonic spinal neuronitis, *Journal of Neurology. Neurosurgery and Psychiatry*, **19**, 268–274.

Cohen, L. (1966) Stiff man syndrome. Two patients treated with diazepam. *Journal of the American Medical Association*, **195**, 160–162.

Dalakas, M.C., Fujii, M., Li, M. and McElroy, B. (2000) The clinical spectrum of antiGAD antibody positive patients with stiff person syndrome. *Neurology*, **55**, 1531–1535.

Dalakas, M.C., Fujii, M., Li, M., Lufti, B., Kyhos, J. and McElroy, B. (2001) High dose intravenous immunoglobulin for stiff person syndrome. *New England Journal of Medicine*, **345**, 1870–1876.

Dalakas, M.C., Li, M., Fujii, M. and Jacobowitz, D.M. (2001) Stiff person syndrome: quantification, specificity and intrathecal synthesis of GAD65 antibodies. *Neurology*, **57**, 780–784.

Davis, D. and Jabbari, B. (1993) Significant improvement of stiff person syndrome after paraspinal injection of botulinum toxin A. *Movement Disorders*, **3**, 371–373.

Davis, S.M., Murray, N.M.F., Diengdoh, J.V., Galea-Debono, A. and Kocen, R.S. (1981) Stimulus-sensitive spinal myoclonus. *Journal of Neurology Neurosurgery and Psychiatry*, **44**, 884–888.

Daw, K., Ujihara, N., Atkinson, M. and Powers, A.C. (1996) Glutamic acid decarboxylase autoantibodies in stiff man syndrome and insulin dependent diabetes mellitus exhibit similarities and differences in epitope recognition. *Journal of Immunology*, **156**, 818–825.

Dinkel, K., Meinck, H.M., Jury, K.M., Karges, W. and Richter, W. (1998) Inhibition of gamma-aminobutyric acid synthesis by glutamic acid decarboxylase autoantibodies in stiff man syndrome. *Annals of Neurology*, **44**, 194–201.

Dropcho, E.J. (1996) Antiamphiphysin antibodies with small-cell lung carcinoma and paraneoplastic encephalomyelitis. *Annals of Neurology*, **39**, 659–667.

Floeter, M.K., Valls-Sole, J., Toro, C., Jacobowitz, D. and Hallett, M. (1998) Physiologic studies of spinal inhibitory circuits in patients with stiff-person syndrome. *Neurology*, **51**, 85–93.

Folli, F., Solimena, M., Cofiell, R., Austoni, M., Tallini, G., Fassetta, G. *et al.* (1993) Autoantibodies to a 128-kd synaptic protein in three women with the stiff-man syndrome and breast cancer. *New England Journal of Medicine*, **328**, 546–551.

Harding, A.E., Thompson, P.D., Kocen, R.S., Batchelor, J.R., Davey, N. and Marsden, C.D. (1989) Plasma exchange and immunosuppression in the stiff-man syndrome. *Lancet*, **I**, 915.

Hau, W., Davis, C., Hirsch, I.B., Eng, L.J., Daniels, T., Walsh, D. and Lernmark, A. (1999) Plasmapharesis and immunosuppression in the stiff-man syndrome with type 1 diabetes: a 2 year study. *Journal of Neurology*, **246**, 731–735.

Henningsen, P. and Meinck, H.M. (2003) Specific phobia is a frequent non-motor feature in stiff man syndrome. *Journal of Neurology, Neurosurgery and Psychiatry*, **74**, 462–462.

Honnorat, J., Saiz, A. and Giometto, B. (2001) Cerebellar ataxia associated with antiglutamic acid decarboxylase antibodies. *Archives of Neurology*, **58**, 225–230.

Howell, D.A., Lees, A.J. and Toghill, P.J. (1979) Spinal internuncial neurones in progressive encephalomyelitis with rigidity. *Journal of Neurology Neurosurgery and Psychiatry*, **42**, 773–785.

Kasperek, S. and Zebrowski, S. (1971) Stiff man syndrome and encephalomyelitis. *Archives of Neurology*, **24**, 22–31.

Khasani, S., Becker, K. and Meinck, H.M. (2004) Hyperekplexia and stiff man syndrome: abnormal brainstem reflexes suggest a physiological relationship. *Journal of Neurology. Neurosurgery and Psychiatry*, **75**, 1265–1269.

Koerner, C., Wieland, B., Richter, W. and Meinck, H.M. (2004) Stiff person syndromes: hyperexcitability correlates with anti-GAD autoimmunity. *Neurology*, **62**, 1357–1362.

Leigh, P.N., Rothwell, J.C., Traub, M. and Marsden, C.D. (1980) A patient with reflex myoclonus and muscle rigidity: "the jerking stiff man syndrome". *Journal of Neurology, Neurosurgery and Psychiatry*, **43**, 1125–1131.

Ligouri, R., Medori, R., Marcello, L., Grimaldi, L., Lugaresi, E. and Montagna, P. (1993) Vigabatrin improves rigidity in stiff-person syndrome. *Neurology*, **43**, 311.

Ligouri, R., Cordivari, C., Lugaresi, E. and Montagna, P. (1997) Botulinum toxin A improves muscle spasms and rigidity in stiff person syndrome. *Movement Disorders*, **12**, 1060–1063.

Manto, M.U., Laute, M.A., Aguera, L.T., Rogemond, V., Pandolfo, M. and Honnorat, J. (2007) Effects of antiglutamic acid decarboxylase antibodies associated with neurological diseases. *Annals of Neurology*, **61**, 544–551.

McCombe, P.A., Chalk, J.B., Searle, J.W., Tannenberg, A.E.G. and Smith, J.J. (1989) Pender MP Progressive encephalomyelitis with rigidity: a case report with magnetic resonance imaging findings. *Journal of Neurology Neurosurgery and Psychiatry*, **52**, 1429–1431.

Meinck, H.M. (2000) Immunomodulation in the stiff man syndrome. *Movement Disorders*, **15** (Suppl 3), 252–253.

Meinck, H.M. and Conrad, B. (1986) Neuropharmacological investigations in the stiff-man syndrome. *Journal of Neurology*, **233**, 340–347.

Meinck, H.M., Faber, L., Morgenthaler, N. *et al.* (2001) Antibodies against glutamic acid decarboxylase: prevalence in neurological diseases. *Journal of Neurology, Neurosurgery and Psychiatry* **71**, 100–103.

Meinck, H.M. and Thompson, P.D. (2002) Stiff Man Syndrome and related conditions. *Movement Disorders*, **17**, 853–866.

Meinck, H.M., Ricker, K. and Conrad, B. (1984) The stiff man syndrome: New pathophysiological aspects from abnormal exteroceptive reflexes and the response to clomipramine, clonidine, and tizanidine. *Journal of Neurology Neurosurgery and Psychiatry*, **47**, 280–287.

Meinck, H.M., Ricker, K., Hulser, P.J., Schmid, E., Peiffer, J. and Solimena, M. (1994) Stiff man syndrome: clinical and laboratory findings in eight patients. *Journal of Neurology*, **241**, 157–166.

Mitsumoto, H., Schwartzman, M.J., Estes, M.L. *et al.* (1991) Sudden death and paroxysmal autonomic dysfunction in stiff-man syndrome. *Journal of Neurology*, **238**, 91–96.

Moersch, F.P. and Woltman, H.W. (1956) Progressive fluctuating muscular rigidity and spasm (stiff-man syndrome): report of a case and some observations in 13 other cases. *Mayo Clinic Proceedings*, **31**, 421–427.

Molloy, F.M., Dalakas, M.C. and Floeter, M.K. (2002) Increased brainstem excitability in stiff person syndrome. *Neurology*, **59**, 449–451.

Murinson, B.B. and Rizzo, M. (2001) Improvement of stiff-person syndrome with tiagabine. *Neurology*, **57**, 366.

Murinson, B.B., Butler, M., Marfurt, K., Gleason, S., De Camilli, P. and Solimena, M. (2004) Markedly elevated GAD antibodies in SPS: affects of age and illness duration. *Neurology*, **63**, 2146–2148.

Penn, R.D. and Mangieri, E.A. (1993) Stiff-man syndrome treated with intrathecal baclofen. *Neurology*, **43**, 241–242.

Penry, J.K., Hoefnagel, D., van den Noort, S. and Denny-Brown, D. (1960) Muscle spasm and abnormal postures resulting from damage to interneurones in spinal cord. *Archives of Neurology*, **3**, 500–512.

Prevett, M.C., Brown, P. and Duncan, J.S. (1997) Improvement of stiff man syndrome with vigabatrin. *Neurology*, **48**, 1133–1134.

Raju, R., Foote, J., Banga, J.P., Hall, T.R., Padoa, C.J., Dalakas, M., Ortqvist, E. and Hampe, C.S. (2005) Analysis of GAD 65 autoantibodies in stiff person syndrome patients. *Journal of Immunology*, **175**, 7755–7762.

Roobol, T.H., Kazzaz, B.A. and Vecht, C.J. (1987) Segmental rigidity and spinal myoclonus as a paraneoplastic syndrome. *Journal of Neurology Neurosurgery and Psychiatry*, **50**, 628–631.

Rosin, L., De Camilli, P., Butler, M. *et al.* (1998) Stiff-man syndrome in a woman with breast cancer: an uncommon central nervous system paraneoplastic syndrome. *Neurology*, **50**, 94–98.

Rothwell, J.C., Obeso, J.A. and Marsden, C.D. (1986) Electrophysiology of somatosensory reflex myoclonus. *Advances in Neurology*, **43**, 385–398.

Ruegg, S.J., Steck, A.J. and Fuhr, P. (2004) Levetiracetam improves paroxysmal symptoms in a patient with stiff person syndrome. *Neurology*, **62**, 338.

Saiz, A., Graus, F., Valldeoriola, F., Valls-Sole, J. and Tolosa, E. (1998) Stiff-leg syndrome: a focal form of stiff-man syndrome. *Annals of Neurology*, **43**, 400–430.

Sandbrink, F., Syed, N.A., Fujii, M.D., Dalakas, M.C. and Floeter, M.K. (2000) Motor cortex excitability in stiff person syndrome. *Brain*, **123**, 2231–2239.

Seitz, R.J., Blank, B., Kiwit, J.C.W. and Benecke, R. (1995) Stiff person syndrome with antiglutamic acid decarboxylase antibodies: complete remission of symptoms after intrathecal baclofen administration. *Journal of Neurology*, **242**, 618–622.

Shariatmadar, S. and Noto, T. (2001) Plasma exchange in Stiff Man Syndrome. *Therapeutic Apheresis*, **5**, 64–67.

Silbert, P.L., Matsumoto, J.Y., McManis, P.G., Stolp-Smith, K.A., Elliott, B.A. and McEvoy, K.M. (1995) Intrathecal baclofen therapy in stiff-man syndrome: a double blind placebo controlled trial. *Neurology*, **45**, 1893–1897.

Solimena, M., Folli, F., Aparisi, R., Pozza, G. and De Camilli, P. (1990) Autoantibodies to GABAergic neurons and pancreatic beta cells in stiff-man syndrome. *New England Journal of Medicine*, **322**, 1555–1560.

Souza-Lima, C.F., Ferraz, H.B., Braz, C.A., Araujo, A.M. and Manzano, G.M. (2000) Marked improvement in a stiff limb patient treated with intravenous immunoglobulin. *Movement Disorders*, **15**, 358–359.

Spehlmann, R., Norcross, K., Rasmus, S.C. and Schlageter, N.L. (1981) Improvement of stiff-man syndrome with sodium valproate. *Neurology*, **31**, 1162–1163.

Stayer, C., Tronnier, V., Dressnandt, J. *et al.* (1997) Intrathecal baclofen therapy for stiff-man syndrome and progressive encephalomyelopathy with rigidity and myoclonus. *Neurology*, **49**, 1519–1597.

Stingele, R., Koelmel, H.W., Hilligardt, B., van Maravic, M., De Camilli, P. and Meinck, H.-M. (1998) Two patients with stiff man syndrome, sensory ganglionopathy and cancer. *Movement Disorders*, **13** (Suppl 2): 208.

Tarlov, I.M. (1967) Rigidity in man due to spinal interneuron loss. *Archives of Neurology*, **16**, 536–543.

Vermeij, F.H., Vandoorn, P.A. and Busch, H.F.M. (1996) Improvement of stiff man syndrome with vigabatrin. *Lancet*, **348**, 612.

Vicari, A.M., Folli, F., Pozza, G. *et al.* (1989) Plasmapheresis in the treatment of stiff-man syndrome. *New England Journal of Medicine*, **320**, 1499–1499.

Walikonis, J.E. and Lennon, V.A. (1998) Radioimmunoassay for glutamic acid decarboxylase (GAD65) autoantibodies as a diagnostic aid for stiff man syndrome and a correlate of susceptibility to type 1 diabetes mellitus. *Mayo Clinic Proceedings*, **73**, 1161–1166.

Warren, J.D., Scott, G., Blumbergs, P.C. and Thompson, P.D. (2002) Pathological evidence of encephalomyelitis in the stiff man syndrome with anti GAD antibodies. *Journal of Clinical Neuroscience*, **9**, 328–329.

Whiteley, A.M., Swash, M. and Urich, H. (1976) Progressive encephalomyelitis with rigidity. *Brain*, **99**, 27–42.

Yu, W., Jiang, M., Miralles, C.P., Li, R.W., Chen, G. and de Blas, A.L. (2007) Gephyrin clustering is required for the stability of GABAergic synapses. *Molecular and Cellular Neuroscience*, **36**, 484–500.

Part IV

CHOREA, TICS AND OTHER MOVEMENT DISORDERS

19

Huntington's Disease

Kevin M. Biglan and Ira Shoulson

University of Rochester, Department of Neurology, Rochester, NY, USA

On February 15, 1872, the young Dr George Huntington read his eloquent essay "On Chorea" (Huntington, 1872) before the Meigs and Mason Medical Society in Middleport, Ohio. He described the clinical characteristics of this incurable form of adult-onset chorea, which he appreciated was inherited in an autosomal dominant mode of transmission. Today, Huntington's disease (HD) is recognized as a lethal neurodegenerative disease characterized by disordered movement, intellectual decline and an array of behavioral disturbances. The progressively disabling clinical features result from selective neuronal degeneration and atrophy, especially involving the basal ganglia and cerebral cortex. The neurophathological hallmarks are in turn a consequence of expression of the IT-15 gene on chromosome 4, representing an expansion of an unstable cytosine-adenine-guanine (CAG) trinucleotide repeat (HDCRG, Mar 1993a). Each offspring of an affected family member has a nominal 50% chance of having inherited the HD mutation, which is highly penetrant, but shows some variations in phenotypic expression.

HD represents one of the most important genetic disorders of adulthood. HD was the first disease recognized to arise from a trinucleotide expansion that can be detected by DNA testing. HD is also a model for the experimental therapeutics of adult-onset neurodegenerative diseases.

CLINICAL CHARACTERISTICS

HD is characterized clinically by the triad of an extrapyramidal movement disorder, progressive cognitive decline (dementia) and an array of behavioral disturbances. There is variability in the clinical presentation and major clinical manifestations of the disease. The cause of some of this variability is understood. For example, clinical onset in childhood or adolescence is associated with a larger number of CAG repeat expansions and an akinetic-rigid phenotype in contrast with the lower number of expanded CAG repeats

and more typical hyperkinetic manifestations that are observed in the more common adult-onset HD. Other contributions to the variable clinical expression of HD, including environmental and extragenetic factors, are under investigation.

HD Diagnosis

Traditionally, the clinical diagnosis of HD has been based on the emergence of characteristic extrapyramidal motor abnormalities in the setting of a confirmatory family history (Folstein *et al.*, 1986). Identification of the genetic mutation responsible for HD in 1993 made it possible to accurately make a genetic diagnosis of HD (HDCRG, 1993a). Now, DNA testing for the HD gene may be informative for adults who have developed extrapyramidal motor abnormalities or cognitive impairment, but without a confirmatory family history of HD, or in consenting adults at risk for HD who wish to learn whether or not they have inherited the HD gene. The complex decision to be tested, the currently irreversible consequences of learning of one's HD gene carrier status, and the research implications for pre-manifest HD will be discussed later.

While the clinical recognition is seemingly straightforward, the diagnosis of manifest HD is typically confirmed only months or years after the insidious emergence of signs and symptoms referable to motor, cognitive, behavioral and functional impairments (Greenamyre and Shoulson, 1994; McCusker *et al.*, 2000; Hahn-Barma *et al.*, 1998; Penney *et al.*, 1990; Baxter *et al.*, 1992).

Motor Manifestations

Chorea is the prototypical motor abnormality characteristic of HD, though a wide range of other motor abnormalities occur (Penney *et al.*, 1990; Tian *et al.*, 1991; Carella *et al.*, 1993; Jankovic and Ashizawa, 1995; Leopold and Kagel,

1985; Louis *et al.*, 1999; van Vugt, van Hilten and Roos, 1996; Racette and Perlmutter, 1998). Some of these motor manifestations, such as impaired ocular motility and rapid alternating movements, may antedate the onset of chorea (Penney *et al.*, 1990; Beenen, Buttner and Lange, 1986; Collewijn *et al.*, 1988; Young *et al.*, 1986).

Chorea represents fast, arrhythmic, semi-purposeful involuntary movements and is the most conspicuous and uniform feature of HD, occurring in 90% of affected individuals. While movements may appear stereotyped in an individual patient, they are highly variable from person to person. Subtle slight movement of the fingers and toes in adults at risk for HD predicts gene carrier status, but the relationship is imperfect (McCusker *et al.*, 2000). What begin as quick fleeting movements typically evolve into slower writhing movements in association with axial posturing of the arms, legs or torso (choreoathetosis). Chorea intensifies and progresses early in the disease in association with more overt movements, including facial grimacing, eyelid elevation, head bobbing, and writhing and jerking of the limbs. Parakinesia or the transformation of an involuntary movement into a seemingly voluntary one is frequently seen, often in the forms of crossing and uncrossing of the legs, smoothing of the hair or rubbing of the chin or brow. An associated feature is motor impersistence whereby individuals are unable to maintain tongue protrusion or eye closure.

Oculomotor abnormalities are very common and early findings in HD and may appear before any signs of chorea. Impairment in oculomotor function may be evidenced by increased latency of response, insuppressible eye blinks or head movements associated with saccade initiation and slowing of saccade velocity (Tian *et al.*, 1991; Beenen, Buttner and Lange, 1986; Collewijn *et al.*, 1988; Young *et al.*, 1986; Kirkwood *et al.*, 2000; Oepen, Clarenbach and Thoden, 1981; Blekher *et al.*, 2006). Abnormalities in fine motor coordination may also occur early (Penney *et al.*, 1990; Young *et al.*, 1986; Siemers *et al.*, 1996).

The slower and more sustained abnormal postures of dystonia may be seen early, especially in young individuals who carry a large number of expanded CAG repeats. Dystonia may also develop prominently as typical adult-onset HD advances, and may be exacerbated by anti-dopaminergic therapy (Penney *et al.*, 1990; Louis *et al.*, 1999; Feigin *et al.*, 1995). Other movement disorders occur in HD including bradykinesia, rigidity, myoclonus, tics, bruxism and ataxia (Carella *et al.*, 1993; Jankovic and Ashizawa, 1995; Racette and Perlmutter, 1998; Reuter *et al.*, 2000; Tan, Jankovic and Ondo, 2000; Paulson, 1979). Like dystonia, bradykinesia and rigidity commonly develop as HD progresses. Hypertonicity, representing both pyramidal (spasticity) and extrapyramidal (rigidity) tone abnormalities may be seen, even in the same patient.

Other signs of pyramidal tract dysfunction are also seen, including hyper-reflexia and extensor plantar responses (Paulson, 1979).

Dysarthria can occur at any stage of the illness, tends to progress, and may become severe enough to leave individuals anarthric. Despite severe dysarthria, central (cortical) language is largely unaffected. Dysphagia tends to be most prominent in the terminal stages of the disease, and aspiration is a common cause of death (Leopold and Kagel, 1985; Edmonds, 1966).

Gait, station and balance become increasingly impaired in HD. Superimposed chorea may give the gait a dance-like or lurching appearance. Patients will appear to be thrown off balance by sudden involuntary movements and move in a zig-zag pattern. Station is typically broad based and postural reflexes are eventually lost. Balance problems lead to falls and injury; although it is remarkable how well some patients are able to avoid falling in the face of their involuntary movements.

Cognitive Dysfunction

Cognitive impairment is inevitable in HD, with the possible exception of a few individuals who have a very late onset of illness (Britton *et al.*, 1995). Cognitive impairment typically progresses from selective deficits in psychomotor, executive and visuospatial abilities to more global impairment (Josiassen, Curry and Mancall, 1983; Bamford *et al.*, 1989; Lawrence *et al.*, 1996; Wilson and Garron, 1979; Shelton and Knopman, 1991). A variety of cognitive domains may be involved, including memory, executive function, visuospatial abilities, cognitive speed, sensorimotor function, concentration, and the acquisition and encoding of sensory stimuli (Bamford *et al.*, 1989; Lawrence *et al.*, 1996; Morris, 1995; Pillon *et al.*, 1991; Huber and Paulson, 1987), but higher cortical language and gnostic operations are generally spared. Dementia, as defined by global intellectual performance two standard deviations below the mean for healthy controls, was seen in up to 66% of patients in one study (Pillon *et al.*, 1991), and is characteristic of advanced illness (Josiassen, Curry and Mancall, 1983). Cognitive inflexibility may also be seen, whereby individuals with HD perseverate incessantly about specific and seemingly unimportant issues. This inflexibility, which may be extremely distressing to caregivers, is thought to result from frontostriatal loop dysfunction (Bamford *et al.*, 1989; Watkins *et al.*, 2000; Lawrence *et al.*, 1998a).

Cognitive impairments may antedate the motor manifestations of HD, but the specificity and character of cognitive dysfunction have not yet been established (McCusker *et al.*, 2000; Penney *et al.*, 1990; Kirkwood *et al.*, 2000). Studies evaluating cognitive measures in seemingly unaffected individuals who have inherited the gene show early impairment in psychomotor tasks, memory and frontal executive function, frequently antedating motor symptoms (McCusker *et al.*, 2000; Hahn-Barma *et al.*, 1998; Paulsen *et al.*, 2001; Foroud *et al.*, 1995; Strauss and Brandt, 1990; Diamond *et al.*, 1992; Jason *et al.*, 1988; Rosenberg, Sorenson and Christensen, 1995; Lawrence *et al.*, 1998b). Other studies have failed to show early cognitive impairment in asymptomatic individuals (Giordani *et al.*, 1995; de Boo *et al.*, 1997; Blackmore, Simpson and Crawford, 1995; Rothlind *et al.*, 1993; Wexler, 1979). Two large prospective studies involving individuals at risk for HD who have chosen not to undergo predictive DNA testing (PHAROS) and in individuals who have been tested (PREDICT HD) are in progress and will help clarify the pattern and temporal sequence of the earliest cognitive and motor abnormalities among HD gene carriers (HSG, 2006; Paulsen *et al.*, 2006).

Behavioral Disturbances

Psychiatric illness has been recognized as an important feature of HD since George Huntington's original description. While Huntington focused on the "tendency to insanity and suicide," a wide range of psychiatric and behavioral disturbances are currently recognized (Caine and Shoulson, 1983). Mood disorders, psychosis, anxiety, obsessions, compulsions, aggression, irritability and apathy may be prominent and disabling features of HD.

Affective disorders are an important and potentially treatable manifestation of HD. Depression is common in HD, occurring in as many as half of HD patients (Caine and Shoulson, 1983; Folstein *et al.*, 1987) with manic features in up to 10% of patients (Folstein *et al.*, 1987; Mendez, 1994). The suicide rate is five times more frequent than in the general population and may account for 2% of HD mortality (Schoenfeld *et al.*, 1984). Affective disorders in HD are believed to be primarily related to the disruption of specific frontal-subcortical neural pathways regulating mood (Mayberg *et al.*, 1992). Anxiety disorders seem to be important clinically, though little epidemiological data exists on these conditions. Generalized anxiety, panic attacks, and obsessive and compulsive symptoms are also seen (Guttman *et al.*, 2002).

Psychosis is also more common in HD than in the general population, occurring in up to 15% of HD patients (Caine and Shoulson, 1983; Mendez, 1994) and may be more common in young-onset cases (Folstein *et al.*, 1987). Paranoia is an important and under-recognized manifestation of psychosis in this population; while frank auditory or visual hallucinations are rare (Guttman *et al.*, 2002). The acute onset or presence of hallucinations should alert the clinician to look for other causes of the psychiatric disturbance.

Aggression in HD varies in severity from the overreaction to relatively trivial issues to overt acts of violence. Aggression may represent a feature of other underlying psychopathology such as paranoia, depression or anxiety. Using an aggression rating scale, Burns *et al.* (Burns *et al.*, 1990) found nearly two-thirds of HD patients showed increased indices of aggression. Irritability, reflecting an inability to control temper or a reduced threshold for the development of anger, may be linked to aggressive behavior and not be recognized by patients themselves (Burns *et al.*, 1990). If left untreated, irritability may lead to aggressive behaviors and psychiatric hospitalization (Dewhurst, Oliver and McKnight, 1970).

Apathy is characterized by a loss of emotion resulting in an internal feeling of disinterest or a behavioral state of inaction (Burns *et al.*, 1990). Apathy is a problem commonly mentioned by caregivers of patients with HD, and may occur independent of depression (Levy *et al.*, 1998).

Psychiatric disturbances may occur very early and appear to pre-date motor manifestations of HD. Some reports suggest psychiatric disturbances are more common in at-risk individuals who have inherited the HD gene compared with their counterparts who have not (McCusker *et al.*, 2000; Shiwach and Norbury, 1994). Other reports do not show such differences (Strauss and Brandt, 1990; Rosenberg, Sorenson and Christensen, 1995). Ongoing cohort studies suggest that subtle sub-clinical psychiatric symptoms may develop prior to diagnosis; however, the specificity of these findings to HD has not yet been established (Duff *et al.*, in press).

Body Mass and Metabolism

Weight loss has long been recognized as a clinical characteristic of HD patients in early as well as in more advanced illness (Djousse *et al.*, 2002). The weight loss often occurs in a setting of ravenous appetite with high caloric intake not keeping pace with the steady loss of body mass. Studies using indirect calorimetry find about 14% higher total energy expenditure in HD patients compared with normal controls, attributable in large part to involuntary movements (Pratley *et al.*, 2000; Gaba *et al.*, 2005). A more recent study in a large population of unaffected adults at risk for HD indicates that pre-manifest individuals who have inherited the HD gene have a lower body mass index compared with their counterparts who do not carry the gene (Marder and Huntington Study Group, 2007). The lower body mass index of pre-manifest HD is also associated with increased energy expenditure, either due to physical activity that is clinically unrecognized or to alterations in energy efficiency. It remains unclear whether early brain pathology (Petersen and Bjorkqvist, 2006) leads to early bioenergetic changes, or whether the ubiquitous gene for HD is expressed subtly in peripheral somatic cells.

In spite of the low body mass and weight loss in HD, glucose intolerance and non-insulin dependent diabetes mellitus are not uncommon in HD patients (Podolsky, Leopold and Sax, 1972; Podolsky and Leopold, 1977; Farrer, 1985). Hypothalamic dysfunction, perhaps involving altered growth hormone secretion, has been suggested as a contributing factor (Leopold and Podolsky, 1975). Of investigative interest, transgenic HD mice very commonly develop diabetes as a terminal consequence of progressive disease (Hurlbert *et al.*, 1999). Altered insulin secretion, insulin resistance and subtle pathology in pancreas, liver and skeletal muscle have not been systematically examined as factors leading to the peculiar bioenergetic features of HD.

Natural History

HD is a relentlessly progressive and lethal disorder. Illness may emerge at any time of life, with the peak incidence between 35 to 40 years of age (Farrer and Conneally, 1985). Longitudinal observation of the extensive Venezuela cohort revealed a slightly younger mean age of onset of 33 years in this population compared with a North American population (Penney *et al.*, 1990). The average age of death for HD patients in the US is approximately 60 years (Lanska *et al.*, 1988) compared with 50 years in the Venezuelan cohort (Penney *et al.*, 1990), perhaps reflecting differences in access to medical care. Very early age of onset seems to portend a short duration of illness, especially in juvenile-onset patients (Foroud *et al.*, 1999; van Dijk *et al.*, 1986). However, others have failed to confirm the association between age of onset and disease duration (Josiassen, Curry and Mancall, 1983).

Total functional capacity (TFC) is a standardized rating of functions and disability that has been used extensively in HD research (Shoulson, Kurlan and Rubin, 1989a). This scale ranges from a score of 13 (normal) to 0 (completely incapacitated) and assesses a patient's capacity in five functional areas (Table 19.1) (Shoulson, Kurlan and Rubin, 1989a). Numerous longitudinal studies have shown an annual decline in TFC of approximately 0.8 to 1.0 units per year (Young *et al.*, 1986; Feigin *et al.*, 1995; Shoulson *et al.*, 1989b). This consistency across populations has made TFC a useful tool for the evaluation of potential therapeutic interventions.

The Huntington Study Group (HSG) is an international consortium of clinical investigators who are committed to advancing knowledge and developing better treatments for HD. The HSG has developed a rating scale, the Unified Huntington's Disease Rating Scale (UHDRS), developed by the HSG, measures disease severity across four domains: motor, cognition, behavior and functional capacity. The UHDRS has been shown to have a high degree of internal consistency and inter-rater reliability (Hogarth *et al.*, 2004). Over time, HD patients generally show a worsening of motor function with increasing dystonia and stable chorea

Table 19.1 Total functional capacity scale.

Occupation
0 = Unable
1 = Marginal Work Only
2 = Reduced capacity for usual job
3 = Normal

Finances
0 = Unable
1 = Major assistance
2 = Slight assistance
3 = Normal

Domestic chores
0 = Unable
1 = Impaired
2 = Normal

ADL
0 = Total care
1 = Gross tasks only
2 = Minimal impairment
3 = Normal

Care level
0 = Full-time skilled nursing
1 = Home or chronic care
2 = Home

scores, worsening cognitive performance, increased occurrence of behavioral disorders, and worsening functional status (Siesling *et al.*, 1998). The UHDRS has been used extensively in research to evaluate the impact of experimental therapeutics on disease progression and illness severity in manifest HD. Subtle abnormalities in UHDRS motor and cognitive domains may differentiate at-risk individuals who do or do not carry the HD gene (Saft *et al.*, 2006; Kipps *et al.*, 2005; Snowden *et al.*, 2002; Langbehn *et al.*, 2007).

Juvenile-Onset HD

Young-onset HD is relatively uncommon, accounting for about 10–15% of manifest HD, but has generated research interest because of its unique clinical phenotype that is often associated with 50 or more expanded CAG repeats. The juvenile variant of HD, where age of onset occurs before 20, is typically manifested by an akinetic-rigid phenotype and paternal inheritance (van Dijk *et al.*, 1986; Rasmussen *et al.*, 2000). However, juvenile-onset of HD may not always fit this stereotype. Several reports indicate that cognitive and behavioral changes may well antedate the onset of motor abnormalities, which often emerge as rigidity, dystonia and bradykinesia (van Dijk *et al.*, 1986; Rasmussen *et al.*, 2000; Siesling, Vegter-van der Vlis and Roos, 1997; Gomez-Tortosa *et al.*, 1998; Roos *et al.*, 1991; Cannella *et al.*, 2004; Nance, 1997; Oliva *et al.*, 1993; Laccone *et al.*, 1999; Squitieri *et al.*, 2000; Wexler and Lorimer, 2004; Young *et al.*, 1986; Duesterhus *et al.*, 2004; Squitieri *et al.*, 2003; Ribai *et al.*, 2006). Paternal inheritance of the HD gene is the rule for onset before the age of 10 and still predominates (about 3:1 paternal:maternal) for onset before the age of 20.

EPIDEMIOLOGY

HD is the most common inherited form of chorea, with a worldwide distribution likely reflecting multiple introductions of the gene from European migrations (Giron and Koller, 1994). New mutations are rare and likely represent expansion of the unstable trinucleotide repeat from an intermediated range (30–35 repeats) in the parent to the pathologic range (≥ 36 repeats) in the offspring (HDCRG, 1993b). This tendency for expansion is one example of the "dynamic mutation" of the trinucleotide repeat underlying HD. Another example is the phenotypic variation within families and between generations.

HD is found throughout North America, South America and Australia, especially in Caucasian populations. It has the highest prevalence rates around Lake Maracaibo in Venezuela and the Moray Firth region of Scotland and is relatively rare in Asian countries and amongst African blacks (Harper, 1992; Hayden, MacGregor and Beighton, 1980). Approximately 30 000 people in the United States have clinical manifestations of HD, and an additional 150 000 healthy people are at risk of developing HD (Conneally, 1984; Tanner and Goldman, 1994).

Throughout Europe, with the notable exception of Finland, prevalence rates are relatively uniform ranging from 2 to 8 per 100 000 (Harper, 1992). Finland is believed to be genetically distinct from the rest of the European population and has the lowest prevalence rates in Europe at 0.5 per 100 000 (Harper, 1992). Regions of the world largely populated by individuals of European descent show a similar prevalence to Europe (Folstein *et al.*, 1987; Harper, 1992; Kokmen *et al.*, 1994).

Little is known of the prevalence of HD in Africa. Hayden carried out the only systematic survey of African populations in South Africa (Hayden, MacGregor and Beighton, 1980). Frequencies similar to European populations were found in white and mixed populations. Prevalence in populations of African origin was about 10 times less frequent. In American blacks of African origin, true prevalence rates are difficult to obtain because of under-ascertainment; however, Folstein *et al.* (Folstein *et al.*, 1987) found a rate comparable to European studies. European origin of these cases in African Americans could neither be identified nor clearly excluded. It seems likely that HD occurs at relatively low rates in persons of African origin.

HD has been documented in Asia, with only Japan having systematic data. Detailed studies in Japan reveal frequencies between 0.11 and 0.45 per 100 000 (Harper, 1992). Case reports from China, India, Turkey and previous Soviet republics in central Asia suggest that the disease occurs in these regions, but exact prevalence rates are not known (Harper, 1992).

PATHOLOGY

The neuropathology of HD is characterized by selective neuronal vulnerability, particularly involving the caudate and putamen of the corpus striatum (Vonsattel *et al.*, 1985). Other regions of the brain including deep cortical layers, thalamus and hippocampus are also affected. In advanced HD, there is prominent, overall atrophy of the brain (Vonsattel *et al.*, 1985; Sotrel *et al.*, 1991). Figure illustrates the striking caudate atrophy of an HD brain compared with a normal brain (Figure 19.1).

Microscopically, the pathological hallmark of the disease is the preferential loss of medium-sized spiny neurons projecting from the striatum to the external pallidum (Mitchell, Cooper and Griffiths, 1999). These striatal neurons contain γ-aminobutyric acid (GABA) and enkephalin as their primary neurotransmitters, which are selectively depleted, while neighboring large interneurons are relatively spared (Perry, Hansen and Kloster, 1973; Reiner *et al.*, 1988; Sapp *et al.*, 1995; Richfield *et al.*, 1995). Intraneuronal inclusions are seen within degenerating neurons (Roizin *et al.*, 1974; DiFiglia *et al.*, 1997), most prominently in the nuclei and neuropil of striatal and cortical neurons. The inclusions represent aggregates of the mutant huntingtin protein and ubiquitin (DiFiglia *et al.*, 1997; Davies *et al.*, 1997) and may pre-date the emergence of clinical manifestations (Gomez-Tortosa *et al.*, 2001).

HD PATHOGENESIS

HD results from an expanded cytosine-adenine- guanine (CAG) trinucleotide repeat of the interesting transcript #15 (IT-15) gene near the telomere of the short arm of chromosome 4 (Goldberg, Telenius and Hayden, 1994). The expanded CAG repeat, occurring in the first exon of the $5'$ region of the gene, codes for an expanded polyglutamine region within the mutant protein named huntingtin (HDCRG, 1993a). Wild-type huntingtin, which is approximately 330 kDa in size, is widely expressed throughout the brain and primarily localized to the cytoplasm of neurons (Landwehrmeyer *et al.*, 1995). Highest concentrations are found in the cerebellum, hippocampus, cerebral cortex, substantia nigra-pars compacta and pontine nuclei (Landwehrmeyer *et al.*, 1995; Sapp *et al.*, 1997; Saudou *et al.*, 1998; Jones, 1999).

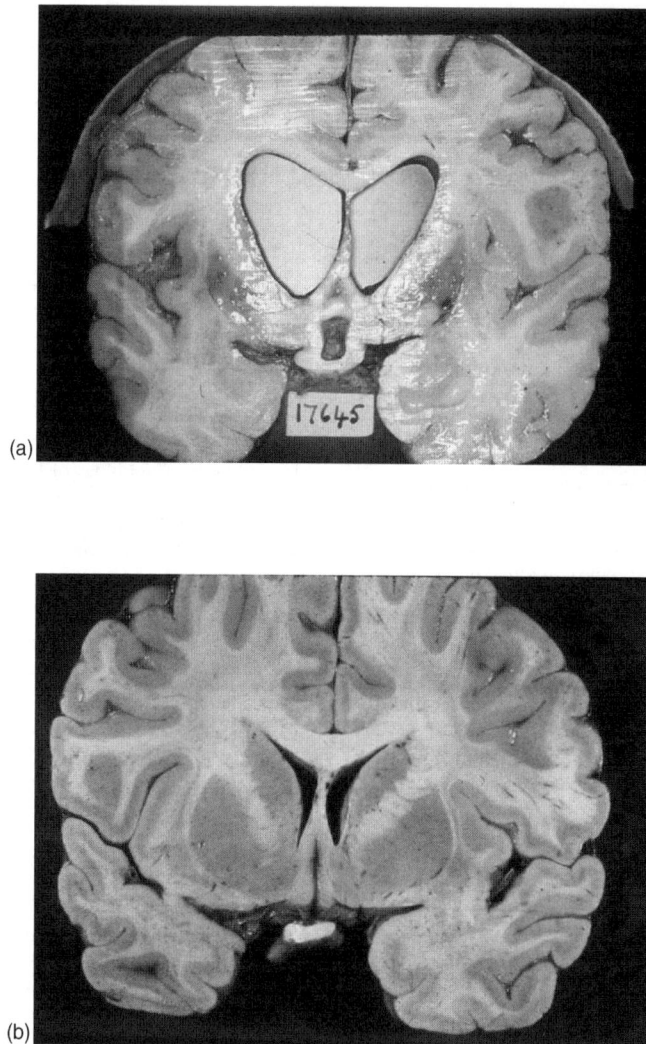

Figure 19.1 HD brain (a) compared with a normal brain (b), demonstrating caudate atrophy.

The expanded CAG mutation is found in all cells of those who have inherited the HD gene, but neuronal cells are conspicuously vulnerable to the ubiquitous expression of the mutant gene. In general, somatic cells of HD patients have the same number of expanded CAG as in brain cells; although, some mosaicism can be detected, particularly in the basal ganglia, cortex and cerebellum of the juvenile HD post-mortem brain (Telenius et al., 1994; Aronin et al., 1995).

The levels of mRNA expression vary from tissue to tissue and within tissues, but there is no correlation between mRNA expression and consequent pathology. In fact, the highest levels of mRNA expression are found in skeletal muscle, kidney and cerebral cortex, and the lowest levels in striatum, pallidum, liver and heart (Landwehrmeyer et al., 1995).

The huntingtin protein product is most abundant in brain paralleling mRNA expression, but regional concentrations vary and do not correlate with specific pathology. Within the cell, huntingtin is concentrated primarily within the cytoplasm, but may also be found in the nucleus of neuronal cells. Huntingtin appears to be a "sticky" protein, interacting with many other proteins, including huntingtin-associated protein and glyceraldehyde 3-phosphate dehydrogenase (GAPDH) which is involved in energy metabolism. The normal function of wild-type huntingtin is unclear, but knocking out both gene alleles in mice experiments proves lethal in the resulting embryos within 10 days post-conception (Duyao et al., 1995; Nasir et al., 1995). At the time of writing, the normal function of huntingtin and how mutant huntingtin leads to neurodegeneration remain a mystery. However, functions and mechanisms are slowly being revealed.

In a transgenic mouse model of HD, mutant huntingtin appears to undergo abnormal cleavage in the cytoplasm, resulting in the translocation of the N-terminal fragment into the nucleus (Wellington, Leavitt and Hayden, 2000). These abnormally cleaved mutant proteins undergo abnormal conformation and form aggregates in the nucleus, as well as deposits in cytoplasm and neurites in other areas of the cell (DiFiglia et al., 1997; Jones, 1999; Mangiarini et al., 1996; Ross, Dec 1997; Scherzinger et al., 1997). Whether these aggregates are byproducts of neurodegeneration or are an important component in the pathogenic process is not known; prevention of the nuclear localization of mutant huntingtin aggregates does inhibit neurodegeneration, suggesting that the altered cleavage and subsequent nuclear translocation represent key steps in the pathogenic cascade leading to neuronal dysfunction and cell death (Saudou et al., 1998). Additionally, the expression of the N-terminal fragment alone can reproduce the pathology and phenotype in HD transgenic mice (Davies et al., 1997; Mangiarini et al., 1996; Cooper et al., 1998).

Many cellular abnormalities have been identified that may contribute to HD pathogenesis, including transcriptional dysregulation (Cha, 2000; Nucifora et al., 2001; Zucker et al., 2005), activation of caspases and cell death pathways, interference with axonal transport, alterations of vesicle recycling, decreased proteasomal function and altered autophagic protein digestion (Ross, 2004; Ross and Poirier, 2004). Altered energy metabolism and mitochondrial dysfunction may contribute to the pathogenesis of HD and may be amenable to experimental treatment (Koroshetz et al., 1997; Beal, 1999).

Evidence for mitochondrial dysfunction and oxidative stress in HD pathogenesis originated with the finding that intracranial injections of the exogenous toxin, 3-nitropropionic acid, in experimental animals causes selective striatal lesions resulting from inhibition of complex 2 of the mitochondrial electron transport chain (Bogdanov et al., 1998; Beal et al., 1993). Abnormalities of mitochondrial function, especially loss of complex 2, have been demonstrated in HD post-mortem brain (Gu et al., 1996). Other evidence for bio-energetic dysfunction include increased lactate production in the cerebral cortex and basal ganglia of patients with HD who have been imaged using ^{1}H NMR spectroscopy (Jenkins et al., 1998), deficits of mitochondrial respiratory chain complexes 2, 3 and 4 in post-mortem caudate nucleus, a

deficiency of complex 1 in circulating platelets of HD patients (Gu et al., 1996; Browne et al., 1997; Tabrizi et al., 1999), and a decrease in ATP to ADP ratios in HD models, suggesting impaired mitochondrial ATP synthesis (Seong et al., 2005).

Several mechanisms have been proposed by which mutant huntingtin may interfere with mitochondrial function and energy metabolism. The N-terminus of huntingtin may directly target mitochondria and impair their function (Panov et al., 2002). There may be actions of huntingtin on glutamate receptors or on inositol trisphospate receptors or other intracellular calcium channels (Zeron et al., 2001; Zeron et al., 2004; Bezprozvanny and Hayden, 2004).

Mutant huntingtin may also impair mitochondrial function indirectly via transcriptional interactions (Bae et al., 2005). For example, mutant huntingtin may act via the transcriptional co-activator PGC1α, which plays a role in regulating mitochondrial biogenesis and activation (Cui et al., 2006; Weydt et al., 2006; Ross and Thompson, 2006) In addition, 8-oxoguanosine DNA glycosylase (OGG1), a DNA repair enzyme that is involved in repairing DNA errors caused by oxidative stress, has been shown to be elevated in several neurodegenerative diseases where oxidative stress is believed to play a role (Fukae et al., 2005). In turn, oxidative damage to DNA promotes OGG1 activity, resulting in enhanced removal of oxidized guanosine species such as 8-hydroxy-2'deoxyguanosine (8OH2'dG). In serum of HD patients, 8OH2'dG has been found elevated almost fourfold compared with controls and may begin to elevate in pre-manifest HD as signs and symptoms emerge (Hersch et al., 2006).

EXPERIMENTAL THERAPEUTICS AND CARE

Overview of Experimental Therapeutics

Experimental therapeutics in manifest HD can be broadly viewed as symptomatic, neuroprotective and restorative approaches. Strickly speaking, symptomatic therapies improve the signs and symptoms of illness without affecting underlying disease progression; therefore, benefits are only temporary in the setting of progressive neurodegeneration. Neuroprotection refers to interventions aimed at producing enduring benefits by favorably influencing underlying etiology or pathogenesis and thereby forestalling onset of illness or clinical decline (Shoulson, 1998). Restorative therapies promote re-growth or repair of areas of neuronal injury or cell loss. Both neuroprotective and restorative treatments exert disease-modifying effects, which could be measured by slowing clinical decline in manifest HD or forestalling onset of illness in pre-manifest HD ("secondary prevention"). The reader is referred to a comprehensive, evidence-based review of symptomatic and disease- modifying pharmacotherapies for HD, by Bonelli and Wenning (2006).

Symptomatic Therapies

Symptomatic therapies in HD have rarely been subjected to rigorous evaluation, with most treatments based on case reports or series and clinical experience. The first rigorous therapeutic research in HD patients was reported by Fahn, who conducted a crossover placebo-controlled study of the anti-psychotic perphenazine in 17 patients and found an appreciable improvement in chorea (Fahn, 1973). Table 19.2 is an overview of recent controlled trials of symptomatic treatments for HD. Most symptomatic treatments in HD have focused on ameliorating chorea, and there have been few controlled studies of symptomatic treatments aimed at ameliorating the cognitive, affective or behavioral disorders of HD.

Tetrabenazine, a selective pre-synaptic depleter of vesicular-stored catecholamines, was evaluated by the HSG in 84 subjects randomized 2:1 to tetrabenazine or placebo for 12 weeks. Chorea scores as measured by the UHDRS and the clinical global impression of the blinded investigators were improved by about 25% in tetrabenazine- vs placebo-treated patients (Huntington Study Group, 2006). However, tetrabenazine treatment was associated with a higher occurrence of parkinsonian features and depression, both predictable and recognizable consequences of catecholamine depletion. Such adverse effects can be managed by reduction in dosage or discontinuation of tetrabenazine.

Amantadine, an anti-viral agent and partial NMDA antagonist, has shown mixed results in treating chorea in randomized, controlled trials (Verhagen Metman *et al.*, 2002; O'Suilleabhain and Dewey, 2003). Riluzole, a drug approved for use in amyotrophic lateral sclerosis that retards pre-synaptic glutamate release, was shown to have a mild beneficial effect on chorea at dosages of 200 mg/day; however, its costs and potential to cause liver function test abnormalities has limited its use (Huntington Study Group, 2003). A number of studies have suggested a beneficial effect of so-called atypical anti-psychotics on chorea; however, only clozapine has been subjected to rigorous assessment, but with mixed results (van Vugt *et al.*, 1997). Levetiracetam showed benefit on chorea in an open-label study vs untreated controls, but has yet to be subjected to a randomized, double-blind placebo-controlled study

Table 19.2 Controlled clinical trials of symptomatic therapies in HD.

Indication	Treatment	Reference	n	Design	Outcome	Results
Chorea	Tetrabenazine	Huntington Study Group, 2006	84	RCT parallel	UHDRS	Reduced Chorea
	Levetiracetam	De Tommaso *et al.*, 2005	22	Open label, untreated controls	UHDRS	Reduced Chorea
	Amantadine	O'Suilleabhain and Dewey, 2003	24	RCT double-blind cross-over	Video Rating	Chorea unchanged, Subjective improvement
	Amantadine	Verhagen Metman *et al.*, 2002	24	RCT double-blind cross-over	UHDRS	Reduced chorea
	Riluzole	Huntington Study Group, 2003	41	RCT parallel	UHDRS	Reduced chorea
	Clozapine	van Vugt *et al.*, 1997	33	RCT parallel	AIMS, UHDRS	Mixed effect on chorea
Cognitive Function	Donepezil	Cubo *et al.*, 2006	30	RCT parallel	AD Assessment Scale, UHDRS	No benefit
	Rivastigmine	De Tommaso *et al.*, 2004	21	Open label, RCT, untreated controls	MMSE, TFC	Trend towards improved MMSE in treated
Behavioral	Fluoxetine	Como *et al.*, 1997	30	RCT, Parallel	TFC UHDRS	No benefit

(De Tommaso *et al.*, 2005). There are no controlled trials evaluating treatment of the akinetic-rigid variant of HD with dopaminergic therapy, whether physical and occupational therapy helps motoric impairment in HD or whether speech therapy improves dysarthria, intelligibility or dysphagia.

Acetylcholinesterase inhibitors have been evaluated in cognitive dysfunction in HD with mixed results. Donepezil was shown to be ineffective in addressing cognitive impairment in HD patients who were randomized to donepezil 10 mg/day or placebo and followed for 12 weeks (Cubo *et al.*, 2006). Rivastigmine has shown a suggestion of benefit in an open-label study (De Tommaso *et al.*, 2004; De Tommaso *et al.*, 2007). Dimebon is a novel anti-histamine that has shown a beneficial effect in experimental models of Alzheimer's disease (Lermontova *et al.*, 2000) and is currently being evaluated for cognitive impairment in HD by the HSG under the sponsorship of Medivation, Inc. (ClinicalTrials.gov Identifier NCT00497159)

Anti-depressants have not been systematically evaluated in depressed HD patients, but both traditional tricyclic and SSRI anti-depressants are widely considered to improve affect. How long the presumed benefits last has not been examined. A randomized placebo-controlled trial of fluoxetine in 30 *non*-depressed HD patients who were followed for four months did not show any benefit on functional, neurological or cognitive batteries, but did suggest a slight improvement in agitation (Como *et al.*, 1997).

Neuroprotective

Neuroprotective experimental therapeutics aim to influence either proximal and/or distal targets in the pathogenic cascade in order to prevent or slow the neurodegenerative process (Hersch and Rosas, 2002). Proximal targets include targeting the transcription, translation, abnormal folding and aggregation of mutant huntingtin, as well as the altered protein–protein interactions, caspase-mediated cleavage and resulting toxic intermediates, transcriptional dysregulation and neurotrophin depletion. These potential proximal targets may be amenable to experimental intervention in the near future. Distal therapeutic targets include final pathways common to neurodegenerative conditions such as excitotoxic and oxidative injury, inflammation and apoptosis. Although less specific and seemingly far from the root cause, experimental therapeutics targeting distal pathways in the pathogenesis of HD may be important in slowing disease progression, even after a cascade of molecular insults have already occurred.

To date, no trials that have demonstrated a slowing of clinical progression in manifest HD (Table 19.3). The multicenter trial evaluating co-enzyme Q10 and remacemide in HD illustrates a determined effort to target distal pathogenetic mechanisms in HD (Huntington Study Group, 2001). Co-enzyme Q10 is an anti-oxidant and co-factor involved in mitochondrial electron transfer, and remacemide is a non-competitive NMDA receptor antagonist. Employing a randomized, double-blind, placebo-controlled, parallel

Table 19.3 Controlled clinical trials of putative neuroprotective therapies in manifest HD.

Treatment	Reference	*n*	Design	Outcome	Results
Creatine	Hersch *et al.*, 2006	64	RCT, parallel	Safety and tolerability	Safe and Tolerable
Creatine	Verbessem *et al.*, 2003	41	RCT, parallel	UHDRS	No benefit
Ethyl EPA	Puri *et al.*, 2005	135	RCT parallel	UHDRS Total Motor Score 4	No benefit in ITT analysis
Minocycline	Huntington Study Group, 2004	60	RCT parallel	Safety and Tolerability	Safe and tolerable
CoQ10/ Remacemide	Huntington Study Group, 2001	347	RCT, 2 × 2 factorial	TFC	Trend towards slowing with CoQ
Lamotrigine	Kremer *et al.*, 1999	64	RCT, parallel	TFC	No benefit
OPC 14 117	Huntington Study Group, 1998	64	RCT, parallel	Safety and Tolerability	Safe and Tolerable
Idebenone QNE	Ranen *et al.*, 1996b No benefit	100	RCT, Parallel	HD-ADL	
Alpha Tocopherol	Peyser *et al.*, 1995	73	RCT, parallel	QNE	No benefit in ITT analysis
Baclofen	Shoulson *et al.*, 1989b	60	RCT, parallel	TFC	No benefit

group 2×2 factorial design, HSG investigators in the US and Canada at 23 sites enrolled and evaluated 347 subjects with early HD for a minimum of 30 months. Research participants were randomized to one of four treatment groups: co-enzyme Q10 600 mg daily, remacemide 600 mg daily, the combination of both active treatments or placebo. Total functional capacity (TFC) was the pre-specified primary outcome. Remacemide did not slow clinical decline; although, a modest anti-choreic effect was observed. Individuals treated with co-enzyme Q10 showed about a 13% slowing in functional decline compared with individuals not receiving co-enzyme Q10 ($p = 0.15$), as well as a benefit on other functional measures. Co-enzyme Q10 600 mg/day was not associated with adverse events of any clinical consequence. Although not statistically significant, these findings are encouraging and represent the first neuroprotective trial to suggest a possible beneficial effect in HD. Studies in early Parkinson' disease patients evaluating dosages of co-enzyme Q10 up to 1200 mg/day have signaled slowing of clinical decline (Shults *et al.*, 2002). Co-enzyme Q10 up to 2400 mg/day has been shown to be well tolerated in HD patients. A long-term placebo-controlled study of co-enzyme Q10 2400 mg/day in early HD patients will soon begin enrolling.

Other experimental compounds are currently in clinical trials. Minocycline, a caspase inhibitor and second-generation tetracycline antibiotic, exerts a variety of anti-apoptotic, anti-oxidant and anti-excitotoxic properties that may be of potential neuroprotective benefit in HD (Chen *et al.*, 2000; Yrjanheikki *et al.*, 1999). Minocycline has been shown to be effective at delaying mortality in mouse models of HD (Chen *et al.*, 2000) and is safe and well tolerated in dosages up to 200 mg/day in HD (Huntington Study Group, 2004). Studies are currently underway to investigate the efficacy of minocycline in subjects with early HD (ClinicalTrials.gov Identifier NCT00277355).

Like co-enzyme Q10, creatine is a nutritional supplement that exerts anti-oxidative effects. Creatine increases brain phosphocreatine, which diffuses through the cytoplasm and buffers energy metabolism by maintaining cellular ATP levels (Hemmer and Wallimann, 1993). Creatine may have neuroprotective effects in a variety of disease processes where altered bioenergetic metabolism plays a pathogenic role. Evidence from animal models suggests a neuroprotective effect of creatine (Ferrante *et al.*, 2000; Matthews *et al.*, 1998). Creatine has been shown to be safe and well tolerated and to reduce serum measures of oxidative DNA injury in HD patients (Hersch *et al.*, 2006). Although earlier studies have not shown a benefit of creatine 5 g/day on HD progression, the study was small ($n = 41$) and higher dosages of creatine seem to be well tolerated and may be more effective (Verbessem *et al.*, 2003). Large longitudinal studies of creatine in

manifest HD to evaluate efficacy are planned and will soon be underway.

Ethyl EPA is an unsaturated fatty acid that targets caspase and mitochondrial function. Ethyl EPA did not show a beneficial response on UHDRS measures of motor function after one year in subjects randomized to ethyl EPA or placebo in the intention-to-treat analysis; although, a post hoc analysis suggested benefit on hyperkinetic motor performance in a sub-group of research participants (Puri *et al.*, 2005). A larger placebo-controlled study of ethyl EPA showed no benefit over six months, although some benefits were detected during the second six-month open-label phase among participants who were assigned to active ethyl EPA during the initial six-month double-blind phase (Dorsey and Huntington Study Group, 2007). Similarly α-tocopherol, a potent anti-oxidant, showed no benefit in slowing HD progression; however, post hoc analysis suggested a potential benefit in individuals with less severe disease (Peyser *et al.*, 1995).

A new therapeutic target involves the potential role of histone de-acetylase (HDAC) inhibitors to favorably influence transcriptional dysregulation in HD. HDAC inhibitors have been shown to be powerful tools in arresting and even reversing polyglutamine-dependent neurodegeneration in *Drosophila* (Steffan *et al.*, 2001). HDAC inhibitors have also been used for the treatment of some types of cancer (Butler *et al.*, 2000; Warrell *et al.*, 1998). Preliminary data suggests that these agents may not be as well tolerated in HD (Hogarth, Lovrecic and Krainc, 2007), but a recently completed study of phenylbutyrate in HD indicates a sufficient level of safety and tolerability to consider further trials of these compounds (Hersch, 2007).

The failure to date of putative neuroprotective agents in HD may be due to the relatively late initiation of treatment after irreversible pathogenic processes have developed. Ideally, neuroprotective therapy would be initiated prior to the onset of symptoms, while neuropathologic mechanisms are potentially more reversible (Gomez-Tortosa *et al.*, 2001). No studies have yet evaluated potential neuroprotective agents in the growing population of pre-manifest HD though studies of co-enzyme Q10 are planned in this population. Two large prospective observational studies are well underway in an attempt to identify sensitive and specific early precursors of HD onset and correlative biomarkers These studies will inform about the feasibility and most efficient methodology for preventive disease-modifying trials in pre-manifest HD.

The Prospective Huntington At Risk Observational Study (PHAROS) enrolled 1001 clinically unaffected adults at risk for HD who have chosen not to undergo predictive DNA testing (HSG, 2006). Employing a de-identified procedure to protect the confidentiality of their genetic status, PHAROS research participants have consented to be followed in a multi-year, double- blinded longitudinal study to examine the precursors of clinical onset and the specificity of emerging phenotype to CAG repeat length.

Neurobiological Predictors of HD (PREDICT-HD) is a similarly large prospective observational study that focuses on unaffected adults who have chosen to undergo predictive DNA testing and been informed that they have inherited the HD gene. PREDICT-HD research participants have consented to be followed prospectively and undergo extensive cognitive assessments and standardized magnetic resonance imaging (MRI) in order to better determine the predictive value of quantitative clinical assessments and emerging biomarkers with respect to the onset of HD (Paulsen et al., 2006). The clinical and biological markers of HD onset defined from these and other longitudinal studies are expected to provide useful endpoints, experience and biomarkers for experimental therapeutic studies aimed at postponing the early onset of HD.

Restorative

Restorative approaches to the treatment of HD have focused on transplantation of fetal tissue (Table 19.4). This research has been prompted by results in animal models of HD where transplanted striatal cells have been demonstrated to survive, differentiate, grow and reverse some motor and behavioral abnormalities (Armstrong et al., 2000; Nakao and Itakura, 2000; Borlongan et al., 1998).

Implantation of striatal fetal tissue allografts has been considered relatively safe in HD patients participating in preliminary, small, uncontrolled trials (Bachoud-Levi et al., 2000a; Philpott et al., 1997; Hauser et al., 2001; Rosser et al., 2002). Functional neuroimaging studies have shown increased metabolic activity in some patients treated with fetal tissue transplantations and long-term follow-up

suggests prolonged survival of these grafts, but not a sustained clinical benefit (Bachoud-Levi et al., 2000b; Bachoud-Levi et al., 2006; Keene et al., 2007). Small improvements in motor, cognitive and behavioral measures were seen in some patients (Philpott et al., 1997; Hauser et al., 2001; Bachoud-Levi et al., 2000). Motor deterioration and mood alterations have also occurred in some patients (Bachoud-Levi et al., 2000a; Hauser et al., 2001). The research experience remains preliminary and has involved small numbers of patients without blinded assessments or controlled interventions to adequately evaluate the safety and efficacy of transplanting fetal tissue. Research guidelines for tissue transplantation in HD have been developed for use in clinical research (Quinn et al., 1996).

Initial attempts at gene transfer studies have focused on the feasibility and safety of these procedures. Ciliary neurotrophic factor (CNTF) has been shown to protect striatal neurons in HD animal models (Emerich and Winn, 2004) and has been administered intraventricularly in HD patients (Bloch et al., 2004). Perhaps, the most innovative approach to restorative therapy has emerged from knowledge about how growth factors, such as brain-derived neurotrophic factor (BDNF), can coax peri-ventricular stem cells to become neurons. This process is made more efficient by overexpressing the Noggin gene that promotes neuronal differentiation. By using intraventricular administration of adenovirus vectors to over-express BDNF and Noggin, investigators have been successful in inducing neurogenesis of medium-sized spiny neurons that have, in turn, enhanced performance and survival in HD transgeneic (R6/2) mice (Cho et al., 2007). Application of this research to HD will depend on replication in other animal experiments and the development of safe and effective methods of vector administration in humans.

Table 19.4 Restorative trials in manifest HD.

Treatment	Reference	n	Design	Outcome	Results
Fetal Neural Transplants	Bachoud-Levi et al., 2000	5	Open label, parallel controls	Standardized neurological, neuro-psychological, behavioral assessments, FDG18 PET	3 with improved function, striatal metabolic activity
Fetal Neural Transplants	Hauser et al., 2001	7	Open label	Feasibility and safety	3 SDH, 1 death
Fetal Neural Transplants	Rosser et al., 2002	4	Open label	Feasibility and safety	Safe, AEs related to immunotherapy
Intraventricular CNTF gene therapy	Bloch et al., 2004	6	Open label	Feasibility and safety	Safe and feasible

Clinical Care

Predictive and Pre-Natal Testing

With the discovery of the gene, it was presumed that adults at risk for inheriting the gene would opt for pre-symptomatic DNA testing. However, since HD genetic testing has become available, less than 10% of individuals who are at immediate risk (50:50) for HD have chosen to be tested, and only about 500 predictive DNA tests are performed in the US annually (Nance *et al.*, 1999). Similar low rates of testing have been observed in central Europe (Laccone *et al.*, 1999). Reasons for deciding not to be tested include an increased risk to offspring if the test were positive, lack of effective treatment, potential loss of health and life insurance, costs of testing and inability to "undo" the test results (Quaid and Morris, 1993). Fears about testing are understandable. The relief from a negative result is offset by the grim reality of a positive one. The impact of the results may affect entire families and reach far beyond the individual tested (Hayes, 1992).

The impact of genetic testing for HD has been evaluated. While Wiggins *et al.* (Wiggins *et al.*, 1992) did not find a negative psychological impact of predictive testing, others (Tibben *et al.*, 1993a) have found negative psychosocial impacts in both those who received positive and negative test results. Of particular interest are the studies that suggest a significant proportion of individuals who undergo predictive genetic testing may fear or experience genetic discrimination, especially if they are refused employment or insurance based merely on genetic risk (Alper *et al.*, 1994; Low, King and Wilkie, 1998; Billings *et al.*, 1992; Lapham, Kozma and Weiss, 1996).

Pre-natal testing involves either a direct or exclusion testing. Direct testing involves detection of the actual CAG expansion and is the most accurate. In exclusion testing, the at-risk grandparent allele is excluded using linkage analysis, leaving the at-risk parent unaware of their gene status, therefore remaining nominally at 50% risk. The implication is that a fetus at high risk will be terminated. Controversy exists regarding the ethics of pre-natal screening for HD as individuals live 30 to 50 years prior to the onset of disease, however, most agree it should remain a personal decision (Post, 1992). Experiences with pre-natal testing are variable; though studies from Europe, Canada and Australia suggest it is uncommon (Simpson *et al.*, 2002; Creighton *et al.*, 2003; Tassicker *et al.*, 2006). In the European experience, 305 individuals underwent pre-natal testing between 1993 and 1998 (Simpson *et al.*, 2002). One hundred thirty-one (43%) of tests were high risk for the mutation, with eight of these pregnancies continuing. These children will grow up knowing their genetic status without being involved in the decision-making. The ramification of such certainty on these individuals is unknown. Pre-implantation genetic diagnosis for HD is an alternative to pre-natal testing that may not carry the same ethical dilemmas (Braude *et al.*, 1998).

Clearly the decision to undergo predictive or pre-natal testing in HD is an exceedingly personal and complex consideration for individuals, families and caregivers. There is probably no more personal and important dilemma than that facing individuals at nominal 50:50 risk for HD, who may choose the irreversible decision to learn of their HD gene carrier status or the emotional burden of undergoing pre-natal testing. Considerable effort and time must be invested in the education, counseling and ongoing care of these individuals at risk for HD. It is essential that individuals undergo skilled genetic and psychological counseling prior to and after the administration of the test (Tibben *et al.*, 1993b; Quaid *et al.*, 1989). Finally, the decision to test must be evaluated within the context of the family because of the far-reaching implications of HD gene test results.

Motor Features

The focus of therapy for motor abnormalities in HD has traditionally been on the control of chorea, which may be disabling for some patients and largely of cosmetic concern for others. The functional impact of chorea also varies from time to time in the same patient. As HD progresses, there is a natural tendancy for chorea to diminish in intensity and for dystonia to emerge and predominate (Feigin *et al.*, 1995). These considerations and the risk of adverse effects make for a cautious approach in deciding to begin and continuing to monitor anti-choreic treatment. Blocking post-synaptic dopaminergic receptors using typical antipsychotics, such as haloperidol, have been the mainstay of treatment for chorea. However the impact of these medications on mood, spontaneity, swallowing, speech, voluntary movements and gait may impair function out of proportion to any improvement in chorea (Shoulson, 1981) At present, it seems prudent to reserve anti-choreic treatment for those individuals with prominent chorea that interferes with functions, activities of daily living, gait and balance, or results in social isolation.

Amantadine appears to be well tolerated and may be a useful agent for disabling chorea in HD (Verhagen Metman *et al.*, 2002). Tetrabenazine, which depletes dopamine storage in pre-synaptic vesicles, is an effective agent for reducing the intensity of chorea, but carries the risks of inducing or exacerbating parkinsonism and depression. These adverse effects are recognizable and favorably responsive to reduction or discontinuation of tetrabenazine dosage (Huntington Study Group, 2006; Jankovic and Beach, 1997; Jankovic, 1982). Close monitoring of patients on tetrabenazine (which is now available in the United States as well as in Europe and Canada) is required. Despite their wide usage, there are few controlled studies of anti-psychotic drugs as anti-choreic agents for HD (Bonelli and Wenning, 2006). Typical or atypical anti-psychotics may be considered as anti-choreic treatments, particularly in individuals with co-morbid psychosis, agitation or irritability.

Some patients with an akinetic-rigid or parkinsonian variant of HD may benefit from dopaminergic therapy (Racette and Perlmutter, 1998; Reuter et al., 2000; Jongen, Renier and Gabreels, 1980). A carbidopa/levodopa preparation started at 25/100 mg daily and increased gradually and as tolerated over several weeks may improve mobility. Co-existing dystonia may intensify, even if chorea remains stable on dopaminergic treatment. There is some evidence to support the use of amantadine in HD patients with the parkinsonian variant of HD (Magnet, Bonelli and Kapfhammer, 2004), Dystonia is difficult to treat, but focal disabling or painful dystonias may be treated judiciously with skeletal muscle relaxants, benzodiazepines and botulinum toxin injections.

Physical therapy, occupational and speech therapy may be useful in HD patients, but there are no systematic studies that address long-term benefits.

Cognitive Impairment

Treatments for cognitive dysfunction are largely ineffective (Peyser et al., 1995; Fernandez et al., 2000; Murman et al., 1997; Shoulson et al., 1978). Acetylcholinesterase inhibitors, for example donepezil, may be considered in patients with memory disturbances. The lowest possible dose should be initiated and titrated slowly.

Behavioral Features

Depression and suicide are common in HD and are an important source of morbidity and mortality (Mendez, 1994). Factors associated with suicide in HD are unknown (Paulsen et al., 2005); however, impulsivity, the fear of abandonment, social isolation and the availability of harmful agents, as well as depression likely contribute to the increased risk of suicide attempts and suicide among those who carry the HD gene. Treatment of depressed HD patients with selective serotonin re-uptake inhibitors (SSRIs) appears to be safe and effective (Patel, Tariot and Asnis, 1996); although, there are no controlled trials to better inform clinicians. SSRIs may suppress chorea and reduce aggression in HD (Como et al., 1997; Fava, 1997). Dosage should be started low and increased as necessary over a several-month period of observation. There are no comparatiuve studies of SSRIs in HD. If a patient fails to respond or does not tolerate one SSRI it may help to switch to another agent. Sertraline, starting at 25 mg/day, may be useful for depression associated with apathy and somnolence. The dosage should be increased gradually and the patient followed closely for signs of agitation. Paroxetine, starting at 10 mg once daily, or, alternatively, given in the evening if sedation arises, may be useful for patients with depression and insomnia. The mixed serotonergic and noradrenergic reuptake inhibitor, venlafaxine, may also be useful; however, gastrointestinal side effects may limit its use. More traditional tricyclic anti-depressants can also be effective in treating depression in HD (Caine and Shoulson, 1983; Shoulson, 1981; Moldawsky, 1984). The major limitations with this class are anti-cholinergic side effects. Mirtazapine may also useful for insomnia associated with depression (Bonelli, 2003).

SSRIs may be effective in treating other psychiatric and behavioral disturbances in HD, including chronic anxiety, obsessive-compulsive symptoms, irritability and agitation, especially in the setting of depression (Como et al., 1997; Fava, 1997; Ranen et al., 1996a; Patzold and Brune, 2002; De Marchi, Daniele and Ragone, 2001). For patients with obsessive rumination and sleep disturbances, clomipramine 25 mg at bedtime may help (Chacko, Corbin and Harper, 2000). Benzodiazepines such as alprazolam may also be useful for the treatment of acute or situational anxiety, or episodic aggressiveness.

Irritability and aggression are common features of the HD and often take the form of poor control of temper or a reduced threshold for the development of anger. Patients may overreact to trivial issues and may be verbally and even physically abusive. In assessing aggression and irritability, secondary causes such as paranoia, depression and anxiety should be sought and treated appropriately (Guttman et al., 2002; Rosenblatt et al., 2002). In addition to SSRIs and as-needed benzodiazepines, the anti-convulsant valproic acid may be useful in treating both aggression and irritability (Grove, Quintanilla and DeVaney, 2000; Kavoussi and Coccaro, 1998). Extended release preparations of valproate allowing twice-daily dosing may enhance compliance. Liver function tests and valproate levels should be monitored, but there is no clear correlation with drug levels, and and improvement may occur at "sub-therapeutic" levels. Propranolol has been reported to reduce aggression in HD associated with frustration (Stewart, 1993).

Psychosis in the form of delusions, paranoia and even frank hallucinations may occur in 10 to 15% of patients. Atypical anti-psychotics including clozapine, quetiapine and olanzapine seem to exert the fewest neuroleptic side effects. More traditional neuroleptics are associated with an increased risk of tardive dyskinesia, the propensity to impair swallowing and gait, and exacerbate dystonia in HD (van Vugt, van Hilten and Roos, 1996; Jankovic, 1995; Schott et al., 1989). Clozapine can be useful in treating psychosis and may improve chorea also (Bonuccelli et al., 1994; Sajatovic et al., 1991). Its use is limited by the necessity for weekly blood monitoring and the rare risk of bone marrow suppression. As with anti-depressants, anti-psychotic treatment should be initiated at low dosage, adjusted gradually, and closely monitored.

Apathy is a common manifestation of HD, but the treatment of apathy has not been systematically evaluated. The removal of medications, such as typical anti-psychotics, may improve apathy. Activating medications, such as methylphenidate or modafinil have not been systematically evaluated in HD.

Participation in Research

In the coming years, many new experimental treatments will be examined in clinical trials involving individuals with pre-manifest HD, as well as patients with manifest HD. The opportunity for research participants and their families to be involved in clinical trials of experimental compounds is key for advancing scientific knowledge and facilitating the development of safe and effective treatments. So far, the HD community has been remarkably willing to participate in clinical research involving multi-year observational studies and interventional trials. In addition to ongoing therapeutic trials in manifest HD and planned trials in pre-manifest HD, the Huntington Study Group (www.huntington-study-group.org), through the sponsorship of the High Q Foundation (New York, NY), is enrolling consenting HD patients and their family members in the COHORT observational study, (see www.huntingtonproject.org and www.clinicaltrials.gov), that aims prospectively to develop biological markers of HD gene expression and disease progression, improve understanding of genotype–phenotype relationships, and identify genetic factors that may modify the onset and course of HD. Among families affected by HD, eligible COHORT research participants include individuals with manifest HD, individuals who have chosen to undergo predictive DNA testing and been found to carry the HD gene (pre-manifest HD) or not, at-risk individuals who have chosen not to be tested, and spouses of individuals with manifest or pre-manifest HD.

SUMMARY

The powerful and singular effect of the HD gene mutation, the associated dose–response effects of the expanded CAG repeats, improved understanding of the pathogenesis of HD and the resulting identification of therapeutic targets, the utility of testing rational agents in animal models of HD and signals emerging from the multi-center co-enzyme Q10 trial (Huntington Study Group, 2001) are accelerating the pace of therapeutic development in HD and spawning more clinical research and trials. In the long term, understanding the complex mechanisms that occur in the pathogenic process of HD will lead to the development of more precise and effective therapeutic weapons to delay the onset or slow the progression of the disease. It is anticipated that safe and

effective treatments will be developed in the coming years to combat the manifold morbidity that is caused by HD. There is an unmet need for symptomatic treatments as well as disease-modifying therapies for both manifest and pre-manifest HD. A rational, comprehensive and scientific approach, where fundamental and clinical research inform each other, remains the cornerstone of therapeutics aimed at relieving the burden and improving the quality of life for patients and families affected by HD.

References

Alper, J.S., Geller, L.N., Barash, C.I., Billings, P.R., Laden, V. and Natowicz, M.R. (1994) Genetic discrimination and screening for hemochromatosis. *Journal of Public Health Policy*, **15**, 345–358.

Armstrong, R.J., Watts, C., Svendsen, C.N., Dunnett, S.B. and Rosser, A.E. (2000) Survival, neuronal differentiation, and fiber outgrowth of propagated human neural precursor grafts in an animal model of Huntington's disease. *Cell Transplantation*, **9**, 55–64.

Aronin, N., Chase, K., Young, C. *et al.* (1995) CAG expansion affects the expression of mutant Huntingtin in the Huntington's disease brain. *Neuron*, **15**, 1193–1201. Abstract.

Bachoud-Levi, A.C., Bourdet, C., Brugieres, P. *et al.* (2000) Safety and tolerability assessment of intrastriatal neural allografts in five patients with Huntington's disease. *Experimental Neurology*, **161**, 194–202.

Bachoud-Levi, A.C., Remy, P., Nguyen, J.P. *et al.* (2000) Motor cognitive improvements in patients with Huntington's disease after neural transplantation. *Lancet*, **356**, 1975–1979.

Bachoud-Levi, A.C., Gaura, V., Brugieres, P. *et al.* (Apr 2006) Effect of fetal neural transplants in patients with Huntington's disease 6 years after surgery: a long-term follow-up study. *The Lancet Neurology*, **5**, 303–309.

Bae, B.I., Xu, H., Igarashi, S. *et al.* (7 Jul 2005) p53 Mediates Cellular Dysfunction and Behavioral Abnormalities in Huntington's Disease. *Neuron*, **47**, 29–41.

Bamford, K.A., Caine, E.D., Kido, D.K., Plassche, W.M. and Shoulson, I. (Jun 1989) Clinical-pathologic correlation in Huntington's disease: a neuropsychological and computed tomography study. *Neurology*, **39**, 796–801.

Baxter, L.R.J., Mazziotta, J.C., Pahl, J.J. *et al.* (Feb 1992) Psychiatric, genetic, and positron emmission tomographic evaluation of persons at risk for Huntington's disease. *Archives of General Psychiatry*, **49**, 148–154.

Beal, M.F. (1999) Coenzyme Q10 administration and its potential for treatment of neurodegenerative diseases. *Biofactors (Oxford, England)*, **9**, 261–266.

Beal, M.F., Brouillet, E., Jenkins, B.G. *et al.* (1 Oct 1993) Neurochemical and histologic characterization of striatal excitotoxic lesions produced by the mitochondrial toxin 3-nitropropionic acid. *The Journal of Neuroscience*, **13**, 4181–4192.

Beenen, N., Buttner, U. and Lange, H.W. (Feb 1986) The diagnostic value of eye movement recordings in patients with Huntington's disease and their offspring. *Electroencephalography and Clinical Neurophysiology*, **63**, 119–127.

Bezprozvanny, I. and Hayden, M.R. (1 Oct 2004) Deranged neuronal calcium signaling and Huntington's disease. *Biochemical and Biophysical Research Communications*, **322**, 1310–1317.

Billings, P.R., Kohn, M.A., de Cuevas, M., Beckwith, J., Alper, J.S. and Natowicz, M.R. (1992) Discrimination as a consequence of genetic testing. *American Journal of Human Genetics*, **50**, 476–482.

Blackmore, L., Simpson, S.A. and Crawford, J.R. (May 1995) Cognitive performance in UK sample of presymptomatic people carrying the gene for Huntington's disease. *Journal of Medical Genetics*, **32**, 358–362.

Blekher, T., Johnson, S.A., Marshall, J. *et al.* (2006) Saccades in presymptomatic and early stages of Huntington's disease. *Neurology*, **67**, 394–399.

Bloch, J., Bachoud-Levi, A.C., Deglon, N. *et al.* (Oct 2004) Neuroprotective gene therapy for Huntington's disease, using polymer-encapsulated cells engineered to secrete human ciliary neurotrophic factor: results of a phase I study. *Human Gene Therapy*, **15**, 968–975.

Bogdanov, M.B., Ferrante, R.J., Kuemmerle, S., Klivenyi, P. and Beal, M.F. (Dec 3 1998) Increased Vulnerability to 3-Nitropropionic Acid in an Animal Model of Huntington's Disease. *Journal of Neurochemistry*, **71**, 2642–2644.

Bonelli, R.M. (1 Mar 2003) Mirtazapine in suicidal Huntington's disease. *Annals of Pharmacotherapy*, **37**, 452.

Bonelli, R.M. and Wenning, G. (2006) Pharmacological management of Huntington's disease: an evidence-based review. *Current Pharmaceutical Design*, **12**, 2701–2720.

Bonuccelli, U., Ceravolo, R., Maremmani, C., Nuti, A., Rossi, G. and Muratorio, A. (1994) Clozapine in Huntington's chorea. *Neurology*, **44**, 821–823.

Borlongan, C.V., Koutouzis, T.K., Poulos, S.G., Saporta, S. and Sanberg, P.R. (1998) Bilateral fetal striatal grafts in the 3-nitropropionic acid-induced hypoactive model of Huntington's disease. *Cell Transplantation*, **7**, 131–135.

Braude, P.R., de Wert, G., Evers-Kiebooms, G., Pettigrew, R.A. and Geraedts, J.P.M. (1998) Non-disclosure preimplantation genetic diagnosis for Huntington's disease: practical and ethical dilemmas. *Prenatal Diagnosis*, **18**, 1422–1426.

Britton, J.W., Uitti, R.J., Ahlskog, J.E., Robinson, R.G., Kremer, B. and Hayden, M.R. (1995) Hereditary late-onset chorea without significant dementia: Genetic evidence for substantial phenotypic variation in Huntington's disease. *Neurology*, **45**, 443–447.

Browne, S.E., Bowling, A.C., MacGarvey, U. *et al.* (1997) Oxidative damage and metabolic dysfunction in Huntington's disease: Selective vulnerability of the basal ganglia. *Annals of Neurology*, **41**, 646–653.

Burns, A., Folstein, S., Brandt, J. and Folstein, M. (1990) Clinical assessment of irritability, aggression, and apathy in Huntington and Alzheimer disease. *Journal of Nervous and Mental Diseases*, **178**, 20–26.

Butler, L.M., Agus, D.B., Scher, H.I. *et al.* (2000) Suberoylanilide hydroxamic acid, an inhibitor of histone deacetylase, suppresses the growth of prostate cancer cells in vitro and in vivo. *Cancer Research*, **60**, 5165–5170.

Caine, E.D. and Shoulson, I. (1983) Psychiatric syndromes in Huntington's disease. *American Journal of Psychiatry*, **140**, 728–733.

Cannella, M., Gellera, C., Maglione, V. *et al.* (2004) The gender effect in juvenile Huntington's disease patients of Italian origin. *American Journal of Medical Genetics Part B (Neuropsychiatric, Genetics)*, **125**, 92–98.

Carella, F., Scaioli, V., Ciano, C., Binelli, S., Oliva, D. and Girotti, F. (1993) Adult onset myoclonic Huntington's disease. *Movement Disorders*, **8**, 201–205.

Cha, J.H. (1 Sep 2000) Transcriptional dysregulation in Huntington's disease. *Trends in Neurosciences*, **23**, 387–392.

Chacko, R.C., Corbin, M.A. and Harper, R.G. (2000) Acquired obsessive-compulsive disorder associated with basal ganglia lesions. *Journal of Neuropsychiatry and Clinical Neurosciences*, **12**, 269–272.

Chen, M., Ona, V.O., Ferrante, R.J. *et al.* (2000) Minocycline inhibits caspase-1 and caspase-3 and delays mortality in a transgenic mouse model of Huntington's disease. *Nature Medicine*, **6**, 797–801.

Cho, S.R., Benraiss, A., Chmielnicki, E., Samdani, A., Economides, A. and Goldman, S.A. (1 Oct 2007) Induction of neostriatal neurogenesis slows disease progression in a transgenic murine model of Huntington's disease. *The Journal of Clinical Investigation*, **117**, 2889–2902.

Collewijn, H., Went, L.N., Tamminga, E.P. and Vegter-Van der Vlis, M. (Sep 1988) Oculomotor deficits in patients with Huntington's disease and their offspring. *Journal of the Neurological Sciences*, **86**, 307–320.

Como, P.G., Rubin, A.J., O'Brien, C.F. *et al.* (1997) A controlled trial of fluoxetine in nondepressed patients with Huntington's disease. *Movement Disorders*, **12**, 397–401.

Conneally, P.M. (1984) Huntington's Disease: Genetics and epidemiology. *American Journal of Human Genetics*, **36**, 506–526.

Cooper, J.K., Schilling, G., Peters, M.F. *et al.* (1998) Truncated N-terminal fragments of huntingtin with expanded glutamine repeats form nuclear and cytoplasmic aggregates in cell culture. *Human Molecular Genetics*, **7**, 783–790.

Creighton, S., Almqvist, S.E., MacGregor, D. *et al.* (2003) Predictive, pre-natal and diagnostic genetic testing for Huntington's disease: the experience in Canada from 1987 to 2000. *Clinical Genetics*, **63**, 462–467.

Cubo, E., Shannon, K.M., Tracy, D. *et al.* (Oct 10 2006) Effect of donepezil on motor and cognitive function in Huntington's disease. *Neurology*, **67**, 1268–1271.

Cui, L., Jeong, H., Borovecki, F., Parkhurst, C.N., Tanese, N. and Krainc, D. (Oct 6 2006) Transcriptional Repression of PGC-1 [alpha] by Mutant Huntingtin Leads to Mitochondrial Dysfunction and Neurodegeneration. *Cell*, **127**, 59–69.

Davies, S., Cozens, B., Turmaine, M. *et al.* (1997) Formation of neuronal intranuclear inclusions underlies the neurological dysfunction in mice transgenic for the HD mutation. *Cell*, **80**, 537–548.

de Boo, G.M., Tibben, A., Lanser, J.B.K. *et al.* (Nov 1997) Early cognitive and motor symptoms in identified carriers of the gene for Huntington's disease. *Archives of Neurology*, **54**, 1353–1357.

De Marchi, N., Daniele, F. and Ragone, M.A. (Jan 9 2001) Fluoxetine in the treatment of Huntington's disease. *Psychopharmacology*, **153**, 264–266.

De Tommaso, M., Specchio, N., Sciruicchio, V., Difruscolo, O. and Specchio, L.M. (2004) Effects of rivastigmine on motor and cognitive impairment in Huntington's disease. *Movement Disorders*, **19**, 1516–1518.

De Tommaso, M., di Fruscolo, O., Sciruicchio, V. *et al.* (2005) Efficacy of Levetiracetam in Huntington's Disease. *Clinical Neuropharmacology*, **28**, 280–284.

De Tommaso, M., Difruscolo, O., Sciruicchio, V., Specchio, N. and Livrea, P. (2007) Two years' follow-up of rivastigmine treatment in Huntington's disease. *Clinical Neuropharmacology*, **30**, 43–46.

Dewhurst, K., Oliver, J.E. and McKnight, A.L. (1970) Sociopsychiatric consequences of Huntington's disease. *British Journal of Psychiatry*, **116**, 255–258.

Diamond, R., White, R.F., Myers, R.H. *et al.* (Nov 1992) Evidence of presymptomatic cognitive decline in Huntington's disease. *Journal of Clinical and Experimental NeuroPsychology*, **14**, 961–975.

DiFiglia, M., Sapp, E., Chase, K. *et al.* (1997) Aggregation of huntingtin in neuronal intranuclear inclusions and dystrophic neurites in brain. *Science*, **277**, 1990–1993.

Djousse, L., Knowlton, B., Cupples, L.A., Marder, K., Shoulson, I. and Myers, R.H. (Nov 12 2002) Weight loss in early stage of Huntington's disease. *Neurology*, **59**, 1325–1330.

Dorsey, E.R. and Huntington Study Group TREND-HD Investigators. (2007) A Randomized, Controlled Trial of Ethyl-EPA for the Treatment of Huntington's Disease – 12-Month Results. *Neurotherapeutics*, **5**, 363 Abstract.

Duesterhus, P., Schimmelmann, B.G., Wittkugel, O. and Schulte-Markwort, M. (2004) Huntington's disease: A case study of early onset presenting as depression. *Journal of the American Academy of Child and Adolescent Psychiatry*, **43**, 1293–1297.

Duff, K., Paulsen, J.S., Beglinger, L.J., Langbehn, D.R. and Stout, J.C., (in press) Psychiatric Symptoms in Huntington's Disease before Diagnosis: The Predict-HD Study. *Biological Psychiatry*, **62**, 1341–1346.

Duyao, M., Auerbach, A.B., Ryan, A. *et al.* (1995) Inactivation of the mouse Huntington's disease gene homolog Hdh. *Science*, **268**, 407–410.

Edmonds, C. (1966) Huntington's chorea, dysphagia and death. *The Medical Journal of Australia*, **2**, 273–274.

Emerich, D.F. and Winn, S.R. (2004) Neuroprotective effects of encapsulated CNTF-producing cells in a rodent model of Huntington's disease are dependent on the proximity of the implant to the lesioned striatum. *Cell Transplantation*, **13**, 253–259.

Fahn, S. (1973) Perphenazine in Huntington's Chorea, in *Advances in Neurology, Volume 1: Huntington's Chorea* (eds A. Barbeau, T.N. Chase and G.W. Paulson), Raven Press, New York, pp. 1872–1972.

Farrer, L.A. (1985) Diabetes mellitus in Huntington's disease. *Clinical Genetics*, **27**, 62–67. Abstract.

Farrer, L.A. and Conneally, P.M. (1985) A genetic model for age at onset in Huntington's disease. *American Journal of Human Genetics*, **37**, 350–357.

Fava, M. (1997) Psychopharmacologic treatment of pathologic aggression. *Psychiatry Clinics of North America*, **20**, 427–451.

Feigin, A., Kieburtz, K., Bordwell, K. *et al.* (1995) Functional decline in Huntington's disease. *Movement Disorders*, **10**, 211–214.

Fernandez, H.H., Friedman, J., Grace, J. and Beason-Hazen, S. (2000) Donepezil for Huntington's disease. *Movement Disorders*, **15**, 173–176.

Ferrante, R.J., Andreassen, O.A., Jenkins, B.G. *et al.* (2000) Neuroprotective effects of creatine in a transgenic mouse. *The Journal of Neuroscience*, **20**, 4389–4397.

Folstein, S.E., Leigh, R.J., Parhad, I.M. and Folstein, M.F. (1986) The diagnosis of Huntington's disease. *Neurology*, **36**, 1279–1283.

Folstein, S.E., Chase, G.A., Wahl, W.E., McDonnell, A.M. and Folstein, M.F. (1987) Huntington's disease in Maryland: clinical aspects of racial variation. *American Journal of Human Genetics*, **41**, 168–179.

Foroud, T., Siemers, E., Kleindorfer, D. *et al.* (May 1995) Cognitive scores in carriers of Huntington's disease gene compared to noncarriers. *Annals of Neurology*, **37**, 657–664.

Foroud, T., Gray, J., Ivashina, J. and Conneally, P.M. (1999) Differences in duration of Huntington's disease based on age at onset. *Journal of Neurology, Neurosurgery, and Psychiatry*, **66**, 52–56.

Fukae, J., Takanashi, M., Kubo, Si. *et al.* (Apr 25 2005) Expression of 8-oxoguanine DNA glycosylase (OGG1) in Parkinson's disease and related neurodegenerative disorders. *Acta Neuropathologica*, **109**, 256–262.

Gaba, A.M., Zhang, K., Marder, K., Moskowitz, C.B., Werner, P. and Boozer, C.N. (Jun 1 2005) Energy balance in early-stage Huntington's disease. *The American Journal of Clinical Nutrition*, **81**, 1335–1341.

Giordani, B., Berent, S., Boivin, M.J. *et al.* (Jan 1995) Longitudinal neuropsychological and genetic linkage analysis of persons at risk for Huntington's disease. *Archives of Neurology*, **52**, 59–64.

Giron, L.T. Jr and Koller, W.C. (1994) A critical survey and update on the epidemiology of Huntington's disease, in *Handbook of Neuroepidemiology* (eds P.B. Gorelick and M. Alter) Marcel Dekker, Inc., New York, pp. 281–292.

Goldberg, Y.P., Telenius, H. and Hayden, M.R. (1994) The molecular genetics of Huntington's disease. *Current Opinion in Neurology*, **7**, 325–332.

Gomez-Tortosa, E., del Barrio, A., Garcia Ruiz, P.J. *et al.* (1998) Severity of cognitive impairment in juvenile and late-onset Huntington's disease. *Archives of Neurology*, **55**, 835–843.

Gomez-Tortosa, E., MacDonald, M.E., Friend, J.C. *et al.* (2001) Quantitative neuropathological changes in presymptomatic Huntington's disease. *Annals of Neurology*, **49**, 29–34.

Greenamyre, J.T. and Shoulson, I. (1994) Huntington's disease, in *Neurodegenerative Diseases* (ed. D.B. Calne), WB Saunders, Philadelphia, pp. 685–704.

Grove, V.E., Quintanilla, J. and DeVaney, G.T. (2000) Improvement of Huntington's disease with olanzapine and valproate. *The New England Journal of Medicine*, **343**, 973–974.

Gu, M., Gash, M.T., Mann, V.M., Javoy-Agid, F., Cooper, J.M. and Schapira, A.H. (1996) Mitochondrial defect in Huntington's disease caudate nucleus. *Annals of Neurology*, **39**, 385–389.

Guttman, M., Alpay, M., Chouinard, S. *et al.* (2002) Clinical management of psychosis and mood disorders in Huntington's disease. in *Mental and Behavioral Dysfunction in Movement Disorders* (eds M.A. Bedard, Y. Agid, G. Chouinardm, S. Fahn, A. Korczyn and P. Lesperance), Totowa, NJ, Humana Press.

Hahn-Barma, V., Deweer, B., Durr, A. *et al.* (Feb 1998) Are cognitive changes the first symptoms of Huntington's disease? A study of gene carriers. *Journal of Neurology, Neurosurgery & Psychiatry*, **62**, 172–177.

Harper, P.S. (1992) The epidemiology of Huntington's disease. *Human Genetics*, **89**, 365–376.

Hauser, R.A., Furtado, S., Cimino, C. *et al.* (2001) Bilateral human fetal striatal transplantation in Huntington's disease. *Neurology*, **58**, 687–695.

Hayden, M.R., MacGregor, J.M. and Beighton, P.H. (1980) The prevalence of Huntington's chorea in South Africa. *South African Medical Journal*, **58**, 193–196.

Hayes, C. (1992) Genetic testing for Huntington's disease – A family issue. *New England Journal of Medicine*, **327**, 1449–1451.

The Huntington's Disease Collaborative Research Group (Mar 1993a) A novel gene containing a trinucleotide repeat that is expanded and unstable on Huntington's disease chromosomes. *Cell*, **26** (72), 971–983.

Huntington's Disease Collaborative Research Group (1993b) A novel gene containing a trinucleotide repeat that is expanded and unstable on Huntington's disease chromosomes. *Cell*, **72**, 971–983.

Hemmer, W. and Wallimann, T. (1993) Functional aspects of creatine kinase in brain. *Developmental Neuroscience*, **15**, 249–260.

Hersch, S.M. and The Huntington Study Group (2008) PHEND-HD: a safety, tolerability, and biomarker study of phenylbutyrate in sympomatic HD. *Neurotherapeutics*, **5**, 363–366.

Hersch, S. and Rosas, H.D. (2002) Neuroprotective therapy for Huntington's disease: new prospects and challenges. *Expert Reviews in Neurotherapeutics*, **1**, 111–118.

Hersch, S.M., Gevorkian, S. and Marder, K. *et al.* (Jan 24 2006) Creatine in Huntington's disease is safe, tolerable, bioavailable in brain and reduces serum 8OH2'dG. *Neurology*, **66**, 250–252.

Hogarth, P., Kayson, E. and Kieburtz, K. *et al.* (2004) Interrater agreement in the assessment of motor manifestations of Huntington's disease. *Movement Disorders*, **20**, 293–297.

Hogarth, P., Lovrecic, L. and Krainc, D. (2007) Sodium phenyl-butyrate in Huntington's disease: A dose-finding study. *Movement Disorders*, **22**, 1962–1964.

The Huntington Study Group (2006) PHAROS Investigators. At risk for Huntington's disease: The PHAROS (Prospective Hungtington At-Risk Observational Study) cohort enrolled. *Archives of Neurology*, **63**, 991–998.

Huber, S.J. and Paulson, G.W. (1987) Memory impairment associated with progression of Huntington's disease. *Cortex; A Journal Devoted to the Study of the Nervous System and Behavior*, **23**, 275–283.

Huntington, G. (Apr 1872) On chorea. *Medical and Surgical Reporter*, **26**, 317–321.

Huntington Study Group (1998) Safety and tolerability of the free-radical scavenger OPC-14117 in Huntington's disease. *Neurology*, **50**, 1366–1373.

Huntington Study Group (2001) A randomized, placebo-controlled trial of coenzyme Q10 and remacemide in Huntington's disease. *Neurology*, **57**, 397–404.

Huntington Study Group (Dec 9 2003) Dosage effects of riluzole in Huntington's disease: a multicenter placebo-controlled study. *Neurology*, **61**, 1551–1556.

Huntington Study Group (Aug 10 2004) Minocycline safety and tolerability in Huntington's disease. *Neurology*, **63**, 547–549.

Huntington Study Group (Feb 14 2006) Tetrabenazine as antichorea therapy in Huntington's disease: a randomized controlled trial. *Neurology*, **66**, 366–372.

Hurlbert, M.S., Zhou, W., Wasmeier, C., Kaddis, F.G., Hutton, J.C. and Freed, C.R. (Mar 1 1999) Mice transgenic for an expanded CAG repeat in the Huntington's disease gene develop diabetes. *Diabetes*, **48**, 649–651.

Jankovic, J. (1982) Treatment of hyperkinetic movement disorders with tetrabenazine: a double-blind crossover study. *Annals of Neurology*, **11**, 41–47.

Jankovic, J. (1995) Tardive syndromes and other drug-induced movement disorders. *Clinical Neuropharmacology*, **18**, 197–214.

Jankovic, J. and Ashizawa, T. (1995) Tourettism associated with Huntington's disease. *Movement Disorders*, **10**, 103–105.

Jankovic, J. and Beach, J. (1997) Long-term effects of tetrabenazine in hyperkinetic movement disorders. *Neurology*, **48**, 358–362.

Jason, G.W., Pajurkova, E.M., Suchowersky, O., Hewitt, J., Hilbert, C. and Hayden, M.R. (Jul 1988) Presymptomatic neuropsychological impairment in Huntington's disease. *Archives of Neurology*, **45**, 769–773.

Jenkins, B.G., Rosas, H.D., Chen, Y. *et al.* (1998) ^{1}H NMR spectroscopy studies of Huntington's disease Correlatioins with CAG repeat numbers. *Neurology*, **50**, 1357–1365.

Jones, A.L. (1999) The localization and interactions of huntingtin. *Philosophical Transactions of the Royal Society of London. Series B, Biological sciences*, **354**, 1021–1027.

Jongen, P.J., Renier, W.O. and Gabreels, F.J. (1980) Seven cases of Huntington's disease in childhood and levodopa induced improvement in the hypokinetic-rigid form. *Clinical Neurology and Neurosurgery*, **82**, 251–261.

Josiassen, R.C., Curry, L.M. and Mancall, E.L. (1983) Development of neuropsychological deficits in Huntington's disease. *Archives of Neurology*, **40**, 791–796.

Kavoussi, R.J. and Coccaro, E.F. (1998) Divalproex sodium for implsive aggressive behavior in patients with personality disorder. *Journal of Clinical Psychiatry*, **59**, 676–680.

Keene, C.D., Sonnen, J.A., Swanson, P.D. *et al.* (Jun 12 2007) Neural transplantation in Huntington's disease: Long-term grafts in two patients. *Neurology*, **68**, 2093–2098.

Kipps, C.M., Duggins, A.J., Mahant, N., Gomes, L., Ashburner, J. and McCusker, E.A. (2005) Progression of structural neuropathology in preclinical Huntington's disease: a tensor based morphometric study. *Journal of Neurology, Neurosurgery, and Psychiatry*, **76**, 650–655.

Kirkwood, S.C., Siemers, E., Bond, C., Conneally, P.M., Christian, J.C. and Foroud, T. (Jul 2000) Confirmation of subtle motor changes among presymptomatic carriers of the Huntington's disease gene. *Archives of Neurology*, **57**, 1040–1044.

Kokmen, E., Özekmeki, S., Beard, M., O'Brien, P.C. and Kurland, L. (1994) Incidence and prevalence of Huntington's disease in Olmsted County. Minnesota (1950 through 1989). *Archives of Neurology*, **51**, 696–698.

Koroshetz, W.J., Jenkins, B.G., Rosen, B.R. and Beal, M.F. (1997) Energy metabolism defects in Huntington's disease and effects of coenzyme Q10. *Annals of Neurology*, **42**, 160–165.

Kremer, B., Clark, C.M., Almqvist, E.W. *et al.* (1999) Influence of lamotrigine on progression of early Huntington's disease. A randomized clinical trial. *Neurology*, **53**, 1000–1011.

Laccone, F., Engel, U., Holinski-Feder, E. *et al.* (1999) DNA analysis of Huntington's disease. Five years of experience in Germany, Austria and Switzerland. *Neurology*, **53**, 801–806.

Landwehrmeyer, G.B., McNeil, S.M., Dure, L.S. *et al.* (Feb 1995) Huntington's disease gene: regional and cellular expression in brain of normal and affected individuals. *Annals of Neurology*, **37**, 218–230.

Langbehn, D.R. and Paulsen, J.S. The Huntington Study Group (May 15 2007) Predictors of diagnosis in Huntington's disease. *Neurology*, **68**, 1710–1717.

Lanska, D.J., Lavine, L., Lanska, M.J. and Schoenberg, B.S. (1988) Huntington's disease mortality in the United States. *Neurology*, **38**, 769–772.

Lapham, E.V., Kozma, C. and Weiss, J.O. (1996) Genetic discrimination: perspectives of consumers. *Science*, **274**, 621–624.

Lawrence, A.D., Sahakian, B., Hodges, J.R., Rosser, A.E., Lange, K.W. and Robbins, T.W. (1996) Executive and mnemonic functions in early Huntington's disease. *Brain*, **119**, 1633–1645.

Lawrence, A.D., Weeks, R.A., Brooks, D.J. *et al.* (1998a) The relationship between striatal dopamine receptor binding and cognitive performance in Huntington's disease. *Brain*, **121**, 1343–1355.

Lawrence, A.D., Hodges, J.R., Rosser, A.E. *et al.* (1998b) Evidence for specific cognitive deficits in preclinical Huntington's disease. *Brain*, **121**, 1329–1341.

Leopold, N. and Kagel, M. (1985) Dysphagia in Huntington's disease. *Archives of Neurology*, **42**, 57–60.

Leopold, N.A. and Podolsky, S. (1975) Exaggerated growth hormone response to arginine infusion in Huntington's disease. *The Journal of Clinical Endocrinology and Metabolism*, **41**, 160–163 Abstract.

Lermontova, N.N., Lukoyanov, N.V., Serkova, T.P., Lukoyanova, E.A. and Bachurin, S.O. (2000) Dimebon improves learning in animals with experimental Alzheimer's disease. *Bulletin of Experimental Biology and Medicine*, **129**, 544–546.

Levy, M.L., Cummings, J.L., Fairbanks, L.A. *et al.* (1998) Apathy is not depression. *Journal of Neuropsychiatry and Clinical Neurosciences*, **10**, 314–319.

Louis, E.D., Lee, P., Quinn, L. and Marder, K. (1999) Dystonia in Huntington's disease: Prevalence and clinical characteristics. *Movement Disorders*, **14**, 95–101.

Low, L., King, S. and Wilkie, T. (1998) Genetic discrimination in life insurance: empirical evidence from a cross sectional survey of genetic support groups in the United Kingdom. *BMJ (Clinical research ed)*, **317**, 1632–1635.

Magnet, M.K., Bonelli, R.M. and Kapfhammer, H.P. (Jul 1 2004) Amantadine in the Akinetic-Rigid Variant of Huntington's Disease. *Annals of Pharmacotherapy*, **38**, 1194–1196.

Mangiarini, L., Sathasivam, K., Seller, M. *et al.* (1996) Exon 1 of the HD gene with an expanded CAG repeat is sufficient to cause a progressive neurological phenotype in transgenic mice. *Cell*, **87**, 493–506.

Marder, K. (2007) Huntington Study Group PHAROS Investigators. Cross-sectional assessment of diet in individuals at risk for Huntington's disease (PHAROS). *Neurology*, **68**, A230. Abstract.

Matthews, R.T., Yang, L., Jenkins, B.G. *et al.* (1998) Neuroprotective effects of creatine and cyclocreatine in animal models of Huntington's disease. *The Journal of Neuroscience*, **18**, 156–163.

Mayberg, H.S., Starkstein, S.E., Peyser, C.E., Brandt, J., Dannals, R.F. and Folstein, S.E. (1992) Paralimbic frontal lobe hypometabolism in depression associated with Huntington's disease. *Neurology*, **42**, 1791–1797.

McCusker, E., Richards, F., Sillence, D., Wilson, M. and Trent, R.J. (Jan 2000) Huntington's disease: neurological assessment of potential gene carriers presenting for predictive DNA testing. *Journal of Clinical Neuroscience*, **7**, 38–41.

Mendez, M.F. (1994) Huntington's disease: update and review of neuropsychiatric aspects. *International Journal of Psychiatry in Medicine*, **24**, 189–208.

Mitchell, I.J., Cooper, A.J. and Griffiths, M.R. (1999) The selective vulnerability of striatopallidal neurons. *Progress in Neurobiology*, **59**, 691–719.

Moldawsky, R.J. (1984) Effect of amoxapine on speech in a patient with Huntington's disease. *American Journal of Psychiatry*, **141**, 150.

Morris, M. (1995) Dementia and cognitive changes in Huntington's disease, in *Behavioral Neurology of Movement Disorders* (eds W.J. Weiner and A.E. Lang), Raven Press, New York, pp. 187–200.

Murman, D.L., Giordani, B., Mellow, A.M. *et al.* (1997) Cognitive, behavioral, and motor effects of the NMDA antagonist ketamine in Huntington's disease. *Neurology*, **49**, 153–161.

Nakao, N. and Itakura, T. (2000) Fetal tissue transplants in animal models of Huntington's disease: the effects on damaged neuronal circuitry and behavioral deficits. *Progress in Neurobiology*, **61**, 313–338.

Nance, M. (1997) Genetic testing of children at risk for Huntington's disease. *Neurology*, **49**, 1048–1053.

Nance, M.A. and Myers, R.H. The US Huntington's Disease Genetic Testing Group (1999) Trends in predictive and prenatal testing for Huntington's disease 1993–1999. *American Journal of Human Genetics*, **65**, A406.

Nasir, J., Floresco, S.B., O'Kusky, J.R. *et al.* (Jun 2 1995) Targeted disruption of the Huntington's disease gene results in embryonic lethality and behavioral and morphological changes in heterozygotes. *Cell*, **81**, 811–823.

Nucifora, F.C., Sasaki, M., Peters, M.F. *et al.* (2001) Interference by huntingtin and atrophin-1 with CBP-mediated transcription leading to cellular toxicity. *Science*, **291**, 2423–2428.

O'Suilleabhain, P. and Dewey, R.B. Jr (Jul 1 2003) A Randomized Trial of Amantadine in Huntington's Disease. *Archives of Neurology*, **60**, 996–998.

Oepen, G., Clarenbach, P. and Thoden, U. (1981) Distrubance of eye movements in Huntington's chorea. *Archiv fur Psychiatrie und Nervenkrankheiten*, **229**, 205–213.

Oliva, D., Carella, F., Savoiardo, M. *et al.* (1993) Clinical and magnetic resource features of the classic and akinetic-rigid variants of Huntington's disease. *Archives of Neurology*, **50**, 17–19.

Panov, A.V., Gutekunst, C.A., Leavitt, B.R. *et al.* (Aug 2002) Early mitochondrial calcium defects in Huntington's disease are a direct effect of polyglutamines. *Nature Neuroscience*, **5**, 731–736.

Patel, S.V., Tariot, P.N. and Asnis, J. (1996) L-Deprenyl augmentation of fluoxetine in a patient with Huntington's disease. *Annals of Clinical Psychiatry*, **8**, 23–26.

Patzold, T. and Brune, M. (2002) Obsessive compulsive disorder in huntington disease: a case of isolated obsessions successfully treated with sertraline. *Neuropsychiatry Neuropsychology and Behavioral Neurology*, **15**, 216–219.

Paulsen, J.S., Zhao, H., Stout, J.C. *et al.* (2001) Clinical markers of early disease in persons near onset of Huntington's disease. *Neurology*, **57**, 658–662.

Paulsen, J.S., Hoth, K.F., Nehl, C. and Stierman, L. (2005) Critical periods of suicide risk in Huntington's disease. *The American Journal of Psychiatry*, **162**, 725–731.

Paulsen, J.S., Hayden, M., Stout, J.C. *et al.* (2006) Preparing for preventive clinical trials: The Predict-HD study. *Archives of Neurology*, **63**, 890.

Paulson, G.W. (1979) Diagnosis of Huntington's disease, in *Huntington's Disease* (eds T.N. Chase, N.S. Wexler and A. Barbeau), Raven Press, New York, pp. 177–184.

Penney, J.B., Young, A.B., Shoulson, I. *et al.* (1990) Huntington's disease in Venezuela: 7 years of follow up on symptomatic and asymptomatic individuals. *Movement Disorders*, **5**, 93–99.

Perry, T.L., Hansen, S. and Kloster, M. (1973) Huntington's chorea. Deficiency of gamma-aminobutyric acid in brain. *New England Journal of Medicine*, **288**, 337–342.

Petersen, A. and Bjorkqvist, M. (Aug 21 2006) Hypothalamic-endocrine aspects in Huntington's disease. *The European Journal of Neuroscience*, **24**, 961–967.

Peyser, C.E., Folstein, M., Chase, G.A. *et al.* (1995) Trial of d-alpha-tocopherol in Huntington's disease. *The American Journal of Psychiatry*, **152**, 1771–1775.

Philpott, L.M., Kopyov, O.V., Lee, A.J. *et al.* (1997) Neuropsychological functioning following fetal striatal transplantation in Huntington's chorea: three case presentations. *Cell Transplantation*, **6**, 203–212.

Pillon, B., Dubois, B., Ploska, A. and Agid, Y. (1991) Severity and specificity of cognitive impairment in Alzheimer's, Huntington's, and Parkinson's diseases and progressive supranuclear palsy. *Neurology*, **41**, 634–643.

Podolsky, S. and Leopold, N.A. (1977) Abnormal glucose tolerance and arginine tolerance tests in Huntington's disease. *Gerontology*, **23**, 55–63, Abstract.

Podolsky, S., Leopold, N.A. and Sax, D.S. (1972) Increased frequency of diabetes mellitus in patients with Huntington's chorea. *Lancet*, **1**, 1356–1358, Abstract.

Post, S.G. (1992) Huntington's disease: prenatal screening for late onset disease. *Journal of Medical Ethics*, **18**, 75–78.

Pratley, R.E., Salbe, A.D., Ravussin, E. and Caviness, J.N. (2000) Higher sedentary energy expenditure in patients with Huntington's disease. *Annals of Neurology*, **47**, 64–70.

Puri, B.K., Leavitt, B.R., Hayden, M.R. *et al.* (Jul 26 2005) Ethyl-EPA in Huntington's disease: A double-blind, randomized, placebo-controlled trial. *Neurology*, **65**, 286–292.

Quaid, K.A. and Morris, M. (1993) Reluctance to undergo predictive testing: the case of Huntington's disease. *American Journal of Medical Genetics*, **45**, 41–45.

Quaid, K.A., Brandt, J., Faden, R.R. and Folstein, S.E. (1989) Knowledge attitude, and the decision to be tested for Huntington's disease. *Clinical Genetics*, **36**, 431–438.

CAPIT-HD committee, Quinn, N., Brown, R. *et al.* (1996) Core assessment program for intracerebral transplantation in Huntington's disease (CAPIT-HD). *Movement Disorder Society*, **11**, 143–150.

Racette, B.A. and Perlmutter, J.S. (1998) Levodopa responsive parkinsonism in an adult with Huntington's disease. *Journal of Neurology, Neurosurgery, and Psychiatry*, **65**, 577–579.

Ranen, N.G., Lipsey, J.R., Treisman, G. and Ross, C.A. (1996a) Sertraline in the treatment of severe aggressiveness in Huntington's disease. *Journal of Neuropsychiatry and Clinical Neurosciences*, **8**, 338–340.

Ranen, N.G., Peyser, C.E., Coyle, J.T. *et al.* (1996b) A controlled trail of idebenone in Huntington's disease. *Movement Disorders*, **11**, 549–554.

Rasmussen, A., Macias, R., Yescas, P., Ochoa, A., Davila, G. and Alonso, E. (2000) Huntington's disease in children: Genotype-Phenotype correlation. *Neuropediatrics*, **31**, 190–194.

Reiner, A., Albin, R.L., D'Amato, C., Penney, J.B. and Young, A. B. (1988) Differential loss of striatal projection neurons in Huntington's disease. *Proceedings of the National Academy of Sciences of the United States of America*, **85**, 5733–5737.

Reuter, I., Hu, M.T., Andrews, T.C., Brooks, D.J., Clough, C. and Chaudhuri, K.R. (2000) Late onset levodopa responsive Huntington's disease with minimal chorea masquerading as Parkinson plus syndrome. *Journal of Neurology Neurosurgery & Psychiatry*, **68**, 238–241.

Ribai, P., Nguyen, K., Hahn-Barma, V. *et al.* (2006) Psychiatric and cognitive difficulties as indicators of juvenile Huntington's disease onset in 29 patients. *Archives of Neurology*, **64**, 813–819.

Richfield, E.K., Maguire-Zeiss, K.A., Vonkemank, H.E. and Voorn, P. (1995) Preferential loss of preproenkephalin versus preprotachykinin neurons from the striatum of Huntington's disease patients. *Annals of Neurology*, **38**, 852–861.

Roizin, L., Stellar, S., Willson, N., Whittier, J. and Liu, J.C. (1974) Electron microscope and enzyme studies in cerebral biopsies of Huntington's chorea. *Transactions of the American Neurological Association*, **99**, 240–243.

Roos, R.A., Vegter-Van der Vlis, M., Hermans, J. *et al.* (1991) Age at onset in Huntington's disease: Effect of line of inheritance of patient's sex. *Medizinische Genetik: Mitteilungsblatt des Berufsverbandes Medizinische Genetik eV*, **28**, 515–519.

Rosenberg, N.K., Sorenson, S.A. and Christensen, A.L. (Aug 1995) Neuropsychological characteristics of Huntington's disease carriers: a double blind study. *Journal of Medical Genetics*, **32**, 600–604.

Rosenblatt, A., Anderson, K., Goumeniouk, D. *et al.* (2002) Clinical management of aggression and frontal syndromes in Huntington's disease. In: Bedard M.A., Agid Y., Chouinard S., Fahn S., Korczyn A. and Lesperance P. (eds.), Mental and Behavioral Dysfunction in Movement Disorders, Totowa, NJ: Humana Press.

Ross, C.A. (Dec 1997) Intranuclear Neuronal Inclusions: A Common Pathogenic Mechanism for Glutamine-Repeat Neurodegenerative Diseases? *Neuron*, **19**, 1147–1150.

Ross, C.A. (Jul 9 2004) Huntington's Disease: New Paths to Pathogenesis. *Cell*, **118**, 4–7.

Ross, C.A. and Poirier, M.A. (2004) Protein aggregation and neurodegenerative disease. *Nature Medicine*, **10**, S10–S14, Abstract.

Ross, C.A. and Thompson, L.M. (Nov 2006) Transcription meets metabolism in neurodegeneration. *Nature Medicine*, **12**, 1239–1241.

Rosser, A.E., Barker, R.A., Harrower, T. *et al.* (Dec 1 2002) Unilateral transplantation of human primary fetal tissue in four patients with Huntington's disease: NEST-UK safety report ISRCTN no 36485475. *Journal of Neurology, Neurosurgery, and Psychiatry*, **73**, 678–685.

Rothlind, J.C., Brandt, J., Zee, D., Codori, A.M. and Folstein, S. (Aug 1993) Unimpaired verbal memory and oculomotor control in asymptomatic adults with the genetic marker for Huntington's disease. *Archives of Neurology*, **50**, 799–802.

Saft, C., Andrich, J., Meisel, N.M., Przuntek, H. and Muller, T. (2006) Assessment of simple movements reflects impairment in Huntington's disease. *Movement Disorders*, **21**, 1208–1212.

Sajatovic, M., Verbanac, P., Ramirez, L.F. and Meltzer, H.Y. (1991) Clozapine treatment of psychiatric symptoms resistant to neuroleptic treatment in patients with Huntington's chorea. *Neurology*, **41**, 156.

Sapp, E., Ge, P., Aizawa, H. *et al.* (1995) Evidence for a preferential loss of enkephalin immunoreactivity in the external globus pallidus in low grade Huntington's disease using high resolution image analysis. *Neuroscience*, **64**, 397–404.

Sapp, E., Schwarz, C., Chase, K. *et al.* (1997) Huntingtin localization in brains of normal and Huntington's disease patients. *Annals of Neurology*, **42**, 604–612.

Saudou, F., Finkbeiner, S., Devys, D. and Greenberg, M.E. (1998) Huntingtin acts in the nucleus to induce apoptosis but death does not correlate with the formation of intranuclear inclusions. *Cell*, **95**, 55–66.

Scherzinger, E., Lurz, R., Turmaine, M. *et al.* (Aug 8 1997) Huntingtin-encoded polyglutamine expansions form amyloid-like protein aggregates in vitro and in vivo. *Cell*, **90**, 549–558.

Schoenfeld, M., Myers, R.H., Cupples, L.A., Berkman, B., Sax, D. S. and Clark, E. (1984) Increased rate of suicide among patients with Huntington's disease. *Journal of Neurology, Neurosurgery, and Psychiatry*, **47**, 1283–1287.

Schott, K., Ried, S., Stevens, I. and Dichgans, J. (1989) Neuroleptically induced dystonia in Huntington's disease: a case report. *European Neurology*, **29**, 39–40.

Seong, I.S., Ivanova, E., Lee, J.M. *et al.* (Oct 1 2005) HD CAG repeat implicates a dominant property of huntingtin in mitochondrial energy metabolism. *Human Molecular Genetics*, **14**, 2871–2880.

Shelton, P.A. and Knopman, D.S. (1991) Ideomotor apraxia in Huntington's disease. *Archives of Neurology*, **48**, 35–41.

Shiwach, R.S. and Norbury, C.G. (Oct 1994) A controlled psychiatric study of individuals at risk for Huntington's disease. *British Journal of Psychiatry*, **165**, 500–505.

Shoulson, I. (1981) Huntington's disease: Functional capacities in patient's treated with neuroleptic and antidepressant drugs. *Neurology*, **31**, 1333–1335.

Shoulson, I. (1998) DATATOP: a decade of neuroprotective inquiry. Parkinson Study Group. Deprenyl and tocopherol antioxidative therapy of parkinsonism. *Annals of Neurology*, **44**, S160–S166.

Shoulson, I., Goldblatt, D., Charlton, M. and Joynt, R.J. (1978) Huntington's disease: treatment with muscimol; a GABA-mimetic drug. *Annals of Neurology*, **4**, 279–284.

Shoulson, I., Kurlan, R. and Rubin, A. (1989a) Assessment of functional capacity in neurodegenerative movement disorders: Huntington's disease as a prototype, in *Quantification of Neurologic Deficit* (ed. T.L. Munsat) Butterworths, Boston, pp. 285–306.

Shoulson, I., Odoroff, C., Oakes, D. *et al.* (1989b) A controlled clinical trial of baclofen as protective therapy in early Huntington's disease. *Annals of Neurology*, **25**, 252–259.

Shults, C.W., Oakes, D., Kieburtz, K. *et al.* (2002) Effects of coenzyme Q10 in early Parkinson' disease: evidence of slowing of the functional decline. *Archives of Neurology*, **59**, 1541–1550.

Siemers, E., Foroud, T., Bill, D.J. *et al.* (Jun 1996) Motor changes in presymptomatic Huntington's disease gene carriers. *Archives of Neurology*, **53**, 487–492.

Siesling, S., Vegter-van der Vlis, M. and Roos, R.A.C. (Jul 1997) Juvenile Huntington's disease in the Netherlands. *Pediatric Neurology*, **17**, 37–43.

Siesling, S., van Vugt, J.P., Zwinderman, A.H., Kieburtz, K. and Roos, R.A. (1998) Unified Huntington's Disease Rating Scale: A follow up. *Movement Disorders*, **13**, 915–919.

Simpson, S.A., Zoeteweij, M.W., Nys, K. *et al.* (2002) Prenatal testing for Huntington's disease: a European collaborative study. *European Journal of Human Genetics*, **10**, 689–693.

Snowden, J.S., Craufurd, D., Thompson, J. and Neary, D. (2002) Psychomotor executive and memory function in preclinical Huntington's disease. *Journal of Clinical and Experimental NeuroPsychology*, **24**, 133–145.

Sotrel, A., Paskevich, P.A., Kiely, D.K., Bird, E.D., Williams, R.S. and Myers, R.H. (1991) Morphometric analysis of the prefrontal cortex in Huntington's disease. *Neurology*, **41**, 1117–1123.

Squitieri, F., Berardelli, A., Nargi, E. *et al.* (2000) Atypical movement disorders in the early stages of Huntington's disease: clinical and genetic analysis. *Clinical Genetics*, **58**, 50–56.

Squitieri, F., Pustorino, G., Cannella, M. *et al.* (2003) Highly disabling cerebellar presentation in Huntington's disease. *European Journal of Neurology*, **10**, 443–444.

Steffan, J.S., Bodai, L., Pallos, J. *et al.* (2001) Histone deacetylase inhibitors arrest polyglutamine-dependent neurodegeneration in Drosophila. *Nature*, **413**, 739–743.

Stewart, J.T. (1993) Huntington's disease and propanolol. *American Journal of Psychiatry*, **150**, 166–167.

Strauss, M.E. and Brandt, J. (Aug 1990) Are there neuropsychologic manifestations of the gene for Huntington's disease in asymptomatic, at-risk individuals? *Archives of Neurology*, **47**, 905–908.

Tabrizi, S.J., Cleeter, M.W.J., Xuereb, J., Taanman, J.W., Cooper, J.M. and Schapira, A.H. (1999) Biochemical abnormalities and excitotoxicity in Huntington's disease brain. *Annals of Neurology*, **45**, 25–32.

Tan, E., Jankovic, J. and Ondo, W. (2000) Bruxism in Huntington's disease. *Movement Disorders*, **15**, 171–173.

Tanner, C.M. and Goldman, S.M. (1994) Epidemiology of movement disorders. *Current Opinion in Neurology*, **7**, 340–345 Abstract.

Tassicker, R.J., Marshall, P.K., Liebeck, T.A., Keville, M.A., Singaram, B.M. and Richards, F.H. (2006) Predictive pre-natal testing for Huntington's Disease in Australia: results and challenges encountered during a 10-year period [1994–2003]. *Clinical Genetics*, **70**, 480–489.

Telenius, H., Kremer, B., Goldberg, Y.P. *et al.* (Apr 1994) Somatic and gonadal mosaicism of the Huntington's disease gene CAG repeat in brain and sperm. *Nature Genetics*, **6**, 409–414.

Tian, J.R., Zee, D., Lasker, A.G. and Folstein, S. (1991) Saccades in Huntington's disease: Predictive tracking and interaction between release of fixation and initiation of saccades. *Neurology*, **41**, 875–881.

Tibben, A., Frets, P., van de Kamp, J. *et al.* (1993a) On attitudes and appreciation 6 months after predictive DNA testing for

Huntington's disease in the Dutch program. *American Journal of Medical Genetics*, **48**, 103–111.

Tibben, A., Duivenvoorden, H., Vegter-Van der Vlis, M. *et al.* (1993b) Presymptomatic DNA testing for Huntington's disease: Identifying the need for psychological intervention. *American Journal of Medical Genetics*, **48**, 137–144.

van Dijk, G., Van der Velde, E.A., Roos, R.A. and Bruyn, G. (1986) Juvenile Huntington's disease. *Human Genetics*, **73**, 235–239.

van Vugt, J.P., van Hilten, B.J. and Roos, R.A. (1996) Hypokinesia in Huntington's disease. *Movement Disorders*, **11**, 384–388.

van Vugt, J.P.P., Siesling, S., Vergeer, M., Van der Velde, E.A. and Roos, R.A.C. (Jul 1 1997) Clozapine versus placebo in Huntington's disease: a double blind randomised comparative study. *Journal of Neurology, Neurosurgery, and Psychiatry*, **63**, 35–39.

Verbessem, P., Lemiere, J., Eijnde, B.O. *et al.* (Oct 14 2003) Creatine supplementation in Huntington's disease: A placebo-controlled pilot trial. *Neurology*, **61**, 925–930.

Verhagen Metman, L., Morris, M.J., Farmer, C. *et al.* (Sep 10 2002) Huntington's disease: A randomized, controlled trial using the NMDA-antagonist amantadine. *Neurology*, **59**, 694–699.

Vonsattel, J.P., Myers, R.H., Stevens, T.J., Ferrante, R.J., Bird, E. D. and Richardson, E.P. Jr, (1985) Neuropathological classification of Huntington's disease. *Journal of Neuropathology and Experimental Neurology*, **44**, 559–577.

Warrell, R.P., He, L., Richon, V., Calleja, E. and Pandolfi, P.P. (1998) Therapeutic targeting of transcription in acute promyelocytic leukemia by use of an inhibitor of histone deacetylase. *Journal of the National Cancer Institute*, **90**, 1621–1625.

Watkins, L., Rogers, R.D., Lawrence, A.D., Sahakian, B., Rosser, A. and Robbins, T.W. (2000) Impaired planning but intact decision making in early Huntington's disease: implications for specific fronto-striatal pathology. *Neuropsychologia*, **38**, 1112–1125.

Wellington, C.L., Leavitt, B.R. and Hayden, M.R. (2000) Huntington's disease: new insights on the role of huntingtin cleavage. *Journal of Transmission supp*, **58**, 1–17.

Wexler, N.S. (1979) Perceptual-motor, cognitive, and emotional characteristics of persons at risk for Huntington's disease, in *Huntington's Disease* (eds T.N. Chase, N.S. Wexler and A. Barbeau), Raven Press, New York, pp. 257–271.

The U.S.-Venezuela Collaborative Research Project, Wexler, N.S. and Lorimer, J. *et al.*, (Mar 9 2004) Venezuelan kindreds reveal that genetic and environmental factors modulate Huntington's disease age of onset. *PNAS*, **101**, 3498–3503.

Weydt, P., Pineda, V.V., Torrence, A.E. *et al.* (Nov 2006) Thermoregulatory and metabolic defects in Huntington's disease transgenic mice implicate PGC-1[alpha] in Huntington's disease neurodegeneration. *Cell Metabolism*, **4**, 349–362.

Wiggins, S., Whyte, P., Huggins, M. *et al.* (1992) The psychological consequences of predicitve testing for Huntington's disease. *New England Journal of Medicine*, **327**, 1401–1405.

Wilson, R.S. and Garron, D.C., (1979) Cognitive affective aspects of Huntington's disease, in *Huntington's Disease* (eds T.N. Chase, N.S. Wexler and A. Barbeau), Raven Press, New York, pp. 193–201.

Young, A.B., Shoulson, I., Penney, J.B. *et al.* (1986) Huntington's disease in Venezuela: neurologic features and functional decline. *Neurology*, **36**, 244–249.

Yrjanheikki, J., Tikka, T., Keinanen, R., Goldsteins, G., Chan, P.H. and Koistinaho, J. (1999) A tetracycline derivative, minocycline, reduces inflammation and protects against focal cerebral ischemia with a wide therapeutic window. *Proceedings of the National Academy of Sciences of the United States of America*, **96**, 13496–13500.

Zeron, M.M., Chen, N., Moshaver, A. *et al.* (Jan 2001) Mutant Huntingtin Enhances Excitotoxic Cell Death. *Molecular and Cellular Neuroscience*, **17**, 41–53.

Zeron, M.M., Fernandes, H.B., Krebs, C. *et al.* (Mar 2004) Potentiation of NMDA receptor-mediated excitotoxicity linked with intrinsic apoptotic pathway in YAC transgenic mouse model of Huntington's disease. *Molecular and Cellular Neuroscience*, **25**, 469–479.

Zucker, B., Luthi-Carter, R., Kama, J.A. *et al.* (Jan 15 2005) Transcriptional dysregulation in striatal projection- and interneurons in a mouse model of Huntington's disease: neuronal selectivity and potential neuroprotective role of HAP1. *Human Molecular Genetics*, **14**, 179–189.

20

Chorea

Francisco Cardoso

Neurology Service, Internal Medicine Department, The Federal University of Minas Gerais Medical School,
Belo Horizonte, MG, Brazil

INTRODUCTION

Chorea, derived from the Latin choreus meaning "dance," describes a syndrome characterized by brief, abrupt involuntary movements resulting from a continuous flow of random muscle contractions. The pattern of movement may sometimes appear playful, conveying a feeling of restlessness to the observer. When choreic movements are more severe, assuming a flinging, sometimes violent, character, they are called ballism (Cardoso *et al.*, 2006). Regardless of its etiology, chorea has the same features. The differential diagnosis of choreic syndromes thus relies not so much on differences in the phenomenology of the hyperkinesia but the presence of accompanying findings.

First noted in the Middle Ages, the most common illness was perhaps the post-infectious chorea now known as Sydenham chorea (SC). Although the latter was first clearly described by Thomas Sydenham in 1686, the casual relationship of this form of chorea with streptococcal infection was only firmly established in the middle of the twentieth century (Taranta and Stollerman, 1956). There were also outbreaks of "dancing mania," a psychiatric condition coinciding with epidemics of the plague in Central Europe (Goetz, Chmura and Lanska, 2001). In the nineteenth century the concise report by George Huntington on affected families in the state of New York led to a clear recognition of hereditary chorea, which would be later, named after him (Huntington, 1872). The book *On Chorea and Choreiform Affectations*, published in 1894 by William Osler, is a landmark in the study of choreas because of the establishment of distinct clinical differences between SC and Huntington disease (HD) (Goetz, 2000). Currently there is the acknowledgment of the existence of a large number of hereditary and non-hereditary causes of chorea. Table 20.1 lists the most important causes of chorea. The aim of this chapter is to provide an overview of classification, clinical manifestations and pathophysiology, as well as the management of the most important causes of chorea.

CLINICAL PRESENTATION AND PREVALENCE

This section contains a discussion of the clinical features of the most frequent causes of chorea. Although there are no community-based studies available regarding the prevalence and incidence of choreas as a whole, there is information regarding the situation in tertiary care centers. According to a recent study from Pennsylvania, SC accounts for almost 100% of acute cases of chorea seen in children (Zomorrodi and Wald, 2006). In contrast, the situation is quite distinct in adult patients. Although no data are available, it is most likely that levodopa-induced chorea in Parkinson's disease patients is the most common cause of chorea seen by neurologists. This issue, however, is discussed in other chapters of this book. HD is the most frequent cause of genetic chorea with reported prevalence rates in North America and Europe ranging from 3 to 7 per 100 000 (Cardoso *et al.*, 2006). The other genetic conditions causing chorea (Table 20.2) are quite rare. One study of consecutive patients with non-genetic forms of chorea seen at a tertiary hospital found that stroke accounted for 50% of all cases, drug abuse was identified in one-third of the patients, while the remaining patients had chorea related to AIDS and other infections, as well as metabolic problems (Piccolo *et al.*, 2003).

Genetic Causes of Chorea

HD is an illness transmitted in an autosomal-dominant manner, typically characterized by a movement disorder, including chorea, cognitive decline and behavioral changes. Carriers of the mutated HD gene typically first

Table 20.1 Etiological classification of Chorea.

Genetic Choreas (See Table 20.2 for details)
Non-Genetic Choreas

Vascular Choreas
- Vascular chorea in stroke (hemichorea-hemiballism)
- Post-pump chorea

Autoimmune Choreas
- Sydenham chorea and variants (chorea gravidarum and oral contraceptive-induced chorea)
- Systemic lupus erythematosus
- Anti-phospholipid antibody syndrome
- Post-infections/post-vaccinial encephalitis

Infectious Chorea
- HIV encephalopathy
- Toxoplasmosis
- Cysticercosis
- Diphtheria
- Bacterial endocarditis
- Neurosyphilis
- Scarlet fever
- Viral encephalitis (Mumps, Measles, Varicella, Japanese encephalitis, West Nile River encephalitis)

Chorea related to Metabolic/Toxic Encephalopathies
- Hyperglycaemia
- Acute intermittent porphyria
- Hypo/hypernatremia
- Hypocalcemia
- Hyperthyroidism
- Hypoparathyroidism
- Hepatic/renal failure
- Carbon monoxide
- Manganese
- Mercury
- Organophosphate poisoning

Drug-induced choreas (See Table 20.3)

Miscellaneous
- Neoplasms (CNS lymphoma, metastatic brain tumors)
- Multiple sclerosis
- Extrapontine myelinolysis
- Subdural haematoma

including eye movement abnormalities, parkinsonian features and dystonia (particularly in juvenile HD or advanced disease), myoclonus, tics, ataxia, dysarthria and dysphagia, as well as spasticity with hyper-reflexia and extensor plantar responses (Leigh *et al.*, 1983; Carella *et al.*, 1993; Jankovic and Ashizawa, 1995; Reuter *et al.*, 2000; Tan, Jankovic and Ondo, 2000). Behavioral and cognitive impairment is universal in HD and may occasionally antedate motor manifestations. Depression is present in up to 40% of patients and responsible for increased suicide rates in HD. The spectrum of behavioral abnormalities in HD is broad and includes anxiety or panic attacks, obsessive compulsive symptoms, manic features, psychosis, irritability and aggressive behavior, and sexual disinhibition, as well as apathy (Caine and Shoulson, 1983; Mendez, 1994; Schoenfeld *et al.*, 1984; Shiwach, 1994; Rosenblatt and Leroi, 2000; Rosenblatt *et al.*, 2003; Guttman *et al.*, 2003). Patients with HD invariably develop dementia with a subcortical pattern whose clinical features include bradyphrenia, decreased verbal fluency and a frontal dysexecutive syndrome (Lawrence *et al.*, 1996; Kirkwood *et al.*, 2001; Ho *et al.*, 2003). HD is relentlessly progressive with death occurring 15–20 years after symptom onset, with particularly rapid progression in the juvenile Westphal variant. End-stage HD patients are typically rigid and akinetic, demented and mute. Immobility and dysphagia often lead to aspiration pneumonia, the most common cause of death in this illness (Lanska *et al.*, 1988; Sorensen and Fenger, 1992; Marshall, 2004). Further details of HD are provided in Chapter 19 of this book.

Up to 7% of patients with otherwise typical features of HD do not have the Huntington gene mutation (Andrew *et al.*, 1994; Stevanin *et al.*, 2002). Such HD-like disorders are genetically heterogeneous and include some autosomal dominant heredoataxias, Huntington's disease-like 2 (HDL2), neuroacanthocytosis and benign hereditary chorea (BHC) (Breedveld *et al.*, 2002; Stevanin *et al.*, 2002; Margolis and Ross, 2003; Bauer *et al.*, 2004). HDL2 caused by mutations in the gene encoding junctophilin-3 bears striking resemblance to HD. Although generally rare, the prevalence of HDL2 seems to be higher among individuals of African ancestry, and is similarly as common as HD in black South Africans. From a clinical point of view, the diagnosis of HDL2 should be strongly considered in individuals of African descendent with an autosomal dominant HD-like disorder. (Walker *et al.*, 2003; Margolis *et al.*, 2004) The core neuroacanthocytosis syndromes include autosomal recessive chorea-acanthocytosis (ChAc) and the X-linked McLeod syndrome (MLS), although rarely, HDL2 and pantothenate-kinase-associated neurodegeneration (PKAN) can also cause this syndrome (Danek *et al.*, 2005; Walker *et al.*, 2007). Other rare genetic causes of chorea are listed in Table 20.2 (Laplanche *et al.*, 1999; Moore *et al.*, 2001). Recently the incidence of BHC has

develop symptoms in the mid-thirties to mid-forties, but age of onset for HD ranges from early childhood to the seventies and eighties. Childhood- and juvenile-onset of HD, before the age of 20, is known as Westphal variant. Although chorea is the prototypical movement disorder in HD and usually present with middle-age or elderly onset, the motor impairment in HD can be quite heterogeneous,

Table 20.2 Genetic choreas.

Condition	Mode of inheritance	Gene/location	Protein product	Usual age of onset	Clinical pointers
HDL2	AD[a]	JPH3/16q	Junctophilin-3	20–40 yr	HD phenotype, sometimes acanthocytosis; almost exclusively African ethnicity.
SCA17	AD[a]	TBP/6q	TBP	10–30 yr	Cerebellar ataxia, chorea, dystonia, hyper-reflexia, cognitive decline
DRPLA	AD[a]	DRPLA/12p	Atrophin-1	About 20 yr	Variable phenotypic picture including chorea, ataxia, seizures, psychiatric disturbances, dementia; more common in Japan than in Europe or US
SCA3/MJD	AD[a]	MJD/14q	Ataxin-3	35–40 yr	Wide phenotypic variability with cerebellar ataxia, protruded eyes, chorea, dystonia, parkinsonian features, neuropathy, pyramidal tract features
SCA2	AD[a]	Ataxin-2/12q	Ataxin-2	30–35 yr	Cerebellar ataxia, chorea, markedly reduced velocity of saccadic eye movements, hyporeflexia
Chorea-acanthocytosis	AR	VPS13A (formerly CHAC)/9q	Chorein	20–50 yr	Orofacial self-mutilation, dystonia, neuropathy, myopathy, seizures, acanthocytosis
McLeod syndrome	X-linked, recessive	XK/Xp	XK-protein	40–70 yr	Dystonia, neuropathy, myopathy, cardiomyopathy, seizures, acanthocytosis, CK elevation
Neuroferritinopathy	AD	FTL/19q	FTL	20–55 yr	Chorea, dystonia, parkinsonian features; usually reduced serum ferritin; MR abnormalities with cyst formation and increased T2 signal in GP and putamen

(continued)

Table 20.2 (Continued).

Condition	Mode of inheritance	Gene/location	Protein product	Usual age of onset	Clinical pointers
AT and ATLD	AR	ATM/11q (AT), MRE11/11q (ATLD)	ATM (AT), MRE 11 (ATLD)	Childhood	Ataxia, neuropathy, oculomotor apraxia, other extrapyramidal manifestations including chorea, dystonia and myoclonus; in AT: oculocutaneous telangiectasias; predisposition to malignancies IgA and IgG deficiency, elevated serum AFP and CEA levels
AOA 1 and 2	AR	APTX/9p (AOA 1), SETX/9q (AOA 2)	Aprataxin (AOA 1), Senataxin (AOA 2)	Childhood or adolescence (later onset in AOA 2)	Ataxia, neuropathy, oculomotor apraxia, other extrapyramidal manifestations including chorea and dystonia; AOA 1: hypoalbuminemia and hypercholesterolemia; AOA 2: elevated serum AFP
Pantothenate kinase associated neurodegeneration (formerly Hallervorden–Spatz syndrome)	AR	PANK2/20p	Pantothenate kinase 2	Childhood, but also adult-onset subtype	Chorea, dystonia, parkinsonian features, pyramidal tract features; MR abnormalities with decreased T2 signal in the GP and SN, "eye of the tiger" sign (hyperintense area within the hypointense area); sometimes acanthocytosis, abnormal cytosomes in lymphocytes
Lesch–Nyhan disease	X-linked, recessive	HPRT/Xq	Hypoxanthine-guanine phosphoribosyl-transferase	Childhood	Chorea, dystonia, hypotonia, self-injurious behavior with biting of fingers and lips, mental retardation; short stature, renal calculi, hyeruricemia

Disease	Inheritance	Gene/locus	Gene product	Age of onset	Clinical features
Wilson's disease	AR	ATP7B/13q	Copper transporting P-type ATPase	<40 yr	Parkinsonian features, dystonia, tremor, rarely chorea, behavioral and cognitive change, corneal Kayser–Fleischer rings, liver disease
PKC syndrome and ICCA syndrome	AD	Unknown/16p	Unknown	<1–40 yr	Paroxysmal movement disorders with dramatic response to low dose carbamazepine (PKC); recurrent brief episodes of abnormal involuntary movements in association with infantile convulsions (ICCA)
BHC	AD	TITF-1/14q; other	Thyroid transcription factor 1	Childhood	Chorea, mild ataxia; genetically heterogeneous

HDL1, HDL3 and HDL4 are very rare conditions (only one family known) and therefore not integrated in the table.

[a] Disorders based on expanded CAG repeats (HDL2 based on CAG/CTG repeats; SCA 17 based on CAG/CAA repeats); age of symptom onset inversely related to repeat size.

HD, Huntington's disease; HDL, HD-like; SCA, spinocerebellar ataxia; MJD, Machado–Joseph Disease; BHC, benign hereditary chorea; DRPLA, dentatorubropallidoluysian atrophy; AT, ataxia telangiectasia; ATDL, AT-like disorder; AOA, ataxia with oculomotor apraxia; PKD/PKC, Paroxysmal kinesigenic dyskinesias/choreoathetosis; AFP, α-fetoprotein; CEA carcinoembryogenic antigen been growing . Patients with this condition, an autosomal dominant illness, have a mutation in the TITF-1 gene, which codes for a transcription factor essential for the organogenesis of the lung, thyroid, and basal ganglia (Kleiner-Fisman *et al.*, 2003). In fact, the clinical picture of these patients is characterized by a variable combination of chorea, mental retardation, congenital hypothyroidism and chronic lung disease, hence the term Brain-Thyroid-Lung syndrome, proposed for this disease (Willemsen *et al.*, 2005; Devos *et al.*, 2006).

Vascular Choreas

Aside levodopa-induced chorea in Parkinson's disease, cerebro-vascular disease is the most common cause of non-genetic chorea (Piccolo *et al.*, 2003). Nevertheless, chorea is an unusual complication of acute vascular lesion, seen in less than 1% of patients with acute stroke (Cardoso *et al.*, 2006). Vascular hemichorea or hemiballism, is usually related to ischemic or hemorrhagic lesion of the basal ganglia and adjacent white matter in the region of the middle or the posterior cerebral artery. The majority of patients with hemichorea-hemiballism have diabetes mellitus. The association of hyperglycemia in type II diabetes, micro-hemorrhage in the pallidum, seen on MRI scans, and chorea has been particularly described among Asians (Lai *et al.*, 2004). The natural history of hemiballism-hemichorea usually includes spontaneous remission.

An uncommon cause of vascular chorea is Moyamoya disease, an intracranial vasculopathy that presents with ischemic lesion or, less commonly, hemorrhagic stroke of the basal ganglia (Gonzalez-Alegre *et al.*, 2003). Another rare form of vascular chorea is "post-pump chorea"—a complication of extracorporeal circulation. The pathogenesis of this movement disorder is believed to be related to vascular insult of the basal ganglia during the surgical procedure. The natural history of post-pump chorea is benign, with spontaneous remission in most cases (Thobois *et al.*, 2004).

Sydenham Chorea (SC)

SC is the most common form of autoimmune chorea. The usual age at onset of SC chorea is 8–9 years, but there are reports on patients who developed chorea during the third decade of life. In most series, there is a female preponderance (Cardoso, Silva and Mota, 1997). Typically, patients develop this disease 4–8 weeks after an episode of group A β-hemolytic streptococcal pharyngitis. The chorea spreads rapidly and becomes generalized, but 20% of patients remain with hemichorea (Nausieda *et al.*, 1980; Cardoso, Silva and Mota, 1997). Patients display motor impersistence, particularly noticeable during tongue protrusion and

ocular fixation. The muscle tone is usually decreased; in severe and rare cases (1.5% of all patients seen at the Movement Disorders Clinic of the Federal University of Minas Gerais, Brazil) this is so pronounced that the patient may become bedridden (chorea paralytica).

Patients often display other neurologic and non-neurologic symptoms and signs. There are reports of common occurrence of tics in SC (Mercadante *et al.*, 1997). In a cohort of 120 SC patients followed up at the Movement Disorders Clinic of the Federal University of Minas Gerais, we have identified complex tics in fewer than 4% of subjects. There is evidence that many patients with active chorea have hypometric saccades, and a few of them also show oculogyric crisis. Dysarthria, as well as reduction of verbal fluency are common. In a case-control study of patients, we described a pattern of decreased verbal fluency that reflected reduced phonetic, but not semantic, output (Cunningham *et al.*, 2006). Studying adults with SC, we have extended this finding, showing that many functions dependent on the prefrontal area are impaired in these patients. The conclusion of this study is that SC should be included among the causes of dysexecutive syndrome (Cardoso *et al.*, 2005).

Attention has also been drawn to behavioral abnormalities in SC. Swedo and colleagues found obsessive-compulsive behavior in 5 out of 13 SC patients, 3 of whom met criteria for obsessive-compulsive disorder, whereas no patient in the rheumatic-fever group presented with obsessive-compulsive behavior (Swedo *et al.*, 1988). Recently, Maia and colleagues investigated behavioral abnormalities in 50 healthy subjects, 50 patients with rheumatic fever without chorea and 56 patients with SC (Maia *et al.*, 2005). The authors found that obsessive-compulsive behavior, obsessive-compulsive disorder, and attention deficit and hyperactivity disorder were more frequent in the SC group (19%, 23.2%, 30.4%) than in the healthy controls (11%, 4%, 8%) or in the patients with rheumatic fever without chorea (14%, 6%, 8%). In this study, the authors demonstrated that obsessive-compulsive behavior displays little degree of interference in the performance of the activities of daily living. Another study compared the phenomenology of obsessions and compulsions of patients with SC with subjects diagnosed with tic disorders (Asbahr *et al.*, 2005). The authors demonstrated that the symptoms observed among the SC patients were different from those reported by patients with tic disorders, but were similar to those previously noted among samples of pediatric patients with primary obsessive-compulsive disorder. A recent investigation comparing healthy controls with patients with rheumatic fever showed that obsessive-compulsive behavior is more commonly seen in patients with SC with relatives who also have obsessions and compulsions (Hounie *et al.*, 2007). This finding suggests a role for genetic predisposition to the development of behavioral problems in SC. We recently reported that, although rarely, SC may induce psychosis during the acute phase of the illness (Teixeira, Maia and Cardoso, 2007).

Finally, it must be kept in mind that SC is a major manifestation of rheumatic fever. In SC, 60–80% of patients display cardiac involvement, particularly mitral valve dysfunction, whereas the association with arthritis is less common, seen in 30% of patients; however, in approximately 20% of patients, chorea is the sole finding (Cardoso, Silva and Mota, 1997). A prospective follow-up of patients with SC with and without cardiac involvement in the first episode of chorea suggests that the heart remains spared in those without lesion at the onset of the rheumatic fever (Panamonta *et al.*, 2007). The current diagnostic criteria of SC are a modification of the Jones criteria: chorea with acute or sub-acute onset and lack of clinical and laboratory evidence of an alternative cause are mandatory findings. The diagnosis is further supported by the presence of additional major or minor manifestations of rheumatic fever (Guidelines for diagnosis of rheumatic fever, Jones criteria, 1992; Cardoso, Silva and Mota, 1997, Cardoso *et al.*, 1999). Recently, the first validated scale to rate SC was published, the Universidade Federal de Minas Gerais Sydenham Chorea Rating Scale. It comprises 27 items, and each is scored from 0 (no symptom or sign) to 4 (severe disability or finding) (Teixeira, Maia and Cardoso, 2005a).

Other Autoimmune Choreas

Other immunologic causes of chorea are systemic lupus erythematosus (SLE), primary anti-phospholipid antibody syndrome (PAPS), vasculitis and paraneoplastic syndromes. Despite SLE or PAPS being described as the prototypes of autoimmune choreas (Quinn and Schrag, 1998), several reports show that chorea is seen in no more than 1–2% of large series of patients with these conditions (Asherson and Cervera, 2003; Sanna *et al.*, 2003). Autoimmune chorea has rarely been reported in the context of paraneoplastic syndromes associated with anti-Hu and/or anti-CRMP5 antibodies in rare patients with small-cell lung carcinoma (Kinirons *et al.*, 2003; Dorban *et al.*, 2004).

Infectious Choreas

Human immunodeficiency virus (HIV) and its complications has been the most commonly reported infectious cause of chorea. In one series of 42 consecutive patients with non-genetic chorea, for instance, AIDS was found to be the cause in 12% of the subjects (Piccolo *et al.*, 2003). Other infections related to chorea are new variant Creutzfeldt–Jakob disease and tuberculosis (Kalita *et al.*, 2003; McKee and Talbot, 2003).

Drug-Induced Choreas

Probably these are the most commonly encountered types of chorea in neurological practice and in the community (Wenning *et al.*, 2005). Certain drugs seem to require pre-existing basal ganglia dysfunction to induce chorea, whereas others appear to be more universally choreogenic. An example of the former is levodopa (Fahn, 2000), which only induces chorea in patients with idiopathic PD or other parkinsonian disorders. Levodopa-induced chorea develops in more than 40% of PD patients depending on age, and duration and dose of levodopa treatment (Schrag and Quinn, 2000). This issue is tackled in other chapters of this book. On the other hand, dopamine antagonists are capable of inducing dyskinesias without pre-existing basal ganglia abnormality. However, chorea as part of tardive dyskinesia is a rare finding: in a consecutive study of 100 patients with this condition, none of them was found to have chorea (Stacy, Cardoso and Jankovic, 1993). The bucco-linguomasticatory syndrome with repetitive movements of tongue twisting and protusion, lip smacking and chewing movements, so typical of neuroleptic-induced tardive dyskinesia in the elderly, is better defined as stereotypy. Furthermore, a variety of other agents have been associated with chorea in retrospective studies or anecdotal case reports (Table 20.3). These include both trycyclic antidepressants and SSRIs (Miller and Jankovic, 1990; Bharucha and Sethi, 1996; Fox, Ebeid and Vincenti, 1997). Phenytoin may also induce involuntary movements including orofacial chorea, particularly when other antiepileptic drugs are administered (Harrison, Lyons and Landow, 1993). There are occasional reports of chorea induced by other anti-epileptic drugs, such as carbamazepine (Bimpong-Buta and Froescher, 1982) and, more recently, lamotrigine (Zaatreh *et al.*, 2001). Chronic exposure to amphetamines and other stimulants may induce orofacial dyskinesias and choreic movements of the trunk and extremities (Stork and Cantor, 1997; Morgan, Winter and Wooten, 2004).

Pathophysiology

Etiologically diverse types of chorea like HD, levodopa-induced chorea in PD or hemichorea following lesions of the STN could all be explained by deficient GPi inhibitory input to the motor thalamus resulting in excessive thalamocortical motor facilitation. However, there are also inconsistencies between the model and clinical evidence, including the abolition of drug-induced chorea in PD through ablation of the GPi (pallidotomy) which, according to the model, should lead to increased excitatory thalamocortical drive and thus worsening of chorea. Current views therefore maintain that more complex changes in the temporal and spatial firing pattern of the GPi underlie

Table 20.3 Drug-induced choreas.

Dopamine receptor blocking agents
- Phenothiazines
- Butyrophenones
- Benzamides

Antiparkinsonian drugs
- L-Dopa
- DA-agonists
- Anti-cholinergics

Antiepileptic drugs
- Phenytoin
- Carbamazepine
- Valproate

Stimulants
- Amphetamines
- Pemoline
- Cocaine
- Theophylline

Ca^{+2}-channel blockers
- Cinnarizine
- Flunarizine
- Verapamil

Others
- Lithium
- Baclofen
- Digoxin
- Tricyclic anti-depressants
- Cyclosporine
- Steroids

hyperkinetic movement disorders such as chorea (Obeso et al., 2002; Mink, 2003; Moro et al., 2004).

Taranta and Stollerman established the casual relationship between infection with group A β-hemolytic streptococci and occurrence of SC (Taranta and Stollerman, 1956). Based on the assumption of molecular mimicry between streptococcal and central nervous system antigens, it has been proposed that the bacterial infection in genetically predisposed subjects leads to formation of cross-reactive antibodies that disrupt the basal ganglia function. Several studies have demonstrated the presence of such circulating antibodies in 50–90% of patients with SC (Husby et al., 1976; Church et al., 2002). A specific epitope of streptococcal M proteins that cross-reacts with basal ganglia has been identified (Bronze and Dale, 1993). In a study of patients seen at the Movement Disorders Clinic of the Federal University of Minas Gerais, we found that all patients with active SC have anti-basal ganglia antibodies

demonstrated by ELISA and Western Blot. In subjects with persistent SC (duration of disease greater than two years, despite best medical treatment) the positivity was about 60% (Church et al., 2002). It must be emphasized that the biological value of the anti-basal ganglia antibodies remains controversial (Cardoso, 2005). Our finding that there is a linear correlation between the increase of intracellular calcium levels in PC12 cells and anti-basal ganglia antibody titer in the serum from SC chorea patients suggests that these antibodies have a pathogenic value (Teixeira et al., 2005b). Because of the difficulties with the molecular mimicry hypothesis in accounting for the pathogenesis of SC, there have been recent studies suggesting a role of immune cellular mechanisms in this condition. (Teixeira et al., 2004) Some authors have suggested that streptococcal infection induces vasculitis of medium-sized vessels, leading to neuronal dysfunction. Such vascular lesions could be produced by anti-phospholipid antibodies. Currently, the weight of evidence suggests that the pathogenesis of SC is related to circulating cross-reactive antibodies.

Vascular chorea is usually the result of necrotic ischemic lesion of the basal ganglia. However, in contrast to classical textbook concepts of hemiballism, the majority of patients with this type of chorea have lesions outside the subthalamus (Ghika-Schmid et al., 1997). In HIV-positive patients, chorea is the result of either the direct action of the virus or other mechanisms, such as opportunistic infections (toxoplasmosis, syphilis and others) which directly damage the basal ganglia, or drugs which interfere with dopaminergic transmission (Cardoso, 2002). The underlying pathophysiology of tardive chorea remains to be determined, but it may include post-synaptic dopamine hypersensitivity or striatal neuroplastic changes (Poewe, Lees and Stern, 1986; Quinn and Schrag, 1998; Margolese et al., 2005). Details of the pathogenesis of HD are provided in Chapter 19.

MANAGEMENT

With the possible exception of HD, there have been very few controlled studies of treatment of different types of chorea. In each of the items of this section, first a review of controlled clinical trials, followed by open studies, will be given and, finally, practical recommendations by the author. Table 20.4 contains general principles for the management of chorea. One principle that generally guides the choice of anti-choreic agents is their ability to powerfully block D2 receptors. With the exception of amantadine (see below), all drugs effective in providing symptomatic improvement of chorea have high affinity towards this family of dopamine receptors. This explains why atypical agents, such as quetiapine and clozapine, often used to treat psychosis in patients with movement disorders are usually ineffective in controlling chorea.

Table 20.4 Management of chorea—general principles.

Step 1:

Treat underlying condition

o   Drug-induced chorea

Remove/modify offending drug (See also Chapter 10)

o   Infectious chorea

HART for HIV encephalopathy

Sulfadiazin, pyrimethamin, and so on for CNS toxoplasmosis

o   Metabolic chorea

Correct underlying abnormality (See Table 20.1)

o   Autoimmune chorea

LES: Immunosuppression with methylprednisolone (1 g/ day for adults or 25 mg/kg in children/kg/day i.v. for five days) followed by 1 mg/kg per day of prednisone. In refractory cases other agents such as cyclophosphamide or azathioprin may be necessary.

PAPS: Anti-coagulation with warfarin.

Sydenham chorea: See Table 20.5

Step 2:

Introduce symptomatic anti-choreic drug therapy. Risperidone (initial dosage of 1 mg/d which can be increased up to 6 mg/day or intolerable adverse effects, such as acute dystonic reaction, parkinsonism, sedation occur)

Other options are olanzapine, initial daily dosage of 2,5 mg; haloperidol, starting at 1 mg a day; or pimozide, initial dose of 2 mg. Olanzapine is relatively well tolerated although less effective than risperidone. Haloperidol and olanzapine are at least as effective as risperidone, but less well tolerated due to the potential of induction of extrapyramidal side-effects and, in the case of pimozide, cardiac block in children. Amantadine (300 mg daily) or tetrabenazine (25–100 mg a day) may have a role in the management of chorea associated to HD. Options more rarely used as anti-choreic agents are fluphenazine, sulpiride or tiapride.

Step 3:

Consider surgery (posteroventral pallidotomy or GPi stimulation) in severe refractory cases with disabling chorea).

Genetic Choreas

Bonelli and Wenning (2006) recently performed a systematic review of therapeutic trials of HD from 1965 through 2005. They identified 218 publications on pharmacological interventions in HD since 1965. Among them were 20 level-I (randomized clinical trials), 55 level-II (non-randomized, controlled clinical studies) and 54 level-III trials (open-label investigations). They concluded that haloperidol, fluphenazine and olanzapine are "possibly useful" for the treatment of chorea. Other agents, such as amantadine, riluzole and tetrabenazine were considered "investigational" for this purpose. L-dopa and pramipexole were also considered "possibly useful" for the management of rigidity; amitryptiline and mirtazapine, for depression; risperidone for psychosis; and olanzapine, haloperidol, and buspirone for behavioral symptoms. Co-enzyme Q10, minocycline, and unsaturated fatty acids were regarded as "investigational" for possible neuroprotection. Since this publication, a multi-center, placebo-controlled study demonstrated that tetrabenazine is useful in the management of chorea related to HD despite the high dropout rate and frequency of serious adverse events (especially depression) (Huntington Study Group, 2006). Chapter 19 contains further details of the management of HD.

There are no controlled studies of treatment of other genetic causes of chorea. Overall, the principles discussed relating to HD also apply to these conditions. There are, however, peculiarities in some cases. A substantial proportion of patients with chorea-acanthocytosis present with a self-mutilating tongue-biting dystonia. This dyskinesia can be quite disabling, preventing these patients from eating properly, as well as resulting in severe injuries. In the author's experience, botulinum toxin injections of the genioglossus muscle can provide substantial and lasting relief. Another clinical feature common in this condition is seizure disorder, requiring use of anti-epileptic drugs. The kinesigenic paroxysmal dyskinesias are quite sensitive to low doses of anti-epileptic drugs whereas non-kinesigenic dyskinesia (Mount–Reback syndrome) responds to benzodiazepines (Demirkiran and Jankovic, 1995; Bruno et al., 2007). Finally, there is one report suggesting that levodopa can be effective in the treatment of BHC (Asmus et al., 2005).

Sydenham Chorea

With one exception, discussed below, there are no controlled studies of symptomatic treatment of SC. The first choice of the author is valproic acid with an initial dosage of 250 mg per day that is increased over a two-week period to 250 mg three times a day. If the response is not satisfactory, dosage can be increased gradually to 1500 mg per day. As this drug has a rather slow onset of action, one should wait two weeks before concluding that a dosage regimen is ineffective. There is evidence from open-label studies that carbamazepine (15 mg/kg per day) is as affective as valproic acid (20 mg/kg per day to 25 mg/kg per day) to induce remission of chorea (Genel et al., 2002).

If the patient fails to respond to this medication, the next option is to prescribe neuroleptics. Risperidone, a moderately potent dopamine D2 receptor blocker, is usually effective in controlling the hyperkinesias. The usual initial regimen is 1 mg a day. If, two weeks later, the chorea is still troublesome, the dosage is increased to twice a day. Neuroleptics are the first choice of treatment in the rare patients who present with chorea paralytica. Dopamine D2 receptor blockers must be used with great caution in patients with SC. There is evidence that, in comparison with other conditions, such as Tourette syndrome, patients with SC have a higher risk of development of drug-induced parkinsonism and dystonia (Teixeira *et al.*, 2003). There are no published guidelines concerning the discontinuation of anti-choreic agents. The author's policy is to attempt a gradual decrease of the dosage (25% reduction every two weeks) after the patient has remained free of chorea for at least one month. Finally, the most important measure in the treatment of patients with SC is secondary prophylaxis. The World Health Organization recommends penicillin or, if there is allergy, sulfa drugs up to age 21 years. If the onset occurs after this age, the recommendation is to maintain prophylaxis indefinitely (Cardoso *et al.*, 2006). Physicians practicing in areas of the world where rheumatic fever is not an important public health problem tend to maintain the prophylaxis for shorter periods of time (one year or even less).

Some controversy exists as to the role of immunosuppression in the management of SC. Despite mention of the effectiveness of prednisone in suppressing chorea, this drug is generally only used when there is associated severe carditis. There are few reports describing the usefulness of plasma exchange or intravenous immunoglobulin in SC. Because of the efficacy of other therapeutic agents described in the previous paragraph, potential complications and the high cost of the latter treatment modalities, these options are not usually recommended. In the author's practice, intravenous methylprednisolone is reserved for patients with persistent disabling chorea refractory to anti-choreic agents. We have reported that 25 mg/kg per day in children and 1 g/day in adults of methylprednisolone for five days followed by 1 mg/kg per day of prednisone is an effective and well-tolerated treatment for patients with SC refractory to conventional treatment with anti-choreic drugs and penicillin (Cardoso *et al.*, 2003; Teixeira, Maia and Cardoso, 2005c; Barash, Margalith and Matitiau, 2005). Finally, a recent double-blind study showed that oral prednisone (initial dosage of 1 mg/kg/day, gradually decreased depending on the clinical response) is faster than placebo in inducing remission of chorea (Paz, Silva and Marques-Dias, 2006). However, at the end of the follow-up there was no difference in the severity of the chorea or the rate of recurrence between the two groups. Table 20.5 summarizes the management of SC.

Table 20.5 Management of Sydenham chorea.

1. Symptomatic anti-choreic therapy
   Step 1: Valproic acid (start with 250 mg/day, increase to 750–1500/day as needed) (carbamazepine 15 mg/kg per day might be equally effective)
   Step 2: Risperidone (1 mg/d to 2 mg/day)
   (Other options are haloperidol, starting at 1 mg a day, or pimozide, initial dose of 2 mg, although are less well tolerated due to the potential of induction of extrapyramidal side effects and, in the case of the latter, cardiac block in children)
   Step 3: For patients refractary to anti-choreic therapies 5 d of i.v. methylprednisolone (1 g/day for adults or 25 mg/kg in children/kg/day is followed by 1 mg/kg per day per o.s. until chorea resolves when dosage is tapered down)

2. Prophylaxis of streptococcus infection
   Penicillin benzathin (1 200 000U IM every 21 d for at 6 mo or, if in areas where rheumatic fever is endemic, until age 18 yr). If there is allergy to penicillin, sulfadiazine is an option (500 mg every 6 h per o.s. for the same duration as described above for penicillin)

Other Choreas

Spontaneous remission is the rule in vascular choreas. Treatment with anti-choreic drugs, such as neuroleptics or dopamine depletors, however, is often necessary in the acute phase when patients present with hemichorea-hemiballism. A few patients with vascular chorea may remain with persistent movement disorders. In this circumstance, they can be effectively treated with stereotactic surgery, such as thalamotomy or posteroventral pallidotomy (Cardoso *et al.*, 1995; Cubo *et al.*, 2000; Choi *et al.*, 2003; Krauss *et al.*, 2003; Moro *et al.*, 2004). Of note, surgery, pallidotomy and GPi DBS have been reported as effective in treating chorea associated with other causes, such as HD and cerebral palsy (Cubo *et al.*, 2000; Krauss *et al.*, 2003; Moro *et al.*, 2004).

Chorea associated with SLE or PAPS has been treated with immunosuppressive measures, especially i.v. methylprednisolone following a dosage regimen as described for SC. As it is accepted that neurological complications, including chorea, in PAPS are related to ischemic events, anti-platelet agents and even anti-coagulants are often prescribed to treat chorea in this condition (Levine and Brey, 1996). These recommendations are, however, based on reports of open-label studies involving small numbers of patients, as well as the clinical experience of physicians (Cardoso *et al.*, 2006).

Levodopa-induced chorea in PD aside, the most important measure in the management of chorea related to drugs is the withdrawal of the offending agent. As described above, although chorea as part of tardive dyskinesia is a rare phenomenon, its management is an important clinical issue. Guidelines suggested are: (i) immediate discontinuation of the anti-dopaminergic agent thought to cause the dyskinesia; (ii) patients with psychiatric ailments often require pharmacological treatment with neuroleptics, which prevents them from being taken off these drugs. In this case, agents thought to be safe are quetiapine and clozapine. Drugs such as risperidone and olanzapine, despite being considered "atypical neuroleptics," have a sufficient potent D2 blocking action to render them not suitable for use in patients with tardive dyskinesia. There is not enough information available on the safety in terms of the extrapyramidal side effects of newer agents such as ziprasidone and aripripazole. Preliminay data, however, suggest that they also have a pharmacological profile unsafe for the management of this clinical problem (Friedman *et al.*, 2006); (iii) In cases where a drug is required to treat disabling neuroleptic-related chorea, the choice is tetrabenazine (Kenney, Hunter and Jankovic, 2007). This dopamine-depleting agent is not widely available and may induce worrisome side effects, such as depression, sedation, orthostatic hypotension and parkinsonism.

In other situations, such as choreas related to infections and metabolic/endocrine dysfunction, the most important therapeutic measure is the correction of the underlying cause. Symptomatic treatment of the movement disorder may be required in some instances (e.g., hemiballism due to opportunistic infection with lesion of the subthalamus in AIDS). In these cases, the drugs of choice are neuroleptics (Cardoso, 2002).

References

Asbahr, F.R., Garvey, M.A., Snider, L.A. *et al.* (2005) Obsessive-compulsive symptoms among patients with Sydenham chorea. *Biological Psychiatry*, **57**, 1073–1076.

Asherson, R.A. and Cervera, R. (2003) Unusual manifestations of the antiphospholipid syndrome. *Clinical Reviews in Allergy & Immunology*, **25**, 61–78.

Asmus, F., Horber, V., Pohlenz, J. *et al.* (2005) A novel TITF-1 mutation causes benign hereditary chorea with response to levodopa. *Neurology*, **64**, 1952–1954.

Andrew, S.E., Goldberg, Y.P., Kremer, B. *et al.* (1994) Huntington disease without CAG expansion: phenocopies or errors in assignment? *American Journal of Human Genetics*, **54**, 852–863.

Barash, J., Margalith, D. and Matitiau, A. (2005) Corticosteroid treatment in patients with Sydenham's chorea. *Pediatric Neurology*, **32**, 205–207.

Bauer, P., Laccone, F., Rolfs, A. *et al.* (2004) Trinucleotide repeat expansion in SCA17/TBP in white patients with Huntington's disease-like phenotype. *Journal of Medical Genetics*, **41**, 230–232.

Bharucha, K.J. and Sethi, K.D. (1996) Complex movement disorders induced by fluoxetine. *Movement Disorders*, **11**, 324–326.

Bimpong-Buta, K. and Froescher, W. (1982) Carbamazepine-induced choreoathetoid dyskinesias. *Journal of Neurology, Neurosurgery, and Psychiatry*, **45**, 560.

Bonelli, R.M. and Wenning, G.K. (2006) Pharmacological management of Huntington's disease: an evidence-based review. *Current Pharmaceutical Design*, **12**, 2701–2720.

Breedveld, G.J., Percy, A.K., MacDonald, M.E. *et al.* (2002) Clinical and genetic heterogeneity in benign hereditary chorea. *Neurology*, **59**, 579–584.

Bronze, M.S. and Dale, J.B. (1993) Epitopes of streptococcal M proteins that evoke antibodies that cross-react with human brain. *Journal of Immunology (Baltimore, MD: 1950)*, **151**, 2820–2828.

Bruno, M.K., Lee, H.Y., Auburger, G.W., Friedman, A. *et al.* (2007) Genotype-phenotype correlation of paroxysmal nonkinesigenic dyskinesia. *Neurology*, **68**, 1782–1789.

Caine, E.D. and Shoulson, I. (1983) Psychiatric syndromes in Huntington's disease. *The American Journal of Psychiatry*, **140**, 728–733.

Cardoso, F. (2002) HIV-related movement disorders: epidemiology, pathogenesis and management. *CNS Drugs*, **16**, 663–668.

Cardoso, F. (2005) Tourette syndrome: autoimmune mechanism, in *Pediatric Movement Disorders. Progress in understanding* (eds E. Fernández-Alvarez, A. Arzimanoglou and E Tolosa), John Libbey Eurotext, Montrouge, pp. 23–46.

Cardoso, F., Jankovic, J., Grossman, R.G. and Hamilton, W.J. (1995) Outcome after stereotactic thalamotomy for dystonia and hemiballismus. *Neurosurgery*, **36**, 501–507.

Cardoso, F., Silva, C.E. and Mota, C.C. (1997) Sydenham's chorea in 50 consecutive patients with rheumatic fever. *Movement Disorders*, **12**, 701–703.

Cardoso, F., Vargas, A.P., Oliveira, L.D., Guerra, A.A. and Amaral, S.V. (1999) Persistent Sydenham's chorea. *Movement Disorders*, **14**, 805–807.

Cardoso, F., Maia, D., Cunningham, M.C. and Valenca, G. (2003) Treatment of Sydenham chorea with corticosteroids. *Movement Disorders*, **18**, 1374–1377.

Cardoso, F., Beato, R., Siqueira, C.F. and Lima, C.F. (2005) Neuropsychological performance and brain SPECT Imaging in adult patients with Sydenham's chorea. *Neurology*, **64** (Suppl 1), A76.

Cardoso, F., Seppi, K., Mair, K.J., Wenning, G.K. and Poewe, W. (2006) Seminar on choreas. *The Lancet Neurology*, **5**, 589–602.

Carella, F., Scaioli, V., Ciano, C., Binelli, S., Oliva, D. and Girotti, F. (1993) Adult onset myoclonic Huntington's disease. *Movement Disorders*, **8**, 201–205.

Choi, S.J., Lee, S.W., Kim, M.C. *et al.* (2003) Posteroventral pallidotomy in medically intractable postapoplectic monochorea: case report. *Surgical Neurology*, **59**, 486–490.

Church, A.J., Cardoso, F., Dale, R.C. *et al.* (2002) Anti-basal ganglia antibodies in acute and persistent Sydenham's chorea. *Neurology*, **59**, 227–231.

Cubo, E., Shannon, K.M., Penn, R.D. and Kroin, J.S. (2000) Internal globus pallidotomy in dystonia secondary to Huntington's disease. *Movement Disorders*, **15**, 1248–1251.

Cunningham, M.C., Maia, D.P., Teixeira, A.L. and Cardoso, F. (2006) Sydenham's chorea is associated with decreased verbal fluency. *Parkinsonism & Related Disorders*, **12**, 165–167.

Danek, A., Jung, H.H., Melone, M.A., Rampoldi L., Broccoli, V. and Walker, R.H. (2005) Neuroacanthocytosis: new developments in a selected group of dementing disorders. *Journal of Neurological Science*, **229–230**, 171–186.

Demirkiran, M. and Jankovic, J. (1995) Paroxysmal dyskinesias: clinical features and classification. *Annals of Neurology*, **38**, 571–579.

Devos, D., Vuillaume, I., de Becdelievre, A. *et al.* (2006) New syndromic form of benign hereditary chorea is associated with a deletion of TITF-1 and PAX-9 contiguous genes. *Movement Disorders*, **21**, 2237–2240.

Dorban, S., Gille, M., Kessler, R., Pieret, F., Declercq, I. and Sindic, C.J. (2004) Chorea-athetosis in the anti-Hu syndrome. *Revue Neurologique*, **160**, 126–129.

Fahn, S. (2000) The spectrum of levodopa-induced dyskinesias. *Annals of Neurology*, **47**, S2–S9.

Fox, G.C., Ebeid, S. and Vincenti, G. (1997) Paroxetine-induced chorea. *Br J Psychiatry*, **170**, 193–194.

Friedman, J.H., Berman, R.M., Goetz, C.G., Factor, S.A., Ondo, W.G., Wojcieszek, J., Carson, W.H. and Marcus, R.N. (2006) Open-label flexible-dose pilot study to evaluate the safety and tolerability of aripiprazole in patients with psychosis associated with Parkinson's disease. *Movement Disorders*, **21**, 2078–2081.

Genel, F., Arslanoglu, S., Uran, N. and Saylan, B. (2002) Sydenham's chorea: clinical findings and comparison of the efficacies of sodium valproate and carbamazepine regimens. *Brain & Development*, **24**, 73–76.

Ghika-Schmid, F., Ghika, J., Regli, F. and Bogousslavsky, J. (1997) Hyperkinetic movement disorders during and after acute stroke: the Lausanne Stroke Registry. *Journal of the Neurological Sciences*, **146**, 109–116.

Goetz, C.G. (2000) William Osler: On chorea: on Charcot. *Annals of Neurology*, **47**, 404–407.

Goetz, C.G., Chmura, T.A. and Lanska, D.J. (2001) History of movement disorders as a neurological specialty: Part 14 of the MDS-sponsored History of Movement Disorders exhibit, Barcelona, June 2000. *Movement Disorders*, **16**, 954–959.

Gonzalez-Alegre, P., Ammache, Z., Davis, P.H. and Rodnitzky, R.L. (2003) Moyamoya-induced paroxysmal dyskinesia. *Movement Disorders*, **18**, 1051–1056.

Guidelines for the diagnosis of rheumatic fever, Jones criteria (1992) 1992 update. Special Writing Group of the Committee of Rheumatic Fever, Endocarditis, and Kawasaki Disease of the Council on Cardio-Vascular Disease of the Young of the American Heart Association . Guidelines for the diagnosis of rheumatic fever. *Journal of the American Medical Association*, **268**, 2069–2073.

Guttman, M., Alpay, M. and Chouinard, S. *et al.* (2003) Clinical management of psychosis and mood disorders in Huntington's disease, in *Mental and Behavioral Dysfunction in Movement Disorders* (eds M.A. Bédard, Y. Agid, S. Chouinard, S. Fahn, A.D. Korczyn and P. Lesperance), Humana Press, Totowa, New Jersey, pp. 409–426.

Harrison, M.B., Lyons, G.R. and Landow, E.R. (1993) Phenytoin and dyskinesias: a report of two cases and review of the literature. *Movement Disorders*, **8**, 19–27.

Ho, A.K., Sahakian, B.J., Brown, R.G. *et al.* (2003) Profile of cognitive progression in early Huntington's disease. *Neurology*, **61**, 1702–1706.

Hounie, A.G., Pauls, D.L., do Rosario-Campos, M.C. *et al.* (2007) Obsessive-compulsive spectrum disorders and rheumatic fever: a family study. *Biological Psychiatry*, **61**, 266–272.

Huntington, G. (1872) On Chorea. *The Medical and Surgical Reporter: A Weekly Journal*, **26**, 317–321.

Huntington Study Group (2006) Tetrabenazine as antichorea therapy in Huntington disease: a randomized controlled trial. *Neurology*, **66**, 366–372.

Husby, G., Van De Rijn, U., Zabriskie, J.B., Abdin, Z.H. and Williams, R.C., Jr (1976) Antibodies reacting with cytoplasm of subthalamic and caudate nuclei neurons in chorea and acute rheumatic fever. *The Journal of Experimental Medicine*, **144**, 1094–1110.

Jankovic, J. and Ashizawa, T. (1995) Tourettism associated with Huntington's disease. *Movement Disorders*, **10**, 103–105.

Kalita, J., Ranjan, P., Misra, U.K. and Das, B.K. (2003) Hemichorea: a rare presentation of tuberculoma. *Journal of the Neurological Sciences*, **208**, 109–111.

Kenney, C., Hunter, C. and Jankovic, J. (2007) Long-term tolerability of tetrabenazine in the treatment of hyperkinetic movement disorders. *Movement Disorders*, **22**, 193–197.

Kinirons, P., Fulton, A., Keoghan, M., Brennan, P., Farrell, M.A. and Moroney, J.T. (2003) Paraneoplastic limbic encephalitis (PLE) and chorea associated with CRMP-5 neuronal antibody. *Neurology*, **61**, 1623–1624.

Kirkwood, S.C., Su, J.L., Conneally, P. and Foroud, T. (2001) Progression of symptoms in the early and middle stages of Huntington disease. *Archives of Neurology*, **58**, 273–278.

Kleiner-Fisman, G., Rogaeva, E., Halliday, W. *et al.* (2003) Benign hereditary chorea: clinical, genetic, and pathological findings. *Annals of Neurology*, **54**, 244–247.

Krauss, J.K., Loher, T.J., Weigel, R., Capelle, H.H., Weber, S. and Burgunder, J.M. (2003) Chronic stimulation of the globus pallidus internus for treatment of non-dYT1 generalized dystonia and choreoathetosis: 2-year follow up. *Journal of Neurosurgery*, **98**, 785–792.

Lai, S.L., Tseng, Y.L., Hsu, M.C. and Chen, S.S. (2004) Magnetic resonance imaging and single-photon emission computed tomography changes in hypoglycemia-induced chorea. *Movement Disorders*, **19**, 475–478.

Lanska, D.J., Lanska, M.J., Lavine, L. and Schoenberg, B.S. (1988) Conditions associated with Huntington's disease at death. A case-control study. *Archives of Neurology*, **45**, 878–880.

Laplanche, J.L., Hachimi, K.H., Durieux, I. *et al.* (1999) Prominent psychiatric features and early onset in an inherited prion disease with a new insertional mutation in the prion protein gene. *Brain: A Journal of Neurology*, **122** (Pt 12), 2375–2386.

Lawrence, A.D., Sahakian, B.J., Hodges, J.R., Rosser, A.E., Lange, K.W. and Robbins, T.W. (1996) Executive and mnemonic functions in early Huntington's disease. *Brain: A Journal of Neurology*, **119** (Pt 5), 1633–1645.

Leigh, R.J., Newman, S.A., Folstein, S.E., Lasker, A.G. and Jensen, B.A. (1983) Abnormal ocular motor control in Huntington's disease. *Neurology*, **33**, 1268–1275.

Levine, S.R. and Brey, R.L. (1996) Neurological aspects of antiphospholipid antibody syndrome. *Lupus*, **5**, 347–353.

Maia, D.P., Teixeira, A.L., Jr, Cunningham, M.C.Q. and Cardoso, F. (2005) Obsessive Compulsive Behavior, Hyperactivity and Attention Deficit Disorder in Sydenham's Chorea. *Neurology*, **64**, 1799–1801.

Margolese, H.C., Chouinard, G., Kolivakis, T.T., Beauclair, L. and Miller, R. (2005) Tardive dyskinesia in the era of typical and atypical antipsychotics. Part 1: pathophysiology and mechanisms of induction. *Canadian Journal of Psychiatry-Revue Canadienne De Psychiatrie*, **50**, 541–547.

Margolis, R.L., Holmes, S.E., Rosenblatt, A. *et al.* (2004) Huntington's Disease-like 2 (HDL2) in North America and Japan. *Annals of Neurology*, **56**, 670–674.

Margolis, R.L. and Ross, C.A. (2003) Diagnosis of Huntington disease. *Clinical Chemistry*, **49**, 1726–1732.

Marshall, F. (2004) Clinical features and treatment of Huntington's disease, in *Movement Disorders: Neurological Principles and Practice* (eds R.L. Watts and W.C. Koller), McGraw-Hill, pp. 589–601.

McKee, D. and Talbot, P. (2003) Chorea as a presenting feature of variant Creutzfeldt-Jakob disease. *Movement Disorders*, **18**, 837–838.

Mendez, M.F. (1994) Huntington's disease: update and review of neuropsychiatric aspects. *International Journal of Psychiatry in Medicine*, **24**, 189–208.

Mercadante, M.T., Campos, M.C., Marques-Dias, M.J. *et al.* (1997) Vocal tics in Sydenham's chorea. *Journal of the American Academy of Child and Adolescent Psychiatry*, **36**, 305–306.

Miller, L.G. and Jankovic, J. (1990) Neurologic approach to drug-induced movement disorders: a study of 125 patients. *Southern Medical Journal*, **83**, 525–532.

Mink, J.W. (2003) The Basal Ganglia and involuntary movements: impaired inhibition of competing motor patterns. *Archives of Neurology*, **60**, 1365–1368.

Moore, R.C., Xiang, F., Monaghan, J. *et al.* (2001) Huntington disease phenocopy is a familial prion disease. *American Journal of Human Genetics*, **69**, 1385–1388.

Morgan, J.C., Winter, W.C. and Wooten, G.F. (2004) Amphetamine-induced chorea in attention deficit-hyperactivity disorder. *Movement Disorders*, **19**, 840–842.

Moro, E., Lang, A.E., Strafella, A.P. *et al.* (2004) Bilateral globus pallidus stimulation for Huntington's disease. *Annals of Neurology*, **56**, 290–294.

Nausieda, P.A., Grossman, B.J., Koller, W.C., Weiner, W.J. and Klawans, H.L. (1980) Sydenham's chorea: an update. *Neurology*, **30**, 331–334.

Obeso, J.A., Rodríguez-Oroz, M.C., Rodríguez, M., Arbizu, J., and Giménez-Amaya, J.M. (2002) The basal ganglia and disorders of movement: pathophysiological mechanisms. *News in Physiological Science*, **17**, 51–55.

Panamonta, M., Chaikitpinyo, A., Auvichayapat, N. *et al.* (2007) Evolution of valve damage in Sydenham's chorea during recurrence of rheumatic fever. *International Journal of Cardiology*, **119**, 73–79.

Paz, J.A., Silva, C.A. and Marques-Dias, M.J. (2006) Randomized double-blind study with prednisone in Sydenham's chorea. *Pediatric Neurology*, **34**, 264–269.

Piccolo, I., Defanti, C.A., Soliveri, P. *et al.* (2003) Cause and course in a series of patients with sporadic chorea. *Journal of Neurology*, **250**, 429–435.

Poewe, W.H., Lees, A.J. and Stern, G.M. (1986) Low-dose L-dopa therapy in Parkinson's disease: a 6-year follow-up study. *Neurology*, **36**, 1528–1530.

Quinn, N. and Schrag, A. (1998) Huntington's disease and other choreas. *Journal of Neurology*, **245**, 709–716.

Reuter, I., Hu, M.T., Andrews, T.C., Brooks, D.J., Clough, C. and Chaudhuri, K.R. (2000) Late onset levodopa responsive Huntington's disease with minimal chorea masquerading as Parkinson plus syndrome. *Journal of Neurology, Neurosurgery, and Psychiatry*, **68**, 238–241.

Rosenblatt, A. and Leroi, I. (2000) Neuropsychiatry of Huntington's disease and other basal ganglia disorders. *Psychosomatics*, **41**, 24–30.

Rosenblatt, A., Abbott, M.H., Gourley, L.M., Troncoso, J.C., Margolis, R.L., Brandt, J. and Ross, C.A. (2003) Predictors of neuropathological severity in 100 patients with Huntington's disease. *Annals of Neurology*, **54**, 488–493.

Sanna, G., Bertolaccini, M.L., Cuadrado, M.J. *et al.* (2003) Neuropsychiatric manifestations in systemic lupus erythematosus: prevalence and association with antiphospholipid antibodies. *The Journal of Rheumatology*, **30**, 985–992.

Schoenfeld, M., Myers, R.H., Cupples, L.A., Berkman, B., Sax, D.S. and Clark, E. (1984) Increased rate of suicide among patients with Huntington's disease. *Journal of Neurology, Neurosurgery, and Psychiatry*, **47**, 1283–1287.

Schrag, A. and Quinn, N. (2000) Dyskinesias and motor fluctuations in Parkinson's disease. A community-based study. *Brain: A Journal of Neurology*, **123** (Pt 11), 2297–2305.

Shiwach, R. (1994) Psychopathology in Huntington's disease patients. *Acta Psychiatrica Scandinavica*, **90**, 241–246.

Sorensen, S.A. and Fenger, K. (1992) Causes of death in patients with Huntington's disease and in unaffected first degree relatives. *Journal of Medical Genetics*, **29**, 911–914.

Stacy, M., Cardoso, F. and Jankovic, J. (1993) Tardive stereotypy and other movement disorders in tardive dyskinesias. *Neurology*, **43**, 937–941.

Stevanin, G., Camuzat, A., Holmes, S.E. *et al.* (2002) CAG/CTG repeat expansions at the Huntington's disease-like 2 locus are rare in Huntington's disease patients. *Neurology*, **58**, 965–967.

Stork, C.M. and Cantor, R. (1997) Pemoline induced acute choreoathetosis: case report and review of the literature. *Journal of Toxicology-Clinical Toxicology*, **35**, 105–108.

Swedo, S.E., Leonard, H.L., Garvey, M. *et al.* (1988) Pediatric autoimmune neuropsychiatric disorders associated with streptococcal infections: clinical description of the first 50 cases. *The American Journal of Psychiatry*, **155**, 264–271.

Tan, E.K., Jankovic, J. and Ondo, W. (2000) Bruxism in Huntington's disease. *Movement Disorders*, **15**, 171–173.

Taranta, A. and Stollerman, G.H. (1956) The relationship of Sydenham's chorea to infection with group A streptococci. *The American Journal of Medicine*, **20**, 1970.

Teixeira, A.L., Cardoso, F., Maia, D.P. and Cunningham, M.C. (2003) Sydenham's chorea may be a risk factor for drug induced parkinsonism. *Journal of Neurology, Neurosurgery, and Psychiatry*, **74**, 1350–1351.

Teixeira, A.L., Jr, Cardoso, F., Souza, A.L.S. and Teixeira, M.M. (2004) Increased serum concentrations of monokine induced by interferon-y/CXCL9 and interferon-y-inducible protein 10/CXCL-10 in Sydenham's chorea patients. *Journal of Neuroimmunology*, **150**, 157–162.

Teixeira, A.L., Jr, Maia, D.P. and Cardoso, F. (2005a) UFMG Sydenham's chorea rating scale (USCRS): Reliability and consistency. *Movement Disorders*, **20**, 585–591.

Teixeira, A.L., Jr, Guimarães, M.M., Romano-Silva, M.A. and Cardoso, F. (2005b) Serum from Sydenham's chorea patients modifies intracellular calcium levels in PC12 cells by a complement independent mechanism. *Movement Disorders*, **20**, 843–845.

Teixeira, A.L., Jr, Maia, D.P. and Cardoso, F. (2005c) Treatment of acute Sydenham's chorea with methyl-prednisolone pulse-therapy. *Parkinsonism & Related Disorders*, **11**, 327–330.

Teixeira, A.L., Jr, Maia, D.P. and Cardoso, F. (2007) Psychosis following acute Sydenham's chorea. *European Child & Adolescent Psychiatry*, **16**, 67–69.

Thobois, S., Bozio, A., Ninet, J., Akhavi, A. and Broussolle, E. (2004) Chorea after cardiopulmonary bypass. *European Neurology*, **51**, 46–47.

Walker, R.H., Rasmussen, A., Rudnicki, D. *et al.* (2003) Huntington's disease-like 2 can present as chorea-acanthocytosis. *Neurology*, **61**, 1002–1004.

Walker, R.H., Jung, H.H., Dobson-Stone, C., Rampoldi, L., Sano, A., Tison, F. and Danek, A. (2007) Neurologic phenotypes associated with acanthocytosis. *Neurology*, **68**, 92–98.

Wenning, G.K., Kiechl, S., Seppi, K. *et al.* (2005) Prevalence of movement disorders in men and women aged 50–89 years

(Bruneck Study cohort): a population-based study. *The Lancet Neurology*, **4**, 815–820.

Willemsen, M.A., Breedveld, G.J., Wouda, S. *et al.* (2005) Brain-Thyroid-Lung syndrome: a patient with a severe multisystem disorder due to a de novo mutation in the thyroid transcription factor 1 gene. *European Journal of Pediatrics*, **164**, 28–30.

Zaatreh, M., Tennison, M., D'Cruz, O. and Beach, R.L. (2001) Anticonvulsants-induced chorea: a role for pharmacodynamic drug interaction? *Seizure: The Journal of the British Epilepsy Association*, **10**, 596–599.

Zomorrodi, A. and Wald, E.R. (2006) Sydenham's chorea in western Pennsylvania. *Pediatrics*, **117**, e675–e679.

21

Treatment of Tics and Tourette Syndrome

Harvey S. Singer and Erika L.F. Hedderick

Johns Hopkins University School of Medicine, Baltimore, Maryland, USA

INTRODUCTION TO TIC DISORDERS

Tourette syndrome (TS) is named after Georges Gilles de la Tourette, who, in 1885, described a series of nine patients with the diagnosis of tic convulsif (Gilles de la Tourette, 1885). Initially felt to be a rare, psychological disorder, Tourette syndrome is now viewed as a common disorder with a prevalence of 1–10/1000 children and a genetic and biochemical basis. This syndrome represents one end of the spectrum of tic disorders, which includes the much more common transient tic disorder, chronic motor and vocal tic disorders and Tourettisms.

Tics, the hallmark component, are sudden, stereotypic, repetitive, rapid, involuntary movements or phonations. Correct diagnosis is based on careful history and observation, either directly or by video taped recording. Tics can be divided into simple and complex behaviors. Simple motor tics are brief, sudden, meaningless movements that include eye blinking, shoulder shrugging and head turning. Complex motor tics are longer in duration, involve a variety of muscle groups and can appear to be purposeful. Examples of complex motor tics are touching, facial or truncal contortions, brushing hair back or dystonic movements. Simple phonic tics include throat clearing, grunting, barking or sniffing, whereas complex vocalizations include the use of words, that is, echolalia, palilalia and coprolalia. It is important to note that coprolalia occurs in only 10% of patients. Tics can occur at any time throughout the day, but are generally not present in sleep and are less prominent during periods of concentration. Patients often report that tics are more severe in times of stress, anxiety, fatigue or following periods of intense activity. Tics tend to have a waxing and waning course with initial tics being replaced or added to others. Older patients often describe a premonitory urge prior to performing the tic. This urge may be suppressed for a period of time, but is then relieved by performance of the tic behavior.

Tics usually appear in the first decade of life, with a peak onset at approximately six to seven years of age. They tend to be most severe the between 7 and 12 years of age, after which there is a decline in tic severity (Leckman et al., 1998). One follow-up study of 58 teenagers and young adults, age 15 to 25 years, found that by self-report, tics almost disappeared in 26%, diminished substantially in 46%, were stable in 14% and were increased in 14% (Erenberg, Cruse and Rothner, 1987). Nevertheless, other studies show that 50% of adults with a history of tics in childhood who report tic freedom as adults, had tics on direct observation (Pappert et al., 2003).

Tic disorders are classified based on the types of tics present, as well as the duration of symptoms and are broadly separated into transient and chronic tic disorders:

- *Transient Tic Disorders.* Transient tic disorders are either motor or vocal tics or both, occurring for less than twelve months. This is the most common and least severe category.
- *Chronic Tic Disorders.* Chronic tic disorders are characterized by tics for greater than 12 months. The tics are either solely motor, both motor and vocal, or, less commonly, only vocal in nature.

TOURETTE SYNDROME

Formal diagnostic criteria, established by the Tourette Syndrome Classification Study Group, include the following:

1. Onset prior to age 21;
2. Multiple motor and at least one vocal tic must be present at some time, though not necessarily concurrently;
3. Waxing and waning course with progressive evolution;
4. Presence of tics for greater than 12 months;

Therapeutics of Parkinson's Disease and Other Movement Disorders   Edited by Mark Hallett and Werner Poewe
© 2008 John Wiley & Sons, Ltd.

5. Absence of precipitating illness (e.g., encephalitis, stroke or degenerative disease) or association with potential tic-inducing medication;
6. Observation by a knowledgeable individual.

The incidence of TS or other tic disorders is significantly elevated in family members suggesting a genetic basis for this syndrome. Support for a genetic basis is provided by twin studies, which show an 86% concordance rate for chronic tic disorders in monozygotic twins compared with 20% in dizygotic twins (Price *et al.*, 1985; Hyde *et al.*, 1992). However, neither a clear mode of inheritance nor a specific genetic linkage has been identified.

Associated Problems

Psychiatric co-morbidities are very common in TS, affecting more than half of all children and adolescents (Gaze, Kepley and Walkup, 2006). Often these associated conditions are more impairing than the tics themselves. A comprehensive evaluation for tics should include a thorough assessment for the following co-morbidities.

- *Attention Deficit Hyperactivity Disorder.* Attention deficit hyperactivity disorder (ADHD) is common in children and adolescents with TS. It is reported to affect 50–70% of patients (Comings and Comings, 1985, 1987). Whether there is a common genetic link between TS and ADHD remains controversial. This disorder generally presents at age 4–5 and often precedes the onset of tics. In children with tics, the addition of ADHD symptoms is associated with increased psychosocial problems, academic difficulties, disruptive behavior and functional impairment (Carter *et al.*, 2000; Spencer *et al.*, 2001; Stephens and Sandor, 1999; Sukhodolsky *et al.*, 2003).
- *Obsessive-Compulsive Disorder.* Obsessive-compulsive behaviors are also common in individuals with TS. In some patients it may be difficult to separate complex tics from compulsions. The incidence of obsessive-compulsive behaviors in TS is reported to be 20–89% (Grad *et al.*, 1987; Robertson, 1995). Symptoms generally manifest several years after the onset of tics, often in adolescence.
- *Affective Disorders: Anxiety and Depression.* Increased rates of both anxiety disorder and depression have been reported in patients with TS. The prevalence of depression has ranged from 13 to 76% in different studies. Some investigators believe depression positively correlates with earlier onset and longer duration of tics, whereas others find no correlations between depression and the number of tics.
- *Episodic Outbursts and Self-Injurious Behavior.* Episodic outbursts or rage attacks are also observed in individuals with TS. In a study comparing children with TS, 37 with co-morbid rage attacks and 31 without this symptom, children with rage attacks were more likely to have ADHD, obsessive-compulsive disorder and oppositional defiant disorder (Budman *et al.*, 2003). Self-injurious behavior is also common in TS. One study of 300 patients with TS found that 27% had mild or moderate and 4% had severe self-injurious behavior (Mathews *et al.*, 2004).
- *Academic Difficulties.* In a study of 200 children with TS, 36% had learning problems, including learning disabilities (22%), poor grades (18%), repeated grade level (12%) and assignment to full-time (8%) or part-time (12%) special education classes (Erenberg, Cruse and Rothner, 1986). Individuals with TS typically have normal intellectual functioning, although there may be executive dysfunction, discrepancies between performance and verbal IQ, impairments of visual perceptual achievement, or a decrease in visual-motor skills.

NEUROBIOLOGICAL BASIS FOR TICS

There is convincing evidence that cortico-striato-thalamo-cortical (C-S-T-C) circuits are involved in the pathogenesis of TS and its associated neuropsychiatric problems. Nevertheless, the precise location and the nature of the abnormality remain topics of active debate within the field. Many investigators have focused on the striatal component of this circuit, likely influenced by the association between basal ganglia dysfunction and other movement disorders (Singer *et al.*, 1993; Peterson *et al.*, 2003). However, evidence is building for a primary cortical dysfunction in TS.

Of direct relevance to pharmacotherapy is the presence of a wide variety of synaptic neurotransmitter systems within the C-S-T-C circuits, that is, dopaminergic, glutaminergic, GABAergic, serotoninergic, noradrenergic and opioid systems. Although, in theory, each individual neurotransmitter could have a pathophysiological role, recognizing the interdigitation between systems, it is possible that imbalances within several systems contribute to the pathobiology of TS. As described in the treatment section, pharmacotherapy for tics has, to date, focused on dopaminergic, adrenereric and GABAergic modulating drugs. In order to provide a background for understanding the rationale behind the use of these medications and possible newer therapeutic approaches, we will briefly discuss the role of each transmitter within the C-S-T-C circuit and some evidence supporting its role in TS.

Dopamine

Excitatory D1 dopamine receptors are expressed predominantly on medium-sized spiny neurons in the striatum as part of the direct pathway (striatum to globus pallidus interna and substantia nigra pars reticulata), whereas inhibitory D2 receptors are found on striatal medium-sized spiny neurons within the indirect pathway (striatum to globus pallidus externa). Activation of the D1 receptors is excitatory to the movement-releasing direct pathway, while activation of D2 receptors inhibits the indirect pathway, which functions to inhibit movement. Thus, activation of D1 and D2 receptors leads to disinhibition of the excitatory glutamatergic neurons in the thalamus, which in turn results in greater excitation to cortical motor areas. In addition to the dopaminergic input from the substantia nigra pars compacta to the striatum, the ventral tegmental area also provides dopaminergic innervation to pyramidal neurons and interneurons in the frontal cortex. The direct innervation of glutamatergic corticostriatal pyramidal neurons enhances their excitatory output, whereas interneurons have the opposite effect. Dopamine proposals have included supersensitive post-synaptic dopamine receptors (Wolf *et al.*, 1996; Wong *et al.*, 1997), dopamine hyperinnervation (Albin *et al.*, 2003) and a pre-synaptic dopamine abnormality (Ernst *et al.*, 1999); however, recent evidence favors enhanced phasic dopamine release (Singer and Minzer, 2003).

Glutamate

Glutamate is the primary excitatory neurotransmitter of corticostriatal neurons, subthalamic nucleus output neurons, thalamostriatal and thalamocortical projections. Significant interactions exist between the dopaminergic and glutamatergic systems that may have therapeutic relevance (de Bartolomeis, Fiore and Iasevoli, 2005). For example, it has been suggested that the beneficial effects of haloperidol in schizophrenia are associated with its inhibition of pre-synaptic dopaminergic inputs on corticostriatal glutamatergic afferent terminals. Reduced levels of glutamate were detected in four post-mortem TS samples in the globus pallidus interna and externa and the substantia nigra pars reticulata (Anderson *et al.*, 1992). Based, in part, on this close relationship, preliminary studies are in progress using therapies directed at glutamate rather than dopaminergic agents, the latter noted to be associated with significant side effects.

GABA

The inhibitory neurotransmitter GABA is the primary output of both the direct and indirect striatum to thalamic circuits. There are two hypotheses for the role of GABA in TS. A decrease in striatal GABAergic projections in both the direct and indirect pathway would cause decreased inhibition of excitatory thalamocortical neurons resulting in increased glutamatergic cortical excitation. A second hypothesis proposes an impairment of cortical inhibition of thalamocortical afferent signals secondary to reduced activity of GABAergic interneurons. One recent study showed marked alterations in the number and density of GABAergic neurons in the basal ganglia structures of TS patients (Kalanithi *et al.*, 2005).

Norepinephrine

α-2 Adrenergic receptors are present in the locus ceruleus. Binding at these sites reduces norepinephrine release and turnover. In addition, there are post-synaptic α-2 receptors in the prefrontal cortex which have been shown to modulate dopamine release (Ventura, Morrone and Puglisi-Allegra, 2007). Norepinephrine has been implicated in TS, based upon the beneficial effects of treatment with α-adrenergic agonists including clonidine and guanfacine (The Tourette's Syndrome Study Group, 2002).

Serotonin

Although some investigators have suggested a direct role for serotonin in tic disorders, most treatment with serotonin-related medications is reserved for co-morbid conditions, for example, obsessive-compulsive disorder, anxiety, episodic outbursts and depression. Serotonin levels can down-regulate dopamine release.

GENERAL PRINCIPLES OF TREATMENT

Although approaches to the assessment and treatment of individuals with TS may vary, there are several important steps (see Table 21.1). All patients with tics should be evaluated to assure the proper diagnosis and to eliminate the possibility that tics are secondary to another medical condition. Direct personal interview of the patient and parent and the use of standardized parent/teacher questionnaires are helpful in identifying the presence of co-morbid psychopathology and academic difficulties. Further, it is

Table 21.1 General principles of treatment.

(1) Document tics, assure proper diagnosis
(2) Assess for co-morbid psychopathology and academic problems
(3) Identify degree of impairment and extent of distress for tics and each co-morbid condition. Often best discussed separately
(4) Educate the patient and family
(5) Establish consensus about need for treatment
(6) Discuss available therapy and treatment goals
(7) Emphasize a comprehensive multi-disciplinary approach and your continued availability

essential to clarify the level of adaptive functioning, degree of impairment, and extent of distress associated with tics, as well as each co-morbid condition. Hence, the physician must determine, based on functional impairment, whether it is the patient's tics, or associated problems that require initial attention. In general, we find that discussion of tic symptoms and co-morbid diagnoses (e.g., ADHD, OCD, behavioral and learning problems) as separate entities enables the family, as well as other health care workers, to focus more accurately on individual needs.

The physician should educate the patient and family about the characteristics of the disorder. More specifically, that tics wax and wane, have periodic fluctuations, are variable and frequently improve in the teenage/early adulthood years. It should be emphasized that tics are involuntary and often exacerbated during periods of anticipation, anxiety, excitement and fatigue. It should be explained that tics are caused by biological factors (genetic with environmental influences) and although exacerbated by stress, are not due emotional etiologies. The effect of environmental factors should be clarified. For example, although acute infections may be associated with increased tics, a preceding β-hemolytic streptococcal infection and/or a diagnosis of PANDAS (pediatric autoimmune neuropsychological disorder associated with streptococcal infections), as an etiology for TS, is controversial.

Treatment goals should be carefully reviewed and the goal of symptomatic therapy defined. For example, the aim of tic-suppressing pharmacotherapy is to reduce tics to a level where they no longer cause a significant psychosocial disturbance, not complete suppression of all motor and phonic tic activity. Lastly, treatment of a child with TS requires a chronic commitment and at times a comprehensive multi-disciplinary approach.

TREATMENT OF TICS

Treatment for tics is available and generally effective. Nevertheless, recognizing the frequency of medication-related side effects, specific criteria should be fulfilled prior to the initiation of pharmacotherapy (see Table 21.2).

Decisions regarding treatment of tics or TS need to be individualized to each patient (see Table 21.3). In addition to the documentation of tics, the physician must assess the severity of the tics, as well as the emotional and psychosocial impact of the tics. For many families, education regarding the diagnosis, natural history, outcome and treatment options obviates or at least delays the need for medical treatment.

Non-Pharmacological Treatment

Although pharmacotherapy is usually considered first-line therapy, recognizing the possibility of medication side

Table 21.2 Possible indications for tic therapy.

(1) Psychosocial impairment: psychosocial difficulties include the loss of self-esteem, comments from peers, excessive worries about tics, failure to participate in family, social or after-school activities.

(2) Functional impairment: rarely tics may interfere with physical skills such as penmanship, reading, concentration and so on.

(3) Classroom disruption: usually due to vocal tics.

(4) Musculoskeletal discomfort: repetitive movements can lead to muscle strain/soreness or bone dislocation.

(5) Persistence of impairing tic symptoms: tics have a waxing and waning course and a proposed fractal pattern. Hence, decisions to treat should be based on the presence and persistence of significantly impairing tics.

effects, some parents and patients prefer alternative psychosocial treatments. A variety of behavioral approaches have been used, although most have not been adequately investigated. If utilized, the treating physician must recognize that these therapies do not negate ongoing educational and supportive care.

1. *Contingency Management*: This approach maintains that tics have the potential to be modified by the contingencies that surround them, for example, positive reinforcement (praise, rewards) for the reduction

Table 21.3 Points for consideration prior to tic treatment.

(1) Most patients with Tourette syndrome have few difficulties secondary to their tics.

(2) The majority of cases are mild and less than 40% require tic-suppressing medication.

(3) Parents are often more concerned about tics than the affected child.

(4) Tics have a waxing and waning course.

(5) Most patients improve during teenage to young adulthood years.

(6) Treatment is symptomatic, not curative.

(7) Studies have suggested the presence of a placebo response.

(8) Other co-morbid conditions will influence the clinical course.

(9) All tic-suppressing medications have associated side effects.

(10) Few drugs have received adequate evaluation as tic-suppressing agents.

of tics or punishment (electric shock, time out) for tic recurrence. In general, contingency management has not been recommended based on the following concerns: limited number of studies, evaluations obtained only as components of additional approaches, benefits that have not been persistent and concerns that exist regarding the ethics of punishment (Peterson, 2007)

2. *Massed Practice:* Massed practice is the purposeful repetition of tics for a specified time period. This method is generally not recommended.

3. *Relaxation Training:* Since tics are exacerbated by stress, several approaches have been used to promote relaxation, including biofeedback, breathing exercises, muscle relaxation, maintaining postures and autogenic training. Relaxation training may be beneficial for individual patients, but values failed to reach significance and were short-lived (Bergin *et al.*, 1998).

4. *Self-Monitoring:* This behavioral approach is based on the systematic observation and recording of tic activities. Generally recommended as part of a standard treatment program.

5. *Habit Reversal:* Habit reversal training (HRT) is the most extensively researched technique and consists of training the individual to become aware of his/her tics (response description and detection, premonitory urges, self-monitoring, situation awareness) and per-

forming a physically competing response to prevent or interrupt their occurrence (competing response training, contingency management). Six randomized, controlled trials of HRT have been conducted since 1980, all of which reported improved tic control (Himle *et al.*, 2006). The three most recent trials, using the standardized Yale Global Tic Severity Scale (YGTSS) as the primary outcome measure, found significantly lower YGTSS scores with HRT, the effects of which persisted at follow-up (Wilhelm *et al.*, 2003; Verdellen *et al.*, 2004; Deckersback *et al.*, 2006). These results are encouraging and support HRT as a potential therapy for individuals with refractory tics or those patients who prefer to defer pharmacologic therapy.

Pharmacologic Treatment

Once the decision to use tic-suppressing medication has been reached, we recommend a staged approach aimed at using the medications with the least side effects first and progressing to second-tier medications, if necessary (see Figure 21.1 and Tables 21.4 and 21.5). Our first-tier medications are designated as such, not based on efficacy, but rather on the lack of long-term side effects (i.e. tardive dyskinesia). If these medications are ineffective or tics are very severe, second-tier medications may be needed. A

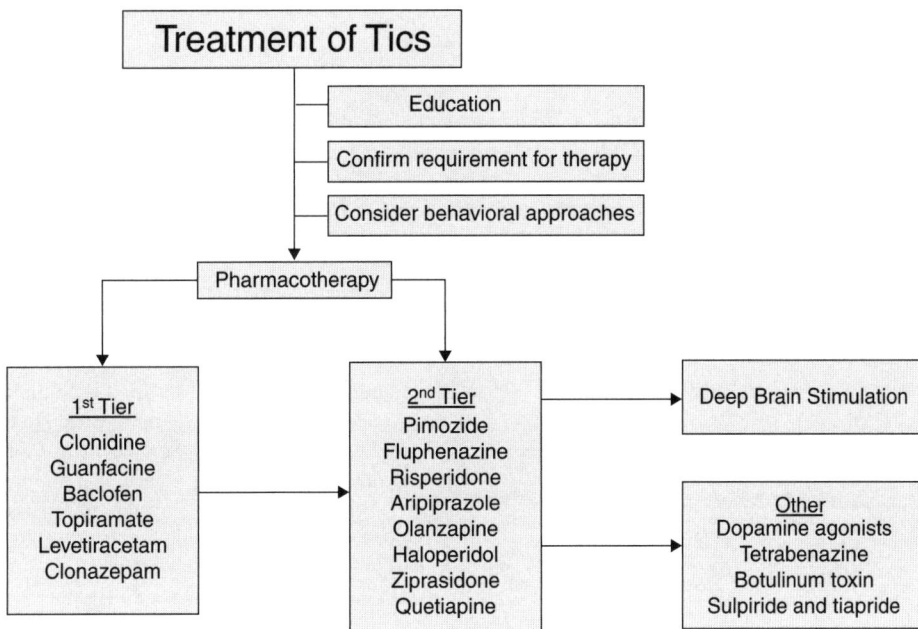

Figure 21.1 Tiered approach to pharmacologic treatment of tics.

Table 21.4 First-tier medications.

Drug	Starting dose	Dosage range	Personal experience
Clonidine	0.05 mg daily	0.1–0.4 mg/day divided BID	Especially with co-morbid ADHD, must be tapered
Guanfacine	0.5 mg daily	1.5–3 mg/day divided BID	Possibly less sedating than clonidine
Levetiracetam	250 mg daily	1–2 g/day divided BID	Conflicting evidence for efficacy
Topiramate	15 mg daily	50–200 mg/day	Some evidence for efficacy
Baclofen	10 mg daily	60 mg/day	Not first line
Clonazepam	0.5 mg daily	0.5–4 mg/day divided BID/TID	Reserved for patients with significant anxiety

wide range of medications have been used for the treatment of tics, however, only pimozide and haloperidol are approved by the United States Food and Drug Administration for the treatment of TS. Other medications, including tiapride and sulpride, are not available in the United States, but have been used with some success in Europe (discussed below). Hence, it should be apparent that most medications have not had efficacy documented in adequate double-blind trials, and only a limited number have been evaluated in direct comparison protocols. Further, in studies showing drug superiority to placebo, the percent improvement of tics ranged from only 30 to 65% (Scahill *et al.*, 2006). Investigators have attempted to classify medications based on short-term safety and efficacy, but results typically represent the extent of evaluation and not necessarily the relative degree of improvement.

A major point, often forgotten, is that the goal of treatment is not to suppress tics completely, but to eliminate the specific indication for initiating treatment, that is, psychological or physical problems. In general, medications should be started at the lowest dose and gradually increased as necessary. Monotherapy should be used whenever possible. After several months of successful treatment, it is appropriate to consider a gradual taper of medication. This is generally scheduled during a less stressful period, for example over summer vacation.

Table 21.5 Second-tier medications.

Drug	Starting dose	Dosage range	Personal experience
Pimozide	0.5–1 mg QHS	2–8 mg divided BID	Good efficacy, need ECG for QT prolongation
Fluphenazine	1 mg QHS	2–5 mg/day	Comparable to haloperidol, personally favored, fewer side-effects
Risperidone	0.5 mg QHS	1–4 mg/day	Favored if co-morbid psychiatric issues
Aripiprazole	2.5–5 mg QHS for adults	10–20 mg/day	Some evidence for efficacy
Olanzapine	2.5 mg QHS	5–10 mg/day QD or BID	Concerns for weight gain and endocrine issues
Haloperidol	0.5 mg daily	1–5 mg/day QD or BID	Efficacious but frequent side-effects
Ziprasidone	5 mg QHS	10–40 mg/day	Need ECG for QT prolongation
Quetiapine	25 mg daily	75–500 mg/day	Least effective

First-Tier Medications (see Table 21.4)

Clonidine

Clonidine is an α-2 adrenergic receptor agonist that primarily activates pre-synaptic autoreceptors in the locus ceruleus and reduces norepinephrine release and turnover. Despite its frequent use, there is a paucity of evidence for the use of clonidine in TS or other tic disorders. There are two small studies evaluating the use of clonidine in a placebo-controlled fashion. The first found no difference between clonidine and placebo (Goetz *et al.*, 1987), while the second showed improvement in both clonidine and placebo with a greater response in those patients treated with clonidine (Leckman *et al.*, 1991). A third trial, also a blinded, placebo-controlled study, showed a significant decrease in tic severity for clonidine vs placebo (The Tourette's Syndrome Study Group, 2002). Clonidine is often used as the first agent and is particularly useful for patients with co-morbid ADHD (The Tourette's Syndrome Study Group, 2002).

The starting dose is 0.05 mg daily. If tolerated, the dose may be increased to 0.05 mg twice daily with subsequent increases every week to a total daily dose of 0.1 to 0.4 mg. Since the drug has a short half-life, some investigators suggest a more frequent dosage schedule for tics. Clearly, when used for treatment of co-morbid ADHD, it should be given four times daily. Side effects include sedation, irritability, dizziness, dry mouth, headache and sleep disturbance. The sedating effects are usually self-limited. A transdermal patch is also available, but not recommended because of local skin irritation and the fact that patches may fall off. Clonidine should be gradually tapered to avoid rebound hypertension and tic exacerbation.

Guanfacine

Guanfacine is a longer acting α-2 adrenergic receptor agonist and one that is thought to be more selective for receptors in the prefrontal cortex. There have been two placebo-controlled trials of guanfacine in children with tic disorders and TS. One study showed a statistically significant improvement in tics compared to placebo (Scahill *et al.*, 2001). Although the second study showed a 30% decrease in the total tic score for guanfacine compared with 11% reduction with placebo, this difference did not reach significance (Cummings *et al.*, 2002). Similar to clonidine, guanfacine has also been used successfully in patients with co-morbid ADHD (Scahill *et al.*, 2001).

The initial dose is 0.5 mg once daily and may be increased to a total daily dose of 1.5 to 3 mg divided twice daily. The side-effect profile is similar to that of clonidine, with sedation and headache being the most common, though generally guanfacine is less sedating than clonidine.

Levetiracetam

Levetiracetam is a broad-spectrum anti-epileptic agent that has been used effectively for a variety of seizure types in the pediatric population. Although its precise mechanism of action remains unclear, studies have suggested that it binds to SV2a, a synaptic vesicle protein found in neurons, and has an atypical GABAergic effect by enhancing chloride ion influx at the $GABA_A$ receptor complex (Poulain and Margineanu, 2002; Rigo *et al.*, 2002). An open-label clinical trial has suggested that levetiracetam may be a useful treatment for tics. All 60 children and adolescents treated with levetiracetam in doses of 1 to 2 g/day showed significant clinical improvements in their vocal and motor tics (Awaad, Michon and Minarik, 2005). In a four-year follow-up of that open-label study, levetiracetam remained 100% effective for tic-suppression and 70% of patients showed improvement in behavior and school performance (Awaad and Minarik, 2005). Despite these reports, a recent double-blind, placebo-controlled trial in 20 children showed no difference between levetiracetam and placebo in the treatment of tics (Smith-Hicks *et al.*, 2007). Although the evidence for levetiracetam is conficting, it is included in our first tier, given the absence of long-term side effects.

Patients are usually started on 10 to 15 mg/kg/day divided twice daily and increased on a weekly basis to a total dose of 30 to 40 mg/kg/day. Side effects are usually limited, with the most prominent being mood changes.

Topiramate

Topiramate, a newer anti-epileptic medication also used for headache prophylaxis, has been reported to have some benefit for tic control. One of the proposed mechanisms is as a $GABA_A$ receptor agonist, potentiating the activity of the inhibitory neurotransmitter. Topiramate is also hypothesized to inhibit the kainate sub-type of the glutamate receptor. One open-label study of two patients suggested a potential benefit (Abuzzahab and Brown, 2001). As with levetiracetam, topiramate is included in the first tier, given its lack of long-term side effects. The effective adult dose in this report of two patients was between 50 and 200 mg per day.

Topiramate dosing may be started as low as 15 mg per day and is increased as necessary. Side effects include weight loss, nephrolithiasis, metabolic acidosis, memory impairment, difficulty with concentration, paresthesias and angle-closure glaucoma. The presence of obesity may be an indication for a trial of topiramate prior to the use of neuroleptics.

Baclofen

Baclofen is a $GABA_B$ receptor agonist used in the treatment of spasticity. Its binding reduces the release of the excitatory neurotransmitters glutamine and aspartate. It has been used in the treatment of other disorders including spasticity, dystonia and chorea in Huntington's disease. There are two open-label studies and one small placebo-controlled crossover study. Shapiro *et al.* evaluated baclofen in a small number of patients and demonstrated no benefit (Shapiro *et al.*, 1988), whereas Awaad reported a beneficial effect in 95% of children (Awaad, 1999). In the only double-blind placebo-controlled crossover study, baclofen (20 mg three times daily) showed statistically significant improvements in total scores based on established rating scales (Leckman *et al.*, 1989; Singer *et al.*, 2001). However, further analysis showed that the benefit was associated with improvement in an overall impairment score rather than a reduction in motor or vocal tics.

Baclofen is initiated at 10 mg three times daily and increased every 3–7 days to a maximum total daily dose of 60 mg. Side effects are generally mild and include gastrointestinal upset, somnolence, weakness, dizziness and headache.

Clonazepam

Clonazepam is a benzodiazepine, which acts as a $GABA_A$ receptor agonist, α-2 adrenergic receptor agonist and up-regulates $5\text{-}HT_1$ binding sites. There are no placebo-controlled trials to date; however, small open-label trials have shown some benefit for tic control (Gonce and Barbeau, 1977; Steingard *et al.*, 1994). One study suggested that clonazepam is superior to clonidine (Drtilkova *et al.*, 1994). Clonazepam is probably best reserved for those patients with significant co-morbid anxiety.

Clonazepam dosing is usually 0.5 to 4 mg per day, divided in two or three doses. Side effects include sedation, dizziness, short-term memory problems and disinhibition. Side effects may be particularly limiting in children. As with other benzodiazepines, this medication should be weaned to avoid withdrawal symptoms.

Second-Tier Medications (see Table 21.5)

If an individual fails initial therapy or presents with severe tics, medications in the second-tier category (classical neuroleptic or atypical neuroleptic category) should be initiated. Medications in this category may be more beneficial than first-tier treatments, but side effects often limit their usefulness. *Classical neuroleptics* (pimozide, fluphenazine, haloperidol, trifluoperazine) are D2 dopamine receptor antagonists. These drugs act to block dopaminergic input from the substantia nigra to the basal ganglia and from the ventral tegmentum to the frontal cortex. They are the most effective at suppressing tics (70–80%) but have more severe side effects, which limit their usefulness. *Atypical neuroleptics* (risperidone, olanzapine, ziprasidone, quetiapine) have a greater affinity for 5HT2 receptors than for D2 receptors. At least some of the difference in efficacy of between the different atypical neuroleptics is likely related to their relative potency of dopamine blockade.

Adverse effects with anti-psychotics may occur even with low doses and include sedation, parkinsonism, acute dystonic reactions, bradykinesia, akathisia, tardive and withdrawal dyskinesias, cognitive blunting, depression, aggression, "fog states," weight gain, prolonged cardiac conduction times (QTc), endocrine dysfunction, and poor school performance, with or without school phobia. Neurological side effects occur with use of atypical neuroleptics, but possibly less frequently than seen with some typical neuroleptics. Recent studies have emphasized the incidence of weight gain and insulin resistance with all atypical anti-psychotics.

Pimozide

Pimozide, a diphenylbutylpiperidine derivative, is a D2 receptor antagonist which also blocks calcium channels. Two studies have shown pimozide to be superior to placebo (Shapiro *et al.*, 1989; Sallee *et al.*, 1997) for tic suppression. Double-blind, placebo-controlled trials of pimozide vs haloperidol have shown mixed results, with one trial showing equal efficacy (Ross and Moldofsky, 1978), one showing haloperidol slightly more effective than pimozide (Shapiro *et al.*, 1989) and the third showing pimozide to be superior to haloperidol (Sallee *et al.*, 1997). In addition, pimozide has been generally associated with fewer side effects including sedation (Ross and Moldofsky, 1978) and extrapyramidal symptoms (Sallee *et al.*, 1997).

Initial dosing is at 0.5 to 1 mg daily at bedtime. This may be gradually increased on a weekly basis in 1 mg increments to a dose of 2 to 8 mg divided twice daily. A baseline electrocardiogram should be obtained prior to initiating therapy with pimozide as it has been associated with QT prolongation. The QTc interval should not exceed 0.47 s in children, 0.52 s in adults or demonstrate a more than 25% increase from the patient's baseline value. Additionally, the use of macrolide antibiotics, azole anti-fungals and protease inhibitors should be avoided, as concurrent administration of these medications may increase pimozide levels, as well as increase QT prolongation.

Fluphenazine

Fluphenazine, a traditional neuroleptic, acts as both a D1 and D2 receptor antagonist. Small studies have shown fluphenazine to be effective in tic control and associated with fewer side effects compared with haloperidol (Singer, Gammon and Quaskey, 1986; Goetz, Tanner and Klawans, 1984).

Dosing should begin at 1 mg daily at bedtime and may be increased by 1 mg per day every week to a goal daily dose of 2 to 5 mg. The two studies above also showed fewer side effects with fluphenazine when compared with haloperidol

(Singer, Gammon and Quaskey, 1986; Goetz, Tanner and Klawans, 1984).

Risperidone

Risperidone is an atypical neuroleptic that acts as a 5-HT$_2$ receptor antagonist at low doses and a D2 antagonist at higher doses. It also has moderate to high affinity for α1-adrenergic, D3, D4 and H1-histamine receptors. It was the first atypical anti-psychotic approved by the FDA for the first-line treatment of schizophrenia, and the most widely evaluated for tic-suppression. It has been shown to be superior to placebo in two randomized, double-blind, placebo-controlled trials for tics (Scahill et al., 2003; Dion et al., 2002). It was equally effective to pimozide in one randomized, double-blind crossover study (Bruggeman et al., 2001) and superior in another (Gilbert et al., 2004).

Risperidone is usually started at 0.5 mg given once daily at night. The dose may be titrated as needed to a total daily dose of 1 to 4 mg divided twice daily (Scahill et al., 2003). Side effects have included sedation, increased appetite and weight gain, acute social phobia, increased prolactin levels, depression and dysphoria.

Aripiprazole

Aripiprazole is a novel partial dopamine (D2) and 5-HT1A receptor agonist. Case reports and open-label studies have supported its efficacy in treating tics (Kastrup et al., 2005; Davies et al., 2006; Yoo, Kim and Kim, 2006). To date, there have been no published blinded, placebo-controlled trials of aripiprazole.

The starting dose in adults is 2.5 to 5 mg daily with a goal dose of 10 to 20 mg daily. In an open-label study in children and adolescents with TS, the mean dose was 0.22 mg/kg (range 0.083 to 0.55 mg/kg).

Olanzapine

Olanzapine is an atypical neuroleptic with moderate to high affinity for D2, D4, 5-HT2A, 5-HT2C and α-1 adrenergic receptors, as well as D1 receptors. Two open-label trials have shown improvement in tic scores (Stamenkovic et al., 2000; Budman et al., 2001). A double-blind, crossover study of olanzapine vs pimozide found that olanzapine was superior to low-dose pimozide in producing tic reduction in four patients with severe tics (Onofrj et al., 2000).

Olanzapine is started at 2.5 mg once daily at bedtime and increased as needed to a total daily dose of 5 to 10 mg divided once or twice daily. Weight gain, insulin resistance and new-onset dyslipidemia may be problematic.

Haloperidol

Haloperidol, a butyrophenone, was the first traditional neuroleptic shown to be effective for tic suppression.

Concerns regarding side effects have limited its use to within the second-tier category of medications. Haloperidol has been shown to be superior to both placebo and to pimozide in one double-blind, placebo-controlled trial (Shapiro et al., 1989).

The therapeutic tic effect with haloperidol is seen at low doses (Singer et al., 1981) and the usual starting dose is 0.5 mg daily. If needed, medication is increased by 0.25 to 0.5 mg on a weekly basis to a goal dose of 1 to 5 mg per day, given either once or twice daily. As previously discussed, some studies have shown a higher incidence of side effects with haloperidol compared with alternative typical neuroleptics.

Ziprasidone

Ziprasidone, an atypical neuroleptic, antagonizes D2 and 5HT2 receptors, but also has widespread effects on other neurotransmitter systems, for example, blocking effects on norepinephrine and serotonin transporters, α-1 adrenergic receptor antagonism, and moderate affinity for histamine H1 receptors. It has been shown to be more effective than placebo in suppressing tic symptoms in patients with TS (Sallee et al., 2000).

Dosing should be started at 5 mg in the evening and increased gradually to 40 mg daily in divided doses. A baseline electrocardiogram should be obtained prior to initiating therapy, as ziprasidone is also associated with prolongation of the QT interval.

Quetiapine

Quetiapine is an atypical neuroleptic that antagonizes 5HT1A, 5HT2, D1, D2, histamine H1, α-1 and α-2 adrenergic receptors. To date, its use for tic suppression is based on case reports. One open-label trial with 12 children and adolescents with TS found a significant reduction in tic scores with quetiapine (Mukaddes and Abali, 2003), as did a retrospective review of 12 patients (Copur et al., 2007).

Quetiapine is initially dosed at 25 mg daily and may be increased as tolerated to relatively high doses of 200 to 500 mg daily.

Other Medications

Pergolide

Pergolide is a mixed dopamine (D1/D2/D3) agonist used primarily for the treatment of Parkinson's disease. Its low-dose use in TS is somewhat counterintuitive, given the finding that the most effective treatments for tic-suppression are dopamine antagonists (neuroleptics). Its hypothesized mechanism of action is the reduction of dopamine release secondary to stimulation of pre-synaptic dopamine autoreceptors. There have been two double-blind placebo-controlled trials of pergolide in TS, both of which showed significant improvement of total tic scores as compared to placebo (Gilbert *et al.*, 2000, 2003).

Despite reports of potential benefit, pergolide was voluntarily withdrawn from the US market in March 2007 secondary to its ergot-induced pleural, retroperitoneal, and peri-cardial fibrosis, vasospasm and concerns of cardiac valvular disease with long-term use.

Tetrabenazine

Tetrabenazine depletes pre-synaptic storage of catecholamines by blocking vesicular monoamine transporters and is also a mild post-synaptic dopamine receptor antagonist. It is used for the treatment of dyskinetic disorders, including chorea in Huntington's disease. There have been two open-label studies of tetrabenazine for tics (Jankovic and Orman, 1988; Jankovic and Beach, 1997). The second demonstrated a "marked improvement in abnormal movements" in 57% of 47 patients with TS (Jankovic and Beach, 1997).

Dosing is started at 12.5 mg daily and increased to 12.5 to 25 mg twice daily in children and 25 to 100 mg per day for adults. Side effects include sedation, depression, parkinsonism, insomnia, anxiety, postural hypotension and akathisia. Tetrabenazine is now available in the United States as well as the rest of the world.

Botulinum toxin

Botulinum toxin, which blocks acetylcholine release at the neuromuscular junction is generally reserved for specific troublesome tics that are not treated by conventional medications (Kwak, Hanna and Jankovic, 2000). One randomized, double-blind, controlled trial of botulinum toxin injection for motor tics showed a 39% reduction in tic frequency with treatment compared to placebo (Marras *et al.*, 2001). Benefits appeared in 3–4 days and lasted a mean of 14 weeks.

Injection is given into the muscle group affected by the motor tic or into the laryngeal folds for vocal tics. Treatment is generally repeated every 3–9 months. Adverse effects include soreness at the injection site, weakness of the injected muscle and dysphasia or hypophonia for laryngeal injections.

Sulpiride and Tiapride

Tiapride and sulpride are substituted benzamides and selective D2 antagonists which appear to lack effects on norepinephrine, acetylcholine, serotonin, histamine, or GABA receptors. Neither is available in the United States, but studies in Europe have shown improvement in tics. One retrospective study of 63 patients with TS treated with sulpiride showed beneficial effects in 59% (Robertson, Schnieden and Lees, 1990). Tiapride is also commonly used in Europe and is supported by a positive therapeutic

effect in a double-blind, placebo-controlled trial of 17 children (Eggers, Rothenberger and Berghaus, 1988).

Marijuana

δ-9-Tetrahydrocannabinol (THC), the major psychoactive substrate in marijuana, has been reported to be effective in tic suppression. Initial interest in THC was based on interview results of 17 patients with TS, 14 of whom reported a reduction in tics with marijuana use (Muller-Vahl *et al.*, 1998). There has been one randomized, double-blind, placebo-controlled study of THC, which showed a significant difference ($p < 0.05$) or a trend toward a significant difference ($p < 0.10$) in tics during the treatment period (Muller-Vahl *et al.*, 2003). THC is not available for clinical use in the United States.

Surgical Approaches

Deep Brain Stimulation

For patients with severe tics refractory to medical management, surgical interventions affecting the proposed cortico-striato-thalamo-cortical circuits involved in TS have been attempted (Neimat, Patil and Lozano, 2006). More recently, deep brain stimulation, a modern stereotactic treatment used in other movement disorders has been proposed as a potential therapy for tics. There have been several recent reports of deep brain stimulation surgery for TS. Targets have included intralaminar thalamic nuclei (Vandewalle *et al.*, 1999; Visser-Vandewalle *et al.*, 2003), globus pallidus interna (Diederich *et al.*, 2005; Shahed *et al.*, 2007) and both globus pallidus interna and thalamus (Houeto *et al.*, 2005; Ackermans et al., 2006). Although the number of cases is small, there has been a reduction in tic frequency by 70 to 90% that persisted over follow-up periods of 8 to 60 months. Recommendations for the use of DBS in TS have been published (Mink *et al.*, 2006).

Potential Future Therapies

Based upon pathophysiological hypotheses involving various neurotransmitter systems with cortico-striatal-thalamo-cortical pathways, a variety of therapeutic options have been proposed, some of which are currently being evaluated in preliminary trials. For example, recognizing that glutamate is the major excitatory transmitter in the central nervous system and has major interactions with dopaminergic systems, preliminary trials with glutamatergic-modulating agents (agonists/antagonists) are in progress. Non-ergot dopamine agonists, such as pramipexole, are being studied, given the positive results with pergolide and the fact that ergot-related side effects should not be present. Transcranial magnetic stimulation (TMS) is a neurophysiologic technique that has been used to probe neural inhibitory circuitry by applying varying frequencies of stimulation to a given brain region. Results of TMS used to suppress tics have been variable (Chae *et al.*, 2004; Orth *et al.*, 2005), but response may be based on coil placement and current flow (Mantovani *et al.*, 2006).

TREATMENT OF CO-MORBIDITIES

Argumentativeness, disruptive behaviors, conduct problems, episodic outbursts (rage), anxiety and mood disorders are relatively common in patients with TS. In many, these difficulties are co-mingled with tics, ADHD and OCD and present a major challenge for the family and physician. In complex cases, it is essential that the affected patient receives the proper evaluation and care from a multidisciplinary team of specialists.

Attention Deficit Hyperactivity Disorder

Stimulant medications are considered to be the treatment of choice for ADHD. Their use, however, in children with TS or other tic disorders has been controversial. Concerns were largely based on early reports, which suggested that stimulant medications had the potential to provoke or intensify tics and that this effect might persist despite medication withdrawal (Barkley *et al.*, 1990; Borcherding *et al.*, 1990; Pollack, Cohen and Friedhoff, 1977). More recently, the Tourette's Syndrome Study Group preformed a multicenter, randomized, double-blind controlled clinical trial of clonidine, methylphenidate, clonidine and methylphenidate in combination, and placebo in children with tics and ADHD (The Tourette's Syndrome Study Group, 2002). Results showed that both clonidine and methylphenidate were associated with significant improvement in ADHD symptoms, with the greatest benefit for combined clonidine and methylphenidate therapy. Data also showed that, compared with placebo, tic severity was reduced in all treatment groups, including those treated with methylphenidate alone. When treatment groups were compared for "worsening of tics," the rates (20–26%) were no different among the groups, including placebo. Hence, stimulants did not exacerbate tics. Given the significant adverse impact on quality of life and social/school functioning in children with ADHD, we recommend treatment and do not believe stimulants are contraindicated in children with tics. Alternative medications for the treatment of ADHD in children with tic disorders include the α-2 adrenergic agonists clonidine and guanfacine, discussed above, as well as atomoxetine, desipramine, and nortriptyline. Atomoxetine, a selective norepinephrine reuptake inhibitor, is used in doses of 1.0–1.5 mg/kg/day, and given in two divided doses. Common adverse effects of atomoxetine include nausea, emesis, diminished appetite, and insomnia. Several placebo-controlled studies have documented the efficacy of the tricyclic anti-depressent desipramine in children and adolescents with ADHD only and TS plus ADHD (Singer *et al.*, 1995; Biederman *et al.*, 1995; Spencer *et al.*, 2002).

Obsessive-Compulsive Disorder

Selective serotonergic reuptake inhibitors (SSRIs) are first-line therapy for obsessive-compulsive disorder and are often used for disabling symptoms. Cognitive-behavioral therapy and the tricyclic anti-depressant clomipramine are also effective treatments for OCD. Empirical support for treatment in children is best with clomipramine, fluoxetine, sertraline and fluvoxamine. All medications should be started in low doses and increased gradually. It is important to note that a black box warning has been issued by the US Food and Drug Administration regarding increased suicidal ideation and suicidality in children and adolescents for SSRIs.

Affective Disorders: Anxiety and Depression

Increased rates of both anxiety disorder and depression have been reported in patients with TS. An important early step is to determine whether these symptoms are derived from, or are independent of the tic disorder. Safety of the individual should be established, especially if the patient is suicidal. Cognitive behavioral therapy and pharmacotherapy should be considered in conjunction with consultation from professionals in psychology and psychiatry.

Episodic Outbursts and Self-Injurious Behavior

Since it is unclear whether these problems are etiologically related to TS or its other co-morbid conditions, a formal psychiatric evaluation is often required. Some investigators believe these behaviors may be related to obsessive-compulsive disorder and suggest treatment with SSRIs and cognitive behavioral therapy.

Academic Difficulties

A variety of factors, including severe tics, medication side effects, co-morbid behavioral/psychiatric disorders (ADHD, obsessive-compulsive behaviors and depression), psychosocial problems, learning disabilities and executive dysfunction can contribute to poor school performance. A comprehensive neuropsychological assessment is often beneficial in defining underlying issues and therapy should be directed at the identified pathology.

References

Abuzzahab, F.S. and Brown, V.L. (2001) Control of Tourette's syndrome with topiramate. *American Journal of Psychiatry*, **158**, 968.

Ackermans, L., Temel, Y., Cath, D., van der Linden, C., Bruggeman, R., Kleijer, M., Nederveen, P., Schruers, K., Colle, H., Tijssen, M.A., Visser-Vandewalle, V., Dutch Flemish Tourette Surgery Study Group (2006) Deep brain stimulation in Tourette's syndrome: two targets? *Movement Disorders*, **21**, 709–713.

Albin, R.L., Koeppe, R.A., Bohnen, N.I. *et al.* (2003) Increased ventral striatal monoaminergic innervation in Tourette syndrome. *Neurology*, **61**, 310–315.

Anderson, G.M., Pollak, E.S., Chatterjee, D., Leckman, J.F., Riddle, M.A. and Cohen, D.J. (1992) Postmortem analysis of subcortical monoamines and amino acids in Tourette syndrome. *Advances in Neurology*, **58**, 123–133.

Awaad, Y. (1999) Tics in Tourette syndrome: new treatment options. *Journal of Child Neurology*, **14**, 316–319.

Awaad, Y., Michon, A.M. and Minarik, S. (2005) Use of levetiracetam to treat tics in children and adolescents with Tourette syndrome. *Movement Disorders*, **20**, 714–718.

Awaad, Y. and Minarik, S. (2005) Long-term follow-up use of levetiracetam to treat tics in children. *Annals of Neurology*, **58**, S112.

Barkley, R.A., McMurray, M.B., Edelbrock, C.S. and Robbins, K. (1990) Side effects of methylphenidate in children with attention deficit hyperactivity disorder: A systemic, placebo-controlled evaluation. *Pediatrics*, **86**, 184–192.

Bergin, A., Waranch, H.R., Brown, J., Carson, K. and Singer, H.S. (1998) Relaxation therapy in Tourette syndrome: a pilot study. *Pediatric Neuorlogy*, **18**, 136–142.

Biederman, J., Baldessarini, R.J., Wright, V., Knee, D. and Harmatz, J.S. (1995) A double-blind placebo controlled study of desipramine in the treatment of ADD: I. Efficacy. *Journal of the American Academy of Child and Adolescent Psychiatry*, **28**, 777–784.

Borcherding, B.G., Keysor, C.S., Rapoport, J.L. *et al.* (1990) Motor/vocal tics and compulsive behaviors on stimulant drugs: Is there a common vulnerability? *Psychiatry Research*, **33**, 83.

Bruggeman, R., van der Linden, C., Buitelaar, J.K. *et al.* (2001) Risperidone versus pimozide in Tourette's disorder: a comparative double-blind parallel-group study. *Journal of Clinical Psychiatry*, **62**, 50–56.

Budman, C.L., Gayer, A., Lesser, M. *et al.* (2001) An open-label study of the treatment efficacy of olanzapine for Tourette's disorder. *Journal of Clinical Psychiatry*, **62**, 290–294.

Budman, C.L., Rockmore, L., Stokes, J. *et al.* (2003) Clinical phenomenology of episodic rage in children with Tourette syndrome. *Journal of Psychosom Research*, **55**, 59.

Carter, A.S., O'Donnell, D.A., Schultz, R.T. *et al.* (2000) Social and emotional adjustment in children affected with Gilles de la Tourette's syndrome: associations with ADHD and family functioning. Attention deficit hyperactivity disorder. *Journal of Child Psychol Psychiatry*, **41**, 215.

Chae, J.H., Nahas, Z., Wassermann, E., Li, X., Sethuraman, G., Gilbert, D., Sallee, F.R. and George, M.S. (2004) A pilot safety study of repetitive transcranial magnetic stimulation (rTMS) in Tourette's syndrome. *Cognitive and Behavioral Neurology*, **17**, 109–117.

Comings, D.E. and Comings, B.G. (1985) Tourette syndrome: Clinical and psychological aspects of 250 cases. *American Journal of Human Genetics*, **37**, 435.

Comings, D.E. and Comings, B.G. (1987) A controlled study of Tourette syndrome: I. Attention-deficit disorder, learning disorders and school problems. *American Journal of Human Genetics*, **41**, 701.

Copur, M., Arpaci, B., Demir, T. and Narin, H. (2007) Clinical effectiveness of quetiapine in children and adolsecents with Tourette's syndrome: a retrospective case-note study. *Clinical Drug Investigation*, **27**, 123–130.

Cummings, D.D., Singer, H.S., Krieger, M., Miller, T.L. and Mahone, E.M. (2002) Neuropsychiatric effects of guanfacine in children with mild Tourette syndrome: a pilot study. *Clinical Neuropharmacology*, **25**, 325–332.

Davies, L., Stern, J.S., Agrawal, N. and Robertson, M.M. (2006) A case series of patients with Tourette's syndrome in the United Kingdom treated with aripiprazole. *Human Psychopharmacology*, **21**, 447–453.

de Bartolomeis, A., Fiore, G. and Iasevoli, F. (2005) Dopamine-glutamate interaction and antipsychotics mechanism of action: implication for new pharmacological strategies in psychosis. *Current Pharmaceutical Design*, **11**, 3561–3594.

Deckersback, T., Rauch, S., Buhlmann, U. and Wilhelm, S. (2006) Habit reversal versus supportive psychotherapy in Tourette's disorder: A randomized controlled trial and predictors of treatment response. *Behavior Research and Therapy*, **44**, 1079–1090.

Diederich, N.J., Kalteis, K., Stamenkovic, M., Pieri, V. and Alesch, F. (2005) Efficient internal pallidal stimulation in Gilles de la Tourette syndrome: A case report. *Movement Disorders*, **20**, 1496–1499.

Dion, Y., Annable, L., Sandor, P. and Chouinard, G. (2002) Risperidone in the treatment of Tourette syndrome: a double-blind, placebo-controlled trial. *Journal of Clinical Psychopharmacology*, **22**, 31–39.

Drtilkova, I., Balaotkova, B., Lemanova, H. and Zak, J. (1994) Therapeutical effects of clonidine and clonazepam in children with tic syndome. *Homeostasis in Health and Disease*, **35**, 296.

Eggers, C., Rothenberger, A. and Berghaus, U. (1988) Clinical and neurobiological findings in children suffering from tic disease following treatment with tiapride. *European Archives of Psychiatry and Neurological, Sciences* **237**, 223–229.

Erenberg, G., Cruse, R.P. and Rothner, A.D. (1986) Tourette Syndrome: an analysis of 200 pediatric and adolescent cases. *Cleveland Clinic Quarterly*, **53**, 127–131.

Erenberg, G., Cruse, R.P. and Rothner, A.D. (1987) The natural history of Tourette syndrome: A follow-up study. *Annals of Neurology*, **22**, 383–385.

Ernst, M., Zametkin, A.J., Jons, P.H., Matochik, J.A., Pascualvaca, D. and Cohen, R.M. (1999) High presynaptic domainergic activity in children with Tourette's disorder. *Journal of the American Academy of Child and Adolescent Psychiatry*, **38**, 86–94.

Gaze, C., Kepley, H.O. and Walkup, J.T. (2006) Co-occurring psychiatric disorders in children and adolescents with Tourette syndrome. *Journal of Child Neurology*, **21**, 657–664.

Gilbert, D.L., Sethuraman, G., Sine, L., Peters, S. and Sallee, F.R. (2000) Tourette's syndrome improvement with pergolide in a randomized, double-blind, crossover trial. *Neurology*, **54**, 1310–1315.

Gilbert, D.L., Dure, L., Sethuraman, G., Raab, D., Lane, J. and Sallee, F.R. (2003) Tic reduction with pergolide in a randomized controlled trial in children. *Neurology*, **60**, 606–611.

Gilbert, D.L., Batterson, J.R., Sethuraman, G. and Sallee, F.R. (2004) Tic reduction with risperidone versus pimozide in a randomized, double-blind crossover trial. *Journal of the American Academy of Child and Adolescent Psychiatry*, **43**, 206–214.

Gilles de la Tourette, G. (1885) Étude sur une affection nerveuse caracterisee par de l'incoordination motrice accompagnee d'echolalie et de copralalie. *Archives of Neurology*, **19**, 158.

Goetz, C.G., Tanner, C.M. and Klawans, H.L. (1984) Fluphenazine and multifocal tic disorders. *Archives Neurology*, **41**, 271–272.

Goetz, C.G., Tanner, C.M., Wilson, R.S. *et al.* (1987) Clonidine and Gilles de la Tourette's syndrome: double-blind study using objective rating methods. *Annals of Neurology*, **21**, 307–310.

Gonce, M. and Barbeau, A. (1977) Seven cases of Gilles de la Tourette's syndrome: partial relief with clonazepam. A pilot study. *The Canadian Journal of Neurological Sciences. Le journal canadien des sciences neurologiques*, **3**, 279–283.

Grad, L.R., Pelcovitz, D., Olson, M. *et al.* (1987) Obsessive-compulsive symptomatology in children with Tourette's syndrome. *Journal of the American Academy of Child and, Adolescent Psychiatry*, **26**, 69.

Himle, M.B., Woods, D.W., Piacentini, J.C. and Walkup, J.T. (2006) Brief review of habit reversal training for Tourette syndrome. *Journal of Child Neurology*, **21**, 719–725.

Houeto, J.L., Karachi, C., Mallet, L., Pillon, B. *et al.* (2005) Tourette's syndrome and deep brain stimulation. *Journal of Neurology Neurosurgery and Psychiatry*, **76**, 992–995.

Hyde, T.M., Aaronson, B.A., Randolph, C., Rickler, K.C. and Weinberger, D.R. (1992) Relationship of birth weight to the phenotypic expression of Gilles de la Tourette's syndrome in monozygotic twins. *Neurology*, **42**, 652–658.

Jankovic, J. and Orman, J. (1988) Tetrabenazine therapy of dystonia, chorea, tics and other dyskinesias. *Neurology*, **38**, 391–394.

Jankovic, J. and Beach, J. (1997) Long-term effects of tetrabenazine in hyperkinetic movement disorders. *Neurology*, **48**, 358–362.

Kalanithi, P.S., Zheng, W., Kataoka, Y. *et al.* (2005) Altered parvalbumin-positive neuron distribution in basal ganglia of individuals with Tourette syndrome. *Proceedings of the National Academy of Sciences of the United States of America*, **102**, 13307–13312.

Kastrup, A., Schlotter, W., Plewnia, C. and Bartels, M. (2005) Treatment of tics in Tourette syndrome with aripiprazole. *Journal of Clinical Psychopharmacology*, **25**, 94–96.

Kwak, C.H., Hanna, P.A. and Jankovic, J. (2000) Botulinum toxin in the treatment of tics. *Archives of Neurology*, **57**, 1190–1193.

Leckman, J.F., Riddle, M., Al Hardin, M.T. *et al.* (1989) The Yale Global Tic Severity Scale: initial testing of a clinician-rated scale of tic severity. *Journal of the American Academy of Child and Adolescent Psychiatry*, **28** 566–573.

Leckman, J.F., Hardin, M.T., Riddle, M.A.c. *et al.* (1991) Clonidine treatment of Gilles de la Tourette's syndrome. *Archives of General Psychiatry*, **48**, 324–328.

Leckman, J.F., Zhang, H., Vitale, A. *et al.* (1998) Course of tic severity in Tourette syndrome: the first two decades. *Pediatrics*, **102**, 14–19.

Mantovani, A., Lisanby, S.H., Pieraccini, F., Ulivelli, M., Castrogiovanni, P. and Rossi, S. (2006) Repetitive transcranial magnetic stimulation (rTMS) in the treatment of obsessive-compulsive disorder (OCD) and Tourette's syndrome (TS). *The International Journal of Neuropsychopharmacology*, **9**, 95–100.

Marras, C., Andrews, D., Sime, E. and Lang, A.E. (2001) Botulinum toxin for simple motor tics. *Neurology*, **56**, 605–610.

Mathews, C.A., Waller, J., Glidden, D. *et al.* (2004) Self injurious behaviour in Tourette syndrome: Correlates with impulsivity and impulse control. *Journal of Neurology, Neurosurgery and Psychiatry*, **75**, 1149.

Mink, J.W., Walkup, J., Frey, K.A., Como, P. *et al.* (2006) Patient selection and assessment recommendations for deep brain stimulation in Tourette syndrome. *Movement Disorders*, **21**, 1831–1838.

Mukaddes, N.M. and Abali, O. (2003) Quetiapine treatement of children and adolescents with Tourette's disorder. *Journal of Child and Adolescent Psychopharmacology*, **13**, 295–299.

Muller-Vahl, K.R., Kolbe, H., Schneider, U. and Emrich, H.M. (1998) Cannabinoids: possible role in patho-physiology and therapy of Gilles de la Tourette syndrome. *Acta Psychiatrica Scandinavica*, **98**, 502–506.

Muller-Vahl, K.R., Prevedel, H., Theloe, K., Kolbe, H., Emrich, H.M. and Schneider, U. (2003) Treatment of Tourette syndrome with delta-9-tetrahydrocannabinol (delta 9-THC): no influence on neuropsychological performance. *Neuropsychopharmacology*, **28**, 384–388.

Neimat, J.S., Patil, P.G. and Lozano, A.M. (2006) Novel surgical therapies for Tourette syndrome. *Journal of Child Neurology*, **21**, 715–718.

Onofrj, M., Paci, C., D'Andreamatteo, G. and Toma, L. (2000) Olanzapine in severe Gilles de la Tourette syndrome: a 52-week double blind cross over study vs. low-dose pimozide. *Journal of Neurology*, **247**, 443–446.

Orth, M., Kirby, R., Richardson, M.P., Snijders, A.H., Rothwell, J.C., Trimble, M.R., Robertson, M.M. and Münchau, A. (2005) Subthreshold rTMS over pre-motor cortex has no effect on tics in patients with Gilles de la Tourette syndrome. *Clinical Neurophysiology*, **116**, 764–768.

Pappert, ElJ., Goetz, C.G., Louis, E.D., Blasucci, L. and Leurgans, S. (2003) Objective assessments of longitudinal outcome in Gilles de la Tourette's syndrome. *Neurology*, **61**, 936–940.

Peterson, A.L. (2007) Psychosocial management of tics and intentional repetitive behaviors associated with Tourette syndrome, in *Treating Tourette Syndrome and Tic Disorder A Guide for Practitioners*, (eds D.W. Woods, J.C. Piacentini and J.T. Walkup), Guilford Press, New York, pp. 154–184.

Peterson, B.S., Thomas, P., Kane, M.J. *et al.* (2003) Basal ganglia volumes in patients with Gilles de la Tourette syndrome. *Achieves of General Psychiatry*, **60**, 415–424.

Pollack, M.A., Cohen, N.L. and Friedhoff, A.J. (1977) Gilles de la Tourette's syndrome. Familial occurrence and precipitation by methylphenidate therapy. *Archives of Neurology*, **34**, 630.

Poulain, P. and Margineanu, D.G. (2002) Levetiracetam opposes the action of $GABA_A$ antagonists in hypothalamic neurones. *Neuropharmacology*, **42**, 346–352.

Price, R.A., Kidd, K.K., Cohen, D.J., Pauls, D.L. and Leckman, J.F. (1985) A twin study of Tourette syndrome. *Achieves of General Psychiatry*, **42**, 815–820.

Rigo, J.M., Hans, G., Nguyen, L., Rocher, V., Belachew, S., Malgrange, B., Leprince, P., Moonen, G., Selak, I., Matagne, A. and Klitgaard, H. (2002) The anti-epileptic drug levetiracetam reverses the inhibition by negative allosteric modulators of neuronal GABA- and glycine-gated currents. *British Journal of Pharmacology*, **136**, 659–672.

Robertson, M.M., Schnieden, V. and Lees, A.J. (1990) Management of Gilles de la Tourette syndrome using sulpiride. *Clinical Neuropharmacology*, **13**, 229–235.

Robertson, M. (1995) The relationship between Gilles de la Tourette's syndrome and obsessive compulsive disorder. *Journal Serotonin Research*, **1** (Suppl), 49.

Ross, M.S. and Moldofsky, H. (1978) A comparison of pimozide and haloperidol in the treatment of Gilles de la Tourette syndrome. *American Journal of Psychiatry*, **135**, 585–587.

Sallee, F.R., Nesbitt, L., Jackson, C., Sine, L. and Sethuraman, G. (1997) Relative efficacy of haloperidol and pimozide in children and adolescents with Tourette's disorder. *American Journal of Psychiatry*, **154**, 1057–1062.

Sallee, F.R., Kurlan, R., Goetz, C.G. *et al.* (2000) Ziprasidone treatment of children and adolescents with Tourette's syndrome:

a pilot study. *Journal of American Academy of Child and Adolescent, Psychiatry*, **39**, 292–299.

Scahill, L., Chappell, P.B., Kim, Y.S. *et al.* (2001) Guanfacine in the treatment of children with tic disorders and ADHD: a placebo-controlled study. *American Journal of Psychiatry*, **158**, 1067–1074.

Scahill, L., Leckman, J.F., Schultyz, R.T. *et al.* (2003) A placebo-controlled trial of risperidone in Tourette syndrome. *Neurology*, **60**, 1130–1135.

Scahill, L., Erenberg, G., Berlin, C.M. *et al.* (2006) Contemporary Assessment and Pharmacotherapy of Tourette Syndrome. *NeuroRx: The Journal of the American Society for Experimental NeuroTherapeutics*, **3**, 192–206.

Shahed, J., Poysky, J., Kenney, C., Simpson, R. and Jankovic, J. (2007) GPi deep brain stimulation for Tourette syndrome improves tics and psychiatric comorbidities. *Neurology*, **68**, 159–160.

Shapiro, A.K., Shapiro, E.S., Young, J.G. and Feinberg, T.E. (1988) *Gilles de la Tourette syndrome*, 2nd edn, Raven Press, New York.

Shapiro, E., Shapiro, A.K., Fulop, G. *et al.* (1989) Controlled study of haloperidol, pimozide, and placebo for the treatment of Gilles de la Tourette's syndrome. *Archives of General Psychiatry*, **46**, 722–730.

Singer, H.S., Rabins, P., Tune, L.E. and Coyle, J.T. (1981) Serum haloperidol levels in Gilles de la Tourette syndrome. *Biological Psychiatry*, **16**, 79–84.

Singer, H.S., Gammon, K. and Quaskey, S. (1986) Haloperidol, fluphenazine and clonidine in Tourette syndrome: controversies in treatment. *Pediatric Neurosciences*, **12**, 71–74.

Singer, H.S., Reiss, A.L., Brown, J.E. *et al.* (1993) Volumetric MRI changes in basal ganglia of children with Tourette's syndrome. *Neurology*, **43**, 950–956.

Singer, H.S., Brown, J., Quaskey, S., Rosenberg, L.A., Mellits, E. D. and Denckla, M.B. (1995) The treatment of attention-deficit hyperactivity disorder in Tourette's syndrome: a double-blind placebo-controlled study with clonidine and desipramine. *Pediatrics*, **95**, 74–81.

Singer, H.S., Wendlandt, J.T., Krieger, M. and Giuliano, J. (2001) Baclofen treatment in Tourette syndrome: a double-blind, placebo-controlled, crossover clinical trial. *Neurology*, **56**, 599–604.

Singer, H.S. and Minzer, K. (2003) Neurobiology of Tourette's syndrome: concepts of neuroanatomic localization and neuro-chemical abnormalities. *Brain and Development*, **25** (Suppl 1), S70–S84.

Smith-Hicks, C.L., Bridges, D.D., Paynter, N.P. and Singer, H.S. (2007) A double blind randomized placebo control trial of levetiracetam in Tourette syndrome. *Movement Disorders*, **22**, 1764–1770.

Spencer, T.J., Biederman, J., Faraone, S. *et al.* (2001) Impact of tic disorders on ADHD outcome across the life cycle: Findings from a large group of adults with and without ADHD. *American Journal of Psychiatry*, **158**, 611.

Spencer, T., Biederman, J., Coffey, B., Geller, D., Crawford, M., Bearman, S.K., Tarazi, R. and Faraone, S.V. (2002) A double-blind comparison of desipramine and placebo in children and adolescents with chronic tic disorder and comorbid attention-deficit/hyperactivity disorder. *Archives of General Psychiatry*, **59**, 649–656.

Stamenkovic, M., Schindle, S.D., Aschauser, H.N. *et al.* (2000) Effective open-label treatment of Tourette disorder with olanzapine. *International Clinical Psychopharmacology*, **15**, 23–28.

Steingard, R.J., Goldberg, M., Lee, D. *et al.* (1994) Adjunctive clonazepam treatment of tic symptoms in children with comorbid tic disorders and ADHD. *Journal of American Acad Child and Adolescent, Psychiatry*, **33**, 394.

Stephens, R.J. and Sandor, P. (1999) Aggressive behaviour in children with Tourette syndrome and comorbid attention-deficit hyperactivity disorder and obsessive-compulsive disorder. *Canadian Journal of Psychiatry*, **44**, 1036.

Sukhodolsky, D.G., Scahill, L., Zhang, H. *et al.* (2003) Disruptive behavior in children with Tourette's syndrome: Association with ADHD comorbidity, tic severity and functional impairment. *Journal of the American Academy of Child and, Adolescent Psychiatry*, **42**, 98.

The Tourette's Syndrome Study Group (2002) Treatment of ADHD in children with tics: a randomized controlled trial. *Neurology*, **58**, 527–536.

Vandewalle, V., Van der Linden, C., Groenewegen, H.J. and Caemaert, J. (1999) Stereotactic treatment of Gilles de la Tourette syndrome by high frequency stimulation of thalamus. *Lancet*, **353**, 724.

Ventura, R., Morrone, C. and Puglisi-Allegra, S. (2007) Prefrontal/ accumbal catecholamine system determines motivational salience attribution to both reward- and aversion-related stimuli. *PNAS*, **104**, 5181–5186.

Verdellen, C.W.J., Keijsers, G.P.J., Cath, D.D. and Hoogduin, C.A. L. (2004) Exposure with response prevention versus habit reversal in Tourette's syndrome: A controlled study. *Behaviour Research and Therapy*, **42**, 501–511.

Visser-Vandewalle, V., Temel, Y., Boon, P., Vreeling, F. *et al.* (2003) Chronic bilateral thalamic stimulation: a new therapeutic approach in intractable Tourette syndrome. *Journal of Neurosurgery*, **99**, 1094–1100.

Wilhelm, S., Deckersback, T., Coffey, B.J. *et al.* (2003) Habit reversal versus supportive psychotherapy for Tourette's disorder: A randomized controlled trial. *American Journal of Psychicatry*, **160**, 1175–1177.

Wolf, S.S., Jones, D.W., Knable, M.B. *et al.* (1996) Tourette syndrome: prediction of phenotypic variation in monozygotic twins by caudate nucleus D2 receptor binding. *Science*, **273**, 1225–1227.

Wong, D.F., Singer, H.S., Brandt, J. *et al.* (1997) D2-like dopamine receptor density in Tourette syndrome measured by PET. *Journal of Nuclear Medicine*, **38**, 1243–1247.

Yoo, H.K., Kim, J.Y. and Kim, C.Y. (2006) A pilot study of aripiprazole in children and adolescents with Tourette's disorder. *Journal of Child and Adolescent Psychopharmacology*, **16**, 505–506.

22

Therapeutics of Paroxysmal Dyskinesias

Shyamal H. Mehta and Kapil D. Sethi

Movement Disorders Program, Department of Neurology, Medical College of Georgia, Augusta, Georgia, USA

INTRODUCTION

Paroxysmal dyskinesias (PxD) are a group of rare movement disorders characterized by their recurrent and episodic nature, arising from a background of normal motor activity and behavior. These abnormal movements can manifest in the form of ballism, dystonia, chorea and athetosis or a combination of these (Sethi, 2000). This interesting sub-set of movement disorders has been further classified into four types, based on the events which precipitate the abnormal movements: (i) paroxysmal kinesigenic dyskinesias (PKD): PxD precipitated by sudden voluntary movements, (ii) paroxysmal non-kinesigenic dyskinesias (PNKD) are the PxD which occur at rest, in the absence of sudden movements, (iii) paroxysmal exertion-induced dyskinesias (PED) occur in the setting of *prolonged* exercise, instead of sudden movements and (iv) paroxysmal hypogenic dyskinesias (PHD), which occur during sleep (however this remains a matter of controversy). PxD can be sporadic, familial (autosomal dominant inheritance) or secondary to other disorders such as multiple sclerosis, stroke and so on. As far as PxD due to a secondary etiology are concerned, one study reports an identifiable cause of PxD in ~22% patients (Blakeley and Jankovic, 2002). Understandably, the age of onset of secondary PxD is highly variable depending on the underlying etiology. The various causes of secondary PxD are listed in Table 22.1. All probable secondary causes should be ruled out before a diagnosis of primary PxD is made.

Early literature on PxD involved the use of specific terminology such as paroxysmal choreoathetosis or paroxysmal dystonic choreoathetosis implying that in all attacks, movements were easily characterized. However, because of the brevity of the attacks, most often these are not witnessed by the diagnosing physician. Also, the movements may be very complex and variable and, as such, not amenable to simple nomenclature. Hence, recent reviews have stressed on the usage of the general term "dyskinesias" for their description (Sethi, 2000; Demirkiran and Jankovic, 1995).

HISTORY OF PAROXYSMAL DYSKINESIAS

From a historical perspective, these rare movement disorders were initially reported as a type of epilepsy or seizures. Spiller recognized paroxysmal movements and called them striatal or subcortical epilepsy. In 1924, Sterling described abnormal movements not precipitated by action and then a year later short-lasting non-kinesigenic attacks were described by Wimmer, but called striatal epilepsy. It was not until 1940, when Mount and Reback described a family with 28 members, that the term *familial paroxysmal choreoathetosis* first appeared in the literature. In this family, the proband had PxD induced, not by movement, but by alcohol and coffee. The spells would begin with an aura of a tight sensation around the neck and abdomen followed by involuntary dystonic posturing of the arms and legs, choreoathetotic movements and dysarthria with preservation of consciousness (Mount and Reback, 1940). Kertesz (1967) reported a group of patients with choreoathetosis precipitated by sudden movement and coined the term *paroxysmal kinesigenic choreoathetosis* (Kertesz, 1967). Lance (1977) reported attacks of intermediate duration in a family, precipitated by prolonged exercise, which are now recognized as PED (Lance, 1977). In 1969, Horner and Jackson described nine members of a family under the label familial paroxysmal choreoathetosis. However, seven of these had only nocturnal attacks. It was not until 1981 that the term nocturnal or hypnogenic dystonia was introduced by Lugaresi and Cirignotta (Lugaresi and Cirignotta, 1981) to describe this disease entity now known as PHD. Further discussion of the history of PxD is beyond the scope of this chapter; for a detailed review of the history please refer to the review by Fahn (1994).

Therapeutics of Parkinson's Disease and Other Movement Disorders   Edited by Mark Hallett and Werner Poewe
© 2008 John Wiley & Sons, Ltd.

Table 22.1 Paroxysmal dyskinesias—secondary causes.

Demyelinating disease—multiple sclerosis

Vascular causes—cerebral infarction, hemorrhage, moya-moya disease and anti-phospholipid antibody syndrome.

Infectious causes—encephalitis, CMV, HIV

Myelopathy and/or radiculopathy

Basal ganglia calcification

Central and peripheral nervous system trauma

Neurodegenerative conditions—Huntington's disease, Parkinson's disease, Progressive supranuclear palsy

Metabolic conditions—diabetes mellitus, hypothyroidism, hypoparathyroidism, pseudohypoparathyroidism, Wilson's disease, mitochondrial cytopathies and kernicterus.

CNS neoplasms

Migraine

Drugs—methylphenidate

PAROXYSMAL KINESIGENIC DYSKINESIAS (PKD)

Clinical Features

PKD onset is typically during childhood, between 5 and 15 years of age, males being more commonly affected then females, with ratios ranging from 2:1 to 4:1 (Sethi, 2002; Lotze and Jankovic, 2003). The condition may be familial or sporadic. Most commonly, the condition is inherited in an autosomally dominant fashion, however there are some reports of autosomal recessive inheritance as well (Goodenough et al., 1978). The attacks are typically precipitated by startle or a sudden movement after a period of rest. There is a refractory period after an attack during which sudden movement may not provoke an attack. The abnormal movements are usually unilateral, however they may proceed to become bilateral. Most patients have dystonia, but some have a combination of chorea and dystonia and, rarely, ballism. Extremities are more commonly involved, as compared to the face, neck and trunk, although the patient can have dysarthria secondary to the dystonia, affecting the speech (Sethi, 2002; Lotze and Jankovic, 2003). Patients may have auras preceding the attacks. The auras have been described as a crawling or tingling sensation, dizziness and paresthesias in the affected body part (Lotze and Jankovic, 2003). The attacks are typically short lived in duration ranging usually from seconds to five minutes, and rarely as long as few hours (Demirkiran and Jankovic, 1995). The frequency of attacks can range from ~100 per day to less than one per month and the neurologic exam in between attacks is usually normal (Lotze and Jankovic, 2003).

In a recent study, Bruno et al. evaluated 121 individuals with idiopathic PKD from 73 families to establish strict diagnostic criteria for the disorder. They found that ~79% of the affected individuals had similar clinical features distinguishable from other diseases. Hence, they proposed the following clinical criteria, based on their results (Bruno et al., 2004b):

(1) Identifiable kinesigenic trigger for the attacks
(2) Short duration of attacks (<1 minute)
(3) No loss of consciousness or pain during the attack
(4) Exclusion of other organic diseases and normal neurologic exam in between attacks
(5) Control of attacks with phenytoin or carbamazepine, if tried
(6) Age at onset between 1 and 20 years, if no family history of PKD.

In their study, nearly 100% of the familial PKD patients satisfied the proposed criteria; however, some of the sporadic PKD patients did not.

There have also been cases of PKD associated with interictal myoclonus. De Grandis et al. reported a 10-year-old boy with PKD along with interictal myoclonus and dystonia, who did not respond to carbamazepine (DeGrandis et al., 2007). Two other patients with PKD have also been reported to have interictal myoclonus; however, in this case, both the patients responded well to carbamazepine (Cochen De Cock et al., 2006).

Genetics

Most cases of PKD are primary and probably of genetic etiology. Several families with PKD have been linked to the pericentromic region of chromosome 16 (Swoboda et al., 2000). PKD has shown to be associated or overlaps clinically with other syndromes as well. A syndrome characterized by a combination of infantile convulsions and paroxysmal choreoathetosis—ICCA syndrome—has also been mapped to a 10 cM region around the centromere on chromsosme 16 (Szepetowski et al., 1997). It appears that there is a great degree of clinical overlap between the two conditions, as some families with PKD have had a history of childhood convulsions as well. Another syndrome, RE-PED-WCcharacterized by rolandic epilepsy, paroxysmal exercise-induced dyskinesias and writer's cramp has also been mapped to a 6 cM region on chromosome 16 (Guerrini et al., 1999). In fact, ICCA syndrome entirely includes the critical region involved in RE-PED-WC syndrome. A locus for PKD (EKD1) has been mapped to 16p11.2-q12.1 in eight Japanese families, and an 18 cM region on chromosome 16p11.2-q11.2 in an Afro-Caribbean family (Tomita et al., 1999; Bennett, Roach and Bowcock, 2000). Interestingly, RE-PED-WC, which also maps to the chromosome

16p12-11.2 region, does not overlap with the PKD localizations (Spacey et al., 2002). Valente et al. have identified a unique PKD locus (EKD2) telomeric to the ICCA and EKD1 loci, indicating a separate gene for the pure PKD phenotype (Valente et al., 2000). An additional British family has been identified, where the PKD locus in this family did not map to the previously identified PKD loci on chromosome 16, probably representing a new gene, EKD3 (Spacey et al., 2002). Thus, it seems that there is significant clinical and genetic heterogeneity in PKD. Despite the strong linkage of PKD to the chromosome 16p11-q21, analysis of the 157 genes was unsuccessful at identifying any mutations responsible for PKD in a recent study of seven families with varying ethnic backgrounds (Kikuchi et al., 2007). Since other paroxysmal neurologic conditions, such as episodic ataxias and some epilepsies have been linked to mutations in ion-channel genes, it may be possible that some of the mutations in the critical region for PKD on chromosome 16 may play a role in ion-channel function. However, the function of mutated genes involved in PKD has to be determined before these disorders can be labeled as channelopathies (Margari et al., 2005).

Treatment of PKD

PKD is characterized by brief attacks of dystonia and choreoathetosis precipitated by sudden movement. Overall, PKD responds well to anti-convulsants, which are the mainstay of therapy. PKD has a relatively benign prognosis, as the attacks gradually diminish in adulthood. Carbamazepine is the drug of choice (Schneider and Bhatia, 2007). In a Taiwanese study, four out of seven patients with PKD were started on low-dose carbamazepine (1.5–2 mg/kg/day). All four patients became episode-free, without decline in school performance, over a follow-up period of 14–30 months (Tsai et al., 2005). From past experience, other anti-convulsants, such as barbiturates, oxcarbazepine and phenytoin have also been proven to be efficacious (Schneider and Bhatia, 2007). In adults, a low dose may be effective in controlling the episodes. One study with eight patients showed that topiramate at doses of 100–200 mg/day was effective in controlling the episodes of PKC with minimal side effects. The patients were followed up for a period ranging from eight months to two years (Huang et al., 2005). In a case series of three children with PKC from Germany, lamotrigine was used to treat the episodes. They found complete elimination of the episodes with doses between 4.5–5 mg/kg/day (Uberall and Wenzel, 2000). In general, treatment recommendations have favored AEDs, which act on voltage-gated neuronal ion channels (i.e., carbamazepine and phenytoin). Lamotrigine, which acts via a use-dependent blockade of voltage-gated sodium channels, may have an important place in the treatment of PKD, if proven to be effective,

based on future, controlled studies (Uberall and Wenzel, 2000). Not too many other options besides anti-convulsants exist for the treatment of PKD. One case report showed that risperidone was effective and could be used as an alternative treatment for PKD (Karakurum, Karatas and Yildirim, 2003). Other drugs that have been helpful include anti-cholinergics, levodopa, flunarizine and tetrabenazine (Lotze and Jankovic, 2003).

As far as secondary PKD is concerned, the response rate is similar to primary PKD. Treatment of the underlying condition causing PKD is helpful in reducing the attacks for obvious reasons. PKD secondary to demyelinating lesions responds favorably to treatment with acetozolamide (Sethi et al., 1992) and benzodiazepines have been used with success in treating PKD in HIV patients (Schneider and Bhatia, 2007). Also Blakeley and Jankovic have reported that injecting botulinum toxin into the agonist muscles was effective in the treatment of secondary PKD with dystonia (Blakeley and Jankovic, 2002).

PKD – Salient Features Recapped:

- Usually of autosomal-dominant etiology, typical onset during childhood (age range 5–15 yr). Frequency of attacks gradually decreases in adulthood
- Attacks precipitated by startle or sudden movements, most common presentation involves dystonia in the extremities
- Attacks are short lasting from seconds to minutes, frequency: ~100/day
- Locus for mutations related to PKD is near the pericentromic region of chromosome 16
- Carbamazepine is the drug of choice, but barbiturates and phenytoin have also proven to be useful
- Lamotrigine and topamax have shown to be useful in a small number of patients.

PAROXYSMAL NON-KINESIGENIC DYSKINESIAS (PNKD)

Clinical Features

PNKD is typically inherited in an autosomal-dominant manner with a high penetrance of 80% (Zorzi et al., 2003). The attacks occur more frequently in males; however, it is not as consistently seen as in PKD. The attacks in PNKD usually begin during childhood, with a mean age of about eight years, but may start up until the early 20s. Attacks occur at rest and may be precipitated by alcohol, coffee, cola, tobacco, emotional excitement and fatigue (Mount and Reback 1940). Typically, attacks begin with a sensation of tightness or tugging, followed by involuntary movements of the mouth or one limb and may spread to involve all the extremities including the face without any loss of awareness (Lance, 1977). Some families have predominantly dystonia, while others have predominantly choreoathetosis (Mount and Reback, 1940). The frequency of episodes may vary from two to three per day to two per year, the episodes are long lasting, with a usual duration of 30 minutes to 3–4 hours (Fink *et al.*, 1996) although some may only last for seconds (Demirkiran and Jankovic, 1995). Occurrence of attacks during rest, the lower frequency and the longer duration of the episodes are key features that distinguish PNKD from PKD. The attacks are usually aborted by sleep. PNKD has been reported to occur concomitantly with familial ataxia, and in one family PNKD was accompanied by myokymia (Sethi, 2000).

Genetics

Lee *et al.* reported mutations in the myofibrillogenesis regulator 1 (MR-1) gene on the long arm of chromosome 2 (2q32-36 locus) causing PNKD in 50 individuals from eight families (Lee *et al.*, 2004). Since then, mutations in the MR-1 gene have been identified in 10 unrelated PNKD kindred (Spacey *et al.*, 2006). Several reports have confirmed the presence of alanine-to-valine substitutions in the MR-1 gene being responsible for the PNKD phenotype (Lee *et al.*, 2004; Chen *et al.*, 2005). Bioinformatic analysis has shown that the MR-1 gene is homologous to the hydroxyacylglutathione hydrolase (HAGH) gene. HAGH functions in a pathway to detoxify methylglyoxal, a compound present in coffee and alcoholic beverages, which may explain why both coffee and alcohol reliably precipitate attacks in PNKD (Lee *et al.*, 2004). Alcohol and caffeine precipitated attacks in 98% of patients with the MR-1 mutation (Bruno *et al.*, 2007). However, there may be some genetic heterogeneity in PNKD, as Spacey *et al.* have described a Canadian PNKD family with 14 members, who did not have mutations in the MR-1 gene. Affected family members presented with episodes of dystonia primarily affecting hands and feet symmetrically, but alcohol, caffeine and excitement were not obvious triggers in this family. Linkage analysis in this pedigree identified a novel gene locus (PNKD-2) at chromosome 2q31, between markers D2S335 and D2S152. One of the interesting genes in this locus is the glutamate decarboxylase gene, which codes for glutamic acid decarboxylase. Glutamate decarboxylase is expressed in the mammalian brain and catalyzes the conversion of glutamic acid to γ-aminobutyric acid (GABA), which is the main inhibitory neuropeptide in the basal ganglia (Spacey *et al.*, 2006). In a recent study, Bruno *et al.* conclude that patients with classic PNKD phenotype, as described by Mount and Reback, are more likely to have MR-1 mutations while the "PNKD-like" kindred with atypical features may not have MR-1 mutations, as some of them may actually have PED (Bruno *et al.*, 2007).

Treatment of PNKD

In PNKD, the paroxysms last longer and are not triggered by movement, but by fatigue, stress, alcohol or caffeine. Avoidance of the precipitating factors can be helpful. Unlike PKD, PNKD does not respond to anti-convulsants, and medical treatment is less rewarding (Dressler and Benecke, 2005). However, anti-convulsants should be tried in every case and an occasional patient may respond to carbamazepine (Bhatia, 1999). Other drugs that have been tried include clonazepam, haloperidol, alternate-day oxazepam, and anti-cholinergics such as benztropine and trihexyphenidyl without consistent success (Sethi, 2000), however, clonazepam may benefit one-third of patients treated (Bhatia 1999). A recent case report showed that sublingual lorazepam was successfully used to treat two children with PNKD from a large kindred (Dooley and Brna, 2004). Deep brain stimulation (DBS) is also being explored as a potential therapeutic option in the treatment of medically refractory PNKD. Loher *et al.* have assessed the effect of chronic stimulation of the ventrointermediate (Vim) thalamus for treatment of dystonic PNKD. Chronic stimulation through a stereotactically implanted monopolar electrode in the left Vim resulted in a decrease of the frequency, duration and intensity of the dystonic paroxysmal movement disorder and the benefit of stimulation was maintained over four years of follow-up (Loher *et al.*, 2001). In another case, stimulation of globus pallidus internus produced immediate and sustained relief of PNKD, secondary to rotator cuff tears (Yamada *et al.*, 2006). Similar to PKD, secondary PNKD may also improve with treatment of the underlying etiology, as seen in the case of PNKD secondary to celiac disease. The patient's neurologic symptoms resolved upon the institution of a gluten-free diet (Hall, Parsons and Benke, 2007). Another patient had a seven-year history of episodes resembling PNKD, secondary to idiopathic hyperparathyroidism. This patient was refractory to valproate, but responded to levetiracetam (Alemdar *et al.*, 2007). In one study, six patients with HIV had PxD, 2/6 patients had PKD and 4/6 patients had PNKD. Benzodiazepines appeared to be of symptomatic benefit in 3/4 patients with PNKD (Mirsattari *et al.*, 1999).

PNKD – Salient Features Recapped:

- Usually autosomal-dominant pattern, typically begins in childhood; mean age ~8 yr
- Attacks occur at rest and are precipitated by alcohol, tobacco, coffee, excitement and fatigue. Clinical manifestations vary from dystonia to choreoathetosis
- Duration of attacks: 30 min – 3–4 h (longer than PKD), frequency of attacks from 2 to 3/day to 2/year (less frequent than PKD)

- Most cases of classical PNKD due to Ala to Val substitution or other mutations in the MR-1 gene on the long arm of chromosome 2
- Patients with atypical PNKD may not have mutations in the MR-1 gene
- Less amenable to treatment as compared to PKD, however, anti-convulsants must be tried in every patient
- Benzodiazepines, anti-cholinergics and haloperidol have been tried with inconsistent responses
- Anecdotal reports of efficacy of DBS in treating PNKD are present in the literature, but larger studies are lacking.

PAROXYSMAL EXERCISE-INDUCED DYSKINESIAS (PED)

Clinical Features

PED is a rare form of PxD, usually inherited in an autosomal-dominant manner, although some sporadic cases have been reported (Sethi, 2000; Bhatia et al., 1997). Male to female predominance is in a ratio 2:3. Mean age of onset of attacks is about five years, ranging from 2 to 30 years. Classically, the attacks are brought on by prolonged exercise, although passive movements, electrical nerve stimulation and exposure to cold have also been reported to precipitate attacks (Wali, 1992). Although the episodes can be variable, in a review of 20 cases by Bhatia et al. dystonia affecting the feet was the most common presentation, with a hemidystonic distribution being the next most common (Bhatia, 1999). Also, exercise limited to a particular body part may provoke dystonia in that body part alone (Plant et al., 1984). The frequency of the attacks varies from one per day to two per month and the usual duration is from minutes to two hours. Attacks usually cease within 10 minutes of stopping the exercise (Nardocci et al., 1989).

PED has also been reported in combination with migraines, different forms of epilepsy and dystonia. Kamm et al. reported a German family with four affected members, who exhibit the above mentioned conditions in variable combinations (Kamm et al., 2007). DeGrandis et al. have also reported a case of PED with the presence of interictal myoclonus and dystonia; however, they did not check for the ε-sarcoglycan mutation in the patient to rule out myoclonus dystonia (DeGrandis et al., 2007). Several case reports have also suggested that PED can be the presenting symptom in patients with young-onset or the familial form of Parkinson's disease (Bozi and Bhatia, 2003; Bruno et al., 2004b; Katzenschlager et al., 2002).

Genetics

PED is much less common compared to PKD and PNKD, hence little genetic information is available regarding this condition. In the study by Bruno et al. ∼68% patients

negative for MR-1 mutation may actually have had PED, as their attacks of dyskinesias were provoked by exercise (Bruno et al., 2007). Phenotypically variant forms of PED have revealed significant heterogeneity; however, the underlying genetic mutations remain currently unidentified. Genetic studies in a family with PED and migraines did not show any linkage to the loci on chromosome 16 (PKD and ICCA), chromosome 2 (PNKD) or chromosome 19p (familial hemiplegic migraine) (Münchau et al., 2000). Another study in a family with typical exercise-induced dystonia, different types of epilepsy (absence and primary generalized seizures), developmental delay and migraine, in variable combinations, also did not reveal linkage to loci on chromosome 2 and 16 (Kamm et al., 2007).

Treatment of PED

These are attacks most commonly of dystonia precipitated by prolonged exercise in addition to some other triggers. Avoidance of prolonged exercise may help diminish the frequency of attacks. Anti-convulsants, such as carbamazepine have been used with limited success in the treatment of PED. Levodopa has been reported to be efficacious in some instances (McGrath and Dure, 2003). Benzodiazepines and anti-cholinergic agents have not benefited most of the patients treated with them. In one case report, Guimaraes et al. described a 40-year-old woman, whose condition worsened on treatment with acetazolamide, whereas gabapentin greatly reduced the frequency and severity of the attacks (Guimarães and Vale Santos, 2000). In cases of medically refractory PED, Bhatia et al. have reported successful amelioration of episodes of PED with unilateral posteroventral medial pallidotomy and the patient remained attack free at the six-month follow-up (Bhatia, Marsden and Thomas, 1998). In a case of secondary PED due to an insulinoma, hypoglycemia precipitated the episodes, which resolved during hyper- or euglycemia. Removal of the tumor abolished the attacks (Tan et al., 2002). Although dystonia following trauma is common, a Chinese individual had PED following a back injury after a motorcycle accident, which had an excellent response to low-dose baclofen (Lim and Wong, 2003). As mentioned earlier, PED can be a presenting symptom of young-onset Parkinson's disease; in the two patients reported by Bozi and Bhatia, both patients improved after treatment of their Parkinson's disease with benzhexol and levodopa (Bozi and Bhatia, 2003).

PED – Salient Features Recapped:

- Usually of an autosomal-dominant etiology with a mean age of onset ∼5 yr (age range 2–30 yr)
- Attacks precipitated by prolonged exercise and exposure to cold

- Frequency of attacks: 1/day to 2/month; duration of attacks: minutes to 2 h. Attacks usually cease within 10 min of stopping exercise
- Exercise limited to one part of the body may provoke dystonia in that body part alone
- Genetic mechanisms of the disease remain to be elucidated
- Avoidance of prolonged exercise and other triggers is the most effective method of preventing the attacks
- Carbamazepine and benzodiazepines have been used with limited success; levodopa has been useful in a few cases
- A case report of successful treatment with unilateral posteroventral medial pallidotomy is present in the literature, but more studies are needed.

Miscellaneous Paroxysmal Movement Disorders

Besides the classic syndromes described by Demerkiran and Jankovic, there are some other paroxysms with dystonia, tremor and ataxia as their main features. These are briefly mentioned in Table 22.2. For a more detailed description, please refer to the review by Schneider and Bhatia (Schneider and Bhatia, 2007). In addition, Pourfar et al. have reported four cases of their own, with four other cases that do not fit into the above mentioned categories. They propose that, instead of the distinct categories as put forth by Demerkiran and Jankovic, they represent a continuum with most cases presenting with predominant features of one or the other (Pourfar et al., 2005).

Also, in recent years, significant advances have been made in understanding the genetic etiology of these disorders, if a clear genetically based etiology is found, it may lead to a new genetically based re-classification of these disorders.

PAROXYSMAL HYPNOGENIC DYSKINESIA (PHD): A FORM OF EPILEPSY?

In 1981, Lugaresi et al. reported five patients with nocturnal episodes characterized by intermittent attacks of dystonia, chorea or ballism during non-REM sleep, in particular stages 2 and 3. The attacks occured in clusters up to 20 times a night, each lasting about 30–60 seconds. The

Table 22.2 Miscellaneous paroxysmal movement disorders.

Benign torticollis of infancy
Sandifer's syndrome
Paroxysms of the tongue
Tonic spasms of multiple sclerosis

involuntary movements could be localized to one limb, involve all the extremities or the trunk as well (Lugaresi and Cirignotta, 1981). Patients could also have automatisms, vocalizations and subsequent sleep disturbances. The disorder did not spontaneously improve over the years, however almost all patients responded to even low doses of carbamazepine. The stereotypic pattern of movements, short duration and response to anti-epileptics suggested an epileptic etiology of the events; however, the absence of ictal and interictal EEG abnormalities made it difficult to classify it as epilepsy (Provini, Plazzi and Lugaresi, 2000). Hence, the disorder was thought of as a movement disorder. However, using zygomatic and sphenoidal electrodes Tinuper et al. found mesial frontal lobe origin of the attacks in three patients (Tinuper et al., 1990). Also the phenotype of the EEG negative patients was clinically indistinguishable from the patients with frontal lobe onset of seizures, suggesting that PHD may actually represent nocturnal frontal lobe epilepsy (NFLE) (Hirsch et al., 1994). Video polysomnography with EEG monitoring may be necessary for the diagnosis of NFLE to detect the stereotypical abnormal movements during the attacks (Provini, Plazzi and Lugaresi, 2000).

However, clinically one encounters patients that have both daytime and night-time attacks of paroxysmal dyskinesia and some are hard to classify using the current classification schemes (Pourfar et al., 2005). In this setting it is useful to remember that the first case of PHD was described by Joynt and Greene in a patient who had multiple sclerosis, and daytime attacks as well (Joynt and Green, 1962). Horner and Jackson described a family with PHD in which some members had daytime attacks (Horner and Jackson, 1969). The presence of daytime attacks in these earlier case reports makes it less likely that these patients would have had NFLE. However, it is possible that most patients with PHD represent a form of epilepsy, but this will not be covered in detail in the context of this chapter.

References

Alemdar, M., Iseri, P., Selekler, M. and Komsuoglu, S.S. (2007) Levetiracetam-responding paroxysmal nonkinesigenic dyskinesia. *Clinical Neuropharmacology*, **30**, 241–244.

Bennett, L.B., Roach, E.S. and Bowcock, A.M. (2000) A locus for paroxysmal kinesigenic dyskinesia maps to human chromosome 16. *Neurology*, **54**, 125–130.

Bhatia, K.P., Soland, V.L., Bhatt, M.H. et al. (1997) Paroxysmal exercise induced dystonia: eight new sporadic cases and a review of literature. *Movement Disorders*, **12**, 1007–1012.

Bhatia, K.P., Marsden, C.D. and Thomas, D.G. (1998) Posteroventral pallidotomy can ameliorate attacks of paroxysmal dystonia induced by exercise. *Journal of Neurology, Neurosurgery, and Psychiatry*, **65**, 604–605.

Bhatia, K.P. (1999) The paroxysmal dyskinesias. *Journal of Neurology*, **246**, 149–155.

Blakeley, J. and Jankovic, J. (2002) Secondary paroxysmal dyskinesias. *Movement Disorders*, **17**, 726–734.

Bozi, M. and Bhatia, K.P. (2003) Paroxysmal exercise-induced dystonia as a presenting feature of young-onset Parkinson's disease. *Movement Disorders*, **18**, 1545–1547.

Bruno, M.K., Hallett, M., Gwinn-Hardy, K. *et al.* (2004b) Clinical evaluation of idiopathic paroxysmal kinesigenic dyskinesia: new diagnostic criteria. *Neurology*, **63**, 2280–2287.

Bruno, M.K., Ravina, B., Garraux, G. *et al.* (2004a) Exercise-induced dystonia as a preceding symptom of familial Parkinson's disease. *Movement Disorders*, **19**, 228–230.

Bruno, M.K., Lee, H.Y., Auburger, G.W. *et al.* (2007) Genotype-phenotype correlation of paroxysmal nonkinesigenic dyskinesia. *Neurology*, **68**, 1782–1789.

Chen, D.H., Matsushita, M., Rainier, S. *et al.* (2005) Presence of alanine-to-valine substitutions in myofibrillogenesis regulator 1 in paroxysmal nonkinesigenic dyskinesia: confirmation in 2 kindreds. *Archives of Neurology*, **62**, 597–600.

Cochen De Cock, V., Bourdain, F., Apartis, E. *et al.* (2006) Interictal myoclonus with paroxysmal kinesigenic dyskinesia. *Movement Disorders*, **21**, 1533–1535.

DeGrandis, E., Mir, P., Edwards, M.J. *et al.* (Nov 23, 2007) Paroxysmal dyskinesia with interictal myoclonus and dystonia: A report of two cases. Parkinsonism Relat Disord. [Epub ahead of print].

Demirkiran, M. and Jankovic, J. (1995) Paroxysmal dyskinesias: clinical features and classification. *Annals of Neurology*, **38**, 571–579.

Dooley, J.M. and Brna, P.M. (2004) Sublingual lorazepam in the treatment of familial paroxysmal nonkinesigenic dyskinesia. *Pediatric Neurology*, **30**, 365–366.

Dressler, D. and Benecke, R. (2005) Diagnosis and management of acute movement disorders. *Journal of Neurology*, **252**, 1299–1306.

Fahn, S. (1994) The paroxysmal dyskinesias, in *Movement Disorders*, 3rd edn (eds C.D. Marsden and S. Fahn), Butterworth Heinemann, Woburn, MA, pp. 310–346.

Fink, J.K., Rainer, S., Wilkowski, J. *et al.* (1996) Paroxysmal dystonic choreoathetosis: tight linkage to chromosome 2q. *American Journal of Human Genetics*, **59**, 140–145.

Goodenough, D.J., Fariello, R.G., Annis, B.L. and Chun, R.W. (1978) Familial and acquired paroxysmal dyskinesias: a proposed classification with delineation of clinical features. *Archives of Neurology*, **35**, 827–831.

Guerrini, R., Bonanni, P., Nardocci, N. *et al.* (1999) Autosomal recessive rolandic epilepsy with paroxysmal exercise-induced dystonia and writer's cramp: delineation of the syndrome and gene mapping to chromosome 16p12-11.2. *Annals of Neurology*, **45**, 344–352.

Guimarães, J. and Vale Santos, J. (2000) Paroxysmal dystonia induced by exercise and acetazolamide. *European Journal of Neurology*, **7**, 237–240.

Hall, D.A., Parsons, J. and Benke, T. (2007) Paroxysmal nonkinesigenic dystonia and celiac disease. *Movement Disorders*, **22**, 708–710.

Hirsch, E., Sellal, F., Maton, B. *et al.* (1994) Nocturnal paroxysmal dystonia: a clinical form of focal epilepsy. *Neurophysiologie Clinique*, **24**, 207–217.

Huang, Y.G., Chen, Y.C., Du, F. *et al.* (2005) Topiramate therapy for paroxysmal kinesigenic choreoathetosis. *Movement Disorders*, **20**, 75–77.

Horner, F.H. and Jackson, L.C. (1969) Familial paroxysmal choreoathetosis, in *Progress in Neurogenetics* (eds A. Barbeau and J-.R. Brunette), Excerpta Medica Foundation, Amsterdam, pp. 745–751.

Joynt, R.J. and Green, D. (1962) Tonic seizures as a manifestation in multiple sclerosis. *Archives of Neurology*, **6**, 293–299.

Kamm, C., Mayer, P., Sharma, M. *et al.* (2007) New family with paroxysmal exercise-induced dystonia and epilepsy. *Movement Disorders*, **22**, 873–877.

Karakurum, B., Karatas, M. and Yildirim, T. (2003) Risperidone as an alternative treatment for paroxysmal kinesigenic dyskinesias. *Neurological Sciences*, **24**, 92–93.

Katzenschlager, R., Costa, D., Gacinovic, S. and Lees, A.J. (2002) [(123)I]-FP-CIT-SPECT in the early diagnosis of PD presenting as exercise-induced dystonia. *Neurology*, **59**, 1974–1976.

Kertesz, A. (1967) Paroxysmal kinesigenic choreoathetosis: an entity within paroxysmal choreoathetosis syndrome. Description of ten cases including one autopsied. *Neurology*, **17**, 680–690.

Kikuchi, T., Nomura, M., Tomita, H. *et al.* (2007) Paroxysmal kinesigenic choreoathetosis (PKC): confirmation of linkage to 16p11-q21, but unsuccessful detection of mutations among 157 genes at the PKC-critical region in seven PKC families. *Journal of Human Genetics*, **52**, 334–341.

Lance, J.W. (1977) Familial paroxysmal dystonic choreoathetosis and its differentiation from related syndromes. *Annals of Neurology*, **2**, 285–293.

Lee, H.Y., Xu, Y., Huang, Y., Ahn, A.H. *et al.* (2004) The gene for paroxysmal non-kinesigenic dyskinesia encodes an enzyme in a stress response pathway. *Human Molecular Genetics*, **13**, 3161–3170.

Lim, E.C. and Wong, W.S. (2003) Post-traumatic paroxysmal exercise-induced dystonia: case report and review of the literature. *Parkinsonism & Related Disorders*, **9**, 371–373.

Loher, T.J., Krauss, J.K., Burgunder, J.M. *et al.* (2001) Chronic thalamic stimulation for treatment of dystonic paroxysmal nonkinesigenic dyskinesia. *Neurology*, **56**, 268–270.

Lotze, T. and Jankovic, J. (2003) Paroxysmal Kinesigenic Dyskinesias. *Seminars in Pediatric Neurology*, **10**, 68–79.

Lugaresi, E. and Cirignotta, F. (1981) Hypnogenic paroxysmal dystonia: epileptic seizure or a new syndrome? *Sleep*, **4**, 129–138.

Margari, L., Presicci, A., Ventura, P. *et al.* (2005) Channelopathy: hypothesis of a common pathophysiologic mechanism in different forms of paroxysmal dyskinesia. *Pediatric Neurology*, **32**, 229–235.

McGrath, T.M. and Dure, D.S. (2003) Paroxysmal dyskinesias in children. *Current Treatment Options in Neurology*, **5**, 275–278.

Mirsattari, S.M., Berry, M.E., Holden, J.K. *et al.* (1999) Paroxysmal dyskinesias in patients with HIV infection. *Neurology*, **52**, 109–114.

Mount, L.A. and Reback, S. (1940) Familial paroxysmal choreoathetosis: preliminary report on a hitherto undescribed clinical syndrome. *Archives of Neurology and Psychiatry*, **44**, 841–847.

Münchau, A., Valente, E.M., Shahidi, G.A. *et al.* (2000) A new family with paroxysmal exercise induced dystonia and migraine: a clinical and genetic study. *Journal of Neurology, Neurosurgery, and Psychiatry*, **68**, 609–614.

Nardocci, N., Lamperti, E., Rumi, V. and Angelini, L. (1989) Typical and atypical forms of paroxysmal choreoathetosis. *Developmental Medicine and Child Neurology*, **31**, 670–674.

Plant, G.T., Williams, A.C., Earl, C.J. *et al.* (1984) Familial paroxysmal dystonia induced by exercise. *Journal of Neurology, Neurosurgery, and Psychiatry*, **47**, 275–279.

Pourfar, M.H., Guerrini, R., Parain, D. and Frucht, S.J. (2005) Classification conundrums in Paroxysmal dyskinesias: A new subtype or variations on classic themes? *Movement Disorders*, **20**, 1047–1051.

Provini, F., Plazzi, G. and Lugaresi, E. (2000) From nocturnal paroxysmal dystonia to nocturnal frontal lobe epilepsy. *Clinical Neurophysiology*, **111** (Suppl 2), S2–S8.

Schneider, S.A. and Bhatia, K.P. (2007) Paroxysmal dyskinesias: An overview, in *Parkinson's Disease and Movement Disorders*, 5th edn (eds J. Jankovic and E. Tolosa), Lippincott, Williams, and Wilkins, Philadelphia, pp. 459–467.

Sethi, K.D., Hess, D.C., Huffnagle, V.H. and Adams, R.J. (1992) Acetazolamide treatment of paroxysmal dystonia in central demyelinating disease. *Neurology*, **42**, 919–921.

Sethi, K.D. (2000) Paroxysmal Dyskinesias. *The Neurologist*, **6**, 77–85.

Sethi, K.D. (2002) Paroxysmal dyskinesias, in *Parkinson's Disease and Movement Disorders*, 4th edn (eds J. Jankovic and E. Tolosa), Lippincott, Williams, and Wilkins, Philadelphia, pp. 430–437.

Spacey, S.D., Valente, E.M., Wali, G.M. *et al.* (2002) Genetic and clinical heterogeneity in paroxysmal kinesigenic dyskinesia: evidence for a third EKD gene. *Movement Disorders*, **17**, 717–725.

Spacey, S.D., Adams, P.J., Lam, P.C. *et al.* (2006) Genetic heterogeneity in paroxysmal nonkinesigenic dyskinesia. *Neurology*, **66**, 1588–1590.

Swoboda, K.J., Soong, B., McKenna, C. *et al.* (2000) Paroxysmal kinesigenic dyskinesia and infantile convulsions: clinical and linkage studies. *Neurology*, **55**, 224–230.

Szepetowski, P., Rochette, J., Berquin, P. *et al.* (1997) Familial infantile convulsions and paroxysmal choreoathetosis: a new neurological syndrome linked to the pericentromeric region of human chromosome 16. *American Journal of Human Genetics*, **61**, 889–898.

Tan, N.C., Tan, A.K., Sitoh, Y.Y. *et al.* (2002) Paroxysmal exercise-induced dystonia associated with hypoglycaemia induced by an insulinoma. *Journal of Neurology*, **249**, 1615–1616.

Tinuper, P., Cerullo, A., Cirignotta, F. *et al.* (1990) Nocturnal paroxysmal dystonia with short-lasting attacks: three cases with evidence for an epileptic frontal lobe origin of seizures. *Epilepsia*, **31**, 549–556.

Tomita, H., Nagamitsu, S., Wakui, K. *et al.* (1999) Paroxysmal kinesigenic choreoathetosis locus maps to chromosome 16p11.2-q12.1. *American Journal of Human Genetics* **65** 1688–1697.

Tsai, J.D., Chou, I.C., Tsai, K.J. *et al.* (2005) Clinical manifestation and carbamazepine treatment of patients with paroxysmal kinesigenic choreoathetosis. *Acta Paediatr Taiwan*, **46**, 138–142.

Uberall, M.A. and Wenzel, D. (2000) Effectiveness of lamotrigine in children with paroxysmal kinesigenic choreoathetosis. *Developmental Medicine and Child Neurology*, **42**, 699–700.

Valente, E.M., Spacey, S.D., Wali, G.M. *et al.* (2000) A second paroxysmal kinesigenic choreoathetosis locus (EKD2) mapping on 16q13-q22.1 indicates a family of genes which give rise to paroxysmal disorders on human chromosome 16. *Brain: A Journal of Neurology*, **123** (Pt 10), 2040–2045.

Wali, G.M. (1992) Paroxysmal hemidystonia induced by prolonged exercise and cold. *Journal of Neurology, Neurosurgery, and Psychiatry*, **55**, 236–237.

Yamada, K., Goto, S., Soyama, N. *et al.* (2006) Complete suppression of paroxysmal nonkinesigenic dyskinesia by globus pallidus internus pallidal stimulation. *Movement Disorders*, **21**, 576–579.

Zorzi, G., Conti, C., Erba, A. *et al.* (2003) Paroxysmal dyskinesias in childhood. *Pediatric Neurology*, **28**, 168–172.

23

Treatment of Miscellaneous Disorders

Marie Vidailhet, Emmanuel Roze and David Grabli

Fédération du Système Nerveux, Salpêtrière Hospital, Assistance Publique Hôpitaux de Paris,
Université Paris 6 – Pierre et Marie Curie and INSERM U679, Paris, France

A wide range of movement disorders cannot be classified into the classical sub-categories of syndromes. According to the body localization, these miscellaneous syndromes can be divided into four groups: face, neck, trunk and limb disorders. When available, an etiologic treatment can be proposed in these disorders considering the benefit/risk ratio, but the cause often remains undetermined. Due to the small number of patients and the nosologic difficulties, randomized, controlled therapeutic trials are lacking in most of these disorders. Symptomatic treatment strategy is therefore based mainly on open-labeled observations and personal experience. Botulinum toxin is a safe and efficient therapeutic option in facial disorders, including hemifacial spasm, facial hemidystonia, tonic spasm and may be occasionally used in geniospasm, bruxism, chronic myokymia, myoclonic dystonia, or dystonic tics of the face. Neck tongue syndrome and bobble-head doll syndrome are important to identify as they may require additional investigations and can be improved with surgical treatment. Treatment of movement disorders of the trunk including spinal and propriospinal myoclonus, and belly dancing are disappointing. However, treatment with benzodiazepines or various anti-epileptic drugs, and in some cases botulinum toxin injections, may result in partial improvement in these conditions. Among limb movement disorders, symptomatic treatment can be alternatively proposed in the absence of possible etiologic treatment. Painful legs and moving toes are often resistant to analgesic treatment and may respond to epidural block or epidural spinal cord stimulation. Stump dyskinesias can be improved with baclofen, gabapentin or anti-depressant treatment, whereas paroxysmal movement disorders may respond to anti-epileptic drugs or benzodiazepines. Treatment of causalgia dystonia syndrome is challenging and includes a combination of physiotherapy and psychotherapy.

INTRODUCTION

Besides the various movement disorders that can be classified into one of the "classical" sub-categories of syndromes (e.g., chorea, dystonia, myoclonus, etc. . . .), a myriad of individual movement disorders is observed and requires appropriate diagnosis and treatment. In order to avoid a fastidious list of miscellaneous diseases and syndromes, a proposed strategy is to consider these movements with a double approach:

(1) According to the body localization (face/neck, upper or lower limbs, trunk and stance)
(2) According to the provoking factor and/or the accompanying signs.

For each type of movement, a brief description and differential diagnosis will be provided, then available treatments and algorithms for management will be proposed. In these disorders, a strong consistent body of evidence for beneficial effects of the treatments, based on randomized, controlled trials, is rarely available and most of the results are based on open-labeled observations or expert opinion, clinical experience and personal expertise.

FACIAL MOVEMENT DISORDERS (TABLE 23.1)

Jerky Movements

The most frequent movement disorder is hemifacial spasm, which is characterized by unilateral involuntary contraction of muscles innervated by the facial nerve (see Chapter 17 on cramps and spasms). The symptoms often predominate around the eye (orbicularis oculi), with syncinetic contractions of the jaw and lips. The platismus

Table 23.1 Treatment approaches to facial movement disorders.

Syndrome	Clinical features	Causes	Management
Hemifacial spasm	Unilateral jerky movements of muscles innervated by the facial nerve (rarely bilateral).	Neurovascular contact	Local botulinum toxin type A
			Injections into orbicularis oculi muscle (rarely, lower facial muscles, in addition), see Chapter 17
Facial myokymia	Fine vermicular muscle contractions localized (e.g., chin, eyelid);	Brain stem tumor	Local botulinum toxin type A injections
	multiplets (electrophysiology)	Multiple sclerosis irradiations (benign when limited to the eyelid)	Low-dose carbamazepine oxcarbazepine, gabapentin
Geniospasm	Isolated chin tremor	Idiopathic Autosomal dominant	Local botulinum toxin type A Into the chin muscle
Oculomasticatory myorythmia	Slow, rhythmic tremor/ myoclonus of the face and jaw pendular vergence oscillations of the eyes	Whipple's disease	Treatments for Whipple's disease
Bruxism	Tooth grinding and tooth clenching	Idiopathic (rarely, secondary to radiotherapy, drug addicts)	Local botulinim toxin injections into the masseter and temporalis muscles
	Hypertrophy of the masseter and temporatis muscles		

muscle is frequently involved with unaesthetic prominent contractions of the muscle bundles. Most of the time, as defined, hemifacial spasm is unilateral, but bilateral spasms have been reported. In that case, the contractions of both sides of the face are neither simultaneous nor synchronous.

The theoretical differential diagnosis is blepharospasm. In contrast to hemifacial spasm, muscle contractions are bilateral, although sometimes slightly asymmetrical, and contractions of peri-ocular muscles are synchronous and may spread to the eyebrows, forehead, lower face (Meige syndrome) and neck (craniocervical dystonia).

A more tricky differential diagnosis is "epilepsia partialis continua" restricted to the face. Depending on the somatotopic representation of the face on the primary motor cortex, the clonic spasms may involve one side of the face. Two clues are helpful in this differential diagnosis: (i) the clonic movements may be predominantly on the lower part of the face or equally involve the upper and lower face; (ii) clonic movements may spread to the contralateral eyebrow or forehead muscles; this never happens in case of primary or secondary (post-paralytic) hemifacial spasm, and only syncinetic movements (blink) can be observed.

Facial hemidystonia is more a theoretical than a real differential diagnosis, as it is most of the time related to secondary dystonia (e.g., secondary to a basal ganglia lesion or stroke).

Tonic spasm of the lower face is sometimes more difficult to recognize, with forced closure of the mouth or lateral deviations of the jaw. Although the main cause may be psychogenic (with modification or alteration with distraction maneuvers) one should be careful about brain stem lesions (tumors or inflammatory lesions, such as in multiple sclerosis). In any case, brain MRI should be done.

Except in the case of epilepsia partialis continua, the common features of these different movement disorders is the occurrence of clonic or tonic spasms in a relatively localized part of the face, with the involvement of easily identifiable muscles.

Botulinum toxin (Costa *et al.*, 2005) is effective and safe for treating hemifacial spasm, as attested by extensive literature (see Chapter 17) concordant with the results of open-label studies (Costa *et al.*, 2005). In contrast, there are no specific data on the use of botulinum toxin in facial hemidystonia or in tonic spasms of the lower face, but the analogy with the beneficial effects in blepharospasm and Meige syndrome allows the use of botulinum toxin injections in the range of the doses used for facial muscles in those with focal dystonia (Balash and Giladi, 2004; Naumann et al., 2006).

Myokymias are defined by continuous fine vibrating muscle contractions (motor unit potential discharges). They are often observed in post-paralytic facial syndrome, (featuring muscle synkinesis, myokimia and involuntary rhythmic contractions). In addition, patients with facial palsy may exhibit, in the early stages, an increase in their spontaneous blinking rate, as well as a sustained low-level contraction of the muscles of the most paralyzed side, mimicking controlateral facial spasm or even "blepharospasm-like" muscle activity (Valls-Sole and Montero, 2003). Unlike post-paralytic facial hemispasm (plus myokymia), this early manifestation does not require botulinum toxin injections and is rapidly self-resolving.

In brief, the presence of myokymia, combined with the electrophysiological detection of multiplets and neuromyotonia suggests an increase of motor axonal membrane excitability and/or peripheral denervation/re-inervation.

Among the various causes of focal myokymias (masseter, mentalis, muscles, tongue) (Sedano et al., 2000), tumor irradiation (Liu, Chen and Chang, 2007) or brainstem tumors are the most frequent. Focal myokymia of the superior oblique muscle are characterized by episodic monocular oscillopsia. Low doses of cabamazepine, oxcarbazepine or gabapentine have a partial beneficial effect in 2/3 patients, whereas the effects of valproic acid are rarely reported, but may be interesting in individual cases.

Chronic myokymia limited to the eyelid is a benign condition, lasting from a few months up to 20 years and is unilateral. Very seldom (1/15) this symptom progresses to ipsilateral hemifacial spasm, but it does not progress to other types of facial movement disorders. In a few cases, botulinum toxin injections relieve discomfort and improve the abnormal movement (Banik and Miller, 2004).

Rhythmic Movements

The frequency and the localization of rhythmic movements are important clues for diagnosis and subsequent treatment. As Chapter 11 specifically addresses the topic, only two types of tremors will be briefly mentioned.

A fast, intermittent tremor localized on the chin is characteristic of chin tremor or geniospasm (Devetag Chalaupka et al., 2006; Papapetropoulos and Singer, 2007). In this benign condition, patients may present chin tremor from infancy, with a benign evolution throughout life and with intermittent fluctuations of the tremor. In most cases, this condition does not require any treatment. Nevertheless, some patients may be treated with low-dose botulinum toxin injections for aesthetic reasons (Bakar et al., 1998; Gordon, Cadera and Hinton, 1993). A slow, rhythmic tremor of the face and jaw, with pendular vergence

oscillations of the eyes (oculomasticatory myorythmia) is highly evocative of Whipple's disease (Schwartz et al., 1986).

Appropriate explorations (brain MRI, lumbar puncture, Whipple's PCR, intestinal biopsy, etc. . . .) should be performed. Even in the absence of anatomic or biological confirmations of the diagnosis, patients with oculomasticatory myoryhtmia should be treated presumptively for Whipple's disease with appropriate antibiotics (Hausser-Hauw et al., 1988).

In some cases of Whipple disease, additional movement disorders such as bruxism (Tison et al., 1992) or leg myoclonus may be observed (Rajput and McHattie, 1997).

Rare cases of facial myoclonus may require specific treatments:

- Myoclonus involving tongue, face, pharynx and sometimes legs has been described in infants with a neurological syndrome of infantile cobalamin (vitamin B12) deficiency. When vitamin B12 is introduced there is spontaneous improvement.
- Progressive continuous myoclonus of the face with ipsilateral spastic hemiparesis (over a period of three years) related to Rasmussen encephalitis has been treated with injections of botulinum toxin in the zygomaticus muscle.
- Myoclonic dystonia of the face is a rare condition (when isolated). A case of myoclonic dystonia has been described in a patient with putaminal lesion related to progressive multi-focal leucoencephalopathy. In this case, botulinum toxin could have been proposed to the patient as symptomatic relief.

Intermittent Tonic Contractions

Bruxism is defined by tooth grinding and tooth clenching with hypertrophy of the masseter and temporalis muscles and imbalance between opening and closing muscles of the jaw (Chikhani and Dichamp, 2003). Most frequently observed during the night, this condition may generate severe pain and lead to alterations in the temporomandibular joints, and tooth destruction. Although bruxism is often a primary condition (including oromandibular dystonia), it can be observed in cases of peripheral lesions or more widespread brain alteration (secondary to head injury, radiotherapy (Lou, Pleninger and Kurlan, 1995), Huntington's disease (Nash et al., 2004), amphetamine addiction (Tan and Jankovic, 2000). Although no randomized trials of botulinum toxin have been conducted in this condition, open-label studies confirm the efficacy and innocuousness of local (masseter and temporalis muscles) injections.

Sub-groups of patients with bruxisms belong to the group of patients with orofacial dystonia (see Chapters 13 and 14).

Dystonic tics, in contrast to "usual" tics, are more often slow, with temporarily sustained spasms. They may mimic blepharospasm or spasmodic torticollis (Jankovic and Stone, 1991) (with twisting or pulling movements of the neck). In patients with true Gilles de la Tourette syndrome, they may be difficult to distinguish from tardive dystonia or tardive tics (Singh and Jankovic, 1988). Nevertheless, voluntary control of the tics may be obtained for at least one minute. Open-label studies report that botulinum toxin injections in the muscle involved in the tonic spasms may be efficacious, both for the involuntary movements and for the premonitory sensory component associated with the tics (Jankovic, 1994).

In contrast to dystonia, the treatment of dystonic tics may require only a few injections, as tics may evolve and change throughout time.

NECK AND TRUNK MOVEMENT DISORDERS (TABLE 23.2)

Neck

Most of the movement disorders of the neck can be included in the three main categories: dystonia (including dystonic tremor and myoclonic dystonia, tardive dystonia), tremor (mainly heat tremor as part of essential tremor) and tics; they have been discussed in previous chapters.

Other types of movement disorders of the neck are part of more widespread diseases. Among them, tremor can be observed as part of Parkinson's diseases, with a slow 6 Hz

postural and rest head tremor, which may be partially improved by anti-parkinsonian treatment (L-dopa). Slow, 2–4 Hz, tremor is observed in lesions of the cerebellar pathway, including severe multiple sclerosis, leucodystrophies, midbrain lesions or severe heat injury. In most of these cases, there is no efficient pharmacological treatment and botulinum toxin injections may be proposed to the patient with only partial relief.

Three particular movements may be important to mention because of specific therapeutic and diagnostic implications:

• *Neck tongue syndrome* is defined by severe neck pain, torticollis and tongue atrophy (O'Meara and Wise, 1995). This symptom may reveal atlantoaxial osteoarthritis (sometimes of tuberculosis origin), especially in children. Treatment is related to the cause of the neck-tongue syndrome.

  In adults, the syndrome may be less spectacular, without movement disorders and nuccal and occipital pain with ipsilateral numbness of the tongue. This is related to a compression of the second cervical root in the atlantoaxial space on sharp rotation of the neck. Recently, a familial form of neck tongue syndrome has been described, without any lesion (Lewis, Frank and Toor, 2003).

• *Bobble-head doll syndrome* is a movement disorder present in childhood, characterized by stereotypical head movements (up and down) at a frequency of 2 to

Table 23.2 Treatment approaches to neck and trunk movement disorders.

Syndrome	Clinical features	Causes	Management
Bobble-head doll syndrome (childhood)	Stereotypical head movements (2–3 Hz)	Third ventricle tumors with hydrocephalus; Dandy–Walker malformations; shunt dysfunctions (hydrocephalus)	Surgical treatment of the underlying lesion
Head banging (9 mo–10 yr old) Rarely persist during adulthood	Rhythmic movements of the neck, body rocking	Sleep onset Sleep (stage II or REM sleep)	Low-dose benzodiazepines
Spinal myoclonus	Bilateral often symmetrical synchronous trunk movements (usually 3–5 Hz)	Focal spinal cord lesions	Benzodiazepines
Propriospinal myoclonus	Axial jerks involve several metameres. Predominantly in lying position; specific EMG propagation pattern	Most often no visible lesions Rarely spinal cord lesions	Benzodiazepines
Belly dancing	Undulating abdominal movements of the abdominal muscles associated with pain	Recurrent abdominal surgery	Transcutaneous electrical nerve stimulation (?)

3 Hz (Mussell *et al.*, 1997; Goikhman *et al.*, 1998). This movement disorder is usually associated with lesions of the third ventricle and ventricle dilatation (Tomasovic, Nellhaus and Moe, 1975). Dandy–Walker malformation (de Brito Henriques *et al.*, 2007), supra or intrasellar arachnoïd cysts or third ventricular tumors with hydrocephalus may present with this particular intermittent movement disorder (differential diagnosis stereotypy and tics). As bobble-head doll syndrome is a surgically curable entity, patients require MR imaging and neuroendocrinological explorations. Moreover, in patients with hydrocephalus treated with a subduroperitoneal shunt, the occurrence of abnormal movements may be symptomatic of shunt dysfunction (Ahn, Cho and Wang, 1997).

- *Head banging.* Rhythmic movement disorders of the neck may be observed as sleep-related disorders. They include head banging and body rocking at sleep onset or during the night (sleep stage II or REM sleep). These are benign conditions. The average age of onset is nine months and by the age of 10 years of age, the majority of the subjects no longer present head banging. In some normal adults, it may persist and become troublesome to the bed partner (Mendez and Mirea, 1998). In such cases, low dose benzodiazepines (0.5 to 2 mg) may be efficacious. Head banging and other various stereotypes may be part of psychiatric manifestations (e.g., in autistic or psychotic subjects) or self-injurious behavior (e.g., in Lesch–Nyhan disease (Robey *et al.*, 2003) or in severe Gilles de la Tourette syndrome). In such cases, sedative or anti-psychotic treatments may be proposed.

Trunk

Trunk movement disorders can be separated in tonic-dystonic postures and more mobile, rhythmic or arrhythmic movement disorders.

In the first sub-group, dystonia of the trunk is the most important feature (primary, related to tardive dystonia, parkinsonism or camptocormia). The various problems are detailed in the chapters on dystonia (Chapter 12 and neuroleptic-induced movement disorders (Chapter 25).

In the second sub-group, spinal myoclonus and belly dancing are the most frequent presentations.

Spinal Myoclonus

Spinal myoclonus may be limited to one or few segments of the spinal cord and jerking is more commonly bilateral, symmetrical and synchronous, although it may be unilateral. The contraction rate is 3 to 5 Hz (0.2–8 Hz) and occasionally the jerks are increased in the lying position or with the legs flexed. In most of the cases, the myoclonus may persist during sleep. Spinal myoclonus has been described, with a wide variety of focal and diffuse lesion, including (in a non-exhaustive list), spinal cord lesions, myelites, viral infections and parainfection causes, post-radiotherapy lesions, arteriovenous malformations, syrinx, Hashimoto's encephalopathy, interferon treatment, vitamin B12 deficiency and so on. A variant of spinal myoclonus, propriospinal myoclonus is characterized by axial jerks that are non-rhythmic and involve several metameres (flexion of the neck, trunk, proximal part of legs and arms). Jerks are spontaneous or stimulus-induced and EMG studies demonstrate that the myoclonus starts at a thoracic level (most often) and propagates slowly, both rostrally and caudally (see Chapter 24).

Treatments for spinal and propriospinal myoclonus are mainly symptomatic: benzodiazepines (clonazepam) have been reported to be partially efficient in various forms of spinal myoclonus, either related to lesions or "primary" forms. It may be of particular interest in cases that get worse during light sleep or rest.

A large number of drugs (including tetrabenazine, trihexyphenidyl, L-dopa, topiramate, piracetam (Ikeda *et al.*, 1996)) have been tested, but there are only a few reports of beneficial effects. Botulinum toxin has been also proposed as a treatment for localized myoclonus, but rarely. Overall, few effects of medical treatments are known. In contrast, it is worth knowing the iatrogenic causes of spinal and propriospinal myoclonus, including intrathecal morphinic agents and selective serotonin re-uptake inhibitors.

Intrathecal anaesthetics (diamorphine, fentanyl) may lead to the emergence of myoclonic spasms, mainly affecting the lower part of the body. Adaptation of doses may help to control the occurrence of myoclonus in patients who are treated via an implanted system for pain control. Systemic tramadol may also be implicated (one case) in spinal myoclonus.

Serotonin syndrome developing after a treatment with selective serotonin re-uptake inhibitors (SSRIs) may induce confusion, agitation, headache, fever, hypertension and myoclonus and the symptoms disappear after discontinuation of the drug. Low doses of SSRIs may induce spinal myoclonus in patients with pre-existing spinal lesion.

Finally, propriospinal myoclonus related to Hashimoto's syndrome is worth knowing (Roze *et al.*, 2007), as treatment with *steroids* may improve the symptoms.

Belly Dancing

Focal uncontrolled abdominal movements, mimicking a belly dancer, have been reported, mainly associated with abdominal pain and a medical history of recurrent abdominal surgery (see Chapter 17). More recently, painless abdominal dyskinesia has been reported after an intramedullary tumor (Shamim and Hallett, 2007) or centropontine mylinolysis (Roggendorf *et al.*, 2007).

Although benzodiazepines, analgesic treatments and botulinum toxin injections have been proposed to a few patients, no marked improvement has been obtained. In patients with severe pain, transcutaneous electrical nerve stimulation is worth trying (Linazasoro *et al.*, 2005).

LIMB MOVEMENT DISORDERS (TABLE 23.3)

Movement disorders of the limbs are extensively covered in the previous chapters and odd movement disorders are either hyperkinetic movements (proximal or distal) or fixed postures.

Hyperkinetic Movement Disorders

Most hyperkinetic movement disorders could be considered to be "induced" movement disorders and may be related either to peripheral or central lesions or to various types of trauma or surgery.

Peripherally Induced Movement Disorders

Painful Legs and Moving Toes

Painful legs and moving toes consists of pain in the affected limb(s) associated with spontaneous wriggling movements of the toes (see Chapter 17). They may also occur in the upper limbs (painful arms and moving fingers) (Spillane *et al.*, 1971). Although pain is the most disabling and persisting part of the syndrome, painless legs and moving toes have also been described (Walters *et al.*, 1993).

In the vast majority of cases, the patients mainly complain of pain and discomfort and rarely mention the movements. Unfortunately most treatment modalities related to pain have incomplete results and little effect on the moving toes (Villarejo *et al.*, 2004). Occasional success in treating both pain and movement disorders has been obtained with lumbar epidural block (Okuda *et al.*, 1998), as a treatment of pain, or with epidural spinal cord stimulation (Takahashi *et al.*, 2002; Raina, Piedimonte and Micheli, 2007).

Most often, these beneficial effects are reported in single cases or small series (open-labeled). When movement disorders are bothersome, local botulinum toxin injections into the toes exterior and flexor muscles may be helpful (Singer and Papapetropoulos, 2007).

Focal Myoclonus

Focal myoclonus of peripheral origin is a rare disorder and may be considered as a differential diagnosis of painful leg and moving toes. However, in peripheral myoclonus, jerks are observed in the muscles corresponding to the territory of

the affected nerve or root. (e.g., traumatic or tumoral lesion in the femoral nerve). In such cases, the movements are improved after surgical treatment and liberation of the femoral nerve (Shin *et al.*, 2007).

Rippling Muscles

Rippling muscles (see Chapter 17) is a rare condition associated with caveolin-3 mutations (Kubisch *et al.*, 2003). Associated symptoms are muscle stiffness, exercise-induced myalgia and cramp-like sensations. Rapid muscle contractions and "wavelets" (rippling muscles) are observed either spontaneously or after muscle percussions (Kubisch *et al.*, 2003). To date, no specific treatment has been proposed. However, rippling muscle syndrome can be revealed by simvastatin and may be improved after discontinuation of the treatment.

Peripheral factors have also been suggested in unusual focal dyskinesia (shoulder movements). There are focal or segmental movements with a slow, sinuous and semi-rhythmic character with long-duration bursts (Caviness *et al.*, 1994). Pain is often present in the affected region (with sometimes a past history of local and often benign peripheral trauma). Local injections of botulinum toxin may help to improve the muscle contractions and may partially relieve the pain.

Stump Dyskinesias

Complex autonomous movements of the proximal extremity (stump) may develop after amputation (Kulisevsky, Marti-Fabregas and Grau, 1992). These continuous movements are often associated with pain and "phantom limb" phenomena (see Chapter 17). Baclofen may be useful for involuntary movements in post-amputation patients. In one case, deep brain stimulation of the thalamus (Cm-pf) improved both abnormal movements and pain (Krauss *et al.*, 2002). Occasionally, autonomous stump movements have been improved by gabapentin (Mera *et al.*, 2004) or anti-depressant treatments.

Hyperkinetic Movement Disorders Related to Central Lesions

Several types of hyperkinetic movement disorders have been associated with spinal cord lesions or injury. In most of the cases, sensory dysfunctions are present, although the importance of sensory disturbances is not always sufficient to explain the diversity of movement disorders.

Pseudo Athetosis

Pseudo athetosis has been described with spinal cord lesions, syrinx or cervical disc herniations. In the latter case, improvement of the movement disorders may be obtained after

Table 23.3 Treatment approaches to limb movement disorders.

Syndrome	Clinical features	Causes	Management
Painful legs and moving toes	Wriggling movements of the toes + pain and discomfort	Peripheral neuropathy	See Chapter 17
		Discal protrusion and root compression	Transcutaneous electrical nerve stimulation (TENS); epidural spinal cord stimulation (rare); botulinum toxin (rare)
Focal myoclonus of peripheral origin	Jerks in the muscles corresponding to the muscles related to the affected nerve or root	Peripheral nerve lesions	none
Rippling muscles	Rapid muscle contractions ("wavelets") spontaneously or after muscle percussion associated with muscular stiffness and exercise. Induced myalgia	Caveolin-3 mutations	None
Unusual focal dyskinesia (e.g., shoulder movements)	Slow sinuous semi rhythmic movements with long duration bursts on EMG. Often associated with pain	Sometimes local trauma	Botulinum toxin
Stump dyskinesias	Autonomous movements of the strump. Often associated with pain or "phantom limb"	After amputations	See Chapter 17 Little treatment
			Baclofen; gabapentin; Cm.pf deep brain stimulation (1 case).
Paroxysmal movement disorders	Paroxysmal	Multiple sclerosis	Carbamazepine (low dose).
	Kinesigenic dyskinesia* Chorea/dystonia		Gabapentin Benzodiazepine
Tonic spasms of the limbs	Spontenaous or stimulus induced tonic spasms (flexion or extension or upper/lower limb)	Spinal cord lesions	Phenyloin
	(several seconds to minutes) + pain	Rarely lesions of internal capsule or brainstem	Baclofen
Causalgia dystonia syndrome	Fixed posture (dystonia) + pain and trophic changes (reflex sympathetic dystrophy).	Peripheral injury	
		Psychogenic	

surgery. In line with this idea, cervical dystonia related to spinal cord lesions may be improved after surgery (e.g., atlantoaxial subluxation).

Paroxysmal Movement Disorders

Paroxysmal movement disorders are rare in multiple sclerosis and may be related to spinal or brain demyelinating plaques (Tranchant, Bhatia and Marsden, 1995). The triggering factors may be sudden movement (paroxysmal kinesigenic dyskinesia) or spontaneous appearance (chorea/dystonia). A useful clue is the triggering of paroxysmal phenomenon following prolonged hyperventilation.

Paroxysmal movements are often improved with low doses of carbamazepine, gabapentin or benzodiazepines (Viallet *et al.*, 2001; Yetimalar, Gurgor and Basoglu, 2004).

Tonic Spasms and Abnormal Postures

Painful, tonic/dystonic spasms of the limbs (either flexion or extension postures) are rare. Spontaneous or stimulus-induced tonic spasms are observed over several seconds or minutes and are highly evocative of a spinal cord origin (Cherrick and Ellenberg, 1986). They have been described in various types of severe inflammatory lesions of the spinal cord, including Sjögren's disease (Taguchi *et al.*, 2006; Jabbari and Salardini, 1999) (attacks may occur up to 25 times/day). The painful spasms may respond to phenytoin or to baclofen. Tonic spasms (also called "tonic seizures") may be related to lesions of the internal capsule or of the brain stem (in relation to demyelinating disease or inflammatory diseases, including post-infection myelitis). Occasional improvements have been reported with carbamazepine or valproate therapy (Libenson, Stafstrom and Rosman, 1994).

Fixed postures of the limbs may be observed in causalgia dystonia syndrome (Bhatia, Bhatt and Marsden, 1993; Schrag *et al.*, 2004), and may be triggered by peripheral injury. Various combinations have been reported and dystonia may follow peripheral injury, may occur in isolation, associated with other movement disorders such as tremor or associated with other signs, from pain to vasomotor, sudomotor and trophic changes up to a full-blown reflex sympathetic dystrophy (RDS).

There is extensive literature on the role of trauma in the development of these fixed postures.

Sympathetic blocks have been said to improve the symptoms temporarily, but this cannot be considered as a treatment. Sympathectomies are unhelpful and are not recommended. Moreover, a wide range of medical treatments, including botulinum toxin have been proposed with little benefit (Bhatia, Bhatt and Marsden, 1993; Schrag *et al.*, 2004; Birklein *et al.*, 2000).

Many patients fulfill the criteria for somatoform disorders and in some cases they may be improved with a combination of physiotherapy and psychotherapy (Schrag *et al.*, 2004). In a recent case, fixed dystonia was treated with pallidal stimulation without any benefit and was subsequently improved by motor cortex stimulation (Romito *et al.*, 2007), but this single observation has to be confirmed (Espay *et al.*, 2007).

CONCLUSION

For these rare movement disorders, in most of the cases treatments were either related to the etiologic factor (especially in case of spinal cord lesions) or no specific treatments were proposed, depending on the clinical presentation.

Benzodiazepines were proposed to most of the patients and botulinum toxin was the second most frequently used treatment in patients with focal abnormal muscle contractions.

Various types of anti-epileptic drugs were proposed for hyperkinetic or paroxysmal movement disorders, especially when additional pain was observed.

In all cases, therapeutic strategies were based on single observations or small series and no prospective controlled trial was available, as the movement disorders are both rare and heterogeneous.

References

Ahn, Y., Cho, B.K. and Wang, K.C. (1997) Bobble-head doll syndrome associated with subduroperitoneal shunt malfunction. *Child's Nervous System*, **13**, 234–237.

Bakar, M., Zarifoglu, M., Bora, I., Turan, F., Sen, C. and Ogul, E. (1998) Treatment of hereditary trembling chin with botulinum toxin. *Movement Disorders*, **13**, 845–846.

Balash, Y. and Giladi, N. (2004) Efficacy of pharmacological treatment of dystonia: evidence-based review including meta-analysis of the effect of botulinum toxin and other cure options. *European Journal of Neurology*, **11**, 361–370.

Banik, R. and Miller, N.R. (2004) Chronic myokymia limited to the eyelid is a benign condition. *Journal of Neuro-Ophthalmology*, **24**, 290–292.

Bhatia, K.P., Bhatt, M.H. and Marsden, C.D. (1993) The causalgia-dystonia syndrome. *Brain: A Journal of Neurology*, **116** (Pt 4), 843–851.

Birklein, F., Riedl, B., Sieweke, N., Weber, M. and Neundorfer, B. (2000) Neurological findings in complex regional pain syndromes – analysis of 145 cases. *Acta Neurologica Scandinavica*, **101**, 262–269.

Caviness, J.N., Gabellini, A., Kneebone, C.S., Thompson, P.D., Lees, A.J. and Marsden, C.D. (1994) Unusual focal dyskinesias: the ears, the shoulders, the back, and the abdomen. *Movement Disorders*, **9**, 531–538.

Cherrick, A.A. and Ellenberg, M. (1986) Spinal cord seizures in transverse myelopathy: report of two cases. *Archives of Physical Medicine and Rehabilitation*, **67**, 1074–1075.

Chikhani, L. and Dichamp, J. (2003) [Bruxism, temporo-mandibular dysfunction and botulinum toxin]. *Ann Readapt Med Phys*, **46**, 333–337.

Costa, J., Espirito-Santo, C., Borges, A. *et al.* (2005) Botulinum toxin type A therapy for hemifacial spasm. *Cochrane Database of Systematic Reviews*, CD004899.

de Brito Henriques, J.G., Henriques, K.S., Filho, G.P., Fonseca, L.F., Cardoso, F. and Da Silva, M.C. (2007) Bobble-head doll syndrome associated with Dandy-Walker syndrome. Case report. *Journal of Neurosurgery*, **107**, 248–250.

Devetag Chalaupka, F., Bartholini, F., Mandich, G. and Turro, M. (2006) Two new families with hereditary essential chin myoclonus: clinical features, neurophysiological findings and treatment. *Neurological Sciences*, **27**, 97–103.

Espay, A.J., Chen, R., Moro, E. and Lang, A.E. (2007) Fixed dystonia unresponsive to pallidal stimulation improved by motor cortex stimulation. *Neurology*, **69**, 1062–1063.

Goikhman, I., Zelnik, N., Peled, N. and Michowiz, S. (1998) Bobble-head doll syndrome: a surgically treatable condition manifested as a rare movement disorder. *Movement Disorders*, **13**, 192–194.

Gordon, K., Cadera, W. and Hinton, G. (1993) Successful treatment of hereditary trembling chin with botulinum toxin. *Journal of Child Neurology*, **8**, 154–156.

Hausser-Hauw, C., Roullet, E., Robert, R. and Marteau, R. (1988) Oculo-facio-skeletal myorhythmia as a cerebral complication of systemic Whipple's disease. *Movement Disorders*, **3**, 179–184.

Ikeda, A., Shibasaki, H., Tashiro, K., Mizuno, Y. and Kimura, J. (1996) Clinical trial of piracetam in patients with myoclonus: nationwide multiinstitution study in Japan. The Myoclonus/ Piracetam Study Group. *Movement Disorders*, **11**, 691–700.

Jabbari, B. and Salardini, A. (1999) Painful tonic/dystonic spasms in Sjogren's syndrome. *Movement Disorders*, **14**, 860–864.

Jankovic, J. (1994) Botulinum toxin in the treatment of dystonic tics. *Movement Disorders*, **9**, 347–349.

Jankovic, J. and Stone, L. (1991) Dystonic tics in patients with Tourette's syndrome. *Movement Disorders*, **6**, 248–252.

Krauss, J.K., Pohle, T., Weigel, R. and Burgunder, J.M. (2002) Deep brain stimulation of the centre median-parafascicular complex in patients with movement disorders. *Journal of Neurology, Neurosurgery, and Psychiatry*, **72**, 546–548.

Kubisch, C., Schoser, B.G., von During, M. *et al.* (2003) Homozygous mutations in caveolin-3 cause a severe form of rippling muscle disease. *Annals of Neurology*, **53**, 512–520.

Kulisevsky, J., Marti-Fabregas, J. and Grau, J.M. (1992) Spasms of amputation stumps. *Journal of Neurology, Neurosurgery, and Psychiatry*, **55**, 626–627.

Lewis, D.W., Frank, L.M. and Toor, S. (2003) Familial neck-tongue syndrome. *Headache*, **43**, 132–134.

Libenson, M.H., Stafstrom, C.E. and Rosman, N.P. (1994) Tonic "seizures" in a patient with brainstem demyelination: MRI study of brain and spinal cord. *Pediatric Neurology*, **11**, 258–262.

Linazasoro, G., Van Blercom, N., Lasa, A., Fernandez, J.M. and Aranzabal, I. (2005) Etiological and therapeutical observations in a case of belly dancer's dyskinesia. *Movement Disorders*, **20**, 251–253.

Liu, L.H., Chen, C.W. and Chang, M.H. (2007) Post-irradiation myokymia and neuromyotonia in unilateral tongue and mentalis muscles: report of a case. *Acta Neuroligica Taiwanica*, **16**, 33–36.

Lou, J.S., Pleninger, P. and Kurlan, R. (1995) Botulinum toxin A is effective in treating trismus associated with postradiation myokymia and muscle spasm. *Movement Disorders*, **10**, 680–681.

Mendez, M.F. and Mirea, A. (1998) Adult head-banging and stereotypic movement disorders. *Movement Disorders*, **13**, 825–828.

Mera, J., Martinez-Castrillo, J.C., Mariscal, A., Herrero, A. and Alvarez-Cermeno, J.C. (2004) Autonomous stump movements responsive to gabapentin. *Journal of Neurology*, **251**, 346–347.

Mussell, H.G., Dure, L.S., Percy, A.K. and Grabb, P.S. (1997) Bobble-head doll syndrome: report of a case and review of the literature. *Movement Disorders*, **12**, 810–814.

Nash, M.C., Ferrell, R.B., Lombardo, M.A. and Williams, R.B. (2004) Treatment of bruxism in Huntington's disease with botulinum toxin. *Journal of Neuropsychiatry and Clinical Neurosciences*, **16**, 381–382.

Naumann, M., Albanese, A., Heinen, F., Molenaers, G. and Relja, M. (2006) Safety and efficacy of botulinum toxin type A following long-term use. *European Journal of Neurology*, **13** (Suppl 4), 35–40.

Okuda, Y., Suzuki, K., Kitajima, T., Masuda, R. and Asai, T. (1998) Lumbar epidural block for 'painful legs and moving toes' syndrome: a report of three cases. *Pain*, **78**, 145–147.

O'Meara, M. and Wise, G. (1995) Painful torticollis with tongue atrophy – a different neck-tongue syndrome. *Neuropediatrics*, **26**, 276–280.

Papapetropoulos, S. and Singer, C. (2007) Sporadic geniospasm (chin trembling): report of a case. *Movement Disorders*, **22**, 434.

Raina, G.B., Piedimonte, F. and Micheli, F. (2007) Posterior spinal cord stimulation in a case of painful legs and moving toes. *Stereotactic and Functional Neurosurgery*, **85**, 307–309.

Rajput, A.H. and McHattie, J.D. (1997) Ophthalmoplegia and leg myorhythmia in Whipple's disease: report of a case. *Movement Disorders*, **12**, 111–114.

Robey, K.L., Reck, J.F., Giacomini, K.D., Barabas, G. and Eddey, G.E. (2003) Modes and patterns of self-mutilation in persons with Lesch-Nyhan disease. *Developmental Medicine and Child Neurology*, **45**, 167–171.

Roggendorf, J., Burghaus, L., Liu, W.C. *et al.* (2007) Belly dancer's syndrome following central pontine and extrapontine myelinolysis. *Movement Disorders*, **22**, 892–894.

Romito, L.M., Franzini, A., Perani, D. *et al.* (2007) Fixed dystonia unresponsive to pallidal stimulation improved by motor cortex stimulation. *Neurology*, **68**, 875–876.

Roze, E., Apartis, E., Vidailhet, M. *et al.* (2007) Propriospinal myoclonus: utility of magnetic resonance diffusion tensor imaging and fiber tracking. *Movement Disorders*, **22**, 1506–1509.

Schrag, A., Trimble, M., Quinn, N. and Bhatia, K. (2004) The syndrome of fixed dystonia: an evaluation of 103 patients. *Brain: A Journal of Neurology*, **127**, 2360–2372.

Schwartz, M.A., Selhorst, J.B., Ochs, A.L. *et al.* (1986) Oculo-masticatory myorhythmia: a unique movement disorder occurring in Whipple's disease. *Annals of Neurology*, **20**, 677–683.

Sedano, M.J., Trejo, J.M., Macarron, J.L., Polo, J.M., Berciano, J. and Calleja, J. (2000) Continuous facial myokymia in multiple sclerosis: treatment with botulinum toxin. *European Neurology*, **43**, 137–140.

Shamim, E.A. and Hallett, M. (2007) Intramedullary spinal tumor causing "belly dancer syndrome". *Movement Disorders*, **22**, 1673–1674.

Shin, H.W., Ye, B.S., Kim, J., Kim, S.M. and Sohn, Y.H. (2007) The contribution of a spinal mechanism in developing peripheral myoclonus: a case report. *Movement Disorders*, **22**, 1350–1352.

Singer, C. and Papapetropoulos, S. (2007) A case of painless arms/ moving fingers responsive to botulinum toxin a injections. *Parkinsonism & Related Disorders*, **13**, 55–56.

Singh, S.K. and Jankovic, J. (1988) Tardive dystonia in patients with Tourette's syndrome. *Movement Disorders*, **3**, 274–280.

Spillane, J.D., Nathan, P.W., Kelly, R.E. and Marsden, C.D. (1971) Painful legs and moving toes. *Brain: A Journal of Neurology*, **94**, 541–556.

Taguchi, Y., Takashima, S., Dougu, N. and Tanaka, K. (2006) Two cases of myelitis associated with Sjogren syndrome without xerosis: characteristic MRI findings. *No to Shinkei*, **58**, 701–707.

Takahashi, H., Saitoh, C., Iwata, O., Nanbu, T., Takada, S. and Morita, S. (2002) Epidural spinal cord stimulation for the treatment of painful legs and moving toes syndrome. *Pain*, **96**, 343–345.

Tan, E.K. and Jankovic, J. (2000) Treating severe bruxism with botulinum toxin. *J Am Dent Assoc*, **131**, 211–216.

Tison, F., Louvet-Giendaj, C., Henry, P., Lagueny, A. and Gaujard, E. (1992) Permanent bruxism as a manifestation of the oculo-facial syndrome related to systemic Whipple's disease. *Movement Disorders*, **7**, 82–85.

Tomasovic, J.A., Nellhaus, G. and Moe, P.G. (1975) The bobble-head syndrome: an early sign of hydrocephalus. Two new cases and a review of the literature. *Developmental Medicine and Child Neurology*, **17**, 777–783.

Tranchant, C., Bhatia, K.P. and Marsden, C.D. (1995) Movement disorders in multiple sclerosis. *Movement Disorders*, **10**, 418–423.

Valls-Sole, J. and Montero, J. (2003) Movement disorders in patients with peripheral facial palsy. *Movement Disorders*, **18**, 1424–1435.

Viallet, F., Witjas, T., Gayraud, D., Pelletier, J. and Regis, J. (2001) Tremor and abnormal movement in multiple sclerosis: symptomatic therapeutic indications. *Revue Neurologique*, **157**, 1079–1084.

Villarejo, A., Porta-Etessam, J., Camacho, A., Gonzalez De La Aleja, J., Martinez-Salio, A. and Penas, M. (2004) Gabapentin for painful legs and moving toes syndrome. *European Neurology*, **51**, 180–181.

Walters, A.S., Hening, W.A., Shah, S.K. and Chokroverty, S. (1993) Painless legs and moving toes: a syndrome related to painful legs and moving toes? *Movement Disorders*, **8**, 377–379.

Yetimalar, Y., Gurgor, N. and Basoglu, M. (2004) Clinical efficacy of gabapentin for paroxysmal symptoms in multiple sclerosis. *Acta Neurologica Scandinavica*, **109**, 430–431.

24

Myoclonus

Shu-Ching Hu[1], Steven J. Frucht[1] and Hiroshi Shibasaki[2]

[1] Department of Neurology, Columbia University Medical Center, New York, NY, USA
[2] Takeda General Hospital, Ishida, Fushimi-ku, Kyoto, Japan

CLINICAL MANIFESTATIONS AND LOCALIZATION OF MYOCLONUS

Myoclonus is a phenomenologic term for sudden, brief, shock-like involuntary movements caused by muscular contractions or inhibitions (Fahn, 2002). Myoclonus disorders are uncommon, with the annual incidence and lifetime prevalence estimated to be 1.3 and 8.6 cases per 100 000 population, respectively (Caviness et al., 1999). Myoclonus can arise from the cerebral cortex, subcortical nuclei, brain stem, spinal cord or peripheral nerve, and myoclonic movements of different origins carry dissimilar phenomenological features (Shibasaki, 2006). Therefore, a logical approach in evaluating a myoclonus disorder is to start with localization before contemplating a syndrome or etiology.

Phenomenologically, myoclonus is characterized by distribution, provocability, rhythmicity, persistency in sleep and relation to muscle contractions. Distribution of myoclonus can be focal, segmental, axial, multi-focal or generalized. Regarding provocability, myoclonus may occur at rest (spontaneous myoclonus) or with voluntary action (action myoclonus), or is triggered by various stimuli (stimulus-sensitive or reflex myoclonus). Myoclonus is usually irregular, but can be periodic or rhythmic, resembling tremor. In sleep, cortical myoclonus ceases unless it is epileptic, whereas certain myoclonus of subcortical origin may persist. Most myoclonic movements are due to active muscular contractions. However, myoclonus also occurs due to sudden muscular inhibitions, and this type of myoclonus is called asterixis or negative myoclonus (Obeso, Arteida and Burleigh, 1995).

Complementing phenomenological analysis, other neurological findings and neuroimaging studies also help localize the myoclonus generator. The most conclusive localization comes from electrophysiological studies (Shibasaki and Hallett, 2005). The electrophysiologic definition of myoclonus is a movement of short duration with a consistent, physiologic, temporospatial pattern. The duration of cortical myoclonus on electromyography (EMG) is usually less than 50 ms. In certain types of subcortical myoclonus, or when larger muscles are involved, the duration may be longer. Electrophysiological studies of myoclonus utilize the techniques of EMG and electroencephalography (EEG). A polymyographic recording by surface electrodes can determine whether a movement is myoclonic or not. The location of a myoclonus generator is additionally inferred by the pattern of activation on polymyography. EEG probes the other end of the motor pathway, and is indispensable in diagnosing cortical myoclonus.

Cortical myoclonus manifests in a variety of distributions and provocability. Action or reflex myoclonus in a multi-focal distribution is characteristic of cortical myoclonus. Cortical myoclonus is epileptic when jerky movements occur with epileptiform discharges on EEG. However, considering the limited sensitivity of EEG and pathophysiology of myoclonus, distinction between epileptic and non-epileptic cortical myoclonus is not always clear (Krauss and Mathews, 2003). For cortical myoclonus that is not accompanied by obvious epileptiform discharges, its cortical origin is evidenced electrophysiologically by the presence of a cortical signal preceding the jerky movement. This finding is best revealed by the technique of jerk-locked back averaging. An exaggerated cortical response in the somatosensory-evoked potential study is also specific to cortical myoclonus.

There are several forms of brain stem myoclonus, for example, palatal myoclonus (also called palatal tremor), brain stem reticular myoclonus and startle syndromes. Palatal myoclonus or tremor is caused by rhythmic contractions of the palatal muscles (Deuschl and Wilms, 2002). This syndrome is covered in more detail in Chapter 11. Brain stem reticular myoclonus presents as axial or generalized jerks (Hallett, 2002). It is typically stimulus-sensitive, and is also referred to as reticular reflex myoclonus. The generator of brain stem reticular myoclonus is in the lower brain stem, and on polymyography, the movement starts in muscles innervated by the lower brain stem before spreading up the brain stem and down the spinal cord. In startle syndromes, the movement is an exaggerated form of physiologic startle response, which is a generalized myoclonic movement triggered by unexpected stimuli (Shibasaki, 2007). The generator of the startle response is mapped to the medial bulbopontine reticular formation. In hereditary startle syndrome, that is hyperekplexia, most cases are caused by mutations in the α1 sub-unit of the glycine receptor.

Two types of myoclonus arise from the spinal cord, spinal segmental myoclonus and propriospinal myoclonus (Rothwell, 2002). Spinal segmental myoclonus presents as segmental jerks, and is sometimes rhythmic or periodic. The distribution of myoclonus in a single or a few adjacent myotomes points to the location of its generator in the spinal cord. Propriospinal myoclonus presents as axial jerks, and may be position-dependent. On polymyography, propriospinal myoclonus usually starts in the abdominal muscles, and propagates at a speed corresponding to that of a slow-conducting propriospinal pathway.

At the peripheral end of the neuraxis, myoclonus occasionally emerges from the nerve root, plexus or nerve. Hemifacial spasm is the prototypic peripherally generated myoclonus, although duration of the movement is at times beyond the myoclonic range (Nielsen, 1985). Myoclonus has been reported to occur after damage to peripheral nerves, and is considered a peripherally induced movement disorder (Jankovic, 2001). In those instances, the myoclonus generator may still reside centrally and not necessarily in the peripheral nervous system (Shin *et al.*, 2007).

ETIOLOGY OF MYOCLONUS

In view of the vast heterogeneity in etiology, causes of myoclonus are first classified into four broad categories—epileptic, physiologic, essential and symptomatic (Fahn, 2002). Epileptic myoclonus is a fragment of epilepsy, and is evaluated and managed in the context of a seizure disorder. Physiologic myoclonus refers to myoclonus that is a normal motor phenomenon, for example, the startle response, hypnic jerk and hiccup. However, when a pathological process invades the circuitry of physiologic myoclonus, it can produce excessive jerks phenomenologically similar to physiologic myoclonus.

Essential myoclonus is a monosymptomatic condition that is often early-onset, non-progressive, and familial. Essential myoclonus shares many features with myoclonus-dystonia, a hereditary movement disorder with myoclonus

and dystonia (Asmus and Gasser, 2004). In myoclonus-dystonia, alcohol-responsive myoclonus is the defining feature, and has a predilection for the upper body. Dystonia may be subtle or absent. Patients with myoclonus-dystonia have no other neurological abnormalities, but have an increased risk of developing obsessive-compulsive disorder and other anxiety disorders (Hess *et al.*, 2007). Two loci, DYT11 and DYT15, have been linked to myoclonus-dystonia, and ε-sarcoglycan is the disease-causing gene in DYT11.

The majority of myoclonus disorders fall into the symptomatic category, in which a cause can be identified across the spectrum of neurological diseases (Table 24.1). When the cause is not apparent, a syndromic diagnosis is a useful intermediate step. Most types of myoclonus of subcortical origin constitute myoclonus syndromes, because each has a characteristic manifestation and a finite number of causes. There exist a number of myoclonus syndromes containing cortical myoclonus, such as progressive myoclonic ataxia, post-hypoxic myoclonus, epilepsia partialis continua, and myoclonus accompanying dementia or parkinsonism.

Progressive myoclonic ataxia (Ramsay Hunt syndrome) is a heterogeneous group of early-onset, progressive disorders with myoclonus and ataxia. Progressive myoclonic ataxia overlaps in clinical presentations and causes with progressive myoclonus epilepsy, an epileptic syndrome dominated by epileptic myoclonus (Marseille Consensus Group, 1990). Inborn errors of metabolism and neurodegenerative disorders account for most causes of progressive myoclonic ataxia. Post-hypoxic myoclonus (Lance–Adams syndrome) occurs as the brain recovers from acute hypoxic damage. A variety of types of myoclonus occur in post-hypoxic myoclonus, especially multi-focal action myoclonus, negative myoclonus and brain stem myoclonus (Frucht, 2002). Epilepsia partialis continua is a myoclonus syndrome of focal cortical origin (Cockerell *et al.*, 1996). Despite its name, epileptiform discharges are not always detected in this condition. Epilepsia partialis continua is mostly caused by Rasmussen's encephalitis and other focal cortical lesions. Myoclonus is a non-specific finding in dementing or parkinsonian disorders, often in their advanced stage (Caviness, 2003). However, in the early stage of such disorders, presence of focal myoclonus is suggestive of corticobasal degeneration, and presence of periodic or quasi-periodic myoclonus should be an alert to a diagnosis of Creutzfeldt–Jakob disease. Opsoclonus-myoclonus syndrome is another myoclonus syndrome, in which myoclonus is likely of brain stem origin (Gwinn and Caviness, 1997). It can be paraneoplastic or due to other causes. The paraneoplastic opsoclonus-myoclonus syndrome is associated with neuroblastoma in children and with lung, breast or ovarian cancer in adults (Wong, 2007).

Table 24.1 Selected causes of symptomatic myoclonus.

Inborn errors of metabolism
    Unverricht–Lundburg disease
    Lafora disease
    Neuronal ceroid lipofuscinosis
    Sialidosis
    Mitochondrial disorders

Metabolic
    Hepatic failure
    Renal failure
    Dialysis disequilibrium syndrome
    Hyponatremia
    Hypoglycemia
    Non-ketotic hyperglycemia
    Vitamin E deficiency

Toxin-induced
    Mercury
    Bismuth
    Aluminum
    Tetra-ethyl lead
    Organochlorine insecticides
    Dichoroethane
    Toluene

Drug- or substance-induced
    Narcotics
    Neuroleptics
    Anti-depressants
    Lithium
    Buspirone
    Anti-epileptics
    Levodopa
    Anesthetics
    Anti-microbials
    Calcium channel blockers
    Anti-arrhythmics
    Contrast media
    Pseudoephedrine
    Cocaine
    Marijuana
    Methylenedioxymethamphetamine (Ecstasy)

Neurodegenerative: parkinsonian or dementing
    Corticobasal degeneration
    Creutzfeldt–Jakob disease
    Parkinson's disease
    Progressive supranuclear palsy
    Multi-system atrophy
    Huntington's disease
    Wilson's disease
    Hallervorden–Spatz disease
    Alzheimer's disease
    Dementia with Lewy body

Neurodegenerative: ataxic
    Friedreich's ataxia
    Ataxia-telangiectasia
    Spinocerebellar ataxia
    Dentatorubropallidoluysian atrophy

Other structural lesions: diffuse or multi-focal
    Post-hypoxic
    Post-traumatic
    Infectious
    Inflammatory
    Paraneoplastic
    Whipple's disease
    Celiac disease

Other structural lesions: focal
    Stroke
    Tumor
    Abscess
    Demyelinating
    Developmental

Lesions in the nerve root, plexus and peripheral nerve

Psychogenic

TREATMENT OF MYOCLONUS: GENERAL PRINCIPLES AND COMMONLY USED MEDICATIONS

Treatment of myoclonus should first focus on the cause, whenever it is treatable. A treatable pathogenic mechanism also provides opportunities for therapeutic interventions; for example, opsoclonus-myoclonus syndrome in children is known to respond to immunotherapies (Wong, 2007). Symptomatic treatment of myoclonus is indicated when myoclonus inflicts discomfort, interferes with care or interrupts voluntary activities. There are a number of pharmacological and non-pharmacological anti-myoclonic therapies. Several factors are considered in selecting appropriate treatment for individual patients. Of primary importance is the origin of the myoclonus, since treatment suitable for cortical myoclonus may not be effective for brain stem or spinal myoclonus, and vice versa. Some anti-myoclonic medications can affect the mental status or balance, so the tolerability of patients needs to be weighed. The elderly and those who are already cognitive or neurologically impaired are particularly vulnerable to these adverse effects. Treatment of myoclonus is often challenging, and significant lessening of myoclonus may not always be feasible. A realistic portrait of the outcome of anti-myoclonic treatment for the patients helps avoid disappointment in difficult situations.

Fundamentally, at the cellular level, myoclonus and epilepsy are similar in that both are generated by abnormal, hyperexcitable neural circuits (Krauss and Mathews, 2003). Therefore, drugs with known anti-epileptic effects have been the prime source of anti-myoclonics. Anti-epileptics have diverse pharmacological mechanisms, and certain anti-epileptics are more potent anti-myoclonics than others.

Benzodiazepines are agonists of the type A receptor of γ-aminobutyric acid (GABA), and have been widely used to treat myoclonus. Among scores of benzodiazepines with different pharmacokinetics, clonazepam is the most commonly used anti-myoclonic. Benzodiazepines have the broadest range of effectiveness for myoclonus of all origins, including cortical, brain stem and spinal myoclonus (Caviness and Brown, 2004; Nirenberg and Frucht, 2005). Valproate is another frequently used anti-myoclonic. It enhances the inhibitory action of GABA, but the exact mechanism is unclear. Valproate is effective for cortical myoclonus, but less so for myoclonus of subcortical origin (Caviness and Brown, 2004; Nirenberg and Frucht, 2005).

In the newer generation of anti-epileptics, levetiracetam is the most notable anti-myoclonic. Levetiracetam binds to synaptic vesicle protein 2A, and modulates GABA-mediated neurotransmission (Lynch et al., 2004). Another structurally related drug, piracetam, has a similar anti-myoclonic effect, although its mechanism may be different from that of levetiracetam (Genton and Van Vleymen, 2000). Levetiracetam is effective for cortical myoclonus (Genton and Gélisse, 2000; Krauss et al., 2001; Frucht et al., 2001; Lim and Ahmed, 2005; Striano et al., 2005). For brain stem myoclonus, the effectiveness of levetiracetam is less certain. For spinal myoclonus, levetiracetam has been reported to have a substantial effect in a case series (Keswani et al., 2002). Similar to levetiracetam, piracetam is effective for cortical myoclonus (Brown et al., 1993; Koskiniemi et al., 1998), but is less or not effective for brain stem myoclonus and for spinal myoclonus (Obeso et al., 1988; Ikeda et al., 1996; Pranzatelli et al., 2001).

TREATMENT OF MYOCLONUS: LESS COMMONLY USED MEDICATIONS AND EMERGING OPTIONS

The effects of other anti-epileptics on non-epileptic myoclonus have not been systemically investigated. Primidone and acetazolamide were described as useful adjuncts in treating severe myoclonus (Obeso et al., 1989; Vaamonde et al., 1992). Ethosuximide was found effective for negative myoclonus (Oguni et al., 1998; Capovilla et al., 1999). Topiramate was shown to be helpful in a case of spinal segmental myoclonus (Siniscalchi et al., 2004). Zonisamide suppresses epileptic myoclonus, but little is known about its

effect on non-epileptic myoclonus (Uthman and Reichl, 2002; Ohtahara, 2006). Paradoxically, a few anti-epileptics have been noticed to be pro-myoclonic rather than anti-myoclonic, for example, vigabatrin, lamotrigine and gabapentin (Gordon, 2002).

γ-Hydroxybutyrate (GHB) is a fatty acid derivative with an anti-myoclonic effect. Initially synthesized as an analog of GABA, GHB was subsequently found to be an endogenous neurotransmitter or neuromodulator that binds to both GABA-B and its bona fide GHB receptors (Crunelli, Emri and Leresche, 2006). The anti-myoclonic potential of GHB had been shown in an animal model of myoclonus (Menon, 1982), before it was confirmed in clinical trials of several alcohol-responsive myoclonus syndromes, including myoclonus-dystonia, post-hypoxic myoclonus and progressive myoclonus epilepsy (Priori et al., 2000; Frucht, Bordelon and Houghton, 2005a; Frucht et al., 2005b). The effect of GHB on other myoclonus disorders is yet to be defined, and its role as an anti-myoclonic remains experimental at present. Prescription of GHB is strictly regulated, due to concern about illicit use.

In general, GABAergic drugs are more effective for cortical myoclonus than for myoclonus of subcortical origin. This discrepancy in effectiveness may reflect differences in the neurochemistry of cortical and subcortical neurotransmission: GABA is the major inhibitory neurotransmitter in the cerebral cortex, whereas glycine is the major inhibitory neurotransmitter in the brain stem and spinal cord. Since glycine also regulates the activity of the glutamate receptor, the few glycinergic drugs were tested mainly under this consideration for disorders like schizophrenia and strokes. Except for two negative studies that the glycine precursor milacemid was ineffective for myoclonus (Brown et al., 1991; Gordon et al., 1993), glycinergic drugs have not been fully explored for their anti-myoclonic effects.

Another neurotransmitter, serotonin, has been implicated in the pathophysiology of post-hypoxic myoclonus (Goetz et al., 2002; Welsh et al., 2002). Post-hypoxic myoclonus improved with serotoninergic therapies, such as 5-hydroxytryptophan, combination of 5-hydroxytryptophan and a peripheral decarboxylase inhibitor, and monoamine oxidase inhibitors (Van Woert and Rosenbaum, 1979; Thal et al., 1980). However, despite their anti-myoclonic efficacy, serotonin replacement therapies are not well tolerated because of significant adverse effects. Outside the context of post-hypoxic myoclonus, serotonin replacement therapies were occasionally reported useful for progressive myoclonus epilepsy, brain stem myoclonus and spinal myoclonus (Chadwick et al., 1977; Jimenez-Jimenez et al., 1991; Pranzatelli et al., 1995).

Medications of other pharmacological mechanisms are less frequently deployed as anti-myoclonics. Tetrabenazine, a monoamine depleter, has also been found effective for myoclonus (Hoehn and Cherington, 1977; Kenney, Hunter and Jankovic, 2007). Tizanidine, an α2-adrenergic agonist, was reported beneficial for cortical myoclonus, and for spinal myoclonus when combined with valproate and baclofen (Mukand and Giunti, 2004; Ray *et al.*, 2005).

Botulinum toxin injection is a well-established therapy for hemifacial spasm, a form of peripherally generated myoclonus, and has replaced medications and surgeries as the front-line treatment of hemifacial spasm (Jost and Kohl, 2001; Defazio *et al.*, 2002). In addition to hemifacial spasm, botulinum toxin injections have been performed with success in other types of focal myoclonus, including palatal myoclonus (Penney, Bruce and Saeed, 2006), facial myoclonus (Browner, Azher and Jankovic, 2006), chin myoclonus (Devetag Chalaupka *et al.*, 2006) and spinal segmental myoclonus (Polo and Jabbari, 1994; Lagueny *et al.*, 1999; Campos *et al.*, 2003; Vivancos-Matellano *et al.*, 2006). Regular use of botulinum toxin injection for focal myoclonus at these locations awaits further validating studies.

In recent years, deep brain stimulation has been performed in several patients with myoclonus-dystonia who had severe medication-refractory myoclonus, dystonia or both. The globus pallidus internus was the most frequently selected target (Vercueil *et al.*, 2001; Liu *et al.*, 2002; Yianni *et al.*, 2003; Cif *et al.*, 2004; Magarinos-Ascone *et al.*, 2005; Foncke *et al.*, 2007). The ventral intermediate thalamic nucleus was chosen in a single case (Trottenberg *et al.*, 2001). In most cases of pallidal stimulation, both myoclonus and dystonia improved substantially. In the case of thalamic stimulation, myoclonus improved, but dystonia did not. Besides myoclonus-dystonia, it is currently unknown whether deep brain stimulation can remedy other myoclonus disorders.

TREATMENT OF MYOCLONUS: CONCLUSION

The concept of evidence-based medicine has permeated every aspect of clinical practice, and treatment of myoclonus is no exception. As a group of uncommon and heterogeneous disorders, there has been a void in large-scale, well-designed studies of treatment of myoclonus. Nevertheless, principles in treatment of myoclonus have been proposed, based on available evidence (Caviness and Brown, 2004; Nirenberg and Frucht, 2005). Pharmacological treatment remains the mainstay in treatment of myoclonus, and a combination of medications of different mechanisms is often more effective than monotherapies (Figure 24.1). The anchors of the combinational approach are benzodiazepines, levetiracetam, piracetam and valproate (Table 24.2). A benzodiazepine, such as clonazepam, is effective for myoclonus of any origin. Levetiracetam, piracetam and valproate are most useful for cortical

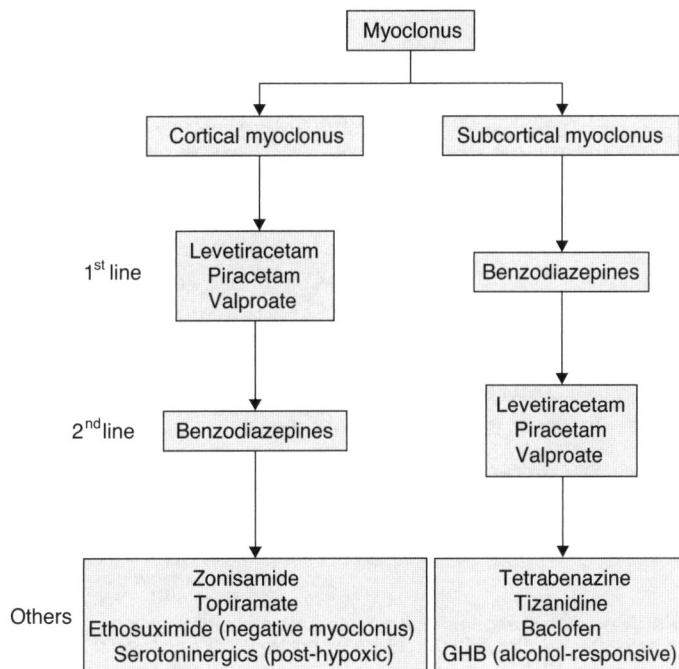

Figure 24.1 Algorithm for pharmacological treatment of myoclonus.

Table 24.2 Medications commonly used in the treatment of myoclonus.

Drug	Total daily dose	Frequency
Clonazepam	1–20 mg (0.01–0.2 mg/kg in children)	2–4 times daily
Levetiracetam	1000–3000 mg (20–60 mg/kg in children)	Twice daily
Piracetam	1.6–24 g	3 times daily
Valproate	10–60 mg/kg	2–4 times daily
Zonisamide	100–600 mg (4–8 mg/kg in children)	Once or twice daily

myoclonus, and selection among them depends largely on their availability and the susceptibility of individual patients to the adverse effects.

For cortical myoclonus, treatment can begin with a monotherapy of levetiracetam, piracetam or valproate, but addition of clonazepam will become necessary in most cases. If cortical myoclonus stays refractory to this combination, zonisamide and topiramate are worth consideration. Other medications may also be considered for selected indications, for example, ethosuximide for negative myoclonus and serotoninergic therapies for post-hypoxic myoclonus.

For brain stem and spinal myoclonus, treatment options are more limited, and results of treatment are generally less satisfactory. Often, treatment needs to start with clonazepam in order to control myoclonus adequately. Adding valproate, levetiracetam or piracetam is a reasonable next step, but the benefit is likely to be limited. Tetrabenazine, tizanidine and baclofen may be considered for spinal myoclonus resistant to clonazepam. For alcohol-responsive myoclonus, GHB is emerging as a promising option.

At this moment, non-pharmacological interventions are deemed experimental in treatment of myoclonus, although some hold potential under certain circumstances, such as botulinum toxin injection for focal myoclonus at amenable sites. As the understanding of myoclonus advances on clinical, electrophysiological and molecular fronts, treatment of myoclonus is expected to be increasingly science and evidence based.

References

Asmus, F. and Gasser, T. (2004) Inherited myoclonus-dystonia, in *Advances in Neurology, volume 94, Dystonia 4* (eds S. Fahn, M. Hallett and M.R. DeLong), Lippincott Williams & Wilkins, Philadelphia, pp. 113–119.

Brown, P., Thompson, P.D., Rothwell, J.C. *et al.* (1991) A therapeutic trial of milacemide in myoclonus and the stiff-person syndrome. *Movement Disorders*, **6**, 73–75.

Brown, P., Steiger, M.J., Thompson, P.D. *et al.* (1993) Effectiveness of piracetam in cortical myoclonus. *Movement Disorders*, **8**, 63–68.

Browner, N., Azher, S.N. and Jankovic, J. (2006) Botulinum toxin treatment of facial myoclonus in suspected Rasmussen encephalitis. *Movement Disorders*, **21**, 1500–1502.

Campos, C.R., Limongi, J.C., Machado, F.C. and Brotto, M.W. (2003) A case of primary spinal myoclonus: clinical presentation and possible mechanisms involved. *Arquivos de Neuro-Psiquiatria*, **61**, 112–114.

Capovilla, G., Beccaria, F., Veggiotti, P. *et al.* (1999) Ethosuximide is effective in the treatment of epileptic negative myoclonus in childhood partial epilepsy. *Journal of Child Neurology*, **14**, 395–400.

Caviness, J.N. (2003) Myoclonus and neurodegenerative disease – what's in a name? *Parkinsonism and Related Disorders*, **9**, 185–192.

Caviness, J.N. and Brown, P. (2004) Myoclonus: current concepts and recent advances. *Lancet Neurology*, **3**, 598–607.

Caviness, J.N., Alving, L.I., Maraganore, D.M. *et al.* (1999) The incidence and prevalence of myoclonus in Olmsted County, Minnesota. *Mayo Clinic Proceedings*, **74**, 565–569.

Chadwick, D., Hallett, M., Harris, R. *et al.* (1977) Clinical, biochemical and physiological features distinguishing myoclonus responsive to 5-hydroxytryptophan, tryptophan with a monoamine oxidase inhibitor, and clonazepam. *Brain: A Journal of Neurology*, **100**, 455–487.

Cif, L., Valente, E.M., Hemm, S. *et al.* (2004) Deep brain stimulation in myoclonus-dystonia syndrome. *Movement Disorders*, **19**, 724–727.

Cockerell, O.C., Rothwell, J., Thompson, P.D. *et al.* (1996) Clinical and physiological features of epilepsia partialis continua. Cases ascertained in the UK. *Brain: A Journal of Neurology*, **119**, 393–407.

Crunelli, V., Emri, Z. and Leresche, N. (2006) Unravelling the brain targets of gamma-hydroxybutyric acid. *Current Opinion in Pharmacology*, **6**, 44–52.

Defazio, G., Abbruzzese, G., Girlanda, P. *et al.* (2002) Botulinum toxin A treatment for primary hemifacial spasm: a 10-year multicenter study. *Archives of Neurology*, **59**, 418–420.

Deuschl, G. and Wilms, H. (2002) Clinical spectrum and physiology of palatal tremor. *Movement Disorders*, **17** (Suppl), S63–S66.

Devetag Chalaupka, F., Bartholini, F., Mandich, G. and Turro, M. (2006) Two new families with hereditary essential chin myoclonus: clinical features, neurophysiological findings and treatment. *Neurological Sciences*, **27**, 97–103.

Foncke, E.M., Bour, L.J., Speelman, J.D. *et al.* (2007) Local field potentials and oscillatory activity of the internal globus pallidus in myoclonus-dystonia. *Movement Disorders*, **22**, 369–376.

Fahn, S. (2002) Overview, history, and classification of myoclonus, in *Advances in Neurology, volume 89, Myoclonus and Paroxysmal Dyskinesias* (eds S. Fahn, S.J. Frucht, M. Hallett and D.D. Truong), Lippincott Williams & Wilkins, Philadelphia, pp. 13–17.

Frucht, S.J. (2002) The clinical challenge of posthypoxic myoclonus, in *Advances in Neurology, volume 89, Myoclonus and Paroxysmal Dyskinesias* (eds S. Fahn, S.J. Frucht, M. Hallett and D.D. Truong), Lippincott Williams & Wilkins, Philadelphia, pp. 85–88.

Frucht, S.J., Louis, E.D., Chuang, C. and Fahn, S. (2001) A pilot tolerability and efficacy study of levetiracetam in patients with chronic myoclonus. *Neurology*, **57**, 1112–1114.

Frucht, S.J., Bordelon, Y. and Houghton, W.C. (2005a) Marked amelioration of alcohol-responsive posthypoxic myoclonus by gamma-hydroxybutyric acid (Xyrem). *Movement Disorder*, **20**, 745–751.

Frucht, S.J., Houghton, W.C., Bordelon, Y. *et al.* (2005b) A single-blind, open-label trial of sodium oxybate for myoclonus and essential tremor. *Neurology*, **65**, 1967–1969.

Genton, P. and Gélisse, P. (2000) Antimyoclonic effect of levetiracetam. *Epileptic Disorders*, **2**, 209–212.

Genton, P. and Van Vleymen, B. (2000) Piracetam and levetiracetam: close structural similarities but different pharmacological and clinical profiles. *Epileptic Disorders*, **2**, 99–105.

Goetz, C.G., Carvey, P.M., Pappert, E.J. *et al.* (2002) The role of the serotonin system in animal models of myoclonus, in *Advances in Neurology, volume 89, Myoclonus and Paroxysmal Dyskinesias* (eds S. Fahn, S.J. Frucht, M. Hallett and D.D. Truong), Lippincott Williams & Wilkins, Philadelphia, pp. 241–248.

Gordon, M.F. (2002) Toxin and drug-induced myoclonus, in *Advances in Neurology, volume 89, Myoclonus and Paroxysmal Dyskinesias* (eds S. Fahn, S.J. Frucht, M. Hallett and D.D. Truong), Lippincott Williams & Wilkins, Philadelphia, pp. 49–76.

Gordon, M.F., Diaz-Olivo, R., Hunt, A.L. and Fahn, S. (1993) Therapeutic trial of milacemide in patients with myoclonus and other intractable movement disorders. *Movement Disorders*, **8**, 484–488.

Gwinn, K.A. and Caviness, J.N. (1997) Electrophysiological observations in idiopathic opsoclonus-myoclonus syndrome. *Movement Disorders*, **12**, 438–442.

Hallett, M. (2002) Neurophysiology of brainstem myoclonus, in *Advances in Neurology, volume 89, Myoclonus and Paroxysmal Dyskinesias* (eds S. Fahn, S.J. Frucht, M. Hallett and D.D. Truong), Lippincott Williams & Wilkins, Philadelphia, pp. 99–102.

Hess, C.W., Raymond, D., de Carvalho Aguiar, P. *et al.* (2007) Myoclonus-dystonia, obsessive-compulsive disorder, and alcohol dependence in SGCE mutation carriers. *Neurology*, **68**, 522–524.

Hoehn, M.M. and Cherington, M. (1977) Spinal myoclonus. *Neurology*, **27**, 942–946.

Ikeda, A., Shibasaki, H., Tashiro, K. *et al.* (1996) Clinical trial of piracetam in patients with myoclonus: nationwide multiinstitution study in Japan. The Myoclonus/Piracetam Study Group. *Movement Disorders*, **11**, 691–700.

Jankovic, J. (2001) Can peripheral trauma induce dystonia and other movement disorders? Yes!. *Movement Disorders*, **16**, 7–12.

Jimenez-Jimenez, F.J., Roldan, A., Zancada, F. *et al.* (1991) Spinal myoclonus: successful treatment with the combination of sodium valproate and L-5-hydroxytryptophan. *Clinical Neuropharmacology*, **14**, 186–190.

Jost, W.H. and Kohl, A. (2001) Botulinum toxin: evidence-based medicine criteria in blepharospasm and hemifacial spasm. *Journal of Neurology*, **248** (Suppl), 21–24.

Kenney, C., Hunter, C. and Jankovic, J. (2007) Long-term tolerability of tetrabenazine in the treatment of hyperkinetic movement disorders. *Movement Disorders*, **22**, 193–197.

Keswani, S.C., Kossoff, E.H., Krauss, G.L. and Hagerty, C. (2002) Amelioration of spinal myoclonus with levetiracetam. *Journal of Neurology, Neurosurgery and Psychiatry*, **73**, 457–458.

Koskiniemi, M., Van Vleymen, B., Hakamies, L. *et al.* (1998) Piracetam relieves symptoms in progressive myoclonus epilepsy: a multicentre, randomised, double blind, crossover study comparing the efficacy and safety of three dosages of oral piracetam with placebo. *Journal of Neurology, Neurosurgery and Psychiatry*, **64**, 344–348.

Krauss, G.L. and Mathews, G.C. (2003) Similarities in mechanisms and treatments for epileptic and nonepileptic myoclonus. *Epilepsy Currents*, **3**, 19–21.

Krauss, G.L., Bergin, A., Kramer, R.E. *et al.* (2001) Suppression of post-hypoxic and post-encephalitic myoclonus with levetiracetam. *Neurology*, **56**, 411–412.

Lagueny, A., Tison, F., Burbaud, P. *et al.* (1999) Stimulus-sensitive spinal segmental myoclonus improved with injections of botulinum toxin type A. *Movement Disorders*, **14**, 182–185.

Lim, L.L. and Ahmed, A. (2005) Limited efficacy of levetiracetam on myoclonus of different etiologies. *Parkinsonism and Related Disorders*, **11**, 135–137.

Liu, X., Griffin, I.C., Parkin, S.G. *et al.* (2002) Involvement of the medial pallidum in focal myoclonic dystonia: a clinical and neurophysiological case study. *Movement Disorders*, **17**, 346–353.

Lynch, B.A., Lambeng, N., Nocka, K. *et al.* (2004) The synaptic vesicle protein SV2A is the binding site for the antiepileptic drug levetiracetam. *Proceedings of the National Academy of Sciences of the, United States of America* **101**, 9861–9866.

Magarinos-Ascone, C.M., Regidor, I., Martinez-Castrillo, J.C. *et al.* (2005) Pallidal stimulation relieves myoclonus-dystonia syndrome. *Journal of Neurology, Neurosurgery, and Psychiatry*, **76**, 989–991.

Marseille Consensus Group (1990) Classification of progressive myoclonus epilepsies and related disorders. *Annals of Neurology*, **28**, 113–116.

Menon, M.K. (1982) Gamma-hydroxybutyrate in experimental myoclonus. *Neurology*, **32**, 434–437.

Mukand, J.A. and Giunti, E.J. (2004) Tizanidine for the treatment of intention myoclonus: a case series. *Archives of Physical Medicine and Rehabilitation*, **85**, 1125–1127.

Nielsen, V.K. (1985) Electrophysiology of the facial nerve in hemifacial spasm: ectopic/ephaptic excitation. *Muscle and Nerve*, **8**, 545–555.

Nirenberg, M.J. and Frucht, S.J. (2005) Myoclonus. *Current Treatment Options in Neurology*, **7**, 221–230.

Obeso, J.A., Artieda, J., Quinn, N. *et al.* (1988) Piracetam in the treatment of different types of myoclonus. *Clinical Neuropharmacology*, **11**, 529–536.

Obeso, J.A., Artieda, J., Rothwell, J.C. *et al.* (1989) The treatment of severe action myoclonus. *Brain: A Journal of Neurology*, **112**, 765–777

Obeso, J.A., Arteida, J. and Burleigh, A.L. (1995) Clinical aspects of negative myoclonus, in *Advances in Neurology, volume 67, Negative Motor Phenomena* (eds S. Fahn, M. Hallett, H.O. Lüders and C.D. Marsden), Lippincott-Raven Publishers, Philadelphia, pp. 1–7.

Oguni, H., Uehara, T., Tanaka, T. *et al.* (1998) Dramatic effect of ethosuximide on epileptic negative myoclonus: implications for the neurophysiological mechanism. *Neuropediatrics*, **29**, 29–34.

Ohtahara, S. (2006) Zonisamide in the management of epilepsy–Japanese experience. 1. *Epilepsy Research*, **68** (Suppl 2), 25–33.

Penney, S.E., Bruce, I.A. and Saeed, S.R. (2006) Botulinum toxin is effective and safe for palatal tremor: a report of five cases and a review of the literature. *Journal of Neurology*, **253**, 857–860.

Polo, K.B. and Jabbari, B. (1994) Effectiveness of botulinum toxin type A against painful limb myoclonus of spinal cord origin. *Movement Disorders*, **9**, 233–235.

Pranzatelli, M.R., Tate, E., Huang, Y. *et al.* (1995) Neuropharmacology of progressive myoclonus epilepsy: response to 5-hydroxy-L-tryptophan. *Epilepsia*, **36**, 783–791.

Pranzatelli, M.R., Tate, E.D., Galvan, I. and Wheeler, A. (2001) Controlled pilot study of piracetam for pediatric opsoclonus-myoclonus. *Clinical Neuropharmacology*, **24**, 352–357.

Priori, A., Bertolasi, L., Pesenti, A. *et al.* (2000) γ-Hydroxybutyric acid for alcohol-sensitive myoclonus with dystonia. *Neurology*, **54**, 1706.

Ray, B.K., Guha, G., Misra, A.K. and Das, S.K. (2005) Involuntary jerking of lower half of the body (spinal myoclonus). *Journal of the Association of Physicians of India*, **53**, 141–143.

Rothwell, J.C. (2002) Pathophysiology of spinal myoclonus, in *Advances in Neurology, volume 89, Myoclonus and Paroxysmal Dyskinesias* (eds S. Fahn, S.J. Frucht, M. Hallett and D.D. Truong), Lippincott Williams & Wilkins, Philadelphia, pp. 137–144.

Shibasaki, H. (2006) Myoclonus, in *Neurology and Clinical Neuroscience* (ed. A.H.V. Schapira), Mosby, Philadelphia, pp. 435–442.

Shibasaki, H. (2007) Myoclonus and startle syndromes, in *Parkinson's Disease and Movement Disorders* (eds J. Jankovic and E. Tolosa), Lippincott Williams and Wilkins, Philadelphia, pp. 376–386.

Shibasaki, H. and Hallett, M. (2005) Electrophysiological studies of myoclonus. *Muscle and Nerve*, **31**, 157–174.

Shin, H.W., Ye, B.S., Kim, J. *et al.* (2007) The contribution of a spinal mechanism in developing peripheral myoclonus: A case report. *Movement Disorders*, **22**, 1350–1352.

Siniscalchi, A., Mancuso, F., Russo, E. *et al.* (2004) Spinal myoclonus responsive to topiramate. *Movement Disorders*, **19**, 1380–1381.

Striano, P., Manganelli, F., Boccella, P. *et al.* (2005) Levetiracetam in patients with cortical myoclonus: a clinical and electrophysiological study. *Movement Disorders*, **20**, 1610–1614.

Thal, L.J., Sharpless, N.S., Wolfson, L. and Katzman, R. (1980) Treatment of myoclonus with L-5-hydroxytryptophan and carbidopa: clinical, electrophysiological, and biochemical observations. *Annals of Neurology*, **7**, 570–576.

Trottenberg, T., Meissner, W., Kabus, C. *et al.* (2001) Neurostimulation of the ventral intermediate thalamic nucleus in inherited myoclonus-dystonia syndrome. *Movement Disorders*, **16**, 769–771.

Uthman, B.M. and Reichl, A. (2002) Progressive Myoclonic Epilepsies. *Current Treatment Options in Neurology*, **4**, 3–17.

Vaamonde, J., Legarda, I., Jimenez-Jimenez, J. and Obeso, J.A. (1992) Acetazolamide improves action myoclonus in Ramsay Hunt syndrome. *Clinical Neuropharmacology*, **15**, 392–396.

Van Woert, M.H. and Rosenbaum, D. (1979) L-5-hydroxytryptophan therapy in myoclonus, in *Advances in Neurology, volume 26, Cerebral Hypoxia and Its Consequences* (eds S. Fahn, J.N. Davis and L.P. Rowland), Lippincott-Raven Publishers, Philadelphia, pp. 107–115.

Vercueil, L., Pollak, P., Fraix, V. *et al.* (2001) Deep brain stimulation in the treatment of severe dystonia. *Journal of Neurology*, **248**, 695–700.

Vivancos-Matellano, F., Arpa-Gutierrez, F.J., Perez-Conde, M.C. *et al.* (2006) The effectiveness of Botulinum toxin Type A in two cases of abdominal myoclonias refractory to conventional therapy. *Revista de Neurología*, **42**, 59–61.

Welsh, J.P., Placantonakis, D.G., Warsetsky, S.I. *et al.* (2002) The serotonin hypothesis of myoclonus from the perspective of neuronal rhythmicity, in *Advances in Neurology, volume 89, Myoclonus and Paroxysmal Dyskinesias* (eds S. Fahn, S.J. Frucht, M. Hallett and D.D. Truong Lippincott Williams & Wilkins, Philadelphia, pp. 307–329.

Wong, A. (2007) An update on opsoclonus. *Current Opinion in Neurology*, **20**, 25–31.

Yianni, J., Bain, P., Giladi, N. *et al.* (2003) Globus pallidus internus deep brain stimulation for dystonic conditions: a prospective audit. *Movement Disorders*, **18**, 436–442.

Part V

DRUG-INDUCED MOVEMENT DISORDERS

25

Neuroleptic-Induced Movement Disorders

S. Elizabeth Zauber and Christopher G. Goetz

Parkinson's Disease and Movement Disorders Program, Department of Neurological Sciences,
Rush University Medical Center, Chicago, IL , USA

INTRODUCTION

Anti-psychotic drugs were introduced in the 1950s and revolutionized the field of psychiatry. However, it was not long before a number of acute and chronic side effects of these medicines were noted, many of them involving involuntary movements. These agents all share dopamine receptor-site blockade as their primary mechanism of action. They include phenothiazines, divided into piperazine-, piperadine-, and aliphatic-based compounds, butyrophenones, including the archetypical drug, haloperidol, and other heterocyclic compounds including benzamides (Table 25.1). A new generation of compounds, termed "atypical anti-psychotic drugs" has been developed, and these drugs have a variety of chemical structures. While the risk of movement disorders is lower with these latter agents, the same gamut of disorders potentially exists for all agents. In addition to neuroleptics, a number of other medicines cause movement disorders and these will be covered in Chapter 26. Whereas, medicines like metoclopramide are not neuroleptics, they share dopamine-receptor blockade actions and therefore can be considered similar to neuroleptic-induced movement disorders. This chapter describes the most common neuroleptic-induced movement disorders, their pharmacological mechanisms, and their treatment. Because the disorders are directly caused by drugs, the obvious first-line treatment is withdrawal of the neuroleptic, but in many instances, psychiatric illness does not permit this intervention and other treatments must be introduced. Even with withdrawal of neuroleptics, some of these movement disorders do not resolve. In these cases, knowledge of pharmacological interactions between the dopaminergic and other neurotransmitter systems helps the clinician in selecting the best treatments. The chapter is organized by the temporal evolution of movement disorders relative to exposure to neuroleptics: acute reactions seen shortly after drug initiation; sub-acute reactions

occurring within weeks of usage; and chronic or tardive syndromes that emerge after months of neuroleptic exposure (Table 25.2).

ACUTE DYSTONIA

Description

Dystonia refers to a movement disorder typified by tonic contractions of muscles, often with a twisting component. Acute, neuroleptic-induced dystonia typically involves the neck and face, although it can involve any part of the body. The most serious manifestation is laryngeal dystonia, which can lead to respiratory failure (Flaherty and Lahmeyer, 1978). Oculogyric crisis is drug-induced dystonia in which the eyes deviate upwards. The trunk can also be involved with painful back arching, termed opisthotonus.

Most dystonic reactions occur very early in the course of treatment with anti-psychotic drugs, 85% within the first four days (Swett, 1975). Males develop acute dystonic reactions twice as frequently as females (Magnuson, Roccaforte and Wengel, 1999). In the past, patients with an underlying psychiatric diagnosis of mania were considered at higher risk for acute dystonia than treated schizophrenics, but this difference likely relates to the higher peak doses used in managing acute manic and hypomanic episodes (Khanna, Das and Damodaran, 1992). The propensity of a given drug to cause acute dystonic reactions parallels the drug's propensity to induce sub-acute parkinsonism (see below). The piperazine group has the highest likelihood of precipitating dystonic reactions, and the piperidine (thioridazine) group and the newer generation neuroleptics, like clozapine, have a low propensity. Cocaine has been shown to increase the risk of acute dystonic reactions (van Harten, van Trier and Horwitz, 1998), and can cause dystonic reactions alone, without neuroleptics.

Therapeutics of Parkinson's Disease and Other Movement Disorders   Edited by Mark Hallett and Werner Poewe
© 2008 John Wiley & Sons, Ltd.

Table 25.1 Commonly prescribed neuroleptics.

Phenothiazines:
    Chlorpromazine (Thorazine)
    Fluphenazine (Prolixin)
    Perphenazine (Trilafon)
    Prochlorperazine (Compazine)
    Thioridazine (Mellaril)
    Trifluoperazine (Stelazine)

Butyrophenones:
    Haloperidol (Haldol)
    Droperidol
    Pimozide (Orap)

Atypical anti-psychotics:
    Clozapine (Clozaril)
    Olanzapine (Zyprexa)
    Risperidone (Risperdal)
    Quetiapine (Seroquel)
    Ziprasidone (Geodon)
    Amisulpride (Solian)

Prevalance

The incidence varies from 2% in large series to 50% in a smaller study of neuroleptic-naive patients treated with typical neuroleptics (Ayd, 1961; Mazurek and Rosebush, 1991). This variation may be due to the age distribution of subjects, since young people are most susceptible to drug-induced dystonic reactions. The relative risk in people younger than 30 years old is 77%, compared to 14% for those older than 40 years old (Mazurek and Rosebush, 1991).

Pathophysiology

Because dystonias in other medical contexts are thought to involve primarily the putamen and its outflow pathways, most of the focus on understanding a biological basis of acute dystonic reactions has been on the dopamine–acetylcholine balance implicit to striatal function and D2 receptor activity. Multiple hypotheses have been offered. Suddenly enhanced dopamine turnover in response to dopamine receptor blockade could theoretically explain this adverse event, but treatment with a dopamine-depleting agent, α-methyl-paratyrosine, fails to prevent acute dystonic reactions. These observations, therefore, cast serious doubt on pre-synaptic dopaminergic release as a primary pathophysiological mechanism (Gershanik, 2002; McCann, Penetar and Belenky, 1990). It is also possible that the dopamine receptor blockers induce other neurochemical changes besides cholinergic disruption, for example,

secondary involvement of γ-amino-butyric acid in the putaminopallidal pathway and resultant enkaphalin enhancement (Matsumoto and Pouw, 2000). In support of this hypothesis, dopamine-receptor antagonists with a high likelihood of acute dystonic reactions, like piperazine-based neuroleptics, also have high binding affinities for σ-1 and σ-2 receptors (Matsumoto and Pouw, 2000). Regardless of these observations, the prevailing concept for the biological basis of acute dystonic reactions from dopamine receptor antagonists, is a direct disruption of striatal dopamine–acetylcholine homeostasis. As such, with D2 and possibly some D1 receptors blocked, acetylcholine acts in relative, though not absolute, higher striatal concentrations and precipitates the dystonic behaviors seen. This theory is supported by a low incidence of acute dystonia with neuroleptic agents with high anti-cholinergic properties, like thioridazine and clozapine. It is further supported by the reduced risk of acute dystonia when neuroleptics are started with an anti-cholinergic agent.

Management

The treatment of acute dystonia has not been rigorously studied in clinical trials. One small double-blind study compared intravenous diazepam to intravenous diphenhydramine and found no difference in benefit or side effects between the two treatments (Gagrat, Hamilton and Belmaker, 1978).

In addition to anti-cholinergics and benzodiazepines, anti-histamines are also used. Some authors suggest that benzodiazepines should be the first-line treatment because neurologists and other physicians are more familiar with the use of intravenous benzodiazepines than anti-cholinerg or anti-histamines.

Patients with acute neuroleptic-induced dystonia may have a recurrence in the first few days and should be treated with oral anti-cholinergics for this time period. Whether or not to treat all patients who are starting on anti-psychotics with prophylactic anti-cholinergics is controversial, because anti-cholinergics may increase the risk of TD. However, for patients who are at highest risk of acute dystonia, prophylaxis seems warranted.

SUB-ACUTE NEUROLEPTIC MALIGNANT SYNDROME

Description

Neuroleptic malignant syndrome (NMS) is an infrequent, but life-threatening complication of neuroleptic drugs. Symptoms of NMS include elevated temperature, muscle rigidity, autonomic dysfunction and mental status changes. Temperature reaches a peak in 48 hours after the syndrome begins. Rigidity can be severe enough to limit chest wall

Table 25.2 Most common neuroleptic-induced movement disorders.

Time course[a]	Syndrome	Symptoms	Treatment
Hours to days	Acute dystonia	Tonic contractions of agonist and antagonist muscles, often in face or trunk	Benzodiazepine Anti-cholinergics
Days to weeks	NMS	Fever, autonomic dysfunction, rigidity	Dantrolene Bromocriptine
Days to weeks	Neuroleptic-induced parkinsonism	Tremor, rigidity, bradykinesia	Anti-cholinergics Amantadine
Weeks	Akathisia	Subjective restlessness with objective purposeful movements	Propranolol
Months to years	Tardive dystonia	Tonic contractions of agonist and antagonist muscles, often in face or trunk	Anti-cholinergics Botulinum toxin
Three months to years	Tardive dyskinesia	Repetitive movements, usually of the face, mouth, and tongue	Reserpine/ Tetrabenazine

[a] Time course refers to the onset of movement disorders relative to the starting of a neuroleptic or to an increase in daily dose.

movement and lead to hypoventilation. A prospective analysis (Rosebush and Stewart, 1989) found that rigidity was present in 95%, tremulousness in 92%, chorea or dystonia in 59% and muteness or hypophonia in 96%. Laboratory values include elevated CK in 71% (Rosenberg and Green, 1989). The diagnostic criteria according to DSM-IV require rigidity and fever plus two of the following: diaphoresis, dysphagia, tremor, incontinence, altered mental status, mutism, tachycardia, labile blood pressure, elevated white blood-cell count and elevated creatine kinase.

Symptoms occur within 10–20 days of neuroleptic introduction or a dosage increase, but may occur after 1–2 months, in patients taking depot drugs. Whereas NMS by definition relates to neuroleptic exposure, a similar syndrome can be seen with a sudden withdrawal of dopaminergic drugs in Parkinson's disease (PD) or with the use of dopamine depleting drugs such as reserpine and tetrabenazine (Bhanushali and Tuite, 2004). Standard and atypical anti-psychotics are associated with this potentially fatal disorder (Hasan and Buckley, 1998). A recent report describes a case of NMS in a pediatric patient treated with aripiprazole (Palakurthi, Parvin and Kaplan, 2007). In a prospective study of 24 cases of NMS, 65% of patients had been given a neuroleptic medicine for first time, had the medicine restarted after a drug free period or had the dose increased. Dehydration was thought to be the precipitating event for most patients whose doses had not changed (Rosebush and Stewart, 1989).

Risk factors, besides dehydration, include a prior episode of NMS, agitation and intramuscular route of medication administration (Bhanushali and Tuite, 2004). Affective disorders were more represented in one prospective study (Rosebush and Stewart, 1989), but this diagnostic propensity was not replicated in a review of 64 case reports (Rosenberg and Green, 1989).

Symptoms typically last 7–14 days after the offending drug has been stopped.

Life-threatening complications occur in 30% of patients (Rosenberg and Green, 1989), including respiratory failure, renal failure, cardiac arrhythmias and complications of immobility, such as pulmonary embolus.

A number of other conditions should be considered in the differential of NMS. Possible CNS infection should be evaluated with a lumbar puncture. The symptoms of malignant hyperthermia, an inherited disorder of muscle, which occurs after exposure to halogenated inhaled anesthetics are very similar to those of NMS. However, the two conditions can be usually differentiated based on exposure history and family history. Catatonia presents with symptoms of mutism and immobility, but patients rarely have fever or autonomic instability. Heat stroke can be distinguished from NMS because patients with heat stroke usually do not sweat, while those with NMS are diaphoretic. Nonetheless, psychotic patients are prone to overdressing, often suffer from overexposure to environmental heat in the summer and take neuroleptic medications, so they are at risk for both heat stroke and NMS. Patients with serotonin syndrome often have prominent gastrointestinal symptoms, such as nausea, vomiting and diarrhea. Ataxia, myoclonus and hyperreflexia are more common in serotonin syndrome than NMS (Bhanushali and Tuite, 2004). Status epilepticus can mimic NMS in rare cases (Rosebush and Stewart, 1989).

Prevalance

While the incidence of NMS among patients treated with neuroleptics is rare, published rates vary from 0.02 to 2.4% (Caroff and Mann, 1993). Prospective studies typically examine hospitalized patients and the rate of NMS among these patients may not represent the rate in all patients treated with neuroleptics. Exact measures of incidence are further complicated by the fact that the diagnoses may be unrecognized. In an attempt to control for some of these confounding factors, one study compared the incidence among hospitalized patients in one institution at two different time points. They concluded that the incidence may be declining from 1.1 to 0.1% over a period of 10 years (Keck, Pope and McElroy, 1991).

Pathophysiology

The observation that NMS could also be caused by the withdrawal of dopamine drugs in patients with Parkinson's disease led to the hypothesis that NMS represents a state of dopamine deficiency (Henderson and Wooten, 1981). Nisijima and Ishiguro have studied the dopamine metabolite HVA in the CSF of patients with NMS and found a significant decrease compared to controls. NMS likely results from a disruption of both nigrostiatal and hypothalamic dopaminergic pathways. Rigidity and akinesia result from nigrostriatal dysfunction, while dysregulation of blood pressure and heart rate result from hypothalamic dysfunction. Dopamine activity in the pre-optic area in the hypothalamus is involved in temperature control, and may be responsible for thermal dysregulation in NMS (Factor, 2005). Dopamine under-activity alone is too simplistic an explanation since dopamine-depleting drugs are infrequently associated with NMS. Under-activity of GABA- or GAGAergic systems directly involved or secondarily diminished by dopaminergic-receptor blockade has been suggested by CSF studies (Nisijima and Ishiguro, 1995).

Treatment

Because it occurs infrequently and is life threatening, NMS has not been studied in large treatment trials. Most of the published data on treatment involve case reports or very small series The mainstay of treatment is to first withdraw the neuroleptic and provide supportive care, including ICU monitoring, IV fluids, temperature control and cardiac monitoring (Bhanushali and Tuite, 2004).

Bromocriptine, a dopamine agonist, and dantrolene have been used to treat NMS. Dantrolene acts on skeletal muscle to inhibit contraction by sequestration of calcium in the sarcoplasmic reticulum, and may also have central effects (Caroff and Mann, 1993). Suggested doses of dantrolene are 1–2 mg/kg i.v. daily, in four divided doses,

which can be changed to oral after temperature and rigidity decrease. However, dantrolene can be hepatotoxic at high or prolonged doses. These conclusions are largely based on clinical experience.

In fact, there is conflicting evidence about the efficacy of dantrolene and bromocriptine in the treatment of NMS. In favor of these medicines, one case series of patients treated with dantrolene or bromocritptine improved sooner (one day compared to seven days) than those treated with supportive care alone (Rosenberg and Green 1989). The authors evaluated treatment success by measuring the time from initiation of the therapy until the beginning of clinical improvement, defined as a persistent decrease in either temperature or rigidity. These drugs have also been shown to reduce mortality. In a retrospective analysis of published cases, investigators compared the death rate of patients receiving a particular drug therapy to rates in those who received only supportive care. They found that both dantrolene and bromocriptine reduced the death rate from 22 to 8%; however, there was no added benefit to using both drugs together (Sakkas *et al.*, 1991). In contrast, a prospective series of 24 cases, in which half the patients received either bromocriptine or dantrolene, there was no difference in NMS duration or mortality in treated vs untreated patients (Rosebush and Stewart, 1989). Treatment assignment was not randomized, making conclusions difficult because it is possible that the patients who were treated with dantrolene or bromocriptine had more severe disease than those given supportive care and therefore no difference in mortality was detected.

Case reports also exist for a response to ECT, but several cases have been complicated by cardiac arrhythmias. Some recommend ECT if patients are refractory to supportive care and medicine, or when the differential diagnosis includes catatonia (Factor, 2005).

Patients who have had NMS are at increased risk of developing NMS when neuroleptics are restarted. However this risk appears to be significantly reduced when medicines are restarted at least two weeks after the resolution of NMS. In a prospective study of 15 patients, 12 of 13 patients had no relapse when neuroleptics were reintroduced after two weeks, while 6 of 7 patients whose neuroleptics were restarted in the first two weeks had a relapse of NMS (Rosebush, Stewart and Gelenberg, 1989).

With the paucity of evidence, the best approach to the treatment of NMS is treatment targeted to the individual patient and situation. All patients should be treated with fluids, temperature control and cardiac monitoring; however, not all patients will require ICU level care. Mild patients may do well with supportive care alone. Benzodiazepines are useful for patients who are agitated. Patients with more severe or continuing symptoms of hyperthermia, rigidity and rhabdomyolysis should be continued on dantrolene or bromocritptine therapy. Patients who are refractory to those medicines, or who have continued psychosis, may benefit from ECT (Caroff, Mann and Keck, 1998).

SUB-ACUTE AKATHISIA

Description

Akathisia is a common side effect of first-generation neuroleptic drugs. It can occur in sub-acute and tardive forms. The sub-acute form occurs within the first weeks of starting neuroleptics or a dose increase (Sachdev, 2005). In contrast, tardive akathisia occurs after prolonged treatment. This temporal pattern suggests that tardive akathisia likely has a different pathophysiology than the sub-acute form, and the two are further differentiated by their management responses (see below). The term akathisia literally means "inability to remain seated." Akathisa causes significant distress to the patient and can contribute to medicine non-adherence (Adler, Rotrosen and Angrist, 2005). Outside of Parkinson's disease and neuroleptic-induced syndromes, akathisia is not a prominent symptom of most other primary medical or neurological disorders. The differential diagnosis, however, includes restless leg syndrome that can be associated with iron deficiency. Iron deficiency can be seen in cases with structural putaminal or pallidal lesions (Barton, Bowie and Ebmeier, 1990), so that iron and ferritin levels should be assayed in appropriate cases.

The severe subjective sense of restlessness, often associated with pronounced anxiety, provokes the akathitic patient to move incessantly in order to relieve symptoms (Gershanik, 2002). The syndrome is defined by the presence of both the subjective sensation of inner restlessness and the objective presence of volitional movements, such as moving about while seated or rocking back from one foot to the other while standing. The patient may also demonstrate repetitive hand movements, truncal rocking and panting respirations (Sunami, Nishikawa and Yorogi, 2000). Akathisia may be difficult to distinguish from other disorders, as it can resemble the psychomotor agitation seen in depression, mania or psychosis, or anxiety. Restless leg syndrome is also in the differential diagnosis of akathisia, but can be distinguished by the nocturnal predominance of symptoms in restless legs syndrome (RLS), and the fact that akathisia is not made specifically worse when the patient is lying down. Typical tardive dyskinesia (TD) is distinguished from akathisia by the phenomenology of movements and by the fact that patients with TD do not experience a feeling of unease that leads to the abnormal movement.

The most significant risk factor for the development of akathisia is the dose of neuroleptics used and rate of increase (Sachdev and Kruk, 1994). Some atypical antipsychotics are associated with lower risk of akathisia. In newly treated patients on olanzapine 7%, and haldol 21% (Tran *et al.,*1997). However, others have risk equal to that of haldol (Rosebush and Mazurek, 1999). Though not firmly established, the development of sub-acute akathisia has been suggested to predict a risk for poor treatment outcome and a higher risk of tardive dyskinesia among schizophrenics (Nair, Josiassen and Abraham, 1999; Eichhammer, Albus and Borrmann-Hassenbach, 2000).

Prevalance

Reported incidence rates vary from 25% up to 75%; a rate of 20% comes from a large survey of over 3000 patients (Ayd, 1961). A prospective study reports a 20% incidence of moderate to severe akathisia (Sachdev and Kruk, 1994). The large variability in these rates is most likely due to differences in diagnostic criteria, and the difficulty in distinguishing akathisia from other related disorders.

Pathophysiology

The biological basis of sub-acute neuroleptic-induced akathisia is poorly understood, but the occurrence of akathisia in other conditions suggests some clues. The frequent association of drug-induced parkinsonism with akathisia and the frequently spontaneous occurrence of akathisia in Parkinson's disease itself suggest that the nigrostiatal dopaminergic system plays a direct role. Cases with structural subcortical lesions associated with akathisia have most damage in the putamen or outflow tracts to the globus pallidus. Subcortical-spinal networks or mesocortical pathways may be pathophysiologically involved. Whereas traditionally, D2 dopaminergic-receptor blockade was hypothesized to be at the core of akathisia, this disorder has a less predictable pharmacology than acute dystonia. Noradrenergic and opioid influences play a likely role in the pathophysiology, because β-noradrenergic blockers and opioid antagonists are often effective therapies if the neuroleptic cannot be withdrawn (Kompoliti and Horn, 2003).

These secondary chemical influences likely involve brainstem nuclei or mesospinal pathways. Serotonergic/dopaminergic imbalance has also been suggested to play a role in akathisia, based on evidence that some of the newly developed neuroleptics with high affinity for 5HT3 receptors have a low index of akathisia (Hirsch, Kissling and Bauml, 2002). The link of akathisia to iron metabolism has been studied, and at least in some studies, neuroleptic-treated patients with and without akathisia have both lower iron and lower ferritin plasma levels than healthy controls (Kuloglu, Atmaca and Ustundag, 2003). Those with akathisia tend to have lower levels than non-akathitic subjects, but the iron and ferritin levels still fall within the normal range (Hofmann, Seifritz and Botschev, 2000). Though iron levels influence dopamine D1 and D2 receptor numbers and sensitivity in rats, exact cellular effects caused by dopamine receptor antagonists in humans have not been identified

(Erikson, Jones and Hess, 2001). RLS has some clinical features in common with akathisia (see description above). There is good evidence that low serum iron increases the risk for RLS and that these patients have lower basal ganglia iron concentration than controls (Earley *et al.,*2000).

Treatment

The anguish experienced by patients with akathisia prompts the need for clinicians to diagnose and treat this condition immediately. Lowering the dose of neuroleptics can be adequate or a switch to a more low potency neuroleptic may resolve the problem without sacrificing necessary control of psychosis. In the event that these solutions are not successful, other medicines may be added, although the evidence for some of these treatments is conflicting.

β-Blockers are the most effective treatment for akathisia. Lipophilic drugs are more effective than other β-blockers, because of their ability to cross the blood–brain barrier. Data from case reports as well as from small randomized, double-blind studies show that low doses of propranolol (20–60 mg/day) reduce akathisia and do not significantly affect blood pressure (Adler *et al.*, 1986; Lipinski *et al.*, 1983).

One three-armed study compared propranolol, an anticholinergic (benztropine) and placebo. Patients in both treatment arms had a similar mean magnitude of improvement (about 30%) a similar portion of patients improved (about 40%) with either treatment. However, in the anticholinergic group, several patients experienced drug-related confusion that limited treatment (Adler *et al.,*1993).

A small double-blind, placebo-controlled trial of clonazepam in a group of hospitalized adolescents with neuroleptic-induced akathisia found a significant improvement (Kutcher *et al.*, 1989). Clonidine improved akathisia, but clinical usefulness was limited by hypotension and sedation. A 5HT2 antagonist (ritanserin) has been used to treat patients who have not responded to β-blockers, benzodiazepines or anti-cholinergics. A prospective study of 10 patients given ritanserin for 2–4 days, found a decrease in subjective and objective measures of akathisia, compared to baseline scores (Miller *et al.*, 1990).

Finally, it is important to determine if the patient has both akathisia and drug-induced parkinsonism with tremor, rigidity and bradykinesia, because in these cases, amantadine or anti-cholinergic agents may treat both syndromes (Gershanik, 2002).

SUB-ACUTE PARKINSONISM

Description

The realization that dopamine-receptor blocking drugs cause drug-induced parkinsonism (DIP) helped lead to the discovery that dopamine depletion was involved in idiopathic PD (Hirose, 2006). For some time, it was incorrectly thought that parkinsonism was required for the antipsychotic effect of neuroleptics. This syndrome usually begins several days or weeks after starting or increasing the daily dose of dopamine receptor antagonists. Patients experience the gradual development of bradykinesia, rigidity, gait and balance instability, and resting tremor. When these signs appear in unison and rigidity is documented on the neurological examination, the diagnosis of parkinsonism is not difficult. However, often the early signs are subtle with more vague symptoms of increasing slowness and difficulty with movement (Kompoliti and Horn, 2003). In these cases where tremor is not prominent, the clinician, family and patient may misinterpret drug-induced parkinsonism as a global over-medication effect or as a sign of impending depression, especially in subjects with bipolar affective disorders. Tremor is seen when the patient's hands are relaxed in the lap, and the movement disorder abates as the patient moves and executes tasks of daily living (resting tremor). Fine motor movements like buttoning, opening envelops, manipulating an eating utensil become slow and difficult, although there is no weakness (bradykinesia). On examination, while the patient remains relaxed, the clinician can detect hypertonicity with a ratchet-like quality (cogwheel rigidity). Difficulty rising from a chair, initiating walking, pivoting smoothly to turn and resisting a postural threat, usually tested by pulling abruptly on the shoulders to assess if patients can right themselves without falling backwards, all are indicative of gait and postural reflex impairment. All signs may be present simultaneously, but often the syndrome only partially develops, so that the physician must be sensitive to all clinical features.

While the symptoms of DIP resemble those of PD and are clinically indistinguishable from those of PD, some studies have noted differences on a population level. While differences may exist they are not significant enough to be helpful in clinical diagnosis, since they apply to groups and not to individuals. For example, tremor is less likely in DIP, (44%) compared to 70% of patients with PD (Hassin-Baer *et al.*, 2001). This study also noted that parkinsonian signs were more marked in the upper extremities compared to lower extremities in DIP, and that freezing of gait is less common in DIP than in PD. Others have suggested that signs in DIP are rarely asymmetric, but a study designed to answer this question did not support that claim, 25% of patients had notable asymmetry (Sethi and Zamrini, 1990).

The onset of DIP is subacute and occurs within 30 days of starting a neuroleptic in 50% of patients and within 72 days in 90% of patients (Ayd, 1961). Symptoms typically improve in 7–8 weeks if the dose of neuroleptic is decreased; however, 50% have persistent symptoms, despite anti-cholinergic treatment. Some patients improve after medicine is withdrawn and then have re-emergence of the parkinsonian symptoms months later without further exposure to neuroleptics. It is hypothesized that those patients had sub-clinical Parkinson's disease which was unmasked by the neuroleptics (Goetz, 1983). Similarly, (Burn and Brooks, 1993) investigated the idea that patients who do not improve after drug withdrawal have sub-clinical Parkinson's disease using ^{18}F-dopa PET. They imaged 13 patients who had been off neurolpetics for at least two weeks, then re-examined them after two years. Those with normal ^{18}F-dopa uptake were more likely to recover from DIP. However an abnormal scan did not necessarily predict persistent symptoms; the majority, 75%, of subjects with abnormal ^{18}F-dopa uptake also had remission.

Prevalance

DIP is thought to represent 20% of all incident cases of parkinsonism (Bower *et al.*, 1999), and may be under-recognized in the elderly. In one study of 3512 patients, patients aged 65–99, who were identified using a Medicaid drug database, patients taking neuroleptics were five times more likely to be prescribed drugs to treat parkinsonism. Further, 37% of patients taking drugs for parkinsonism were also taking neuroleptics (Avorn *et al.*, 1995). Elderly patients are thought to be at higher risk for this side effect than younger patients, but there is no established gender predominance.

Pathophysiology

Because Parkinson's disease and drug-induced parkinsonism are phenotypically indistinguishable, similar biochemical bases for the two disorders have been proposed (Klawans, 1973). In Parkinson's disease, the primary degenerative lesion is loss of the dopaminergic cells projecting from the pars compacta of the substantia nigra in the mesencephalon to the putamen and caudate nucleus (striatum). These cells interact primarily with D2 receptors (Jankovic, 2003). The primary site of action for neuroleptics precipitating drug-induced parkinsonism is this same post-synaptic dopamine D2 receptor population within the striatum.

Treatment

The most commonly used treatments are anti-cholinergics and amantadine. One study of 112 patients taking conventional neuroleptics found that about 80% of patients had improvement in parkinsonism with anti-cholinergics. The magnitude of response, however, was not reported (Kruse, 1960). Several studies have compared anti-cholinergics to amantadine. One double-blind crossover study of 39 patients showed equal efficacy of amantadine and trihexyphenidyl, but amantadine had fewer side effects (Fann and Lake, 1976). Another double-blind crossover study of 38 patients found benztropine to be more effective than amantadine (Kelly *et al.*, 1974).

The first step in treatment of DIP is to discontinue the offending drug, if possible. If the underlying disease for which the neuroleptic is prescribed does not permit changes in the neuroleptic, the next step is to change to a drug with a lower risk of EPS. Because neuroleptic metabolism often involves the generation of several intermediate or end products with dopamine antagonist properties, drug clearance should be not be presumed until three or four months after cessation. The addition of medicine to treat DIP should be reserved for symptomatic patients, since the treatments have only modest benefit and have significant side effects.

TARDIVE DYSKINESIA

Description

Tardive dyskinesia (TD) has been called tardive stereotypy and oral buccal lingual dyskinesia. It was first described in the 1950s within five years of the first anti-psychotic drug chlorpromazine becoming widely available (Fernandez and Friedman, 2003).

The movements of TD usually involve the tongue, lip or jaw, for example, tongue twisting and protrusion, lip smacking and puckering, and chewing. These movements may be unsightly and disruptive to social interactions, dental hygiene and vocal communication (Joseph and Young, 1999). When the diaphragmatic muscles and vocal apparatus are involved, irregular gasping respirations and noises may also occur. The movements occur in a repetitive and stereotyped manner and this fact can help to distinguish them from the dyskinesias seen in Huntington's disease, which are more random and unpredictable (Fernandez and Friedman, 2003). Forehead and eyebrow movements that are seen in Huntington's disease are not typical of TD (Jankovic, 1995). Movements may also involve the upper and lower extremities, as well as the axial muscles and diaphragm (Klawans, Goetz and Perlik, 1980). Movements in TD are increased by distraction or stress, and suppressed by voluntary action of the involved body part. They disappear in sleep (Sachdev, 2005). By definition, tardive dyskinesia is related to chronic neuroleptic exposure and the minimal exposure time is considered to be three months.

Many potential risk factors have been hypothesized, but the most consistently identified is age. Older patients have a higher incidence and lower remission rate (Tarsy and Baldessarini, 2006). Only 5% of exposed young adults develop tardive syndromes, whereas in patients over 45, the rate exceeds 30%, and in older institutionalized subjects the prevalence is 60% (Byne, White and Parella, 1998). Within the elderly population, a reduced rate of dyskinesia occurs in very old subjects, an observation that can be explained by documented late age-related loss of striatal dopamine receptors (Sweet, Mulsant and Rifai, 1992). A history of acute dystonic reactions to neuroleptics and affective disorders has also been proposed as a risk factor (Kane, Woerner and Lieberman, 1988). Intermittent treatment is thought to be more likely than continuous treatment to cause TD. Drug holidays do not prevent TD and may even increase the risk (van Harten, Hoek and Matroos, 1998).

The choice of neuroleptic drug is likely important to the risk of tardive dyskinesia. Although not extensively studied with carefully controlled trials, traditional neuroleptics of the piperazine group and the butyrophenone, haloperidol, are thought to have the highest risk of causing tardive dyskinesia, followed by the piperidine compounds, like chlorpromazine, and lastly by the piperidine neuroleptics, like thioridazine and the newer generation compounds, including clozapine, olanzapine, quetiapine, ziprasidone and aripiprazole (Meltzer, 1987). Even with these latter agents, however, a risk of tardive dyskinesia is present, and risk is thought to be dose and duration related (Glazer, Morgenstern and Doucette, 1993).

About half of patients with TD experience a waxing and waning course of mild to moderate symptoms, despite continued neuroleptic treatment. In this context, 10–30% of patients have a reduction in symptoms or remission over time, approximately 30–40% remain with the same movements and 10–30% worsen. The risk factors for worsening are the same as the risk factors for TD: age, gender, affective disorders, duration of exposure (Hyde et al., 2005). TD may transiently worsen when neuroleptic dose is decreased, but stabilize or improve afterwards (withdrawal dyskinesia). Remission rates vary, depending on the follow-up observation time, and it is clear that some cases resolve as late as five years after cessation of the causative drug (Gershanik, 2002).

Prevalance

Incidence and prevalence are difficult to study in TD for several reasons.

First, the severity of movements fluctuates spontaneously and with emotional arousal so that assessment determinations in cross-sectional surveys can be misleading. Further, although neuroleptics cause TD, when neuroleptic doses are acutely increased, the movements may actually abate and even disappear, so that frequency assessments need to take into account recent changes in medication dosage (Tarsy and Baldessarini, 2006). Measurements of incidence and prevalence are also complicated by the observation that spontaneous dyskinesias can occur in the absence of neuroleptic exposure. In a study of 2250 subjects, dyskinesias were observed in 1.3% of healthy

elderly and 4.8% of in-patient medical geriatric patients. Among psychiatric patients who were never exposed to neuroleptics, 0–2% had dyskinesias compared to 13–36% of chronic hospitalized psychiatric patients (Kane, 2004). The most accepted data suggest a prevalence of 20% among people treated with standard neuroleptics, and an incidence about 5% per year (Sachdev, 2005). The risk of developing TD does not appear to decline over time. In a nine-year cohort study of patients who had remained free of TD despite taking first generation anti-psychotics for a mean duration of 18 years, the subsequent annual incidence of TD was 10.2% (van Harten et al., 2006).

Pathophysiology

Many mechanisms have been proposed, and while the exact mechanism is unknown, it is likely that several interacting factors are involved. The main categories of interest are the balance between dopamine and cholinergic striatal activity, dysfunction of GABA neurons, excitotoxicity related to glutamatergic and other systems, and endogenous opioids.

At the level of the striatum, the dopaminergic and cholinergic systems have a competitive neurochemical balance of activities. The classic model of TD posits that chronic neuroleptics block striatal dopamine D2 receptors and causes denervation hypersensitivity after chronic receptor antagonism. This hypersensitivity then leads to an eventual hyperdopaminergic behavior in the form of stereotypic, choreic movements (Casey, 2004). Rodent models of TD have shown that after two weeks of exposure to neuroleptics, the number of D2 receptors increases. This model does not accurately reflect some of the major features of TD, however, because all animals are affected, while only a fraction of people exposed to neuroleptics develop TD. Furthermore, animals must be stimulated with dopamine agonists before symptoms appear, and the findings in the animals are reversible once medicines are stopped.

Despite these caveats, there is evidence from PET studies that D2 receptor binding increases in the striatum after withdrawal from chronic antipsychotic treatment. Nine subjects with schizophrenia who were eligible for drug withdrawal were studied with PET imaging. After a 14-day drug washout, the D2 receptor binding patterns were measured and compared to binding potentials from antipsychotic-naive subjects with schizophrenia. On average, the patients chronically exposed to anti-psychotic drugs had a higher D2 receptor binding potential than the untreated patients, and those with the highest D2 receptor upregulation (98%) also had severe TD at the time of the examination (Silvestri et al., 2000).

New interest has focused on neuroleptic effects on D1 receptors, those linked to adenyl cyclase enzymatic activity. Whereas typical neuroleptics primary block D2 receptors, leaving D1 variably affected, high turnover rates of dopamine consequent to the D2 receptor blockade could abnormally activate D1 receptors. In an animal model of tardive dyskinesia, rats with genetically mediated inactivated D1 receptor expression developed fewer abnormal movements when treated with chronic neuroleptics than those with full D1 function (van Kampen and Stoessl, 2000).

The observation that anti-cholinergics increase choreic dyskinetic movements of tardive dyskinesia, but improve tardive dystonia suggests that the cholinergic system is involved in the pathophysiological mechanisms related to phenotypic expression of tardive dyskinesia, but it is not clear that there is a direct relationship to pathogenesis.

Regarding glutamate and excitotoxicity, thalamocortical activity could theoretically cause a wide variety of movement disorders affecting descending corticospinal, corticobrain stem, and especially corticosubcortical networks (Mitchell, Crossman and Limigna, 1992). Excessive activation of thalamocortical function primarily involves the neurotransmitter glutamate, and tardive dyskinesia has also been suggested to relate to excitotoxic effects of glutamate and related compounds (Naidu and Kulkarni, 2001). In addition to excitotoxcitiy, neuroleptic medications themselves may have a toxic effect. The medicines inhibit complex I of the electron transport chain, which may lead to oxidative stress and cell injury (Burkhardt et al.,1992).

A complementary hypothesis focuses on the opioid system, because animals treated with chronic neuroleptics have reduced activity of the medial globus pallidus, ventral anterior and ventral lateral thalamic nuclei, as well as markedly increased subcortical metenkephalin levels. Drugs associated with low frequencies of tardive dyskinesia, like clozapine, do not induce metenkephalin-like immunoreactivity responses, whereas a more traditional neuroleptic, haloperidol, causes significant enhancement (Bester and Harvey, 2000).

The fourth area of interest for the pathophysiology of TD is GABA. The major inhibitory component of basal ganglia pathways is GABA. Investigators studied the activity of glutamic acid decarboxylase (GAD), the rate-limiting step in GABA synthesis, in a post-mortem study of patients with tardive dyskinesia. They reported decreased activity in the subthalamic nucleus of affected individuals compared to controls (Andersson et al., 1989). These authors also reported that GAD activity is reduced in the STN of primates with neuroleptic-induced dyskinesia compared to neuroleptic-exposed primates without dyskinesia, suggesting that this finding may be specific to dyskinesia and not a result of the neuroleptic exposure.

Treatment

Prevention of TD is the best treatment and the most important guidelines are to use neuroleptics only when needed, and to limit the dose and duration of therapy. When the first signs of TD emerge, the first step in treatment of TD is to stop the offending medicine, if possible. In a review of 285 treatment studies, involving 3000 patients, Jeste and Wyatt found that neuroleptic withdrawal reversed TD in 37% of patients, but patients often showed an initial worsening that peaked about 1–2 weeks after the dose of neuroleptic was decreased or stopped (Jeste and Wyatt, 1982). If neuroleptics cannot be withdrawn because of the underlying psychotic illness, changing to atypical antipsychotic drugs should be considered.

A number of other treatments have been studied for managing TD in patients who are already on the lowest possible anti-psychotic medication dose or who have stopped neuroleptics, but persist with residual involuntary movements. First, for patients with choreic movements, anti-cholinergic drugs should be withdrawn because they exacerbate the symptoms of TD (Jeste and Wyatt, 1982). Agents that decrease the synthesis or pre-synaptic release of dopamine have been studied as treatments for TD. α-Methyldopa and reserpine were studied in a randomized, placebo-controlled trial of 30 patients with TD and psychosis in remission. Neuroleptic doses were not changed during the two-week study and TD movements were scored as absent, mild, moderate or severe. Both active treatment groups had a 50% decrease in severity scores compared to an 18% decrease in the placebo group (Huang et al., 1981). Hypotension is a potential complication of both drugs, and reserpine is associated with the risk of drug-induced depression.

Tetrabenazine depletes pre-synaptic monoamines and blocks post-synaptic dopamine receptors. In an open study of 526 patients followed for an average of 28.9 months, 89% of patients treated with tetrabenazine had improvement defined as a marked reduction in abnormal movements and excellent improvement in function, as scored by patients, caregivers and physicians. However, this high estimate of treatment response selected for patients more likely to respond, by excluding subjects who dropped out because of lack of treatment response in the first two weeks. Side effects included fatigue or drowsiness in 36%, parkinsonism in 28% and depression in 15%. Side effects were reversible with dose reduction (Jankovic and Beach, 1997).

Because of its low risk of causing TD, clozapine has been studied in the treatment of TD. Lieberman et al. (1991) studied the effects of clozapine on 30 patients with TD and found that 43% had >50% improvement in TD symptoms. Patients with dystonic movements were most likely to improve. However, 50% of patients originally started on clozapine dropped out because of side effects, and they were not included in the analysis.

Clozapine was used in an 18-week study of 20 neuroleptic-resistant schizophrenics with TD, neuroleptic-induced parkinsonism or neuroleptic-induced akathisia.

The investigators reported a 74% improvement in TD, 69% improvement in PD and 78% improvement in akathisia with clozapine. Subjects started clozapine after a two-week washout of their prior neuroleptics. If patients were taking a conventional neuroleptic, the improvement in symptoms could simply be caused by the change to an atypical antipsychotic. There was no control group that had previous medicines stopped, but did not start on clozapine (Spivak *et al.*, 1997), so that the results are difficult to attribute directly to clozapine. However, in general, studies in TD after withdrawal of conventional anti-psychotics show a more modest improvement, suggesting that at least part of the improvement response can be attributed to clozapine.

A review of the results of 14 studies of clozapine for TD suggests that there is no clear evidence that clozapine is effective as a treatment for TD, once abnormal movements have developed. Certainly it has a lower risk than other drugs for causing TD so it is a reasonable choice for treating psychosis in patients who have TD, although blood monitoring is important and some psychotic patients may not be reliable enough to co-operate with regular toxicity monitoring (Factor and Friedman, 1997).

Given the anti-dyskinetic effect of amantadine in levodopa-induced parkinsonism, amantadine has been used to treat TD. One double-blind, crossover study of 16 patients showed a 15% improvement in TD movements with amantadine. However, one-quarter of the patients had an increase in their abnormal movements (Angus *et al.*, 1997).

The fact that GABA deficiency may be involved in TD has led to the use of GABAergic drugs. Evidence for the use of benzodiazepines in TD was reviewed in a Cochrane Review, and no studies with conclusive evidence for efficacy were found (Bhoopathi and Soares-Weiser, 2006). In another observational study, 30 patients with TD started on gabapentin were followed for one year, and a 47.5% reduction in movements based on one rating scale occurred. Side effects included sedation, dizziness and confusion and no control or comparator group data were reported (Hardoy *et al.*, 2002).

The exact mechanism of action of levetiracetam is unknown, but it may involve blockade of N-type calcium channels (Lukyanetz, Shkryl and Kostyuk, 2002) and may have indirect effects on GABA and glycine receptors through zinc and β-carbolines (Rigo *et al.*, 2000). Levetiracetam was studied in 16 patients with chronic psychosis and TD, enrolled consecutively in an open-label, observational study. Doses were increased up to 2000 mg/day or to benefit. Patients were followed for three months and rated by the Abnormal Involuntary Movement Scale which showed a significant improvement during the open label trial. Side effects included drowsiness and confusion (Meco *et al.*, 2006).

Vitamin E has been investigated in many small, two-week long, double-blind studies. Doses of 1200–1600 mg/ day were compared to placebo and showed a 24–43% benefit (as reviewed in Pierre, 2005). However, the largest and longest study of vitamin E (Adler *et al.*, 1999) did not replicate these results. It was a multi-centered, prospective, randomized trial of 158 subjects followed for two years. Because prior studies had suggested that patients with shorter duration of symptoms were more likely to improve, patients with TD for more than 10 years were not included. This study may have selected for more treatment-resistant patients since many patients were on atypical neuroleptics at the time of study enrollment.

If a patient remains refractory to all other treatments or cannot safely use one of the above therapies, resuming or even increasing the causative neuroleptic may be necessary to suppress TD and to provide symptomatic benefit. In this context, higher doses of neuroleptics or treatment re-initiation led to improvement in more than 60% of treated patients (Jeste and Wyatt, 1982). In this context, informed consent is particularly important, since the patient and physician are using the causative agent to treat TD.

TARDIVE DYSTONIA

Description

Tardive dystonia (Tdt) is a form of tardive dyskinesia, but is considered separately because there are several clinical, epidemiological and pathophysiological differences that distinguish it from the traditional form of TD. Moreover, drugs that improve tardive dystonia can exacerbate traditional TD. Often the two problems co-exist and the clinician must assess the prominent features of a given patient to decide on what primary clinical problem to treat.

The phenomenology of tardive dystonia in its pure form is clinically indistinguishable from idiopathic torsion dystonia. The movements may include focal, segmental or generalized dystonia with muscle spasms and twisting postures that are often painful. They most commonly involve the cranial-cervical area, occurring in this region among 87% of cases (Kiriakakis *et al.*, 1998).

Similar to patients with idiopathic dystonia, patients with tardive dystonia report sensory tricks (Kang, Burke and Fahn, 1986), where touching a body part can transiently relieve dystonic spasms. Studies of tardive dystonia suggest that retrocollis and anterocollis as well as head turning are more common in tardive dystonia compared to idiopathic torsion dystonia (Kiriakakis *et al.*, 1998; Kang, Burke and Fahn, 1986). Other manifestations of tardive dystonia can include blepharospasm, jaw deviation, trismus, torticollis or oculogyric crisis (Jankovic, 1995). Particularly prominent are back arching movements (opistotonus).

One feature that can help distinguish tardive dystonia from idiopathic dystonia is the frequent co-existence of typical choreic or stereotypic movements of TD.

Burke *et al.* found that 16 of 42 patients had other movements such as chorea of mouth, or myoclonous (Burke *et al.,*1982). Another series reported that 37 of 67 Tdt subjects had concominant TD movements (Kang, Burke and Fahn, 1986).

The majority of patients, 83%, begin their tardive dystonia with focal onset dystonia. Thereafter, the symptoms progress to become segmental or generalized, such that only about 15% remain focal over a prolonged period (Kang, Burke and Fahn, 1986; Kiriakakis *et al.*, 1998). Generalized dystonia is more likely to develop in younger patients (Kang, Burke and Fahn, 1986).

Duration of exposure to neuroleptics may be shorter for tardive dystonia than for TD. In one study, 21% of patients had been exposed to drugs for less than one year (Kang, Burke and Fahn, 1986). In a series of 42 patients, the duration of treatment was not correlated with severity of dystonia (Burke *et al.,*1982). Compared to women, men develop dystonia at a younger age (Kang, Burke and Fahn, 1986) and after a shorter duration of exposure (Kiriakakis *et al.*, 1998).

Tardive dystonia has an insidious onset. It is progressive for months then persistent and static for years (Burke *et al.,*1982). Few patients (14%) have remission. Remission is four times more likely if neuroleptics are stopped, and five times more likely in patients who have had less than 10 years of drug exposure, compared to those with more than 10 years of drug exposure (Kiriakakis *et al.*, 1998). Kang, Burke and Fahn also reported that remission is more common in people with the shortest exposure and with prompt medicine withdrawal after symptom onset (Kang, Burke and Fahn, 1986). However, withdrawal of neuroleptic did not impact the likelihood of a treatment response to medicine (Kang, Burke and Fahn, 1986).

Prevalance

Reports of prevalence vary considerably depending on the population studied and the clinical criteria used for dystonia. When only studies that include uniform diagnostic criteria, as described in (Burke *et al.,*1982), are included, the average prevalence rate is found to be 3% (van Harten and Kahn, 1999).

Pathophysiology

While little is known about the exact pathophysiology of tardive dystonia, the fact that it resembles idiopathic dystonia, suggests that the two may share the same mechanism. The exact pathophysiology of idiopathic dystonia has not been fully elucidated. PET studies show abnormal activity in both sensory and motor cortex in subjects with dystonia (Jankovic, 2007). The role of dopamine in dystonia is suggested by the knowledge of dopa-responsive dystonia,

which is due to a mutations in genes involved in dopamine synthesis. Furthermore, PET studies have shown reduced D2 receptor density in idiopathic dystonia (Perlmutter *et al.*, 1997).

Treatment

Studies of treatment of tardive dystonia have not been randomized or controlled. Most data come from retrospective reviews or case series. Anti-cholinergics have been shown to provide some benefit in 39–46% of patients, while tetrabenezine has showed benefit in 63–68% of patients (Burke *et al.,*1982; Kang, Burke and Fahn, 1986). The use of anti-cholinergics may aggravate choreic/stereotypic movements, whereas tetrabenazine improves both dystonic and more rapid movements.

Botoulinum toxin A has been studied in patients with focal or segmental tardive dystonia who fail to respond to oral medicines. In a retrospective review of these patients, 29/34 had moderate to marked improvement (Tarsy *et al.*, 1997).

Since deep brain stimulation (DBS) is effective for idiopathic torsion dystonia (see Chapter 15) it has also been studied for tardive dystonia. Trottenberg *et al.* 2005 reported on five patients with intractable Tdt treated with high-frequency stimulation of the globus pallidus. All patients had improvement in 12–72 hours. Dystonia rating scale scores decreased by 83% and the effects were reversible in minutes to hours after turning stimulators off.

As with other forms of TD, the most important preventative treatment is to use neuroleptics only when absolutely necessary, to use low doses and to limit the exposure to the minimum amount of time to treat psychotic behaviors. When tardive dystonic symptoms develop, removing the causative agent is particularly important if psychiatric disease permits, because of the data cited above. If neuroleptics cannot be stopped or the doses reduced, the treatment options for tardive dystonia can be divided into oral agents and other treatments. For patients with focal or segmental dystonia that is amenable to botulinum toxin injection, this treatment can provide meaningful benefit without significant systemic side effects (Tarsy *et al.,*1997) that run the risk of aggravating psychiatric treatment. For patients with generalized dystonia, or focal dystonia that is not amenable to botulinum toxin injection, oral agents may be used.

OTHER TARDIVE SYNDROMES

The tardive syndromes described below are rare. There have been no studies that specifically examine the prevalence, pathophysiology or treatment of these disorders. Information about these syndromes comes from case reports or case series.

Tardive Akathisa

Tardive akathisia occurs during or after exposure to chronic neuroleptics. The features of this disorder have been described in a retrospective review and are similar in clinical presentation to sub-acute akathisia (see above), but appear after chronic exposure to anti-psychotics. Tardive dystonia and TD often co-exist with tardive akathisia. Younger patients were most likely to have remission or response to therapy. Reserpine and tetrabenazine were effective in most patients, while some patients improved with benzodiazepines (Burke *et al.*, 1989). A case report of two patients showed improvement with propranolol (Yassa, Iskandar and Cristina, 1988).

Tardive Tourettism

Several case reports of tardive tourettism or tic movements that are stereotypic motor and vocal tics, exist in the literature. One example involved a 45-year-old patient who developed symptoms of a tic disorder after 10 years of chronic neuroleptic treatment for schizophrenia. He had complex motor and vocal tics, but no symptoms of attention deficit disorder (ADD), or obsessive-compulsive disorder (OCD). The absence of co-morbid ADD and OCD in tardive Tourettism has been noted by other authors (Bharucha and Sethi, 1995). In a series of 12 patients with neuroleptic-induced tics, five had concominant TD with oro-facial-lingual choreic movements. Pimozide and clonidine were used with some success (Bharucha and Sethi, 1995). Another case report and review of prior case reports suggested that patients may improve with clonazepam (Reid, 2004).

Tardive Myoclonus

Myoclonic movements have infrequently been reported in patients exposed to chronic neuroleptic drugs. One case series described arrhythmic, shock-like contractions of the muscles in the upper extremities. Movements were not affected by action, rest or posture, but disappeared in sleep. The authors used EMG to provide electrophysiological data distinguishing myoclonus from chorea. Clonazepam was helpful (Fukuzako *et al.*, 1990). Face and neck myoclonus have been described in a single case report (Little and Jankovic, 1987).

FUTURE DIRECTIONS

Significant progress has been made in the understanding of neuroleptic-induced movement disorders, but many unanswered questions remain. Future research should be directed towards a better understanding of which patients are likely to develop movement disorders when exposed to various medications to treat underlying psychiatric diseases. The field of pharmacogenetics may help elucidate whether an individual patient is likely to respond to a particular medicine, and whether or not a patient is at a high risk of developing side effects. Genetic studies may also help elucidate the mechanism of neuroleptic-induced movement disorders. Are the same genetic abnormalities involved in idiopathic dystonia or parkinsonism, involved in drug-induced parkinsonism or tardive dystonia, for example.

For treatment, new pharmacological discoveries and better understanding of the physiological basis of dyskinesias may allow better treatment options. The challenge is great, however, in that researchers working on the other main condition where dyskinesias are prominent, that is PD, have failed to identify new treatments.

References

Adler, L.A., Angrist, B., Peselow, E. *et al.* (1986) A controlled comparison of Propranolol in the treatment of neuroleptic-induced akathisia. *British Journal of Psychiatry*, **149**, 42–45.

Adler, L.A., Peselow, E., Rosenthal, M. and Angrist, B. (1993) A controlled comparison of the effects of Propranolol, Benztropine, and Placebo on akathisia: an interim analysis. *Psychopharmacology Bulletin*, **29**, 283–286.

Adler, L.A., Rotrosen, J., Edson, R. *et al.* (1999) Vitamin E treatment for tardive dyskinesia. *Archives of General Psychiaatry*, **56**, 836–841.

Adler, L.A., Rotrosen, J. and Angrist, B. (2005) Acute drug-induced akathisia, in *Drug Induced Movement Disorders* (eds S.A. Factor, A.E. Lang and W.J. Weiner), Blackwell Publishing, Massachusetts, pp. 140.

Andersson, U., Haggstrom, J., Levin, E.D. *et al.* (1989) Reduced glutamde decarboxylase activity in the subthalamic nucleus in patients with tardive dyskinesia. *Movement Disorders*, **4**, 37–46.

Angus, S., Sugars, J., Boltezar, R., Koskewich, S. and Schneider, N. M. (1997) A controlled trial of amantadine hydrochloride and neuroleptics in the treatment of tardive dyskinesia. *Journal of Clinical Psychopharmacology*, **17**, 88–91.

Avorn, J., Bohn, R.L., Mogun, H. *et al.* (1995) Neuroleptic drug exposure and treatment of parkinsonism in the elderly: a case-control study. *The American Journal of Medicine*, **99**, 48–54.

Ayd, F.J. (1961) A survey of drug-induced extrapyramidal reactions. *The Journal of the American Medical Association*, **175**, 1054–1060.

Barton, A., Bowie, J. and Ebmeier, K. (1990) Low plasma iron status and akathisia. *Journal of Neurology and Neurosurgery and Psychiatry*, **53**, 671–674.

Bester, A.M. and Harvey, B.H. (2000) Early suppression of striatal cyclic GMP may predetermine the induction and severity of chronic haloperidol-induced vacuous chewing movements. *Metabolic Brain Disease*, **15**, 275–285.

Bhanushali, M.J. and Tuite, P.J. (2004) The evaluation and management of patients with neuroleptic malignant syndrome. *Neurology Clinics of North America*, **22**, 389–411.

Bharucha, K.J. and Sethi, K.D. (1995) Tardive tourettism after exposure to neuroleptic therapy. *Movement Disorders*, **10**, 791–793.

Bhoopathi, P.S. and Soares-Weiser, K. (2006) Benzodiazepines for neuroleptic-induced tardive dyskinesia. *Cochrane Database of Systemic Reviews*, **4**, 1–20.

Bower, J.H., Maraganore, D.M., McDonnel, S.K. and Rocca, W.A. (1999) Incidence and distribution of parkinsonism in Olmstead county, Minnesota, 1976–1990. *Neurology*, **52**, 1214–1220.

Burke, R.E., Fahn, J.J., Marsden, C.D. *et al.* (1982) Tardive Dystonia: Late-onset and persistent dystonia caused by antipsychotic drugs. *Neurology*, **32**, 1335–1346

Burke, R.E., Kang, U.J., Jankovic, J. *et al.* (1989) Tardive akathisia: an analysis of clinical features and response to open therapeutic trials. *Movement Disorders*, **4**, 157–175.

Burkhardt, C., Kelly, J.P., Lim, Y. *et al.* (1992) Neuroleptic medications inhibit complex I of the electron transport chain. *Annals of Neurology*, **33**, 512–517.

Burn, D.J. and Brooks, D.J. (1993) Nigral dysfunction in drug-induced parkinsonism: an ^{18}F-dopa PET study. *Neurology*, **43**, 552–556.

Byne, W., White, L. and Parella, M. (1998) Tardive dyskinesias in a chronically institutionalized population of elderly schizophrenic patients. *International Journal of Geriatric Psychiatry*, **13**, 473–479.

Caroff, S.N. and Mann, S.C. (1993) Neuroleptic malignant syndrome. *Contemporary Clinical Neurology*, **77**, 185–202.

Caroff, S.N., Mann, C.S. and Keck, P.E. (1998) Specific treatment of the neuroleptic malignant syndrome. *Biological Psychiatry*, **44**, 378–381.

Casey, D.E. (2004) Pathophsiology of antippsychotic drug-induced movement disorders. *Journal of Clinical Psychiatry*, **65** (Suppl 9), 25–28.

Earley, C.J., Allen, R.P., Beard, J.L. and Connor, J.R. (2000) Insight into the pathophysiology of restless legs syndrome. *Journal of Neuroscience Research*, **62**, 623–628.

Eichhammer, P., Albus, M. and Borrmann-Hassenbach, M. (2000) Association of dopamine D3-recetpor gene variants with neuroleptic induced akathisia in schizophrenic patients. *American Journal of Medical Genetics*, **96**, 187–191.

Erikson, K.M., Jones, B.C. and Hess, E.J. (2001) Iron deficiency decreases dopamine D1 and D2 receptors in rat brain. *Pharmacology Biochemistry and Behavior*, **69**, 409–418.

Factor, S.A. (2005) Neuroleptic Malignant Syndrome, in *Drug Induced Movement Disorders* (eds S.A. Factor, A.E. Lang and W.J. Weiner), Blackwell Publishing, Massachusetts, pp. 202–203.

Factor, S.A. and Friedman, J.H. (1997) The emerging role of clozapine in the treatment of movement disorders. *Movement Disorders*, **12**, 483–496.

Fann, W. and Lake, W. (1976) Amantadine versus trihexyphenidyl in the treatment of neuroleptic-induced parkinsonism. *American Journal of Psychiatry*, **133**, 940–943.

Fernandez, H.H. and Friedman, J.H. (2003) Classification and treatment of tardive syndromes. *The Neurologist*, **9**, 16–27.

Flaherty, J.A. and Lahmeyer, H.W. (1978) Laryngeal-pharyngeal dystonia as a possible cause of asphyxia with Haloperidol treatment. *American Journal of Psychiatry*, **135**, 1414–1415.

Fukuzako, H., Tominagoa, H., Izumi, K. *et al.* (1990) Postural myoclonus associated with long-term administration of neurolpetics in schizophrenic patients. *Biological Psychiatry*, **27**, 1116–1126.

Gagrat, D., Hamilton, J. and Belmaker, R.H. (1978) Intravenous diazepam in the treatment of neuroleptic-induced acute dystoni and akathisia. *American Journal of Psychiatry*, **135**, 1232–1233.

Gershanik, O.S. (2002) Drug-Induced Dyskinesia, in *Parkinson's Disease and Movement Disorders*, 4th edn (eds J. Jankovic and E. Tolosa), Lippincott, Williams and Wilkins, Philadelphia, pp. 365–379.

McCann, U.D., Penetar, D.M. and Belenky, G. (1990) Acute dystonic reaction in normal humans caused by catecholamine depletion. *Clinal Neuropharmacology*, **13**, 565–568.

Goetz, C.G. (1983) Drug-induced parkinsonsism and idiopathic parkinson's disease. *Archives of Neurology*, **40**, 325–326.

Glazer, W.M., Morgenstern, H. and Doucette, J.T. (1993) Predicting the long-term risk of tardive dyskinesias in outpatients maintained on neuroleptic medications. *Journal of Clinical Psychiatry*, **54**, 4–6.

Hardoy, M.C., Carta, M.G., Carpiniello, B. *et al.* (2002) Gabapentin in antipsychotic-induced tardive dyskinesia: results of 1-year follow-up. *Journal of Affective Disorders*, **75**, 125–130.

Hasan, S. and Buckley, P. (1998) Novel Antipsychotic and the neuroleptic malignant syndrome: A review and critique. *American Journal of Psychiatry*, **155**, 1113–1116.

Hassin-Baer, S., Sirota, P., Korczyn, A.D. *et al.* (2001) Clinical characteristics of neuroleptic-induced parkinsonism. *Journal of Neural Transmission*, **108**, 1299–1308.

Henderson, V.W. and Wooten, G.F. (1981) Neuroleptic malignant syndrome: A pathogenetic role for dopamine receptor blockade? *Neurology*, **31**, 132–137.

Hirose, G. (2006) Drug inducded parkinsonism: a review. *Journal of Neurology*, **253** (Suppl 3), 22–24.

Hirsch, S.R., Kissling, W. and Bauml, J. (2002) A 28-week comparison of ziprasidone and haloperidol in outpatients with stable schizophrenia. *J Clin Psychiatry*, **63**, 516–523.

Hofmann, M., Seifritz, E. and Botschev, C. (2000) Serum iron and ferritin in acute neuroleptic akathisia. *Psychiatry Research*, **93**, 201–207.

Huang, C.C., Wang, R.I.H., Hasegawa, A. and Alverno, L. (1981) Reserpine and Alpha-methyldopa in the treatment of tardive dyskinesia. *Psychopharmacology*, **73**, 359–362.

Hyde, T.M., Apud, J.A., Fisher, W.C. and Egan, M.F. (2005) Tardive Dyskinesia, in *Drug Induced Movement Disorders* (eds S.A. Factor, A.E. Lang and W.J. Weiner), Blackwell Publishing, Massachusetts, pp. 219.

Jankovic, J. (1995) Tardive syndromes and other drug-induced movement disorders. *Clinical Neuropharmacology*, **18**, 197–214.

Jankovic, J. (2003) Movement Disorders, in *Textbook of Clinical Neurology*, 2nd edn (ed. C.G. Goetz), WB Saunders, Philadelphia, pp. 713–740.

Jankovic, J. (2007) Dystonic Disorders, in *Parkinson's Disease and Movement Disorders*, 5th edn (eds J. Jankovic and E. Tolosa Lippincott Williams and Wilkins, Philedelphia, pp. 321–347.

Jankovic, J. and Beach, J. (1997) Long-term effects of tetrabenazine in hyperkinetic movement disorders. *Neurology*, **48**, 358–362.

Jeste, D.V. and Wyatt, R.J. (1982) Theraputic strategies against tardive dyskinesia. *Archives of General Psychiatry*, **39**, 803–816.

Joseph, A.B. and Young, R.R. (1999) *Movement Disorders in Neurology and Neuropsychiatry*, Blackwell Science, Oxford, UK.

Kane, J.M. (2004) Tardive dyskinesia rates with atypical antipsychotics in adults: prevalence and incidence. *Journal of Clinical Psychiatry*, **65** (Suppl 9), 15–20.

Kane, J.M., Woerner, M. and Lieberman, J. (1988) Tardive Dyskinesia: prevalence, incidence, and risk factors. *Journal of Clinical Psychophramacology*, **8**, 52S–56.

Kang, U.J., Burke, R.E. and Fahn, S. (1986) Natural History and treatment of tardive dystonia. *Movement Disorders*, **1**, 193–208.

Keck, P.E., Pope, H.G. and McElroy, S.L. (1991) Declining frequency of neuroleptic malignant syndrome in a hospital population. *American Journal of Psychiatry*, **148**, 880–882.

Kelly, J.T., Zimmermann, R.L., Abuzzahab, F.S. and Schiele, B.C. (1974) A double-blind study of amantadine hydrochloride versus benztropine mesylate in drug-induced parkinsonism. *Pharmacology*, **12**, 65–73.

Khanna, R., Das, A. and Damodaran, S.S. (1992) Prospective study of neuroleptic-induced dystonia in mania and schizophrenia. *American Journal of Psychiatry*, **149**, 511–513.

Kiriakakis, V., Bhatia, K.P., Quinn, N.P. and Marsden, D. (1998) The natural history of tardive dystonia: a long-term follow-up study of 107 cases. *Brain*, **121**, 2053–2066.

Kompoliti, K. and Horn, S.S. (2003) Drug-induced and iatrogenic neurological disorders, in *Textbook of Clinical Neurology*, 2nd edn (ed. C.G. Goetz), WB Saunders, Philadelphia, pp. 1225–1254.

Klawans, H.L. (1973) *The Pharmacology of Extrapyramidal Movement Disorders*, S. Karger, Basal.

Klawans, H.L., Goetz, C.G. and Perlik, S. (1980) Tardive dyskinesia: review and update. *American Journal of Psychiatry*, **137**, 900–907.

Kruse, W. (1960) Treatment of Drug-induced extrapyramidal symptoms. *Diseases of the Nervous System*, **1**, 79–81.

Kuloglu, M., Atmaca, M. and Ustundag, B. (2003) Serum iron levels in schizophrenic patients with or without akathisia. *European Neuropsychological Pharmacology*, **13**, 67–71.

Kutcher, S., Williamson, P., MacKenzie, S. *et al.* (1989) Successful Clonazepam treatment of neuroleptic-induced akathisia in older adolescents and young adults: a double-blind, placebo-controlled study. *Journal of Clinical Psychopharmacology*, **9**, 403–406.

Lieberman, J.A., Saltz, B.L., Johns, C.A. *et al.* (1991) The effects of Clozapine on tardive dyskinesia. *British Journal of Psychiatry*, **158**, 503–510.

Lipinski, J.F., Zubenko, G.S., Barreira, P. and Cohen, B. (1983) Propranolol in the treatment of the neuroleptic-induced akathisia. *The Lancet*, **2**, 685–686.

Little, J.T. and Jankovic, J. (1987) Tardive myoclonus. *Movement Disorders*, **2**, 307–311.

Lukyanetz, E.A., Shkryl, V.M. and Kostyuk, P.G. (2002) Selective blockade of N-type calcium channels by levetiracetam. *Epilepsia*, **43**, 9–18.

Magnuson, T.M., Roccaforte, W.H. and Wengel, S.P. (1999) Medication-induced dystonias in nine patients with dementia. *Journal of Neuropsychopharmacology*, **19**, 219–225.

Matsumoto, R.R. and Pouw, B. (2000) Correlation between neuroleptic binding to sigma 1 and sigma 2 receptors and acute dystonic reactions. *European Journal of Pharmacology*, **401**, 155–160.

Mazurek, M.F. and Rosebush, M.I. (1991) A prospective study of neuroleptic-induced dystonia: incidence and relationship to age, sex, medications, and concurrent parkinsonism. *Neurology*, **41** (Suppl 1), 274.

Meco, G., Fabrizio, E., Epifanio, A. *et al.* (2006) Levetiracetam in tardive dyskinesia. *Clinical Neuropharmacology*, **29**, 265–268.

Meltzer, H.Y. (1987) *Psychopharmacology: the third generation of progress*, Raven Press, New York.

Miller, C.H., Fleischhacker, W.W., Ehrmann, H. and Kane, J.M. (1990) Treatment of neuroleptic induced akathisia with the 5-HT$_2$ antagonist Ritanserin. *Neurology*, **41** (Suppl 1), 374.

Mitchell, I.J., Crossman, A.R. and Limigna, U. (1992) Regional changes in 2-deoxyglucose uptake associated with neuroleptic-induced tardive dyskinesias in the Cebus monkey. *Movement Disorders*, **1**, 32–37.

Naidu, P.S. and Kulkarni, S.K. (2001) Excitatory mechanisms in neuroleptic-induced vacuous chewing movements. *Behavioural Pharmacology*, **12**, 209–216.

Nair, C.J., Josiassen, R.C. and Abraham, G. (1999) Does akathisia influence psychopathology in psychotic patients treated with clozapine? *Biological Psychiatry*, **45**, 1376–1383.

Nisijima, K. and Ishiguro, T. (1995) Cerebrospinal fluid levels of monoamine metabolites and gamma-aminobutyric acid in neuroleptic malignant syndrome. *Journal of Psychiatry Research*, **29**, 233–244.

Palakurthi, H.B., Parvin, M.M. and Kaplan, S. (2007) Neuroleptic malignant syndrome from ariprazole in an agitated pediatric patient. *Clinical Neurophamacology*, **30**, 47–51.

Perlmutter, J.S., Stambuk, M.K., Markham, J. *et al.* (1997) Decrease [18F]spiperone binding in putamen in idiopathic focal dystonia. *Neuroscience*, **17**, 843–850.

Pierre, J.M. (2005) Extrapyramidal Symptoms with Atypical Antipsychotics. *Drug Safety*, **28**, 191–208.

Reid, S.D. (2004) Neuroleptic-induced tardive tourette treated with clonazepam. *Clinical Neuropharmacology*, **27**, 101–104.

Rigo, J.M., Nguyen, L., Belachew, S. *et al.* (2000) Levetiracetam: novel modulation of ionotropic inhibitory receptors. *Epilepsia*, **41**, (suppl 3). 35.

Rosebush, P.I. and Mazurek, M.F. (1999) Neurologic side effects in neuroleptic-naïve patients treated with haloperidol or risperidone. *Neurology*, **52**, 782–785.

Rosebush, P. and Stewart, T. (1989) A prospective analysis of 24 episodes of neuroleptic malignant syndrome. *American Journal of Psychiatry*, **146**, 717–725.

Rosebush, P.I., Stewart, T.D. and Gelenberg, A.J. (1989) Twenty neuroleptic rechallenges after neuroleptic malignant syndrome in 15 patients. *Journal of Clinical Psychiatry*, **50**, 295–298.

Rosenberg, M.R. and Green, M. (1989) Neuroleptic malignant syndrome: reivew of response to therapy. *Archives of Internal Medicine*, **149**, 1927–1931.

Sachdev, P. and Kruk, J. (1994) Clinical characteristics and predisposing factors in acute drug-induced akathisia. *Archives of General Psychiatry*, **51**, 963–974.

Sachdev, P.S. (2005) Neuroleptic-induced Movement Disorders: An Overview. *Psychiatry Clinics of North America*, **28**, 255–274.

Sakkas, P., davis, J.M., Janicak, P.G. and Wang, Z. (1991) Drug treatment of the neuroleptic malignant syndrome. *Psychopharmacology Bulletin*, **27**, 381–384.

Sethi, K.D. and Zamrini, E.Y. (1990) Asymmetry in clinical features of drug-induced parkinsonism. *Journal of Neruopsychiatry*, **2**, 64–66.

Silvestri, S., Seeman, M.V., Negrete, J. *et al.* (2000) Increased dopamine D2 receptor binding after long-term treatment with antipsychotics in humans: a clinical PET study. *Psychopharmacology*, **152**, 174–180.

Spivak, B., Mester, R., Abesgaus, J. *et al.* (1997) Clozapine treatment for neuroleptic-induced tardive dyskinesia, parkinsonism, and chronic akathisia in scizophrenic patients. *Journal of Clinical Psychiatry*, **58**, 318–322.

Sunami, M., Nishikawa, T. and Yorogi, A. (2000) Intravenous administration of levodopa ameliorated a refractory akathisia: case induced by interferon-alpha. *Clinical Neuropharmacology*, **23**, 59–61.

Swett, C. (1975) Drug-induced dystonia. *American Journal of Psychiatry*, **132**, 532–534.

Tarsy, D. and Baldessarini, R.J. (2006) Epidemiology of tardive dyskinesia: Is risk declining with modern antipsychotics? *Movement Disorders*, **21**, 589–598.

Sweet, R.A., Mulsant, B.H. and Rifai, A.H. (1992) Relation of age to prevalence of tardive dyskinesias. *American Journal of Psychiatry*, **149**, 141–145.

Tarsy, D., Kaufman, K.D., Sethi, M.H. *et al.* (1997) An open-label study of botulinum toxin a for the treatment of tardive dystonia. *Clinical Neuropharmacology*, **20**, 90–93.

Tran, P.V., Dellva, M.A., Tollefson, G.D. *et al.* (1997) Extrapyramidal symptoms and tolerability of Olanzapine versus haloperidol in the acute treatment of schizophrenia. *Journal of Clinical Psychiatry*, **58**, 205–211.

Trottenberg, T., Volkmann, J., Deuschl, G. *et al.* (2005) Treatment of Severe Tardive Dystonia with pallidal deep brain stimulation. *Neurology*, **64**, 344–346.

van Harten, P.N., Hoek, H.W. and Matroos, G.E. (1998) Intermittent neuroleptic treatment and risk for tardive dyskinesias. *American Journal of Psychiatry*, **155**, 565–567.

van Harten, P.N., van Trier, J.C. and Horwitz, E.H. (1998) Cocaine as a risk factor for neuroleptic-induced acute dystonia. *Journal of Clinical Psychiatry*, **59**, 128–130.

van Harten, P.N. and Kahn, R.N. (1999) Tardive dystonia. *Schizophrenia Bulletin*, **25**, 741–748.

van Harten, P.N., Hoek, H.W., Matroos, G.E. and van Os, J. (2006) Incidence of tardive dyskinesia and tardive dystonia in African Caribbean patients on long-term antipsychotic treatment: the Curacao extrapyramidal syndromes study. *Journal of Clinical Psychiatry*, **67**, 1920–1927.

van Kampen, J.M. and Stoessl, A.J. (2000) Dopamine D1A receptor function in a rodent model of tardive dyskinesias. *Neuroscience*, **101**, 629–635.

Yassa, R., Iskandar, H. and Cristina, N. (1988) Propranolol in the treatment of tardive akathisa: a report of two cases. *Journal of Clinical Psychopharmacology*, **88**, 283–285.

26

Other Drug-Induced Dyskinesias

Oscar S. Gershanik

Department of Neurology-Centro Neurologico-Hospital Frances, Scientific Director, Institute for Neuroscience, Fundacion Favaloro, Director, Laboratory of Experimental Parkinsonism, Ininfa-Conicet, Buenos Aires, Argentina

INTRODUCTION

Drug-induced dyskinesias are recognized as one of the frequent types of secondary movement disorders; neuroleptics or dopamine (DA)-blocking agents in general are the main offenders and most commonly induce parkinsonism, tardive dyskinesia and acute dystonic reactions (Goetz, Chapter 25). Due to the widespread use of these drugs in the treatment of psychiatric disorders, a large body of information is available regarding neuroleptic-induced dyskinesia. Other drugs, like central nervous system stimulants, certain anti-convulsants, tricyclic anti-depressants, estrogens, antibiotics, immunosuppressive agents and so on, are also capable of inducing movement disorders, through different pathogenetic mechanisms and with a quite variable clinical expression.

DRUGS INVOLVED IN THE PRODUCTION OF DYSKINESIAS

Asterixis, chorea, dystonia, myoclonus and tremor are the most common clinical presentations of dyskinesias induced by drugs other than neuroleptics and DA blocking agents (Table 26.1, modified from Kipps et al., 2005), but their overall prevalence is rather low.

Most of the information available is based on isolated anecdotal reports, small series or data collected from the safety information reported in clinical trials of some of the offending drugs. As many of these drugs may cause different types of movement disorders it is advisable to analyze the problem by drug category rather than by type of dyskinesia (see Table 26.2).

The different dyskinesias caused by levodopa are discussed in Chapter 5.

Anti-Epileptic Drugs

Of all anti-epileptic agents, phenytoin is the drug most frequently associated with the development of movement disorders. It has been reported to induce orofacial chorea, ballismus, dystonia, tremor, asterixis and myoclonus (Harrison, Lyons and Landow, 1993; Duarte et al., 1996; Chi, Chua and Kong, 2000). In the review of the literature by Harrison, Lyons and Landow (1993), there were 77 cases reported up to 1993. Involuntary movements have occurred in some patients with high plasma-phenytoin levels, while in 23% of the cases phenytoin levels were within the therapeutic range; however, phenytoin-induced movement disorders most often develop in patients on polytherapy, or after increasing dosage. In one series (Harrison, 1993) 68% of the patients who developed movement disorders were taking other anti-epileptic drugs in combination with phenytoin. The dyskinesias observed with phenytoin usually disappear with dose reduction or drug withdrawal. The most common type of hyperkinesia observed in these patients is choreoathetosis, present in 91% of cases. In some of the cases reported in the literature the presentation is episodic and paroxysmal with long bouts of dyskinesias and periods of almost disappearance of the involuntary movement (Dravet et al., 1980; Saito et al., 2001). In one of the patients reported by Saito et al. (2001), an ictal SPECT was performed, showing basal ganglia hypoperfusion contralateral to the dyskinesia. More than one type of movement disorder can be present in the same patient. It has been suggested that a pre-existing lesion in the basal ganglia might be an important predisposing factor for the development of phenytoin-induced dyskinesias. However, in only 12% of the patients reported in the literature a focal structural lesion of the brain was identified. Phenytoin is believed to decrease high-frequency repetitive firing of action potentials by enhancing sodium-channel inactivation. Whether this mechanism is related or not to the capacity of this drug for producing dyskinesias remains to be established (Macdonald and Kelly, 1995).

Carbamazepine (CBZ) has also been found to beresponsible for the development of a variety of dyskinesias,

Table 26.1 Drug-induced dyskinesias.

Type of dyskinesias	Drugs
Chorea	*Common:*L-Dopa *Uncommon:* Phenytoin, carbamazepine, tricyclic anti-depressants, estrogen, cocaine, baclofen, trazodone, anti-cholinergics, ciprofloxacine
Myoclonus	*Common:* SSRIs *Uncommon:* Tricyclic anti-depressants, lithium, MAO inhibitors, carbamazepine, penicillin and cephalosporin antibiotics, cocaine, opiates, amantadine, L-dopa, bromocriptine
Tremor	*Common:* Neuroleptics, valproate, alcohol, sympathomimetics *Uncommon:* Opiates, SSRIs, immunosuppressives, hypoglycemic agents, antibiotic and anti-viral agents, other anti-convulsants, anti-arrhythmics, anti-depressants, xanthines, corticosteroids, thyroxine, amiodarone
Dystonia	*Common:* Neuroleptics and other DA-agonists (anti-emetics), L-dopa *Uncommon:* Dopamine agonists, phenytoin, carbemazepine, SSRI and tricyclic anti-depressants, cocaine, erythromycin, buspirone, ranitidine, nefazadone, benztropine, diphenhydramine
Parkinsonism	*Common:* Neuroleptics and other DA-agonists (anti-emetics) *Uncommon:* Flunarizine, cinnarizine, tricyclic anti-depressants, tacrine, chemotherapeutic agents, carbamazepine, phenytoin, valproate, lamotrigine, MPTP
Tics	*Uncommon:* Carbamazepine, phenytoin, lamotrigine, dexamphetamine, methylphenidate, cocaine
Akathisia	*Common:* Neuroleptics *Uncommon:* Tricyclic anti-depressants; calcium channel antagonists; SSRIs; MAO, monoamine oxidase; MPTP

Adapted from Kipps C.M., Fung V.S., Grattan-Smith P., de Moore G.M., Morris J.G. Movement disorder emergencies. *Mov. Disord.*, 2005 Mar; 20(3):322–34.

Table 26.2 Non-neuroleptic drug-induced dyskinesias.

Type of drug	Type of dyskinesias
Anti-convulsants (phenytoin, carbamazepine, gabapentin, pregabaline, valproate, lamotrigine, ethosuximide, tiagabine, topiramate, vigabatrin, felbamate)	Asterixis, chorea, dystonia, myoclonus, tics, tremor
Tricyclic anti-depressants (amitryptiline, impipramine)	Chorea, myoclonus, dystonia, akathisia, tremor
SSRIs	Myoclonus, tremor, dystonia, akathisia
Psychostimulants (cocaine, atomoxetine, methylphenidate, dexamphetamine, pemoline)	Chorea, myoclonus, tics
Sympathomimetics (ephedrine, pseudoephedrine, phenylpropanolamine, beta-adrenergic bronchodilators, etc.)	Tremor
Anti-histamines (diphenidramine, hydroxizine, cetrizine, cyclizine, cimetidine, ranitidine)	Dystonia, tremor, chorea
Antibiotics (penicillin, ciprofloxacin, erythromycin)	Myoclonus, tremor
Immunosuppressive agents (cyclosporin A, tacrolimus)	Myoclonus, tremor
Miscellaneous (amantadine, baclofen, benzodiazepines, bupropion, buspirone, diazoxide, digoxin, estrogens, fentanyl, lithium, opiates, propofol, tumor necrosis factor)	Chorea, dystonia myoclonus, tics, tremor

including tics and dystonia. Tics, both motor and vocal, are perhaps the most frequently reported dyskinesias with CBZ. They have been reported in patients without pre-existing evidence of Tourette syndrome (TS) or tics, or as an exacerbation of TS; both in normal or brain-damaged children, and in patients with Huntington's disease and tardive dyskinesia (Neglia, Glaze and Zion, 1984; Kurlan *et al.*, 1989; Robertson *et al.*, 1993; Holtmann, Korn-Merker and Boenigk, 2000). Dystonia secondary to the use of CBZ is less frequent than tics; oculogyric crisis, segmental cranio-cervical dystonia and generalized axial dystonia with opisthotonus have all been described. The mode of presentation of dystonic phenomena is frequently sub-acute (2–3 weeks after the introduction of the drug), or as an acute dystonic reaction coincident with a sudden increase in dosage. Most of these phenomena resolve with dose reduction or discontinuation of the drug (Jacome, 1979; Soman *et al.*, 1994; Bradbury, Bentick and Todd, 1982; Gorman and Barkley, 1995; Crosley and Swender, 1979; Stryjer *et al.*, 2002). Brain damage has been proposed as a predisposing factor in come cases (Crosley and Swender, 1979). There is only one report of choreiform movements and myoclonus with CBZ (Go, 1999). Although CBZ probably exerts its anti-epileptic effect by the stabilization of sodium channels, it is possible that the induction of dyskinesias is related to its ability to increase acetylcholine in the striatum and inhibit dopamine neurotransmission. Studies in rats have demonstrated that although therapeutic concentrations of carbamazepine increase dopamine neurotransmission in specific areas, supratherapeutic concentrations of carbamazepine may inhibit dopamine transmission (Okada *et al.*, 1997).

Gabapentin (GBP) belongs to the newer generation of anti-epileptic drugs and has also been reported to induce different movement disorders. Choreoathetosis, and dystonia in the form of oculogyric crisis, dystonic jerking or acute segmental dystonic reactions, have been reported with the use of GBP for epilepsy, neuropathic pain and essential tremor (Reeves *et al.*, 1996; Chudnow, Dewey and Lawson, 1997; Pina and Modrego, 2005). It has been speculated that predisposing factors may facilitate the development of dyskinesia, as reported in mentally retarded patients given GBP who developed choreoathetosis (Chudnow, Dewey and Lawson, 1997). In all cases resolution was observed after discontinuation of the drug. Newly developed choreoathetoid dyskinesias have also been reported in Parkinson's disease patients receiving GBP for neuropathic pain, which resolved upon discontinuation of the drug (Norton and Quarles, 2001; Raju, Walker and Lee, 2007). Perhaps the most frequent dyskinesia observed in patients under treatment with GBP is myoclonus. Asconape, Diedrich and DellaBadia (2000) found that 13 out of 104 patients under treatment with GBP for epilepsy presented with myoclonus, of which 10 had newly developed multifocal myoclonus, three had focal myoclonus contralateral to

their epileptic focus, and in two there was exacerbation of pre-existing myoclonus. Not all cases required treatment or withdrawal of GBP, as in most, the dyskinesia was subtle and did not interfere with daily life. Myoclonus completely disappeared in those cases in which the drug was discontinued. In patients with impaired renal function or end-stage renal disease, GBP has been found to induce myoclonus when given for the treatment of neuropathic pain (Holtkamp *et al.*, 2006; Zhang *et al.*, 2005). In these cases it was speculated that impairment of renal function was responsible for the elevation of GBP plasma levels, leading to toxicity and myoclonus, as pharmacokinetic studies in humans have shown that GBP is not metabolized, is not bound to serum proteins and is cleared by renal excretion alone. Asterixis or negative myoclonus characterized by brief, sudden lapses of posture has also been reported in patients receiving GBP for neuropathic pain (Jacob, Chand and Omeima, 2000; Sechi *et al.*, 2004; Babiy *et al.*, 2005), and in some cases this phenomenon was responsible for postural instability and frequent falls. The pathophysiological mechanisms by which GBP induces dyskinesia are not very well understood. GBP is structurally related to γ-aminobutyric acid (GABA), may alter the synthesis and release of GABA in the brain and has high-affinity binding to the α-2-δ subunit of voltage-activated calcium channels. It is also known to increase the release of DA in central pathways as well as serotonin and noradrenaline, while decreasing levels of glutamic acid (Raju, Walker and Lee, 2007). Pregabaline (isobutyl-GABA) and vigabatrine (γ-vinyl-GABA), both structurally similar drugs to GBP, are also known for their capacity to induce asterixis and/or myoclonus (Neufeld and Vishnevska, 1995; Huppertz, Feuerstein and Schulze-Bonhage, 2001; Heckmann *et al.*, 2005). Tiagabine is another anti-epileptic drug acting through GABA-mediated mechanisms (inhibition of GABA uptake) that has been linked to the occurrence of abnormal involuntary movements. Tremor is perhaps the most frequent of these, and has been reported to be present in 9–31% of patients treated with this drug (Fakhoury, Uthman and Abou-Khalil, 2000; Leppik *et al.*, 1999). In addition, transient acute dystonic reactions (focal limb dystonia, oromandibular dystonia, writer's cramp) or sustained athetoid limb movements have been reported with tiagabine (Wolanczyk and Grabowska-Grzyb, 2001; Tombini *et al.*, 2006).

Valproic acid or valproate (VPA) is a first-line anti-epileptic drug and one of the most widely prescribed. Postural tremor induced by VPA has been reported to occur in 6–45% of cases (Perucca, 2002). Such a wide variability can be explained by the use of different ascertainment methods. VPA-induced postural tremor has the typical characteristics of enhanced physiological tremor, and its frequency and severity are dose-related (Rinnerthaler *et al.*, 2005). In addition to tremor, VPA has been related to the development of choreiform movements. All cases of VPA-induced chorea were observed in patients with brain damage (vascular lesions, traumatic brain injury, non-ketotic hyperglycemia) (Lancman, Asconape and Penry, 1994; Gunal, Guleryuz and Bingol, 2002; Morrison, Sankar and Shields, 2006). As with other drug-induced dyskinesias, valproate withdrawal resulted in either improvement or disappearance of the abnormal involuntary movements. Its pharmacological effects involve a variety of mechanisms, including increased GABA-ergic transmission, reduced release and/or effects of excitatory amino acids, blockade of voltage-gated sodium channels and modulation of dopaminergic and serotoninergic transmission (Perucca, 2002).

Lamotrigine (LTG), is another new-generation anti-epileptic drug which has been associated with drug-induced dyskinesias of variable presentation, including tics and tourettism, tremor, chorea, dystonia and myoclonus. "De novo" occurrence of motor and phonic tics in at least eight children without prior history of Tourette syndrome has been reported with LTG therapy after several months of treatment (Lombroso, 1999; Sotero de Menezes et al., 2000). In those patients in whom LTG could be withdrawn, the symptoms disappeared after a few weeks; re-challenge with the drug resulted in re-emergence of tics in two cases. Myoclonus is the second most frequently reported dyskinesia with LTG, both as exacerbation of pre-existing myoclonic phenomena or in patients without prior history of abnormal involuntary movements (Janszky et al., 2000; Crespel et al., 2005). In some cases it can become a severely disabling symptom, and in one patient it lead to the development of myoclonic status. It has been related to high plasma levels of the drug and improvement was observed in all cases with dose reduction; in one case complete withdrawal of the drug was necessary. Blepharospasm in one case and chorea and tremor in another are uncommon dyskinesias observed with the use of LTG (Verma et al., 1999; Das et al., 2003). LTG is believed to block excessive pre-synaptic release of excitatory amino acids (EAAs). EAAs can also interfere with striatal dopamine uptake. Conceivably, LTG may cause dyskinesias by failing, at high doses, to properly regulate the pre-synaptic release of EAAs in the striatum (Macdonald and Kelly, 1995; Lombroso, 1999).

There are occasional reports of dyskinesias induced by other anti-epileptic drugs, such as ethosuximide (Kirschberg, 1975) and felbamate (chorea and dystonia) (Kerrick et al., 1995).

Anti-depressants (Tricyclic and Selective Serotonin Reuptake Inhibitors (SSRIs)

Tricyclic anti-depressants (TCAs), such as amitryptiline and imipramine, have been associated infrequently with the occurrence of movement disorders. However, a comprehensive review of the literature published 10 years ago (Vandel et al., 1997) suggested that they were more common than previously believed. Since the publication of that review, very little has been added in terms of knowledge of their true prevalence or clinical phenomenology. One of the earliest published papers is that of Fann, Sullivan and Richman (1976) reporting on one case of buccolingual dyskinesias and another with more widespread choreoathetoid movements, which were clearly attributable to the use of a TCA. A further important contribution, published in 1987 (Garvey and Tollefson, 1987) reported on the presence of myoclonus in almost 40% of cases receiving TCAs, in nine of which it became so bothersome as to require withdrawal of the medication. In addition to chorea (predominantly buccolingual) and myoclonus, there have been reports of akathisia, alone or in association with myoclonus or dystonia, both focal and segmental. There are only a few publications specifically addressing the issue of tremor induced by TCAs (Kronfol, Greden and Zis, 1983; Raethjen et al., 2001). However, in several of the reports of clinical trials evaluating TCAs alone, or in comparison with other anti-depressants, tremor is mentioned as a frequent side effect, sometimes disabling enough to warrant discontinuation of the drug (Watanabe et al., 1978; Smith et al., 1990; Morgan and Sethi, 2005). Dyskinesia secondary to the use of TCAs may appear acutely or after chronic use, usually several months. In the majority of cases, reported TCAs had been prescribed at therapeutic doses. In a few instances TCAs were given at very high doses or in combination with other psychotropic drugs (Vandel et al., 1997). It has been suggested that both the anti-cholinergic and serotonin-reuptake inhibiting properties of the tricyclic anti-depressants could be related to the development of abnormal movements (Vandel et al., 1997). In the case of tremor induced by TCA, it has been shown that it is the consequence of an enhancement of the central component of physiological tremor (Raethjen et al., 2001).

Selective serotonin reuptake inhibitors (SSRIs) have also been associated with the development of movement disorders (Gerber and Lynd, 1998; Schillevoort et al., 2002; Hedenmalm et al., 2006). In their comprehensive review, Gerber and Lynd (1998) were able to compile all available data on SSRI-induced movement disorders at the time of their analysis. They reviewed a total of 127 published reports involving 30 cases of akathisia, 19 of dystonia, 12 of dyskinesia, 6 of tardive dyskinesia (TD), 25 of parkinsonism and 15 cases of mixed disorders. Ten isolated cases of bruxism were also identified, and 10 additional reports could not be classified. In addition, manufacturers of these drugs provided 49 reports of akathisia, 44 of dystonia, 208 of dyskinesia, 76 of TD, 516 of parkinsonism and 60 of bruxism. More recently, two pharmacovigilance reports from the Netherlands and Sweden tried to estimate the risk and risk factors involved in the development of extrapyramidal symptoms in patients under treatment with SSRIs, based on spontaneous reporting of adverse events

(Schillevoort *et al.*, 2002; Hedenmalm *et al.*, 2006). The Dutch pharmacovigilance study concluded that SSRIs were associated with a twofold increase in extrapyramidal adverse events compared to other anti-depressants. Parkinsonism and dystonia were the most frequently reported (59.0 and 21.3%, respectively). However, tremor often was the only sign of parkinsonism (83.3%). Only one report described akathisia. In most cases, other factors contributed to the increased risk (advanced age, concomitant treatment with anti-psychotics, pre-existing Parkinson's disease, etc.) (Schillevoort *et al.*, 2002). In the Swedish study, in addition to estimating the relative frequency of these adverse events, the authors obtained blood samples to identify possible genetic risk factors. The risk of extrapyramidal adverse events with SSRIs seems to increase with advanced age and with the presence of the A1 allele of DRD2 Taq1A polymorphism (Hedenmalm *et al.*, 2006). Curiously, in none of these publications is tremor mentioned specifically, except as a symptom of parkinsonism, despite being one of the most common movement disorders induced by these drugs (Edwards and Anderson, 1999). Almost 20% of patients started on SSRIs develop tremor in the absence of a previous history of tremor (Wernicke, 1985; Diaz-Martinez *et al.*, 1998). In a systematic analysis of tremor induced by the use of fluoxetine, Serrano-Duenas (2002) reported on the findings in 21 cases. Contrary to the interpretation of the adverse event reports included in the Dutch pharmacovigilance study, which attributed tremor to drug-induced parkinsonism, in this study, tremor was clearly postural or action in nature and with a frequency much higher (6–12 Hz) than typical parkinsonian rest tremor (Schillevoort *et al.*, 2002; Serrano-Duenas, 2002). The mechanisms involved in SSRI-induced movement disorders are not fully understood, but it has been suggested that serotonin may have an inhibitory influence on dopaminergic neurotransmission (Leo, 1996).

Myoclonus and tremor can be part of a more serious adverse effect observed with SSRIs, the serotonin syndrome (Boyer and Shannon, 2005). This is a potentially fatal disorder linked to excessive serotonergic activity. It is characterized by changes in mental status, hypertension, restlessness, myoclonus, hyper-reflexia, diaphoresis, diarrohea, shivering and tremor. The combined use of an MAO-B inhibitor plus an SSRI may lead to the development of serotonin syndrome, thus physicians are warned of the potential danger of this combination. Estimates of its incidence in this context are however quite low, 0.24% of parkinsonian patients in a survey had experienced symptoms compatible with this syndrome, while in only 0.04% they were considered to be serious (Richard *et al.*, 1997).

In addition to SSRIs, there are other anti-depressants acting on the serotonergic system, but with a different mechanism of action. Trazodone is an atypical anti-depressant with a mixed mechanism of action (antagonist/agonist at the 5HT receptor). There have been very few reports of movement disorders induced by this drug, including two cases of dystonia and one case each of myoclonus and chorea (McNeill, 2006). Nefazodone, another 5HT2 receptor antagonist anti-depressant has been involved in the production of an acute dystonic reaction appearing 2 h after the patient took the first dose of the drug (Burda *et al.*, 1999).

Treatment strategies include discontinuation of the SSRI, dosage reduction or the addition of a benzodiazepine, β-blocker or anti-cholinergics. Complete disappearance of the movement disorder after discontinuation of SSRIs may take several months (Serrano-Duenas, 2002). Buspirone, a drug acting as a full agonist at the 5-HT1A receptor, has been proposed as the preferred treatment for SSRI-induced bruxism (Bostwick and Jaffee, 1999).

Psychostimulants

Central nervous system stimulants are also known to induce dyskinetic movements (Weiner *et al.*, 2001). Amphetamine, or methamphetamine-induced chorea has been reported in the setting of acute or chronic abuse/addiction, generally associated with hyperactivity and repetitive behaviors (Rylander, 1972; Lundh and Tunving, 1981; Rhee, Albertson and Douglas, 1988; Sperling and Horowitz, 1994), however, it has been reported only rarely with therapeutic uses of the drug. There have been a few reports including that of a woman taking an amphetamine precursor for weight loss, and a man who developed chorea temporally related to an increase in the dose of mixed amphetamine salts he was receiving as treatement for his attention deficit hyperactivity disorder (ADHD) (Morgan, Winter and Wooten, 2004). The mechanism by which amphetamine causes choreiform dyskinesias is thought to be related to its capacity to stimulate the release of dopamine from pre-synaptic striatal terminals. Elevated nigrostriatal dopamine, especially involving the D2 receptor system, leads to a decrease in striatopallidal GABA level. This can, in turn, produce a loss of inhibitory regulation leading to the development of hyperkinetic movements. (Caligiuri and Buitenhuys, 2005). Stereotypies observed in rodents after administration of high doses of amphetamine are believed to be the equivalent to hyperactivity and choreiform dyskinesias in humans.

Cocaine as a drug of abuse has also been held responsible for the development of abnormal involuntary movements. Hyperactivity and repetitive stereotyped behaviors (punding), as previously mentioned with amphetamine, are also observed among cocaine addicts. In addition, there have been reports of multi-focal tics, akathisia, dystonia, exacerbation of neuroleptic-induced dystonic reactions, myoclonus and choreiform movements (Rylander, 1972; Pascual-Leone and Dhuna, 1990; Kumor, Sherer and Jaffe, 1986; Daras, Koppel and Atos-Radzion, 1994; Bartzokis *et al.*, 1999).

In most instances reported in the medical literature, patients developing abnormal involuntary movements with cocaine had predisposing factors, such as previous exposure to neuroleptics or pre-existent brain disease. Writhing body movements of a choreoathetoid nature are refered to among cocaine-abusing individuals as "crack-dancing" (Daras, Koppel and Atos-Radzion, 1994). "Crack-dancing" appears to be fairly prevalent within this population, although due to its transient nature, with a typical duration of 2–6 days, few of these individuals seek medical care for this disorder. This may explain the scarcity of published reports on this phenomenon. There are, however, a few examples of persisting dyskinesias after a long period of abstinence. In addition to acute or sub-acute choreic dyskinesias, the presence of choreic movements in chronic cocaine-dependent (CD) individuals has also been evaluated. Compared to normal controls, a large sample of ($n = 71$) CD subjects scored significantly higher using an abnormal involuntary movements scale, particularly in the limbs and body components of the scale, reflecting the presence of subtle choreoathetoid movements in these individuals (Bartzokis et al., 1999). Cocaine is a dopamine-uptake blocker acting on the pre-synaptic dopamine transporter system, leading to increased dopaminergic stimulation at the striatal level, similar to what is observed with amphetamine. The presence of persistent dyskinesias in chronic cocaine abusers, as well as the persistence of these abnormal involuntary movements in CD subjects even after prolonged periods of abstinence, raises the possibility of either a toxic effect of psychostimulant substances or their ability to induce enduring plastic changes in basal ganglia circuitry (Weiner et al., 2001).

Pemoline is another psychostimulant used mainly for the treatment of ADHD that was withdrawn from the US market in 2005 due to the risks of liver toxicity, which outweighed its potential therapeutic benefits. As this drug is still available in several countries outside the US, it is still important to consider its potential ability to induce dyskinesias. Although infrequently, pemoline has been associated with the development of choreoathetoid movements and tics, both in the acute and chronic setting (Stork and Cantor, 1997). In some cases the development of abnormal involuntary movements was quite abrupt and appeared minutes after pemoline was first ingested. In all cases withdrawal of the medication resulted in disappearance of the movement disorder, usually within 24 h (Sallee et al., 1989; Stork and Cantor, 1997). Pemoline causes catecholamine re-uptake inhibition in the central nervous system, and has also been shown to enhance sodium potassium ATPase activity at low concentration while inhibiting its activity at high concentrations in rats. The end result of these mechanisms is a higher concentration of norepinephrine, epinephrine and dopamine in central neuronal synapses (Stork and Cantor, 1997). The mechanism of action of pemoline shares some similarities with cocaine.

Other central nervous system stimulants used in the treatment of ADHD have also been implicated in many instances in the development of tics or other dyskinesias, and the close association of treatment and exacerbation of symptoms in some Tourette syndrome cases has been reported. Methylphenidate, one of the most widely used drugs within this category, has been reported to induce generalized choreoathetoid movements, isolated orofacial dyskinesias and rabbit syndrome (Extein, 1978; Senecky et al., 2002; Mendhekar and Duggal, 2006). A cross-sectional analysis of a clinic cohort of children with ADHD under treatment with stimulant drugs revealed that approximately 9% of them developed a tic disorder, predominantly transient in nature, with less than 1% having development of chronic tics or Tourette syndrome (Lipkin, Goldstein and Adesman, 1994). Atomoxetine is a norepinephrine reuptake inhibitor, and one of the more recently introduced drugs for the treatment of ADHD, apparently lacking stimulant properties. Little published information is available on the neurologic side effects of atomoxetine or the possibility of drug interaction. Four cases of tics originally noted on stimulant medication that re-emerged on atomoxetine and resolved with withdrawal of atomoxetine were reported in a recent letter (Lee et al., 2004). Two other cases, ascertained from poison center telephone reports, identified "myoclonus" associated with atomoxetine (Spiller, Lintner and Winter, 2004). In one case, myoclonus was associated with acute unintentional ingestion in an atomoxetine-naive child. The other case occurred on the second day of therapeutic use. Bond, Garro and Gilbert (2007) recently reported two cases of reversible movement disorders associated with the addition of atomoxetine to regimens that included other psychoactive drugs. A nine-year-old taking clonidine and dextroamphetamine developed psychosis, abnormal involuntary movements and insomnia. An 18-year-old also initiating venlafaxine developed facial tics, tremors and speech disturbance. Acute symptoms did not respond to diphenhydramine in either case, but resolved after atomoxetine and other medications were discontinued. Possible explanations included atypical atomoxetine effect, excess atomoxetine or metabolites due to poor metabolizer status (CYP 2D6 polymorphism/deficiency), a drug–drug interaction leading to elevated drug levels, or to excess synaptic norepinephrine or dopamine. Serotonin syndrome was considered as a possibility in the second case, but not the first (Bond et al., 2007).

In most instances, the movement disorders seen with these drugs are transient. The risk of developing chronic tics with the use of central nervous system stimulants in patients with ADHD has not been firmly established, and there are a number of well-controlled studies that failed to find a significant association (Law and Schachar, 1999; Palumbo *et al.*, 2004; Roessner *et al.*, 2006).

Sympathomimetics

Among the sympathomimetics, β-adrenergic agonists used in the treatment of respiratory disorders are also known to produce involuntary movements. Tremor is the most frequent movement disorder seen with drugs like terbutaline, bambuterol, albuterol, salbutamol and others (Sears, 2002). The incidence of tremor, however, is low with the use of these drugs and is more frequently reported with oral therapy than with inhaled therapy. It has been hypothesized that tremor is the result of an imbalance between the fast- and slow-twitch muscle groups of the extremities (Sears, 2002). Severity varies greatly between individuals, and is a dose-related phenomenon. Normal subjects, as well as asthmatic individuals, may develop tremor when exposed to β-adrenergic agonists. The more potent full agonists are more likely to produce tremor than partial or less potent agonists. It is important to be aware that these drugs may exacerbate pre-existing essential tremor, as they possess the opposite effects of β-antagonists used in the treatment of this condition. Withdrawal of the medication is the best therapeutic strategy, although, in many instances, tolerance may develop with continued use.

Pseudoephedrine and phenyl-propanolamine, drugs possessing sympathomimetic and amphetamine-like properties, commonly included in over-the-counter cold medications, have also been reported to induce either myoclonus or tremor (Dietz, 1981; Lopez Lois *et al.*, 2005).

Anti-Histamines

Anti-histamines are widely used for a number of indications, including sedation, treatment of allergic reactions, rhinitis and use as anti-emetics (Simons, 2004). The designation anti-histamine is used almost exclusively for drugs acting as antagonists or inverse agonists at the H-1 receptor site (Leurs, Church and Taglialatela, 2002). Other drugs, like ranitidine and cimetidine, acting at different histamine receptor sites (H-2) are used as inhibitors of gastric secretion (Simons, 2004). Despite their availability in numerous over-the-counter medications leading to uncontrolled use, there are not as many reports on movement disorders induced by these drugs as one would have expected. Dystonia is the type of dyskinesia most frequently experienced by patients receiving this type of medication. Cetrizine has been linked to the development of generalized dystonic tics in one case and oculogyric crises in at least nine patients (Fraunfelder and Fraunfelder, 2004). Onset of the movement disorder in these cases has been mostly subacute, although in a few the problem developed either acutely or chronically. All of the cases reported were children receiving the usually prescribed dose of the medication, and in all cases the problem resolved with withdrawal of the offending drug. In a number of cases there was a positive rechallenge, which confirmed the causative relationship with the suspected drug (Fraunfelder and Fraunfelder, 2004; Rajput and Baerg, 2006). With most of the other first-generation H-1 type anti-histamines there are isolated reports of acute dystonic reactions in the majority of cases. They have been reported with diphenhydramine, cyclizine, promethazineand azatadine (Joske, 1984; DeGrandi and Simon, 1987; Etzel, 1994; King *et al.*, 2003). There is only one report involving the development of a tardive dyskinesia-like syndrome (buccolingual dyskinesias) in a patient under chronic treatment with a common cold medicine containing clorpheniramine (Thach, Chase and Bosma, 1975).

There are also reports of acute intoxication with diphenhydramine, seen in the emergency room involving 68 non-fatal and 55 fatal cases (Pragst, Herre and Bakdash, 2006). Fatality was in these cases related to higher plasma concentrations of the drug. The intoxication symptoms reported during emergency admission were quite variable and included somnolence, sedation in some cases, while in others the clinical presentation included tachycardia, anti-cholinergic syndrome, agitation, hallucinations, confusion, tremor, convulsions, delirium and coma. This is the only instance in which the presence of tremor has been reported as a side effect of anti-histamines (Pragst, Herre and Bakdash, 2006).

Ranitidine and cimetidine, with histamine-blocking properties at the H-2 receptor, as mentioned above, have also been linked to acute dystonic reactions, chorea and postural and action tremor, in a few isolated reports (Bateman *et al.*, 1981; Romisher, Felter and Dougherty, 1987; Lehmann, 1988; Davis *et al.*, 1994; Wilson, Woodward and Ferrara, 1997; Kapur, Barber and Peddireddy, 1999; Peiris and Peckler, 2001). Onset of the acute dystonic reaction has been within minutes of first exposure to these drugs in some cases, or after repeated administration (Romisher, Felter and Dougherty, 1987; Kapur, Barber and Peddireddy, 1999; Peiris and Peckler, 2001). Withdrawal of the medication, and, in some cases, administration of i.v. diphenhydramine, alone or in combination with lorazepam, diazepam or benzotropine, brought, in all cases, rapid reversal of the situation (Romisher, Felter and Dougherty, 1987; Kapur, Barber and Peddireddy, 1999; Peiris and Peckler, 2001).

The majority of second- and third-generation H-1 antagonists are almost devoid of central nervous system penetration and therefore less likely to produce movement disorders (Simons, 2004).

The relative low frequency of drug-induced dyskinesias observed with these drugs despite their widespread use, is probably justified by the existence of predisposing factors in those few individuals that actually develop them (Rajput and Baerg, 2006).

The mechanism by which anti-histamines induce the appearance of abnormal involuntary movements is poorly understood. It has been hypothesized that in some cases the piperazinic structure of these compounds, similar to that of D2 dopamine receptor-blocking drugs, could account for their capacity to induce acute dystonic reactions (Rajput and Baerg, 2006). Other effects on basal ganglia circuitry mediated through histamine receptors, cholinergic receptors or additional neurotransmitter systems cannot be ruled out (Fraunfelder and Fraunfelder, 2004).

Antibiotics

Among the antibiotics, penicillin was one of the first to be associated with the development of dyskinesias, specifically myoclonus, usually in the context of encephalopathy (Sackellares and Smith, 1979). Penicillin-induced myoclonus is believed to be caused by generators at the cortical, subcortical or even at the lower brain stem/spinal level (Sackellares and Smith, 1979). Within the fluoroquinolones, ciprofloxacin is the most frequently reported in the literature as responsible for the occurrence of a variety of movement disorders, including propriospinal myoclonus, generalized myoclonus, palatal tremor, tremor and chorea (Pastor et al., 1996; Post, Koelman and Tijssen, 2004; Azar et al., 2005; Cheung et al., 2007). Episodic Tourette-like symptomatology (motor and vocal tics, coprolalia, echolalia and echopraxia) has been reported in an elderly patient with encephalopathy under treatment with ofloxacin (Thomas and Reagan, 1996). The presence of limb automatisms, hypersalivation and post-episode amnesia in this case raises the possibility that the episodes were in fact frontal-onset complex partial seizures. (Thomas and Reagan, 1996). Tremor is probably the most commonly encountered hyperkinetic movement disorder in patients under ciprofloxacine treatment with an incidence of up to 3% of the cases (Azar et al., 2005; Cheung et al., 2007) Levofloxacion, another representative of the fluoroquinolones, has been reported to induce chorea, myoclonus and tremor in two patients; in one shortly after starting treatment, while in the second the movement disorder appeared two months after being put on this drug for the treatment of chronic bronchitis (Yasuda et al., 1999). Cephalosporins, such as ceftazidime, have also been implicated in the development of dyskinesias, including asterixis, and encephalopathy with myoclonic jerks (Hillsley and Massey, 1991; Chan et al., 2006; Martin, 2007). Imipenem, an antibiotic of the carbapenem class, in addition to lowering the convulsive threshold leading to 1.5% of seizure cases in patients receiving this drug, has been linked to the development of myoclonus in at least two cases (Frucht and Eidelberg, 1997). An acute dystonic reaction involving the neck muscles, occurring 5 h. after first exposure to the drug has been reported with erythromycin; symptoms abated almost immediately after receiving parenteral diphenydramine; however, they recurred after 30 minutes, requiring an additional dose of diphenydramine, this time together with benztropine (Brady and Hall, 1992). This is the only instance of an abnormal involuntary movement caused by an antibiotic of the macrolide class that is found in the literature.

All of these are either isolated cases or reports involving a limited number of cases, as movement disorders are not the most common adverse events encountered with these drugs. Therefore we lack information on the overall incidence of abnormal involuntary movements in patients receiving antibiotics. In the majority of cases the development of the movement disorder occurred in conjunction with an encephalopathic disorder, frequently associated with drug-induced epileptic seizures (Hillsley and Massey, 1991; Pastor et al., 1996; Post, Koelman and Tijssen, 2004; Azar et al., 2005; Chan et al., 2006; Martin, 2007; Cheung et al., 2007). In all patients, cessation of the causative agent promoted complete recovery within a few days to two weeks. In the case of a patient who developed propriospinal myoclonus a few days after the introduction of ciprofloxacin, withdrawal of the medication did not lead to complete recovery until several months later, which led the authors to propose that the drug might have triggered a spinal myoclonic generator that continued to be active even after the drug had been stopped (Post, Koelman and Tijssen, 2004).

The pathophysiology of movement disorders secondary to the use of antibiotics is not completely understood. It is hypothesized that β-lactams (penicillin and cephalosporins), carbapenems (imipenem) and fluoroquinolones (ciprofloxacin, levofloxacin, oxofloxacin) probably exert both their convulsive threshold-lowering effect and their dykinesia-inducing effect through interactions with the GABA system (inhibition of GABA-receptor binding or reduction of GABA release from nerve terminals) (De Sarro et al., 1995). It must be emphasized that in the majority of cases in which these effects have been observed, there were significant predisposing factors, such as advanced age, pre-existing seizure disorder, encephalopathy, renal impairment, liver disease and so on (Pastor et al., 1996; Yasuda et al., 1999; Martin, 2007).

Immunosupressants

Calcineurin inhibitors, like cyclosporin A and tacrolimus, routinely used as immunosupressants in organ transplantation, are a frequent cause of neurological adverse events both at the central nervous system and the peripheral nervous system level. Estimates of the overall frequency of neurotoxic effects of these drugs in transplant recipients ranges from 10 to 28% (Bechstein, 2000). Between 20 and 40% of the cases developing neurological adverse events experience tremor, thus making this symptom the most frequent side effect in patients under immunosuppressive therapy. Tremor is mainly observed either in action or while sustaining a posture. In the majority of cases the severity is relatively mild and most patients report no interference with activities of daily life (Munhoz et al., 2005). In some studies, a higher incidence of tremor was reported for tacrolimus, than for cyclosporin A (35% vs 12%) (Bechstein, 2000). There appears to be a significant variability in the incidence of neurological adverse events according to the type of transplanted organ. For cyclosporin A, the incidence of tremor in kidney transplant is 21%, while in bone marrow transplantation is 16% (Walker and Brochstein, 1988). In the case of tacrolimus, the incidence of neurotoxic effects is significantly higher in patients with liver transplantation than in heart or lung transplanted cases (Bechstein, 2000). In a recent study from Brazil, up to 48% of patients receiving cyclosporin A experienced tremor at some point in their treatment (Munhoz et al., 2005). In most cases, tremor tends to diminish or disappear with continued treatment or with reduction or cessation of therapy.

The pathophysiology of neurotoxic adverse events of calcineurin inhibitors is quite complex and probably involves a wide range of different mechanisms to account for the diversity of both central and peripheral side effects. In the case of tremor, both cyclosporin A and tacrolimus are believed to modulate the activity of both excitatory (NMDA) and inhibitory (GABA) receptors via calcineurin (Bechstein, 2000). It is possible to hypothesize that an imbalance between excitatory and inhibitory influences at the basal ganglia and related nuclei could lead to the development of tremor. Peripheral factors, however, cannot be completely ruled out.

Miscellaneous

Buspirone, a non-benzodiazepine anxiolytic drug with serotonergic and dopaminergic properties, has been associated with isolated reports of akathisia, orofacial dyskinesias, transient myoclonus, tremor, vocalizations and transient or persistent dystonia (LeWitt et al., 1993). Benzodiazepines, such as diazepam, bromazepam, clorazepate and lorazepam, although rarely, have been found to worsen or even induce dyskinesias, including acute dystonic reactions and tardive dyskinesias (Rosenbaum and de la Fluente, 1979; Hooker and Danzl, 1988; Perez Trullen et al., 1992). A case of acute dystonic reaction (lingual dyskinesias and akathisia) has been reported with the use of intravenous midazolam, requiring flumazenil, which completely abolished it (Stolarek and Ford, 1990). As benzodiazepines modulate GABA transmission it is possible that an imbalance between excitatory and inhibitory mechanisms at the basal ganglia level is responsible for the development of abnormal involuntary movements with these drugs (Perez Trullen et al., 1992).

Oral contraceptives (OC) are occasionally responsible for the development of choreatic movements. The associa-tion of chorea and OC was first described by Fernando in 1966, and since then 50 or more cases have been reported in the literature (Vela et al., 2004). The movement disorder usually appears 9–60 days after the onset of treatment. The existence of predisposing factors has been discussed, as some patients developing chorea with the use of oral contraceptives had a history of rheumatic fever, encephalitis or chorea gravidarum; in other cases a diagnosis of systemic lupus erythematosus or the presence of antiphospholipid antibodies were believed to be contributing factors (Vela et al., 2004). However, there are some patients without any other known risk factor (Miranda et al., 2004). It is almost the rule that the involuntary movements disappear a few days after drug withdrawal. OC-induced dyskinesias are probably related to effects of estrogens both on dopamine-receptor sensitivity and their effect on the number of D2 dopamine-receptor binding sites at the striatal level (Hruska and Silbergeld, 1980; Di Paolo et al., 1982). Two recent reports have provided new insights into the pathophysiology of this disorder. In one case a positron emission tomography (PET) study with ^{18}F-fluorodeoxyglucose demonstrated a dense focus of increased glucose metabolism involving the body of the left caudate nucleus in a young patient with OC-induced chorea in the absence of any known predisposing factor (Vela et al., 2004). Miranda et al. (2004), a propos of a case without evidence of pre-existing rheumatic disease and in the absence of a recent streptoccocal infection, who developed chorea after one year of treatment with OC and had positive anti-basal ganglia antibodies did a thorough review of the literature and revitalized the concept of an immune-mediated mechanism for this disorder. Gamboa, Isaacs and Harter, 1971 were, in fact, the first to postulate an immunological mechanism in the pathogenesis of this condition, or at least the need for the presence of a compromised immune system on top of which OC would be able to induce chorea. It remains to be proven whether or not the majority of OC-induced choreas are positive for anti-basal ganglia antibodies.

Other drugs that occasionally have been reported to induce dyskinesias are amantadine (vocal myoclonus in a Parkinsonian patient) (Pfeiffer, 1996), baclofen (generalized chorea in an Alzheimer's disease patient) (Crystal, 1990), bupropion (exacerbation of tics in patients with Tourette and ADHD; buccolingual dyskinesias in 63 year-old man with recurrent depression) (Spencer et al., 1993; Kohen and Sarcevic, 2006), diazoxide (rigidity, tremor, oculogyric crises in 15% of patients treated with this drug) (Pohl, 1975), digoxin (chorea in a seven-year-old girl with congenital heart disease) (Sekul, Kaminer and Sethi, 1999), fentanyl (myoclonus and facial dyskinesias in a 59-year old myasthenic man) (Petzinger, Mayer and Przedborski, 1995), lithium (choreoathetosis in at least 14 cases reported in the literature; myoclonus of apparently

Is the disorder of common occurrence with the suspected medication?

YES   NO

| 1. Reduce or withdraw (whenever possible) medication and monitor reduction of symptomatology.
 2. Evaluate predisposing factors or alternative diagnoses.
 3. Simplify therapeutic regime if there is polypharmacy.
 4. If symptoms persist assess need for symptomatic medication. | 1. Evaluate first alternative diagnoses.
 2. If no other explanations for the dyskinesias are found, reduce or withdraw medication.
 3. Eventually, rechallenge with the suspected medication to confirm causality.
 4. If symptoms persist assess need for symptomatic medication. |

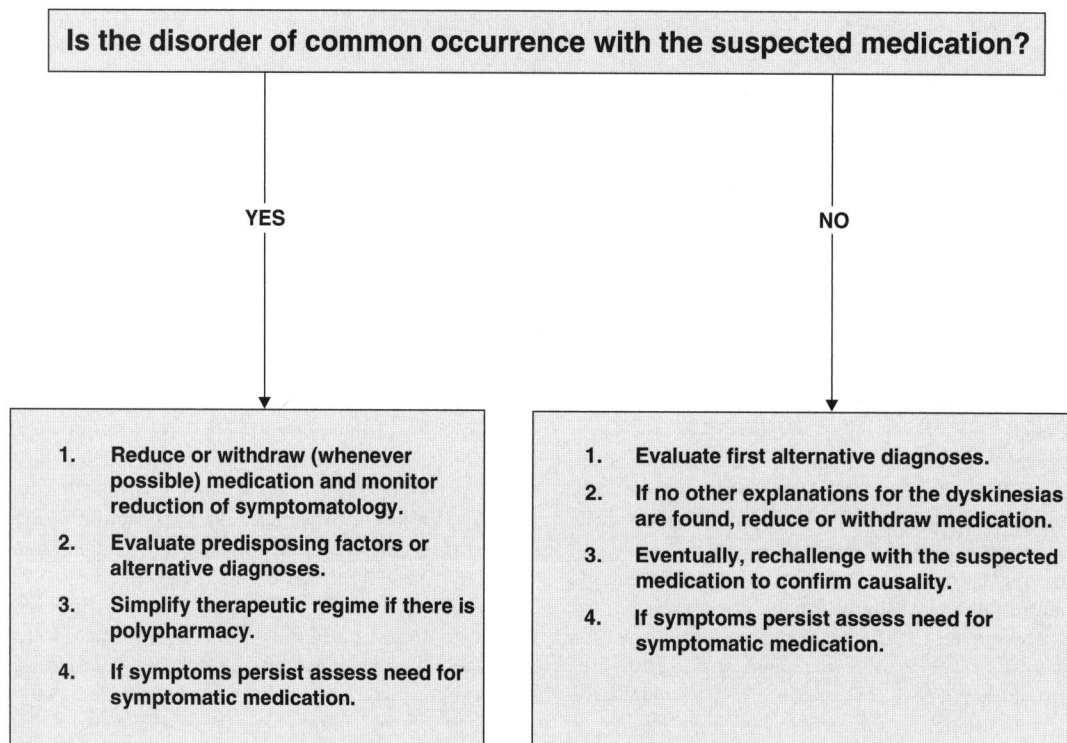

Figure 26.1 Diagnostic and therapeutic algorithm for the management of drug-induced dyskinesias.

cortical origin in several patients) (Reed, Wise and Timmerman, 1989; Caviness and Evidente, 2003; Stemper *et al.*, 2003), methadone (choreoathetoid movements in addicts given this mu opioid agonist) (Wasserman and Yahr, 1980; Bonnet *et al.*, 1998), propofol (choreoathetosis in a seven-year-old boy given this drug for anaesthesia induction) (Diltoer *et al.*, 1996) and tumor necrosis factor (myoclonus and tremor in a 20 year-old woman with Ehlers–Danlos syndrome) (Ferbert *et al.*, 1993).

PRINCIPLES OF MANAGEMENT

One of the major challenges one faces when tackling the problem of drug-induced dyskinesias is the diversity of the clinical phenomenology and the variety of drugs involved in their production. In addition, in some of the isolated reports found in the literature involving drugs rarely or infrequently causing dyskinesias, it is often difficult to inequivocally find a causative relationship and even harder at times to provide a rational explanation for their occurrence in terms of pathophysiological mechanisms. Thus it becomes necessary to approach the problem of drug-induced dyskinesia in a systematic fashion, as provided in the following paragraphs (see also Figure 26.1):

1. Dyskinesia caused by non-neuroleptic medications is an infrequent adverse event (AE). However the treating physician confronted with a patient in whom dyskinesias develop in the course of treatment with any medication, should be suspicious and must consider the possibility of a causal relationship between the abnormal involuntary movement and the drug the patient is receiving. It is important to remember that an AE is defined as any unfavorable and unintended sign (including an abnormal laboratory finding), symptom or disease temporally associated with the use of a medicinal product. Therefore a causal relationship should be suspected in cases in which the dyskinesia appears soon after the introduction of any new medication or in the course of a prolonged treatment.

2. Bearing in mind what has been defined in the preceding paragraph, there are different levels of suspicion in considering the possibility of a drug-induced origin of dyskinesia. First, when the dyskinesia observed in a patient is a well-known and frequent AE of the medication in question (e.g., chorea and phenytoin; myoclonus and penicillin; tremor and sympathomimetics, immunosuppressants, or valproate; akathisia, tardive dyskinesias, and parkinsonism with SSRIs;

etc.) the level of suspicion should be high. In all other cases it is important to be aware that although infrequent, dyskinesias can occur with a wide variety of medications and steps should be taken to confirm or rule out a causal relationship. Hopefully, the list of medications and the different types of dyskinesias reported as causally related to them, provided in Table 26.2, will be helpful.

3. In all cases it is important to rule out other possible causes responsible for the development of dyskinesias (structural, infectious, metabolic, etc.). One should bear in mind, however, that in the development of drug-induced dyskinesias, structural lesions, infectious disorders, metabolic disturbances, as well as polypharmacy may be contributing factors.

4. Withdrawal, whenever possible, or dose reduction of the medication suspected to be the cause of the dyskinesias is the first step necessary to elucidate the nature of the problem. In the majority of cases this results in prompt abatement of the dyskinesias. In some cases it may take longer for the dyskinesias to disappear and it may become necessary to resort to symptomatic medication until the problem disappears and its secondary cause is ascertained. Parentheral anti-cholinergics and diphenhydramine in acute dystonic reactions; anti-myoclonic agents such as clonazepam, valproate or levetiracetam in myoclonus; benzodiacepines, β-blockers, primidone or gabapentin in postural tremor; amantadine in parkinsonism; are some of the therapeutic agents most frequently used.

5. In some cases confirmation of causality is brought about by re-challenging with the offending drug and re-emergence of the dyskinesia.

We believe comprehensive reviews such as this are important to provide the readers with as much information as possible on such a complex issue. They should be always attentive to the possibility of having to deal with some of the problems exemplified here or even discover new drugs with the ability to induce dyskinesias that have not yet been reported.

References

Asconape, J., Diedrich, A. and DellaBadia, J. (2000) Myoclonus associated with the use of gabapentin. *Epilepsia*, **41** (4), 479–481.

Azar, S., Ramjiani, A. and Van Gerpen, J.A. (2005) Ciprofloxacin-induced chorea. *Movement Disorders*, **20** (4), 513–514.

Babiy, M., Stubblefield, M.D., Herklotz, M. and Hand, M. (2005) Asterixis related to gabapentin as a cause of falls. *American Journal of Physical Medicine & Rehabilitation*, **84** (2), 136–140.

Bartzokis, G., Beckson, M., Wirshing, D.A., Lu, P.H., Foster, J.A. and Mintz, J. (1999) Choreoathetoid movements in cocaine dependence. *Biological Psychiatry*, **45** (12), 1630–1635.

Bateman, D.N., Bevan, P., Longley, B.P., Mastaglia, F. and Wandless, I. (1981) Cimetidine induced postural and action tremor. *Journal of Neurology, Neurosurgery, and Psychiatry*, **44** (1), 94.

Bechstein, W.O. (2000) Neurotoxicity of calcineurin inhibitors: impact and clinical management. *Transpl Int.* **13** (5), 313–326.

Bond, G.R., Garro, A.C. and Gilbert, D.L. (2007) Dyskinesias associated with atomoxetine in combination with other psychoactive drugs. *Clinical Toxicology (Phila)*, **45** (2), 182–185.

Bonnet, U., Banger, M., Wolstein, J. and Gastpar, M. (1998) Choreoathetoid movements associated with rapid adjustment to methadone. *Pharmacopsychiatry*, **31** (4), 143–145.

Bostwick, J.M. and Jaffee, M.S. (1999) Buspirone as an antidote to SSRI-induced bruxism in 4 cases. *Journal of Clinical Psychiatry*, **60** (12), 857–860.

Boyer, E.W. and Shannon, M. (2005) The serotonin syndrome. *The New England Journal of Medicine*, **352** (11), 1112–1120.

Bradbury, A.J., Bentick, B. and Todd, P.J. (1982) Dystonia associated with carbamazepine toxicity. *Postgraduate Medical Journal*, **58** (682), 525–526.

Brady, W. and Hall, K. (1992) Erythromycin-related dystonic reaction. *American Journal of Emergency Medicine*, **10** (6), 616.

Burda, A., Webster, K., Leikin, J.B., Chan, S.B. and Stokes, K.A. (1999) Nefazodone-induced acute dystonic reaction. *Veterinary and Human Toxicology*, **41** (5), 321–322.

Caligiuri, M.P. and Buitenhuys, C. (2005) Do preclinical findings of methamphetamine-induced motor abnormalities translate to an observable clinical phenotype? *Neuropsychopharmacology*, **30** (12), 2125–2134.

Caviness, J.N. and Evidente, V.G. (2003) Cortical myoclonus during lithium exposure. *Archives of Neurology*, **60** (3), 401–404.

Chan, S., Turner, M.R., Young, L. and Gregory, R. (2006) Cephalosporin-induced myoclonus. *Neurology*, **66**, 20.

Cheung, Y.F., Wong, W.W., Tang, K.W., Chan, J.H. and Li, P.C. (2007) Ciprofloxacin-induced palatal tremor. *Movement Disorders*, **22** (7), 1038–1043.

Chi, W.M., Chua, K.S. and Kong, K.H. (2000) Phenytoin-induced asterixis—uncommon or under-diagnosed? *Brain Injury*, **14** (9), 847–850.

Chudnow, R.S., Dewey, R.B. Jr, and Lawson, C.R. (1997) Choreoathetosis as a side effect of gabapentin therapy in severely neurologically impaired patients. *Archives of Neurology*, **54** (7), 910–912.

Crespel, A., Genton, P., Berramdane, M., Coubes, P., Monicard, C., Baldy-Moulinier, M. and Gelisse, P. (2005) Lamotrigine associated with exacerbation or de novo myoclonus in idiopathic generalized epilepsies. *Neurology*, **65** (5), 762–764.

Crystal, H.A. (1990) Baclofen therapy may be associated with chorea in Alzheimer's disease. *Annals of Neurology*, **28** (6), 839.

Crosley, C.J. and Swender, P.T. (1979) Dystonia associated with carbamazepine administration: experience in brain-damaged children. *Pediatrics*, **63** (4), 612–615.

Daras, M., Koppel, B.S. and Atos-Radzion, E. (1994) Cocaine-induced choreoathetoid movements ("crack dancing"). *Neurology*, **44**, 751–752.

Das, K.B., Harris, C., Smyth, D.P. and Cross, J.H. (2003) Unusual side effects of lamotrigine therapy. *Journal of Child Neurology*, **18** (7), 479–480.

Davis, B.J., Aul, E.A., Granner, M.A. and Rodnitzky, R.L. (1994) Ranitidine-induced cranial dystonia. *Clinical Neuropharmacology*, **17** (5), 489–491.

DeGrandi, T. and Simon, J.E. (1987) Promethazine-induced dystonic reaction. *Pediatric Emergency Care*, **3** (2), 91–92.

De Sarro, A., Ammendola, D., Zappala, M., Grasso, S. and De Sarro, G.B.(Jan 1995) Relationship between structure and convulsant properties of some beta-lactam antibiotics following intracerebroventricular microinjection in rats. *Antimicrobial Agents and Chemotherapy*, **39** (1), 232–237.

Diaz-Martinez, A., Benassinni, O., Ontiveros, A., Gonzalez, S., Salin, R., Basquedano, G. and Martinez, R.A. (1998) A randomized, open-label comparison of venlafaxine and fluoxetine in depressed outpatients. *Clinical Therapeutics*, **20** (3), 467–476.

Dietz, A.J., Jr (1981) Amphetamine-like reactions to phenylpropanolamine. *The Journal of the American Medical Association*, **245** (6), 601–602.

Diltoer, M.W., Rosseneu, S., Ramet, J., De Wolf, D., Spapen, H.D., De Turck, B.J. and Huyghens, L.P. (1996) Anticholinergic treatment for choreoathetosis in a child after induction with propofol. *Anesthesia and Analgesia*, **82** (3), 670.

Di Paolo, T., Bedard, P.J., Dupont, A., Poyet, P. and Labrie, F. (1982) Effects of estradiol on intact and denervated striatal dopamine receptors and on dopamine levels: a biochemical and behavioral study. *Canadian Journal of Physiology and Pharmacology*, **60** (3), 350–357.

Dravet, C., Dalla Bernardina, B., Mesdjian, E., Galland, M.C. and Roger, J. (1980) Paroxysmal dyskinesia during treatment with diphenylhydantoin. *Revue Neurologique*, **136** (1), 1–14.

Duarte, J., Sempere, A.P., Cabezas, M.C., Marcos, J. and Claveria, L.E. (1996) Postural myoclonus induced by phenytoin. *Clinical Neuropharmacology*, **19** (6), 536–538.

Edwards, J.G. and Anderson, I. (1999) Systematic review and guide to selection of selective serotonin reuptake inhibitors. *Drugs*, **57**, 507–533.

Etzel, J.V. (1994) Diphenhydramine-induced acute dystonia. *Pharmacotherapy*, **14** (4), 492–496.

Extein, I. (1978) Methylphenidate-induced choreoathetosis. *The American Journal of Psychiatry*, **135** (2), 252–253.

Fakhoury, T., Uthman, B. and Abou-Khalil, B. (2000) Safety of long-term treatment with tiagabine. *Seizure: The Journal of the British Epilepsy Association*, **9** (6), 431–435.

Fann, W.E., Sullivan, J.L. and Richman, B.W. (1976) Dyskinesias associated with tricyclic antidepressants. *British Journal of Psychiatry*, **128**, 490–493.

Ferbert, A., Biniek, R., Kindler, J. and Maurin, N., (1993) Myoclonus and tremor induced acutely by administration of tumor necrosis factor in a patient with Ehlers-Danlos syndrome. *Movement Disorders*, **8** (2), 232–233.

Fraunfelder, F.W. and Fraunfelder, F.T. (2004) Oculogyric crisis in patients taking cetirizine. *American Journal of Ophthalmology*, **137** (2), 355–357.

Frucht, S. and Eidelberg, D. (1997) Imipenem-induced myoclonus. *Movement Disorders*, **12** (4), 621–622.

Gamboa, E., Isaacs, G. and Harter, D. (1971) Chorea associated with oral contraceptive therapy. *Archives of Neurology*, **25**, 112–114.

Garvey, M.J. and Tollefson, G.D. (1987) Occurrence of myoclonus in patients treated with cyclic antidepressants. *Archives of General Psychiatry*, **44** (3), 269–272.

Gerber, P.E. and Lynd, L.D. (1998) Selective serotonin-reuptake inhibitor-induced movement disorders. *Annals of Pharmacotherapy*, **32** (6), 692–698.

Go, T. (1999) Carbamazepine-induced involuntary movements in a girl with localization-related epilepsy. *No To Hattatsu*, **31** (4), 366–369.

Gorman, M. and Barkley, G.L. (1995) Oculogyric crisis induced by carbamazepine. *Epilepsia*, **36** (11), 1158–1160.

Gunal, D.I., Guleryuz, M. and Bingol, C.A. (2002) Reversible valproate-induced choreiform movements. *Seizure: The Journal of the British Epilepsy Association*, **11** (3), 205–206.

Harrison, M.B., Lyons, G.R. and Landow, E.R. (1993) Phenytoin and dyskinesias: a report of two cases and review of the literature. *Movement Disorders*, **8** (1), 19–27.

Heckmann, J.G., Ulrich, K., Dutsch, M. and Neundorfer, B. (2005) Pregabalin associated asterixis. *American Journal of Physical Medicine & Rehabilitation*, **84** (9), 724.

Hedenmalm, K., Guzey, C., Dahl, M.L., Yue, Q.Y. and Spigset, O. (2006) Risk factors for extrapyramidal symptoms during treatment with selective serotonin reuptake inhibitors, including cytochrome P-450 enzyme, and serotonin and dopamine transporter and receptor polymorphisms. *Journal of Clinical Psychopharmacology*, **26** (2), 192–197.

Hillsley, R.E. and Massey, E.W. (1991) Truncal asterixis associated with ceftazidime, a third-generation cephalosporin. *Neurology*, **41** (12), 2008.

Holtkamp, M., Halle, A., Meierkord, H. and Masuhr, F. (2006) Gabapentin-induced severe myoclonus in a patient with impaired renal function. *Journal of Neurology*, **253** (3), 382–383.

Holtmann, M., Korn-Merker, E. and Boenigk, H.E. (2000) Carbamazepine-induced combined phonic and motor tic in a boy with Down's syndrome. *Epileptic Disorders*, **2** (1), 39–40.

Hooker, E.A. and Danzl, D.F. (1988) Acute dystonic reaction due to diazepam. *The Journal of Emergency Medicine*, **6** (6), 491–493.

Hruska, R.E. and Silbergeld, E.K. (1980) Increased dopamine receptor sensitivity after estrogen treatment using the rat rotation model. *Science (New York, NY)*, **208** (4451), 1466–1468.

Huppertz, H.J., Feuerstein, T.J. and Schulze-Bonhage, A. (2001) Myoclonus in epilepsy patients with anticonvulsive add-on therapy with pregabalin. *Epilepsia*, **42** (6), 790–792.

Jacob, P.C., Chand, R.P. and Omeima, el-S. (2000) Asterixis induced by gabapentin. *Clinical Neuropharmacology*, **23** (1), 53.

Jacome, D. (1979) Carbamazepine-induced dystonia. *The Journal of the American Medical Association*, **241** (21), 2263.

Janszky, J., Rasonyi, G., Halasz, P., Olajos, S., Perenyi, J., Szucs, A. and Debreczeni, T. (2000) Disabling erratic myoclonus during lamotrigine therapy with high serum level–report of two cases. *Clinical Neuropharmacology*, **23** (2), 86–89.

Joske, D.J. (1984) Dystonic reaction to azatadine. *The Medical Journal of Australia*, **141** (7), 449.

Kapur, V., Barber, K.R. and Peddireddy, R. (1999) Ranitidine-induced acute dystonia. *American Journal of Emergency Medicine*, **17** (3), 258–260.

Kerrick, J.M., Kelley, B.J., Maister, B.H., Graves, N.M. and Leppik, I.E. (1995) Involuntary movement disorders associated with felbamate. *Neurology*, **45** (1), 185–187.

King, H., Corry, P., Wauchob, T. and Barclay, P. (2003) Probable dystonic reaction after a single dose of cyclizine in a patient with a history of encephalitis. *Anaesthesia*, **58** (3), 257–260.

Kipps, C.M., Fung, V.S., Grattan-Smith, P., de Moore, G.M. and Morris, J.G. (2005) Movement disorder emergencies. *Movement Disorders*, **20** (3), 322–334.

Kirschberg, G.J. (1975) Dyskinesia-an unusual reaction to ethosuximide. *Archives of Neurology*, **32**, 137–138.

Kohen, I. and Sarcevic, A. (2006) Mirtazapine in bupropion-induced dyskinesias: a case report. *Movement Disorders*, **21** (4), 584–585.

Kronfol, Z., Greden, J.F. and Zis, A.P. (1983) Imipramine-induced tremor: effects of a beta-adrenergic blocking agent. *Journal of Clinical Psychiatry*, **44** (6), 225–226.

Kumor, K., Sherer, M. and Jaffe, J. (1986) Haloperidol-induced dystonia in cocaine addicts. *Lancet*, **2**, 1341–1342.

Kurlan, R., Kersun, J., Behr, J., Leibovici, A., Tariot, P., Lichter, D. and Shoulson, I. (1989) Carbamazepine-induced tics. *Clinical Neuropharmacology*, **12** (4), 298–302.

Lancman, M.E., Asconape, J.J. and Penry, J.K. (1994) Choreiform movements associated with the use of valproate. *Archives of Neurology*, **51** (7), 702–704.

Law, S.F. and Schachar, R.J. (1999) Do typical clinical doses of methylphenidate cause tics in children treated for attention-deficit hyperactivity disorder? *Journal of the American Academy of Child and Adolescent Psychiatry*, **38** (8), 944–951.

Lee, T.S.W., Lee, T.D., Lombroso, P.J. and King, R.A. (2004) Atomoxetine and tics in ADHD. *Journal of the American Academy of Child and Adolescent Psychiatry*, **43**, 1068–1069.

Lehmann, A.B. (1988) Reversible chorea due to ranitidine and cimetidine. *Lancet*, **2** (8603), 158.

Leo, R.J. (1996) Movement disorders associated with the serotonin selective reuptake inhibitors. *Journal of Clinical Psychiatry*, **57**, 449–454.

Leppik, I.E., Gram, L., Deaton, R. and Sommerville, K.W. (1999) Safety of tiagabine: summary of 53 trials. *Epilepsy Research*, **33** (2–3), 235–246.

Leurs, R., Church, M.K. and Taglialatela, M. (2002) H1-antihistamines: inverse agonism, anti-inflammatory actions and cardiac effects. *Clinical and Experimental Allergy*, **32** (4), 489–498.

LeWitt, P.A., Walters, A., Hening, W. and McHale, D. (Jul 1993) Persistent movement disorders induced by buspirone. *Movement Disorders*, **8** (3), 331–334.

Lipkin, P.H., Goldstein, I.J. and Adesman, A.R. (1994) Tics and dyskinesias associated with stimulant treatment in attention-deficit hyperactivity disorder. *Archives of Pediatrics & Adolescent Medicine*, **148** (8), 859–861.

Lombroso, C.T. (1999) Lamotrigine-induced tourettism. *Neurology*, **52** (6), 1191–1194.

Lopez Lois, G., Gomez Carrasco, J.A. and Garcia de Frias, E. (2005) Adverse reaction of pseudoephedrine. *Anales de Pediatría (Barcelona)*, **62** (4), 378–380.

Lundh, H. and Tunving, K. (1981) An extrapyramidal choreiform syndrome caused by amphetamine addiction. *Journal of Neurology, Neurosurgery, and Psychiatry*, **44** (8), 728–730.

Macdonald, R.L. and Kelly, K.M. (1995) Antiepileptic drug mechanisms of action. *Epilepsia*, **36** (Suppl 2), S2–S12.

Martin, M.G. (2007) Encephalopathy with myoclonic jerks resulting from ceftazidime therapy: an under-recognized potential side-effect when treating febrile neutropenia. *Leukemia & Lymphoma*, **48** (2), 413–414.

McNeill, A. (2006) Chorea induced by low-dose trazodone. *European Neurology*, **55** (2), 101–102.

Mendhekar, D.N. and Duggal, H.S. (2006) Methylphenidate-induced rabbit syndrome. *Annals of Pharmacotherapy*, **40** (11), 2076.

Miranda, M., Cardoso, F., Giovannoni, G. and Church, A. (2004) Oral contraceptive induced chorea: another condition associated with anti-basal ganglia antibodies. *Journal of Neurology, Neurosurgery, and Psychiatry*, **75** (2), 327–328.

Morgan, J.C. and Sethi, K.D. (2005) Drug-induced tremors. *The Lancet Neurology*, **4**, 866–876.

Morgan, J.C., Winter, W.C. and Wooten, G.F. (2004) Amphetamine-induced chorea in attention deficit-hyperactivity disorder. *Movement Disorders*, **19** (7), 840–842.

Morrison, P.F., Sankar, R. and Shields, W.D. (2006) Valproate-induced chorea and encephalopathy in atypical nonketotic hyperglycinemia. *Pediatric Neurology*, **35** (5), 356–358.

Munhoz, R.P., Teive, H.A., Germiniani, F.M., Gerytch, J.C. Jr, Sá, D.S., Bittencourt, M.A., Pasquini, R., Camargo, C.H. and Werneck, L.C. (2005) Movement disorders secondary to long-term treatment with cyclosporine A. *Arq Neuropsiquiatr*, **63** (3A), 592–596.

Neglia, J.P., Glaze, D.G. and Zion, T.E. (1984) Tics and vocalizations in children treated with carbamazepine. *Pediatrics*, **73**, 841–844.

Neufeld, M.Y. and Vishnevska, S. (1995) Vigabatrin and multifocal myoclonus in adults with partial seizures. *Clinical Neuropharmacology*, **18** (3), 280–283.

Norton, J.W. and Quarles, E. (2001) Gabapentin-related dyskinesia. *Journal of Clinical Psychopharmacology*, **21** (6), 623–624.

Okada, M., Hirano, T., Mizuno, K., Chiba, T., Kawata, Y., Kiryu, K., Wada, K., Tasaki, H. and Kaneko, S. (1997) Biphasic effects of carbamazepine on the dopaminergic system in rat striatum and hippocampus. *Epilepsy Research*, **28** (2), 143–153.

Palumbo, D., Spencer, T., Lynch, J., Co-Chien, H. and Faraone, S.V. (2004) Emergence of tics in children with ADHD: impact of once-daily OROS methylphenidate therapy. *Journal of Child and Adolescent Psychopharmacology*, **14** (2), 185–194.

Pascual-Leone, A. and Dhuna, A. (1990) Cocaine-associated multifocal tics. *Neurology*, **40**, 999–1000.

Pastor, P., Moitinho, E., Elizalde, I., Cirera, I. and Tolosa, E. (1996) Reversible oral-facial dyskinesia in a patient receiving ciprofloxacin hydrochloride. *Journal of Neurology*, **243** (8), 616–617.

Peiris, R.S. and Peckler, B.F. (2001) Cimetidine-induced dystonic reaction. *Emergency Medicine*, **21** (1), 27–29.

Perez Trullen, J.M., Modrego Pardo, P.J., Vazquez Andre, M. and Lopez Lozano, J.J. (1992) Bromazepam-induced dystonia. *Biomedicine & Pharmacotherapy*, **46** (8), 375–376.

Perucca, E. (2002) Pharmacological and therapeutic properties of valproate: a summary after 35 years of clinical experience. *CNS Drugs*, **16** (10), 695–714.

Petzinger, G., Mayer, S.A. and Przedborski, S. (1995) Fentanyl-induced dyskinesias. *Movement Disorders*, **10** (5), 679–680.

Pfeiffer, R.F. (1996) Amantadine-induced "vocal" myoclonus. *Movement Disorders*, **11** (1), 104–106.

Pina, M.A. and Modrego, P.J. (2005) Dystonia induced by gabapentin. *Annals of Pharmacotherapy*, **39** (2), 380–382.

Pohl, J.E. (1975) Development and management of extrapyramidal symptoms in hypertensive patients treated with diazoxide. *American Heart Journal*, **89** (3), 401–402.

Post, B., Koelman, J.H. and Tijssen, M.A. (2004) Propriospinal myoclonus after treatment with ciprofloxacin. *Movement Disorders*, **19** (5), 595–597.

Pragst, F., Herre, S. and Bakdash, A. (2006) Poisonings with diphenhydramine–a survey of 68 clinical and 55 death cases. *Forensic Science International*, **161** (2–3), 189–197.

Raethjen, J., Lemke, M.R., Lindemann, M., Wenzelburger, R., Krack, P. and Deuschl, G. (Jan 2001) Amitriptyline enhances the central component of physiological tremor. *Journal of Neurology, Neurosurgery, and Psychiatry*, **70** (1), 78–82.

Rajput, A. and Baerg, K. (2006) Cetirizine-induced dystonic movements. *Neurology*, **66** (1), 143–144.

Raju, P.M., Walker, R.W. and Lee, M.A. (2007) Dyskinesia induced by gabapentin in idiopathic Parkinson's disease. *Movement Disorders*, **22** (2), 288–289.

Reed, S.M., Wise, M.G. and Timmerman, I. (1989) Choreoathetosis: a sign of lithium toxicity. *Journal of Neuropsychiatry and Clinical Neurosciences*, **1** (1), 57–60.

Reeves, A.L., So, E.L., Sharbrough, F.W. and Krahn, L.E. (1996) Movement disorders associated with the use of gabapentin. *Epilepsia*, **37** (10), 988–990.

Rhee, K.J., Albertson, T.E. and Douglas, J.C. (1988) Choreoathetoid disorder associated with amphetamine-like drugs. *American Journal of Emergency Medicine*, **6** (2), 131–133.

Richard, I.H., Kurlan, R., Tanner, C., Factor, S., Hubble, J., Suchowersky, O. and Waters, C. (1997) Serotonin syndrome and the combined use of deprenyl and an antidepressant in Parkinson's disease. Parkinson Study Group. *Neurology*, **48** (4), 1070–1077.

Rinnerthaler, M., Luef, G., Mueller, J., Seppi, K., Wissel, J., Trinka, E., Bauer, G. and Poewe, W. (2005) Computerized tremor analysis of valproate-induced tremor: a comparative study of controlled-release versus conventional valproate. *Epilepsia*, **46** (2), 320–323.

Robertson, P.L., Garofalo, E.A., Silverstein, F.S. and Komarynski, M.A. (1993) Carbamazepine-induced tics. *Epilepsia*, **34** (5), 965–968.

Roessner, V., Robatzek, M., Knapp, G., Banaschewski, T. and Rothenberger, A. (2006) First-onset tics in patients with attention-deficit-hyperactivity disorder: impact of stimulants. *Developmental Medicine and Child Neurology*, **48** (7), 616–621.

Romisher, S., Felter, R. and Dougherty, J. (1987) Tagamet-induced acute dystonia. *Annals of Emergency Medicine*, **16** (10), 1162–1164.

Rosenbaum, A.H. and de la Fluente, J.R. (1979) Benzodiazepines and tardive dyskinesia. *Lancet*, **2** (8148), 900.

Rylander, G. (1972) Psychosis and the punding and choreiform syndromes in addiction to central stimulant drugs. *Psychiatria Neurologia Neurochirurgia*, **75**, 203–212.

Sackellares, J.C. and Smith, D.B. (1979) Myoclonus with electrocerebral silence in a patient receiving penicillin. *Archives of Neurology*, **36** (13), 857–858.

Saito, Y., Oguni, H., Awaya, Y., Hayashi, K. and Osawa, M. (2001) Phenytoin-induced choreoathetosis in patients with severe myoclonic epilepsy in infancy. *Neuropediatrics*, **32** (5), 231–235.

Sallee, F.R., Stiller, R.L., Perel, J.M. and Everett, G. (1989) Pemoline-induced abnormal involuntary movements. *Journal of Clinical Psychopharmacology*, **9** (2), 125–129.

Schillevoort, I., van Puijenbroek, E.P., de Boer, A., Roos, R.A., Jansen, P.A. and Leufkens, H.G. (2002) Extrapyramidal syndromes associated with selective serotonin reuptake inhibitors: a case-control study using spontaneous reports. *International Clinical Psychopharmacology*, **17** (2), 75–79.

Sears, M.R. (2002) Adverse effects of beta-agonists. *The Journal of Allergy and Clinical Immunology*, **110** (6 Suppl), S322–S328.

Sechi, G., Murgia, B., Sau, G., Peddone, L., Tirotto, A., Barrocu, M. and Rosati, G. (2004) Asterixis and toxic encephalopathy induced by gabapentin. *Progress in Neuro-Psychopharmacology & Biological Psychiatry*, **28** (1), 195–199.

Sekul, E.A., Kaminer, S. and Sethi, K.D. (1999) Digoxin-induced chorea in a child. *Movement Disorders*, **14** (5), 877–879.

Senecky, Y., Lobel, D., Diamond, G.W., Weitz, R. and Inbar, D. (2002) Isolated orofacial dyskinesia: a methylphenidate-induced movement disorder. *Pediatr Neurology*, **27** (3), 224–226.

Serrano-Duenas, M. (2002) Fluoxetine-induced tremor: clinical features in 21 patients. *Parkinsonism & Related Disorders*, **8** (5), 325–327.

Simons, F.E. (2004) Advances in H1-antihistamines. *The New England Journal of Medicine*, **351** (21), 2203–2217.

Smith, W.T., Glaudin, V., Panagides, J. and Gilvary, E. (1990) Mirtazapine vs. amitriptyline vs. placebo in the treatment of major depressive disorder. *Psychopharmacology Bulletin*, **26** (2), 191–196.

Soman, P., Jain, S., Rajsekhar, V., Vineeta, S. and Sharma, B.K. (1994) Dystonia–a rare manifestation of carbamazepine toxicity. *Postgraduate Medical Journal*, **70** (819), 54–55.

Sotero de Menezes, M.A., Rho, J.M., Murphy, P. and Cheyette, S. (2000) Lamotrigine-induced tic disorder: report of five pediatric cases. *Epilepsia*, **41** (7), 862–867.

Spencer, T., Biederman, J., Steingard, R. and Wilens, T. (1993) Bupropion exacerbates tics in children with attention-deficit hyperactivity disorder and Tourette's syndrome. *Journal of the American Academy of Child and Adolescent Psychiatry*, **32** (1), 211–214.

Sperling, L.S. and Horowitz, J.L. (1994) Methamphetamine-induced choreoathetosis and rhabdomyolysis. *Annals of Internal Medicine*, **121** (12), 986.

Spiller, H.A., Lintner, C.P. and Winter, M.L. (2004) Atomoxetine (Strattera) exposure in children (abstract). *Journal of Toxicology-Clinical Toxicology*, **42**, 720.

Stemper, B., Thurauf, N., Neundorfer, B. and Heckmann, J.G. (2003) Choreoathetosis related to lithium intoxication. *European Journal of Neurology*, **10** (6), 743–744.

Stolarek, I.H. and Ford, M.J. (1990) Acute dystonia induced by midazolam and abolished by flumazenil. *BMJ (Clinical Research Ed)*, **300** (6724), 614.

Stork, C.M. and Cantor, R. (1997) Pemoline induced acute choreoathetosis: case report and review of the literature. *Journal of Toxicology-Clinical Toxicology*, **35** (1), 105–108.

Stryjer, R., Strous, R.D., Bar, F., Ulman, A.M. and Rabey, J.M. (2002) Segmental dystonia as the sole manifestation of carbamazepine toxicity. *General Hospital Psychiatry*, **24** (2), 114–115.

Thach, B.T., Chase, T.N. and Bosma, J.F. (1975) Oral facial dyskinesia accociated with prolonged use of antihistaminic decongestants. *The New England Journal of Medicine*, **293** (10), 486–487.

Thomas, R.J. and Reagan, D.R. (1996) Association of a Tourette-like syndrome with ofloxacin. *Annals of Pharmacotherapy*, **30** (2), 138–141.

Tombini, M., Pacifici, L., Passarelli, F. and Rossini, P.M. (2006) Transient athetosis induced by tiagabine. *Epilepsia*, **47** (4), 799–800.

Vandel, P., Bonin, B., Leveque, E., Sechter, D. and Bizouard, P. (1997) Tricyclic antidepressant-induced extrapyramidal side effects. *European Neuropsychopharmacology: The Journal of the European College of Neuropsychopharmacology*, **7** (3), 207–212.

Vela, L., Sfakianakis, G.N., Heros, D., Koller, W. and Singer, C. (2004) Chorea and contraceptives: case report with pet study and review of the literature. *Movement Disorders*, **19** (3), 349–352.

Verma, A., Miller, P., Carwile, S.T., Husain, A.M. and Radtke, R.A. (1999) Lamotrigine-induced blepharospasm. *Pharmacotherapy*, **19** (7), 877–880.

Walker, R.W. and Brochstein, J.A. (1988) Neurologic complications of immunosuppressive agents. *Neurologic Clinics*, **6** (2), 261–278.

Wasserman, S. and Yahr, M.D. (1980) Choreic movements induced by the use of methadone. *Archives of Neurology*, **37** (11), 727–728.

Watanabe, S., Yokoyama, S., Kubo, S., Iwai, H. and Kuyama, C. (1978) A double-blind controlled study of clinical efficacy of maprotiline and amitriptyline in depression. *Folia Psychiatrica Et Neurologica Japonica*, **32** (1), 1–31.

Weiner, W.J., Rabinstein, A., Levin, B., Weiner, C. and Shulman, L.M. (2001) Cocaine-induced persistent dyskinesias. *Neurology*, **56** (7), 964–965.

Wernicke, J.F. (1985) The side effect profile and safety of fluoxetine. *Journal of Clinical Psychiatry*, **46**, 59–67.

Wilson, L.B., Woodward, A.M. and Ferrara, J.J. (1997) An acute dystonic reaction with long-term use of ranitidine in an intensive care unit patient. *Journal of the Louisiana State Medical Society*, **149** (1), 36–38.

Wolanczyk, T. and Grabowska-Grzyb, A. (2001) Transient dystonias in three patients treated with tiagabine. *Epilepsia*, **42** (7), 944–946.

Yasuda, H., Yoshida, A., Masuda, Y., Fukayama, M., Kita, Y. and Inamatsu, T. (1999) Levofloxacin-induced neurological adverse effects such as convulsion, involuntary movement (tremor, myoclonus and chorea like), visual hallucination in two elderly patients. *Nippon Ronen Igakkai Zasshi*, **36** (3), 213–217.

Zhang, C., Glenn, D.G., Bell, W.L. and O'Donovan, C.A. (2005) Gabapentin-induced myoclonus in end-stage renal disease. *Epilepsia*, **46** (1), 156–158.

Part VI

ATAXIA AND DISORDERS OF GAIT AND BALANCE

27

Ataxia

Thomas Klockgether

Department of Neurology, University Hospital of Bonn, Germany

INTRODUCTION

The ataxias comprise a wide spectrum of disorders with ataxia as the leading symptom. In most of these disorders, ataxia is due to degeneration of the cerebellar cortex and its afferent or efferent fiber connections. A classification of ataxia that distinguishes between hereditary and non-hereditary ataxias is given in Table 27.1.

Diagnostic tests are selected according to the clinical situation. In patients with a disease onset before the age of 25 years and a disease affecting only one generation, autosomal recessive ataxias have to be considered. If one of the parents had a similar disease, an autosomal dominantly inherited spinocerebellar ataxia (SCA) is probable. Patients with a sporadic disease starting in adulthood may have an acquired ataxia, such as alcoholic cerebellar degeneration (ACD) or paraneoplastic cerebellar degeneration (PCD), or a sporadic degenerative ataxia, such as multiple system atrophy (MSA) or sporadic adult-onset ataxia (SAOA). Since 20% of patients with sporadic adult-onset ataxia have a causative gene mutation, despite a negative family history, molecular tests for Friedreich's ataxia (FRDA) and SCA are recommended in these patients if there is no evidence for an acquired ataxia or MSA.

GENERAL PRINCIPLES OF THERAPY

Although the genetic defects of many hereditary ataxias are known etiologic treatment approaches are available only for some rare forms of ataxia, such as ataxia with isolated vitamin E deficiency (AVED), cerebrotendinous xanthomatosis or Refsum's disease. In most other types of hereditary and non-hereditary degenerative ataxia only supportive treatment is possible. The situation is different in the acquired ataxias, which are due to defined exogenous or endogenous causes. In several of them, treatment approaches are available that improve ataxia or at least prevent further progression.

In general, it is assumed that physiotherapy and speech therapy are helpful in ataxia disorders, although this has not been proven in controlled trials (Armutlu, Karabudak and Nurlu, 2001; Perez-Avila et al., 2004). The goal should be to maintain the highest possible level of autonomy, to cope with physical disability and to prevent secondary complications. In some patients with prominent tremor, the application of weight to the wrist may lead to some functional improvement of hand function (McGruder et al., 2003). With progression of the disease, many patients will require walking aids and a wheelchair.

It has been repeatedly claimed that a number of centrally acting drugs, such as 5-hydroxy-tryptophan, buspirone, physostigmine and D-cycloserine have an anti-ataxic action and temporarily improve cerebellar ataxia (Trouillas et al., 1995). However, the efficacy of these anti-ataxic drugs has not been proven in randomized, controlled studies so that such drugs cannot be recommended (Ogawa, 2004).

There are numerous neurological and non-neurological symptoms that may occur in association with certain ataxia disorders. Well-known examples are cardiomyopathy and diabetes mellitus in FRDA. These accompanying symptoms require conventional medical and neurological treatment, if not otherwise stated.

FRIEDREICH'S ATAXIA (FRDA)

With a prevalence of 1.7–4.7: 100 000, FRDA is the most frequent recessively inherited ataxia. Mean age at onset is 15 years (Dürr et al., 1996). FRDA is a progressive disease leading to disability and premature death. Median latency to become wheelchair-bound after disease onset is 11 years. Life expectancy after disease onset is estimated at 35–40 years (Klockgether et al., 1998; Ribai et al., 2007). Clinically, FRDA is characterized by gait and limb ataxia, dysarthria, lower limb areflexia, loss of proprioception and cardiomyopathy. A minority of FRDA patients develop diabetes mellitus (Dürr et al., 1996).

Therapeutics of Parkinson's Disease and Other Movement Disorders   Edited by Mark Hallett and Werner Poewe
© 2008 John Wiley & Sons, Ltd.

Table 27.1 Classification of ataxias.

Hereditary ataxias
  Autosomal recessive ataxias
    Friedreich's ataxia (FRDA)
    Ataxia telangiectasia (AT)
    Autosomal recessive ataxia with oculomotor apraxia
      type 1 (AOA1)
    Autosomal recessive ataxia with oculomotor apraxia
      type 2 (AOA2)
    Spinocerebellar ataxia with axonal neuropathy
      (SCAN1)
    Autosomal recessive spastic ataxia of Charlevoix-
      Saguenay (ARSACS)
    Abetalipoproteinemia
    Ataxia with isolated vitamin E deficiency (AVED)
    Refsum's disease
    Cerebrotendinous xanthomatosis
    Other autosomal recessive ataxias
  Autosomal dominant ataxias
    Spinocerebellar ataxias (SCA)
    Episodic ataxias (EA)
Non-hereditary degenerative ataxias
  Multiple system atrophy, cerebellar type (MSA-C)
  Sporadic adult-onset ataxia of unknown origin (SAOA)
Acquired ataxias
  Alcoholic cerebellar degeneration
  Ataxia due to other toxic reasons
  Ataxia caused by acquired vitamin deficiency or
    metabolic disorders
  Paraneoplastic cerebellar degeneration
  Immune-mediated ataxias

FRDA is caused by a homozygous, intronic GAA repeat expansion of the frataxin gene (Campuzano *et al.*, 1996). Due to the mutation, tissue frataxin levels are severely reduced. Frataxin is a mitochondrial protein that is involved in the assembly of iron–sulfur clusters. As several enzymes of the mitochondrial respiratory chain contain iron–sulfur clusters, mitochondrial respiration is impaired and free radical production increased. This is associated with accumulation of mitochondrial iron (Pandolfo, 2002). The neurodegeneration in FRDA starts in the dorsal root ganglion cells and spreads to ascending and descending spinal pathways.

Therapeutic trials in FRDA used compounds that are assumed to improve mitochondrial function and decrease free radical production. In an open trial in 10 FRDA patients extended over 47 months, co-enzyme Q10 (400 mg per day) and vitamin E (2100 IU per day) improved cardiac and skeletal muscle bioenergetics, as well as cardiac function assessed by echocardiography. In some patients, ataxia

scores were better than predicted from historical controls, but clear evidence for a beneficial effect of the compounds on neurological function was lacking (Hart *et al.*, 2005). Idebenone is a short-chain quinone analog of co-enzyme Q10 that acts as a free radical-scavenger and improves mitochondrial function. At a dose of 5 mg/kg per day, idebenone was found to decrease the left ventricular mass of FRDA patients in a number of small, non-randomized and uncontrolled studies (Rustin *et al.*, 1999; Hausse *et al.*, 2002; Buyse *et al.*, 2003). This was confirmed in a randomized, placebo-controlled study of 29 FRDA patients. However, idebenone had no action on cardiac and neurological function (Mariotti *et al.*, 2003; Ribai *et al.*, 2007). A recent study found that idebenone in doses up to 75 mg/kg is well tolerated by FRDA patients. A 6 month placebo-controled phase II clinical trial that used doses ranging from 5 to 45 mg/kg found a trend towards dose-dependent improvement of neurological function in juvenile FRDA patients (Di Prospero *et al.*, 2007). Currently, a phase III clinical trial of high dose idebenone in FRDA is ongoing.

Other candidates for a therapy of FRDA are histone deacetylase inhibitors that increase frataxin expression and iron chelators that reduce mitochondrial iron. None of these compounds have so far been tested in patients.

As there is no evidence for clinical efficacy of any drug in FRDA, drug treatment is not recommended.

ATAXIA TELANGIECTASIA (AT)

AT is an autosomal recessively inherited multi-system disorder with an estimated prevalence of 1.2: 100 000. AT starts in early childhood and leads to premature death, often around the age of 20 years. Clinically, AT is characterized by cerebellar ataxia, oculocutaneous telangiectasias, a high incidence of neoplasia, radiosensitivity and recurrent infections. Almost all patients have increased α-fetoprotein serum levels. An almost definite diagnosis can be made by a lymphocyte radiosensitivity assay. The gene affected in AT, ATM (ataxia telangiectasia mutated), encodes a member of the phosphoinositol-3 kinase family involved in cell cycle checkpoint control and DNA repair (Savitsky *et al.*, 1995). More than 200 distinct mutations distributed over the entire gene have been reported. In the central nervous system, the mutations result in degeneration of the cerebellar cortex.

There is no effective treatment for AT. Treatment of infections should be initiated early and maintained over a prolonged time. Administration of immunoglobulins can be considered in patients with repeated infections. Treatment of malignant neoplasias is a particular problem because AT patients have increased sensitivity to radiation and chemotherapy. Therefore, conventional radiotherapy should be avoided, and chemotherapy should be administered only on an individual basis (Sandoval and Swift, 1998).

AUTOSOMAL RECESSIVE ATAXIA WITH OCULOMOTOR APRAXIA TYPE 1 (AOA1)

AOA1 is a rare autosomal recessively inherited ataxia caused by mutations in the aprataxin gene. Aprataxin is involved in the repair of single-strand DNA breaks (Sano et al., 2004).

Disease onset of AOA1 is around seven years. AOA1 patients present with progressive ataxia and oculomotor apraxia, often accompanied by chorea, neuropathy and mental retardation. With progression of the disease, neuropathy becomes increasingly disabling (Le Ber et al., 2003) and serum albumin levels decrease. AOA1 takes a progressive course leading to severe disability and premature death, usually in mid adulthood. Two independent studies found a decreased co-enzyme Q10 content in striated muscle of AOA1 patients (Quinzii et al., 2005; Le Ber et al., 2007). Prompted by these observations, a therapeutic trial of co-enzyme Q10 supplementation may be warranted in AOA1. However, clinical data on the efficacy of co-enzyme Q10 in AOA1 are lacking.

AUTOSOMAL RECESSIVE ATAXIA WITH OCULOMOTOR APRAXIA TYPE 2 (AOA2)

AOA2 is an autosomal receessively inherited ataxia caused by mutations in the senataxin gene (Moreira et al., 2004). Like aprataxin, senataxin is involved in the repair of single-strand DNA breaks. It has been suggested that AOA2 is the second most frequent recessive ataxia after FRDA in Europe (Le Ber et al., 2004).

Disease onset of AOA2 is around 15 years. Clinical presentation is characterized by ataxia and neuropathy. Only half of the patients have oculomotor apraxia. α-Fetoprotein is always increased in AOA2 (Le Ber et al., 2004). To distinguish AOA2 from AT a lymphocyte radiosensitivity assay is required. There is no effective treatment for AOA2.

SPINOCEREBELLAR ATAXIA WITH AXONAL NEUROPATHY (SCAN1)

A homozygous mutation in tyrosyl-DNA phosphodiesterase 1 (TDP1), an enzyme that is essential for preventing the formation of double-strand DNA breaks in yeast, was shown to cause an autosomal recessive ataxia associated with axonal neuropathy, SCAN1 (Takashima et al., 2002). There is no effective treatment for SCAN1.

AUTOSOMAL RECESSIVE SPASTIC ATAXIA OF CHARLEVOIX–SAGUENAY (ARSACS)

ARSACS is a rare autosomal recessive disorder clinically characterized by progressive ataxia and spasticity. Molecular genetic studies in an isolated population in Quebec, Canada, identified causative mutations in a gene encoding sacsin, a large protein with a heat-shock domain (Engert et al., 2000). Sacsin mutations have been also found in a European and Japanese ataxia patients (Grieco et al., 2004). There is no effective therapy for ARSACS. A minority of patients with pronounced spasticity may benefit from anti-spastic drugs.

ABETALIPOPROTEINEMIA

Abetalipoproteinemia is a rare autosomal recessively inherited disorder characterized by onset of diarrhea soon after birth and slow development of a neurological syndrome thereafter. The neurological syndrome consists of ataxia, weakness of the limbs with loss of tendon reflexes, disturbed sensation and retinal degeneration. Abetalipoproteinemia is caused by mutations in the gene encoding a sub-unit of a microsomal triglyceride transfer protein (Sharp et al., 1993). As a consequence, circulating apoprotein B-containing lipoproteins are almost completely missing, and the patients are unable to absorb and transport fat and fat-soluble vitamins. The neurological symptoms are due to vitamin E deficiency.

Management of abetalipoproteinemia consists of a diet with reduced fat intake and vitamin supplementation. Intake of dietary fat should be restricted to 25% of the total daily calories. One-third of daily fat should stem from food sources, two-thirds should be given as medium-chain triglycerides. Patients should receive an adequate supply of essential fatty acids (Kohlschuetter, 2000).

Despite the principal absorption defect, vitamin E can be supplemented orally, since patients are able to secrete very small amounts of apoprotein B-containing lipoproteins. Recommended doses are 50–100 mg/kg per day. In addition, vitamin A (200–400 IU/kg per day) and vitamin K (5 mg every 2 weeks) are given. Levels of vitamin E and A should be closely monitored. Vitamin supplementation should be started as early as possible. Restoration of normal vitamin E levels will lead to clinical improvement or arrest of further deterioration (Kohlschuetter, 2000).

ATAXIA WITH ISOLATED VITAMIN E DEFICIENCY (AVED)

AVED is a rare autosomal recessively inherited disorder with a phenotype resembling FRDA. AVED patients carry homozygous mutations of the gene encoding α-tocopherol transport protein, a liver-specific protein that incorporates vitamin E into very low-density lipoproteins (Ouahchi et al., 1995). As a consequence, vitamin E is rapidly eliminated.

Since there is no absorption deficit, oral supplementation of vitamin E at a dose of 800–2000 mg per day is recommended (Martinello *et al.*, 1998). Vitamin E concentrations should be closely monitored to guarantee that vitamin E is restored to normal levels.

REFSUM'S DISEASE

Refsum's disease is a rare autosomal recessively inherited disorder due to mutations in the gene encoding phytanoyl-CoA hydroxylase, which is involved in the α-oxidation of phytanic acid (Jansen *et al.*, 1997). The clinical phenotype of Refsum's disease is caused by accumulation of phytanic acid in body tissues. Clinically, Refsum's disease is characterized by ataxia, demyelinating sensorimotor neuropathy, pigmentary retinal degeneration, deafness, cardiac arrhythmias and ichthyosis-like skin changes. Whereas ocular and hearing problems are usually slowly progressive, there may be acute exacerbations that are precipitated by low caloric intake and mobilization of phytanic acid from adipose tissue.

Refsum's disease is treated by dietary restriction of phytanic acid from the 50 to 100 mg contained in a normal Western diet, to less than 10 mg per day. The diet should provide adequate caloric intake to prevent mobilization of phytanic acid from adipose stores (Gibberd *et al.*, 1985). With good dietary supervision ataxia and neuropathy may improve. In contrast, the progressive loss of vision and hearing cannot be prevented.

In acute exacerbations, plasma exchange (four sessions over a period of 7–21 days) is effective in lowering phytanic acid levels and improving neurological and cardiac function. Plasmapheresis may also be considered in patients in whom dietary control is insufficient (Harari *et al.*, 1991).

CEREBROTENDINOUS XANTHOMATOSIS (CTX)

CTX is a rare autosomal recessive lipid storage disorder with accumulation of cholestanol in various tissues. The disorder is due to mutations of the gene encoding 27-hydroxylase (Leitersdorf *et al.*, 1993). The clinical syndrome includes ataxia, spasticity, cognitive decline and cataracts. Xanthomatous swelling of the tendons is highly characteristic, but not present in all patients.

CTX is treated by oral administration of chenodeoxycholate (750 mg per day) (Berginer, Salen and Shefer, 1984). This treatment results in a marked drop in plasma cholestanol levels and prevents further progression of the neurological syndrome. In early stages of the disease, clinical improvement may be achieved. Cataracts and xanthomatous swelling of the tendons are not affected by this treatment. Treatment can be further improved by addition of HMG CoA reductase inhibitors, such as 8 (Peynet *et al.*, 1991).

MARINESCO–SJOGREN SYNDROME (MSS)

MSS is characterized by ataxia, mental retardation, myopathy and cataracts. It is caused by mutations that disrupt the protein function of SIL1, a nucleotide exchange factor for the Hsp70 chaperone BiP, which is a key regulator of the main functions of the endoplasmic reticulum (Senderek *et al.*, 2005). There is no effective treatment for MSS.

SPINOCEREBELLAR ATAXIAS (SCAs)

The SCAs are a genetically heterogeneous group of autosomal dominantly inherited progressive ataxia disorders. Up to now, almost 30 different gene loci have been found. Of the known mutations, SCA1,2,3,6,7 and 17 are translated CAG repeat expansions coding for an elongated polyglutamine tract within the respective proteins (Table 27.2). These diseases belong to a larger group of polyglutamine disorders that also include Huntington's disease, dentatorubro-pallidoluyisian atrophy and spinobulbar muscular atrophy. Three SCAs, SCA8,10 and 12 are caused by untranslated repeat expansions in non-coding regions of the respective genes. In SCA5 (beta-III spectrin, SPTBN2), SCA13 (potassium channel), SCA14 (protein kinase Cγ, PKCγ), SCA27 (fibroblast growth factor 14, FGF14) and 16q22-linked ADCA (puratrophin), point mutations have been found in the respective genes. In all other SCAs, the affected genes and mutations have not yet been identified.

The molecular pathogenesis of the diverse SCAs is incompletely understood. In the SCAs caused by expanded CAG repeat expansions, it is assumed that the abnormal polyglutamine-containing proteins encoded by the mutated genes acquire a novel toxic function and exert deleterious effects on specific neuronal populations. In this respect, these disorders resemble other CAG repeat disorders, such as Huntington's disease and spinobulbar muscular atrophy (Zoghbi and Orr, 2000). With the exception of SCA6 (α_{1A} voltage-dependent calcium channel sub-unit, CACNA1A) and SCA17 (TATA binding protein, TBP), the functions of the disease proteins of all SCAs of the polyglutamine group were completely unknown when the respective gene mutations were discovered. The physiological roles of these proteins, which have been named ataxins, are currently under intense investigation. Recent research suggested that the pathogenesis of each of the polyglutamine SCAs critically depends on the specific properties of the respective proteins.

The neuropathology of the SCAs is diverse. Many forms have widespread degeneration involving the cerebellum, brain stem, spinal cord and parts of the basal ganglia. A characteristic ultrastructural hallmark of the SCAs caused by translated CAG repeat mutations is the occurrence of neuronal intranuclear inclusions.

Table 27.2 Mutations and clinical phenotypes of the spinocerebellar ataxias (SCA) caused by CAG repeat expansions.

Disorder	Mutation	Gene product	Clinical phenotype
SCA1	Translated CAG repeat expansion	Ataxin-1	Ataxia, pyramidal signs, neuropathy, dysphagia, restless legs syndrome
SCA2	Translated CAG repeat expansion	Ataxin-2	Ataxia, slow saccades, neuropathy, restless legs syndrome
SCA3 (Machado–Joseph disease)	Translated CAG repeat expansion	Ataxin-3	Ataxia, pyramidal signs, ophthalmoplegia, neuropathy, dystonia, restless legs syndrome
SCA6	Translated CAG repeat expansion	Calcium channel subunit (CACNA1A)	Almost pure cerebellar ataxia
SCA7	Translated CAG repeat expansion	Ataxin-7	Ataxia, ophthalmoplegia, visual loss
SCA17	Translated CAG repeat expansion	TATA binding protein (TBP)	Ataxia, chorea, dystonia, dementia

The prevalence of the dominant ataxias is estimated 3.0:100 000 (van de Warrenburg *et al.*, 2002). The majority of SCAs, including the frequent types SCA1, SCA2 and SCA3, have a complex clinical phenotpye characterized by progressive ataxia in association with a variety of additional extracerebellar symptoms, including pyramidal signs, dysphagia, ophthalmoplegia, dystonia, restless legs syndrome and neuropathy. In a minority of SCAs, clinical presentation is almost pure cerebellar. The most frequent type in this category is SCA6. SCA7 is unique in that ataxia is associated with progressive visual loss due to retinal degeneration (Table 27.2).

The mean age of onset of SCA1, 2 and 3 is 30–40 years with considerable variation between and within families. SCA6 has a later disease onset with an average of 50 years (Schöls *et al.*, 1998). Most patients require a wheelchair at about 15 years and die 20–25 years after disease onset (Klockgether *et al.*, 1998). The less common SCAs that are caused by point mutations usually take a more benign course.

At present, there are no rational treatment approaches for the SCAs. Accompanying symptoms, such as restless legs syndrome are treated in the standard manner. In animal models of SCA1, local application of specific RNAi that knock down ataxin-1 expression, and lithium treatment improved ataxia (Watase *et al.*, 2007; Xia *et al.*, 2004).

EPISODIC ATAXIAS (EAs)

EAs are rare autosomal dominant disorders characterized by intermittent attacks of ataxia. To date, two different genetic and clinical variants are known. Missense mutations in a brain potassium channel gene, KCNA1 result in EA1 (Browne *et al.*, 1994). EA1 is characterized by brief attacks of ataxia and dysarthria often provoked by movements and startle, with onset in early childhood. EA1 is associated with interictal myokymia, that is, twitching of small muscles around the eyes or in the hands.

Truncating mutations of the CACNA1A gene encoding the α_{1A} voltage-dependent calcium channel sub-unit have been found in families with EA2 (Ophoff *et al.*, 1996). A translated CAG repeat mutation of this gene is the cause of SCA6. Compared with EA1, attacks in EA2 start later, last longer and are precipitated by emotional stress and exercise, but not by startle. Some individuals who may or may not suffer from episodic ataxia have slowly progressive ataxia and cerebellar atrophy.

In both disorders acetazolamide is used to prevent attacks. The effect of acetazolamide is more reliable in EA2 than in EA1. If treatment is necessary, patients are typically started on a low dose (125 mg per day), which is then gradually increased (500–700 mg per day) until a satisfactory suppression of attacks is achieved (Griggs and Nutt, 1995). Paraesthesias, which frequently occur under acetazolamide may be reduced by oral potassium supplementation. Alternatively, 4-aminopyridine (15 mg per day), carbamazepine or phenytoin may be used (Strupp *et al.*, 2004).

MULTIPLE SYSTEM ATROPHY (MSA)

MSA is a sporadic, adult-onset disease encompassing the former disease categories striatonigral degeneration, sporadic olivopontocerebellar atrophy and Shy–Drager syndrome.

The prevalence of MSA is 4.4:100 000 (Schrag, Ben Shlomo and Quinn, 1999). Mean age at disease onset is 55 years. MSA takes an unrelentingly progressive course. After a median latency of six years, MSA patients become wheelchair-bound. The median life expectancy after disease onset is nine years (Klockgether *et al.*, 1998). Clinically, MSA patients present with various combinations of parkinsonism, cerebellar ataxia and autonomic failure (orthostatic hypotension, urinary incontinence) (Gilman *et al.*, 1999).

The etiology of MSA is unknown. To date, no genetic or environmental risk factors have been found. MSA brains shown widespread degeneration encompassing the basal ganglia, brainstem, cerebellum and intermediolateral cell columns of the spinal cord. The ultrastructural hallmark of MSA is the presence of ubiquitinated oligodendroglial cytoplasmic inclusions containing α-synuclein.

There is no curative or preventive treatment for MSA. Recent trials with minocycline and riluzole failed to demonstrate a beneficial effect of these compounds on the course of this disease. Parkinsonian symptoms respond to dopaminergic medication, although the response is less robust than in idiopathic Parkinson's disease (Colosimo *et al.*, 1995). Autonomic symptoms are treated in the standard manner. There is no effective symptomatic treatment for ataxia.

SPORADIC ADULT-ONSET ATAXIA OF UNKNOWN ORIGIN (SAOA)

Even with extensive work-up, the underlying cause cannot be elucidated in many sporadic ataxia patients. It is assumed that these patients suffer from a sporadic degenerative cerebellar disorder, which has been tentatively denoted as SAOA. SAOA is estimated to be twice as frequent as the cerebellar type of MSA (Abele *et al.*, 2007). Age of onset is around 47 years, and life expectancy is almost normal. Most of the patients have isolated cerebellar atrophy with little or no involvement of the brainstem.

In most patients of this group, cerebellar ataxia is the prominent symptom. However, pyramidal signs and sensory disturbances may occur. SAOA can be differentiated from MSA by the lasting absence of severe autonomic failure. There are no specific treatment approaches.

ALCOHOLIC CEREBELLAR DEGENERATION

Alcoholic cerebellar degeneration is probably the most common form of chronic cerebellar ataxia, although reliable estimates of prevalence are not available. Clinically, ataxia due to alcoholism is characterized by ataxic gait and stance without major involvement of the upper extremities. Ataxia occurs sub-acutely in heavy drinkers, and may then stabilize for years. Symptoms may progress particularly in those who continue to drink. The pathological changes consist of a loss of the Purkinje cell layer of the vermis and the anterior parts of the cerebellar hemispheres.

It is not entirely clear whether alcoholic cerebellar degeneration is due to nutritional deficiency of vitamin B1 (thiamine), as in Wernicke's encephalopathy, or whether it is due to the toxic actions of alcohol or both (Butterworth, 1995). Strict abstinence improves ataxia, whereas ataxia progresses in patients who continue to drink (Diener *et al.*, 1984). It is therefore essential that patients undergo an alcoholism cure. In addition, vitamin B1 is supplemented. Initially, 50 mg are given intravenously and intramuscularly. Intramuscular injections are repeated for several days until supplementation is continued with an oral vitamin B1 preparation. In addition to vitamin B1 a multivitamin preparation is recommended.

ATAXIA DUE TO OTHER TOXIC REASONS

There are a number of compounds that may lead to cerebellar degeneration and persistent ataxia after chronic intake. These compounds include phenytoin, anti-cancer drugs (5-fluouracil, cytosine arabinoside), lithium salts and solvents. Anti-convulsants other than phenytoin are generally considered safe although many of them cause reversible ataxia at higher doses. In cases of toxic cerebellar damage, further exposition to the toxic agent should be stopped. In acute lithium intoxication, hemodialysis is the treatment of choice.

ATAXIA CAUSED BY ACQUIRED VITAMIN DEFICIENCY AND METABOLIC DISORDERS

Vitamin B1

Wernicke's encephalopathy is an acute or sub-acute encephalopathy caused by deficiency of vitamin B1 (thiamine) typically occurring in chronic alcoholics. Wernicke's encephalopathy may also result from excessive fasting, repeated vomiting and prolonged parenteral nutrition without adequate vitamin supplementation. In addition to ataxia, the clinical syndrome includes eye muscle paresis, peripheral neuropathy, seizures and mental confusion. If not treated adequately, Wernicke's encephalopathy may result in a chronic amnesic state, Korsakov's psychosis. There is close relationship between Wernicke's encephalopathy and alcoholic cerebellar degeneration, since vitamin B1 plays a prominent role in both disorders. Immediate parenteral application of high doses of vitamin B1 is necessary.

Initially, 50 mg are given intravenously and intramuscularly. Intramuscular injections are repeated for several days until supplementation is continued with an oral vitamin B1 preparation. In addition to vitamin B1 a multi-vitamin preparation is recommended.

Vitamin B12

Vitamin B12 deficiency leads to macrocytic anemia, polyneuropathy and sub-acute combined degeneration of the spinal cord. Sensory ataxia is usually the prominent symptom of vitamin B12 deficiency. The most frequent cause is reduced absorption from lack of intrinsic factor due to gastric disease.

Vitamin B12 (hydroxycobalamin) is given intramuscularly at a dose of 1000 μg per day until neurological symptoms improve. Subsequently, the interval between applications is expanded to 3–4 days for a year, followed by life-long application of 1000 μg per month. Since 1% of orally given vitamin B12 is absorbed, even in the absence of intrinsic factor, high-dose oral vitamin B12 supplementation (1000 μg per day) is an alternative approach for maintenance therapy after initial parenteral supplementation (Adachi et al., 2000). Serum levels of homocysteine and methyl malonic acid are useful to monitor therapy.

Vitamin E

Acquired vitamin E deficiency may occur as a consequence of malabsorption in gastrointestinal diseases such as celiac disease, cystic fibrosis, short-bowel syndrome, biliary atresia and intrahepatic cholestasis. Patients present with ataxia of gait and stance, dysarthria and sensory neuropathy, with loss of tendon reflexes (Harding et al., 1982). To stop further progression, intramuscular application of vitamin E at a dose of 100–200 mg per day should be initiated as early as possible. Most patients are also deficient in other vitamins which should be supplemented together with vitamin E.

Hypothyroidism

Cerebellar ataxia is a rare neurological complication of hypothyroidism. The pathogenesis of this syndrome is unclear. Ataxia is completely relieved after adequate substitution of thyroid hormone.

PARANEOPLASTIC CEREBELLAR DEGENERATION (PCD)

PCD is an immune-mediated sub-acute degeneration of the cerebellar cortex that may occur in association with almost every tumor. Most frequently, however, small-cell lung cancer, cancer of the breast and ovary, and lymphoma are involved. A rapidly evolving pancerebellar syndrome is the typical clinical manifestation of PCD. However, ataxia may also be the presenting clinical feature in other paraneoplastic syndromes, such as paraneoplastic encephalomyelitis/sensory neuronopathy.

In many, but not all, patients with PCD, antibodies are found in the serum and CSF that react with antigens expressed by the nervous system and the tumor. These antibodies do not cause cerebellar degeneration. Rather, they are disease markers. Anti-Hu antibodies are found in association with small-cell lung cancer, anti-Yo antibodies mainly with ovarian cancer, anti-Tr with lymphoma and anti-Ri antibodies with various malignancies (Shams'ili et al., 2003).

Ataxia in PCD has a sub-acute onset and rapidly progresses to severe disability. In most cases, ataxia precedes the detection of the underlying tumor. Ataxia involves upper and lower extremities and is accompanied by dysarthria and variable degrees of dysphagia. The clinical syndrome is similar in all types of PCD with the exception of PCD associated with anti-Ri antibodies. A highly characteristic feature of this disorder is the presence of opsoclonus leading to oscillopsia.

At disease onset, CT or MRI do not show major cerebellar atrophy. However, cerebellar atrophy usually develops in the further disease course. A suspected diagnosis of PCD is confirmed by demonstration of specific antibodies. However, absence of antibodies does not rule out a diagnosis of PCD. In cases with suspected or proven PCD, a careful search for the underlying tumor is required. If this search is negative it has to be repeated every six months for three years.

Tumor treatment has been shown to be the only factor predicting improvement or stabilization of ataxia (Candler et al., 2004). In contrast, efficacy of immunosuppressive treatment has been shown only in single cases (Paone and Jeyasingham, 1980; David et al., 1996). This may be because irreversible damage to the cerebellum occurs rather quickly.

IMMUNE-MEDIATED ATAXIAS

Neurological disorders including ataxia may occur in celiac disease. Although known for years it has not been established whether neurological manifestations are immune-mediated or due to malnutrition. More recently, it was claimed that ataxia may occur as a result of immune-mediated damage to the cerebellum in patients with cryptic gluten sensitivity and circulating anti-gliadin antibodies. It has been proposed to label this disorder "gluten ataxia" (Hadjivassiliou et al., 1998). However, anti-gliadin antibodies are also frequently found in healthy controls and in patients with inherited ataxias making it questionable that they cause ataxia (Abele et al., 2003). There are some uncontrolled reports of improvement on a gluten-free diet, but this has not been demonstrated in controlled trials. Therefore, a gluten-free diet cannot be recommended for patients with ataxia and anti-gliadin antibodies.

Very rarely, ataxia is part of a polyglandular endocrine autoimmune syndrome in patients with circulating anti-glutamic acid decarboxylase antibodies (Honnorat *et al.*, 2001). Ataxia may improve in response to application of immunoglobulins or steroids (Abele *et al.*, 1999; Kim *et al.*, 2006).

References

Abele, M., Minnerop, M., Urbach, H., Specht, K. and Klockgether, T. (2007) Sporadic adult onset ataxia of unknown etiology. A clinical, electrophysiological and imaging study. *Journal of Neurology*, **254**, 1384–1389.

Abele, M., Schöls, L., Schwartz, S. and Klockgether, T. (2003) Prevalence of antigliadin antibodies in ataxia patients. *Neurology*, **60**, 1674–1675.

Abele, M., Weller, M., Mescheriakov, S., Burk, K., Dichgans, J. and Klockgether, T. (1999) Cerebellar ataxia with glutamic acid decarboxylase autoantibodies. *Neurology*, **52**, 857–859.

Adachi, S., Kawamoto, T., Otsuka, M., Todoroki, T. and Fukao, K. (2000) Enteral vitamin B12 supplements reverse postgastrectomy B12 deficiency. *Annals of Surgery*, **232**, 199–201.

Armutlu, K., Karabudak, R. and Nurlu, G. (2001) Physiotherapy approaches in the treatment of ataxic multiple sclerosis: a pilot study. *Neurorehabil Neural Repair*, **15**, 203–211.

Berginer, V.M., Salen, G. and Shefer, S. (1984) Long-term treatment of cerebrotendinous xanthomatosis with chenodeoxycholic acid. *The New England Journal of Medicine*, **311**, 1649–1652.

Browne, D.L., Gancher, S.T., Nutt, J.G. *et al.* (1994) Episodic ataxia/myokymia syndrome is associated with point mutations in the human potassium channel gene, *KCNA1*. *Nature Genetics*, **8**, 136–140.

Butterworth, R.F. (1995) Pathophysiology of alcoholic brain damage: synergistic effects of ethanol, thiamine deficiency and alcoholic liver disease. *Metabolic Brain Disease*, **10**, 1–8.

Buyse, G., Mertens, L., Di Salvo, G. *et al.* (2003) Idebenone treatment in Friedreich's ataxia: neurological, cardiac, and biochemical monitoring. *Neurology*, **60**, 1679–1681.

Campuzano, V., Montermini, L., Moltò, M.D. *et al.* (1996) Friedreich's ataxia: Autosomal recessive disease caused by an intronic GAA triplet repeat, expansion. *Science (New York, NY)*, **271**, 1423–1427.

Candler, P.M., Hart, P.E., Barnett, M., Weil, R. and Rees, J.H. (2004) A follow up study of patients with paraneoplastic neurological disease in the United Kingdom. *Journal of Neurology, Neurosurgery, and Psychiatry*, **75**, 1411–1415.

Colosimo, C., Albanese, A., Hughes, A.J., De Bruin, V.M.S. and Lees, A.J. (1995) Some specific clinical features differentiate multiple system atrophy (striatonigral variety) from Parkinson's disease. *Archives of Neurology*, **52**, 294–298.

David, Y.B., Warner, E., Levitan, M., Sutton, D.M., Malkin, M.G. and Dalmau, J.O. (1996) Autoimmune paraneoplastic cerebellar degeneration in ovarian carcinoma patients treated with plasmapheresis and immunoglobulin. A case report. *Cancer*, **78**, 2153–2156.

Di Prospero, N.A., Baker, A., Jeffries, N. and Fischbeck, K.H. (2007) Neurological effects of high-dose idebenone in patients with Friedreich's ataxia: a randomised, placbo-controlled trial. *Lancet neurology*, **6**, 878–886.

Diener, H.C., Dichgans, J., Bacher, M. and Guschlbauer, B. (1984) Improvement of ataxia in alcoholic cerebellar atrophy through alcohol abstinence. *Journal of Neurology*, **231**, 258–262.

Dürr, A., Cossee, M., Agid, Y. *et al.* (1996) Clinical and genetic abnormalities in patients with Friedreich's ataxia. *The New England Journal of Medicine*, **335**, 1169–1175.

Engert, J.C., Berube, P., Mercier, J. *et al.* (2000) ARSACS, a spastic ataxia common in northeastern Quebec, is caused by mutations in a new gene encoding an 11.5-kb ORF. *Nature Genetics*, **24**, 120–125.

Gibberd, F.B., Billimoria, J.D., Goldman, J.M. *et al.* (1985) Heredopathia atactica polyneuritiformis: Refsum's disease. *Acta Neurologica Scandinavica*, **72**, 1–17.

Gilman, S., Low, P.A., Quinn, N. *et al.* (1999) Consensus statement on the diagnosis of multiple system atrophy. *Journal of the Neurological Sciences*, **163**, 94–98.

Grieco, G.S., Malandrini, A., Comanducci, G. *et al.* (2004) Novel SACS mutations in autosomal recessive spastic ataxia of Charlevoix-Saguenay type. *Neurology*, **62**, 103–106.

Griggs, R.C. and Nutt, J.G. (1995) Episodic ataxias as channelopathies. *Annals of Neurology*, **37**, 285–287.

Hadjivassiliou, M., Grunewald, R.A., Chattopadhyay, A.K. *et al.* (1998) Clinical, radiological, neurophysiological, and neuropathological characteristics of gluten ataxia. *Lancet*, **352**, 1582–1585.

Harari, D., Gibberd, F.B., Dick, J.P. and Sidey, M.C. (1991) Plasma exchange in the treatment of Refsum's disease (heredopathia atactica polyneuritiformis). *Journal of Neurology, Neurosurgery, and Psychiatry*, **54**, 614–617.

Harding, A.E., Muller, D.P., Thomas, P.K. and Willison, H.J. (1982) Spinocerebellar degeneration secondary to chronic intestinal malabsorption: a vitamin E deficiency syndrome. *Annals of Neurology*, **12**, 419–424.

Hart, P.E., Lodi, R., Rajagopalan, B. *et al.* (2005) Antioxidant treatment of patients with Friedreich ataxia: four-year follow-up. *Archives of Neurology*, **62**, 621–626.

Hausse, A.O., Aggoun, Y., Bonnet, D. *et al.* (2002) Idebenone and reduced cardiac hypertrophy in Friedreich's ataxia. *Heart (British Cardiac Society)*, **87**, 346–349.

Honnorat, J., Saiz, A., Giometto, B. *et al.* (2001) Cerebellar ataxia with anti-glutamic acid decarboxylase antibodies: study of 14 patients. *Archives of Neurology*, **58**, 225–230.

Jansen, G.A., Ofman, R., Ferdinandusse, S. *et al.* (1997) Refsum disease is caused by mutations in the phytanoyl-CoA hydroxylase gene. *Nature Genetics*, **17**, 190–193.

Kim, J.Y., Chung, E.J., Kim, J.H., Jung, K.Y. and Lee, W.Y. (2006) Response to steroid treatment in anti-glutamic acid decarboxylase antibody-associated cerebellar ataxia, stiff person syndrome and polyendocrinopathy. *Movement Disorders*, **21**, 2263–2264.

Klockgether, T., Lüdtke, R., Kramer, B. *et al.* (1998) The natural history of degenerative ataxia: a retrospective study in 466 patients. *Brain*, **121**, 589–600.

Kohlschuetter, A. (2000) Abetalipoproteinemia, in *Handbook of Ataxia Disorders* (ed. T. Klockgether), M. Dekker, New York, pp. 205–221.

Le Ber, I., Bouslam, N., Rivaud-Pechoux, S. *et al.* (2004) Frequency and phenotypic spectrum of ataxia with oculomotor apraxia 2: a clinical and genetic study in 18 patients. *Brain*, **127**, 759–767.

Le Ber, I., Moreira, M.C., Rivaud-Pechoux, S. *et al.* (2003) Cerebellar ataxia with oculomotor apraxia type 1: clinical and genetic studies. *Brain*, **126**, 2761–2772.

Le Ber, I., Dubourg, O., Benoist, J.F. *et al.* (2007) Muscle coenzyme Q10 deficiencies in ataxia with oculomotor apraxia 1. *Neurology*, **68**, 295–297.

Leitersdorf, E., Reshef, A., Meiner, V. *et al.* (1993) Frameshift and splice-junction mutations in the sterol 27- hydroxylase gene cause cerebrotendinous xanthomatosis in Jews or Moroccan origin. *The Journal of Clinical Investigation*, **91**, 2488–2496.

Mariotti, C., Solari, A., Torta, D., Marano, L., Fiorentini, C. and Di Donato, S. (2003) Idebenone treatment in Friedreich patients: one-year-long randomized placebo-controlled trial. *Neurology*, **60**, 1676–1679.

Martinello, F., Fardin, P., Ottina, M. *et al.* (1998) Supplemental therapy in isolated vitamin E deficiency improves the peripheral neuropathy and prevents the progression of ataxia. *Journal of the Neurological Sciences*, **156**, 177–179.

McGruder, J., Cors, D., Tiernan, A.M. and Tomlin, G. (2003) Weighted wrist cuffs for tremor reduction during eating in adults with static brain lesions. *American Journal of Occupational Therapy*, **57**, 507–516.

Moreira, M.C., Klur, S., Watanabe, M. *et al.* (2004) Senataxin, the ortholog of a yeast RNA helicase, is mutant in ataxia-ocular apraxia 2. *Nature Genetics*, **36**, 225–227.

Ogawa, M. (2004) Pharmacological treatments of cerebellar ataxia. *Cerebellum*, **3**, 107–111.

Ophoff, R.A., Terwindt, G.M., Vergouwe, M.N. *et al.* (1996) Familial hemiplegic migraine and episodic ataxia type-2 are caused by mutations in the Ca^{2+} channel gene CACNL1A4. *Cell*, **87**, 543–552.

Ouahchi, K., Arita, M., Kayden, H. *et al.* (1995) Ataxia with isolated vitamin E deficiency is caused by mutations in the α-tocopherol transfer protein. *Nature Genetics*, **9**, 141–145.

Pandolfo, M. (2002) Iron metabolism and mitochondrial abnormalities in Friedreich ataxia. *Blood Cells, Molecules & Diseases*, **29**, 536–547.

Paone, J.F. and Jeyasingham, K. (1980) Remission of cerebellar dysfunction after pneumonectomy for bronchogenic carcinoma. *The New England Journal of Medicine*, **302**, 156.

Perez-Avila, I., Fernandez-Vieitez, J.A., Martinez-Gongora, E., Ochoa-Mastrapa, R. and Velazquez-Manresa, M.G. (2004) Effects of a physical training program on quantitative neurological indices in mild stage type 2 spinocerebelar ataxia patients. *Revue Neurologique*, **39**, 907–910.

Peynet, J., Laurent, A., De Liege, P. *et al.* (1991) Cerebrotendinous xanthomatosis: treatments with simvastatin, lovastatin, and chenodeoxycholic acid in 3 siblings (see comments). *Neurology*, **41**, 434–436.

Quinzii, C.M., Kattah, A.G., Naini, A. *et al.* (2005) Coenzyme Q deficiency and cerebellar ataxia associated with an aprataxin mutation. *Neurology*, **64**, 539–541.

Ribai, P., Pousset, F., Tanguy, M.L. *et al.* (2007) Neurological, cardiological, and oculomotor progression in 104 patients with Friedreich ataxia during long-term follow-up. *Archives of Neurology*, **64**, 558–564.

Rustin, P., vonKleistRetzow, J.C., ChantrelGroussard, K., Sidi, D., Munnich, A. and Rotig, A. (1999) Effect of idebenone on cardiomyopathy in Friedreich's ataxia: a preliminary study. *Lancet*, **354**, 477–479.

Sandoval, C. and Swift, M. (1998) Treatment of lymphoid malignancies in patients with ataxia-telangiectasia (see comments). *Medical and Pediatric Oncology*, **31**, 491–497.

Sano, Y., Date, H., Igarashi, S. *et al.* (2004) Aprataxin, the causative protein for EAOH is a nuclear protein with a potential role as a DNA repair protein. *Annals of Neurology*, **55**, 241–249.

Savitsky, K., Bar-Shira, A., Gilad, S. *et al.* (1995) A single ataxia telangiectasia gene with a product similar to PI- 3 kinase. *Science (New York, NY)*, **268**, 1749–1753.

Schöls, L., Krüger, R., Amoiridis, G., Przuntek, H., Epplen, J.T. and Riess, O. (1998) Spinocerebellar ataxia type 6: genotype and phenotype in German kindreds. *Journal of Neurology, Neurosurgery, and Psychiatry*, **64**, 67–73.

Schrag, A., Ben Shlomo, Y. and Quinn, N.P. (1999) Prevalence of progressive supranuclear palsy and multiple system atrophy: a cross-sectional study. *Lancet*, **354**, 1771–1775.

Senderek, J., Krieger, M., Stendel, C. *et al.* (2005) Mutations in SIL1 cause Marinesco-Sjogren syndrome, a cerebellar ataxia with cataract and myopathy. *Nature Genetics*, **37**, 1312–1314.

Shams'ili, S., Grefkens, J., de Leeuw, B. *et al.* (2003) Paraneoplastic cerebellar degeneration associated with antineuronal antibodies: analysis of 50 patients. *Brain*, **126**, 1409–1418.

Sharp, D., Blinderman, L., Combs, K.A. *et al.* (1993) Cloning and gene defects in microsomal triglyceride transfer protein associated with abetalipoproteinaemia. *Nature*, **365**, 65–69.

Strupp, M., Kalla, R., Dichgans, M., Freilinger, T., Glasauer, S. and Brandt, T. (2004) Treatment of episodic ataxia type 2 with the potassium channel blocker 4-aminopyridine. *Neurology*, **62**, 1623–1625.

Takashima, H., Boerkoel, C.F., John, J. *et al.* (2002) Mutation of TDP1, encoding a topoisomerase I-dependent DNA damage repair enzyme, in spinocerebellar ataxia with axonal neuropathy. *Nature Genetics*, **32**, 267–272.

Trouillas, P., Serratrice, G., Laplane, D. *et al.* (1995) Levorotatory form of 5-hydroxytryptophan in Friedreich's ataxia: Results of a double-blind drug-placebo cooperative study. *Archives of Neurology*, **52**, 456–460.

van de Warrenburg, B.P., Sinke, R.J., Verschuuren-Bemelmans, C.C. *et al.* (2002) Spinocerebellar ataxias in the Netherlands: prevalence and age at onset variance analysis. *Neurology*, **58**, 702–708.

Watase, K., Gatchel, J.R., Sun, Y. *et al.* (2007) Lithium therapy improves neurological function and hippocampal dendritic arborization in a spinocerebellar ataxia type 1 mouse model. *PLoS Medicine*, **4**, e182.

Xia, H., Mao, Q., Eliason, S.L. *et al.* (2004) RNAi suppresses polyglutamine-induced neurodegeneration in a model of spinocerebellar ataxia. *Nature Medicine*, **10**, 816–820.

Zoghbi, H.Y. and Orr, H.T. (2000) Glutamine repeats and neurodegeneration. *Annual Review of Neuroscience*, **23**, 217–247.

28

Treatment of Gait and Balance Disorders

Bastiaan R. Bloem[1], Alexander C. Geurts[2], S. Hassin-Baer[3] and Nir Giladi[4]

[1] Department of Neurology and Parkinson Center Nijmegen (ParC), Donders Center for Neuroscience
Radboud University Nijmegen Medical Centre, Nijmegen, The Netherlands
[2] Department of Rehabilitation, Radboud University Nijmegen Medical Centre, Nijmegen, The Netherlands
[3] Movement Disorders Clinic, Department of Neurology, Sheba Medical Center,
Sackler School of Medicine, Tel-Aviv, Israel
[4] Movement Disorders Unit, Department of Neurology, Tel-Aviv Sourasky Medical Centre, Sackler School of Medicine,
Tel-Aviv University, Tel-Aviv, Israel

INTRODUCTION

This chapter deals with the treatment of axial mobility deficits: gait impairment, postural instability and falls. Axial mobility deficits in patients with neurological diseases are both common and devastating. The prevalence of gait disorders increases with age. At the age of 60 years, gait is abnormal in about 15% of people (Sudarsky, 2001), and this increases to around 80% at the age of 85 years (Bloem et al., 1992). These gait disorders can usually be ascribed to underlying diseases of the nervous system or musculoskeletal system, even when gait impairment appears to be present in isolation, without concurrent neurological signs during routine neurological examination. The prevalence of gait disorders is particularly high among neurological patients, and this is true for disorders affecting the central nervous system, the peripheral nervous system, or both. Gait is often an early and sometimes even the presenting sign, as is the case in, for example, patients with hereditary degenerative ataxias. For other disorders, gait may initially be unaffected, but becomes almost inevitably impaired with disease progression, as can be seen in patients with Parkinson's disease (PD).

Gait and balance disorders often have devastating consequences (Table 28.1), the most significant being falls and fall-related injuries. The risk of falls increases with aging: about 30% of elderly subjects over 65 years of age fall at least once a year, and about half of them even more than once (Nevitt et al., 1989). Up to 25% of elderly fallers sustain physical injuries that are severe enough to warrant some sort of medical attention (Luukinen et al., 1995). Injuries caused by accidental falls range from relatively innocent bruises to major fractures of long pipe bones or head trauma. Hip fractures are common and widely feared, because secondary complications are frequent and because the associated mortality rate is high. Another important consequence is a reduced mobility, which leads to loss of independence. This immobility is often compounded by a fear of falling, which further limits patients in their movements and thus affects the quality of life (Jorstad et al., 2005). For some patients, this fear of falling is appropriate because balance is severely disturbed, but for others the degree of fear is disproportionate and leads to unnecessary immobility, loss of independence or social isolation. Secondary immobility also promotes development of osteoporosis, which in turn increases the risk of future fractures following falls. Importantly, gait disturbances are also a marker for future development of cardiovascular disease and dementia (Bloem et al., 2000; Verghese et al., 2002; Marquis et al., 2002). Up to 50% of elderly fallers are unable to get up after a fall, not only due to injury, but more commonly due to physical frailty and proximal muscle weakness (Tinetti, Wen-Liang and Claus, 1993). Patients who lie on the ground for a long time after a fall may develop dehydration, pressure sores, rhabdomyolysis, hypothermia or pneumonia, which eventually may cause death. Falling and fall-related injuries are also a prominent reason for nursing-home admission. Not surprisingly, quality of life among fallers is markedly impaired (Tinetti and Williams, 1997). Finally, gait disorders are associated with a reduced survival, due to a combination of fatal falls (e.g., an epidural haematoma following head trauma), reduced cardiovascular fitness and death from underlying disease (Wilson et al., 2002; Scarmeas et al., 2005). Falls also represent a major health problem for the public health system due to the immense costs associated with falls and the resultant injuries.

Therapeutics of Parkinson's Disease and Other Movement Disorders   Edited by Mark Hallett and Werner Poewe
© 2008 John Wiley & Sons, Ltd.

Table 28.1 Negative consequences of gait and balance disorders.

- Falls and near-falls
- Fall-related injuries
- Fear of falling
- Reduced mobility
  o Loss of independence
  o Social isolation
  o Osteoporosis

- Inability to rise after a fall
- Impaired quality of life
- Nursing home admission
- Reduced survival
  o Fatal falls
  o Reduced cardiovascular fitness
  o Death from underlying disease

- Financial burden for the public health system

Proper recognition of these aspects serves as a basis for individualized treatment, tailored to specific problems in individual patients.

PATHOPHYSIOLOGY

The pathophysiology of axial mobility deficits is complex, and a detailed discussion of the many contributing factors is beyond the scope of this chapter. Note that gait disorders, balance impairment and the resultant falls typically have a multi-factorial pathophysiology, where multiple risk factors jointly contribute in each individual patient. The clinical work-up should therefore not stop when a single risk factor or contributing disease has been identified.

In order to plan an optimal treatment strategy, it is essential to scrutinize four main components: "extrinsic" factors (situated in the environment, such as poor lighting in the house); "intrinsic" (patient-related) factors; compensatory strategies and specific protective factors (Table 28.2).

Inappropriate footwear (high heels, slippery soles or loosely fitting shoes) is an example of a common, but frequently overlooked, extrinsic factor. Domestic hazards are also important. For example, pets (dogs or cats) are notorious sources of stumbling in the household (Pluijm *et al.*, 2006).

Intrinsic risk factors include, not only the presence of a wide range of neurological disorders, but also the use of drugs, alcohol or both. Medication is a prominent risk factor for falls and hip fractures, due to a combination of sedation, cognitive impairment, carotid sinus syndrome, orthostatic hypotension, urinary incontinence, behavioral abnormalities, extrapyramidal side effects, ataxia and muscle weakness. Particularly notorious are benzodiazepines or anti-depressants, recent initiation of new medication and

Table 28.2 The four main components of the pathophysiology underlying gait impairment, postural instability and falls.

Component	Example of intervention
1. *Extrinsic factors (situated in the environment)*	
• Poor lighting in the house	Home visit by occupational therapist
2. *Intrinsic factors (related directly to the patient)*	
• Polypharmacy	Reduce number of drugs
3. *Compensatory strategies*	
• Beneficial, for example, gait slowing	Promote and incorporate into therapeutic approach
• Maladaptive	Discourage and train alternative strategies
4. *Protective factors (see also Table 28.4)*	
• Use of walking aids	Choose proper device and train its use

The list of items in each component is long, and this table merely provides a few examples to illustrate how a systemic work-up can lead to a multi-factorial therapeutic intervention.

polypharmacy (if a patient daily takes at least one drug with an established risk of increasing falls) (Ensrud *et al.*, 2002; Ziere *et al.*, 2006). Neuroleptics, anti-hypertensive medication and anti-arrhythmics also increase the risk of falls.

It is important to ascertain the patients' abilities to adapt to their deficits and the environment, for several reasons. First, part of the signs observed in patients could reflect compensatory adaptation that may help to reduce the risk of falls. For example, gait slowing could be a sign of underlying disease (e.g., bradykinesia in Parkinson patients), but may also represent a purposeful strategy to reduce the risk of tripping and falling. Such strategies should be stimulated as part of the therapeutic approach. But other strategies may be maladaptive and should be discouraged. In this respect, it is necessary to search for cognitive dysfunction, as this may impede the subject's ability to adjust for their impairments. The role of cognition becomes obvious when people perform multiple actions simultaneously, or need to quickly shift attention from one task to another. To perform such actions, cognitive abilities are needed to effectively monitor the environment, choose flexible response patterns to appearing threats and to make appropriate motor responses. Frontal executive functions are particularly important for maintaining walking stability (Hausdorff *et al.*, 2005; Springer *et al.*, 2006). Falls are therefore common in subjects with both motor deficits and concurrent cognitive decline (Bloem *et al.*, 2004a), perhaps because gait and balance are affected from both the cognitive and motor end of the control spectrum. For example, compared to cognitively normal elderly fallers, elderly patients with dementia have a twofold higher rate of falls, sustain more fractures and have a reduced life expectancy (Shaw and Kenny, 1998; Shaw, 2002). This may also explain why demented patients are vulnerable to dual task performance while walking or maintaining balance (Sheridan et al., 2003; Camicioli et al., 1997). The range of "mixed" disorders is broad: progressive supranuclear palsy, dementia with Lewy bodies, normal pressure hydrocephalus, Huntington's disease, to mention but a few. Even lesions in "subcortical" structures, such as the cerebellum may lead to cognitive impairment (Schmahmann and Sherman, 1998). Adverse effects on cognition may also explain the high incidence of falls and injuries in subjects taking psychoactive medication (Leipzig, Cumming and Tinetti, 1999). A specific concern includes patients who—despite a sometimes severe balance or gait deficit—are overly confident, causing a degree of recklessness. Such "motor recklessness" can be found in, for example, patients with progressive supranuclear palsy and is associated with a high incidence of falls and injuries, typically including fractures of long pipe bones and head traumas (Bloem et al., 2004a). Note that identifying cognitive impairment is important when planning therapeutic interventions, as the chances of successful rehabilitation are less in patients with cognitive impairment (Friedman, Baskett and Richmond, 1989; Oude Voshaar et al., 2006).

ASSESSMENT OF GAIT AND BALANCE

Determining the optimal treatment strategy and evaluating the outcome requires a careful clinical assessment. This is not always straightforward in clinical practice where a wide variety of available tests are available. Test execution and scoring is inconsistent across different physicians, and essential clinimetric properties (such as sensitivity, specificity or responsiveness) are insufficiently known. For example, all prospective, controlled, double-blind studies which assessed gait disturbances in PD used the Unified Parkinson's Disease Rating Scale (UPDRS) as the outcome measure. However, the gait sub-scale of the UPDRS, which involves subjective report by the patient (Part 2) and objective impression by the examiner (Part 3), has never been validated for the independent assessment of gait. Another example is ascertainment of falls, which is usually done retrospectively (hence subject to recall problems) and not based on prospectively completed diaries. As a result, there are no good data about the effect of drugs on the risk of falling.

A considerable problem is the assessment of patients who suffer from "episodic" gait disturbances. These are easily missed in the office, but represent notorious causes of falls, because the episodic nature makes it difficult for patients to adapt their walking behavior (Snijders et al., 2007). One striking example is freezing of gait (FOG) in parkinsonian disorders, which is often suppressed by the anxiety associated with a doctor's visit. The only validated tool to assess FOG is the FOG Questionnaire, which is subjective and based on the patient's perception (Giladi et al., 2000). The questionnaire has been used in prospective, double-blind, placebo-controlled drug studies, where FOG severity was the primary outcome (Gurevich et al., 2007). An improved version is underway, featuring, among others, a video with characteristic freezing episodes as a tool to enhance the patient's and their carer's understanding of what FOG really is (Nieuwboer et al., 2006). Another semi-objective assessment of FOG severity is based on video segments that can be assessed blindly by unbiased, blinded observers (Schaafsma et al., 2003a). Such a method can effectively assess short-term interventions like the effect of levodopa or apomorphine, but not a long-term effect on daily activities or general mobility.

In clinical practice, it is best to use a battery of complementary tests, with emphasis on functional everyday tasks, such as rising from a chair or turning while walking. Use of validated rating scales such as the Berg Balance Scale or Tinetti Mobility Index helps to systematically score several relevant domains. A pragmatic gait classification system has recently been proposed that can serve as a basis to plan further tailored treatment (Snijders et al., 2007). Various quantitative electrophysiological techniques are available to study gait and balance in more detail. Commonly used tools are ambulatory goniometers or accelerometers—to quantify movement of the limbs or trunk (Allum and Carpenter, 2005)—and shoes with pressure-sensitive insoles (Hausdorff, Rios and Edelberg, 2001; Plotnik et al., 2005) or a carpet with pressure sensitive sensors (Nelson et al., 2002)—to measure subtle changes in locomotion rhythmicity, variability or left–right synchronization. It remains unclear whether the currently available equipment can support clinical decision-making in individual patients. Possible exceptions include detailed EMG studies in spastic or dystonic patients to fine-tune treatments with, for example, botulinum toxin; and kinematic gait analyses to assist rehabilitation specialists in choosing specific segmental orthoses or adjusted footwear (Carlson et al., 1997; Buurke et al., 2005; Minns, 2005; den Otter et al., 2007).

GENERIC VS DISEASE-SPECIFIC TREATMENT STRATEGIES

Treatment of axial mobility deficits consists of two complementary approaches: generic strategies that are common to all patients, irrespective of the underlying disorder

(Table 28.3); and disease-specific interventions tailored to the specific pathophysiology of the underlying condition. The generic strategy typically includes a multi-disciplinary and multi-factorial approach, often aimed at eliminating generic risk factors (e.g., sedative medication or domestic hazards) and providing support. Disease-specific strategies usually include a combination of pharmacotherapy and surgery, sometimes supported by specific physiotherapeutic interventions (e.g., external cueing for gait disorders in PD). Several disease-specific treatments have already been covered in the preceding chapters. Here, we will highlight some therapies that are specifically aimed at improving gait or balance. This will be done for patients with parkinsonism or spasticity. Note that this field is generally characterized by a lack of good randomized, controlled trials, so the emphasis will mainly be placed on a pragmatic approach for use in clinical practice.

GENERIC TREATMENT STRATEGIES

Prevention of Falls

Optimal prevention calls for a reliable strategy to identify subjects at risk of falling, but this proves difficult, particularly identifying potential fallers before they have sustained their very first fall. The best predictor for falls appears to be the presence of prior falls, which is somewhat unsatisfactory, because subjects are already falling before prevention is initiated. Asking about fear of falling may have some potential as an early predictor of falling (Pickering *et al.*, 2007). The cumulative number of concurrent risk factors is also important, preventive strategies being warranted in persons who have two or more risk factors for falls (Nevitt *et al.*, 1989; Tinetti, 2003; Tinetti, Speechley and Ginter, 1988; Campbell, Borrie and Spears, 1989).

Prevention of falls and injuries can take place at three different levels. Primary prevention focuses on elderly people who have not yet fallen, and aims to eliminate risk factors that are common in the elderly, such as osteoporosis or use of psychoactive drugs. Tackling risk factors that are only weakly associated with falls may still be rewarding if they are sufficiently prevalent in the general population. Patients may have to be actively recruited for such a fall-prevention program, as a recent study showed that PD patients in the United States adhered poorly to an annual fall-prevention program (Swarztrauber, Graf and Cheng, 2006). Secondary prevention focuses on elderly patients who have fallen at least once and aims to avoid recurrent falls. Here, the emphasis is on treatment of specific underlying disorders and eliminating intrinsic or extrinsic risk factors that are strongly associated with falls (Tinetti, 2003; Boers *et al.*, 2001; Kannus *et al.*, 2005). The proposed interventions should be practical and easy to implement, and this calls for optimal co-operation with the patient and

Table 28.3 Summary of generic treatment strategies for gait, balance and falls.

- Optimize medication
  - Withdraw drugs
    - Psychoactive drugs (mainly benzodiazepines and anti- depressants)
    - Cardiovascular drugs
    - Avoid polypharmacy
    - Avoid daily alcohol use
  - Specific treatments
    - Analgesics (for antalgic gait)
    - Anxiolytics (for excessive fear)
    - Others (see specific chapters)
  - Secondary prevention (cardiovascular prophylaxis)
    - Anti-hypertensive
    - Anti-platelet agents
- Physiotherapy
  - Gait or balance training
  - Extrapolation to demanding (complex) conditions
  - Exercise therapy
  - Balance confidence training (but no proven efficacy to date)
  - Training use of walking aids
- Occupational therapy
  - Integrating acquired basic skills into relevant personal activities
  - Advice with regard to transport
  - Behavioral adaptations (at home, or at work)
  - Eliminating domestic hazards for falls[a]
  - Installing handrails (e.g., in toilet or bathroom)
- Treadmill training
  - Independent walking
  - With body weight support
  - With robotic support
- Technical aids
  - Orthoses
    - Ankle-foot orthosis
    - knee-ankle-foot orthosis
  - Functional electric stimulation
  - Proper (orthopedic) footwear
- Virtual reality training
- Mental imagery training

These strategies can be applied to all patients, irrespective of the specific underlying disorder.
[a] Only effective when delivered as part of a multi-factorial intervention.

family, who should receive both verbal and written information on the preventive measures. Tertiary prevention concerns measures that benefit elderly patients who frequently fall, who have sustained recurrent injuries and have risk factors for falls that are only just amenable to secondary prevention. This includes frail elderly patients in nursing homes, those with dementia and patients with severe sensorimotor disabilities.

Details of specific interventions will be described below. Note that we will restrict ourselves to falls *without* preceding loss of consciousness, because falls caused by syncope represent a completely different category, with its own specific treatment (Bloem *et al.*, 2004b; Voermans *et al.*, 2007).

Drugs

The best intervention is usually to withdraw medication, particularly psychoactive drugs (mainly benzodiazepines and anti-depressants) or cardiovascular drugs, and to avoid polypharmacy. For example, in patients with PD who already have a considerably increased risk of falling, use of psychotropic drugs must be avoided because this further increases the risk of falls by about fivefold (Bloem *et al.*, 2001). The pharmacist can play an active role in preventing falls. A recent randomized, controlled trial showed that when a pharmacist reduced the number of drugs in elderly care home residents, the number of falls was reduced by 40% (Keller and Slattum, 2003). Another "drug" that should be targeted is alcohol, because daily alcohol increases the falling risk (Gray and Hildebrand, 2000).

Depending on the underlying gait disorder, specific drugs may be beneficial, sometimes with dramatic improvements of gait. For example, analgesics can improve antalgic gait, while anxiolytics can be used judiciously in patients with excessive fear. Disease-specific drug treatments can be found in the preceding chapters, such as the use of anti-cholinergics or botulinum toxin injections for the treatment of dystonia.

Secondary prevention of gait disorders includes evaluation of cardiovascular risk factors, especially for patients with spastic gait after stroke, hypokinetic-rigid gait due to vascular disease and cautious gait. For example, patients with treated hypertension have less white matter lesions than untreated patients (de Leeuw *et al.*, 2002). Prophylactic treatment with anti-platelet agents should be considered in gait disorders based on hypoxic-ischemic disease. However, the efficacy and cost-efficiency of these interventions have not been demonstrated in elderly patients.

Surgery

There are no generic surgical treatments for gait, but we will discuss three examples where surgery can be considered for

specific gait disorders that are not discussed elsewhere in this chapter. The relatively high operation risks must always be weighed against the expected benefits, certainly in elderly patients. For mild to moderate cervical spondylotic myelopathy, decompressive surgery is no better than conservative treatment (Kadanka *et al.*, 2000; Fouyas, Statham and Sandercock, 2002). Recent findings suggest that dystonic gait can respond to bilateral stimulation of the internal globus pallidus, sometimes producing a spectacular improvement (Krack and Vercueil, 2001), but well-controlled studies are needed to further delineate the merits of this intervention. Finally, for patients with normal pressure hydrocephalus, most clinicians would currently exclude patients with prominent white matter lesions from ventricular shunting. Although some patients improve dramatically after ventricular shunt placement, the most difficult aspect is to select those patients who will benefit most. Several predictors have been proposed, ranging from a diagnostic lumbar puncture (tapping cerebrospinal fluid to evaluate the effect of lowering pressure) to magnetic resonance spectroscopy of N-acetyl aspartate (Shiino *et al.*, 2004; Relkin *et al.*, 2005). No single test has adequate predictive ability, although ancillary testing can increase the predictive accuracy for prognosis to greater than 90% (Marmarou *et al.*, 2005). Measuring the success of treatment is hampered by the lack of a standard for outcome assessment of shunt treatment (Klinge *et al.*, 2005). Improvements are usually temporary, lasting, at best, several years. Cognitive problems tend to be refractory to treatment (Bloem *et al.*, 2005), hence patients with severe cognitive decline are usually excluded from surgery.

Physiotherapy

Several neurologically oriented training methods have been advocated based on theoretical grounds, but the literature has failed to show the superiority of any one particular method over another (Pollock *et al.*, 2007; van Peppen *et al.*, 2007). In fact, it appears that many different methods are potentially effective, as long as they comply with several generic training and learning principles. Thus, studies that addressed the effectiveness of physiotherapy in different central neurological diseases have consistently yielded two important prerequisites for efficacy, irrespective of the stage of rehabilitation.

First, training effects greatly depend on the intensity, both in terms of frequency and duration (van Peppen *et al.*, 2007; Kwakkel, 2006). Second, the effects of training are highly task-specific (van Peppen *et al.*, 2007; French *et al.*, 2007; Macko, Ivey and Forrester, 2005), which implies that physiotherapy should be targeted at individually relevant activities in a meaningful environment. Task-specificity is consistent with the principle of "ecological validity," which is well known from theories of motor learning (Mulder and

Hochstenbach, 2001). Based on these theories, balance and gait training should also adhere to another principle, namely that it should incorporate sufficient "variability of practice." Because daily life activities are never performed in exactly the same way and under the same environmental circumstances, relevant activities should be pursued under various mechanical, visual and cognitive constraints. In other words, it is not sufficient to regain normal level walking skills under optimal conditions. Instead, standing and walking should also be trained under demanding complex conditions, such as reduced vision, while performing a secondary task, while negotiating obstacles or when exposed to a slippery surface (Mulder and Geurts, 1993). The emphasis should thus be placed on mastering independent and safe practical ambulation skills with sufficient speed and endurance, if necessary with the assistance of technical aids (Barbeau et al., 1998), allowing subjects to regain the more complex skills necessary to meet the demands of daily life. These principles of ecological validity and variability of practice are relevant for the training of complex balance and gait skills, as well as for the prevention of falls, as was demonstrated in a recent trial (Weerdesteyn et al., 2006).

Exercise therapy is a key element in the rehabilitation of balance and gait in patients with central neurological disorders. Exercise focuses primarily on improving muscle force, coordination and endurance to restore basic balance and gait skills, within biological limits. For example, augmented exercise therapy has a favorable effect on gait speed and activities of daily living in stroke patients (Kwakkel et al., 2004). Exercise also helps to counter the many risks that are associated with sedentary lifestyle. A scientific statement of the American Heart Association underscored that a sedentary lifestyle is one of the leading preventable causes of death, and that an inverse linear relationship exists between volume of physical activity and all-cause mortality (Marcus et al., 2006). Participation in regular physical activity is highly desirable, as a tool to prevent complications of immobility (decreased risk of cardiovascular disease, type 2 diabetes mellitus, osteoporosis, depression, obesity, breast cancer and colon cancer) and mortality (Hakim et al., 1998; Manson et al., 2002; Marcus et al., 2006; Bloem, van Vugt and Beckley, 2001). Moreover, physical activity can positively influence sleep disturbances and constipation, and postpone or reduce depression (Dunn et al., 2005; Regan et al., 2005). Importantly, even moderate exercise can slow cognitive decline (van Gelder et al., 2004; Yaffe et al., 2001) and postpone dementia (Larson et al., 2006; Laurin et al., 2001), but there is a dose–response relationship: people who walk longer distances have a greater protective effect on cognitive decline (Weuve et al., 2004; Abbott et al., 2004). Interestingly, animal studies suggest that physical activity might slow down disease progression in disorders such as PD

(Tillerson et al., 2003; Steiner et al., 2006), but whether such disease-modifying effects can be extended to humans remains to be determined.

Finally, it is felt that physiotherapists could deliver balance confidence training and thereby reduce the fear of falling (Tennstedt et al., 1998; Hauer et al., 2001). Fear of falling can be substantial in patients with severe balance impairment, and the resultant restriction of mobility is sometimes beneficial as it can serve as an adequate tertiary preventive measure. However, for many patients, the fear is disproportional to the actual degree of balance impairment and risk of falls. Reduction of fear and regaining confidence is important for these persons, as it helps restore mobility and promotes independence. Group treatment using a behavioral-cognitive approach aimed to change attitudes as well as training with a physical therapist might be helpful (Rucker et al., 2006). However, these effects diminish as patients become more frail (Faber et al., 2006). Moreover, two recent studies failed to show a beneficial effect of post-fall counseling (Rucker et al., 2006) or exercise (Arai et al., 2007) on fear and balance confidence, perhaps because participants were not fearful enough at baseline.

Occupational Therapy

Occupational therapists (OTs) often operate in concert with physiotherapists to achieve similar goals, albeit through different means. The OT can help the patient to integrate acquired basic skills into relevant personal activities that require "parallel" information processing, for example, by proposing and training feasible action plans. OTs can also advise the patient with regard to transport or domestic and occupational behavioral adaptations, to prevent secondary complications such as falls.

Asking the OT to eliminate domestic hazards is theoretically attractive because most falls occur indoors. For example, proper lighting should be installed for people who frequently fall during night-time visits to the toilet. A potty chair next to the bed or a condom catheter in men obviates the need for a risky nightly travel to the toilet. Home visits seemed effective when delivered as part of a multi-factorial intervention to those with an increased risk of falls (Gillespie et al., 2004). Individual patients with obvious extrinsic falls are most likely to benefit. However, this strategy proved ineffective when delivered in isolation (van Haastregt et al., 2000a, 2000b; Day et al., 2002; Stevens et al., 2001), presumably because only a minority of falls can be ascribed solely to environmental factors. Another explanation is that even intensive programs delivered by dedicated health professionals achieve only modest reductions in the prevalence of targeted hazards (Day et al., 2002; Stevens et al., 2001). Compliance of elderly persons is often disappointing, simply because many refuse to adapt their homes. Therefore, patients need to agree to any proposed preventive measure (Cumming *et al.*, 2001). Another aspect is that home visits are generally costly and time consuming (Robertson *et al.*, 2001).

Treadmill Training

Treadmill training is an effective means to intensify gait rehabilitation. Patients with independent-level walking skills may profit from treadmill training by increasing their walking speed and walking distance (or endurance). For example, treadmill training results in reduction of falls and improvement of gait in patients with PD (Protas *et al.*, 2005). A drawback of treadmill training is its limited ecological validity and the fact that it allows almost no variability of practice. As such, it cannot replace dynamic balance and gait exercises under real-life circumstances. However, treadmill walking creates two important training possibilities for patients with poor balance and gait skills.

First, it permits application of body weight support (BWS) during gait training in patients with insufficient weight-bearing capacity or poor dynamic balance. Patients can be supported by a parachute harness attached to the ceiling with a spring, which can give way in the direction of walking. BWS can range from 0 to 30–40% (Hesse *et al.*, 2001). During walking, one or two physiotherapists can facilitate movements of the legs, depending on the level of voluntary control and muscle tone. Gradually, in the course of rehabilitation, the amount of manual assistance is decreased, as is the amount of BWS, in order to achieve independent walking. Although the advantage of body-weight supported treadmill training has not been unambiguously demonstrated (Moseley *et al.*, 2005), clinical experience suggests that it may constitute a pivoting point in the rehabilitation of patients that are not able to walk without BWS.

Second, treadmill training can be combined with a gait robot that imposes external forces on the body to support rhythmic leg movements (Figure 28.1). Using such robots, the intensity of (body-weight supported) treadmill training can easily be enhanced, because the strenuous manual facilitation by therapists is no longer necessary (Mayr *et al.*, 2007). More importantly, modern robots that are currently being developed can sense forces generated by the subject and adjust their imposed movements accordingly (Veneman *et al.*, 2007). Gait training can thus be programmed towards specific body segments, depending on the stage of rehabilitation (e.g., initially at hip movements, whereas knee and ankle movements are targeted in a later phase). A recent Cochrane Review concluded that stroke patients who receive electromechanical-assisted gait training in combination with physiotherapy are more likely to achieve independent walking than patients receiving gait training without these devices (Mehrholz *et al.*, 2007).

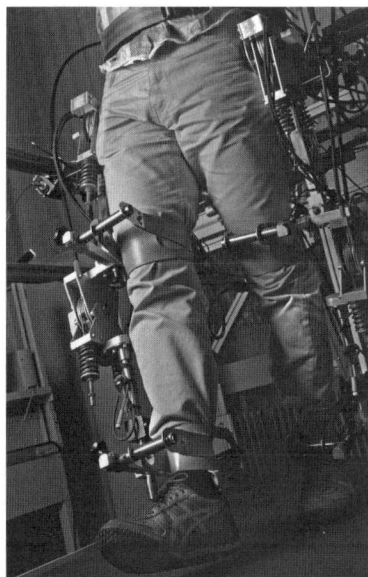

Figure 28.1 Recently developed gait robots, such as the LOwer extremity Powered ExoSkeleton (LOPES), sense the forces generated by the subject and adjust their imposed forces accordingly. In this way, training programs can be administered taking optimal account of the individual functional capacities of the subject. Figure provided courtesy of G. van Ouwerkerk (CTW, University of Twente) and the manufacturers (Dept. of Biomechanical Engineering, Faculty of Engineering Technology, University of Twente, The Netherlands)

Walking Aids

Evaluating the use of walking aids deserves specific attention. Many elderly patients do not use walking aids, either because they are not recommended to do so, or because they are too ashamed to revert to walking aids. However, if patients are instructed accurately, they are often pleased with their regained confidence, mobility and independence. Walking aids should always be prescribed with caution, because they never provide sufficient compensation for involuntary motions or recklessness, for example, in patients suffering from festination, impulsive behavior, or situational misjudgments. Indeed, incorrect use of walking aids can increase the risk of falling (Bateni and Maki, 2005).

A cane or quad cane is the simplest walking aid for patients with dynamic balance problems in the frontal plane. When normal weight-shifting strategies can no longer be applied safely, loss of lateral balance and subsequent lateral falls can be prevented using a cane on the ipsilateral side. When balance problems are predominantly present in the sagittal plane, a walker is the first-choice option. Sufficient bilateral dexterity is, however, necessary to adequately utilize a walker, although individual adaptations for one-handed patients are possible.

Other Technical Aids

Many patients with central neurological disease eventually develop persistent instability of the hip, knee or ankle, limiting their capacity to walk safely. For these patients, technical aids can make a difference between dependency and independency, in particular with regard to outdoor ambulation. Insufficient foot elevation ("foot drop") is often associated with loss of active foot eversion and is the most common abnormality observed in patients with hemiparesis, for example due to stroke (Perry, Waters and Perrin, 1978). However, foot drop is also frequently observed in patients with PD or dystonia of the lower leg, and of course in patients with peroneal neuropathy or L4-5 radiculopathy. In patients with foot drop due to central neurological disease, weakness of ankle dorsiflexion and eversion often coincides with a tendency towards pes equinovarus due to increased muscle tone and decreased muscle length of the ankle plantarflexors and invertors (Perry, Waters and Perrin, 1978; Mauritz, 2002). As a result, foot support and ankle stability are compromised during the stance phase of gait, while foot drop during the swing phase imposes an increased risk of tripping. To compensate for these deficiencies, an ankle-foot orthosis (AFO) can be prescribed (Figure 28.2). Generally, two types of AFO are available: (i) those that can be worn in a normal shoe, which are commonly made of polypropylene or carbon and are non-articulated; and (ii) hinged, metal AFOs that are permanently attached to the outside of the shoe and consist of one or two metal bars with an articulation at ankle level. In patients with structural ankle-foot deformities or with spastic dystonia about the ankle joint, a high orthopedic shoe with an integrated ankle-foot socket may be preferred.

Rarely, a knee-ankle-foot orthosis (KAFO) is required, for example in patients with insufficient quadriceps strength during loading, or in patients with a symptomatic knee hyperextension thrust during the stance phase (Kakurai and Akai, 1996). In such cases, a lightweight KAFO can be prescribed, preferably with an automatic knee lock during late swing/initial contact and a release during pre-swing. Hip instability is usually due to weak hip abductors and rather common in patients with hemiparesis. It is reflected in the frontal plane and can be compensated using a cane at the non-paretic side. By taking weight onto the cane with the non-paretic arm during weight bearing on the paretic leg, pelvic drop and compensatory trunk lateroflexion can be prevented.

In selected patients, motor deficits may be overcome by functional electrical stimulation (FES). Although many

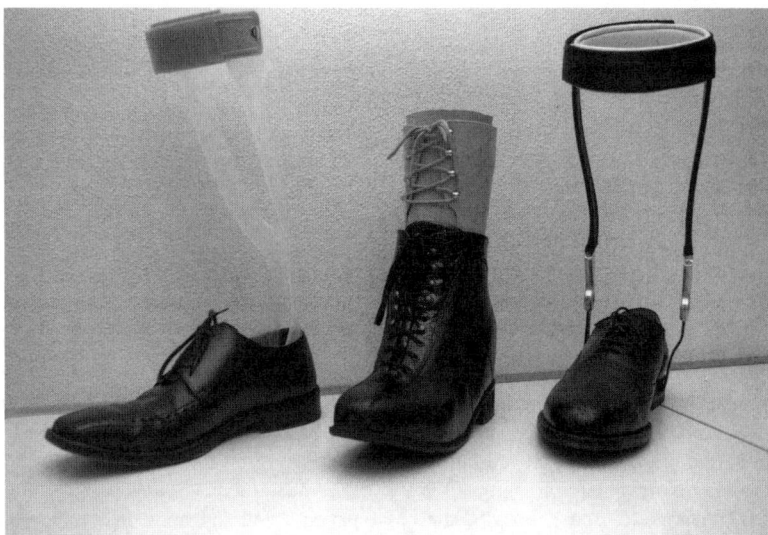

Figure 28.2 Three types of ankle-foot orthosis (AFO): on the left side a polypropylene, non-articulated AFO inserted in a normal shoe, in the middle an ankle-foot socket integrated in an orthopedic (made-to-measure) shoe, and on the right side a metal (double-bar), articulated AFO attached to the outsole of a normal shoe. Figures provided courtesy of OIM Orthopedics, The Netherlands.

types of FES have been advocated for patients with a variety of central neurological disorders (Stein, 1999; Sweeney, Lyons and Veltink, 2000; Kottink et al., 2004), clinical application remains limited due to practical and technical problems. The type of FES for which most problems have been solved is currently undergoing revival, that is, stimulation of the (common) peroneal nerve triggered by heel rise and heel strike during walking (Figure 28.3). Recently, both external and implantable wireless systems for peroneal FES have yielded promising functional results (Kottink et al., 2007; Burridge et al., 2007; Sheffler et al., 2006). Clinical experience shows that peroneal FES not only causes foot elevation, but also facilitates the whole movement of the swing leg in patients with moderate degrees of "stiff knee gait," thus improving step adjustments and obstacle avoidance (Daly et al., 2006). In addition, compared to AFOs, peroneal FES allows better execution of ankle strategies during the stance phase of gait, thereby permitting more normal dynamic balance reactions. Although primarily developed for patients with stroke, peroneal FES is likely also effective for other well-selected patients with disorders such as multiple sclerosis or partial spinal cord lesions.

Other advice relates to footwear. Proper ready-made footwear with sturdy soles can be recommended to reduce the number of falls. In addition, slightly raised heels may help to reduce retropulsion. For patients with foot deformities or a tendency towards varus or valgus deviation or instability at the ankle, custom-made orthopedic footwear should be recommended for recreating an adequate base of support and for providing sufficient ankle stability. When doing so, it is important that useful ankle mobility is preserved as much as possible in order to allow ankle strategies and foot roll-off while standing and walking.

Other Rehabilitation Techniques

Virtual reality (VR) is a promising, computer-assisted method in rehabilitation to improve motor function (You et al., 2005). In general, subjects with locomotor disabilities appear capable of motor learning in VR environments with reasonable transfer of learned capabilities to real-world equivalent motor tasks (Holden, 2005). Recent functional MRI findings suggest that VR can induce cortical reorganization from aberrant ipsilateral to contralateral activation of the supplementary motor cortex in chronic stroke patients. This enhanced cortical reorganization might play an important role in the recovery of locomotor function in these patients (You et al., 2005).

An encouraging new method in neurorehabilitation is the use of mental imagery (MI) (Jackson et al., 2001; Mulder, 2007). Recent studies indicate that MI may promote the relearning of both trained and untrained daily life tasks in stroke patients (Daly et al., 2006; de and Mulder, 2007; Liu et al., 2004; Krakauer, 2006). For locomotor training after

stroke, promising case studies have been reported (Dunsky et al., 2006). In addition, a randomized, controlled trial has shown that mirror therapy combined with conventional stroke rehabilitation may enhance lower-extremity motor recovery in sub-acute stroke patients (Sutbeyaz et al., 2007). Overall, evidence for the efficacy of both VR and MI on walking ability in stroke patients has yet to be strengthened.

Protective Measures

When gait and balance problems become difficult to treat and falls can no longer be prevented, the priority shifts towards prevention of secondary consequences, such as avoiding injuries. Several protective measures are available (Table 28.4). Wearing special hip protectors sewn into undergarments were initially thought to reduce hip fractures (Kannus et al., 2000), but recent work suggests that currently used designs are not very effective, even among patients with good compliance (which is in itself often problematic and further reduces the clinical utility of hip protectors) (Kiel et al., 2007). Other patient-worn protective devices include wrist protectors or helmets. An alternative for indoor falls is the use of shock-absorbing floors, and the use of handrails in toilets and bathrooms.

Patients must be asked about their self-confidence in performing everyday activities. Excessive fear leads to unnecessary immobilization, but patients who are overly confident (possibly due to co-existent cognitive deficits) are at risk of falls due to hazardous behavior. In the latter group, the benefit of restricting the patient's activities (which may help to reduce falls) must be weighed against the loss of mobility and independence. In nursing homes, restriction of unsupervised activities should not be routinely prescribed, but must be restricted as a last resort treatment in patients with severe cognitive impairment, extreme recklessness or frequent wandering due to disorders such as progressive supranuclear palsy or Alzheimer's disease (Bloem et al., 2005; Capezuti et al., 1996; Buchner and Larson, 1987; Sullivan-Marx et al., 1999).

Osteoporosis is a risk factor for fractures, and can be treated in various ways (Sato et al., 1999). Promoting physical activity has a beneficial effect on bone mineral density and reduces the risk of hip fractures (Grahn Kronhed et al., 2006). Use of the pro-vitamin 1α-hydroxyvitamin D3, calcium supplementation, risedronate and alendronate/raloxifene arrests progression of osteoporosis and reduces hip fractures (Close, Neuprez and Reginster, 2006; Sato, Honda and Iwamoto, 2007).

Multi-disciplinary Rehabilitation

Optimal rehabilitation of axial mobility deficits is really a multi-disciplinary concern, and multi-faceted interventions

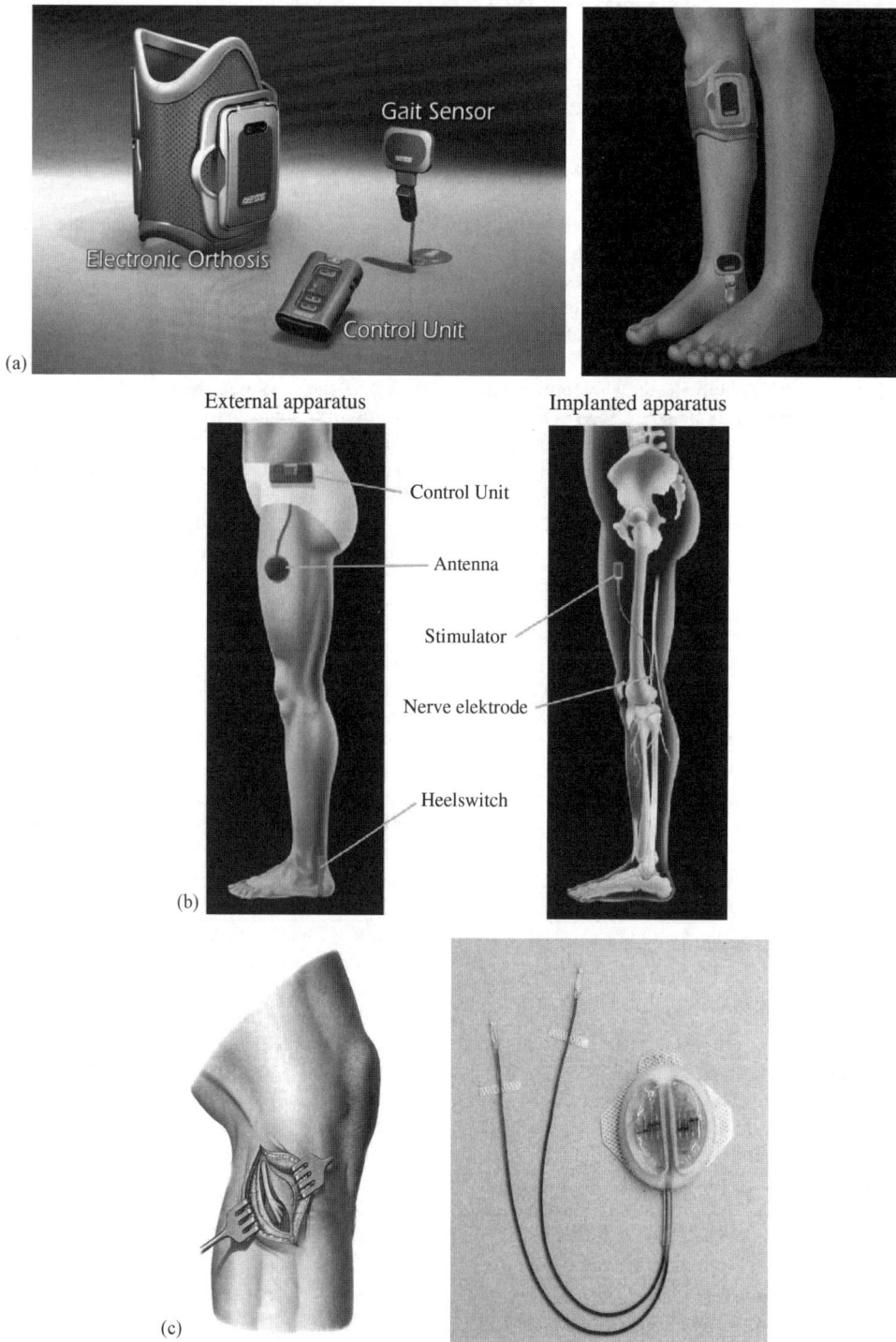

Figure 28.3 Three commercially available systems for functional electrical stimulation (FES) of the peroneal nerve: (a) The L300 system (TM by Ness) provides external stimulation of the common peroneal nerve and the anterior tibial muscle through two skin electrodes; (b) The ActiGait system (TM by Otto Bock) provides direct stimulation of the common peroneal nerve through a four-channel cuff electrode; (c) The StimuStep system (TM by Finetech-Medical) stimulates the superficial and deep peroneal nerves separately, through two epineural electrodes. Each system has its specific characteristics and (dis) advantages that need to be further elucidated through clinical trials and long-term follow-up studies.

Table 28.4 Tertiary measures to prevent the complications of falls.

Consequence of falls	Potential intervention
Hip fractures	• Protective hip pads[a] • Shock-absorbent carpets
Other injuries	• Wrist pads • Protective helmets
Osteoporosis	• Promoting physical activity • Drug treatment (1α-hydrosyvitamin D3, calcium suppletion, risedronate, alendronate/raloxifene)
Immobility/reduced fitness	• Promote physical exercise • Physiotherapy
Inability to stand up after falling	• Electronic warning system around the neck or wrist
Disproportional fear of falling	• Group treatment using behavioral-cognitive therapy[b] • Physiotherapy to regain confidence
Recklessness in cognitively impaired patients	• Restrain activities if untreatable dangerous behavior

[a] Not very effective, according to latest evidence.
[b] No beneficial effect shown in recent trials, at least not among patients with low baseline levels of fear.

are more effective than single therapeutic measures (Tinetti, 2003; American Geriatrics Society, 2001). Even patients with cognitive impairment can benefit, but injuries are more difficult to prevent than falls themselves (Oliver *et al.*, 2007). The overall goal is to extend elementary balance and gait training to rehabilitation of complex activities of daily living, for example related to self-care, household activities or going outdoors. The multi-disciplinary team should include medical specialists (a neurologist, a rehabilitation specialist, and—for older people with complex co-morbidity—a geriatrician), a physiotherapist, an occupational therapist and a specialized nurse. The physician is the primarily responsible for considering pharmacological or surgical interventions. During admission to a rehabilitation clinic, the rehabilitation nurse provides 24-hour supervision and care, and assists in the training of basic self-care activities. The neuropsychologist may assist the team in finding adequate cognitive strategies for improving ambulatory abilities in terms of action plans and executive functions, or with regard to facilitating

techniques such as mental imagery. In addition, the neuropsychologist can provide diagnostic information concerning cognitive and behavioral deficits.

DISEASE-SPECIFIC TREATMENT STRATEGIES

Parkinson's Disease

Treating gait and balance in PD has two main objectives: (i) to improve mobility, gait speed and independency; and (ii) to reduce postural instability and decrease the risk of falling. These two treatment goals are interconnected and will therefore be discussed together, even though some drugs might have a more specific effect on postural control and others on locomotion. A further reason for lumping both treatment goals is the lack of detailed research that has specifically examined how drugs influence locomotion or postural responses.

Pathophysiology and Classification of Parkinsonian Gait and Balance Disorders

Treatment should be tailored to the pathophysiology of parkinsonian gait and balance disorders. Comprehensive reviews have been published (Bloem *et al.*, 2004c; Morris, 2000; Nutt, Hammerstad and Gancher, 1992; Giladi, Bloem and Hausdorff, 2007), and we will only highlight several key aspects here. Many factors play a role in the development and worsening of gait and balance disturbances in parkinsonism (Table 28.5). When examining a patient, the neurologist would mark the most significant gait disturbance and aim to treat this problem specifically. For example, a different approach should be taken to improve gait problems associated with fear, cognitive decline, misjudgment, dysexecutive syndrome, distractibility or difficulties with dual tasking. Also, beneficial effects on one domain of gait or balance may be countered by adverse effects in other domains. For example, treating bradykinesia and rigidity with levodopa might have also disadvantages due to cognitive or autonomic side effects.

Of particular importance is the relation to the underlying patterns of neurodegeneration and the resultant neurochemical changes. Three main groups of symptoms can be identified (Figure 28.4). First, gait impairment and postural instability may partially reflect the progressive loss of dopamine-producing cells in the substantia nigra. One compelling argument to support this is the fact that patients with "selective" hypodopaminergic syndromes such as MPTP-induced parkinsonism can present with gait and balance abnormalities that are all characteristic for PD (Bloem and Roos, 1995). Second, non-dopaminergic lesions are likely to play a role in the pathophysiology, and

Table 28.5 Disease-specific risk factors that contribute to the pathophysiology of gait impairment, postural instability and falls in Parkinson's disease (PD).

- *Gait impairment*
  - o Reduced step height (creates stumbling risk)
  - o Freezing of gait
- *Stiffness*
  - o Muscle rigidity
  - o Intrinsic muscle changes
  - o Active co-contraction (caused by fear?)
- *Abnormal environmental perception*
  - o Impaired visual feedback due to oculomotor disturbances
  - o Incorrect central processing of visual information
  - o Decreased sensitivity of extensor load receptors
  - o Disturbed central processing of kinaesthetic feedback
- *Impaired automatic postural corrections*
  - o Abnormally large destabilizing responses
  - o Decreased and delayed stabilizing responses
  - o Impaired reflex gain control (postural "inflexibility")
- *Abnormal compensatory stepping movements*
  - o Slowed execution/akinesia
  - o Undersized steps
- *Abnormal protective arm movements*
  - o Improperly directed
  - o Undersized
  - o Absent (arms in pockets due to shame of tremor)
- *Abnormal voluntary postural corrections*
  - o Start problems (akinesia)
  - o Slowing (bradykinesia)
  - o Freezing
  - o Impaired anticipatory postural responses
- *Increased sway beyond limits of stability*
  - o Dyskinesias
  - o Trips due to shuffling gait
- *Reduced muscle strength*
- *Cognitive impairment*
  - o (Subcortical) dementia
  - o Medication-induced psychosis/hallucinations
- *Orthostatic* hypotension/*syncope*
  - o Disease-related (rare)
  - o Medication-induced

Note that "generic" risk factors for falls (e.g., benzodiazepines) can also contribute and aggravate the axial mobility problems, over and above the disease-specific effects of PD itself.

this is particularly true for postural instability and falls (Bonnet *et al.*, 1987; Koller *et al.*, 1989; Bloem *et al.*, 1996; Klawans, 1986). Indeed, both postural instability and non-dopaminergic lesions emerge (and thus coincide) in advanced PD. Furthermore, dynamic posturography studies suggest that several balance problems (mainly the reactive automatic postural responses) in PD are not primarily dopamine-dependent (Bloem *et al.*, 1996; Dietz, Berger and Horstmann, 1988; Horak, Frank and Nutt, 1996; Bloem *et al.*, 1994). In advanced stages of the disease, severe gait impairment and dopamine-resistant freezing of gait may be related to neurodegeneration within the pedunculopontine nucleus in the dorsal brain stem (Jellinger, 1991; Pahapill and Lozano, 2000; Zweig *et al.*, 1989), where step initiation and step maintenance are normally governed. Therefore, pharmacotherapy of gait and balance problems should ideally aim at correction of both dopaminergic and non-dopaminergic deficits. Third, some of the gait and balance problems in PD may in fact be caused by dopaminergic treatment. Adverse drug effects include freezing of gait during the ON state, dyskinesias or orthostatic hypotension (Bloem, van Vugt and Beckley, 2001; Giladi, Kao and Fahn, 1997). In such patients, reducing the dosage or number of anti-parkinson drugs may improve postural control.

Medical Treatment of Parkinsonian Gait and Balance Disorders

Pharmacotherapeutic options to treat gait impairment and postural instability in PD are summarized in Table 28.6.

Levodopa

Multiple studies using different assessment techniques after a single dose or long-term treatment have shown that levodopa improves walking velocity and the spatiotemporal gait parameters in PD (Bowes *et al.*, 1990; Blin *et al.*, 1991; O'Sullivan *et al.*, 1998; Krystkowiak *et al.*, 2003; Vokaer *et al.*, 2003; Lubik *et al.*, 2006). Furthermore, levodopa can improve gait rhythmicity, which is an accepted risk marker for future falls (Schaafsma *et al.*, 2003b). In contrast, clinical experience suggests that postural instability and falls respond poorly to treatment with dopaminergic drugs (Bonnet *et al.*, 1987; Bloem *et al.*, 1996; Klawans, 1986). Dopaminergic medication is also largely ineffective for other axial motor problems, such as turning in bed (Lakke, 1985; Narabayashi *et al.*, 1987). However, controlled experiments showed that some postural abnormalities can in fact partially improve with anti-parkinson medication, albeit usually not to normal levels (Bloem *et al.*, 1996; Beckley *et al.*, 1995; Burleigh-Jacobs *et al.*, 1997; Horak and Frank, 1996). Therefore, increasing

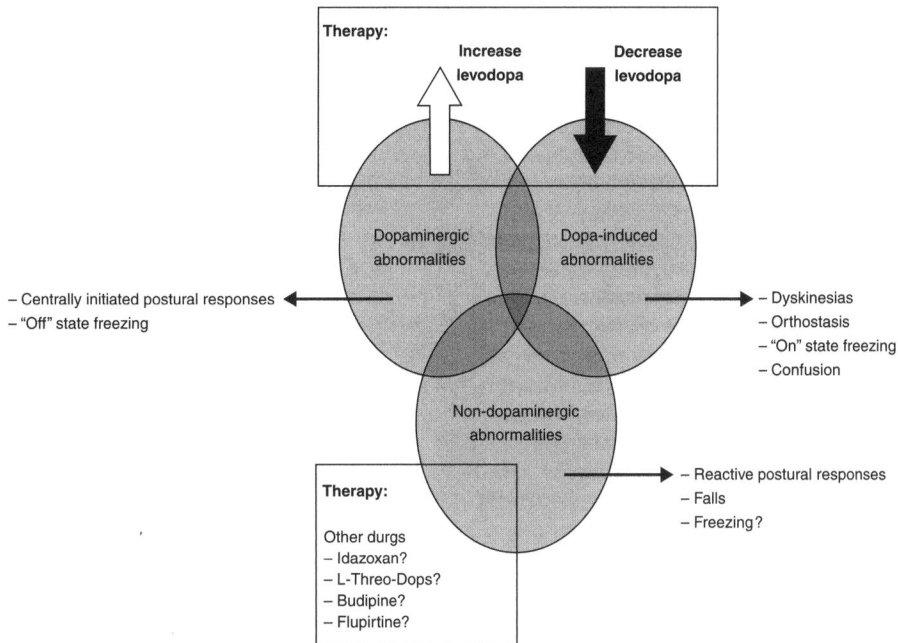

Figure 28.4 Neurochemical abnormalities involved in the pathophysiology of falls and FOG in PD. Three categories can be distinguished (depicted by the three overlapping circles), and each calls for a different treatment strategy (summarized in the two boxes). Dopaminergic abnormalities require an increase of dopaminergic drugs, but the opposite is necessary for dopa-induced abnormalities (caused by excessive dopaminergic medication). The third group of abnormalities is conceivably related to lesions outside the dopaminergic substantia nigra and requires correction of non-dopaminergic neurotransmitter deficits. However, unequivocally effective non-dopaminergic treatments are not yet available for routine clinical practice. Treatment is particularly complex for symptoms with a contribution from multiple domains, such as FOG, which can be a dopaminergic, dopa-induced or a non-dopaminergic feature.

dopaminergic therapy should always be considered. Note that if anti-parkinson medication markedly improves bradykinesia and rigidity, falls may paradoxically increase because the resultant increase in mobility makes some patients more liable to fall.

The issue of freezing of gait (FOG) is a challenging one. Most FOG episodes are related to the OFF state (or hypodopaminergic state) in parkinsonism (Bloem *et al.*, 2004c). Consequently, almost all drugs that improve the severity or duration of OFF periods over 24 h will also improve FOG among patients who are prone to freeze in the OFF phase. Considerably fewer patients have FOG during the ON state, although one must be careful here: most cases considered to be ON freezers are actually patients with good control of bradykinesia, rigidity and frequently even tremor, but who continue to suffer from FOG because of underdosing with respect to FOG. Such patients will stop freezing if dopaminergic treatment is increased. A small group of patients (the exact percentage is unknown) walk normally during the OFF phase

(early in the morning, before the first daily dose) and start to freeze when turning ON. FOG in those patients will improve if dopaminergic treatment is reduced. In general, OFF state FOG responds much better to dopaminergic medication at early stages of the disease. With disease progression, FOG becomes more resistant to levodopa.

Dopamine Agonists

Dopamine agonists (DA) generally have similar, albeit weaker positive effects on gait, as demonstrated in several trials performed in early and later stages of PD (for example, Olanow *et al.*, 1994; Rascol *et al.*, 2000). Curiously, in several prospective, double-blind studies comparing levodopa monotherapy to DA monotherapy, patients randomized to a DA reported a higher frequency of FOG, despite significant improvements in their general motor state (Rascol *et al.*, 2000; Parkinson Study Group, 2000). The exact mechanism behind this observation remains unclear,

Table 28.6 Medical treatment of gait disturbances in parkinsonism.

Drug	Clinical benefits	Evidence of efficacy	
		Gait in general	Freezing of gait[a]
Selegiline	FOG	A	A[b]
Rasagiline	FOG	A	A[b]
Amantadine	Hypokinetic gait	A	B
Dopamine agonists	Hypokinetic gait	A	Might worsen freezing
Levodopa	Hypokinetic gait and FOG	A	A
Botulinum toxin	Dystonic gait	Never tested	Not effective; might increase falls!
L-threo-DOPS	FOG in pure akinesia syndrome; not effective for FOG in PD		C
Cholinesterase inhibitors	Improved FOG and brain perfusion in pure akinesia syndrome		C
Methylphenidate	Improved cognition and locomotion; conflicting results	C	C

[a] Translation of evidence into recommendation, as follows: Level A = At least one class I study or 2 convincing class II studies; Level B = At least one class II study or 3 consistent class III studies; C = At least 2 convincing and consistent class III studies.
[b] Clinical significance is not clear.

and the findings do not necessarily imply that DA *induced* FOG in these patients. An equally plausible explanation is that FOG simply emerged with disease progression, and was better suppressed in the levodopa arm because this afforded a greater symptomatic effect. In clinical practice, when patients develop FOG while on DA monotherapy, a first step is to increase the dose of the agonist. Improvement in FOG would suggest that this was OFF period freezing that had been insufficiently treated; a further worsening of FOG would suggest an adverse effect of the DA and would necessitate a switch to levodopa. Whether some agonists are more effective or safer than others is unknown, and any differences seem clinically irrelevant, although switching between different DAs can be useful in individual patients.

Mono-Amine Oxidase Inhibitors

This class of drugs can enhance dopaminergic stimulation by decreasing dopamine metabolism at the level of the synapse. Additional indirect activities may result from the effect of active metabolites: methamphetamine for selegiline, and amino-indane for rasagiline. Both selegiline and rasagiline can improve gait in early and late stages of PD (Giladi *et al.*, 2001; Shoulson *et al.*, 2002; Zuniga *et al.*, 2006). Of special interest are several prospective, double-blind, placebo-controlled studies, which demonstrated a

beneficial effect of selegiline on FOG in early disease stages (Giladi *et al.*, 2001), and an effect of both selegiline and rasagiline on FOG in more advanced stages of PD (Giladi *et al.*, 2001; Shoulson *et al.*, 2002). However, in these studies, gait was always assessed using the UPDRS gait question and rarely using a direct gait assessment technique. Rasagiline has recently been tested more specifically in a controlled, double-blind sub-study of the LARGO study where FOG severity was the primary outcome (Giladi, Rascol and Brooks, 2004). In this study, rasagiline was better than placebo and as effective as entacapone in decreasing the total score of the FOG questionnaire, but the clinical significance of this finding is not yet clear.

Amantadine

Amantadine improves gait disturbances in PD by reducing OFF period parkinsonian signs (Freedman *et al.*, 1971; Walker *et al.*, 1972). A recent double-blind, crossover study reported that amantadine improved the severity of FOG in seven patients with pure freezing syndrome (Kondo, 2007). Amantadine may also be used to treat parkinsonian gait in patients with atypical parkinsonism. For example, a double blind and placebo-controlled trial showed that when given intravenously for five consecutive days, amantadine was superior to placebo in improving the parkinsonian gait of patients with higher-level gait disorders (Baezner *et al.*, 2001). Although not studied properly, amantadine is also felt to be one of the most effective drugs to improve gait in patients with progressive supranuclear palsy (Bloem *et al.*, 2005).

Specific Drug Treatment for Freezing of Gait

Because most FOG episodes occur in the OFF state and improve with dopaminergic medication, it is difficult to discuss the actual "specific" effect of any drug on FOG unless it does not have any symptomatic effect on parkinsonism in general. Only four such drugs have been assessed for the treatment of FOG: botulinum toxin injected into calf muscles; donepezil (an acetylcholinesterase inhibitor); methylphenidate; and EL-threo-DOPS (a precursor of norepinephrine). None of the trials that examined these drugs met the criteria for level A of the evidence-based medicine criteria (Table 28.6). Perhaps the most interesting compound is methylphenidate, as this may improve both gait and cognitive functioning (Auriel *et al.*, 2006; Devos *et al.*, 2007).

Other Non-Dopaminergic Drugs

Given the likely role for extranigral and non-dopaminergic lesions in the pathophysiology of parkinsonian gait and balance disorders, it would be interesting to test the efficacy of "non-dopaminergic" drugs (aimed at correcting adrenergic, serotonergic or cholinergic deficits). Only very few attempts have been made, including the aforementioned trials with L-threo-DOPS. Theoretically, one may expect acetylcholinesterase inhibitors such as rivastigmine or memantine, as enhancers of attention and memory (by improving cholinergic transmission), to directly and indirectly improve aspects of motor control as well. Furthermore, by reducing visual hallucinations in patients with PD, acetylcholinesterase inhibitors may reduce dangerous wandering behavior and improve motor performance. Unfortunately, there are currently no non-dopaminergic precursors with proven efficacy on gait or balance available for use in clinical practice.

Adverse Effects of Dopaminergic Drug Treatment

In PD, use of dopaminergic medication may paradoxically increase falls by causing violent dyskinesias, FOG (during the "ON" phase), orthostatic hypotension or confusion (Bloem and Bhatia, 2004). In such patients it is necessary to reduce, rather than increase, the dose of anti-parkinson medication.

Drug Treatment for Atypical Parkinsonism

Due to the paucity of well-designed clinical trials, it is unclear to what extent patients with other types of hypokinetic-rigid disorders improve with dopaminergic medication. Our experience suggests that a careful trial of levodopa may be justified, and some patients temporarily improve. For example, about one-third of patients with "vascular parkinsonism" can improve with levodopa (presumably those with a concurrent pre-synaptic dopaminergic lesion), although generally high levodopa dosages are required—up to 1 g/day (Zijlmans *et al.*, 2004). However, a temporary placebo response cannot be excluded, and a gratifying and long-lasting response to levodopa is generally only seen in patients with true idiopathic PD.

Surgery for Parkinson's Disease

Stereotactic neurosurgery of the basal ganglia is a relatively new and promising treatment for mostly young Parkinson patients with dose-limiting adverse effects of drug therapy. Various approaches have been investigated, including different targets (thalamus, internal globus pallidus, subthalamic nucleus and, most recently, the pedunculopontine nucleus (PPN)) and different techniques (lesions vs electrical stimulation; unilateral vs bilateral interventions).

Thalamic surgery occasionally improves gait in PD, but the risk of postural deficits is considerable, particularly following bilateral approaches (Speelman, 1991). In occasional patients, electrical stimulation of the nucleus ventralis intermedius of the thalamus improves postural control, apparently via reduction of tremor in the legs and trunk (Burleigh *et al.*, 1993). Unilateral thalamic lesions result in minor, short-lasting amelioration of balance in up to 30% of patients (Speelman, 1991). However, thalamic procedures generally provide little relief of postural instability or gait (Benabid *et al.*, 1996; Defebvre *et al.*, 1996).

Stereotactic surgery aimed at the internal globus pallidus or subthalamic nucleus effectively reduces appendicular symptoms (tremor, rigidity and akinesia of the extremities) in advanced PD, but the effects on axial symptoms (gait impairment and postural instability) are less well documented. A meta-analysis showed that bilateral internal globus pallidus stimulation, bilateral subthalamic nucleus stimulation and, to a lesser extent, unilateral pallidotomy improved postural instability and gait disability in PD (Bakker *et al.*, 2004). Bilateral subthalamic nucleus stimulation can also improve gait initiation and maintenance in PD, and reduce the stooped posture (Azulay *et al.*, 2001; Faist *et al.*, 2001; Crenna *et al.*, 2006). FOG during the ON state does not improve (Stolze *et al.*, 2001; Davis, Lyons and Pahwa, 2006). Unlike the effects on "appendicular" signs such as reaching, bilateral interventions seem more effective than unilateral interventions, perhaps because the basal ganglia affect walking via bilateral projections to the PPN (Crenna *et al.*, 2006; Yokoyama *et al.*, 1999; Kumar *et al.*, 1999; Bastian *et al.*, 2003).

There are several concerns when planning stereotactic surgery for gait or balance problems in PD. Clinical experience suggests that the axial symptoms of PD respond less consistently than appendicular symptoms. The effects on axial symptoms can vary considerably among individual patients, and some patients do not improve at all (Siegel and Metman, 2000). Also, the duration of improvement for axial symptoms is shorter than for appendicular symptoms, particularly after pallidotomy or pallidal stimulation. After long-term follow-up, balance has deteriorated in most patients due to progression of the underlying disease. A practical concern is that stereotactic interventions occasionally aggravate gait and balance impairment, and this risk seems greatest with bilateral approaches aimed at the globus pallidus. These adverse effects on gait can occur immediately post-operatively, but there is increasing focus on a sub-group of patients with a seemingly selective post-operative deterioration of axial motor control, in the face of persistent improvements in appendicular motor control (van Nuenen *et al.*, 2008). At present, patients with marked gait and balance impairment that respond poorly to antiparkinson medication appear unsuitable candidates for stereotactic neurosurgery. For younger patients with milder axial symptoms that respond well to dopaminergic therapy and no cognitive impairment, deep brain surgery can be considered.

There is an increasing interest in the PPN as a new target for stereotactic surgery, given its presumed role in the initiation and maintenance of gait, and perhaps in regulating balance as well (Pahapill and Lozano, 2000). Several studies have now shown that bilateral stimulation of the PPN is technically feasible and can in fact improve gait during both the ON and OFF state, but all studies were performed in small groups (Mazzone *et al.*, 2005; Plaha and Gill, 2005). PPN stimulation is most effective at much lower frequencies (20–25 Hz) compared to STN stimulation. A recent study included six patients with unsatisfactory pharmacological control of gait and postural stability, and submitted these patients to bilateral implantation of DBS electrodes in the STN and PPN (Stefani *et al.*, 2007). Clinical effects were evaluated 2–6 months after surgery in the OFF and ON medication state, and also with both STN and PPN stimulation switched on or off, or with only one target being stimulated. PPN stimulation was particularly effective for gait and postural items. In the ON medication state, the combination of STN and PPN stimulation provided a significant further improvement when compared to the specific benefit mediated by activating either single target. These findings indicate that, in patients with advanced PD, PPN stimulation associated with standard STN stimulation may be useful in improving gait and in optimizing the dopamine-mediated ON state, particularly in those whose response to isolated STN stimulation has deteriorated over time. However, follow-up was short, assessment of gait and balance was not done in a very detailed manner, and many technical and safety issues remain to be sorted out.

Physiotherapy for Parkinson's Disease

Gait and balance deficits in PD may improve with physiotherapy. Generic physiotherapy strategies have been discussed above. In addition, evidence-based guidelines have been developed, and consist partially of evidence derived from an increasing number of good-quality trials, and partially of expert opinion (Keus *et al.*, 2007). These guidelines provide practical recommendations in several key "domains" of PD where physiotherapy is deemed to be effective, including gait impairment, postural instability, falls and immobility. One clear example includes the use of external rhythmic auditory, visual or tactile cues to ameliorate gait and to reduce FOG in PD (Morris *et al.*, 1997; Rubinstein, Giladi and Hausdorff, 2002; Nieuwboer *et al.*, 2007). Use of external cues to improve gait apparently permits patients to bypass their defective basal ganglia circuitry. A possible explanation is that, for example, the visual cortex can access motor pathways via indirect projections involving the cerebellum, rather than the basal ganglia (Manganotti *et al.*, 2001). Such circuitries could also underlie the phenomenon of kinesia paradoxica. The use of cueing techniques is now supported by high-quality randomized trials (Nieuwboer *et al.*, 2007).

Physiotherapists can make other contributions as well. Patients can be instructed to avoid dual-tasking in daily life, and to split complex movements into sequential components that are easier to execute separately (this segmentation technique is termed "chaining") (Kamsma, Brouwer and Lakke, 1995). Physiotherapists can also teach patients to make safer "transfers" (e.g., getting in and out of bed) and improve cardiovascular fitness (Morris *et al.*, 1997). Further options are to teach patients specific maneuvers to reduce orthostatic hypotension, such as standing with crossed legs and muscles contracted (Mathias and Kimber, 1998), but this is obviously unattractive in patients with severe balance impairment. For this latter group, selectively increasing the inspiratory impedance may also be used to reduce orthostatic hypotension to a similar degree as can be achieved with leg muscle tensing (Thijs *et al.*, 2007). Further research is needed to determine how long the effects of physical therapy last and whether or not some form of chronic maintenance therapy is required. One study showed improvements in FOG with external cueing, but the clinical benefits were short-lasting (Brichetto *et al.*, 2006).

An important role is to facilitate the use of walking aids. Specific designs are available for PD patients, such as the inverted cane. Wheeled walkers occasionally cause or aggravate propulsion because PD patients with impaired hand function cannot use the handbrakes. Caution is also needed when walkers are given to patients with FOG. Wheeled walkers offered no reduction in FOG, while standard walkers can actually increase FOG (Cubo *et al.*, 2003).

Occupational Therapy for Parkinson's Disease

Removing domestic hazards is presumably not effective because most falls in PD are unrelated to environmental circumstances (Bloem *et al.*, 2001). However, individual patients with obvious extrinsic falls may benefit, for example when patients have frequent FOG episodes because the living room is too crowded. Poor illumination may indirectly lead to falls by impairing visual compensation.

Spastic Gait and Balance

Pathophysiology

Spasticity is defined as a velocity-dependent increase in tonic stretch reflexes and is one component of the upper motor neuron syndrome. Common causes of spasticity include multiple sclerosis, cerebral palsy, traumatic brain and spinal injuries, stroke, and sporadic or hereditary spastic paraplegias. Spasticity is described using the terms "negative" and "positive" symptoms (Table 28.7), where negative symptoms include muscle weakness, decreased coordination, loss of dexterity and fatigue. Positive symptoms manifest clinically as increased muscle tone, exaggerated deep tendon reflexes, muscle spasm, persistence of primitive reflexes, clonus, extensor plantar responses, and discordant mass activation of muscles. In addition, secondary complications may develop, such as contractures. The effects of spasticity range from mild muscle stiffness to severe, painful muscle spasms and contractures resulting in postural and joint deformities that reduce mobility and substantially impede activities of daily living.

Spasticity commonly affects gait. Note that not all spasticity is necessarily bad for gait: patients with minimal voluntary control over their legs—but with prominent extensor tone of lower extremities—use their spastic muscle tone to help in ambulation or transfer (Mayer, 1997). A unilateral lesion of the corticospinal tract in the hemisphere or brain stem causes a contralateral spastic, hemiparetic gait. The affected arm is adducted at the shoulder, flexed at the elbow, and flexed at the wrist and fingers. The upper extremity does not swing and is held up against the chest or

Table 28.7 Characteristics of spastic paresis.

- Positive symptoms
  - Hyper-reflexia/clonus
  - Flexion/extension spasms
  - Associated reactions
  - Co-contractions/mass activation of muscles
  - Abnormal posture/spastic dystonia
  - Primitive reflexes
- Negative symptoms
  - Muscle weakness/paresis
  - Loss of dexterity/co-ordination
  - Muscle slowness
  - Increased muscle fatigability
- Secondary symptoms
  - Increased muscle stiffness
  - Loss of muscle length (myogenic contracture)
  - Pain

Recognition of these three main domains serves as a basis for individualized treatment, tailored to specific problems in individual patients.

abdomen. There is decreased flexion of the hip and knee and less ankle dorsiflexion. The affected stiff spastic leg is swept outward to avoid the foot dragging on the floor (circumduction) while the upper body rocks slightly to the contralateral side. There is a decreased cadence and thus slowing of walking velocity. Spasticity affecting both lower limbs is termed spastic paraparesis. Detailed descriptions of the spastic gait have been made in dedicated gait laboratories (Klebe *et al.*, 2004). Treatment must be carefully tailored to the pathophysiology and the specific movement abnormalities in order to optimally enhance mobility, improve posture and increase the range of motion.

Medical Treatment

The pharmacologic treatment of spasticity is limited to oral and intrathecal anti-spastic drugs, or to intramuscular injections for chemodenervation. All treatment modalities must be combined with physiotherapy. A practical algorithm to support treatment decisions is shown in Figure 28.5. Individual treatment options are summarized in Table 28.8.

Oral Anti-Spasticity Agents

Anti-spasticity agents are mainly benzodiazepines, dantrolene, tizanidine and baclofen. These can afford a generalized reduction in body tone and decrease the frequency and severity of muscle spasms. Adverse effects are significant, including sedation, muscle weakness, dizziness, seizures and hepatotoxicity. Efficacy might diminish with prolonged use, necessitating higher doses (and increasing the risk of adverse effects). The effects of oral anti-spastics on gait

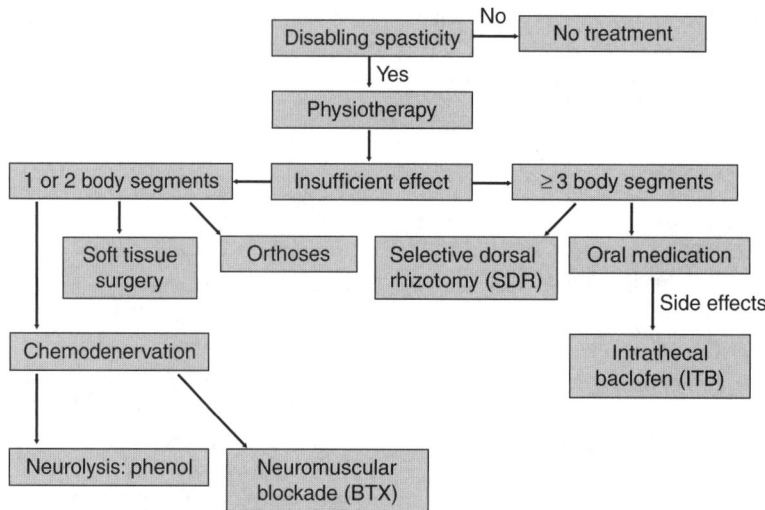

Figure 28.5 A decision algorithm for the treatment of spasticity. Spasticity should only be treated when the disabling consequences overrule the possible beneficial effects, for example, with regard to support function of the legs. The first treatment choice is physiotherapy, in particular regular stretching of affected muscles and adequate positioning of affected limbs during daytime and night-time. In case of insufficient effect and focal spasticity (of one or two body segments), focal measures are warranted. Orthoses may support the efficacy of stretching and provide better positioning of affected joints. Chemodenervation (such as with botulinum toxin, BTX) will result in a decrease in neural activation of spastic muscles. Soft tissue surgery will increase the length and enhance the activation threshold of affected muscles. In case of generalized spasticity (that is, three or more affected body segments), systemic medication is a first choice. Baclofen can be administered more selectively into the cerebrospinal fluid to prevent systemic side effects. Selective dorsal rhizotomy (SDR) is a surgical option for severe generalized spasticity of the lower limbs, especially in children.

have been sparsely studied. One study showed that, despite alleviation of flexor and extensor spasms and a decrease in resistance to passive leg movement, oral baclofen failed to improve gait (Duncan, Shahani and Young, 1976).

Chemodenervation

Chemodenervation may be accomplished with phenol or botulinum toxin (BTX) injections. Both reduce harmful spasticity in one area, while preserving useful spasticity in other areas, thereby preserving useful motor function. Patients with profound weakness of the lower limbs or those with long-lasting fixed contractures are usually not good candidates. In some patients with contractures, chemodenervation may be considered, but usually additional measures such as taping, serial casting or surgical release should follow. All patients should engage in an intensive physiotherapeutic program following this treatment. The main targets in spasticity of the lower limbs are: plantar flexion, foot inversion, thigh adduction (scissoring), hip-knee flexion, hip-knee extension, toe curling and truncal flexion (O'Brien, 2002).

Several studies have examined the effects of BTX on gait. In a randomized, double-blind study, 20 patients with post-stroke spasticity—with ankle plantar flexor and foot invertor spasticity—were randomly assigned to receive either botulinum toxin type A (BTX-A) injected into calf muscles, or a tibial nerve blockade with phenol (Kirazli et al., 1998). Both treatment groups showed significant improvement in spasticity scores. However, scores for eversion and ambulation were improved only in BTX-treated patients, and functional improvements were better overall with BTX therapy. In another open-label study involving patients with hereditary spastic paraplegia, BTX-A was injected into lower limb muscles (because of equinus, varus and pathological hip adduction) (Rousseaux et al., 2007). The results showed a moderate reduction of ankle plantar flexor and hip adductor spasticity, with a partial increase in the range of ankle motion, and an increased gait velocity. In children with cerebral palsy, BTX-A injected into the gastrocnemius muscle (because of a spastic equinus foot) and into the hamstring muscles improved gait, as well as range of motion of the ankle, knee and hip (Corry et al., 1999). This also permitted a delay for corrective surgery. Finally, a recent multi-centre randomized

Table 28.8 Therapeutic interventions to alleviate spastic gait.

Intervention	Effect	Pitfalls
Oral anti-spastics		
• Benzodiazepines	• Generalized reduction in body tone	• Significant adverse effects, including sedation, muscle weakness, dizziness, seizures, tolerance and hepatotoxicity
• Dantrolene	• Decreased frequency and severity of muscle spasms	
• Tizanidine	• No specific effect on gait	
• Baclofen		
Chemodenervation (local i.m. injections)	• Improve range of motion	• Additional measures such as taping, serial casing or surgical release should follow
• Botulinum toxin	• Reduces deformities in lower limbs	• Intensive physiotherapy is necessary
• Phenol	• Improves walking velocity	• Complications mainly with phenol—pain and dysesthesia
	• Permits delay in corrective surgery in children	
Surgical interventions	• Provides a permanent reduction in lower limb tone	• Must be combined with operations on tendons and an intensive postoperative rehabilitative program
• Selective dorsal rhizotomy (for children with CP)	• Increased range of motion	• Can cause muscle weakness
	• Improved posture	
	• Long-lasting improvement in gait dynamics	
• Intrathecal baclofen	• Reduction in tone	• Dizziness, drowsiness, headaches, nausea, and weakness. Infections and device failure.
	• Improved range of motion	
	• Decreased painful muscle spasm	
	• Increased walking velocity	
• Orthopedic surgery	• Surgery for lengthening the Achilles tendon, the hamstrings and the iliopsoas muscle, and release of adductors from the pubis	• Best postponed until later (school) age

study compared multi-level BTX-A plus comprehensive rehabilitation with usual care in 46 children with spastic cerebral palsy (Scholtes *et al.*, 2007). The results demonstrated improved knee extension during gait, increased muscle length and decreased spasticity in the injected muscles after six weeks. The effect on gait lasted less than 24 weeks.

Surgical Interventions

Surgical interventions are a critical element in the rehabilitation of patients with a spastic gait (Boop,

Woo and Maria, 2001). To date, the risks associated with surgical interventions are small, and the chances for immediate and long-lasting improvements high. Currently, the most commonly performed neurosurgical procedures for the treatment of spasticity are selective dorsal rhizotomy and placement of intrathecal baclofen pumps. Other surgical interventions include selective peripheral neurotomy and various orthopedic surgical procedures. Selective peripheral neurotomy is reserved for severe focal spasticity, when BTX injections cannot delay surgery any longer (Sindou and Mertens, 2000).

Selective Dorsal Rhizotomy

Selective dorsal rhizotomy (SDR) is an evidence-based treatment for spasticity in cerebral palsy, and is also used for spasticity caused by other etiologies. Good candidates are patients with spastic diplegia who are still ambulatory with aids, those with good strength, those that demonstrate good muscle group isolation and postural stability, and who do not have fixed contractures. Patients must also be motivated to work with physiotherapists on an intensive rehabilitative program post-operatively (Smyth and Peacock, 2000). Guidelines for surgery in children with cerebral palsy underscore that the surgical indications depend on the pre-operative (dis)abilities, as well as on functional goals (Sindou and Mertens, 2000). For example, in independent ambulatory children, the goal is to improve the efficiency and cosmetics of walking by eliminating abnormally responsive neural circuitries through functional SDR. This is best done when the child can co-operate with the physiotherapist, preferably between three and seven years of age. In contrast, for children who are in the process of developing ambulatory skills and who only temporarily require an assistive device, surgery should be delayed until they have perfected these skills. Spastic children who undergo SDR sustain a permanent reduction in lower extremity tone, increased range of motion in the legs and improved posture while sitting and kneeling. Importantly, these children also experience a long-lasting improvement in gait dynamics, as reflected both clinically and experimentally using computerized gait analysis (Subramanian et al., 1998).

Intrathecal Baclofen

Intrathecal baclofen (ITB) involves a direct infusion of baclofen into the subarachnoid space around the spinal cord, potentiating γ-aminobutyric acid (GABA)-mediated inhibition of spasticity. Appropriate candidates are patients with severe, generalized spasticity that impedes independent function, including ambulation. Ideally, ITB should reduce spasticity, but preserve gait function. An advantage of ITB is its ability to reduce dystonia which is common in patients with cerebral palsy, but which may not respond to SDR (Goldstein, 2001).

Improved tone following a test dose of 50 to 100 μg of baclofen (administered by lumbar puncture) is followed by pump implantation for continuous ITB infusion, with gradual dose adjustments to maximize patient benefit and minimize side effects. Potential side effects include those referable to baclofen (e.g., drowsiness or weakness, but also risk of baclofen overdose and withdrawal syndrome with respiratory failure and coma), technical problems (1% per year, mainly breakage or disconnection of the catheter) and infections.

ITB is very effective in patients with cerebral or spinal spasticity. Positive effects of ITB on gait have been reported after bolus intrathecal injections and in patients with continuous infusion. For example, a one-year follow-up study including ambulatory patients with spasticity showed that ITB improved gait in 20 of 24 patients (Gerszten, Albright and Barry, 1997). In patients with spastic hemiplegia, ITB improved walking and reduced muscle stiffness at the ankles and knees of the affected side (Remy-Neris et al., 2003). ITB has also been tested in patients with traumatic brain injury. Thus, ITB bolus injection reduced spasticity in ambulatory patients with traumatic brain injury, resulting in increased stride length and gait velocity (Horn, Yablon and Stokic, 2005). ITB–given within one year of onset of acquired brain injury—improved gait speed without adverse effects on recovery (Francisco et al., 2005). Finally, ITB has been tested in patients with sporadic and hereditary spastic paraplegia (Klebe et al., 2005). The results showed an increased gait velocity accompanied by larger step length and a reduced step width, but no change in other kinematic gait parameters. Only 50% of the patients initially included actually received continuous ITB because a bolus test showed variable effects and worsening or unmasking of pre-existent weakness.

Orthopedic Surgery

Soft tissue surgery remains a common component in the management of ambulatory patients with spastic gait. The main procedures are aimed at lengthening the achilles tendon, the hamstrings and iliopsoas muscle, and to release the adductors from the pubis (Karol, 2004). Multi-site simultaneous tendon surgery can improve gait by reducing contractures of the hip, knee and ankle, and by enhancing the activation threshold of the lengthened muscles.

Additional Interventions

Physiotherapy is essential to stretch muscles and prevent muscle shortening. Adequate and prolonged stretching may reduce muscle tone as well, both during the stretching and for some time afterwards. In addition, initial muscle relaxation is necessary to facilitate the fit of orthotic devices such as braces. If pain is a major issue, potential sources of pain should be identified and treated accordingly, thereby decreasing the frequency of muscle spasms. Finally, given the complex management of spasticity, with multiple (often complementary) treatment options and a delicate planning of both immediate and long-term ramifications of the interventions, patients are best treated in a multi-disciplinary setting.

CONCLUSIONS

Axial mobility deficits are generally regarded as being difficult to treat. However, this chapter illustrates the broad spectrum of possible therapeutic interventions that is available to alleviate gait and balance problems, and to reduce falls in affected patients. Unfortunately, in most areas, the level of supporting scientific evidence is still insufficient to make very strong recommendations. Therefore, well-designed and adequately powered studies are needed in the forthcoming years to further improve and expand the therapeutic arsenal.

ACKNOWLEDGEMENTS

Dr. B.R. Bloem was supported by a ZonMw VIDI research grant (number 016.076.352).

References

Abbott, R.D., White, L.R., Ross, G.W., Masaki, K.H., Curb, J.D. and Petrovitch, H. (2004) Walking and dementia in physically capable elderly men. *The Journal of the American Medical Association*, **292**, 1447–1453.

Allum, J.H. and Carpenter, M.G. (2005) A speedy solution for balance and gait analysis: angular velocity measured at the centre of body mass. *Current Opinion in Neurology*, **18**, 15–21.

American Geriatrics Society, (2001) Britisch Geriatrics Society, and American Academy of Orthopaedic Surgeons Panels on Falls Prevention. Guideline for the prevention of falls in older persons. *Journal of the American Geriatrics Society*, **49**, 664–672.

Arai, T., Obuchi, S., Inaba, Y. *et al.* (2007) The effects of short-term exercise intervention on falls self-efficacy and the relationship between changes in physical function and falls self-efficacy in Japanese older people: a randomized controlled trial. *American Journal of Physical Medicine & Rehabilitation*, **86**, 133–141.

Auriel, E., Hausdorff, J.M., Herman, T., Simon, E.S. and Giladi, N. (2006) Effects of methylphenidate on cognitive function and gait in patients with Parkinson's disease: a pilot study. *Clinical Neuropharmacology*, **29**, 15–17.

Azulay, J.P., Mesure, S., Freiburger, C. *et al.* (2001) Quantitative effects of levodopa versus bilateral subthalamic stimulation on posture and gait in Parkinson's disease, in Control of Posture and Gait. Maastricht: Symposium of the International Society for Postural and Gait Research (eds J.E. Duysens, B.C.M. Smits-Engelsman and H. Kingma), pp. 718–719.

Baezner, H., Oster, M., Henning, O., Cohen, S. and Hennerici, M. G. (2001) Amantadine increases gait steadiness in frontal gait disorder due to subcortical vascular encephalopathy: a double-blind randomized placebo-controlled trial based on quantitative gait analysis. *Cerebrovascular Diseases*, **11**, 235–244.

Bakker, M., Esselink, R.A., Munneke, M., Limousin-Dowsey, P., Speelman, J.D. and Bloem, B.R. (2004) Effects of stereotactic neurosurgery on postural instability and gait in Parkinson's disease. *Movement Disorders*, **19**, 1092–1099.

Barbeau, H., Norman, K., Fung, J., Visintin, M. and Ladouceur, M. (1998) Does neurorehabilitation play a role in the recovery of walking in neurological populations? *Annals of the New York Academy of Sciences*, **860**, 377–392.

Bastian, A.J., Kelly, V.E., Revilla, F.J., Perlmutter, J.S. and Mink, J.W. (2003) Different effects of unilateral versus bilateral subthalamic nucleus stimulation on walking and reaching in Parkinson's disease. *Movement Disorders*, **18**, 1000–1007.

Bateni, H. and Maki, B.E. (2005) Assistive devices for balance and mobility: benefits, demands, and adverse consequences. *Archives of Physical Medicine and Rehabilitation*, **86**, 134–145.

Beckley, D.J., Panzer, V.P., Remler, M.P., Ilog, L.B. and Bloem, B.R. (1995) Clinical correlates of motor performance during paced postural tasks in Parkinson's disease. *Journal of the Neurological Sciences*, **132**, 133–138.

Benabid, A.-L., Pollak, P., Gao, D. *et al.* (1996) Chronic electrical stimulation of the ventralis intermedius nucleus of the thalamus as a treatment of movement disorders. *Journal of Neurosurgery*, **84**, 203–214.

Blin, O., Ferrandez, A.M., Pailhous, J. and Serratrice, G. (1991) Dopa-sensitive and dopa-resistant gait parameters in Parkinson's disease. *Journal of the Neurological Sciences*, **103**, 51–54.

Bloem, B.R. and Bhatia, K.P. (2004) Gait and balance in basal ganglia disorders, in *Clinical Disorders of Balance, Posture and Gait*, 2 edn (eds A.M. Bronstein, T. Brandt, J.G. Nutt and M.H. Woollacott), Arnold, London, pp. 173–206.

Bloem, B.R., Haan, J., Lagaay, A.M., van Beek, W., Wintzen, A.R. and Roos, R.A. (1992) Investigation of gait in elderly subjects over 88 years of age. *Journal of Geriatric Psychiatry and Neurology*, **5**, 78–84.

Bloem, B.R., Beckley, D.J., van Dijk, J.G. *et al.* (1994) Medium latency stretch reflexes in young-onset Parkinson's disease and MPTP-induced parkinsonism. *Journal of the Neurological Sciences*, **123**, 52–58.

Bloem, B.R. and Roos, R.A. (1995) Neurotoxicity of designer drugs and related compounds, in *Handbook of clinical Neurology, Vol. 21 (65): Intoxications of the Nervous System, Part II* (eds P.J. Vinken, G.W. Bruyn, H.L. Klawans and F.A. de Wolff), Elsevier, Amsterdam, pp. 363–414.

Bloem, B.R., Beckley, D.J., van Dijk, J.G., Zwinderman, A.H., Remler, M.P. and Roos, R.A. (1996) Influence of dopaminergic medication on automatic postural responses and balance impairment in Parkinson's disease. *Movement Disorders*, **11**, 509–521.

Bloem, B.R., Gussekloo, J., Lagaay, A.M., Remarque, E.J., Haan, J. and Westendorp, R.G.J. (2000) Idiopathic senile gait disorders are signs of subclinical disease. *Journal of the American Geriatrics Society*, **48**, 1098–1101.

Bloem, B.R., Grimbergen, Y.A., Cramer, M., Willemsen, M.D. and Zwinderman, A.H. (2001) Prospective assessment of falls in Parkinson's disease. *Journal of Neurology*, **248**, 950–958.

Bloem, B.R., van Vugt, J.P. and Beckley, D.J. (2001) Postural instability and falls in Parkinson's disease. *Advances in Neurology*, **87**, 209–223.

Bloem, B.R., Munneke, M., Mazibrada, G. *et al.* (2004a) The nature of falling in progressive supranuclear palsy. *Movement Disorders*, **19**, 359–360.

Bloem, B.R., Overeem, S. and van Dijk, J.G. (2004b) Syncopal falls, drop attacks and their mimics, in *Clinical Disorders of Balance, Posture and Gait*, 2 edn (eds A.M. Bronstein, T. Brandt, J.G. Nutt and M.H. Woollacott), Arnold, London, pp. 286–316.

Bloem, B.R., Hausdorff, J.M., Visser, J.E. and Giladi, N. (2004c) Falls and freezing in Parkinson's disease: a review of two interconnected, episodic phenomena. *Movement Disorders*, **19**, 871–884.

Bloem, B.R., Korhan, E.K. and de Leeuw, F.E. (2005) Treatment of axial mobility deficits in movement disorders, in *Gait disorders*.

Evaluation and management (eds J.M. Hausdorff and N.B. Alexander), Taylor & Francis, London, pp. 289–308.

Boers, I., Gerschlager, W., Stalenhoef, P.A. and Bloem, B.R. (2001) Falls in the elderly. II. Strategies for prevention. *Wiener Klinische Wochenschrift*, **113**, 398–407.

Bonnet, A.M., Loria, Y., Saint-Hilaire, M.H., Lhermitte, F. and Agid, Y. (1987) Does long-term aggravation of Parkinson's disease result from nondopaminergic lesions? *Neurology*, **37**, 1539–1542.

Boop, F.A., Woo, R. and Maria, B.L. (2001) Consensus statement on the surgical management of spasticity related to cerebral palsy. *Journal of Child Neurology*, **16**, 68–69.

Bowes, S.G., Clark, P.K., Leeman, A.L. *et al.* (1990) Determinants of gait in the elderly parkinsonian on maintenance levodopa/carbidopa therapy. *British Journal of Clinical Pharmacology*, **30**, 13–24.

Brichetto, G., Pelosin, E., Marchese, R. and Abbruzzese, G. (2006) Evaluation of physical therapy in parkinsonian patients with freezing of gait: a pilot study. *Clinical Rehabilitation*, **20**, 31–35.

Buchner, D.M. and Larson, E.B. (1987) Falls and fractures in patients with Alzheimer-type dementia. *The Journal of the American Medical Association*, **257**, 1492–1495.

Burleigh, A.L., Horak, F.B., Burchiel, K.J. and Nutt, J.G. (1993) Effects of thalamic stimulation on tremor, balance, and step initiation: a single subject study. *Movement Disorders*, **8**, 519–524.

Burleigh-Jacobs, A., Horak, F.B., Nutt, J.G. and Obeso, J.A. (1997) Step initiation in Parkinson's disease: influence of levodopa and external sensory triggers. *Movement Disorders*, **12**, 206–215.

Burridge, J.H., Haugland, M., Larsen, B. *et al.* (2007) Phase II trial to evaluate the ActiGait implanted drop-foot stimulator in established hemiplegia. *Journal of Rehabilitation Medicine*, **39**, 212–218.

Buurke, J.H., Hermens, H.J., Erren-Wolters, C.V. and Nene, A.V. (2005) The effect of walking aids on muscle activation patterns during walking in stroke patients. *Gait & Posture*, **22**, 164–170.

Camicioli, R.M., Howieson, D.B., Lehman, S. and Kaye, J.A. (1997) Talking while walking. The effect of a dual task in aging and Alzheimer's disease. *Neurology*, **48**, 955–958.

Campbell, A.J., Borrie, M.J. and Spears, G.F. (1989) Risk factors for falls in a community-based prospective study of people 70 years and older. *Journals of Gerontology*, **44**, M112–M117.

Capezuti, E., Evans, L., Strumpf, N. and Maislin, G. (1996) Physical restraint use and falls in nursing home residents. *Journal of the American Geriatrics Society*, **44**, 627–633.

Carlson, W.E., Vaughan, C.L., Damiano, D.L. and Abel, M.F. (1997) Orthotic management of gait in spastic diplegia. *American Journal of Physical Medicine & Rehabilitation*, **76**, 219–225.

Close, P., Neuprez, A. and Reginster, J.Y. (2006) Developments in the pharmacotherapeutic management of osteoporosis. *Expert Opinion on Pharmacotherapy*, **7**, 1603–1615.

Corry, I.S., Cosgrove, A.P., Duffy, C.M., Taylor, T.C. and Graham, H.K. (1999) Botulinum toxin A in hamstring spasticity. *Gait & Posture*, **10**, 206–210.

Crenna, P., Carpinella, I., Rabuffetti, M. *et al.* (2006) Impact of subthalamic nucleus stimulation on the initiation of gait in Parkinson's disease. *Experimental Brain Research*, **172**, 519–532.

Cubo, E., Moore, C.G., Leurgans, S. and Goetz, C.G. (2003) Wheeled and standard walkers in Parkinson's disease patients with gait freezing. *Parkinsonism & Related Disorders*, **10**, 9–14.

Cumming, R.G., Thomas, M., Szonyi, G., Frampton, G., Salkeld, G. and Clemson, L. (2001) Adherence to occupational therapist recommendations for home modifications for falls prevention. *American Journal of Occupational Therapy*, **55**, 641–648.

Daly, J.J., Roenigk, K., Holcomb, J. *et al.* (2006) A randomized controlled trial of functional neuromuscular stimulation in chronic stroke subjects. *Stroke; A Journal of Cerebral Circulation*, **37**, 172–178.

Davis, J.T., Lyons, K.E. and Pahwa, R. (2006) Freezing of gait after bilateral subthalamic nucleus stimulation for Parkinson's disease. *Clinical Neurology and Neurosurgery*, **108**, 461–464.

Day, L., Fildes, B., Gordon, I., Fitzharris, M., Flamer, H. and Lord, S.R. (2002) Randomised factorial trial of falls prevention among older people living in their own homes. *BMJ (Clinical Research Ed)*, **325**, 128–134.

de, V.S. and Mulder, T.W. (2007) Motor imagery and stroke rehabilitation: a critical discussion. *Journal of Rehabilitation Medicine*, **39**, 5–13.

de Leeuw, F.E., de Groot, J.C., Oudkerk, M. *et al.* (2002) Hypertension and cerebral white matter lesions in a prospective cohort study. *Brain: A Journal of Neurology*, **125**, 765–772.

Defebvre, L., Blatt, J.L., Blond, S., Bourriez, J.L., Gieu, J.D. and Destee, A. (1996) Effect of thalamic stimulation on gait in Parkinson's disease. *Archives of Neurology*, **53**, 898–903.

den Otter, A.R., Geurts, A.C., Mulder, T.W. and Duysens, J. (2007) Abnormalities in the temporal patterning of lower extremity muscle activity in hemiparetic gait. *Gait & Posture*, **25**, 342–352.

Devos, D., Krystkowiak, P., Clement, F. *et al.* (2007) Improvement of gait by chronic, high doses of methylphenidate in patients with advanced Parkinson's disease. *Journal of Neurology, Neurosurgery, and Psychiatry*, **78**, 470–475.

Dietz, V., Berger, W. and Horstmann, G.A. (1988) Posture in Parkinson's disease: impairment of reflexes and programming. *Annals of Neurology*, **24**, 660–669.

Duncan, G.W., Shahani, B.T. and Young, R.R. (1976) An evaluation of baclofen treatment for certain symptoms in patients with spinal cord lesions. A double-blind, cross-over study. *Neurology*, **26**, 441–446.

Dunn, A.L., Trivedi, M.H., Kampert, J.B., Clark, C.G. and Chambliss, H.O. (2005) Exercise treatment for depression: efficacy and dose response. *American Journal of Preventive Medicine*, **28**, 1–8.

Dunsky, A., Dickstein, R., Ariav, C., Deutsch, J. and Marcovitz, E. (2006) Motor imagery practice in gait rehabilitation of chronic post-stroke hemiparesis: four case studies. *International Journal of Rehabilitation Research*, **29**, 351–356.

Ensrud, K.E., Blackwell, T.L., Mangione, C.M. *et al.* (2002) Central nervous system-active medications and risk for falls in older women. *Journal of the American Geriatrics Society*, **50**, 1629–1637.

Faber, M.J., Bosscher, R.J., Chin, A.P.M. and van Wieringen, P.C. (2006) Effects of exercise programs on falls and mobility in frail and pre-frail older adults: A multicenter randomized controlled trial. *Archives of Physical Medicine and Rehabilitation*, **87**, 885–896.

Faist, M., Xie, J., Kurz, D. *et al.* (2001) Effect of bilateral subthalamic nucleus stimulation on gait in Parkinson's disease. *Brain: A Journal of Neurology*, **124**, 1590–1600.

Fouyas, I.P., Statham, P.F. and Sandercock, P.A. (2002) Cochrane review on the role of surgery in cervical spondylotic radiculomyelopathy. *Spine*, **27**, 736–747.

Francisco, G.E., Hu, M.M., Boake, C. and Ivanhoe, C.B. (2005) Efficacy of early use of intrathecal baclofen therapy for treating spastic hypertonia due to acquired brain injury. *Brain Injury*, **19**, 359–364.

Freedman, B.E., Getz, E., MacGregor, J.M. and Ames, F.R. (1971) Amantadine hydrochloride in the treatment of parkinsonism: a placebo-controlled double-blind study. *South African Medical Journal*, **45**, 435–437.

French, B., Thomas, L.H., Leathley, M.J. *et al.* (2007) Repetitive task training for improving functional ability after stroke. *Cochrane Database of Systematic Reviews*, CD006073.

Friedman, P.J., Baskett, J.J. and Richmond, D.E. (1989) Cognitive impairment and its relationship to gait rehabilitation in the elderly. *The New Zealand Medical Journal*, **102**, 603–606.

Gerszten, P.C., Albright, A.L. and Barry, M.J. (1997) Effect on ambulation of continuous intrathecal baclofen infusion. *Pediatr Neurosurg*, **27**, 40–44.

Giladi, N., Kao, R. and Fahn, S. (1997) Freezing phenomenon in patients with parkinsonian syndromes. *Movement Disorders*, **12**, 302–305.

Giladi, N., Shabtai, H., Simon, E.S., Biran, S., Tal, J. and Korczyn, A. (2000) Construction of freezing of gait questionnaire for patients with Parkinson's disease. *Parkinsonism & Related Disorders*, **6**, 165–170.

Giladi, N., Mcdermott, M.P., Fahn, S. *et al.* (2001) Freezing of gait in PD: prospective assessment in the DATATOP cohort. *Neurology*, **56**, 1712–1721.

Giladi, N., Rascol, O. and Brooks, E. (2004) Rasagiline treatment can improve freezing of gait in advanced Parkinson's disease: a prospective randomized, double blind placebo and entacapone controlled study. *Movement Disorders*, **19** (Suppl 9), S191.

Giladi, N., Bloem, B.R. and Hausdorff, J.M. (2007) Gait disturbances and falls, in Neurology and Clinical Neurosciences (ed. A.H. Schapira), Mosby Elsevier, Philadelphia, pp. 455–470.

Gillespie, L.D., Gillespie, W.J., Cumming, R., Lamb, S.E. and Rowe, B.H. (2004) Interventions for preventing falls in the elderly (Cochrane Review). *The Cochrane Library*, **4**, 1–29.

Goldstein, E.M. (2001) Spasticity management: an overview. *Journal of Child Neurology*, **16**, 16–23.

Grahn Kronhed, A.C., Blomberg, C., Lofman, O., Timpka, T. and Moller, M. (2006) Evaluation of an osteoporosis and fall risk intervention program for community-dwelling elderly. A quasi-experimental study of behavioral modifications. *Aging Clinical and Experimental Research*, **18**, 235–241.

Gray, P. and Hildebrand, K. (2000) Fall risk factors in Parkinson's disease. *Journal of Neuroscience Nursing*, **32**, 222–228.

Gurevich, T., Peretz, C., Moore, O., Weizmann, N. and Giladi, N. (2007) The effect of injecting botulinum toxin type a into the calf muscles on freezing of gait in Parkinson's disease: a double blind placebo-controlled pilot study. *Movement Disorders*, **22**, 880–883.

Hakim, A.A., Petrovitch, H., Burchfiel, C.M. *et al.* (1998) Effects of walking on mortality among nonsmoking retired men. *The New England Journal of Medicine*, **338**, 94–99.

Hauer, K., Rost, B., Rutschle, K. *et al.* (2001) Exercise training for rehabilitation and secondary prevention of falls in geriatric patients with a history of injurious falls. *Journal of the American Geriatrics Society*, **49**, 10–20.

Hausdorff, J.M., Rios, D.A. and Edelberg, H.K. (2001) Gait variability and fall risk in community-living older adults: a 1-year prospective study. *Archives of Physical Medicine and Rehabilitation*, **82**, 1050–1056.

Hausdorff, J.M., Yogev, G., Springer, S., Simon, E.S. and Giladi, N. (2005) Walking is more like catching than tapping: gait in the elderly as a complex cognitive task. *Experimental Brain Research*, **164**, 541–548.

Hesse, S., Werner, C., Bardeleben, A. and Barbeau, H. (2001) Body weight-supported treadmill training after stroke. *Current Atherosclerosis Reports*, **3**, 287–294.

Holden, M.K. (2005) Virtual environments for motor rehabilitation: review. *CyberPsychology & Behavior*, **8**, 187–211.

Horak, F.B. and Frank, J.S. (1996) Three separate postural systems affected in parkinsonism, in *Motor Control*, **7** (eds D.G. Stuart, V.S. Gurfinkel and M. Wiesendanger), Motor Control Press, Tucson, pp. 343–346.

Horak, F.B., Frank, J.S. and Nutt, J.G. (1996) Effects of dopamine on postural control in parkinsonian subjects: scaling, set, and tone. *Journal of Neurophysiology*, **75**, 2380–2396.

Horn, T.S., Yablon, S.A. and Stokic, D.S. (2005) Effect of intrathecal baclofen bolus injection on temporospatial gait characteristics in patients with acquired brain injury. *Archives of Physical Medicine and Rehabilitation*, **86**, 1127–1133.

Jackson, P.L., Lafleur, M.F., Malouin, F., Richards, C. and Doyon, J. (2001) Potential role of mental practice using motor imagery in neurologic rehabilitation. *Archives of Physical Medicine and Rehabilitation*, **82**, 1133–1141.

Jellinger, K.A. (1991) Pathology of Parkinson's disease. Changes other than the nigrostriatal pathway. Molecular and Chemical Neuropathology/Sponsored by the International Society for Neurochemistry and the World Federation of Neurology and Research Groups on Neurochemistry and Cerebrospinal Fluid, **14**, 153–197.

Jorstad, E.C., Hauer, K., Becker, C. and Lamb, S.E. (2005) Measuring the psychological outcomes of falling: a systematic review. *Journal of the American Geriatrics Society*, **53**, 501–510.

Kadanka, Z., Bednarik, J., Vohanka, S. *et al.* (2000) Conservative treatment versus surgery in spondylotic cervical myelopathy: a prospective randomised study. *European Spine Journal*, **9**, 538–544.

Kakurai, S. and Akai, M. (1996) Clinical experiences with a convertible thermoplastic knee-ankle-foot orthosis for post-stroke hemiplegic patients. *Prosthetics and Orthotics International*, **20**, 191–194.

Kamsma, Y.P., Brouwer, W.H. and Lakke, J.P.W.F. (1995) Training of compensation strategies for impaired gross motor skills in Parkinson's disease. *Physiotherapy Theory and Practice*, **11**, 209–229.

Kannus, P., Parkkari, J., Niemi, S. *et al.* (2000) Prevention of hip fracture in elderly people with use of a hip protector. *The New England Journal of Medicine*, **343**, 1506–1513.

Kannus, P., Sievanen, H., Palvanen, M., Jarvinen, T. and Parkkari, J. (2005) Prevention of falls and consequent injuries in elderly people. *Lancet*, **366**, 1885–1893.

Karol, L.A. (2004) Surgical management of the lower extremity in ambulatory children with cerebral palsy. *Journal of the American Academy of Orthopaedic Surgeons*, **12**, 196–203.

Keller, R.B. and Slattum, P.W. (2003) Strategies for prevention of medication-related falls in the elderly. *Consultant Pharmacists*, **18**, 248–258.

Keus, S.H., Bloem, B.R., Hendriks, E.J., Bredero-Cohen, A.B. and Munneke, M. (2007) Evidence-based analysis of physical therapy in Parkinson's disease with recommendations for practice and research. *Movement Disorders*, **22**, 451–460.

Kiel, D.P., Magaziner, J., Zimmerman, S. *et al.* (2007) Efficacy of a hip protector to prevent hip fracture in nursing home residents: the HIP PRO randomized controlled trial. *The Journal of the American Medical Association*, **298**, 413–422.

Kirazli, Y., On, A.Y., Kismali, B. and Aksit, R. (1998) Comparison of phenol block and botulinus toxin type A in the treatment of spastic foot after stroke: a randomized, double-blind trial.

American Journal of Physical Medicine & Rehabilitation, **77**, 510–515.

Klawans, H.L. (1986) Individual manifestations of Parkinson's disease after ten or more years of levodopa. *Movement Disorders*, **1**, 187–192.

Klebe, S., Stolze, H., Kopper, F. *et al.* (2004) Gait analysis of sporadic and hereditary spastic paraplegia. *Journal of Neurology*, **251**, 571–578.

Klebe, S., Stolze, H., Kopper, F. *et al.* (2005) Objective assessment of gait after intrathecal baclofen in hereditary spastic paraplegia. *Journal of Neurology*, **252**, 991–993.

Klinge, P., Marmarou, A., Bergsneider, M., Relkin, N. and Black, P.M. (2005) Outcome of shunting in idiopathic normal-pressure hydrocephalus and the value of outcome assessment in shunted patients. *Neurosurgery*, **57** (Suppl), S40–S52.

Koller, W.C., Glatt, S., Vetere-Overfield, B. and Hassanein, R. (1989) Falls and Parkinson's disease. *Clinical Neuropharmacology*, **2**, 98–105.

Kondo, T. (2007) Drug intervention for freezing of gait resistant to dopaminergic therapy: a pilot study. *Parkinsonism & Related Disorders*, **12** (Suppl 2), S63–S66.

Kottink, A.I., Oostendorp, L.J., Buurke, J.H., Nene, A.V., Hermens, H.J. and IJzerman, M.J. (2004) The orthotic effect of functional electrical stimulation on the improvement of walking in stroke patients with a dropped foot: a systematic review. *Artificial Organs*, **28**, 577–586.

Kottink, A.I., Hermens, H.J., Nene, A.V. *et al.* (2007) A randomized controlled trial of an implantable 2-channel peroneal nerve stimulator on walking speed and activity in poststroke hemiplegia. *Archives of Physical Medicine and Rehabilitation*, **88**, 971–978.

Krack, P. and Vercueil, L. (2001) Review of the functional surgical treatment of dystonia. *European Journal of Neurology*, **8**, 389–399.

Krakauer, J.W. (2006) Motor learning: its relevance to stroke recovery and neurorehabilitation. *Current Opinion in Neurology*, **19**, 84–90.

Krystkowiak, P., Blatt, J.L., Bourriez, J.L. *et al.* (2003) Effects of subthalamic nucleus stimulation and levodopa treatment on gait abnormalities in Parkinson's disease. *Archives of Neurology*, **60**, 80–84.

Kumar, R., Lozano, A.M., Sime, E., Halket, E. and Lang, A.E. (1999) Comparative effects of unilateral and bilateral subthalamic nucleus deep brain stimulation. *Neurology*, **53**, 561–566.

Kwakkel, G. (2006) Impact of intensity of practice after stroke: issues for consideration. *Disability and Rehabilitation*, **28**, 823–830.

Kwakkel, G., van, P.R., Wagenaar, R.C. *et al.* (2004) Effects of augmented exercise therapy time after stroke: a meta-analysis. *Stroke; A Journal of Cerebral Circulation*, **35**, 2529–2539.

Lakke, J.P.W.F. (1985) Axial apraxia in Parkinson's disease. *Journal of the Neurological Sciences*, **69**, 37–46.

Larson, E.B., Wang, L., Bowen, J.D. *et al.* (2006) Exercise is associated with reduced risk for incident dementia among persons 65 years of age and older. *Annals of Internal Medicine*, **144**, 73–81.

Laurin, D., Verreault, R., Lindsay, J., MacPherson, K. and Rockwood, K. (2001) Physical activity and risk of cognitive impairment and dementia in elderly persons. *Archives of Neurology*, **58**, 498–504.

Leipzig, R.M., Cumming, R.G. and Tinetti, M.E. (1999) Drugs and falls in older people: a systemic review and meta-analysis: 1. psychotropic drugs. *Journal of the American Geriatrics Society*, **47**, 30–39.

Liu, K.P., Chan, C.C., Lee, T.M. and Hui-Chan, C.W. (2004) Mental imagery for promoting relearning for people after stroke: a randomized controlled trial. *Archives of Physical Medicine and Rehabilitation*, **85**, 1403–1408.

Lubik, S., Fogel, W., Tronnier, V., Krause, M., Konig, J. and Jost, W.H. (2006) Gait analysis in patients with advanced Parkinson's disease: different or additive effects on gait induced by levodopa and chronic STN stimulation. *Journal of Neural Transmission*, **113**, 163–173.

Luukinen, H., Koski, K., Honkanen, R. and Kivela, S.-L. (1995) Incidence of injury-causing falls among older adults by place of residence: a population-based study. *Journal of the American Geriatrics Society*, **43**, 871–876.

Macko, R.F., Ivey, F.M. and Forrester, L.W. (2005) Task-oriented aerobic exercise in chronic hemiparetic stroke: training protocols and treatment effects. *Topics in Stroke Rehabilitation*, **12**, 45–57.

Manganotti, P., Bortolomasi, M., Zanette, G., Pawelzik, T., Giacopuzzi, M. and Fiaschi, A. (2001) Intravenous clomipramine decreases excitability of human motor cortex. A study with paired magnetic stimulation. *Journal of the Neurological Sciences*, **184**, 27–32.

Manson, J.E., Greenland, P., Lacroix, A.Z. *et al.* (2002) Walking compared with vigorous exercise for the prevention of cardiovascular events in women. *The New England Journal of Medicine*, **347**, 716–725.

Marcus, B.H., Williams, D.M., Dubbert, P.M. *et al.* (2006) Physical activity intervention studies: what we know and what we need to know: a scientific statement from the American Heart Association Council on Nutrition, Physical Activity, and Metabolism (Subcommittee on Physical Activity); Council on Cardiovascular Disease in the Young; and the Interdisciplinary Working Group on Quality of Care and Outcomes Research. *Circulation*, **114**, 2739–2752.

Marmarou, A., Bergsneider, M., Klinge, P., Relkin, N. and Black, P.M. (2005) The value of supplemental prognostic tests for the preoperative assessment of idiopathic normal-pressure hydrocephalus. *Neurosurgery*, **57** (Suppl), S17–S28.

Marquis, S., Moore, M.M., Howieson, D.B. *et al.* (2002) Independent predictors of cognitive decline in healthy elderly persons. *Archives of Neurology*, **59**, 601–606.

Mathias, C.J. and Kimber, J.R. (1998) Treatment of postural hypotension. *Journal of Neurology, Neurosurgery, and Psychiatry*, **65**, 285–289.

Mauritz, K.H. (2002) Gait training in hemiplegia. *European Journal of Neurology*, **9** (Suppl 1), 23–29.

Mayer, N.H. (1997) Clinicophysiologic concepts of spasticity and motor dysfunction in adults with an upper motoneuron lesion. *Muscle & Nerve Suppl*, **6**, S1–S13.

Mayr, A., Kofler, M., Quirbach, E., Matzak, H., Frohlich, K. and Saltuari, L. (2007) Prospective, blinded, randomized crossover study of gait rehabilitation in stroke patients using the Lokomat gait orthosis. *Neurorehabil Neural Repair*, **21**, 307–314.

Mazzone, P., Lozano, A., Stanzione, P. *et al.* (2005) Implantation of human pedunculopontine nucleus: a safe and clinically relevant target in Parkinson's disease. *Neuroreport*, **16**, 1877–1881.

Mehrholz, J., Werner, C., Kugler, J. and Pohl, M. (2007) Electromechanical-assisted training for walking after stroke. *Cochrane Database of Systematic Reviews*, CD006185.

Minns, R.J. (2005) The role of gait analysis in the management of the knee. *Knee*, **12**, 157–162.

Morris, M.E. (2000) Movement disorders in people with Parkinson's disease: a model for physical therapy. *Physical Therapy*, **80**, 578–597.

Morris, M.E., Bruce, M., Smithson, F. *et al.* (1997) Physiotherapy strategies for people with Parkinson's disease, in *Parkinson's Disease: A Team Approach* (eds M.E. Morris and R. Iansek), Buscombe Vicprint Ltd, Blackburn, pp. 27–64.

Moseley, A.M., Stark, A., Cameron, I.D. and Pollock, A. (2005) Treadmill training and body weight support for walking after stroke. *Cochrane Database of Systematic Reviews*, CD002840.

Mulder, T.W. (2007) Motor imagery and action observation: cognitive tools for rehabilitation. *Journal of Neural Transmission*, **114**, 1265–1278.

Mulder, T.W. and Geurts, A. (1993) Recovery of motor skill following nervous system disorders: a behavioural emphasis. *Baillieres Clinical Neurology*, **2**, 1–13.

Mulder, T.W. and Hochstenbach, J. (2001) Adaptability and flexibility of the human motor system: implications for neurological rehabilitation. *Neural Plasticity*, **8**, 131–140.

Narabayashi, H., Kondo, T., Yokochi, F. and Nagatsu, T. (1987) Clinical effects of L-threo-3, 4-dihydroxyphenylserine in cases of parkinsonism and pure akinesia. *Advances in Neurology*, **45**, 593–602.

Nelson, A.J., Zwick, D., Brody, S. *et al.* (2002) The validity of the GaitRite and the Functional Ambulation Performance scoring system in the analysis of Parkinson gait. *NeuroRehabilitation*, **17**, 255–262.

Nevitt, M.C., Cummings, S.R., Kidd, S. and Black, D.M. (1989) Risk factors for recurrent nonsyncopal falls. A prospective study. *The Journal of the American Medical Association*, **261**, 2663–2668.

Nieuwboer, A., Herman, T., Rochester, L. and Giladi, N. (2006) Evaluation of freezing of gait severity in patients with Parkinson's disease: the perception of caregivers. *Movement Disorders*, **21** (Suppl 15), S493.

Nieuwboer, A., Kwakkel, G., Rochester, L. *et al.* (2007) Cueing training in the home improves gait-related mobility in Parkinson's disease: the RESCUE trial. *Journal of Neurology, Neurosurgery, and Psychiatry*, **78**, 134–140.

Nutt, J.G., Hammerstad, J.P. and Gancher, S.T. (1992) *Parkinson's disease: 100 maxims*, Edward Arnold, London.

O'Brien, C.F. (2002) Treatment of spasticity with botulinum toxin. *Clinical Journal of Pain*, **18** (Suppl), S182–S190.

O'Sullivan, J.D., Said, C.M., Dillon, L.C., Hoffman, M. and Hughes, A.J. (1998) Gait analysis in patients with Parkinson's disease and motor fluctuations: influence of levodopa and comparison with other measures of motor function. *Movement Disorders*, **13**, 900–906.

Olanow, C.W., Marsden, C.D., Lang, A.E. and Goetz, C.G. (1994) The role of surgery in Parkinson's disease management. *Neurology*, **44**, S17–S20.

Oliver, D., Connelly, J.B., Victor, C.R. *et al.* (2007) Strategies to prevent falls and fractures in hospitals and care homes and effect of cognitive impairment: systematic review and meta-analyses. *BMJ (Clinical Research Ed)*, **334**, 82–88.

Oude Voshaar, R.C., Banerjee, S., Horan, M. *et al.* (2006) Fear of falling more important than pain and depression for functional recovery after surgery for hip fracture in older people. *Psychological Medicine*, **36**, 1635–1645.

Pahapill, P.A. and Lozano, A.M. (2000) The pedunculopontine nucleus and Parkinson's disease. *Brain: A Journal of Neurology*, **123**, 1767–1783.

Parkinson Study Group (2000) Pramipexole vs levodopa as initial treatment for Parkinson's disease: A randomized controlled trial. Parkinson Study Group. *The Journal of the American Medical Association*, **284**, 1931–1938.

Perry, J., Waters, R.L. and Perrin, T. (1978) Electromyographic analysis of equinovarus following stroke. *Clinical Orthopaedics and Related Research*, **131**, 47–53.

Pickering, R., Grimbergen, Y.A., Rigney, U. *et al.* (2007) A meta-analysis of six prospective studies of falls in Parkinson's disease. *Movement Disorders*, **22**, 1892–1900.

Plaha, P. and Gill, S.S. (2005) Bilateral deep brain stimulation of the pedunculopontine nucleus for Parkinson's disease. *Neuroreport*, **16**, 1883–1887.

Plotnik, M., Giladi, N., Balash, Y., Peretz, C. and Hausdorff, J.M. (2005) Is freezing of gait in Parkinson's disease related to asymmetric motor function? *Annals of Neurology*, **57**, 656–663.

Pluijm, S.M., Smit, J.H., Tromp, E.A. *et al.* (2006) A risk profile for identifying community-dwelling elderly with a high risk of recurrent falling: results of a 3-year prospective study. *Osteoporosis International*, **17**, 417–425.

Pollock, A., Baer, G., Langhorne, P. and Pomeroy, V. (2007) Physiotherapy treatment approaches for the recovery of postural control and lower limb function following stroke: a systematic review. *Clinical Rehabilitation*, **21**, 395–410.

Protas, E.J., Mitchell, K., Williams, A., Qureshy, H., Caroline, K. and Lai, E.C. (2005) Gait and step training to reduce falls in Parkinson's disease. *Neurorehabilitation*, **20**, 183–190.

Rascol, O., Brooks, D.J., Korczyn, A.D., De Deyn, P.P., Clarke, C.E. and Lang, A.E. (2000) A five-year study of the incidence of dyskinesia in patients with early Parkinson's disease who were treated with ropinirole or levodopa. 056 Study Group. *The New England Journal of Medicine*, **342**, 1484–1491.

Regan, C., Katona, C., Walker, Z. and Livingston, G. (2005) Relationship of exercise and other risk factors to depression of Alzheimer's disease: the LASER-AD study. *International Journal of Geriatric Psychiatry*, **20**, 261–268.

Relkin, N., Marmarou, A., Klinge, P., Bergsneider, M. and Black, P.M. (2005) Diagnosing idiopathic normal-pressure hydrocephalus. *Neurosurgery*, **57** (Suppl), S4–S16.

Remy-Neris, O., Tiffreau, V., Bouilland, S. and Bussel, B. (2003) Intrathecal baclofen in subjects with spastic hemiplegia: assessment of the antispastic effect during gait. *Archives of Physical Medicine and Rehabilitation*, **84**, 643–650.

Robertson, M.C., Devlin, N., Gardner, M.M. and Campbell, A.J. (2001) Effectiveness and economic evaluation of a nurse delivered home exercise programme to prevent falls. 1: Randomised controlled trial. *BMJ (Clinical Research Ed)*, **322**, 697–701.

Rousseaux, M., Launay, M.J., Kozlowski, O. and Daveluy, W. (2007) Botulinum toxin injection in patients with hereditary spastic paraparesis. *European Journal of Neurology*, **14**, 206–212.

Rubinstein, T.C., Giladi, N. and Hausdorff, J.M. (2002) The power of cueing to circumvent dopamine deficits: a review of physical therapy treatment of gait disturbances in Parkinson's disease. *Movement Disorders*, **17**, 1148–1160.

Rucker, D., Rowe, B.H., Johnson, J.A. *et al.* (2006) Educational intervention to reduce falls and fear of falling in patients after fragility fracture: results of a controlled pilot study. *Preventive Medicine*, **42**, 316–319.

Sato, Y., Manabe, S., Kuno, H. and Oizumi, K. (1999) Amelioration of osteopenia and hypovitaminosis D by 1 alpha-hydroxyvitamin D3 in elderly patients with Parkinson's disease. *Journal of Neurology, Neurosurgery, and Psychiatry*, **66**, 64–68.

Sato, Y., Honda, Y. and Iwamoto, J. (2007) Risedronate and ergocalciferol prevent hip fracture in elderly men with Parkinson's disease. *Neurology*, **68**, 911–915.

Scarmeas, N., Albert, M., Brandt, J. *et al.* (2005) Motor signs predict poor outcomes in Alzheimer disease. *Neurology*, **64**, 1696–1703.

Schaafsma, J.D., Balash, Y., Gurevich, T., Bartels, A.L., Hausdorff, J.M. and Giladi, N. (2003a) Characterization of freezing of gait subtypes and the response of each to levodopa in Parkinson's disease. *European Journal of Neurology*, **10**, 391–398.

Schaafsma, J.D., Giladi, N., Balash, Y., Bartels, A.L., Gurevich, T. and Hausdorff, J.M. (2003b) Gait dynamics in Parkinson's disease: relationship to Parkinsonian features, falls and response to levodopa. *Journal of the Neurological Sciences*, **212**, 47–53.

Schmahmann, J.D. and Sherman, J.C. (1998) The cerebellar cognitive affective syndrome. *Brain: A Journal of Neurology*, **121** (Pt 4), 561–579.

Scholtes, V.A., Dallmeijer, A.J., Knol, D.L. *et al.* (2007) Effect of multilevel botulinum toxin a and comprehensive rehabilitation on gait in cerebral palsy. *Pediatric Neurology*, **36**, 30–39.

Shaw, F.E. (2002) Falls in cognitive impairment and dementia. *Clinics in Geriatric Medicine*, **18**, 159–173.

Shaw, F.E. and Kenny, R.A. (1998) Can falls in patients with dementia be prevented? *Age Ageing*, **27**, 7–9.

Sheffler, L.R., Hennessey, M.T., Naples, G.G. and Chae, J. (2006) Peroneal nerve stimulation versus an ankle foot orthosis for correction of footdrop in stroke: impact on functional ambulation. *Neurorehabil Neural Repair*, **20**, 355–360.

Sheridan, P.L., Solomont, J., Kowall, N. and Hausdorff, J.M. (2003) Influence of executive function on locomotor function: divided attention increases gait variability in Alzheimer's disease. *Journal of the American Geriatrics Society*, **51**, 1633–1637.

Shiino, A., Nishida, Y., Yasuda, H., Suzuki, M., Matsuda, M. and Inubushi, T. (2004) Magnetic resonance spectroscopic determination of a neuronal and axonal marker in white matter predicts reversibility of deficits in secondary normal pressure hydrocephalus. *Journal of Neurology, Neurosurgery, and Psychiatry*, **75**, 1141–1148.

Shoulson, I., Oakes, D., Fahn, S. *et al.* (2002) Impact of sustained deprenyl (selegiline) in levodopa-treated Parkinson's disease: a randomized placebo-controlled extension of the deprenyl and tocopherol antioxidative therapy of parkinsonism trial. *Annals of Neurology*, **51**, 604–612.

Siegel, K.L. and Metman, L.V. (2000) Effects of bilateral posteroventral pallidotomy on gait of subjects with Parkinson's disease. *Archives of Neurology*, **57**, 198–204.

Sindou, M.P. and Mertens, P. (2000) Neurosurgery for spasticity. *Stereotact Funct Neurosurg*, **74**, 217–221.

Smyth, M.D. and Peacock, W.J. (2000) The surgical treatment of spasticity. *Muscle & Nerve*, **23**, 153–163.

Snijders, A.H., van de Warrenburg, B.P., Giladi, N. and Bloem, B.R. (2007) Neurological gait disorders in elderly people: clinical approach and classification. *Lancet Neurology*, **6**, 63–74.

Speelman, J.D. (1991) Parkinson's disease and stereotaxic neurosurgery. Amsterdam: Thesis.

Springer, S., Giladi, N., Peretz, C., Yogev, G., Simon, E.S. and Hausdorff, J.M. (2006) Dual-tasking effects on gait variability: The role of aging, falls, and executive function. *Movement Disorders*, **21**, 950–957.

Stefani, A., Lozano, A.M., Peppe, A. *et al.* (2007) Bilateral deep brain stimulation of the pedunculopontine and subthalamic nuclei in severe Parkinson's disease. *Brain: A Journal of Neurology*, **130**, 1596–1607.

Stein, R.B. (1999) Functional electrical stimulation after spinal cord injury. *Journal of Neurotrauma*, **16**, 713–717.

Steiner, B., Winter, C., Hosman, K. *et al.* (2006) Enriched environment induces cellular plasticity in the adult substantia nigra

and improves motor behavior function in the 6-OHDA rat model of Parkinson's disease. *Experimental Neurology*, **199**, 291–300.

Stevens, M., Holman, C.D., Bennett, N. and de Klerk, N. (2001) Preventing falls in older people: outcome evaluation of a randomized controlled trial. *Journal of the American Geriatrics Society*, **49**, 1448–1455.

Stolze, H., Klebe, S., Poepping, M. *et al.* (2001) Effects of bilateral subthalamic nucleus stimulation on parkinsonian gait. *Neurology*, **57**, 144–146.

Subramanian, N., Vaughan, C.L., Peter, J.C. and Arens, L.J. (1998) Gait before and 10 years after rhizotomy in children with cerebral palsy spasticity. *Journal of Neurosurgery*, **88**, 1014–1019.

Sudarsky, L. (2001) Gait disorders: prevalence, morbidity, and etiology. *Advances in Neurology*, **87**, 111–117.

Sullivan-Marx, E.M., Strumpf, N.E., Evans, L.K., Baumgarten, M. and Maislin, G. (1999) Predictors of continued physical restraint use in nursing home residents following restraint reduction efforts. *Journal of the American Geriatrics Society*, **47**, 342–348.

Sutbeyaz, S., Yavuzer, G., Sezer, N. and Koseoglu, B.F. (2007) Mirror therapy enhances lower-extremity motor recovery and motor functioning after stroke: a randomized controlled trial. *Archives of Physical Medicine and Rehabilitation*, **88**, 555–559.

Swarztrauber, K., Graf, E. and Cheng, E. (2006) The quality of care delivered to Parkinson's disease patients in the U.S. Pacific Northwest Veterans Health System. *BMC Neurology*, **6**, 26.

Sweeney, P.C., Lyons, G.M. and Veltink, P.H. (2000) Finite state control of functional electrical stimulation for the rehabilitation of gait. *Medical & Biological Engineering & Computing*, **38**, 121–126.

Tennstedt, S., Howland, J., Lachman, M., Peterson, E., Kasten, L. and Jette, A. (1998) A randomized, controlled trial of a group intervention to reduce fear of falling and associated activity restriction in older adults. *Journals of Gerontology Series B-Psychological Sciences and Social Sciences*, **53**, 384–392.

Thijs, R.D., Wieling, W., van den Aardweg, J.G. and van Dijk, J.G. (2007) Respiratory countermaneuvers in autonomic failure. *Neurology*, **69**, 582–585.

Tillerson, J.L., Caudle, W.M., Reveron, M.E. and Miller, G.W. (2003) Exercise induces behavioral recovery and attenuates neurochemical deficits in rodent models of Parkinson's disease. *Neuroscience*, **119**, 899–911.

Tinetti, M.E. (2003) Clinical practice. Preventing falls in elderly persons. *The New England Journal of Medicine*, **348**, 42–49.

Tinetti, M.E. and Williams, C.S. (1997) Falls, injuries due to falls, and the risk of admission to a nursing home. *The New England Journal of Medicine*, **337**, 1279–1284.

Tinetti, M.E., Speechley, M. and Ginter, S.F. (1988) Risk factors for falls among elderly persons living in the community. *The New England Journal of Medicine*, **319**, 1701–1707.

Tinetti, M.E., Wen-Liang, L. and Claus, E.B. (1993) Predictors and prognosis of inability to get up after falls among elderly persons. *The Journal of the American Medical Association*, **269**, 65–70.

van Gelder, B.M., Tijhuis, M.A., Kalmijn, S., Giampaoli, S., Nissinen, A. and Kromhout, D. (2004) Physical activity in relation to cognitive decline in elderly men: the FINE Study. *Neurology*, **63**, 2316–2321.

van Haastregt, J.C.M., Diederiks, J.P.M., van Rossum, E., de Witte, L.P. and Crebolder, H.F.J.M. (2000a) Effects of preventive home visits to elderly people living in the community: systematic review. *British Medical Journal*, **320**, 754–758.

van Haastregt, J.C.M., Diederiks, J.P.M., van Rossum, E., de Witte, L.P., Voorhoeve, P.M. and Crebolder, H.F.J.M. (2000b) Effects of a programme of multifactorial home visits on falls and mobility impairments in elderly people at risk: randomised controlled trial. *British Medical Journal*, **321**, 994–998.

van Nuenen, B.F., Esselink, R.A., Munneke, M., Speelman, J.D., van Laar, T. and Bloem, B.R. (2008) Secondary gait deterioration after bilateral subthalamic nucleus stimulation in Parkinson's disease. *Movement Disorders, accepted pending minor revision.*

van Peppen, R.P., van Hendriks, H.J., Meeteren, N.L., Helders, P.J. and Kwakkel, G. (2007) The development of a clinical practice stroke guideline for physiotherapists in The Netherlands: a systematic review of available evidence. *Disability and Rehabilitation*, **29**, 767–783.

Veneman, J.F., Kruidhof, R., Hekman, E.E., Ekkelenkamp, R., van Asseldonk, E.H. and van der, K.H. (2007) Design and evaluation of the LOPES exoskeleton robot for interactive gait rehabilitation. *IEEE Transactions on Neural Systems and Rehabilitation Engineering*, **15**, 379–386.

Verghese, J., Lipton, R.B., Hall, C.B., Kuslansky, G., Katz, M.J. and Buschke, H. (2002) Abnormality of gait as a predictor of non-Alzheimer's dementia. *The New England Journal of Medicine*, **347**, 1761–1768.

Voermans, N.C., Snijders, A.H., Schoon, Y. and Bloem, B.R. (2007) Why old people fall (and how to stop them). *Practical Neurology*, **7**, 158–171.

Vokaer, M., Azar, N.A. and de Beyl, D.Z. (2003) Effects of levodopa on upper limb mobility and gait in Parkinson's disease. *Journal of Neurology, Neurosurgery, and Psychiatry*, **74**, 1304–1307.

Walker, J.E., Albers, J.W., Tourtellotte, W.W., Henderson, W.G., Potvin, A.R. and Smith, A. (1972) A qualitative and quantitative evaluation of amantadine in the treatment of Parkinson's disease. *Journal of Chronic Diseases*, **25**, 149–182.

Weerdesteyn, V., Rijken, H., Geurts, A.C., Smits-Engelsman, B. C., Mulder, T.W. and Duysens, J. (2006) A five-week exercise program can reduce falls and improve obstacle avoidance in the elderly. *Gerontology*, **52**, 131–141.

Weuve, J., Kang, J.H., Manson, J.E., Breteler, M.M., Ware, J.H. and Grodstein, F. (2004) Physical activity, including walking, and cognitive function in older women. *The Journal of the American Medical Association*, **292**, 1454–1461.

Wilson, R.S., Schneider, J.A., Beckett, L.A., Evans, D.A. and Bennett, D.A. (2002) Progression of gait disorder and rigidity and risk of death in older persons. *Neurology*, **58**, 1815–1819.

Yaffe, K., Barnes, D., Nevitt, M., Lui, L.Y. and Covinsky, K. (2001) A prospective study of physical activity and cognitive decline in elderly women: women who walk. *Archives of Internal Medicine*, **161**, 1703–1708.

Yokoyama, T., Sugiyama, K., Nishizawa, S., Yokota, N., Ohta, S. and Uemura, K. (1999) Subthalamic nucleus stimulation for gait disturbance in Parkinson's disease. *Neurosurgery*, **45**, 41–47.

You, S.H., Jang, S.H., Kim, Y.H. *et al.* (2005) Virtual reality-induced cortical reorganization and associated locomotor recovery in chronic stroke: an experimenter-blind randomized study. *Stroke; A Journal of Cerebral Circulation*, **36**, 1166–1171.

Ziere, G., Dieleman, J.P., Hofman, A., Pols, H.A., van der Cammen, T.J. and Stricker, B.H. (2006) Polypharmacy and falls in the middle age and elderly population. *British Journal of Clinical Pharmacology*, **61**, 218–223.

Zijlmans, J.C., Katzenschlager, R., Daniel, S.E. and Lees, A.J. (2004) The L-dopa response in vascular parkinsonism. *Journal of Neurology, Neurosurgery, and Psychiatry*, **75**, 545–547.

Zuniga, C., Lester, J., Cersosimo, M.G., Diaz, S. and Micheli, F.E. (2006) Treatment of primary progressive freezing of gait with high doses of selegiline. *Clinical Neuropharmacology*, **29**, 20–21.

Zweig, R.M., Jankel, W.R., Hedreen, J.C., Mayeux, R. and Price, D.L. (1989) The pedunculopontine nucleus in Parkinson's disease. *Annals of Neurology*, **26**, 41–46.

Part VII

RESTLESS LEGS SYNDROME

29

The Restless Legs Syndrome

Richard P. Allen[1] and Birgit Högl[2]

[1] Dept of Neurology, Johns Hopkins University, Baltimore, MD, USA
[2] Dept of Neurology, University of Innsbruck, Innsbruck, Austria

INTRODUCTION: HISTORY

Restless legs syndrome (RLS) is, for several reasons, a bit of an oddity in a book such as this one, focused on movement disorders. It is, in a sense, both among the oldest and the youngest of these movement disorders. It was well described in the medical literature as a treatable disorder by Willis in1683, at least 230 years before Parkinson described the "shaking palsy." Willis' description of violent limb movements engendered by quiet rest (see Figure 29.1) captures much of our current understanding of the disorder. But RLS remained largely ignored by the medical community for over 270 years, until Ekbom's classic series of clinical studies and his excellent monograph (Ekbom, 1945; Ekbom, 1950) not only established primary features of the disorder, but also anointed it with its current name.

Even after Ekbom's work RLS remained in the shadows until the convergence of three factors forced it into the main stream of medicine. First, the development in the later half of the twentieth century of the field of sleep medicine and Lugaresi's recognition of periodic leg movements disturbing sleep (PLMS) of RLS patients (Lugaresi *et al.*, 1968) alerted clinicians to an unusual movement disorder that, unlike most others discussed in this book, becomes worse with rest and sleep. Second, the development of geriatric medicine included an emphasis on medical management to ensure quality of life for relatively healthy older adults. Medical attention turned to disorders like RLS that, while not directly mortal, profoundly disturb life, particularly for those over 55. Life spans in the fairly recent past in European history were more like that of Willis, who died at age 52. RLS occurs at any age, but becomes a daily distressing symptom mostly for those over age 50. Third, Akpinar's serendipitous discovery that levodopa provides dramatically effective treatment for RLS (Akpinar, 1982) completed this confluence propelling RLS into the main stream of medical consideration.

Now, this common disorder producing abnormal movements in sleep and also profound loss of sleep in otherwise healthy older adults can be effectively treated by the same dopaminergic medications used to treat Parkinson's disease (PD). It is, however, also treated by medications that have little benefit for PD. RLS thus is one of the most recent of the movement disorders to receive significant medical attention. A book such as this written only 30 years ago would have hardly mentioned RLS, perhaps in a section or a paragraph in a chapter on other disorders. While a young field, as hopefully you will partly see in this chapter, it is one producing remarkable scientific and clinical advances with implications beyond the disorder itself.

What makes RLS an oddity in this book is not so much its long gestation, nor its tantalizing treatment overlap with Parkinson's disease, nor even its strange rest-induced abnormal movements, rather RLS is primarily a sensory more than a movement disorder. The sensory experience of the urge to move or akathisia, not the movements themselves, defines the disorder. It is closest to, but quite distinct from neuroleptic-induced akathisia described in Chapter 25 of this book. This unique aspect of RLS makes its neurobiology relevant to understanding the neurobiology of sensory-motor integration, but it also makes the defining symptoms entirely subjective sensory experiences, significantly complicating the diagnosis of RLS.

DIAGNOSIS, CLINICAL PRESENTATION AND EVALUATION

Diagnosis

Diagnosis of RLS requires evaluation of the patient's subjective report of the sensory symptoms defining the disease. Some of the features supporting the diagnosis can be objectively assessed, but while recent genetic, physiological and neurobiological advances hold promise we, at this time,

First Medical Description of RLS: Willis, 1685

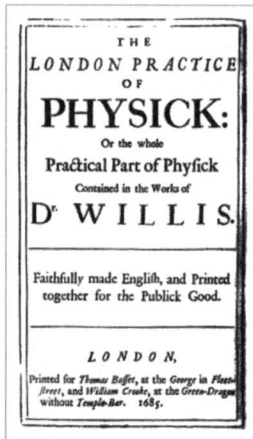

THE

LONDON PRACTICE

OF

PHYSICK:

Or the whole

Practical Part of Physick

Contained in the Works of

D.ʳ WILLIS.

Faithfully made English, and Printed
together for the Publick Good.

LONDON,

Printed for *Thomas Basset*, at the *George in Fleet-
street*, and *William Crooke*, at the *Green-Dragon*
without *Temple-Bar*. 1685.

"Wherefore to some, on being a bed, they **betake themselves to sleep**, presently in the **arms and legs**, leaping and contractions of the tendons, and so great a restlessness and tossings of their members ensue that the diseased are **no more able to sleep than if they were in the place of the greatest torture.**"

Figure 29.1 Willis picture and RLS description.

do not have a biological marker of the disease. The four essential diagnostic criteria for RLS listed in Table 29.1 were set forth at a consensus workshop held in 2002 at the National Institute of Health in Washington DC and formally approved by the International Restless Legs Syndrome Study Group (IRLSSG) (Allen *et al.*, 2003). The simple statement of these criteria, however, somewhat obscures the subtleties embodied in them. These criteria divide into one that specifies the subjective symptom and three that define conditions regulating expression of the symptoms.

Table 29.1 Essential diagnostic criteria for RLS.

(1)   An urge to move the legs, usually accompanied or caused by uncomfortable and unpleasant sensations in the legs. (Sometimes the urge to move is present without the uncomfortable sensations and sometimes the arms or other body parts are involved in addition to the legs)

(2)   The urge to move or unpleasant sensations begin or worsen during periods of rest or inactivity such as lying or sitting

(3)   The urge to move or unpleasant sensations are partially or totally relieved by movement, such as walking or stretching, at least as long as the activity continues

(4)   The urge to move or unpleasant sensations are worse in the evening or night than during the day or only occur in the evening or night. (When symptoms are very severe, the worsening at night may not be noticeable but must have been previously present.)

From Allen, R.P. *et al.* (2003) *Sleep Med.*, **4**, 101–119. Copyright © 2003, Elsevier.

Essential Diagnostic Criteria

Diagnostic Criterion 1 (Defining the RLS Symptom): An Urge to Move the Legs, Usually Accompanied or Caused by Uncomfortable and Unpleasant Sensations in the Legs

The sensory symptom defining RLS can best be conceptualized as an akathisia focused on the legs. Akathisia involves clear awareness of the urge to move. Unconscious or even partially aware habitual movements (e.g., nervous foot tapping) do not constitute RLS symptoms. The unusual sensory symptoms or paresthesias occur typically without any physical signs in the legs and are most often described as some dynamic or moving sensation happening deep in the legs, not like an itch on the surface of the leg (see Table 29.2). The paresthesias should generally concur in time and location with the focal akathisia. The most difficult clinical judgment about this criterion occurs when a patient reports a need to move to reduce the paresthesia. Here the critical question involves deciding if the sensation being reduced is an urge to move or some other pain condition. Often it helps to ask what occurs if the patient does not move. The urge to move may become more pronounced and intense; the legs may even move or "jerk" on their own, but the degree of associated paresthesia will generally not worsen. Development of profound pain with delayed movement indicates possible conditions other than RLS, for example, leg cramps.

Diagnostic Criterion 2: RLS Symptoms Begin or Worsen During Periods of Rest or Inactivity Such as Lying or Sitting

RLS symptoms rarely, if ever, occur spontaneously; rather they are provoked or engendered by quiet resting. The quiet resting involves decreased mental and physical activity.

Table 29.2 Descriptive terms for restless legs syndrome.

Creepy-crawly	Ants crawling
Jittery	Pulling
Worms moving	Soda bubbling in the veins
Electric current	Shock-like feelings
Fidgets	The gotta-moves
Burning	Jimmy legs
Heebie-jeebies	Tearing
Throbbing	Tight feeling
Grabbing sensation	Elvis legs
Itching bones	Crazy legs
Cramping like	Tooth ache in leg
Pain (in 30–50% of	
clinical cases)	

The longer and deeper the quiescent state the more likely and the more intense the occurrence of RLS symptoms. Thus symptoms can be provoked by having patients sit up with legs stretched out for a long period of time, for example, one hour remaining relaxed and awake with minimal mental activity. This describes the suggested immobilization test (SIT) used to evaluate RLS severity and some standardized adaptation of the procedure may be helpful for RLS diagnosis in the future. Note that RLS symptoms should not start when walking or moving about. The symptoms should also be engendered by quiescent states in general and not by particular body positions, such as sitting with legs crossed. Decreased mental activity, for example, relaxation, but also tedium or boredom can also provoke or worsen symptoms, so other activities creating alertness, such as an emotionally intense argument, also relieve the RLS symptoms.

Diagnostic Criterion 3: RLS Symptoms are Partially or Totally Relieved by Movement, Such as Walking or Stretching, at Least as Long as the Activity Continues

RLS symptoms are at least partly if not completely relieved by movement. The patients should report that once they start moving they are more comfortable than if they stop moving, that is there should be some sense that symptoms abate at least somewhat almost immediately or at least shortly after starting movement and this improvement should persist as long as the movement continues. Both real movement and alertness reduce the symptoms. However, since any real movement always produces alertness, the more general diagnostic statement would be that increased alertness relieves the symptoms. But since movement can be directly observed it provides the better diagnostic criteria. It should, however, be clear to the clinician that the level of alertness is the major driving force producing and relieving symptoms and any factor that affects the level of alertness will also affect the expression of RLS symptoms.

Diagnostic Criterion 4: RLS Symptoms are Worse in the Evening or Night Than During the Day or Only Occur in the Evening or Night

Late afternoon and night-times are the worst times for RLS and conversely mid-morning—about the normal time for waking from sleep and the first few hours of waking—appears to be a "protected period" when symptoms rarely occur and if present are less severe than at other times of day. The circadian modulation of RLS symptoms occurs independent of activity. Thus quiet resting engenders more symptoms in the night-time than mid-morning. This pattern appears to follow the body's biological clock and can be disrupted by jet lag, shift work or other circadian rhythm disorders. Diagnosis should attend, not only to worsening symptoms with afternoon and evening rest, but also fewer or no symptoms with resting in the morning at the normal waking time. Patients generally report disrupted sleep during the initial parts of the sleep period with better sleep in the morning.

Features Supporting the Diagnosis of RLS: Response to Dopaminergic Treatment, Periodic Limb Movements in Sleep and Family History of RLS

These three features have differing values. The first two have most significance when not present. A failure to show any clinical response at least initially to a therapeutic trial dose of levodopa (100–200 mg) should raise concern about the accuracy of the diagnosis, since it has been reported that 80–90% or more of RLS patients report improvement with this treatment (Stiasny-Kolster et al., 2006). Unfortunately under normal clinical conditions, as many as 30–50% of patients report a positive subjective response to placebo (Trenkwalder et al., 2004a; Walters et al., 2004) so this fails to be adequately specific, although it may be more specific in situations with standard rest procedures designed to provoke the RLS symptoms. Periodic limb movements in sleep similarly occur at high rates in 80–90% of RLS patients and the failure to find any indication for these casts some doubt on a diagnosis of RLS. Again, however, 30–60% of those without RLS also have high rates of PLMS, particularly for those over age 40 (Pennestri et al., 2006). The PLM rates become more specific for RLS for younger adults and particularly for children and are included in the special diagnostic criteria for children. Finally, family history of RLS when present supports the diagnosis, since the risk of having RLS is 3–5 times greater than expected for first degree relatives of RLS patients (Allen et al., 2002). In contrast to the other supportive features, a lack of a family history has no diagnostic significance, particularly if the age at which the RLS symptoms were first experienced was over 45. The familial form of RLS occurs more with those whose symptoms start earlier in life.

Differential Diagnosis

Although often ignored, the differential diagnosis provides an important counterbalance to the concept that you can simply ask four questions covering the RLS symptoms to make a diagnosis of RLS. Several conditions listed in Table 29.3 can be easily mistaken for RLS and need to be specifically evaluated. Separating peripheral neuropathy from RLS can be difficult, but two critical issues help. RLS, unlike peripheral neuropathy, does not produce numbness and can be significantly relieved almost immediately with movement or increased alertness. Leg cramps are usually easy to distinguish from RLS, except for those who have

Table 29.3 Major conditions to consider in the differential diagnosis of RLS.

Condition	Differential from RLS diagnostic criteria
Positional discomfort	Not any rest position, Mostly only one fixed position
	Relief by a position change, not activity or alertness
Drug (neuroleptic)-induced akathisia:	Not focal, occurs with/after drug use
Painful legs and moving toes;	Not nocturnal or quiescegenic
Pain syndromes:	Not quickly relieved by movement
Sleep starts:	Not quiescegenic, limited to sleep onset
Nocturnal leg cramps:	Not quickly relieved by movement
Anxiety/psychiatric states	Not relieved by movement
	Closely related to stress and mental status

warning feelings that leg cramps are about to happen and respond to these feelings by moving the legs. They may answer positively to all four diagnostic criteria for RLS, feeling they have to move the legs. The difficulty here is separating the need to move to avoid the awful pain of a leg cramp from responding to an internal urge to move. One approach is to ask the patients what would happen if they did not move. If they then describe leg cramps or the pains of leg cramps the diagnosis should not be RLS unless they have other symptoms matching the RLS criteria. Many other leg-pain conditions, including vascular problems may, on the surface, look like RLS. They generally differ by not responding with significant relief occurring rapidly with movement, and also they may come back or occur when the patient is moving. RLS symptoms should not start to occur when the patient is walking. Some individuals develop habits of moving their legs, feet or toes when sitting or lying down for a long time. These unconscious movement habits occur without the patient being aware of them unless someone else notices them. RLS involves a conscious urge to move that the patient is painfully aware of. Unconscious habitual movements do not meet the criteria for RLS diagnosis.

Clinical Presentation

RLS symptom occurrence varies widely, from infrequent (less than monthly) and mildly annoying, to daily and

extremely distressing, even disabling. One group of RLS clinical experts viewed RLS symptoms as clinically significant when they occurred at least twice a week and were moderately or severely disturbing to the patient (Allen et al., 2005b). Mild RLS may only be expressed with prolonged quiescent periods such as riding in a car or plane or sitting watching television in the evening; the duration of lying still before sleep onset may be too short to provoke symptoms. When severe, the RLS symptoms become expressed in any resting situation occurring during the evening or night. Patients may avoid symptoms during the day and evening by maintaining activity, but this obviously fails for sleep. Thus sleep disturbance becomes a major presenting symptom reported by 88% of a sample of primary-care patients with clinically significant RLS (Hening et al., 2004). Sleep is also the primary morbidity for these more severely affected patients and the degree of sleep disturbance appears to be the most significant factor determining several other adverse effects of RLS (Kushida, Allen and Atkinson, 2004). Thus RLS patients often present with complaints of insomnia and RLS must be considered as a diagnosis for every patient complaining of insomnia. It is important to note that the RLS patient may complain of only sleep maintenance or only sleep onset difficulties but in more severe cases is likely to complain of both.

Pain in the legs is the second most common complaint reported by 60% of those with clinically significant RLS symptoms in a general population survey (Allen et al., 2005b). In that survey some significant leg discomfort or pain was reported as one of the primary symptoms in 88% of those with clinically significant RLS symptoms. In another large study, leg complaints were even more frequent than sleep complaints, and nearly two thirds of the patients had been treated with a venotonic (Crochard et al., 2007). A diagnosis of vascular disorder was also frequently given to RLS patients (60.7%) in another study (Tison et al., 2005). It is very important, however, to note that these later studies reporting higher rates of leg pain did not involve either careful training of the physician nor adequate questionnaire screening for the differential diagnosis of RLS and other leg pains, including vascular and cramping leg pains that can often be mistaken for RLS. The four essential criteria for RLS diagnosis are often identified for patients with other leg disorders unless care is given to ensure the full quality of these criteria as described above. Nonetheless, patient complaints of leg pains, leg discomfort or sleep disturbance should be considered for possible RLS and a careful differential diagnosis completed.

Evaluation

RLS Patients need to be evaluated on two different dimensions. First, the subjective symptom report should consider the natural occurrence of the RLS symptoms. The usual number of days in a week or month with symptoms, the usual time of onset of symptoms and the usual severity of symptoms when they occur. These clinical considerations should be balanced with appraisal of the degree of activity of the patient, since this modulates the symptoms occurrence. A symptom and activity diary may be helpful for determining these features of RLS. The second dimension involves obtaining subjective and objective assessments in conditions known to provoke RLS symptoms. Symptoms during resting and sleep deserve special attention since these often cause the most significant adverse effects. Total sleep times, number of awakenings and the time to fall asleep should be clinically evaluated. In addition, patients during resting and sleep have distinctive periodic leg movements each lasting about 1 to 10 s and occurring every 5 to 90 s (Zucconi et al., 2006). These are generally considered to be abnormally excessive when they occur in sleep at rates greater than 15/hr for adults and 5/hr for children (American Academy of Sleep Medicine, 2005). These also occur during the 60 minutes of sitting awake, resting with legs-stretched out in a SIT and are considered abnormal when the rate of occurrence is greater than 12/hr (Michaud et al., 2002). Clinical severity of symptoms relates reasonably well to the rate of PLMS (Garcia-Borreguero et al., 2004; Allen and Earley, 2001), and thus these motor signs of RLS provide a good objective severity assessment, particularly useful for within-subject evaluation of change with treatment or medical/environmental conditions. Subjective rating of leg discomfort or the urge to move during the resting periods, also provides a useful evaluation of symptom severity. This has been done on a simple visual analog scale during SIT tests, but could also be part of a diary or a more general questionnaire on RLS. RLS is primarily a sensory disorder, yet little attention has been given to evaluation of its sensory symptoms. Neither qualitative nor quantitative evaluation of the sensory features of RLS has received as much attention or development as that given to the motor features of RLS, such as the PLMS and PLMW.

Three clinical scales have been developed and validated for rating RLS severity. The Johns Hopkins RLS severity scale was developed mostly for those with daily RLS symptoms and is based upon the usual time of onset of symptoms, either before noon, before evening (6 pm), before bedtime or at or after bedtime (Allen and Earley, 2001). The IRL-6 scale emphasizes evaluation of common symptom occurrence at different times of the day (Oertel et al., 2006). The most commonly used scale is the IRLSSG RLS severity rating scale (IRLS), which has 10 items covering both symptoms and life-impact of RLS (The International Restless Legs Syndrome Study Group, 2003). Each item is rated as 0 to 4 and the scores are considered to indicate symptom severity as mild for less than 10, moderate for 11–20, severe for 21–30 and very

severe for 31–40. (The International Restless Legs Syndrome Study Group, 2003). A copy of the American English version of the scale is available on the IRLSSG web site (http://www.irlssg.org/), and versions for commercial use in several languages are available from MAPI research trust (http://www.mapi-research.fr/t_03_serv_dist_user.htm). This scale can be administered by a trained clinician repeatedly in any clinic setting, but the scale is not designed to be completed by the patient without the clinician reading the items and recording the patients response.

PREVALENCE

Estimates of prevalence of RLS have become somewhat controversial. Two problems have distorted these estimates. First, the methods used to identify those with RLS have often relied upon a single, frequently non-specific question, or a small set of questions, in a large population survey, without any significant validation of the accuracy for detecting those with RLS. Many of these surveys commonly quoted for RLS prevalence did not even cover the four basic diagnostic criteria. But even for the two sets of survey studies with some diagnostic validation of the questions used, the sensitivity and specificity of the questions were generally less than 90%, with an expected positive predictive value of about 60% (Nichols et al., 2003). This means that at least 40% of the patients identified in these surveys as having RLS symptoms did not have RLS. The second problem with the surveys involves the failure to separate any occurrence of symptoms for RLS from those that would be considered clinically significant. Thus, early indications for 15 to 20% prevalence for RLS were both wrong and seriously misleading. Table 29.4 presents the prevalence estimates from general population surveys using full diagnostic criteria for occurrence of any RLS symptoms. The best estimates range from 7 to 10% with 1.5–2 times as many females as males. As noted in Table 29.4 prevalence may be less in southern European countries and in Turkey. In one large population-based study ($n = 16\,202$), including the United States and five European countries, the overall prevalence of any RLS was 7%. But the prevalence of clinically significant RLS (moderately to severely distressing symptoms occurring at least twice a week) was only about 3%, with still about twice as many women as men (Allen et al., 2005b) (See Table 29.4). This 3% figure is closer to that previously estimated in early clinical studies and is somewhat more consistent with general clinical experience. Prevalence generally increases with age, reaching a peak in most studies between 50 and 70 years old and then for unclear reasons decreases in the oldest age groups (see Figure 29.2). A somewhat smaller ($n = 701$) prevalence study in a general population limited to ages 50–89 years determined RLS status by a direct clinical interview (Hogl et al., 2005). This better method

Table 29.4 Prevalence of all RLS from general population-based surveys from America and Europe using the full diagnostic criteria.

Ref.	Location	N	Age range	Method	Min Sx frequency	Prevalence as % of population		
						All	Female	Male
Bjorvatn[a] (2005)	Norway-Denmark	2005	≥18	Telephone interview	Any life time	11.5	13.4	9.4
Berger (2004)	North-East Germany	4107	20–79	interview	Any current	10.6	13.4	7.6
Högl[b] (2005)	South Tyrol	701	50–89	Interview	Any life time	10.6	14.2	6.6
Ulfberg (2001)	Sweden	140	18–64	Qstnr	Any current	—	11.4	—
Ulfberg (2001)	Sweden	2608	18–64	Qstnr	Any current	—	—	5.8
Tison[a] (2005)	France	10 263	≥18	Interview	Any life-time	9.1	—	—
					Any past 12 mo	8.5	10.8	5.8
					≥weekly[c]	4.5	5.5	3.2
Allen (2005)	EU + USA	15 391	≥18	Interview[d]	Any life-time	7.2	9.0	5.4
					≥weekly	5.0	6.2	2.8
					≥2/wk + distress	2.7	3.7	1.7
Sevim[b] (2003)	Mersin Turkey	3234	≥18	Interview	Any past month	3.2	3.9	2.5

Qstnr = Questionnaire completed by the subject.
[a] Diagnosis did not require leg paresthesia other than urge to move.
[b] Diagnosis included self-report of restlessness.
[c] Estimated after adjustment for sample lost before obtaining frequency data.
[d] Interview was face-to-face in Europe and by telephone in USA.

found similar prevalence rates of 10.6% for any RLS with 5% for moderate and 2% for severe RLS, somewhat higher than the clinically significant rates from the larger study, but overall similar, given differences in ages, sample size and criteria determining clinical significance.

Prevalence of RLS in children aged 8–17 has now been determined using a careful structured telephone interview for one child in each family from a large sample (n = 10 523) obtained from the United Kingdom and the United States (Picchietti et al., 2007). Overall, about 2% of these children met the pediatric criteria for diagnosis of RLS and clinically significant RLS symptoms (moderately or severely distressing symptoms occurring at least twice a week) occurred for 0.5% of the children aged 8–11 and 1% of those aged 12–17. Unlike the adult sample, there were no gender differences in prevalence.

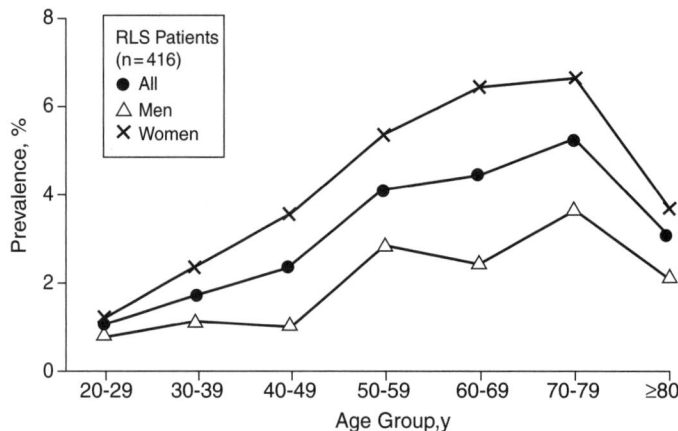

Figure 29.2 Prevalence of clinically significant RLS by age and gender (from Allen, R.P. et al. (2005b) Restless legs syndrome prevalence and impact: REST general population study. *Arch Intern Med*, **165**, 1286–1292. Copyright © 2005, American Medical Association).

Only about 10–20% of those identified as having RLS symptoms in these epidemiological studies had been previously diagnosed with RLS. There remains a potentially large unmet medical need for diagnosis and treatment of RLS in the United States and Europe.

PATHOPHYSIOLOGY

Both the neurobiology and genetics of RLS have made remarkable advances over the past few years and our understanding of the biological basis for this disease has led to some treatment advances. We now know that iron deficiency is one major cause of RLS. All studies that have evaluated CNS iron status have found it reduced in RLS. The CSF ferritin is not only lower than normal, but the relation between serum and CSF ferritin is affected so that a normal level of CSF ferritin appears to occur only for very high levels of serum ferritin, as independently reported by both American and Japanese studies (Earley *et al.*, 2000; Mizuno *et al.*, 2005) (see Figure 29.3). Similarly, imaging studies using MRI (Earley *et al.*, 2006; Allen *et al.*, 2001) or ultrasound (Schmidauer *et al.*, 2005) have shown reduced iron status for the substantia nigra (see Figure 29.4). Autopsy evaluations of the substantia nigra and putamen have found reduced iron, H-ferritin and iron transport proteins DMT1 and ferroportin (Connor *et al.*, 2003; Connor *et al.*, 2004). One of the genetic studies found an association between the gene for neuronal nitric oxide synthase (nNOS) and the severity of RLS. nNOS is in the pathway regulating DMT1 expression. Lower peripheral iron both increases the risk of developing RLS (Akyol *et al.*, 2003) and, for RLS patients in general, makes the symptoms worse (Sun *et al.*, 1998; O'Keeffe *et al.*, 1994; O'Keeffe, 2005b). Moreover, improving iron status reduces RLS symptoms both when done for those with low serum ferritin (O'Keeffe *et al.*, 1994) and even for some with high serum ferritin (O'Keeffe, 2005b). Thus iron status needs to be evaluated in all RLS patients and oral iron treatment is certainly indicated for those with serum ferritin less than 45–50 mcg/L, and possibly all with late-onset RLS (O'Keeffe, 2005a; O'Keeffe, 2005b). i.v. iron treatment may also offer a future treatment for RLS, given the limited absorption of oral iron (Earley *et al.*, 2004), but this treatment is experimental at this time and needs to be reserved for those with clear iron deficiency that fails to respond to oral iron or to patients with gastrectomy-induced iron malabsorption (Tovey and Hobsley, 2000; Shiga *et al.*, 2006).

The dramatic response to dopaminergic treatment strongly suggests a dopamine pathology in RLS, but the nature or extent of this remains unclear. Brain imaging of the striatum has produced conflicting results with dopamine-receptor binding decreased in one PET and one SPECT study, increased in one PET study and not significantly changed in two SPECT studies. Dopamine transporter evaluations were negative in three SPECT studies,

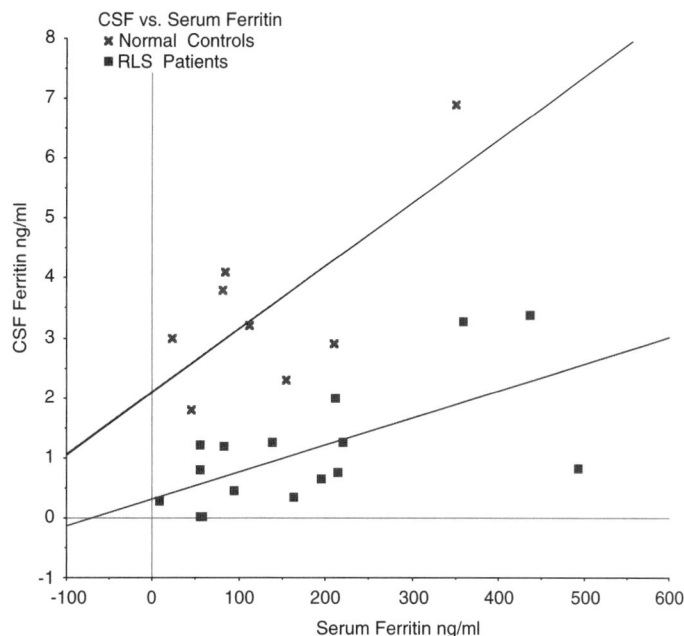

Figure 29.3 CSF ferritin vs serum ferritin for RLS patients and age-gender matched controls. Slightly modified from Earley, C.J. *et al.* (2000) Abnormalities in CSF concentrations of ferritin and transferrin in restless legs syndrome. *Neurology*, **54**, 1698–1700. Copyright © 2000, Lippincott Williams & Wilkins.

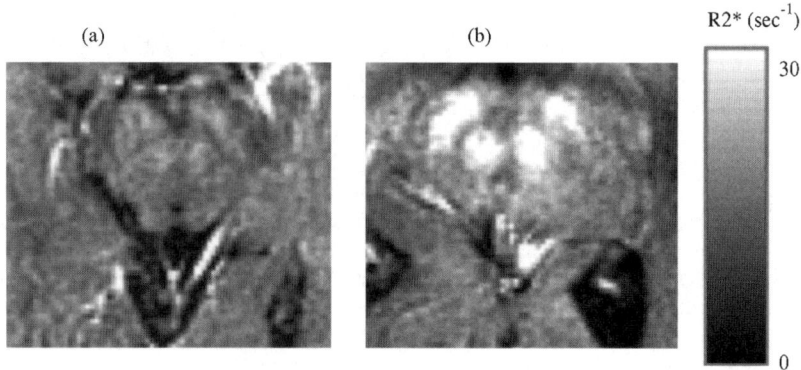

Figure 29.4 R2* images in: (a) a 70-year-old RLS patient; (b) a 71-year-old control subject. Much lower R2* relaxation rates indicating less iron are apparent in the RLS case in both red nucleus and substantia nigra. From Allen, R.P. *et al.* (2001) MRI measurement of brain iron in patients with restless legs syndrome. *Neurology*, **56**, 263–5. Copyright © 2008, Lippincott Williams & Wilkins.

but this has not been evaluated with the better spatial resolution provided by current PET techniques. The animal and cellular models of effects of iron deficiency on dopaminergic systems produced consistent, although somewhat puzzling, results, indicating decreased striatal D2 receptors and impaired DAT functioning (Erikson *et al.*, 2001; Nelson *et al.*, 1997). These would indicate a possible increase in extracellular dopamine and increased nigrostriatal tyrosine hydroxylase activity. The puzzling question becomes how to account for treatment benefits from increased dopaminergic stimulation if the extracellular dopamine level is larger. One possible explanation would be an increased amplitude of the circadian variation compromising the adequacy of post-synaptic adaptation to circadian variation. This could produce inadequate post-synaptic sensitivity at the nadir of the dopamine circadian cycle, during the evening and night-time when RLS symptoms are generally expressed. This post-hoc conceptualization explains the circadian pattern for RLS symptoms, but at this time there are no clinical studies that would support this concept. The autopsy study has shown increased dopamine in the cells of the putamen and increased tyrosine hydroxylase consistent with the patterns suggested by the cellular and animal iron deficiency. Clearly the nature of the dopamine pathology of RLS needs further study. It even remains unclear which of the dopamine systems contribute to the observed symptoms, but it seems likely that the expression of this disorder will involve more than a single DA system. Knowing the specific systems most involved, however, probably offers little useful information for developing treatments or understanding the underlying pathology disrupting these systems.

One interesting aspect of the iron studies is the indication that brain iron deficiency produces disturbances in systems involving other neurotransmitters, including adenosine and glutamate. These may indicate the basis for the treatment benefits from gabapentin (Earley, 207) and may also point to benefits from other treatments, such as adenosine antagonists. The genetic factors contributing to RLS are likely to show other factors besides iron contributing to development of RLS, that may further our understanding of current and possible future treatments for RLS.

GENETICS

The linkage studies of RLS have identified several chromosomal loci for familiar RLS (Chromosomes 12q, 14q, 9q, 2q, 20p, 4q and 17p), but, to date, none of these studies has led to identification of a particular gene related to RLS. Two recent genome-wide association studies based on SNP evaluations comparing RLS patients with large control groups have, however, identified specific genetic variations highly associated with RLS. One study using RLS patients from Europe and Canada reported highly significant associations between RLS and intronic variants in the homeobox gene MEIS 1 (chromosome 2p), the BTBD9 gene encoding a BTB (POZ) domain (chromosome 6p), as well as variants in a third locus containing the genes encoding mitogen-activated protein kinase MAP2K5 and the transcription factor LBXCOR1 (chromosome15q). Each genetic variant was associated with a more than 50% increase in risk for RLS, with the combined allelic variants conferring more than half of the risk. The findings of this carefully done study were based on analyses of both an initial sample of 401 familial RLS patients and 1644 subjects from a population-based cohort and a replication study of 2903 sporadic and familial RLS patients, and 891 control subjects.

A second similar association study conducted on a well-described population in Iceland also found a strong association between RLS and an intron on the BTBD9 gene. That study examined phenotype information for relation to the allele of BTBD9 associated with RLS and reported that both increased PLMS and decreased serum ferritin were associated with occurrence of that allele. Curiously this allelic variation showed no significant association for RLS patients without PLMS, but did for subjects with PLMS, independent of whether or not they were diagnosed with RLS.

The biological meaning of these genetic findings remains at this point largely speculative. The only findings clearly suggesting biological factors associated with RLS involve the phenotype relations reported in the Icelandic study, that is, reduced iron status and increased PLMS. The reduced iron status is consistent with documented neuropathology of RLS patients. The significance of the PLMS remains to be further evaluated.

MANAGEMENT

Management of RLS starts with consideration of, not only the frequency and the time of day that RLS symptoms occur, but also the nature of the symptoms reported by the patient and the results of basic medical evaluation. Figures 29.6–29.8 summarize treatment algoruthms based on these considerations modified from that developed by the medical advisory board of the American Restless Legs Syndrome Foundation (Silber *et al.*, 2004) Although a relatively new field in movement disorders, nonetheless some evidence has been developed supporting components of these various treatments. The following first evaluates the evidence and rationale supporting the recommended treatment components and then presents some practical guidelines for treatment of RLS.

Evidence and Rationale for Treatment Components

Medical Evaluation

For an RLS patient this minimally involves a physical and neurological examination with particular attention to indications for neuropathy. Tests should include a full iron evaluation (see Table 29.5), CBC and fasting glucose or HbA1C, if available. Mental status should include evaluation for depression and anxiety disorders. A medication history should be obtained. Given the well-established relation between peripheral iron status and RLS (Sun *et al.*, 1998; O'Keeffe *et al.*, 1994; O'Keeffe, 2005a), every patient diagnosed with RLS should be presumed likely to have an iron deficiency and thus the criteria for iron deficiency can be set to match that from a population of those referred for evaluation of anemia. The ROC curve for such a population defining iron deficiency by bone marrow aspiration indicates an optimal serum ferritin indicating iron deficiency is about 45 to 50 mcg/L (see Figure 29.5),

Table 29.5 Recommended laboratory Tests for initial evaluation of RLS.

Morning fasting levels of:
  CBC (Hgb, Hct, RDW in particular)
  Glucose
  HbA1C (optional)
  Ferritin
  Transferrin saturation
  Total iron binding capacity
  Total iron
  C-reactive protein

but notice that even a serum ferritin of 100 mcg/L missed nearly 10% of those with no iron in the bone marrow, as indicated recently by an RLS case with a serum ferritin of 84 with no iron in the bone marrow who had complete relief from RLS from oral iron treatment (O'Keeffe, 2005b). An important aspect of this case was an abnormally elevated erythrocyte sedimentation rate (ESR) and such evaluation could be considered with RLS patients, particularly if the ferritin is above 50 mcg/L. A percentage transferrin saturation below 20% can also be considered to indicate likely iron deficiency. An alternative might be the soluble transferrin receptors TR. An increase of the sTR reflects the initial response of the body to iron deficiency (Chang *et al.*, 2007). The sTR has been reported to be a better marker for iron deficiency than ferritin because it is independent of inflammation, and has been used in RLS studies (Hogl *et al.*, 2005). However the high cost may limit its use. The importance of iron evaluation cannot be over-emphasized. Not only does it prove useful for treatment planning, but it may uncover mortal disease, particularly colon cancer that may be treated if caught early. Patients with presumed iron deficiency should receive medical evaluation for possible causes of the iron deficiency. They should generally be placed on oral iron treatment, but since this treatment may require many weeks to be effective they will usually also be given other treatment for RLS, as appropriate.

Pharmacological Treatment

Four major types of drugs are currently used for treatment of RLS: dopamine agonists and levodopa, gabapentin and similar anti-convulsants, opioids and gabanergic hypnotics.

Dopaminergic Treatment, Levodopa

Levodopa combined with a peripheral decarboxylase inhibitor (benserazide or carbidopa) was the first dopaminergic medication shown in clinical cases to be effective in treatment of RLS (Akpinar, 1982; Akpinar, 1987; Von

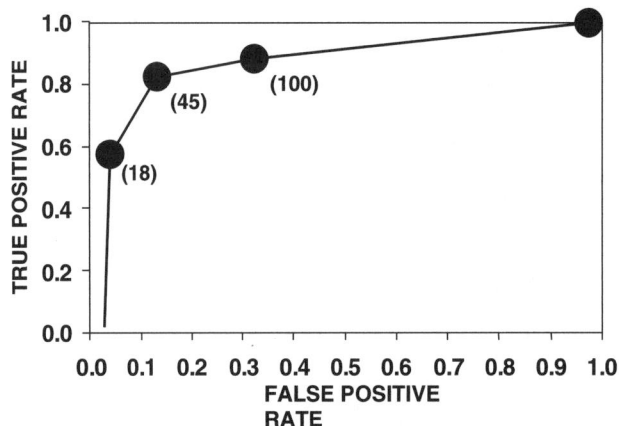

Figure 29.5 Accuracy of serum ferritin for detecting no bone marrow iron in consecutive series of 259 anemic patients over age 65 (serum ferritin values are in parentheses). From Guyatt, G.H. *et al.* (1990) Diagnosis of iron-deficiency anemia in the elderly. *Am. J. Med.*, **88**: 205–209. Copyright © 1990, Elsevier.

Scheele, 1986; Montplaisir *et al.*, 1986). There have been several small- to medium-sized double-blinded, placebo-controlled trials demonstrating efficacy of 100–400 mg of levodopa (Benes *et al.*, 1999; Brodeur *et al.*, 1988; Saletu *et al.*, 2003) and one crossover study demonstrating greater benefit for levodopa then either placebo or propoxyphene (Allen *et al.*, 1992; Kaplan *et al.*, 1993). Levodopa with benserazide was the first drug approved by a government regulatory agency for treatment of RLS, but only in Austria, Switzerland and Germany. It was found to be rapidly effective with little adverse effects, except for the major problem with augmentation noted below. The augmentation involved significant worsening of the RLS condition, occurred in up to 80% of the patients treated and was considered severe enough to warrant avoiding this medication for daily treatment of RLS (Allen and Earley, 1996b; Earley and Allen, 1996).

Dopaminergic Treatment, Dopamine Agonists'

Recent treatment development has focused on the dopaminergic medications and in particular the dopamine agonists. Based on extensive clinical studies these generally provide the first line of treatment and two in particular, pramipexole and ropinirole have been approved for treatment of RLS by local government agencies in the United States, most of Europe and South Korea. The efficacy and safety of both of these medications has been well established, based on sleep laboratory studies showing reduction in PLMS (the movement sign of RLS) (Allen *et al.*, 2004; Partinen *et al.*, 2006) and multiple large (sample sizes for all studies with each drug of about 1000) randomized, double-blinded, placebo-controlled clinical trials lasting 6–12 weeks (Trenkwalder *et al.*, 2004a; Walters *et al.*, 2004; Bogan *et al.*, 2006;

Winkelman *et al.*, 2006; Oertel *et al.*, 2007), with extension evaluations of duration of efficacy lasting 36–39 weeks (Montplaisir *et al.*, 2006; Trenkwalder *et al.*, 2006). Both drugs appear effective with minimal adverse effects and, in some cases, dramatic clinical improvements. Both are approved for treatment of moderate to severe RLS using doses given 1–3 hours before bed (see Table 29.6 for dose and titration schedules). Both drugs are predominately D2, D3 agonists with little binding to D1. Ropinirole has a shorter half-life of about six hours and may require increasing the dose enough to ensure treatment efficacy continues throughout the night, for patients who have some early morning symptoms. Ropinirole is also liver metabolized, primarily involving CYP1A2 and should be used cautiously for patients with hepatic impairment, but has been used successfully in patients on dialysis (Pellecchia *et al.*, 2004). Dose adjustments may be needed for patients on estrogen or CYP1A2 inhibitors (e.g., diproflaxicin). Pramipexole has in young adults a slightly longer half-life of about eight hours, but given its renal excretion without significant metabolism in the liver, the half-life becomes longer for older individuals. Its use is not recommended for those with severe renal impairment. Overall the choice of which of these medications to use depends on consideration of the differences in metabolism/clearance and, to some extent, the desired duration of treatment benefit. For patients with symptoms restricted to the first part of the night, the shorter acting medication may suffice, for those with symptoms starting before bedtime and continuing into the early morning, the longer-acting medication might be preferred. Both of these medications have been officially approved for single doses given 1–3 hours before bed, but, as noted below, they are commonly used in divided doses when RLS symptoms present in the early evening or late afternoon; in

Table 29.6 Non-ergot dopaminergic medications for treatment of RLS.

Rx	Start dose mg	Titration	Maximum dose mg	Minutes to peak plasma levels	Half-life hrs	Receptor activation	% with augmentation	elimination
L-dopa[a,b]	100	100, 3–7 d	400[c]	30	1.5–3	All Dopamine receptors	50–70%	hepatic
Pramipexole	0.125	0.125, 3–7 d	0.75	120	8–12	D2, D3	30%	renal
Ropinirole	0.25	0.25, 3–7 d	4.0	60–120	6–7	D2, D3	unknown	hepatic
Rotigotine (24-hour patch)	1.0/24 hr	1.0/24, 7 d	3.0/24h	N/A	N/A	D1, D2, D3,	unknown	renal (some fecal)

These drugs have mainly hepatic elimination except for pramipexole and rotigotine which have principally renal elimination.
Generally give oral medications 0.5 to 2 hours before times symptom relief is desired.
[a] Not recommended for daily use except at very lowest dose.
[b] With peripheral decarboxylation inhibitor (e.g., carbidopa, benserazide).
[c] Maximum doses have been used over 400 mg with RLS but the risk of augmentation increases with increasing doses.

general, it is recommended that the total daily dose not exceed that approved by the regulatory agencies.

Several ergotamine dopamine agonists have been evaluated for treatment benefit for RLS, pergolide (Earley and Allen, 1996; Trenkwalder *et al.*, 2004b), cabergoline (Stiasny *et al.*, 2000; Stiasny-Kolster *et al.*, 2004; Oertel *et al.*, 2006), lisuride (Benes, 2006) and, in earlier years, bromocriptine(Walters *et al.*, 1988). Both pergolide and cabergoline have been studied in reasonably large double-blind, controlled studies. Since the ergotamine dopamine agonists have been found, in general, to cause problems with cardiac fibrosis and do not appear to have any particular advantage over other dopaminergic treatment, they are not at this time considered a primary treatment for RLS and have not been included in Table 29.6 listing dopaminergic medications. However, it has been reported that fibrotic cardiac valvulopathy is highly unlikely with lisuride. This is based on the hypothesis that cardiac valve fibrosis is not an ergot side affect, but related to 5-HT2B agonist effects of the mentioned ergoline dopamine agonists. Lisuride, however, has 5-HT2B antagonist properties and a retrospective database review did not find any reports of cardiac valve fibroses and a low incidence of other fibrosis (Hofmann *et al.*, 2006). Given the delayed awareness for cardiac valve fibrosis noted only years after therapy with pergolide, the reliability of spontaneous reports must be interpreted with caution.

Two newer dopamine agonists have been reported in the literature and appear likely to be used for RLS treatment. Rotigotine, a new dopamine agonist recently evaluated for treatment of RLS, uses a patch delivery to provide 24-hour dopamine treatment. Rotigotine has active binding on the D1 as well as D2/D3 receptors. One moderate-size pilot study ($n = 63$ divided into four treatment groups) showed treatment benefits for higher doses of rotigotine compared to placebo (Moller *et al.*, 2003). Two large clinical trials evaluating this treatment for RLS have been completed in Europe and the United States. The reports of these trials as presented at professional congresses indicate patients have impressive improvements in clinical ratings, including a significant proportion of patients reporting essentially complete remission from all symptoms. In addition, ropinirole has been made available in both a 24-hour and 14-hour formulation. The latter, while specifically designed for RLS, will probably not be available outside of the United States and possibly South Korea. The 24-hour ropinirole medication will likely be available for treatment of Parkinson's disease and could be used in some countries "off label" for RLS. The reports presented at conferences on the 14-hour formulation of ropinirole include data on standard large-scale clinical trials and show it produces, as expected, effective treatment over a longer duration than the immediate release ropinirole, with about the same adverse effects. This makes the 14-hour ropinirole duration

of treatment benefit somewhat longer than pramipexole for younger adults, but the difference would be less clear for older adults. Adverse effects are similar to other dopamine agonists, except that the patch produces problems that are usually mild, although a significant percentage of patients have a bad skin reaction leading to discontinuing the treatment.

Adverse Effects from Dopaminergic Treatments

The dopamine agonists, as a class, have been found to commonly produce nausea that, while usually transitory, becomes severe enough to require discontinuing treatment in less than 5% of patients. Transitory headaches are also commonly reported (up to 25% of patients), but lead to discontinuing treatment in less than 3% of the patients (Walters *et al.*, 2004; Trenkwalder *et al.*, 2004a) (Winkelman *et al.*, 2006). The somewhat less common, but more significant adverse effects from the dopamine agonists include peripheral edema and daytime sleepiness. The peripheral edema reflects the mild vascular effects of the agonist and may at times limit use of the mediations. The daytime sleepiness problem has been documented to occur for patients with PD accompanied with experiences of sudden onset of sleepiness (Lang *et al.*, 2002), but only one such case has been reported for RLS patients and that occurred when reducing the dose of pergolide (Bassetti *et al.*, 2002). Another survey indicated that while sudden onset of sleep occurred for RLS patients it was somewhat reduced by treatment with dopamine agonists (Moller *et al.*, 2006). Nonetheless, sleepiness occurred as an adverse event in about 12–15% of patients in the large dopamine agonist clinical trials (Walters *et al.*, 2004; Trenkwalder *et al.*, 2004a; Winkelman *et al.*, 2006). Problems of impulsive/compulsive behaviors with dopamine agonist treatment of RLS have been reported for gambling (Evans and Butzkueven, 2007; Quickfall and Suchowersky, 2007; Tippmann-Peikert *et al.*, 2007) and presumably occur for other similar behaviors (e.g., nocturnal eating, hypersexuality), as they do for dopamine agonist treatment of PD (Nirenberg and Waters, 2006). Given the potential risk, patients should be advised of this uncommon adverse effect. Dopaminergic adverse effects noted for PD that have not been reported for RLS include dyskinesias, punding, hallucinations and orthostatic hypotension. These differences may reflect the lower doses used in RLS, or the effects of the interaction of dopamine treatment and the neuropathology of PD.

Augmentation with Medication Treatment of RLS

Augmentation of all RLS symptoms appears to occur for some RLS patients treated with dopaminergic medications or tramadol (Earley and Allen, 2006). Augmentation

Table 29.7 World Association of Sleep Medicine and Max Plank Institute criteria for clinical diagnosis of RLS augmentation.

Augmentation requires meeting conditions A and either B or C below

A. Symptoms considered consistent with augmentation must:
   (1) occur 5 out of 7 d in a week
   (2) not be accounted for by factors not related to continuing medication use, for example, change in medical status or medication changes that exacerbate RLS
   (3) have occurred with some indication of initial positive response to the dopaminergic treatment

B. Persisting (although not immediate) paradoxical response to treatment, for example, RLS symptoms worsen with increasing dopaminergic dose soon after the dose was increased; RLS symptoms improve with decreasing dopaminergic dose in a few days after the dose is deceased.

C. Usual time symptoms start each day occurs earlier than before treatment either:
   (a) at least 4 h earlier
   or
   (b) at least 2 h earlier with one of the following:
      (i) shorter latency to symptoms at rest than before starting treatment
      (ii) involvement of parts of the body in the symptoms not or rarely affected before starting treatment
      (iii) greater intensity of the symptoms when they occur than before stating treatment
      (iv) shorter duration of relief from the treatment than experienced during the initial treatment phase.

Restatement of the criteria presented by Garcia-Borreguero, D. *et al.* (2007), *Sleep Medicine*, **8**, 520–530. Copyright © 2007, Elsevier.

represents a worsening of the underlying RLS process, so that all symptoms become worse to the point that they start occurring earlier in the day and may have greater intensity when they occur, with less duration of rest required to engender them, and may involve more parts of the body. (Allen and Earley, 1996b). A recent consensus conference at the Max Plank Institute in Munich, Germany developed the World Association of Sleep Medicine criteria for clinical diagnosis of augmentation summarized in Table 29.7 (Garcia-Borreguero *et al.*, 2007). Augmentation appears to occur more for shorter- than longer-acting dopamine agonists (see Table 29.6).

Anti-Convulsants (Gabapentin and Carbamazepine)

Only specific anti-convulsants and not the entire class provide effective treatment for RLS. Gabapentin is usually well tolerated and several small open-label trials reported it provided effective treatment (Mellick and Mellick, 1996; Allen and Earley, 1996a; Adler, 1997; Happe *et al.*, 2001). One small ($n = 24$) double-blinded, placebo-controlled crossover trial (Garcia-Borreguero *et al.*, 2002) reported that gabapentin provided effective treatment for about 73% of the patients, with 18% showing mild benefit and 9% showing no response. It was discussed that those with pain associated with the RLS might have a better response to gabapentin. Total sleep time, sleep efficiency and slow-wave sleep showed significant increases for gabapentin

treatment. The gabapentin dose in this study was given twice a day and the final dose average dose was 1855 mg with a maximum of 2400 mg. The major limitation of this medication is the markedly variable, and sometimes limited, absorption and the somewhat short half-life. In patients on dialysis, the gabapentin dose has to be kept very low, for example, 200–300 mg/d, and is generally not recommended for these patients.

A new "pro-drug" for gabapentin has recently been developed that stabilizes the drug absorption and prolongs availability of drug in blood, permitting once a day dosing. Approximately 2 mg of the gabapentin pro-drug provides 1 mg of gabapentin in the blood. Treatment of RLS with this pro-drug has been evaluated in a small ($n = 38$) crossover study with EEG sleep studies at fixed, divided doses of 600 mg at 5 pm and 1200 mg before bed, and in a modest-sized ($n = 95$) parallel-group study with random assignment to placebo, 600 mg or 1200 mg taken with food at 5 pm for two weeks (Kushida, 2007). Both studies showed significant treatment benefits, which were minimal for the lowest dose of 600 mg, but clinically significant and large for the higher doses. Several patients on the higher dose reported essentially complete relief from their RLS symptoms. Sleep parameters showed increased sleep times, increased slow-wave sleep and decreased PLMS. A standard large, double-blinded, placebo-controlled, parallel-group trial evaluating this gabapentin pro-drug has been completed, and preliminary results indicate that it is effective and safe for treatment of moderate to severe RLS. It is not clear, however, if all subjects benefit from this treatment, nor whether or not those with pain with their RLS would benefit more than others. At this point we do not have extensive clinical experience using this drug with RLS patients, nor have the data from the one large clinical trial been published in a peer-reviewed journal. A small double-blind placebo-controlled study with slow-release valproic acid reported some benefits compared to levodopa (Eisensehr *et al.*, 2004). Carbamazepine was the first anti-epileptic to be evaluated in a very small crossover study (Lundvall, Abom and Holm, 1983) and then in a modest-size ($n = 174$) double-blinded, placebo-controlled, parallel-group study, and both studies showed treatment benefits. In current practice, however, carbamazepine does not play a major role in RLS treatment.

Opioids

While it appears from several small studies and clinical experience that all of the opioid analgesics provide some therapeutic benefit for RLS, there have been no large clinical trials evaluating RLS treatment with these drugs. There have been several small open-label clinical reports of RLS treatment benefits for oxycodone (Trezepacz, Violette and Sateia, 1984), codeine (Kavey *et al.*, 1988; Trezepacz, Violette and Sateia, 1984), propoxyphene (Walters *et al.*, 2001), methadone (Ondo, 2005) and one general report of longer-term treatment experience with a wide variety of opioids (Walters *et al.*, 2001). There is one small ($n = 11$) randomized, double-blinded, crossover trial evaluating RLS treatment with oxycodone compared to placebo. The oxycodone dose ranged from 3 to 20 mg/d and the response to oxycodone compared to placebo was much improved for six, somewhat improved for two and there was essentially no improvement for three of the subjects. Overall there is meager data to support the use of the opioids for treatment of RLS. Safety is not established, particularly in terms of problems of dependence and possible respiratory suppression, especially during sleep in the older RLS patients. Nonetheless, these medications have become increasingly used as either an added medication or an alternate medication when the dopaminergic treatment and gabapentin alternative fail to suffice for RLS treatment (Walters *et al.*, 2001), and some have suggested that the longer-acting opioids, such as methadone can be used successfully when other treatments have failed (Ondo, 2005). When choosing opioids for treatment, preference is given to the substances with longer plasma half-life, and transcutaneous treatment is an option. There is some concern that all opioids are not the same with regard to effectiveness in RLS treatment, but results from comparative studies have to date only been published in abstract form or presented at meetings (Becker, 2005).

GABA Active Hypnotics

Benzodiazipines and other gaba-active hypnotics were long used for treatment of PLMS, although the sleep improvement on these medications does not seem to be matched with an equivalent reduction in rate of PLMS (Mitler *et al.*, 1986). Several studies have evaluated clonazepam for treatment of PLMS with mixed results (Oshtory and Vijayan, 1980; Peled and Lavie, 1987; Mitler *et al.*, 1986; Horiguchi *et al.*, 1992; Edinger and Al, 1996), but there have been only a few evaluating clonazepam treatment for RLS. The small open-label studies report that clonazepam improved RLS (Boghen, 1981; Matthews, 1979; Montagna *et al.*, 1984), but one small controlled crossover study found no benefit for clonazepam compared to placebo (Boghen *et al.*, 1986). One study using SITs suggested that daytime use of lorazepam actually increased PLMS compared to placebo (Allen, Lesage and Earley, 2005a). Thus, while there is no reason to assume these medications will not improve the sleep of RLS patients and thereby provide treatment benefit, there is no indication that they actually provide any direct treatment for RLS. One interesting report noted that the rather significant blood pressure increases observed to occur with PLMS were not reduced by temazepam (Ali *et al.*, 1991), despite better sleep. Thus the benefits from these medications may be limited to decreased cortical arousal and better-maintained sleep. They may have a major role to play as an add-on therapy to improve sleep.

Iron Treatment

Despite studies relating decreased peripheral iron status with both increased risk (Akyol *et al.*, 2003) and increased severity of RLS (O'Keeffe *et al.*, 1994, Sun *et al.*, 1998) there have been few studies evaluating treatment benefits from oral iron treatment. An open-label study by O'Keeffe found two months of oral iron treatment reduced RLS symptoms for patients with a serum ferritin below 45 mcg/L (O'Keeffe *et al.*, 1994). One double-blind study failed to find any benefit for oral treatment of RLS, but also had a short treatment period and involved mostly patients with serum ferritin over 45 mcg/L (Davis *et al.*, 2000), so the results are not inconsistent with those from O'Keeffe. A more recent double-blinded, placebo-controlled study included subjects with serum ferritin below 45 mcg/L and showed significant reductions in RLS scores for those treated with oral iron compared to placebo (Wang *et al.*, 2006). The literature includes case presentations of some patients with indications for iron deficiency, who show remarkable improvement of symptoms over 2–6 months of treatment with oral iron (O'Keeffe, 2005b). Thus despite general clinical agreement on the value of iron treatment for RLS and a good theoretical basis supporting this treatment we have little experimental data indicating efficacy of iron treatment for RLS.

Intravenous iron treatment has been studied in two open-label trials. Nordlander in the 1950s first reported a series of 22 patients with 21 showing complete remission of the RLS symptoms when treated with repeated doses of about 200 mg of a formulation of iron dextran (Nordlander, 1953; Nordlander, 1954). A more recent open-label study reported that a single dose of 1000 mg of iron dextran produced complete remission of the RLS for 6 of 10 patients. The duration of symptom relief varied considerably from 3 to over 36 months (Earley *et al.*, 2004). A small placebo-controlled, double-blinded clinical trial of RLS symptoms in patients on dialysis showed significant benefits for a single i.v. dose of 1000 mg of iron dextran ($n = 11$) compared to placebo ($n = 14$) that lasted 2–4 weeks (Sloand *et al.*, 1998). A more recent double-blind trial failed to find benefit for a very slow infusion of a single large (1000 mg) dose of iron sucrose, but the data suggest that this formulation of iron, when given in one infusion has only minimal impact on CSF iron status (Earley *et al.*, 2008). The iron from a single dose of dextran appears to be available for transport to the brain for several days after the injection. The duration of the availability of the iron for transport to the brain may be a critical factor to consider in planning i.v. iron treatments. Overall, despite the appeal of this treatment for RLS, we have only small clinical trials suggesting that in some cases intravenous iron may be an effective treatment, but we do not know basic critical factors for successful i.v. iron treatment of RLS. It is encouraging that none of the trials with either oral or i.v. iron reported significant adverse effects. i.v. iron using the high-molecular-weight dextran, however, is known to produce life-threatening anaphylactic reactions and should be used cautiously. Anaphylactic reactions appear to be less of a problem for the low-molecular weight dextran (Auerbach, Ballard and Glaspy, 2007; Auerbach and Al Talib, 2008) and this formulation should generally be preferred over the high-molecular weight dextran. Anaphylactic reactions also appear to be very rare for the alternate i.v. iron formulations (e.g., iron gluconate, iron sucrose) (Kumpf, 2003)

Non-Pharmacological Treatment

Physical and mental activity must, by definition of the syndrome, provide relief from RLS symptoms. This really requires no experimental evaluation. Many other activities have been reported by patients to provide symptom relief, but none of these have been experimentally evaluated and what works may be largely idiosyncratic to the patient. RLS probably represents a disorder expressed during quiet resting state that permits sleep onset, but also for humans a relaxed state for observation and contemplation. All

activities that appear to wake up or increase alertness also appear to be helpful in reducing RLS symptoms.

Medications and Substances to be Avoided

A limited clinical trial with 12 RLS patients on dopaminergic treatment showed that diphenhydramine severely exacerbates RLS symptoms and should be avoided (Allen, Lesage and Earley, 2005a). Presumably all anti-histamines that reach the brain will have this effect and should be avoided for RLS. One very small study showed that a dopamine antagonist given to untreated RLS patients exacerbated the RLS symptoms, particularly the motor symptoms (Winkelmann *et al.*, 2001). In that same study the opiate antagonist naloxone failed to exacerbate any RLS symptoms. Dopamine antagonists that reach the brain should, in general, not be used by patients with RLS. Most anti-depressants are considered to exacerbate RLS, particularly SSRIs and also the SNRI venlafaxine, but there are few experimental data supporting this position. Nonetheless these should be used with caution, if at all, with RLS patients. The anti-depressants buproprion and trazodone are considered not likely to exacerbate RLS symptoms, but there are few experimental data supporting this clinical impression.

Despite common reports that caffeine and nicotine (tobacco use) should be avoided, there are no data with the currently accepted diagnostic standards for RLS that support this view. The stimulating action of these drugs would be expected to provide transitory relief from RLS symptoms, although there may be increased sleepiness and RLS symptoms with chronic use or when the stimulate effects are abating. In contrast, there is general clinical agreement that low-dose alcohol with its sedative effects significantly exacerbates RLS.

Practical Guidelines for Management

These are summarized in Figures 29.6–29.8, adapted, with some modification from the algorithm for RLS treatment developed by the medical advisory board of the Restless Legs Syndrome Foundation (Silber *et al.*, 2004)

General Major Considerations for Management

All RLS patients should be evaluated for iron status, and if serum ferritin is less than 45–50 mcg/l or % transferrin saturation is less than 20% oral iron treatment can be started using ferrous sulfate and 200 mg of vitamin C. Treatment decisions depend mostly on terms of the number of days with symptoms and then the on time of day symptoms start. All significant iron deficiency should be evaluated for possible causes. Iron deficiency detected at RLS evaluation has sometimes led to detection of gastrointestinal or

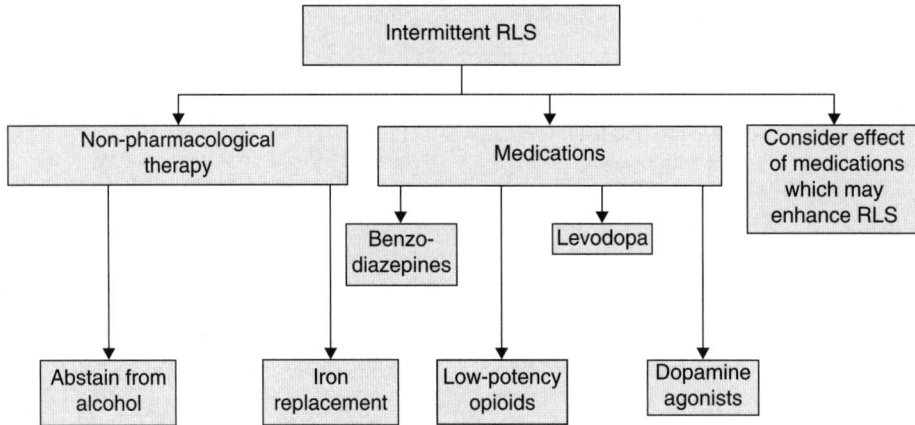

Figure 29.6 Treatment for intermittent RLS (occurring less than twice a week).

other malignancies, when workup of iron deficiency was performed. Particular attention should be paid to iron status when RLS starts fairly abruptly as both nearly daily and severe when present.

Possible medication use or medical causes of the RLS should be evaluated, particularly if the RLS symptoms started after age 45 and there is no family history of the disorder. The age-of-onset of any RLS symptoms, although sometimes hard to obtain from patients, still provides an important guide to determining evaluation of possible secondary causes. Medication uses that exacerbate or even possibly engender RLS symptoms should be avoided, and in particular the use of anti-histamines that reach the brain should not be used by RLS patients. Most anti-depressant medications (except buproprion) should be considered as possible sources of exacerbating RLS. This appears to be particularly the case for SSRIs and even more so for the more activating venlafaxine. These should be removed or reduced as much as possible.

All patient evaluations should cover five symptom factors relevant to treatment decisions: frequency (number of days per week with symptoms), time during the day symptoms occur, severity of symptoms when present, degree of sleep disturbance and the degree of pain associated with the symptoms.

Iron Treatment, Special Management Considerations

Oral iron can be given in tablets containing 25–65 mg of elemental iron (e.g., iron sulfate); generally the larger amount of elemental iron in the ferrous sulfate tablets is preferred. Oral iron should be taken at a time that is two hours after and one hour before meals, and should be taken with 200 mg of vitamin C. If the medication upsets the stomach, it can be taken after a meal, but the amount of iron absorbed will be less. The iron can be taken one to three times a day, depending on the severity of the iron deficiency. Always follow patients on iron with routine blood work at

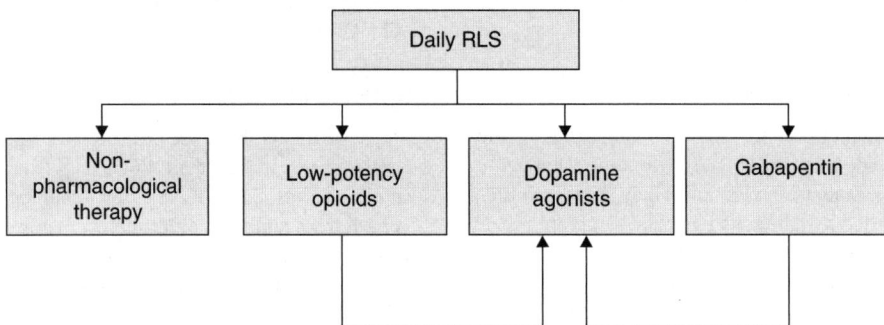

Figure 29.7 Treatment for daily or nearly daily RLS (occurring at least twice a week).

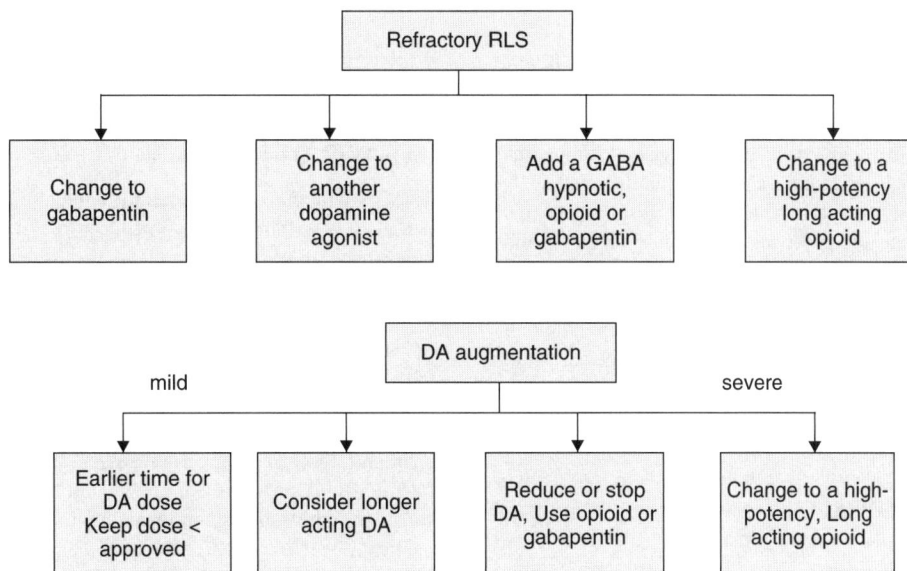

Figure 29.8 Treatment for refractory or difficult RLS (failed to respond adequately or developed adverse effects from first line treatment such as significant augmentation that limited effectiveness of the treatment).

about two months after starting treatment, and then every 6–12 months, to detect possible hemochromotosis as indicated by transferrin saturation at 60% or greater. Once ferritin levels exceed 50 mcg/L the oral iron can be discontinued, but regular annual evaluations should include serum ferritin and transferrin saturation tests.

i.v. iron treatment is not approved for RLS, but can be considered for patients with significant iron deficiency (e.g., serum ferritin < 17 mcg/L) who cannot tolerate or do not respond to a six-month trial of oral iron treatment. Before starting treatment, patients should be carefully evaluated to rule out sources of blood loss maintaining the iron deficiency. Intravenous iron can be given as a series of two or three treatments over a week, using either ferric gluconate or iron sucrose. Current treatment choices include: 10 mL of ferric gluconate (Ferrlicit) (two packages of 62.5 mg each; 125 mg of elemental iron) given by a slow i.v. push over 10–15 minutes or 5 mL of iron sucrose (Venofer) (100 mg of elemental iron) given by a slow i.v. push over 5–10 minutes. (Silverstein and Rodgers, 2004). The series of two or three treatments can be repeated if the serum ferritin or % saturation remains abnormal. Do not start or continue this treatment if the serum ferritin exceeds 50 mcg/L or the % transferrin saturation exceeds 40%.

Treatment Goals

These goals vary greatly between patients, but should cover at least four factors: (i) reducing occurrence of RLS symptoms and, in particular, any pain or discomfort with the RLS; (ii) restoring the ability to rest and partake in sedentary activities while awake; (iii) establishing sleep with adequate duration and quality; (iv) reducing daytime fatigue associated with RLS, if present, although this may be largely improved with better sleep.

Major Management Categories

Mild RLS

Patients who report mild or only somewhat annoying symptoms may only require non-pharmacological treatments. If the mild symptoms disturb them during unusual periods of sustained rest, such as traveling long distances in a car or plane, then consider treatment as described below for intermittent RLS. If the mild symptoms present as a problem mildly disturbing sleep, then consider possible use of a gaba-active hypnotic. These medications promote sleep, permitting the patient to acquire and maintain sleep, despite occurrence of the symptoms. These medications may actually make RLS symptoms worse if the patient stays awake or wakes up after taking them, but if the patient sleeps, the RLS symptoms may no longer be a significant problem. Persisting leg movements not significantly reduced by these medications may, however, disturb the sleep of a bed partner.

Intermittent RLS

Symptoms that occur less than twice a week can often be managed with PRN (taken as needed) medications, either levodopa (depending on the patients body weight, 100 or 200 mg given in a single dose) or a low dose of a dopamine agonist (because dopamine agonists usually need to be titrated up slowly to avoid nausea, PRN doses higher than 0.18 mg pramipexole or 0.5 mg ropinirole should probably be avoided). These patients may sometimes know the situations in which they are likely to experience symptoms and can be advised to take their medication about 30 minutes before that time for levodopa and about one hour before for dopamine agonists. Non-pharmacological management can often benefit these patients. Activities to maintain alertness will likely forestall symptoms occurring during the daytime, although these are obviously counter-productive at bedtime.

Daily RLS: Without Significant Pain

Dopamine agonists (see Table 29.6) provide the currently accepted first-line treatment. If symptoms are only at or after bedtime, then it may be adequate to use a single dose about an hour before symptoms start. If the symptoms start earlier in the evening or afternoon then a divided dose may be appropriate with the first dose taken about one hour before the usual time for symptoms to start. In this regard, the patient needs to define the start of the time period when they are at risk for developing RLS. The longer-acting medications, once available, should permit taking a single dose that will provide effective treatment for the entire time the patient is at risk for RLS symptom occurrence. Alternate medications that can be considered include the opiates and gabapentin or the gabapentin pro-drug. The short-acting opioids and gabapentin would need to be taken once or twice a day, as needed to cover the time at risk for RLS. The longer-acting opioids and the gabapentin pro-drug may be taken once a day to cover the time at risk for RLS.

Daily RLS: With Significant Pain

When RLS presents with pain either associated with the RLS symptoms or because of neuropathy occurring, possibly contributing to the onset or severity of RLS, then the use of either gabapentin or the pro-drug for gabapentin could be considered as an alternative to dopamine agonists as a first-line treatment. Opioids are also an alternate choice here. In such cases the medication may treat both the pain and the RLS. This alternative deserves particular consideration for pain from neuropathy, even though the neuropathy, in general, has no relation to the RLS. The dopamine agonists generally provide little relief for neuropathic pains. Pain that appears as part of the RLS symptoms may, however, be adequately treated by either a dopamine agonist or gabapentin drugs.

Daily RLS: Treatment Resistant

Therapy with one of the dopamine agonists, or with gabapentin, used within the recommended dose limits may fail, either because of unacceptable adverse effects or lack of sufficient efficacy. Exceeding the dose limits is not recommended. This is particularly true for the dopamine agonists, where it will likely lead to augmentation with only transitory benefits for this or any subsequent increases in dose. When adverse effects limit acceptance of a medication, consider using an alternate dopamine agonist or changing type of medication. When the medication is tolerated and provides some, but not sufficient, relief, consider either adding or changing to another type of medication. If treatment suffices for daytime symptoms, but does not adequately improve sleep, then consideration can be given to adding a gaba-active hypnotic. Concerns regarding hypnotic treatment for intervals longer than a month must be kept in mind, but do not appear to be as much a problem for RLS patients as other patients with insomnia. Psychophysiological insomnia may also co-exist with RLS and persist after sufficient treatment of RLS. For psycho-physiological insomnia (not due to RLS), behavioral treatment strategies have been shown to produce very good short- and long-term results. The importance of ensuring adequate sleep needs to be emphasized and included in treatment evaluation since sometimes the patient is satisfied with improved sleep, even when it remains less than adequate. When daytime RLS symptoms persist, then opioids are generally considered the best alternative medication. For more severe cases, with frequent and distressing RLS not adequately controlled by the first-line treatment, the treatment of last resort is often the longer-acting opioids such as methadone or the fentanyl patch.

Augmentation Management

Augmentation of RLS symptoms with treatment using a dopaminergic medication or tramadol can be managed either by adjusting the current medication dosage, adding another type of medication or changing medications all together. If augmentation occurs with a levodopa medication, always change to a dopamine agonist. If the current medication is tramadol, change to another opioid. When augmentation occurs with a dopamine agonist, then the choices depend on the severity of the augmentation, the current dose of the agonist and the time of day the RLS symptoms are occurring. If the augmentation is mild to moderate, the dose of dopamine agonist is not at the maximum approved dose and the time of RLS symptoms remains in the late afternoon or evening, but not early afternoon or morning, then the dopamine agonist dose may be given in divided doses to cover the times of symptoms and, if needed, may be increased. The dose should not exceed that approved for treatment of RLS. If, however, these conditions are not met, then an alternate medication should be added or substituted for the dopamine agonists. In most cases of moderate to severe augmentation, the dopamine agonists should be discontinued gradually, after starting the alternate medication.

References

Adler, C.H. (1997) Treatment of restless legs syndrome with gabapentin. *Clinical Neuropharmacology*, **20**, 148–151.

Akpinar, S. (1982) Treatment of restless legs syndrome with levodopa plus benserazide [letter]. *Archives of Neurology*, **39**, 739.

Akpinar, S. (1987) Restless legs syndrome treatment with dopaminergic drugs. *Clinical Neuropharmacology*, **10**, 69–79.

Akyol, A., Kiylioglu, N., Kadikoylu, G. *et al.* (2003) Iron deficiency anemia and restless legs syndrome: is there an electrophysiological abnormality? *Clinical Neurology and Neurosurgery*, **106**, 23–27.

Ali, N.J., Davies, R.J., Fleetham, J.A. and Stradling, J.R. (1991) Periodic movements of the legs during sleep associated with rises in systemic blood pressure. *Sleep*, **14**, 163–165.

Allen, R., Becker, P.M., Bogan, R. *et al.* (2004) Ropinirole decreases periodic leg movements and improves sleep parameters in patients with restless legs syndrome. *Sleep*, **27**, 907–914.

Allen, R.P., Barker, P.B., Wehrl, F. *et al.* (2001) MRI measurement of brain iron in patients with restless legs syndrome. *Neurology*, **56**, 263–265.

Allen, R.P. and Earley, C.J. (1996a) An open label clinical trial with structured subjective reports and objective leg activity measures comparing gabapentin with alternative treatment in the restless legs syndrome. *Sleep Research*, **25**, 184.

Allen, R.P. and Earley, C.J. (1996b) Augmentation of the restless legs syndrome with carbidopa/levodopa. *Sleep*, **19**, 205–213.

Allen, R.P. and Earley, C.J. (2001) Validation of the Johns Hopkins restless legs severity scale. *Sleep Medicine*, **2**, 239–242.

Allen, R.P., Kaplan, P.W., Buchholz, D.W. *et al.* (1992) Double-blinded, placebo controlled comparison of high dose propoxyphene and moderate dose carbidopa/levodopa for treatment of periodic limb movements in sleep. *Sleep Research*, **21**, 166.

Allen, R.P., La Buda, M.C., Becker, P. and Earley, C.J. (2002) Family history study of the restless legs syndrome. *Sleep Medicine*, **3** (Suppl), S3–S7.

Allen, R.P., Lesage, S. and Earley, C.J. (2005a) Anithistamines and benzodiazipines exacerbate daytime restless legs syndrome (RLS) symptoms (Abstract). *Sleep*, **28**, A279.

Allen, R.P., Picchietti, D., Hening, W.A. *et al.* (2003) Restless legs syndrome: diagnostic criteria, special considerations, and epidemiology. A report from the restless legs syndrome diagnosis and epidemiology workshop at the National Institutes of Health. *Sleep Medicine*, **4**, 101–119.

Allen, R.P., Walters, A.S., Montplaisir, J. *et al.* (2005b) Restless legs syndrome prevalence and impact: REST general population study. *Archives of Internal Medicine*, **165**, 1286–1292.

American Academy of Sleep Medicine (2005) *International Classification of Sleep Disorders: Diagnostic and Coding Manual*, American Academy of Sleep Medicine, Westchester, IL.

Auerbach, M. and Al Talib, K. (2008) Low-molecular weight iron dextran and iron sucrose have comparative safety profiles in chronic kidney disease. *Kidney International*, **73**, 528–530.

Auerbach, M., Ballard, H. and Glaspy, J. (2007) Clinical update: intravenous iron for anaemia. *Lancet*, **369**, 1502–1504.

Bassetti, C., Clavadetscher, S., Gugger, M. and Hess, C.W. (2002) Pergolide-associated "sleep attacks" in a patient with restless legs syndrome. *Sleep Medicine*, **3**, 275–277.

Becker, P.M. (2005) Opiates for RLS: assessing risk vs benefit. *Sleep*, **28**, A272–A274

Benes, H. (2006) Transdermal lisuride: short-term efficacy and tolerability study in patients with severe restless legs syndrome. *Sleep Medicine*, **7**, 31–35.

Benes, H., Kurella, B., Kummer, J. *et al.* (1999) Rapid onset of action of levodopa in restless legs syndrome: a double-blind, randomized, multicenter, crossover trial. *Sleep*, **22**, 1073–1081.

Bogan, R.K., Fry, J.M., Schmidt, M.H. *et al.* (2006) Ropinirole in the treatment of patients with restless legs syndrome: a US-based randomized, double-blind, placebo-controlled clinical trial. *Mayo Clinic Proceedings*, **81**, 17–27.

Boghen, D. (1981) Successful treatment of restless legs with clonazepam. *Annals of Neurology*, **8**, 341.

Boghen, D., Lamothe, L., Elie, R. *et al.* (1986) The treatment of the restless legs syndrome with clonazepam: a prospective controlled study. *The Canadian Journal of Neurological Sciences*, **13**, 245–247.

Brodeur, C., Montplaisir, J., Godbout, R. and Marinier, R. (1988) Treatment of restless legs syndrome and periodic movements during sleep with L-dopa: a double-blind, controlled study. *Neurology*, **38**, 1845–1848.

Chang, J., Bird, R., Clague, A. and Carter, A. (2007) Clinical utility of serum soluble transferrin receptor levels and comparison with bone marrow iron stores as an index for iron-deficient erythropoiesis in a heterogeneous group of patients. *Pathology*, **39**, 349–353.

Connor, J.R., Boyer, P.J., Menzies, S.L. *et al.* (2003) Neuropathological examination suggests impaired brain iron acquisition in restless legs syndrome. *Neurology*, **61**, 304–309.

Connor, J.R., Wang, X.S., Patton, S.M. *et al.* (2004) Decreased transferrin receptor expression by neuromelanin cells in restless legs syndrome. *Neurology*, **62**, 1563–1567.

Crochard, A., El Hasnaoui, A., Pouchain, D. *et al.* (2007) Diagnostic indicators of restless legs syndrome in primary care consultations: The DESYR study. *Movement Disorders*, **22**, 791–797.

Davis, B.J., Rajput, A., Rajput, M.L. *et al.* (2000) A randomized, double-blind placebo-controlled trial of iron in restless legs syndrome. *European Neurology*, **43**, 70–75.

Earley, C. (2007) Iron deficiency and RLS. WASM2007 (World Association of Sleep Medicine Congress, 2007), Bangkok, Thailand.

Earley, C.J. and Allen, R.P. (1996) Pergolide and carbidopa/levodopa treatment of the restless legs syndrome and periodic leg movements in sleep in a consecutive series of patients. *Sleep*, **19**, 801–810.

Earley, C.J. and Allen, R.P. (2006) Restless legs syndrome augmentation associated with tramadol. *Sleep Medicine*, **7**, 592–593.

Earley, C.J., Barker, P.B., Horska, A. and Allen, R.P. (2006) MRI-determined regional brain iron concentrations in early- and late-onset restless legs syndrome. *Sleep Medicine*, **7**, 459–461.

Earley, C.J., Connor, J.R., Beard, J.L. *et al.* (2000) Abnormalities in CSF concentrations of ferritin and transferrin in restless legs syndrome. *Neurology*, **54**, 1698–1700.

Earley, C.J., Heckler, D., Horská, A. *et al.* (2004) The treatment of restless legs syndrome with intravenous iron dextran. *Sleep Medicine*, **5**, 231–235.

Earley, C.J., Horská, A., Mohamed, M.A. *et al.* (2008) A randomized, double-blind, placebo-controlled trial of intravenous iron sucrose in restless legs syndrome. *Sleep Medicine*, (in press).

Edinger, J. and Al, E. (1996) Comparison of cognitive-behavioral therapy and clonazepam for treating periodic limb movement disorder. *Sleep*, **19**, 442–444.

Eisensehr, I., Ehrenberg, G.B.L., Rogge Solti, S. and Niachtar, S. (2004) Treatment of idiopathic restless legs syndrome (RLS) with slow-release valproic acid compared with slow-release levodopa/benserazid. *Journal of Neurology*, **251**, 579–583.

Ekbom, K.A. (1945) *Restless legs*, Ivar Haeggströms, Stockholm.

Ekbom, K.A. (1950) *Restless legs*. A report of 70 new cases. *Acta Medica Scandinavica*, **246**, 64–68.

Erikson, K.M., Jones, B.C., Hess, E.J. *et al.* (2001) Iron deficiency decreases dopamine D1 and D2 receptors in rat brain. *Pharmacology, Biochemistry, and Behavior*, **69**, 409–418.

Evans, A.H. and Butzkueven, H. (2007) Dopamine agonist-induced pathological gambling in restless legs syndrome due to multiple sclerosis. *Movement Disorders*, **22**, 590–591.

Garcia-Borreguero, D., Allen, R.P., Kohnen, R. *et al.* (2007) Diagnostic standards for dopaminergic augmentation of restless legs syndrome: report from a world association of sleep medicine - international restless legs syndrome study group consensus conference at the max planck institute. *Sleep Medicine*, **8**, 520–530.

Garcia-Borreguero, D., Larrosa, O., De La Llave, Y. *et al.* (2004) Correlation between rating scales and sleep laboratory measurements in restless legs syndrome. *Sleep Medicine*, **5**, 561–565.

Garcia-Borreguero, D., Larrosa, O., De La Llave, Y. *et al.* (2002) Treatment of restless legs syndrome with gabapentin: a double-blind, cross-over study. *Neurology*, **59**, 1573–1579.

Guyatt, G.H., Patterson, C., Ali, M. *et al.* (1990) Diagnosis of iron-deficiency anemia in the elderly. *Am. J. Med.*, **88**, 205–209.

Happe, S., Klosch, G., Saletu, B. and Zeitlhofer, J. (2001) Treatment of idiopathic restless legs syndrome (RLS) with gabapentin. *Neurology*, **57**, 1717–1719.

Hening, W., Walters, A.S., Allen, R.P. *et al.* (2004) Impact, diagnosis and treatment of restless legs syndrome (RLS) in a primary care population: the REST (RLS epidemiology, symptoms, and treatment) primary care study. *Sleep Medicine*, **5**, 237–246.

Hofmann, C., Penner, U., Dorow, R. *et al.* (2006) Lisuride, a dopamine receptor agonist with 5-HT2B receptor antagonist properties: absence of cardiac valvulopathy adverse drug reaction reports supports the concept of a crucial role for 5-HT2B receptor agonism in cardiac valvular fibrosis. *Clinical Neuropharmacology*, **29**, 80–86.

Hogl, B., Kiechl, S., Willeit, J. *et al.* (2005) Restless legs syndrome: a community-based study of prevalence, severity, and risk factors. *Neurology*, **64**, 1920–1924.

Horiguchi, J., Inami, Y., Sasaki, A. *et al.* (1992) Periodic leg movements in sleep with restless legs syndrome: effect of clonazepam treatment. *Japanese Journal of Psychiatry and Neurology*, **46**, 727–732.

Kaplan, P.W., Allen, R.P., Buchholz, D.W. and Walters, J.K. (1993) A double-blind, placebo-controlled study of the treatment of periodic limb movements in sleep using carbidopa/levodopa and propoxyphene. *Sleep*, **16**, 717–723.

Kavey, N., Walters, A.S., Hening, W. and Gidro-Frank, S. (1988) Opioid treatment of periodic movements in sleep in patients without restless legs. *Neuropeptides*, **11**, 181–184.

Kumpf, V.J. (2003) Update on parenteral iron therapy. *Nutrition in Clinical Practice*, **18**, 318–326.

Kushida, C. (2007) XP13512 treatment of RLS. WASM2007 (World Association of Sleep Medicine Congress, 2007), Bangkok, Thailand.

Kushida, C.A., Allen, R.P. and Atkinson, M.J. (2004) Modeling the causal relationships between symptoms associated with restless legs syndrome and the patient-reported impact of RLS. *Sleep Medicine*, **5**, 485–488.

Lang, A.E., Hobson, D.E., Martin, W. and Rivest, J. (2002) Excessive daytime sleepiness and sudden onset sleep in Parkinson's disease: A survey from 18 Canadian movement disorders clinics. *Journal of the American Medical Association*, **287**, 455–463.

Lugaresi, E., Coccagna, G., Berti Ceroni, G. and Ambrosetto, C. (1968) Restless legs syndrome and nocturnal myoclonus, in *The Abnormalites of Sleep in Man* (eds H. Gastaut, E. Lugaresi and G. Berti Ceroni), Aulo Gaggi Editore, Bologna.

Lundvall, O., Abom, P.E. and Holm, R. (1983) Carbamazepine in restless legs. A controlled pilot study. *European Journal of Clinical Pharmacology*, **25**, 323–324.

Matthews, W.B. (1979) Treatment of the restless legs syndrome with clonazepam [letter]. *British Medical Journal*, **1**, 751.

Mellick, G.A. and Mellick, L.B. (1996) Management of restless legs syndrome with gabapentin (Neurontin). *Sleep*, **19**, 224–226.

Michaud, M., Paquet, J., Lavigne, G. *et al.* (2002) Sleep laboratory diagnosis of restless legs syndrome. *European Neurology*, **48**, 108–113.

Mitler, M.M., Browman, C.P., Menn, S.J. *et al.* (1986) Nocturnal myoclonus: treatment efficacy of clonazepam and temazepam. *Sleep*, **9**, 385–392.

Mizuno, S., Mihara, T., Miyaoka, T. *et al.* (2005) CSF iron, ferritin and transferrin levels in restless legs syndrome. *Journal of Sleep Research*, **14**, 43–47.

Moller, J.C., Korner, Y., Cassel, W. *et al.* (2006) Sudden onset of sleep and dopaminergic therapy in patients with restless legs syndrome. *Sleep Medicine*, **7**, 333–339.

Moller, J.C., Stiasny, K., Benes, H. *et al.* (2003) Rotigotine CDS (Constant Delivery System) in the Treatment of Moderate to Advanced Stages of Restless Legs Syndrome – A Double-Blind Placebo-Controlled Pilot Study. *Sleep*, **26**, A340.

Montagna, P., Sassoli De Bianchi, L., Zucconi, M. *et al.* (1984) Clonazepam and vibration in restless legs syndrome. *Acta Neurologica Scandinavica*, **69**, 428–430.

Montplaisir, J., Godbout, R., Poirier, G. and Bedard, M.A. (1986) Restless legs syndrome and periodic movements in sleep: physiopathology and treatment with L-dopa. *Clinical Neuropharmacology*, **9**, 456–463.

Montplaisir, J., Karrasch, J., Haan, J. and Volc, D. (2006) Ropinirole is effective in the long-term management of restless legs syndrome: A randomized controlled trial. *Movement Disorders*, **21**, 1627–1635.

Nelson, C., Erikson, K., Pinero, D.J. and Beard, J.L. (1997) In vivo dopamine metabolism is altered in iron-deficient anemic rats. *The Journal of Nutrition*, **127**, 2282–2288.

Nichols, D.A., Kushida, C.A., Allen, R.P. *et al.* (2003) Validation of RLS diagnostic questions in a primary care practice. *Sleep*, **26**, A346.

Nirenberg, M.J. and Waters, C. (2006) Compulsive eating and weight gain related to dopamine agonist use. *Movement Disorders*, **21**, 524–529.

Nordlander, N.B. (1953) Therapy in restless legs. *Acta Medica Scandinavica*, **145**, 453–457.

Nordlander, N.B. (1954) Restless legs. *British Journal of Physical Medicine*, **17**, 160–162.

O'Keeffe, S.T. (2005a) Secondary causes of restless legs syndrome in older people. *Age Ageing*, **34**, 349–352.

O'Keeffe, S.T. (2005b) Iron deficiency with normal ferritin levels in restless legs syndrome. *Sleep Medicine*, **6**, 281–282.

O'Keeffe, S.T., Gavin, K. and Lavan, J.N. (1994) Iron status and restless legs syndrome in the elderly. *Age Ageing*, **23**, 200–203.

Oertel, W.H., Benes, H., Bodenschatz, R. *et al.* (2006) Efficacy of cabergoline in restless legs syndrome: a placebo-controlled study with polysomnography (CATOR). *Neurology*, **67**, 1040–1046.

Oertel, W.H., Stiasny-Kolster, K., Bergtholdt, B. *et al.* (2007) Efficacy of pramipexole in restless legs syndrome: a six-week, multicenter, randomized, double-blind study (effect-RLS study). *Movement Disorders*, **22**, 213–219.

Ondo, W.G. (2005) Methadone for refractory restless legs syndrome. *Movement Disorders*, **20**, 345–348.

Oshtory, M.A. and Vijayan, N. (1980) Clonazepam treatment of insomnia due to sleep myoclonus. *Archives of Neurology*, **37**, 119–120.

Partinen, M., Hirvonen, K., Jama, L. *et al.* (2006) Efficacy and safety of pramipexole in idiopathic restless legs syndrome: A polysomnographic dose-finding study – The PRELUDE study. *Sleep Medicine*, **7**, 407–417.

Peled, R. and Lavie, P. (1987) Double-blind evaluation of clonazepam on periodic leg movements in sleep. *Journal of Neurology, Neurosurgery, and Psychiatry*, **50**, 1679–1681.

Pellecchia, M.T., Vitale, C., Sabatini, M. *et al.* (2004) Ropinirole as a treatment of restless legs syndrome in patients on chronic hemodialysis: an open randomized crossover trial versus levodopa sustained release. *Clinical Neuropharmacology*, **27**, 178–181.

Pennestri, M.H., Whittom, S., Adam, B. *et al.* (2006) PLMS and PLMW in healthy subjects as a function of age: prevalence and interval distribution. *Sleep*, **29**, 1183–1187.

Picchietti, D., Allen, R.P., Walters, A.S. *et al.* (2007) Restless legs syndrome: prevalence and impact in children and adolescents – the Peds REST study. *Pediatrics*, **120**, 253–266.

Quickfall, J. and Suchowersky, O. (2007) Pathological gambling associated with dopamine agonist use in restless legs syndrome. *Parkinsonism & Related Disorders*, **13**, 535–536.

Saletu, M., Anderer, P., Hogl, B. *et al.* (2003) Acute double-blind, placebo-controlled sleep laboratory and clinical follow-up studies with a combination treatment of rr-L-dopa and sr-L-dopa in restless legs syndrome. *Journal of Neural Transmission*, **110**, 611–626.

Schmidauer, C., Sojer, M., Seppi, K. *et al.* (2005) Transcranial ultrasound shows nigral hypoechogenicity in restless legs syndrome. *Annals of Neurology*, **58**, 630–634.

Shiga, K., Nishimukai, M., Tomita, F. and Hara, H. (2006) Ingestion of difructose anhydride III, a non-digestible disaccharide, prevents gastrectomy-induced tron malabsorption and anemia in rats. *Nutrition*, **22**, 786–793.

Silber, M.H., Ehrenberg, B.L., Allen, R.P. *et al.* (2004) An algorithm for the management of restless legs syndrome. *Mayo Clinic Proceedings*, **79**, 916–922.

Silverstein, S.B. and Rodgers, G.M. (2004) Parenteral iron therapy options. *American Journal of Hematology*, **76**, 74–78.

Sloand, J., Shelly, M., Erenstone, A. *et al.* (1998) Safety and efficacy of total dose iron dextran administration in pateints on home renal replacement therapies. *Peritoneal Dialysis International*, **18**, 522–527.

Stiasny, K., Robbecke, J., Schuler, P. and Oertel, W.H. (2000) Treatment of idiopathic restless legs syndrome (RLS) with the D2-agonist cabergoline – an open clinical trial. *Sleep*, **23**, 349–354.

Stiasny-Kolster, K., Benes, H., Peglau, I. *et al.* (2004) Effective cabergoline treatment in idiopathic restless legs syndrome. *Neurology*, **63**, 2272–2279.

Stiasny-Kolster, K., Kohnen, R., Moller, J.C. *et al.* (2006) Validation of the "L-DOPA test" for diagnosis of restless legs syndrome. *Movement Disorders*, **21**, 1333–1339.

Sun, E.R., Chen, C.A., Ho, G. *et al.* (1998) Iron and the restless legs syndrome. *Sleep*, **21**, 371–377.

The International Restless Legs Syndrome Study Group, 2003 Validation of the International Restless Legs Syndrome Study Group rating scale for restless legs syndrome. *Sleep Medicine*, **4**, 121–132.

Tippmann-Peikert, M., Park, J.G., Boeve, B.F. *et al.* (2007) Pathologic gambling in patients with restless legs syndrome treated with dopaminergic agonists. *Neurology*, **68**, 301–303.

Tison, F., Crochard, A., Leger, D. *et al.* (2005) Epidemiology of restless legs syndrome in French adults: a nationwide survey: the INSTANT Study. *Neurology*, **65**, 239–246.

Tovey, F.I. and Hobsley, M. (2000) Post-gastrectomy patients need to be followed up for 20–30 years. *World Journal of Gastroenterology*, **6**, 45–48.

Trenkwalder, C., Garcia-Borreguero, D., Montagna, P. *et al.* (2004a) Ropinirole in the treatment of restless legs syndrome: results from the TREAT RLS 1 study, a 12 week, randomised, placebo controlled study in 10 European countries. *Journal of Neurology, Neurosurgery, and Psychiatry*, **75**, 92–97.

Trenkwalder, C., Hundemer, H.P., Lledo, A. *et al.* (2004b) Efficacy of pergolide in treatment of restless legs syndrome: the PEARLS Study. *Neurology*, **62**, 1391–1397.

Trenkwalder, C., Stiasny-Kolster, K., Kupsch, A. *et al.* (2006) Controlled withdrawal of pramipexole after 6 months of open-label treatment in patients with restless legs syndrome. *Movement Disorders*, **21**, 1404–1410.

Trezepacz, P.T., Violette, E.J. and Sateia, M.J. (1984) Response to opioids in three patients with restless legs syndrome. *The American Journal of Psychiatry*, **141**, 993–995.

Von Scheele, C. (1986) Levodopa in restless legs. *Lancet*, **2**, 426–427.

Walters, A.S., Hening, W.A., Kavey, N. *et al.* (1988) A double-blind randomized crossover trial of bromocriptine and placebo in restless legs syndrome. *Annals of Neurology*, **24**, 455–458.

Walters, A.S., Ondo, W.G., Dreykluft, T. *et al.* (2004) Ropinirole is effective in the treatment of restless legs syndrome. TREAT RLS 2: a 12-week, double-blind, randomized, parallel-group, placebo-controlled study. *Movement Disorders*, **19**, 1414–1423.

Walters, A.S., Winkelmann, J., Trenkwalder, C. *et al.* (2001) Long-term follow-up on restless legs syndrome patients treated with opioids. *Movement Disorders*, **16**, 1105–1109.

Wang, Y., Mysliviec, V., Fischer, C. *et al.* (2006) Efficacy of iron in patients with restless legs syndrome and a low-normal ferritin: A randomized, double-blind, placebo controlled study. Association of professional sleep societies, Sleep 2006, Salt lake City, Utah, USA, Sleep.

Winkelman, J.W., Sethi, K.D., Kushida, C.A. *et al.* (2006) Efficacy and safety of pramipexole in restless legs syndrome. *Neurology*, **67**, 1034–1039.

Winkelmann, J., Schadrack, J., Wetter, T.C. *et al.* (2001) Opioid and dopamine antagonist drug challenges in untreated restless legs syndrome patients. *Sleep Medicine*, **2**, 57–61.

Zucconi, M., Ferri, R., Allen, R. *et al.* (2006) The official World Association of Sleep Medicine (WASM) standards for recording and scoring periodic leg movements in sleep (PLMS) and wakefulness (PLMW) developed in collaboration with a task force from the International Restless Legs Syndrome Study Group (IRLSSG). *Sleep Medicine*, **7**, 175–183.

Part VIII

PEDIATRIC MOVEMENT DISORDERS

Pediatric Movement Disorders

Jonathan W. Mink

University of Rochester, NY, USA

INTRODUCTION

Movement disorders in children constitute a broad spectrum ranging from normal developmental variations to signs of serious degenerative diseases. Movement disorders in children differ from those in adults in several important aspects. The approach to movement disorders in children is complicated by the impact of development on the capacity of the nervous system to manifest signs and symptoms. Furthermore, certain disorders only begin to manifest at specific developmental stages or ages. The same illness may present differently depending upon the age of onset of symptoms. Detection of a progressive disorder may be complicated by superposition of a progressive disorder on the natural improvement of function that is expected throughout childhood. Therefore, a child with a progressive movement disorder may continue to develop new skills despite falling further and further behind age-appropriate behavior. The presence of a movement disorder may affect the current and continuing development of the child's normal motor and cognitive abilities. Thus, an acute illness may have developmental consequences that outlast the duration of the injury itself.

It is important to recognize that movement disorders in childhood are more likely to be secondary symptoms of other diseases, rather than primary (Sanger, 2003; Sanger *et al.*, 2003; Schlaggar and Mink, 2003). In adults, dystonia and parkinsonism are usually due to primary dystonia or idiopathic Parkinson's disease, respectively. However, dystonia or parkinsonism in children are more likely to be features of an underlying static or progressive neurological disorder. Diagnosis in children is complicated by the fact that many symptoms have more than one cause, and any particular underlying pathophysiology may lead to a complex combination of symptoms. The diagnostic workup in children is guided by symptoms, but the existence of a large class of diseases that can lead to the same set of symptoms often necessitates a broad etiologic workup. There may be specific etiologic treatments, as well as symptomatic treatments, both of which may be beneficial in an individual child. In particular, many of the causes of childhood movement disorders do not yet have any specific treatment, yet symptomatic treatment for the resulting movement disorder can be extremely helpful and lead to improvement in quality of life.

Another distinction between movement disorders in adults and children is that many adult neurological disorders can be attributed to anatomically localized pathology, but childhood disorders are frequently due to global or multifocal injury that may affect particular cell types, receptor types or metabolic pathways. Therefore, in children, the injury is often sparse, but global, with manifestations across multiple areas of function, including sensorimotor and cognitive functions.

DIAGNOSIS OF MOVEMENT DISORDERS IN CHILDHOOD

Just as for adult movement disorders, classification of the movement disorder based upon the spatial and temporal pattern is essential for diagnosis. It is also important to define the context in which the movements occur. It is essential that the clinician see the movement abnormalities. If the movements are not apparent during the neurological examination, repeating the examination at another time, or obtaining video recordings of the movements is essential. The widespread availability of video cameras has substantially improved the diagnosis of movement disorders in children.

Most childhood movement disorders are characterized by the presence of abnormal involuntary movements (hyperkinetic disorders). Parkinsonism is much less common. Paroxysmal disorders are more common in children than in adults and thus may be difficult to fully characterize because the presence is intermittent and brief. Finally, children are more likely to have disorders characterized by multiple types of abnormal movement. This is particularly true of neurometabolic disorders that may present with a combination of ataxia, chorea, dystonia and myoclonus for example. Laboratory tests, imaging and other diagnostic testing should be based on the specific movement disorder. There is no "movement disorder workup," since the causes are varied and some movement disorders (e.g., tics) are rarely symptomatic of an underlying disease.

A comprehensive discussion of movement disorders in children is beyond the scope of this chapter. The most commonly encountered movement disorders in children are tics, tremor and the multiple movement disorders seen in children with cerebral palsy. Metabolic disorders can also cause movement disorders, but in those cases the treatment is usually symptomatic for the specific movement disorder. Treatment of chorea, tics, dystonia, myoclonus and tremor are discussed in other chapters of this book. For specific treatment of childhood metabolic disorders and cerebral palsy, readers are referred to more comprehensive texts (Lyon, Kolodny and Pastores, 2006; Maria, 2005; Singer *et al.*, 2005). Many specific movement disorders of childhood are discussed other chapters of this book. The remainder of this chapter will be devoted to the discussion of movement disorders unique to early childhood, with an emphasis on those that are developmentally determined and likely to be transient.

DEVELOPMENTAL MOVEMENT DISORDERS

The presence of a movement disorder in a child usually raises concerns about an underlying serious, progressive, degenerative or metabolic disease. However, many movement disorders are benign and related to normal stages of development. In fact, it may be difficult to justify the term "disorder" in describing many of these movements. The developing nervous system may produce a variety of motor patterns that would be pathological in older children and adults, but are simply a manifestation of CNS immaturity. Like many of the neonatal reflexes (e.g., grasping, rooting, placing, tonic neck reflexes), these motor patterns disappear as neuron connectivity and myelination matures. Examples include the minimal chorea of infants, the mild action dystonia commonly seen in toddlers and the overflow movements that are commonly seen in young children. Other transient or developmental movement disorders may be manifestations of abnormal neural function, but do not correlate with serious underlying pathology. These are typically associated with complete resolution of the abnormal movements and ultimately normal development and neurological function. Most of these conditions occur during infancy or early childhood. It is important to recognize these transient developmental movement disorders, distinguish them from more serious disorders, and be able to provide reassurance when possible.

Benign Neonatal Sleep Myoclonus

Benign neonatal sleep myoclonus is characterized by repetitive myoclonic jerks occurring only during sleep (Coulter and Allen, 1982; Paro-Panjan and Neubauer, 2008). In this condition, myoclonic jerks typically start in the first week of life. The myoclonic jerks are typically in the distal more than proximal limbs and more prominent in the upper than the lower extremities. In some cases, jerks of axial or facial muscles can be seen. The myoclonus can be focal, multi-focal, unilateral or bilateral. The movements can be rhythmic or non-rhythmic. Typically, the movements occur in clusters of jerks at 1–5 Hz over a period of several seconds. An episode of jerking can last from a few seconds up to 20 min. Benign neonatal sleep myoclonus typically diminishes in the second month, and is usually gone before 10 months of age, but has been reported to persist as long as three years in one patient (Egger, Grossmann and Auchterlonie, 2003). Ictal and interictal EEG are typically normal. The movements are most likely to occur during quiet (non-REM) sleep (Resnick *et al.*, 1986). Waking the baby causes the movements to cease. Episodes of myoclonus can be exacerbated by treatment with benzodiazepines (Reggin and Johnson, 1989). Treatment is not required and neurological outcome is normal.

Benign Myoclonus of Early Infancy (Benign Infantile Spasms)

Benign myoclonus of early infancy is characterized by episodes of myoclonic spasms involving flexion of the trunk, neck and extremities, in a manner resembling the infantile spasms of West syndrome (Lombroso, 1990; Lombroso and Fejerman, 1977). The myoclonic spasms typically occur in clusters. In some cases they involve a shuddering movement of the head and shoulders, and in others the movements of the trunk and limbs are extensor. There is no change in consciousness during the spells. Unlike benign neonatal sleep myoclonus, the movements in benign myoclonus of early infancy only occur in the waking state. The onset of these spells is usually between ages three and nine months, but they may begin in the first month of life. The spells usually cease within two weeks to eight months of onset (Maydell *et al.*, 2001), but may persist for 1–2 years (Lombroso, 1990). Both ictal and interictal EEGs are normal, distinguishing this entity from infantile spasms. Treatment is not required. Development and neurological outcome are normal.

Jitteriness

Jitteriness is a movement disorder that is commonly observed in the neonatal period. Jitteriness manifests as generalized, symmetric, rhythmic oscillatory movements that resemble tremor or clonus. Up to 50% of term infants exhibit jitteriness during the first few days of life, especially when stimulated or crying. Jitteriness usually disappears shortly after birth, but can persist for months or recur after being gone for several weeks (Kramer, Nevo and Harel, 1994; Shuper *et al.*, 1991). Persistent jitteriness has been associated with hypoxic-ischemic injury, hypocalcemia, hypoglycemia and drug withdrawal. Jitteriness is highly stimulus sensitive. It can be precipitated by startle and suppressed by gentle passive flexion of the limb. Unlike seizures, there are no associated abnormal eye movements or autonomic changes (Volpe, 1995). Idiopathic jitteriness is usually associated with normal development and neurologic outcome. The outcome of infants with symptomatic jitteriness depends on the underlying cause. No treatment is required.

Shuddering

Shuddering episodes are characterized by periods of rapid tremor of the head, shoulders and arms that resemble shivering (Kanazawa, 2000; Holmes and Russman, 1986). Onset is in infancy or early childhood, but can occur as late as 10 years of age. The episodes last several seconds and can occur up to 100 times/day. During a spell, there is no change in consciousness. Ictal and interictal EEGs are normal. The preservation of consciousness and normal EEG distinguish this entity from seizures. Similarity to benign myoclonus of early infancy has been suggested (Kanazawa, 2000), but shuddering is better classified as tremor than myoclonus. Shuddering episodes typically abate as the child grows older. The prognosis for development and neurological function is uniformly good. No treatment is required.

Paroxysmal Tonic Upgaze of Infancy

Paroxysmal tonic upgaze of infancy is a disorder characterized by repeated episodes of upward gaze deviation, (Ouvrier and Billson, 1988; Ouvrier and Billson, 2005) though downward gaze has also been reported (Wolsey and Warner, 2006). Onset is usually in the first year of life. This condition is characterized by episodes of variably sustained conjugate upward deviation of the eyes that is often accompanied by neck flexion. The gaze deviation can be sustained or intermittent during an episode. The typical episode lasts for hours, but can persist for a few days. Attempts to look downward are accompanied by downbeating nystagmus. Horizontal eye movements are normal during an episode. Spells may resolve with sleep and be aggravated by fatigue or infection. There may be mild ataxia during an episode.

Paroxysmal tonic upgaze is usually idiopathic, but has been reported to have autosomal dominant inheritance. It is uncommonly associated with structural lesions, but reported conditions have included hypomyelination, periventricular leukomalacia, vein of Galen malformation or pinealoma (Ouvrier and Billson, 2005). There is no specific treatment, but there have been a few reports of improvement with levodopa treatment (Ouvrier and Billson, 1988; Campistol, Prats and Garaizar, 1993). Outcome is good in most cases, but persistent ataxia, cognitive impairment and residual minor oculomotor disorders have been reported (Ouvrier and Billson, 2005).

Spasmus Nutans

Spasmus nutans is a condition beginning in late infancy (3–8 months) that is characterized by a slow head tremor (approximately 2 Hz) that can be horizontal ("no-no") or vertical ("yes-yes"). The head movements are accompanied by a small-amplitude nystagmus that can by dysconjugate, conjugate or uniocular (Anthony, Ouvrier and Wise, 1980). When the child is looking at an object, the nodding or nystagmus may increase and if the head is held, the nystagmus typically increases. These observations have led to the suggestion that the head nodding is compensatory for the nystagmus (Gottlob *et al.*, 1992). Spasmus nutans generally resolves within several months, but the majority of patients continue to have a fine, sub-clinical, nystagmus until at least 5–12 years of age (Gottlob, Wizov and Reinecke, 1995). Long-term outcome for visual acuity is good. No treatment is required.

Spasmus nutans must be distinguished from congenital nystagmus (Gottlob *et al.*, 1990). Congenital nystagmus usually begins in the newborn period before six months of age. Congenital nystagmus is usually bilaterally symmetric where spasmus nutans is often asymmetric. Congenital nystagmus persists beyond a few months. Visual acuity is abnormal in about 90% of children with congenital nystagmus. While these features are useful in distinguishing congenital nystagmus from spasmus nutans, some children who clinically appear to have spasmus nutans at the time of presentation, have been found to have retinal abnormalities (Smith *et al.*, 2000; Kiblinger *et al.*, 2007). Neuroimaging abnormalities, including tumor and aplasia of the cerebellar vermis have been described in patients with spasmus nutans, but this is an uncommon association (Kiblinger *et al.*, 2007; Unsold and Ostertag, 2002; Kim, Park and Lee, 2003). Routine neuroimaging in the absence of other evidence for intracranial pathology has limited yield (Arnoldi and Tychsen, 1995).

Head Nodding

Head nodding without accompanying nystagmus can occur as paroxysmal events in older infants and toddlers (Nellhaus, 1983). These head movements can be lateral ("no-no"), vertical ("yes-yes") or oblique. The episodes may occur several times a day. The frequency (1–2 Hz) is slower than that of shuddering. The movements do not occur when the child is lying, but can occur in the sitting or standing position. The movements typically resolve within months, but can persist longer. Some children with head nodding have a prior history of shuddering spells; others may have a family history of essential tremor (DiMario, 2000). Developmental and neurological outcome are benign in this condition. No treatment is required.

Benign Paroxysmal Torticollis

Benign paroxysmal torticollis is an episodic disorder starting in the first year of life. It typically manifests as a head tilt to one side for a few hours or days. Spells can last as little as 10 minutes or as long as two months, but this is uncommon (Giffin, Benton and Goadsby, 2002). The torticollis may occur without any associated symptoms, or may be accompanied by pallor, vomiting, irritability or ataxia. Episodes typically recur with some regularity, up to twice a month initially and becoming less frequent as the child grows older. The spells abate spontaneously, usually by 2–3 years of age but always by age five. The child is normal between spells. Interictal and ictal EEGs are normal.

It has been suggested that benign paroxysmal torticollis is a migraine variant (Al-Twaijri and Shevell, 2002). There is often a family history of migraine. Some older children complain of headache during a spell, and many children go on to develop typical migraine after they have "outgrown" the paroxysmal torticollis (Deonna and Martin, 1981; Roulet and Deonna, 1988). Two patients with benign paroxysmal torticollis have been reported from a kindred with familial hemiplegic migraine linked to a CACNA1A mutation (Giffin, Benton and Goadsby, 2002). Few data exist on treatment of benign paroxysmal torticollis. Treatment is rarely indicated, since the episodes are generally brief and self-limited. Some clinicians provide a trial of cyproheptadine as a migraine prophylactic agent.

The differential diagnosis is broad, and diagnosis of benign paroxysmal torticollis is one of exclusion. Torticollis can be seen as an acute dystonic reaction to medication, as a symptom of a posterior fossa or cervical cord lesion or cervical vertebral abnormalities. In the case of structural lesions, the torticollis tends to be persistent and not paroxysmal. Torticollis can also be a sign of IVth nerve palsy. Congenital muscular torticollis is present from birth, is non-paroxysmal, and is associated with palpable tightness or fibrosis of the sternocleidomastoid muscle unilaterally.

Benign Idiopathic Dystonia of Infancy

Benign idiopathic dystonia of infancy is a rare disorder characterized by a segmental dystonia, usually of one upper extremity, that can be intermittent or persistent (Deonna, Ziegler and Nielsen, 1991; Willemse, 1986). The syndrome usually appears before five months of age and disappears by one year of age. The characteristic posture is of shoulder abduction, pronation of the forearm and flexion of the wrist. The posture occurs when the infant is at rest and goes away completely with volitional movement. Occasionally, both arms, an arm and leg on one side of the body, or the trunk can be involved. In some infants the posture is only apparent with relaxation or in certain positions. In others it may be present during all waking hours. The rest of the neurological examination is normal and the developmental and neurologic outcome is normal. Exclusion of progressive dystonia, brachial plexus injury, infantile hemiplegia and orthopedic abnormalities is important, but can be based on history and examination. Effective treatment has not been described, but reassurance is often sufficient since the outcome is normal.

Posturing During Masturbation

Masturbation is a normal behavior that occurs in the majority of both boys and girls. While masturbation occurs at all ages and has even been observed *in utero*, it is most common at about four years of age and during adolescence (Leung and Robson, 1993). Masturbation in young children may involve unusual postures or movements (Bower, 1981), which may be mistaken for abdominal pain or seizures (Fleisher and Morrison, 1990). Masturbatory movements in boys are usually obvious to the observer due to direct genital manipulation. In girls, they are more subtle and often involves adduction of the thighs, or sitting on a hand or foot and rocking. When the movements are accompanied by posturing of the limbs they are often mistaken for paroxysmal dystonia. Several characteristic features of masturbating girls who present for diagnosis have been identified (Fleisher and Morrison, 1990; Mink and Neil, 1995; Yang *et al.*, 2005): (i) onset after two months of age and before three years of age; (ii) stereotyped posturing with pressure applied to the pubic area; (iii) quiet grunting, diaphoresis or facial flushing; (iv) episode duration of less than a minute to several hours; (v) no alteration of consciousness; (vi) normal findings on examination; (vii) cessation with distraction or engagement of the child in another activity. Unnecessary diagnostics test are commonly performed before the true nature of the behavior is recognized. No imaging or laboratory evaluation is required if the movements abate when the child is distracted, the movements involve irregular rocking, the child remains interactive, there is some degree of volitional control, direct genital stimulation is involved and the neurologic and physical examinations are normal. There appears to be no association with sexual thoughts in the child. Instead, it is probably better to view these movements on the spectrum of other self-comforting behaviors such as thumb sucking or rocking, which have no concerning connotations for the parents (Mink and Neil, 1995; Yang *et al.*, 2005). Masturbation is a normal human behavior, so there is no expectation that this behavior will cease as the child grows older. However, the frequency of the behavior usually decreases as the child gets older and the behavior is less likely to occur under the observation of the parents. Neurological and developmental outcome is normal. No treatment is required, but it is important to educate the parents about the behavior. Reassurance for the family is the key to management, with redirection should the behavior prove embarrassing for the family or occur in public (Leung and Robson, 1993; Fleisher and Morrison, 1990; Yang *et al.*, 2005). The parents should be educated that this is a normal behavior resulting from random exploration of the body by the infant.

Transient Tic Disorder

Transient tic disorder is a disorder of childhood with one or several tics that are indistinguishable from the tics of chronic tic disorder, but that last only several months. The diagnosis is made in retrospect, since only with complete resolution can this be distinguished from a chronic tic disorder or Tourette syndrome. Transient tics can occur at anytime during childhood, but are most commonly seen in pre-school and primary-school age children. Approximately 10% of children may have a transient tic or tics (Robertson, 2003). In most cases, transient tics do not require treatment. If the tics cause impairment or distress, medical treatment may be indicated. Medications for treatment of transient tics are the same as those used for treatment of tics in Tourette syndrome (see Chapter 24). The cause is unknown, but transient tic disorder has been reported in members of a large kindred with Tourette syndrome, suggesting that transient tic disorder is a possible expression of the Tourette syndrome gene(s) (Kurlan *et al.*, 1988). Once the tics have resolved, they usually do not recur and long-term prognosis is excellent.

SUMMARY

Movement disorders in childhood can be complex and worrisome. However, many conditions appear to be developmentally determined and have a uniformly good outcome. Recognition of these conditions in young children is important, to avoid unnecessary invasive testing and undue parental anxiety. Direct observation of the movement is essential, as is consideration of the developmental context.

References

Al-Twaijri, W. and Shevell, M. (2002) Pediatric migraine equivalents: occurrence and clinical features in practice. *Pediatric Neurology*, 26, 365–368.

Anthony, J., Ouvrier, R. and Wise, G. (1980) Spasmus nutans, a mistaken entity. *Archives of Neurology*, 37, 373–375.

Arnoldi, K. and Tychsen, L. (1995) Prevalence of intracranial lesions in children initially diagnosed with disconjugate nystagmus (spasmus nutans). *Journal of Pediatric Ophthalmology and Strabismus*, 32, 296–301.

Bower, B. (1981) Fits and other frightening or funny turns in young people. *Practitioner*, 225, 297–304.

Campistol, J., Prats, J. and Garaizar, C. (1993) Benign paroxysmal tonic upgaze of childhood with ataxia. A neurophthalmological syndrome of familial origin? *Developmental Medicine and Child Neurology*, 35, 436–439.

Coulter, D. and Allen, R. (1982) Benign neonatal myoclonus. *Archives of Neurology*, 39, 191–192.

Deonna, T. and Martin, D. (1981) Benign paroxysmal torticollis in infancy. *Archives of Disease in Childhood*, 56, 956–959.

Deonna, T., Ziegler, A. and Nielsen, J. (1991) Transient idiopathic dystonia in infancy. *Neuropediatrics*, 22, 220–224.

DiMario, F.J. (2000) Childhood head tremor. *Journal of Child Neurology*, 15, 22–25.

Egger, J., Grossmann, G. and Auchterlonie, I.A. (2003) Lesson of the week: benign sleep myoclonus in infancy mistaken for epilepsy. *BMJ*, 326, 975–976.

Fleisher, D.R. and Morrison, A. (1990) Masturbation mimicking abdominal pain or seizures in young girls. *The Journal of Pediatrics*, 116, 810–814.

Giffin, N.J., Benton, S. and Goadsby, P.J. (2002) Benign paroxysmal torticollis of infancy: four new cases and linkage to CACNA1A mutation. *Developmental Medicine and Child Neurology*, 44, 490–493.

Gottlob, I., Zubcov, A., Catalano, R. *et al.* (1990) Signs distinguishing spasmus nutans (with and without central nervous system lesions) from infantile nystagmus. *Ophthalmology*, 97, 1166–1175.

Gottlob, I., Zubcov, A., Wizov, S. and Reinecke, R. (1992) Head nodding is compensatory in spasmus nutans. *Ophthalmology*, 99, 1024–1031.

Gottlob, I., Wizov, S. and Reinecke, R. (1995) Spasmus nutans. A long-term follow-up. *Investigations in Ophthalmology and Visual Sciences*, 36, 2768–2771.

Holmes, G. and Russman, B. (1986) Shuddering attacks. Evaluation using electroencephalographic frequency modulation radiotelemetry and videotape monitoring. *American Journal of Diseases of Children*, 140, 72–73.

Kanazawa, O. (2000) Shuddering attacks-report of four children. *Pediatric Neurology*, 23, 421–424.

Kiblinger, G.D., Wallace, B.S., Hines, M. and Siatkowski, R.M. (2007) Spasmus nutans-like nystagmus is often associated with underlying ocular, intracranial, or systemic abnormalities. *Journal of Neuro-Ophthalmology*, 27, 118–122.

Kim, J.S., Park, S.H. and Lee, K.W. (2003) Spasmus nutans and congenital ocular motor apraxia with cerebellar vermian hypoplasia. *Archives of Neurology*, 60, 1621–1624.

Kramer, U., Nevo, Y. and Harel, S. (1994) Jittery babies: a short term follow-up. *Brain and Development*, 16, 112–114.

Kurlan, R., Behr, J., Medved, L. and Como, P. (1988) Transient tic disorder and the spectrum of Tourette's syndrome. *Archives of Neurology*, 45, 1200–1201.

Leung, A.K.C. and Robson, W.L.M. (1993) Childhood masturbation. *Clinical Pediatrics*, 32, 238–241.

Lombroso, C. (1990) Early myoclonic encephalopathy, early infantile epileptic encephalopathy, and benign and severe infantile myoclonic epilepsies: a critical review and personal contributions. *Journal of Clinical Neurophysiology*, 7, 380–408.

Lombroso, C. and Fejerman, N. (1977) Benign myoclonus of early infancy. *Annals of Neurology*, **1**, 138–148.

Lyon, G., Kolodny, E.H. and Pastores, G.M. (2006) *Neurology of Hereditary Metabolic Diseases of Children*, 3rd edn, McGraw-Hill, New York.

Maria, B.L. (2005) *Current Management in Child Neurology*, 3rd edn, BC Decker, Inc., Hamilton.

Maydell, B.V., Berenson, F., Rothner, A.D., Wyllie, E. and Kotagal, P. (2001) Benign myoclonus of early infancy: an imitator of West's syndrome. *Journal of Child Neurology*, **16**, 109–112.

Mink, J. and Neil, J. (1995) Masturbation mimicking paroxysmal dystonia or dyskinesia in a young girl. *Movement Disorders*, **10**, 518–520.

Nellhaus, G. (1983) Abnormal head movements of young children. *Developmental Medicine and Child Neurology*, **25**, 384–389.

Ouvrier, R. and Billson, F. (1988) Benign paroxysmal upgaze of childhood. *Journal of Child Neurology*, **3**, 177–180.

Ouvrier, R. and Billson, F. (2005) Paroxysmal tonic upgaze of childhood – a review. *Brain & Development*, **27**, 185–188.

Paro-Panjan, D. and Neubauer, D. (2008) Benign neonatal sleep myoclonus: Experience from the study of 38 infants. *European Journal of Paediatric Neurology*, **12**, 14–18.

Reggin, J. and Johnson, M. (1989) Exacerbation of benign sleep myoclonus by benzodiazepine treatment. *Annals of Neurology*, **26**, 455.

Resnick, T.J., Moshe, S.L., Perotta, L. and Chambers, H.J. (1986) Benign neonatal sleep myoclonus. Relationship to sleep states. *Archives of Neurology*, **43**, 266–268.

Robertson, M.M. (2003) Diagnosing Tourette syndrome: Is it a common disorder? *Journal of Psychosomatic Research*, **55**, 3–6.

Roulet, E. and Deonna, T. (1988) Benign paroxysmal torticollis in infancy. *Developmental Medicine and Child Neurology*, **30**, 409–410.

Sanger, T.D. (2003) Pediatric movement disorders. *Current Opinion in Neurology*, **16**, 529–535.

Sanger, T.D., Delgado, M.R., Gaebler-Spira, D., Hallett, M. and Mink, J.W. (2003) Classification and definition of disorders causing hypertonia in childhood. *Pediatrics*, **111**, e89–e97.

Schlaggar, B.L. and Mink, J.W. (2003) Movement disorders in children. *Pediatrics in Review*, **24**, 39–51.

Shuper, A., Zalzberg, J., Weitz, R. and Mimouni, M. (1991) Jitteriness beyond the neonatal period: a benign pattern of movement in infancy. *Journal of Child Neurology*, **6**, 243–245.

Singer, H.S., Kossoff, E.H., Hartman, A.L., and Crawford, T.O. (2005) *Treatment of Pediatric Neurologic Disorders*, Taylor & Francis, Boca Raton.

Smith, D., Fitzgerald, K., Stass-Isern, M. and Cibis, G. (2000) Electroretinography is necessary for spasmus nutans diagnosis. *Pediatric Neurology*, **23**, 33–36.

Unsold, R. and Ostertag, C. (2002) Nystagmus in suprasellar tumors: recent advances in diagnosis and therapy. *Strabismus*, **10**, 173–177.

Volpe, J. (1995) Neurology of the Newborn, 3rd edn, WB Saunders, Philadelphia.

Willemse, J. (1986) Benign idiopathic dystonia in the first year of life. *Developmental Medicine and Child Neurology*, **28**, 355–363.

Wolsey, D.H. and Warner, J.E. (2006) Paroxysmal tonic downgaze in two healthy infants. *Journal of Neuro-Ophthalmology*, **26**, 187–189.

Yang, M.L., Fullwood, E., Goldstein, J. and Mink, J.W. (2005) Masturbation in infancy and early childhood presenting as a movement disorder: 12 cases and a review of the literature. *Pediatrics*, **116**, 1427–1432.

Part IX

PSYCHOGENIC MOVEMENT DISORDERS

31

Psychogenic Movement Disorders

Elizabeth Peckham and Mark Hallett

Human Motor Control Section, NINDS, NIH, Bethesda, USA

INTRODUCTION

The evaluation of patients with a suspected psychogenic etiology is one of the most difficult tasks for a practicing neurologist. Patients do not want to be told that the diagnosis is "psychological," there is no confirmatory "test" to prove that the patients are psychogenic (although there is support through neurophysiology in psychogenic myoclonus and tremor) and the diagnosis is based largely on the clinical experience of the evaluating neurologist. There is always concern for possible litigation in relation to this diagnosis and often these patients are in the process of obtaining or are currently on disability secondary to their condition. The diagnosis of a psychogenic movement disorder (PMD) should only be made in circumstances where the neurologist has specialty training in movement disorders and after other etiologies have been excluded.

EPIDEMIOLOGY

Patients with psychogenic movement disorders are seen in 1–9% of admissions to neurological units (Bhatia and Schneider, 2007; Shill and Gerber, 2006; Hinson and Haren, 2006). In movement disorder specialty clinics, this number has been reported to be around 2–3%, but is as high as 25% in a tertiary referral center (Miyasaki et al., 2003). The type of movement disorder seen varies somewhat, but generally tremor and dystonia are the most common. In one series of over 500 patients, the movements seen were as follows: tremor (39.8%), dystonia (40.6%), myoclonus (17.2%), tics (4.3%), parkinsonism (3.2%), other dyskinesias (1.5%) and chorea (0.6%) (Kim, Pakiam and Lang, 1999). There is a female preponderance (67–81%) and PMDs are more common in younger individuals with a mean age of 44 years (Thomas and Jankovic, 2004). In 10–15% of patients there is an associated organic neurological diagnosis (Kim, Pakiam and Lang, 1999; Hinson and Haren, 2006). Psychiatric diagnoses are commonly

seen in PMD and in one series of 42 patients, 38% had anxiety and 19.1% had major depression (Feinstein et al., 2001). Prognosis is generally poor, with up to 90% of patients continuing to have abnormal movements (Feinstein et al., 2001), and a similar poor prognosis has been seen in functional weakness and sensory disturbances in a follow-up of 12 years (Stone et al., 2003b). Factors that are positive prognostic indicators include a short duration of illness, the presence of an underlying psychiatric illness (anxiety or depression) and when there is a specific trigger that can be identified (Bhatia and Schneider, 2007; Hinson and Haren, 2006).

DIAGNOSTIC CRITERIA

There are four levels of diagnostic certainty, as described by Fahn and Williams (Fahn and Williams, 1998):

1. Documented PMD: the movements are relieved by psychotherapy, psychological suggestion (including physical therapy) or the administration of placebos, or the patient must be witnessed to be free of symptoms when supposedly unobserved.
2. Clinically established PMD: the movements are inconsistent over time, or incongruent with the classical symptomatology (i.e., a patient complaining of posturing of the limb resists passive and active movement, but easily grooms himself daily). In addition, one or more of the following are present: other neurologic signs that are definitely psychogenic (false weakness or sensory findings and self-inflicted injuries), multiple somatizations or a documented psychiatric illness.
3. Probable PMD: the movements are inconsistent or incongruent with the classical disorder, but other features in support of psychogenicity are lacking.
4. Possible PMD: a suspicion for a psychogenic basis for the movements is based only on the presence of an obvious emotional disturbance.

Additional criteria proposed by Shill and Gerber (Shill and Gerber, 2006) included excessive pain or fatigue, the patient's previous exposure to neurological disease (disease modeling) and the factor of secondary gain.

PMDs pose an especially troubling problem for the neurologist. Many different treatments have been proposed, but treatment response is variable and prognosis is poor. An evaluation with a psychiatrist is imperative to establish any underlying element of anxiety, depression or other psychiatric disorder that can be treated with appropriate medications. In conjunction with medical treatment, additional care can be provided through rehabilitation medicine (physical therapy and occupational therapy) and psychotherapy. Alternative treatments, such as biofeedback, hypnosis and acupuncture have been proposed, either in conjunction with or as a primary form of treatment (see Figure 31.1) There are no double-blind, placebo-controlled clinical trials in this area and evidence for treatments is largely based on case reports or is anecdotal.

Neurological Evaluation of the Patient

History

On evaluation of the patient, there are multiple "red flags" in the history that can point to a psychogenic etiology (Table 31.1). The onset of symptoms is generally abrupt and often the symptoms may come and go in severity, possibly even remitting at times (Kim, Pakiam and Lang, 1999). The course of PMDs tends to be static, rather than progressive, as seen in degenerative disorders (Fahn and Williams, 1998; Miyasaki *et al.*, 2003). However, patients may note that their symptoms get acutely worse when they are under stress. Often, prior to the onset of symptoms, there

is a specific trigger, such as an accident or work-related injury (Bhatia and Schneider, 2007). Co-morbid somatizations are commonly seen and include unexplained gastrointestinal symptoms (nausea and vomiting), sexual dysfunction, unexplained sensory loss and pain. In addition, underlying psychiatric diagnoses are often found. Of these, the most common appear to be depression, anxiety and other conversion disorders. Another finding is pronounced fatigue in many patients (Bhatia and Schneider, 2007). Anecdotally, we have found in our clinic that many patients specifically state that fatigue is a result of the excessive amount of the movement that occurs. This is an interesting aspect, since generalized fatigue is reported in patients with underlying organic movement disorders, but usually there is no fatigue reported in correlation with the specific movement itself. PMDs are more commonly reported in health professionals and those that have been witness to other family or friends with a neurological condition (Bhatia and Schneider, 2007). This suggests a role for disease modeling in this group of patients.

Examination

On examination there are additional criteria that are often seen (Table 31.1). The salient feature to describe the examination is inconsistency. The movements themselves usually vary in amplitude, frequency and duration. At times, the movements may stop completely, especially with distraction. They may also increase when attention is paid to the movement (Schrag and Lang, 2005). The movements are often bizarre and not consistent with any previously described neurological condition. Additional findings on examination can include false weakness and

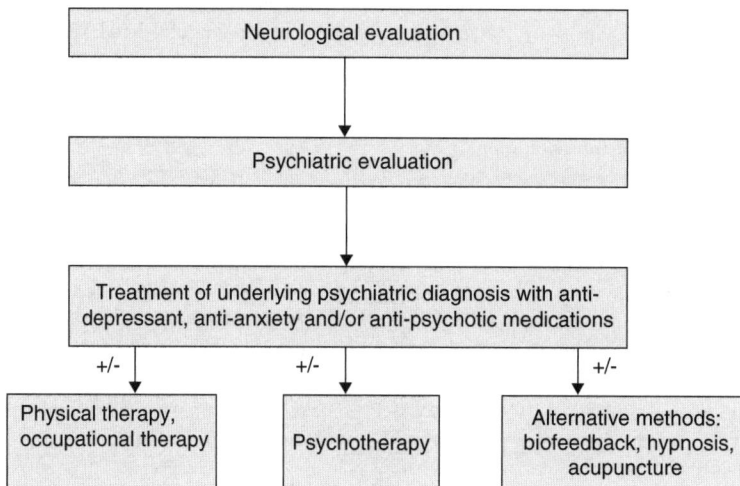

Figure 31.1 Treatment approach.

Table 31.1 Clues to the diagnosis of psychogenic movement disorders (Fahn and Williams, 1998; Miyasaki *et al.*, 2003).

A. Historical
  1. Abrupt onset
  2. Static course
  3. Spontaneous remissions
  4. Obvious psychiatric disturbance
  5. Multiple somatizations
  6. Employed in health profession
  7. Pending litigation or compensation
  8. Presence of secondary gain
  9. Young age

B. Clinical:
  1. Inconsistent character of movement (amplitude, frequency, distribution, selective ability)
  2. Paroxysmal movement disorder
  3. Movements increase with attention or decrease with distraction
  4. Ability to trigger or relieve the abnormal movement with unusual or non-physiological interventions. (e.g., trigger points of the body)
  5. False weakness
  6. False sensory complaints
  7. Self-inflicted injuries
  8. Deliberate slowness of movements
  9. Functional disability out of proportion to exam findings
  10. Movement abnormality that is bizarre, multiple or difficult to classify

C. Therapeutic responses
  1. Unresponsive to appropriate medications
  2. Response to placebo
  3. Remission with psychotherapy

non-physiological sensory loss (Factor, Podskalny and Molho, 1995). This is discussed in more detail below. In general, the disability reported by patients is out of proportion to the examination findings. Often, patients struggle on the examination, as manifest by grimacing, sighing or looking exhausted. When they attempt to perform minor movements, they may use their whole body to do this and seem to put in more effort than is actually required (Bhatia and Schneider, 2007).

TYPES OF PSYCHOGENIC MOVEMENT DISORDERS

Any type of movement can be present on the examination. Most commonly seen are tremor and dystonia, as reported by several groups (Thomas and Jankovic, 2004; Factor, Podskalny and Molho, 1995; Hinson and Haren, 2006). Other diagnoses include myoclonus, parkinsonism, gait disorders and tics. These conditions may occur alone or patients may have multiple movements present.

Tremor

The most common site for tremor is the hand (84%), followed by the leg (28%) (Thomas and Jankovic, 2004). Frequency of the psychogenic tremor is usually less than 6 Hz and the examination shows variability in frequency and amplitude. When attention is drawn to the tremor, the amplitude may increase, and with distraction it is decreased and may resolve completely (Bhatia and Schneider, 2007). The tremor can be present at rest, posture, intention or in combination and may be exhausting for the patient (Thomas and Jankovic, 2004). The most consistent findings to separate a psychogenic cause of tremor from organic tremor are the presence of the co-activation sign and the absence of finger tremor (Deuschl *et al.*, 1998). The co-activation sign can be tested at the bedside by noticing an increased tone in association with the tremor. However, once the tremor disappears, the tone normalizes. In some patients, this finding can be demonstrated on electromyography by tremulous free co-activation of antagonist muscle prior to the onset of tremor (Deuschl *et al.*, 1998). An additional finding that can be seen on examination, and proven with tremor physiology, is entrainment. This occurs when the patient taps one of the hands at a specified frequency. A psychogenic tremor will slow down or speed up based on the frequency tested. An additional bedside test includes having the patient perform a quick ballistic movement with one hand while the opposite hand is held in the position where the tremor is most prominent. There should be a significant reduction in the tremor amplitude or complete cessation of the tremor when the underlying etiology is psychogenic. In contrast, patients with Parkinson's disease and essential tremor will not have any change in their tremor (Kumru *et al.*, 2004).

In the laboratory, neurophysiology testing can be very helpful in this group of patients. Surface electromyography recordings can give an accurate estimation of the frequency and amplitude of the tremor. In addition, the tremor can be evaluated in rest, posture and with a kinetic position of the hands. In accordance with the bedside examination, the tremor of a psychogenic patient often shows great variability in amplitude and may be present in multiple positions. Specific tasks with weighting and entrainment can be tested. Most patients with a psychogenic tremor will have an increase in their tremor amplitude with Weighting, (Deuschl *et al.*, 1998). In contrast, patients with exaggerated physiological or pathological tremors show a decrease or no change with weighting, respectively. Testing entrainment, psychogenic patients have entrainment of the tremor (O'Sulleabhein and Matsumoto, 1998) or an inability to tap at the required frequency (Zeuner *et al.*, 2003). Again, this is in contrast to patients who have underlying essential tremor or Parkinson's disease, where the tremor frequency does not change with this task.

Dystonia

Psychogenic dystonia can be an especially difficult diagnosis to make, as there is no confirmatory physiology test. It is important to be familiar with the features of organic dystonia to make this diagnosis. Features suggestive of a psychogenic etiology include presence of the dystonic posturing at rest, abrupt onset, involvement of the leg or foot in an adult and spontaneous remissions (Thomas and Jankovic, 2004). In addition, this group of patients often exhibits inconsistent bizarre posturing that changes during the course of the examination (Shill and Gerber, 2006). An organic etiology is suspected in patients who have a childhood onset, steadily progressive course, exacerbation by movement and a good response to dopamine (for dopa-responsive dystonia). For focal dystonias, the presence of a sensory trick is suggestive of an organic etiology (although this can be present in psychogenic cases as well) (Shill and Gerber, 2006).

Parkinsonism

The tremor of psychogenic parkinsonism occurs in rest and in posture without the brief pause during the transition between states. Other features of psychogenic tremor described above may also be present. The rigidity present in this group of patients is not a true rigidity, but an inability to relax and resembles voluntary movement (Miyasaki *et al.*, 2003). The slowness in these patients is inconsistent over different portions of the examination and often these patients expend a great deal of effort to do a minor task (Thomas and Jankovic, 2004). Gait is usually stiff and the arm may have an unusual posture. Testing of postural stability shows an exaggerated response, such as flailing of the arms upward, strong retropulsion with a minor pull and no falls (Miyasaki *et al.*, 2003; Thomas and Jankovic, 2004).

Myoclonus

The presentation of psychogenic myoclonus can be variable in distribution, presenting in a generalized, segmental or focal pattern. It usually occurs at rest and commonly increases with movement (Shill and Gerber, 2006). The character of the movements is inconsistent in frequency, amplitude and duration and many patients may experience periods of remission from hours to days (Thomas and Jankovic, 2004).

Physiology studies may be very helpful in patients in differentiating psychogenic vs organic myoclonus. EMG activity with a mean duration of <70 ms is likely to be organic. Patients with stimulus sensitive myoclonus (tapping a specific muscle or area produces jerks) of a psychogenic nature show variability and a long latency to the onset of jerking after the stimulus occurs (Thomas and Jankovic, 2004). One of the most helpful aspects of physiology is the evaluation for the Bereitschaftspotential (BP). The presence of a BP occurs prior to normal voluntary movements and is also present with psychogenic myoclonus. This evaluation is performed by a technique called jerk lock averaging where the myoclonic jerks are time locked with activity on an electroencephalogram. A BP is present when there is a slow negative slope of activity in the one to two seconds preceding the movement. If a BP is found, this is very helpful in diagnosing psychogenic myoclonus, as this is not seen in cortical myoclonus. However, if it is not found, the etiology is still in question. A BP can be absent in normal subjects (Shibasaki and Hallett, 2006).

Gait

Psychogenic gait can be found in isolation or in combination with other psychogenic movement disorders. As in other PMDs, the gait disturbance presents with inconsistency on the examination, unusual phenomena and findings that contradict another neurological diagnosis. In one study, there were six characteristic features of psychogenic gait that were present in 97% of patients. These included: fluctuation of impairment, excessive slowness of movement, psychogenic Romberg, walking on ice, uneconomic postures with wastage of muscle energy, and sudden buckling of movements, either with or without falls (Sudarsky, 2006). Another study compared patients with psychogenic gait disorder in isolation vs a psychogenic gait in combination with other psychogenic movements. In pure psychogenic gait, the most common feature was buckling of the knee, followed by astasia-abasia. In a mixed psychogenic gait, the most common pattern was slowing of gait, followed by a dystonic type of gait (Baik and Lang, 2007). Recently, the "chair test" has been proposed as a way to help evaluate patients with psychogenic gait (Okun *et al.*, 2007). For this test, patients are asked to sit in a swivel chair and propel the chair forward and backward. PMD patients were compared with control subjects who had a diagnosis of Parkinson's disease or multiple system atrophy with an associated gait abnormality. Almost all of the PMD patients were able to propel the chair forward well even though they had abnormalities in their gait. The control subjects, however, had the same amount of difficulty moving in the chair as they did with walking.

PSYCHOGENIC FINDINGS IN THE NEUROLOGIC EXAMINATION THAT MAY BE PRESENT IN THE PSYCHOGENIC MOVEMENT DISORDER PATIENT: (TABLE 31.2)

1. Mental status exam: this part of the examination should be normal. However, severely depressed or anxious patients may have difficulty concentrating.

2. Speech: the sudden onset of a speech disorder without radiological findings (stroke) and normal laryngosopic exam should prompt the clinician to consider a psychogenic etiology. Usually this will present either post-virus or post-trauma and may be a reaction to an event, such as profound loss, death or shock. Patients can present with a variety of complaints, including, but not limited to, total loss of voice, whispering, continuous high pitched voice, high pitched voice with breaks and low pitched, coarse or monotone voice (Baker, 1998). In addition, there is a case report (Verhoeven et al., 2005) and we have seen a patient in our clinic who developed a "foreign accent syndrome" thought to be of psychogenic origin.

3. Cranial nerve examination: psychogenic ophthalmologic syndromes may be present in the psychogenic movement disorder patient. Possible findings include: convergence spasm (Suzuki et al., 2001), ptosis, partial or complete blindness and tunnel vision (Shaibani and Sabbagh, 1998). Convergence spasm is manifest by transient periods of convergence, miosis and accommodation. In general, this is thought to be a finding in psychogenic patients. However, this finding has been reported in other conditions, including tumors of the posterior fossa, prior head trauma, Arnold Chiari malformation, and in vestibulopathy (Dagi, Chrousos and Cogan, 1987). Ptosis can have many different causes; however, an important finding at bedside of a psychogenic ptosis includes unilateral depression of the ipsilateral eyebrow when the patient is asked to open their eyes. This is in contrast to a patient with an organic condition where the unilateral eyebrow will be elevated. Mono-ocular or binocular blindness may be another complaint. A bedside test that can be performed for further evaluation is the mirror test. The clinician can hold a mirror in front of the patient and tilt it from side to side. Humans will either look away from the mirror or follow it reflexively when it is placed in front of them (Shaibani and Sabbagh, 1998). Finally, tunnel vision may be an associated complaint in this group of patients. This is psychogenic when the visual field remains the same regardless of the distance tested. In contrast, funnel vision (an organic condition) will have visual fields that expand in inches proportionate to the distance viewed. This can be evaluated with formal visual field testing.

4. Strength examination: the tone examination should be normal, but the examiner may find it difficult for the patient to relax, which may give a false impression of increased tone. On the strength exam, it is important to look for inconsistency. An example is when the patient appears weak on the examination, but is able to walk across the room without difficulty, or vice versa (Factor, Podskalny and Molho, 1995). Specific signs may include give-way weakness, Hoover's sign and the adductor sign. "Give-way" weakness occurs when the patient gives full power strength followed by quick breaks in the power of the muscle group tested. In organic weakness, this decrement is slow and steady. Testing for a Hoover's sign occurs with having the patient lay in a supine position and cupping each of the patients' heels. When the patient is asked to raise one leg, the contralateral leg should exhibit pressure in the opposite direction. If this pressure is not felt, then the patient has a decreased effort. If the pressure is present and full, then the patient does not have a true paralysis. Finally, the adductor sign occurs with a similar mechanism. When one adductor muscle contracts, the opposite adductor should reflexively contract as well. When this does not occur, the patient may have a decreased effort (Shaibani and Sabbagh, 1998).

5. Sensory examination: patients with PMDs may report many sensory findings that are not reproducible on the examination. In addition, they may report non-physiological sensory loss, such as a hemisensory deficit that affects all modalities (hearing, taste, vision, smell) (Shaibani and Sabbagh, 1998). Again, it is important to look for inconsistencies on the examination. Patients may complain of complete sensory loss of the lower extremities, but are able to tandem walk. Bedside examinations that may help include using a tuning fork at the midline of the forehead to see if one side is felt more strongly than another (should be felt equally on both sides due to bone conduction). Sensation can also be tested with the arms or legs crossed when there is a hemisensory complaint (Shaibani and Sabbagh, 1998).

6. Reflexes: the reflex examination should be symmetrical and normal. Frontal release signs should not be present, except for cases where this may be a normal finding in an elderly patient.

7. Cerebellar: the cerebellar exam may have soft signs on the examination. This is one area where the patient may exhibit a great deal of effort to make minor movements. The effort appears out of proportion to the task presented. The movements may also be slowed; again, this may be out of proportion to the rest of their examination. Finger to nose may be inaccurate with the eyes

Table 31.2 Psychogenic signs that may co-exist in the psychogenic movement disorder patient.

	Possible Exam Finding	Differential diagnosis	Workup
Mental status examination	(1) Difficulty with concentration	(1) Anxiety	* Psychiatric evaluation
		(2) Depression	* Neuropsychological evaluation
		(3) Dementia	
Speech	(1) Total loss of voice	(1) Spasmodic dysphonia	* Nasolaryngoscopy
	(2) Whispering voice	(2) Structural brain lesion (stroke, tumor, multiple sclerosis)	* MRI of the brain
	(3) Continued high pitch voice with or without breaks		
	(4) Low pitched monotone voice		
	(5) Foreign accent syndrome		
Cranial nerves	(1) Convergence spasm	(1) Brain tumor (posterior fossa, pituitary)	* MRI of the brain
	(2) Ptosis	(2) Myasthenia gravis	* Workup for myasthenia if suspected (Ach antibody, EMG)
	(3) Partial or complete blindness	(3–4) Stroke	* Ophthalmology consult for evaluation of the fundus and formal visual fields
	(4) Tunnel vision		* Bedside mirror test
Strength	(1) Inconsistent examination (cannot walk across the room, but muscle group testing is normal)	Broad differential for weakness depending on the rest of the exam: cortical, spinal, neuromuscular, muscle, nerve	* Bedside tests: Hoover's sign, adductor sign
	(2) Give-way weakness		* MRI brain
			* MRI spinal cord
			* EMG
			* Muscle biopsy
Sensory	(1) Non-physiological complaint of sensory loss	Same as above	* Somatosensory evoked potentials
	(2) On examination, splitting of the midline with vibration		* MRI brain
			* MRI spine
Reflexes	(1) Should be normal and symmetric	Same as above	* H reflex
	(2) Frontal release signs should be absent		
Cerebellar	(1) Great deal of effort to make small movements (out of proportion to the task).	(1) Cerebellar lesion–stroke, tumor, multiple sclerosis	* MRI brain: posterior fossa
		(2) Parkinsonism (if slowed, irregular movements	
		(3) Ataxia	
Postural stability	(1) Exaggerated response: swaying, slowed, walking backwards, free fall onto examiner	(1) Parkinsonism	* MRI brain: posterior fossa
		(2) Ataxias	

open, but when the eyes are closed they are able to touch their own nose without difficulty. True cerebellar findings should prompt the clinician for another etiology.

8. Gait: features may be present, as described under the above discussion of psychogenic gait.
9. Postural stability: patients may have an exaggerated reaction to postural testing. This may manifest as marked swaying without falling, slowed movements forward or backwards, flinging both arms upward without falling or an exaggerated startle (Bhatia and Schneider, 2007; Thomas and Jankovic, 2004).

TREATMENT MODALITIES

Medical Treatment

Inpatient

Inpatient hospitalization is currently utilized in specialized centers in Canada, England and some other countries, and consists of a team of neurologists, psychiatrists, psychologists, physical therapists and sometimes therapists that perform alternative treatments. In one case series, 81% of 32 treated patients had complete resolution of their symptoms (Rosebush and Mazurek, 2005). Hospital stay in this group ranged from one week to six months. The remaining patients in this case series had partial resolution of symptoms. In many cases, this is certainly the best option. Unfortunately, inpatient treatment is not an option for most patients in the United States (and some other countries) for several reasons: few centers in the US have this capability; inpatient hospitalizations are very short in the US (couple of weeks) as compared with overseas (several months); and, finally, the US insurance system will not cover it. Because of these limitations, the best option is a multi-modality approach as an outpatient.

Outpatient

Oral Medications

There has been one trial of anti-depressant medications in PMD patients, where patients were started on a dose of paroxetine and citalopram and titrated up to an optimal dose (Voon and Lang, 2005). Those patients who did not respond were switched to venlafaxine. Paroxitine and citalopram are both selective serotonin reuptake inhibitors, while venlafaxine blocks both the reuptake of serotonin and norepinephrine. This drug regimen was chosen by the authors based on routine clinical practice and treating the patients underlying co-morbid symptoms of depression and/or anxiety. Of the patients treated, 67% had a diagnosis of chronic PMD with primary conversion symptoms and

recent or current depression. Of these patients, 7 of 10 responded with a complete remission of symptoms. The remaining 33% had a diagnosis of somatization disorder, hypochondriasis, factitious disorder or malingering and none of these patients improved.

Neuroleptic medications have also been reported to help in hysterical neurosis of the conversion type. Eighteen patients were followed and given either haloperidol or sulpiride (Rampello et al., 1996). Evaluation showed a greater improvement in the sulpiride group. The potency of hyperprolactinemia was theorized to play a role in the superiority of sulpiride over haloperidol. There is a case report evaluating risperidone for a patient with psychogenic stiff neck (Marazziti and Dell'Osso, 2005). In this study, the patient had an underlying history of depression and was treated with sertraline and risperidone. The symptoms of psychogenic stiff neck disappeared completely after treatment with risperidone alone for six months.

Physical Therapy

A retrospective study was performed in 10 patients who received physical therapy for a diagnosis of conversion disorder (Speed, 1996). In all cases, patients with gait difficulty were selected and they were able to ambulate normally at the end of treatment. They also received psychological treatment when appropriate. There is also a case series of physical therapy treatment in patients with conversion disorder in an inpatient hospitalization setting (Ness, 2007). All three of these patients had complete resolution of symptoms. Behavioral modification and shaping techniques were used. Correct patterns of movements were emphasized and praised while abnormal movements were ignored.

Behavioral Modification

A case series evaluated 39 consecutive patients with a combination of behavioral techniques and physical therapy (Shapiro and Teasell, 2004). The patients were admitted to a rehabilitation service and given supervised exercises to perform. At the beginning of treatment, they were told that they had a musculoskeletal problem that could resolve completely. If the patients did not improve after four weeks, behavioral treatment was initiated. The patients were told that the problem was either psychiatric in nature (conversion disorder) or that the treatment needed to be modified. Once the modification plan was implemented, they should improve quickly and completely. If this did not happen, then the diagnosis was conversion disorder and they would not fully recover because of an unconscious need to remain disabled. This behavioral treatment was successful in 8/9 acute patients and 1/28 chronic patients.

Psychotherapy

A single-blind clinical trial evaluated 10 patients with psychodynamic psychotherapy for one hour per week over a 12-week period (Hinson et al., 2006). The psychotherapy focused on early life experiences, personality traits and parenting dynamics, and tried to link these early behaviors with current behaviors. The patients were also given anti-anxiety or anti-depressant medications at the treating psychiatrists' discretion. In seven patients, the total psychogenic movement disorder scale improved to a significant degree.

Biofeedback

There are no published reports of biofeedback for PMD patients. There is one abstract that evaluated electromyography (EMG) biofeedback as a treatment (Rosebush and Mazurek, 2005). In this study 9 of 15 patients (60%) improved with EMG biofeedback. Patients received several sessions of training using biofeedback, where they attempted to decrease the EMG signal of their movements. They were then followed until improvement or resolution of their symptoms. Most patients were on additional pharmacological therapy.

Hypnosis

Hypnosis was used as a treatment in a randomized, controlled clinical trial in 44 patients with conversion disorder, motor type or somatization disorder with motor conversion symptoms (Moene et al., 2003). Patients were either assigned to a waiting-list condition or a hypnosis condition. Improvement was seen in the hypnosis-condition patients, when compared to baseline through objective observation and a subjective interview. Two additional studies evaluated hypnosis in the inpatient setting. One study followed 45 patients and hypnosis was used as a randomized treatment in a sub-set of the patients (Moene et al., 2002). There was no difference in primary outcome when comparing groups that did or did not receive hypnosis. The second study described eight cases of inpatients with conversion disorder, where hypnosis was thought to play a role in improvement of their symptoms (Moene, Hoogduin and Van Dyck, 1988).

Acupuncture

No formal trials have been performed to assess acupuncture in PMD patients. There is one case report that describes a patient with chronic, treatment-resistant PMD that had a dramatic response to acupuncture (Van Nuenen et al., 2007).

Trial of Placebo

There is one case report of one patient where a placebo treatment was tried in a minor with parental consent (Lim, Ong and Seet, 2007). In this case, the patient had psychogenic blepharospasm that was not improved with botulinum toxin. She was given an alternative placebo medication and it was suggested to her that this was a very effective medication for her symptoms and if she improved she would not have to see a psychiatrist. The patient had complete resolution of symptoms. Although a response to placebo was helpful in this case, it is currently considered unethical by many authorities and therefore is not recommended.

Treatment of Somatoform Disorders

Many of the methods discussed above for treatment were studied initially in patients with somatoform disorders other than PMDs. In a review of randomized, controlled trials (Kroenke, 2007) and intervention studies in somatoform disorders (Sumathipala, 2007), cognitive behavioral therapy was found to be the most efficacious treatment. Trials of anti-depressants were thought to hold some promise, but not be a conclusive form of treatment at this time. The term conversion disorder is used when the physical symptoms in a somatoform disorder are neurological in nature (Hurwitz, 2004). In a systematic review of psychosocial interventions for conversion disorder by the Cochrane Collaboration, 260 references were reviewed and of these it was not possible to draw any conclusions about possible benefits, due to poor methodological quality and poor reporting (Ruddy and House, 2005). Future research in this area should be aimed at direct comparison of treatment modalities in a randomized, double-blind research design.

General Guidance

Telling the Patient

The initial phase of treatment is how the patient is told about the diagnosis. This may be the most difficult part, and it is important to be ready for any type of reaction. Surprisingly, some patients are relieved and welcome the thought that psychological triggers may be playing a factor in their diagnosis. Reassurance is a very important factor, and it is important to be unambiguous in the diagnosis. If the doctor expresses uncertainty, the patient will likely not accept the diagnosis. It is important to emphasize that the neurological examination looks intact, the workup is negative for other neurological conditions and there is hope that they can get better.

    The term to use for the diagnosis is controversial. We prefer to start with the phenomenological description, that is, for example, myoclonus or tremor. The second component is the cause. Some experts prefer to use "psychogenic," and this term will almost certainly come out at some point, but we prefer to use "functional." The brain is structurally intact (which is good), but it is malfunctioning. The nature of the malfunction is not yet fully understood, but it can be reversed. The term "functional" may be more acceptable to patients than other terms. In one study in patients with seizure-type movements, the terms "stress-related seizures" or "functional seizures" were found to be less offensive than the terms "psychogenic seizure," "non-epileptic attack disorder" or "pseudoseizures" (Stone *et al.*, 2003a). It is very important to describe the medical condition to the patient in a way that will help ensure trust in the physician, so there is a better chance for recovery. In addition, we generally discuss that stress may play a contributing factor in the development of PMDs and try to identify any possible stressors.

If there is the ability to have long-term care with this patient, it may be best to see them for a couple of appointments, plant the idea early on that this is in the differential diagnosis and that you need to rule out some other conditions. If the patient has seen other physicians they may have been told "it is all in your head," "just stop doing it," and so on. Lack of sympathy for this diagnosis does not help your patient or help you to keep a patient that may actually get better.

Referral to a Psychiatrist

It is very important to refer the patient to a psychiatrist who has an understanding of psychogenic movement disorders. Commonly, the diagnosis is made, the patient is willing to undergo a psychiatric evaluation and then is told by the evaluating psychiatrist that they have an underlying neurological problem (and it can't possibly be psychiatric). This is extremely frustrating for the patient to hear, will lose any credibility that you have with the patient and send them on an endless search for what is the "real cause" of their condition. The psychiatrist has to understand that the referral is not made for the diagnosis of the condition, but for identification and treatment of any underlying psychiatric problem. This should be a principal component of therapy.

CONCLUSION

Psychogenic movement disorders are truly a crisis for neurology (Hallett, 2006). They occur in a relatively young population and can be reversible with early intervention and multi-modality treatment. However, this requires an astute knowledge of this condition and appropriate referral to a psychiatrist and additional therapists. To compound this difficult problem, the medical community at large is poorly educated on this topic, and as a result these patients are misdiagnosed.

References

Baik, J.S. and Lang, A.E. (2007) Gait abnormalities in psychogenic movement disorders. *Movement Disorders*, **22** (3), 395–399.

Baker, J. Psychogenic dysphonia: peeling back the layers. *Journal of Voice*, **12** (4), 527–535.

Bhatia, K.P. and Schneider, S.A. (2007) Psychogenic tremor and related disorders. *Journal of Neurology*, **254** (5), 569–574.

Dagi, L.R.,Chrousos, G.A. and Cogan, D.C. (1987) Spasm of the near reflex associated with organic disease. *American Journal of Ophthalmology*, **103** (4), 582–585.

Deuschl, G., Koster, B., Lucking, C.H. and Scheidt, C. (1998) Diagnostic and pathophysiological aspects of psychogenic tremors. *Movement Disorders*, **13** (2), 294–302.

Factor, S.A., Podskalny, G.D. and Molho, E.S. (1995) Psychogenic movement disorders: frequency, clinical profile and characteristics. *Journal of Neurology, Neurosurgery, and Psychiatry*, **59**, 406–412.

Fahn, S. and Williams, D.T. (1998) Psychogenic dystonia. *Advances in Neurology*, **50**, 431–455.

Feinstein, A., Stergiopoulos, V., Fine, J. and Lang, A.E. (Jul–Sep 2001) Psychiatric outcome in patients with a psychogenic movement disorder: a prospective study. *Neuropsychiatry, Neuropsychology and Behavioral Neurology*, **14** (3), 169–176.

Hallett, M. (2006) Psychogenic movement disorders: A crisis for neurology. *Current Neurology and Neuroscience Reports*, **6**, 269–271.

Hinson, V.K. and Haren, W.B. (2006) Psychogenic movement disorders. *The Lancet Neurology*, **5**, 695–700.

Hinson, V.K.,Weinstein, S., Bernard, B., Leurgans, S.E. and Goetz, C.G. (2006) Single blind clinical trial of psychotherapy for treatment of psychogenic movement disorders. *Parkinsonism and Related Disorders*, **12**, 177–180.

Hurwitz, T.A. (Mar 2004) Somatization and conversion disorder. *Canadian Journal of Psychiatry*, **49** (3), 172–178.

Kim, Y.J., Pakiam, A.S. and Lang, A.E. (1999) Historical and clinical features of psychogenic tremor: A review of 70 cases. *The Canadian Journal of Neurological Sciences*, **26** (3), 190–195.

Kroenke, K. (2007) Efficacy of treatment for somatoform disorders: a review of randomized controlled trials. *Psychosomatic Medicine*, **69** (9), 881–888.

Kumru, H.,Valls-Sole, J.,Valldeoriola, F., Marti, M., Sanegre, M. and Tolosa, E. (2004) Transient arrest of psychogenic tremor induced by contralateral ballistic movements. *Neuroscience Letters*, **370**, 135–139.

Lim, E.C., Ong, B.K. and Seet, R.C. (2007) Is there a place for placebo in management of psychogenic movement disorders? *Annals of the Academy of Medicine, Singapore*, **36** (3), 208–210.

Marazziti, D. and Dell'Osso, B. (2005) Effectiveness of risperidone in psychogenic stiff neck. *CNS Spectrums*, **10** (6), 443–444.

Miyasaki, J.M., Sa, D.S., Galvez-Jimenez, N. and Lang, A.E. (2003) Psychogenic movement disorders. *The Canadian Journal of Neurological Sciences*, **30** (suppl 1), S94–S100.

Moene, F.C., Spinohoven, P., Hoogduin, K.A. and van Dyck, R. (2003) A randomized controlled clinical trial of a hypnosis-based treatment for patients with conversion disorder, motor type. *International Journal of Clinical and Experimental Hypnosis*, **51** (1), 29–50.

Moene, F.C., Hoogduin, K.A. and Van Dyck, R. (1988) The inpatient treatment of patients suffering from (motor) conversion symptoms: a description of eight cases. *International Journal of Clinical and Experimental Hypnosis*, **46** (2), 171–190.

Moene, F.C., Spinhoven, P., Hoogduin, K.A. and van Dyck, R. (2002) A randomized controlled clinical trial on the additional effect of hypnosis in a comprehensive treatment programme for inpatients with conversion disorder of the motor type. *Psychotherapy and Psychosomatics*, **71** (2), 66–72.

Ness, D. (2007) Physical therapy management for conversion disorder. *Journal of Neurologic Physical Therapy*, **31** (1), 30–39.

O'Suilleabhain, P.E. and Matsumoto, J.Y. (1998) Time-frequency analysis of tremors. *Brain*, **121**, 2127–2134.

Okun, M.S., Rodriguez, R.L., Foote, K.D. and Fernandez, H.H. (2007) The "chair test" to aid in the diagnosis of psychogenic gait disorders. *The Neurologist*, **13** (2), 87–91.

Rampello, L., Raffaele, R., Nicoletti, G., Le Pira, F., Malaguarnera, M. and Drago, F. (1996) Hysterical neurosis of the conversion type: therapeutic activity of neuroleptics with different hyperprolactinemic potency. *Neuropsychobiology*, **33** (4), 186–188.

Rosebush, P. and Mazurek, M. (2005) The treatment of conversion disorder, in Psychogenic Movement Disorders (ed. M. Hallett *et al.*), Lippincott Williams & Wilkins, Philadelphia PA, pp. 289–301.

Ruddy, R. and House, A. (2005) Psychosocial interventions for conversion disorder (Review). *Cochrane Database of Systematic Reviews*, (4), CD005331.

Schrag, A. and Lang, A.E. (2005) Psychogenic movement disorders. *Current Opinion in Neurology*, **18**, 399–404.

Shaibani, A. and Sabbagh, M.N. (1998) Pseudoneurologic syndromes: recognition and diagnosis. *American Family Physician*, **57** (10), 2485–2494.

Shapiro, A.P. and Teasell, R.W. (2004) Behavioural interventions in the rehabilitation of acute v. chronic non-organic (conversion/factitious) motor disorder. *British Journal of Psychiatry*, **185**, 140–146.

Shibasaki, H. and Hallett, M. (2006) What is the bereitschaftspotential? *Clinical Neurophysiology*, **117** (11), 2341–2356.

Shill, H. and Gerber, P. (2006) Evaluation of clinical diagnostic criteria for psychogenic movement disorders. *Movement Disorders*, **21** (8), 1163–1168.

Speed, J. (1996) Behavioral management of conversion disorder: retrospective study. *Archives of Physical Medicine and Rehabilitation*, **77**, 147–154.

Stone, J., Campbell, K., Sharma, N., Carson, A., Warlow, C.P. and Sharpe, M. (2003a) What should we call pseudoseizures? The patient's perspective. *Seizure: The Journal of the British Epilepsy Association*, **12** (8), 568–572.

Stone, J., Sharpe, M., Rothwell, P.M. and Warlow, C.P. (2003b) The 12 year prognosis of unilateral functional weakness and sensory disturbance. *Journal of Neurology, Neurosurgery, and Psychiatry*, **74**, 591–596.

Sudarsky, L. (2006) Psychogenic gait disorders. *Seminars in Neurology*, **26**, 351–356.

Sumathipala, A. (2007) What is the evidence for the efficacy of treatments for somatoform disorders? A critical review of previous intervention studies. *Psychosomatic Medicine*, **69** (9), 889–900.

Suzuki, A., Mochizuki, H., Kajiyama, Y., Kimura, M., Furukawa, T., Ichikawa, G., Arai, H. and Mizuno, Y. (2001) A case of convergence spasm in hysteria improved with a brief psychiatric assessment. *No To Shinkei*, **53** (12), 1141–1144.

Thomas, M. and Jankovic, J. (2004) Psychogenic movement disorders: diagnosis and management. *CNS Drugs*, **18** (7), 437–452.

Van Nuenen, B.F., Wohlgemuth, M., Wong Chung, R.E., Abdo, W.F. and Bloem, B.R. (2007) Acupuncture for psychogenic movement disorders: Treatment or diagnostic tool. *Movement Disorders*, **22**, 1353–1355.

Verhoeven, J., Marien, P., Engelborghs, S., D'Haenen, H. and DeDeyn, P. (2005) A foreign speech accent in a case of conversion disorder. *Behavioural Neurology*, **16** (4), 225–232.

Voon, V. and Lang, A.E. (2005) Antidepressant treatment outcomes of psychogenic movement disorder. *Journal of Clinical Psychiatry*, **66** (12), 1529–1534.

Zeuner, K.E., Shoge, R.O., Goldstein, S.R., Dambrosia, J.M. and Hallett, M. (2003) Accelerometry to distinguish psychogenic from essential or parkinsonian tremor. *Neurology*, **61**, 548–550.

Index

Note: Page references in *italics* refer to figures; those in **bold** refer to Tables

Therapeutics of Parkinson's Disease and Other Movement Disorders   Edited by Mark Hallett and Werner Poewe
© 2008 John Wiley & Sons, Ltd.